Increase Your Chance of Passing the *NCLEX-PN®* with the Attached Bonus CD-ROM.

Get Familiar with Test Taking on Screen

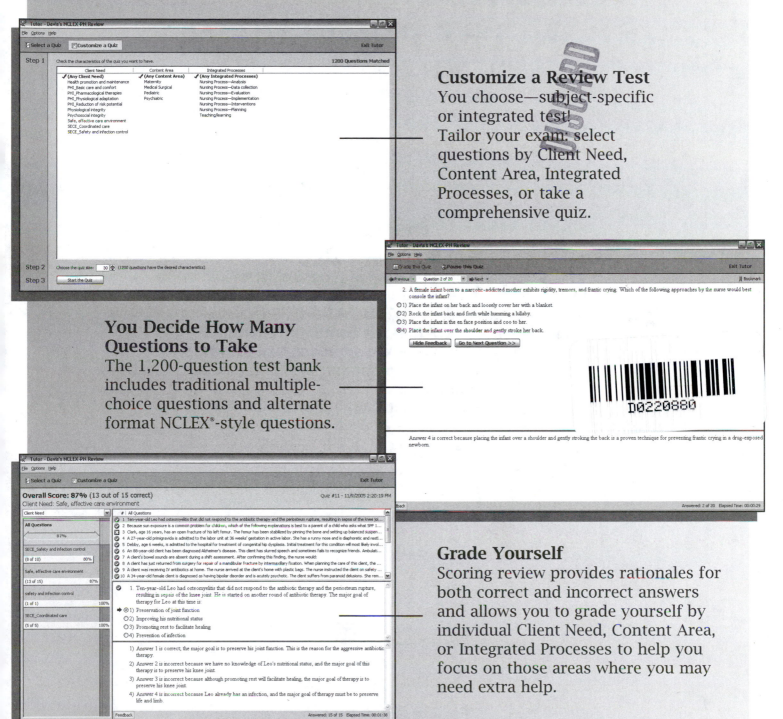
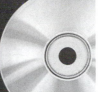

Customize a Review Test
You choose—subject-specific or integrated test! Tailor your exam: select questions by Client Need, Content Area, Integrated Processes, or take a comprehensive quiz.

You Decide How Many Questions to Take
The 1,200-question test bank includes traditional multiple-choice questions and alternate format NCLEX®-style questions.

Grade Yourself
Scoring review provides rationales for both correct and incorrect answers and allows you to grade yourself by individual Client Need, Content Area, or Integrated Processes to help you focus on those areas where you may need extra help.

Your success is guaranteed!

DAVIS'S
NCLEX-PN® REVIEW
THIRD EDITION

Money
Back Guarantee

If you are a graduate of a nursing program accredited in the United States, take the NCLEX-PN® for the first time, and do not pass after using *Davis's NCLEX-PN® Review,* return the book to **F. A. Davis Company, Customer Service, 404-420 N. 2nd Street, Philadelphia, PA 19123.** Enclose your original receipt for purchase of the book and copies of your official test results notification and your certification of graduation. We will refund the price you paid for the book. If you have any questions, please call 800-323-3555.

NCLEX-PN® is a registered trademark of National Council of State Boards of Nursing, Inc. (NCSBN).

DAVIS'S
NCLEX-PN® REVIEW
THIRD EDITION

GOLDEN M. TRADEWELL, RN, PhD

Chair
Associate Professor
Department of Nursing
Southern Arkansas University
Magnolia, Arkansas

PATRICIA GAUNTLETT BEARE, RN, PhD

Professor
Louisiana State University Medical Center
School of Nursing
New Orleans, Louisiana

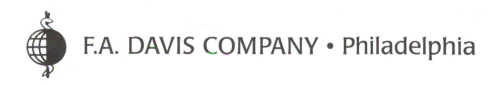 F.A. DAVIS COMPANY • Philadelphia

ֿ Company
Street
PA 19103
.com

Printed in the United States of America

Last digit indicates print number: 10 9 8 7 6 5 4 3 2 1

Publisher, Nursing: Robert G. Martone
Developmental Editor: Alan Sorkowitz
Project Editor: Tom Ciavarella
Design Manager: Carolyn O'Brien

As new scientific information becomes available through basic and clinical research, recommended treatments and drug therapies undergo changes. The authors and publisher have done everything possible to make this book accurate, up-to-date, and in accord with accepted standards at the time of publication. The authors, editors, and publisher are not responsible for errors or omissions or for consequences from application of the book, and make no warranty, expressed or implied, in regard to the contents of the book. Any practice described in this book should be applied by the reader in accordance with professional standards of care used in regard to the unique circumstances that may apply in each situation. The reader is advised always to check product information (package inserts) for changes and new information regarding dose and contraindications before administering any drug. Caution is especially urged when using new or infrequently ordered drugs.

Library of Congress Cataloging-in-Publication Data

Davis's NCLEX-PN review/[edited by] Golden M. Tradewell, Patricia Gauntlett Beare.–3rd ed.
   p. ; cm.
Includes index.
ISBN 0-8036-1459-4
1. Practical nursing–Examinations, questions, etc. 2. Practical nursing–Outlines, syllabi, etc. 3. National Council Licensure Examination for Practical/Vocational Nurses–Study guides.
  [DNLM: 1. Nursing, Practical–United States–Examination Questions. WY 18.2 D265 2006] I. Title: NCLEX-PN review. II. Tradewell, Golden M. III. Beare, Patricia Gauntlett.
RT62.D38 2006
610.73076–dc22

2005026772

Illustration Credits

Pages 148 and 161: Modified from Basic Life Support for Healthcare Providers. American Heart Association, 1997, reproduced with permission. Pages 148 and 161: Modified from Scanlon, VC and Sanders, T: Student Workbook for Essentials of Anatomy and Physiology, ed 4. Philadelphia, FA Davis Company, 2003, p 73, with permission. Pages 284 and 308: From Williams, LS and Hopper, PD: Understanding Medical-Surgical Nursing, ed 2. Philadelphia, FA Davis Company, 2003, p 328, with permission. Pages 284 and 309: From Williams, LS and Hopper, PD: Understanding Medical-Surgical Nursing, ed 2. Philadelphia, FA Davis Company, 2003, p 417, with permission. Pages 285 and 310: From Dillon, PM: Nursing Health Assessment: A Critical Thinking, Case Studies Approach. Philadelphia, FA Davis Company, 2003, p 459, with permission. Pages 552 and 570: From Williams, LS and Hopper, PD: Understanding Medical-Surgical Nursing, ed 2. Philadelphia, FA Davis Company, 2003, p 480, with permission. Pages 578 and 594: Modified from Scanlon, VC and Sanders, T: Student Workbook for Essentials of Anatomy and Physiology, ed 4. Philadelphia, FA Davis Company, 2003, p 149, with permission. Pages 614 and 630: Modified from Scanlon, VC and Sanders, T: Student Workbook for Essentials of Anatomy and Physiology, ed 4. Philadelphia, FA Davis Company, 2003, p 263, with permission. Pages 650 and 667: Modified from Basic Life Support for Healthcare Providers. American Heart Association, 1997, reproduced with permission.

DEDICATION

I would like to dedicate this third edition to my children, Kim and Aaron, for their love and support through my educational endeavors. They both realize that the reality of this book is only one of many accomplishments that occurred as a result of the long years of graduate school.

Golden M. Tradewell, RN, PhD

PREFACE

This book's purposes are to provide the candidate for practical/vocational nurse licensure with a concise review of the information necessary to pass the NCLEX-PN licensing examination and to assist the candidate to apply this information in simulated clinical situations by using effective test-taking skills. Chapters 1 and 2 (Unit I) provide basic information on the development, administration, and scoring of the NCLEX-PN and how to prepare for and take the examination. The new alternative test items are discussed, such as innovative item types that require calculation, identification of more than one correct answer, identification of a location on a figure, or filling in the blank.

Clinical Specialties Content Reviews and Tests (Unit II)

In Chapters 3 through 7, recognized nursing authors and experts have prepared the nursing content reviews in outline form. These include reviews of maternity nursing, pediatric nursing, medical-surgical nursing, gerontological nursing, and psychiatric–mental health nursing. The nursing content has been organized according to the nursing process to enable the student to study according to client needs. Cultural aspects of client care are included within each nursing content review. Test questions have been formulated to apply this content in typical clinical situations. The test answer section of each chapter includes the correct answer, rationales for the correct and incorrect answer choices, the relevant step of the nursing process, integrated processes, and the general category of client need based on the revision of categories in the new NCLEX-PN test plan. There are 800 content review questions in this section, including the new alternative test items.

Related Sciences Reviews and Tests (Unit III)

Chapter 8, on procedures for the licensed practical nurse, has been updated. Chapter 9, Leadership, Management, and Delegation, is new, reflecting the increased emphasis these subjects are receiving on the NCLEX-PN. Major revisions and additions have been made to the chapters containing pharmacology and nutrition, which are now Chapters 10 and 11, respectively. Cultural aspects of client care are included within the content review found in Chapters 10 and 11. This section includes 425 questions, including questions in the new alternative formats.

Comprehensive Integrated Practice Tests (Unit IV)

Because the NCLEX-PN test is intended to measure the ability to practice as a licensed practical/vocational nurse, these four tests are designed to apply nursing knowledge to health-care situations that require nursing intervention. Test items have been prepared by nurse-clinicians and educators who have written items for the NCLEX-PN examination. Within this section, questions using the new alternative test formats have been included. Each of the four tests contains 205 questions, the maximum number included on the NCLEX-PN itself, for a total of 820 questions in this section. A CD-ROM with 1200 additional questions, including new alternative test items not found in the book, accompanies this text.

Summary

The content as presented in this book will enable the NCLEX-PN candidate to review essential nursing knowledge and apply this knowledge to test questions in the examination. The number of test questions has been greatly expanded, and questions in the new alternative formats have been added. These questions are designed to give the candidate more practice in applying content to simulated clinical practice settings. Through careful review, candidates will no longer fear the unknown as they review and understand the content and skills necessary to pass the examination.

Golden M. Tradewell
Patricia Gauntlett Beare

ACKNOWLEDGMENTS

Many people have helped make this third edition a reality:

To Alan Sorkowitz, for his patience and support of the changes that were suggested;

To our contributors, whose expertise has added value and integrity; and

To the members of the F. A. Davis team, who guided this book through the production process.

CONTRIBUTORS

Lizabeth L. Carlson, RN, DNS, BC
Dean of Nursing
Assistant Professor of Nursing
Delta State University School of Nursing
Cleveland, Mississippi

Valecia Carter-Vaughn, RN, MSN
Clinical Nursing Instructor
Louisiana State University Health Sciences Center School of
   Nursing
New Orleans, Louisiana

Jennifer Couvillion, RN, PhD
Instructor of Nursing
Louisiana State University Health Sciences Center School of
   Nursing
New Orleans, Louisiana

Kathleen R. Culliton, RN, CS, MS, GNP
Assistant Professor
Weber State University
Ogden, Utah

Jerry Denny, RN, MS, MSN
Assistant Professor
McNeese State University College of Nursing
Lake Charles, Louisiana

Deborah Garbee, RN, APRN, MN, BC
Instructor of Nursing
Louisiana State University Health Sciences Center School of
   Nursing
New Orleans, Louisiana

Judith Gentry, RN, APRN, MSN, OCN
Assistant Professor of Clinical Nursing
Louisiana State University Health Sciences Center School of
   Nursing
New Orleans, Louisiana

Cynthia Bowers Howard, RN, APRN, MSN, BC, CNS
Assistant Professor
McNeese State University College of Nursing
Lake Charles, Louisiana

Eileen W. Keefe, RN.C, MS
Assistant Professor of Clinical Nursing
School of Nursing, Retired
Louisiana State University Health Sciences Center
New Orleans, Louisiana

Demetrius J. Porche, RN, CCRN, DNS
Associate Dean of Research & Evaluation
Louisiana State University Health Sciences Center School of
   Nursing
New Orleans, Louisiana

Larry D. Purnell, RN, PhD
Professor
College of Health and Nursing Sciences
University of Delaware
Newark, Delaware

Susan I. Ray, RN, MS
Nursing Faculty
Copiah-Lincoln Community College
Wesson, Mississippi

Kara Schmitt, PhD
Director, BOPR—Testing Services
State of Michigan CIS/Office of Health Services
Lansing, Michigan

Karen Silady, RN, MN
Instructor of Nursing
Louisiana State University Health Sciences Center School of
   Nursing
New Orleans, Louisiana

Nora F. Steele, RN.C, DNS, PNP
Delgado Community College Charity School of Nursing
New Orleans, Louisiana

Danny G. Willis, RN, DNSc
Assistant Professor
Boston College
Chestnut Hill, Massachusetts

CONTENTS

What You Need to Know About the NCLEX-PN

CHAPTER 1

Development, Administration, and Scoring of the NCLEX-PN™*

Patricia Gauntlett Beare, RN, PhD
Nora F. Steele, RN.C, DNS, PNP

The National Council Licensure Examination for Practical Nurses (NCLEX-PN), prepared by the National Council of State Boards of Nursing (NCSBN), is designed to measure a candidate's knowledge, skills, and abilities essential to the safe and effective practice of practical nursing. The examination is comprehensive in terms of testing a candidate's ability to work as a practical nurse without harming clients. The results determine whether a candidate can react and respond appropriately to various clinical situations typically encountered by a practical nurse. Candidates who pass the examination are viewed by their boards of nursing as being competent to protect the health, safety, and welfare of clients.

Overview of the NCLEX Examination Testing Process

Since 1994, nurse licensure candidates have been taking the National Council Licensure Examination (NCLEX) on computers at many conveniently located test centers across the United States and its territories. The change to computerized adaptive testing (CAT) for the nurse licensure examination came about as a result of a decision made in August 1991 by the NCSBN. Pearson VUE provides test administration services.

To sit for the examination, you, as a practical nurse licensure candidate, must first complete an examination application and submit it, along with the appropriate fee(s) and other required documents, such as a certificate of graduation from a school of nursing, to the relevant board of nursing before the deadline date.

Because each state has different procedures and deadlines, you must be thoroughly familiar with the requirements of the

jurisdiction in which you wish to be licensed. In most instances, the nursing program that you attended will instruct you regarding the forms that must be completed as well as the procedures to follow. If the school does not provide you with this information, or if you wish to be licensed in another jurisdiction, it is your responsibility to contact the specific board office for information. (All state boards of nursing, their addresses, and their phone numbers are listed in Appendix A.)

Eligibility Requirements

To take the NCLEX, candidates must satisfy these requirements:
- Apply for licensure in the state or territory in which you wish to be licensed.
- Meet all of the board of nursing's eligibility requirements to take the NCLEX.
- Register for the examination with Pearson VUE.
- Bring the *Authorization to Test* and acceptable forms of identification to the Pearson Professional Testing Center for NCLEX administration. Each candidate will receive an Authorization to Test in the mail from Pearson VUE after the board of nursing declares the candidate eligible to sit for the examination.

When completing the NCLEX-PN application, be certain that you do so legibly and correctly, as this information will be used in printing your admission card, recording results, providing cumulative data to nursing programs, and perhaps even printing the eventual license. Foreign-trained candidates should recognize that additional documentation of education and proof of English-language proficiency may be required when a licensure application is submitted to a board of nursing office. For this reason, if you were educated outside the United States, you should send your application as early as possible. It is essential that you contact the jurisdiction in which you wish to be licensed to learn what specific

---

*NCLEX, NCLEX-PN, and NCLEX-RN are trademarks of the National Council of State Boards of Nursing.

documentation or additional examination results, or both, are required. In addition, you should contact the Commission on Graduates of Foreign Nursing Schools (CGFNS) for detailed information about the requirements that you may have to meet, using the following address and phone number:

Commission on Graduates
of Foreign Nursing Schools
3600 Market Street Suite 400
Philadelphia, PA 19104-2651
215-222-8767
www.cgfns.org

Basis for the Examination Content

A job analysis of tasks performed by practical nurses entering the profession is used to develop the NCLEX-PN. The NCLEX-PN administered in October 1990 was the first to use the results of a job analysis.[1] A new job analysis was completed in 2003.[2] The purpose of the job analysis was to determine the frequency with which certain tasks are performed by practical nurses entering the profession, as well as the criticality of these tasks (i.e., which tasks, if performed incorrectly, could do serious or critical harm to a client). Nurses throughout the country and in a variety of clinical settings completed a survey that listed several hundred tasks typically performed by practical nurses. The respondents' answers, in terms of the frequency and criticality of these tasks, formed the basis for the NCLEX-PN.

Components of the Examination

The examination is not designed merely to measure a candidate's ability to recall or recognize certain facts. Rather the purpose of the examination is to determine how well a candidate can relate learned facts to common nursing situations. Most items in the examination deal with a candidate's ability to (1) apply information or knowledge learned in one situation and correctly transfer it to another situation, or (2) analyze a relationship by breaking it into simpler components, by making comparisons, or by identifying the relationships between and among certain pieces of information. Remember, the examination is designed to determine how well you will respond in typical, real-life clinical situations and not just whether you are able to recall facts learned in school.

The test plan or specifications for constructing each form of the examination is based on four major categories of client needs.[3] Integrated throughtout the NCLEX-PN items are beliefs about people and nursing, the nursing process (data collection, planning, implementation, and evaluation), caring, communication and documentation, and teaching and learning. Items are developed to reflect standards of care and the scope of practice of the practical nurse.

Client Needs

The four broad categories of client needs serve as the framework for the NCLEX-PN (Table 1–1). The categories and subcategories identify the health needs of clients across the life span in a variety of settings which provide the foundations for nursing actions. A brief description of these needs follows,

Table 1–1. **NCLEX-PN Test Plan**	
Client Health Needs	Percentage
Safe & effective care environment	13%–25%
Coordinated care	11%–17%
Safety and infection control	8%–14%
Health promotion/maintenance	7%–13%
Psychosocial integrity	8%–14%
Physiological integrity	39%–63%
Basic care and comfort	11%–17%
Pharmacological therapies	9%–15%
Reduction of risk potential	10%–16%
Physiological adaptation	12%–18%

along with the percentage of items covering each. The percentages reflect the number of test items from each category you may expect to see in your exam. You can use this information to help plan your studies.

Safe and Effective Care Environment (13%–25%)

The practical nurse assists in meeting client needs in this area by providing nursing care in the categories of (1) coordination of care (11%–17%) and (2) safety and infection control for clients and health care personnel (8%–14%).

Health Promotion and Maintenance (7%–13%)

The practical nurse participates as a member of the health-care team to assist in promoting fulfillment of the client's (1) growth and development through the life span and (2) prevention and/or early detection of disease.

Psychosocial Integrity (8%–14%)

Practical nursing care is provided to promote achievement of the client's emotional, mental, and social well-being at all stages of development. Mental health and cultural awareness concepts are incorporated into care.

Physiological Integrity (39%–63%)

The practical nurse provides care to promote achievement of the client's needs in the areas of (1) basic care and comfort (11%–17%), (2) pharmacological therapies (9%–15%), (3) reduction of risk potential (10%–16%), and (4) physiological adaptation (12%–18%).

Computerized Adaptive Testing

The NCLEX, administered by computer, uses the methodology called computerized adaptive testing (CAT), mentioned on page 3. With CAT, the computer selects the questions you will answer during the examination to give you the best opportunity to demonstrate your competence.

There are four types of items (questions) on the NCLEX. The majority are multiple-choice questions where you are presented with information and asked to select the one best answer from four choices. The other types are referred to as alternative item types. Innovative item types may require calculation, identification of more than one correct answer, identification of a location on a figure, or filling in the blank. With CAT, a drop-down calculator is available to assist with the accuracy of calculations. Items are scored as correct or incorrect; there is no partial credit on any item.

Multiple-choice: In this type of item, there is a stem and you are asked to select the best answer from one of four options. The majority of items (98%–99%) are multiple-choice.

Fill in the blank: In this type of item, there is a stem and you are asked to complete a calculation or put a list of options in order. You may be presented with a situation in the stem and asked to calculate and enter the answer. A drop-down calculator may be used with the NCLEX. The NCLEX tutorial directions state: "Type a number as your answer. Do not use spaces or commas to separate the numbers. Do not type words or anything else, such as units of measure (e.g., milliliters, grams)."[3] Punctuation and letters are not required as a part of the answer. For example, "cc" would be included in the information presented and must not be repeated. If the student is asked to put options in order, the NCLEX tutorial directions state: "To record your answer … type the number sequence. Do not type in spaces, commas, or slashes to separate the number sequence."

Hotspot identification: In this type of item, a question is presented and you are directed to identify an area of a figure. The answer is recorded as the location selected on a diagram or figure.

Multiple-response: In this type of item, there is a stem and list of options, usually six options/choices. You are asked to select all the answers that are correct. The stem indicates that more than one option may be correct.

Any type of item may include a table, chart, or graphic image.

The questions are presented to you one at a time on a computer screen. You can view each question as long as you like, but you cannot go back to previous questions once you have recorded your answer choices, nor can you leave a question unanswered.

Using the Computer

Although the NCLEX is given on a computer, you are not expected to know how to use a computer before you take the examination. Only two keys—the space bar and the enter key—are used to highlight and record your answer. You will be instructed how to record answers at the test center, and you will have an opportunity to practice on three sample questions before the examination begins. Even after the examination starts, you will be able to request help regarding the use of the computer. The computer practice disk that accompanies this book operates using the same combination of keys that you will use on the test itself, giving you more than 1000 questions on which to practice using the computer (there are 1200 questions).

Examination Format

The examination typically presents a situation or incident involving a client, family members, or both. Following each situation is a question pertaining to this information. Because this examination is designed to assess a candidate's ability to practice safely in the work setting, the test items generally relate to various real-life situations in which the practical nurse would be involved. Although candidates must possess basic nursing knowledge to answer the questions, the primary focus is on the ability to apply the basic knowledge to a variety of clinical settings.

Each test item consists of an introductory statement or problem known as the *stem*. The stem is followed by choices or possible responses to the problem. The incorrect choices are known as *distractors*. Distractors are created in such a way that they may seem correct to someone who is unfamiliar with the terminology, procedure, or general practice. The distractors are not designed to "trick" candidates, but rather to discriminate between those candidates who are qualified to enter the profession and those who are not.

Examination Length

Practical/vocational nurse (PN/VN) candidates take a minimum of 85 questions. The maximum number of questions a PN/VN candidate will answer is 205 during the 5-hour maximum testing period. As you take the examination, questions are selected for you based on your responses to previous questions. Testing stops when a candidate's performance is estimated as being either above or below the passing standard with a predetermined level of certainty regardless of the number of questions taken or the amount of testing time elapsed. Depending on individual patterns of correct and incorrect responses, different candidates will answer varying numbers of questions and use varying amounts of time. The examination also stops when the maximum number of questions have been answered (205) or the 5-hour time limit has been reached.

It is important to understand that the length of your examination does not indicate a pass-or-fail result. The number of questions answered is not related to a pass-or-fail decision. A candidate with a relatively short examination may pass or fail the same as a candidate with a long examination. Each candidate, no matter what the length of the examination, has ample opportunity to demonstrate true competence and is given an examination that conforms to the NCLEX test plan.

Guessing

You must answer every question even if you are not sure of the right answer. The computer will not allow you to go on to the next question without answering the question on the screen. If you are not sure of the correct answer, make your best guess and move on to the next question.

Reviewing Answers

After you select an answer to a question, you will have a chance to think about your answer and change it as many times as you like. However, once you confirm your answer and go on to the next question, you will not be allowed to go back to any previous question.

The Passing Standard

To ensure a consistent standard of competence in nursing practice, the National Council uses a criterion-referenced standard. This means that passing or failing depends solely on a candidate's level of performance in relation to the established point that represents entry-level competence. There is no fixed percentage of candidates that pass or fail each examination.

Diagnostic Profile

A diagnostic profile is provided to candidates who fail the examination. The diagnostic profile is mailed to candidates by their respective board of nursing, along with the results of the examination. Using this information, failing candidates can determine their areas of relative strength and weakness based on the test plan and design their study accordingly before retaking the NCLEX.

Reporting Results

Although the NCLEX is scored as the candidate completes each question, *no results* are released at the test center. NCLEX results, available *only* from your board of nursing, will be mailed to candidates approximately 1 month after the examination. *Do not call* your board of nursing, Pearson VUE, or the National Council for NCLEX results.

Retake Policy

The National Council's retake policy states that candidates must wait a minimum of 91 days between examinations. In addition, each board of nursing may establish its own retake policies, with retakes permitted no more frequently than the policy established by the National Council. This is an important policy that allows the National Council to be certain that all candidates receive a valid examination.

Personal Identification and Examination Security

Because of the importance of the NCLEX, numerous security measures are enforced during the administration of the examination. Strict candidate identification (ID) requirements have been established.

Identification Requirements

When you arrive at the test center, you will be required to present two forms of ID and your Authorization to Test. You will not be admitted to the examination without the proper ID and your Authorization to Test.
- Both pieces of ID must be signed and one must bear a recent photograph of you. The name on the ID with the photograph must be the same as the name that appears on your Authorization to Test.
- Candidates wishing to make a legal name change or an address change must contact their board of nursing.

Please note the following examples of acceptable forms of ID. At least one of your forms of ID must be from the list of primary forms of ID. The ID form must be current (not expired). Examples of acceptable forms of primary ID (must include your signature and photograph) are:
- Driver's license with photograph
- Employee ID card with photograph
- School ID card with photograph
- State ID card with photograph
- Passport

Secondary forms of ID must include your signature. Examples of acceptable forms of secondary ID include your Social Security card, valid credit cards, and bank automated teller machine cards.

Additional Precautions

Additional security measures that will be taken at the test centers include the following:
- Your thumbprint and photograph will be taken. Your photograph will be included on the report of your results. In some cases, your thumbprint may be used to confirm your identity by the board of nursing in the jurisdiction in which you have applied for licensure. You cannot be tested without having your thumbprint and picture taken.
- You will not be allowed to take any personal items into the testing room. This includes such items as watches, cell phones, and wallets. You may put personal items, including your identification forms, in a locker outside the testing area. Scratch paper will be provided if you need it.
- You will be observed at all times while taking the examination. This observation will include direct observation by test center staff, as well as video and audio recording of your examination session.

Special Testing Circumstances

Testing accommodations for candidates with disabilities will be made only with the authorization of your board of nursing. To ensure that adequate time is available to evaluate any request for an accommodation, contact your board of nursing as early as possible, preferably before submitting your registration to Pearson VUE.

Procedure for Requesting Special Accommodations

To request special accommodations, you must do the following:
- Request information from your board of nursing concerning its requirements for requesting testing accommodations.
- Make a request for accommodations to your board of nursing. Your request must comply with requirements established by your board of nursing for persons requesting testing accommodations. Typically, boards of nursing require documentation of past accommodations, if any, and a specific diagnosis by an appropriate health-care professional that includes a

Table 1-2. Communicating about the NCLEX

Questions About:	Answers
• Registering to take the NCLEX • Authorization to Test (ATT) • Name corrections on your ATT • Lost Authorization to Test • Acceptable forms of identification • Comments about the test center	*Visit:* http://www.vue.com/nclex *Call:* 1-866-496-2539 8 AM to 8 PM Eastern Time. Candidates with hearing impairments who use a Telecommunications Device for the Deaf (TDD) may call 1-800-627-3529 24 hours/day 7 days/week *Write:* NCLEX Exam Program Pearson Professional Testing 5601 Green Valley Drive Bloomington, MN 55437-1099 *E-Mail:* vuepearsonprofesssionaltesting@vue.com
• NCLEX development • General NCLEX information • Unresolved concerns related to administration	*Write:* National Council of State Boards of Nursing 111 E. Wacker, Suite 2900 examination Chicago, IL 60601-4277 *Call:* NCSBN Testing 866-293-9600 *Fax:* NCSBN 312-279-1036
• Name or address changes • Licensure • Endorsement • Interpretation of results • Diagnostic profiles • Scheduling an appointment to test	Write or call your board of nursing.
• Rescheduling or canceling your testing appointment	Wait until you receive your Authorization to Test and the bulletin that will accompany it entitled *Scheduling and Taking Your NCLEX.* Follow directions in the bulletin.
• Examination results	Examination results are sent to you by your board of nursing. Wait a minimum of 4 weeks after your examination for your results to arrive in the mail.

description of the accommodations appropriate for your condition.

- Send your request to your board of nursing as early as possible so that, if approved by the board of nursing, the special accommodations can be made in a timely manner.

Overview of the NCLEX Examination Testing Process*

To be licensed as a practical nurse (PN) (sometimes referred to as a licensed [LPN], vocational nurse [VN], or licensed vocational nurse [LVN]), a candidate must take the NCLEX. To take this examination, candidates must generally go through the following steps, which are listed in chronological order:

1. The candidate applies to the board of nursing for a license, following instructions from that board.
2. The candidate gets an *NCLEX Candidate Bulletin* from the board of nursing.
3. The candidate submits a registration form to Pearson VUE (the National Council's contracted testing service). Pearson VUE will acknowledge the candidate's registration by mail.
4. The board of nursing communicates the candidate's eligibility to test to Pearson VUE.
5. Pearson VUE sends the candidate an Authorization to Test (ATT) with a booklet called *Scheduling and Taking Your NCLEX* and a list of testing centers.
6. The candidate will contact a Pearson Testing Center and schedule an appointment to test. You decide which testing center you prefer; it may be closer to home, work, or a study group.
7. On the appointed day, the candidate takes the test at the selected Pearson Testing Center.
8. The Pearson Testing Center transmits the test results to Pearson VUE. After verifying the accuracy of the results, Pearson VUE transmits them to the designated board of nursing.
9. The board of nursing sends results to the candidate.

Table 1–2 lists telephone and fax numbers and addresses where you may request more information about the NCLEX.

REFERENCES

1. Kane, M and Colton, D: Job Analysis of Newly Licensed Practical/Vocational Nurses, 1986–87. National Council of State Boards of Nursing, Chicago, 1988.
2. Smith, JE and Crawford, LH: Report of Findings from the 2003 LPN/VN Practice Analysis: Link the NCLEX-PN Examination to Practice. National Council of State Boards of Nursing, Chicago, 2003.
3. 2005 NCLEX-PN Test Plan for the National Council Licensure Examination for Practical Nurses. National Council of State Boards of Nursing, Chicago, 2004.

*The information in this section is copyright by the National Council of State Boards of Nursing, Inc., Chicago, Illinois, 1998. Available at: http://www.ncsbn.org.

CHAPTER 2

Preparing for and Taking the NCLEX-PN

Kara Schmitt, PhD
Golden M. Tradewell, RN, PhD

While preparing for and taking the NCLEX-PN, you must constantly remember that you have the ability to pass the examination. Although the manner in which you respond to items may be different, and although the number of items may be more than in other tests you have taken during your studies, the examination is still just an examination. To do well, you have to be both psychologically and intellectually prepared.

Test Anxiety

Although stress and anxiety are *not* really the same, these terms are used to mean the same in this chapter. Stress and anxiety are normal reactions to situations such as preparing for and taking the NCLEX-PN. If you were to ask your friends who have already passed the examination if they were anxious before and during the test, the answer would certainly be "yes." In fact, some amount of anxiety is actually *good* for you and has been found to improve test-taking ability. On the other hand, uncontrollable anxiety hurts your ability to do well. It has been said that stress is "the spice of life or the kiss of death—depending on how we cope with it."[1]

By learning how to handle stress effectively, you can use it to your advantage. Stress or anxiety and the manner in which you recognize and respond to it (your ability to react positively) are personal. No one method works for everyone; therefore, the information given in this chapter is merely designed to give you some ideas of ways in which you might be able to reduce large amounts of stress. The best way to deal with stress is to take specific steps to cope with and reduce the stress-producing situation. Studying and preparing for an examination is the *best* way to reduce the stress felt before an examination. An inappropriate approach, which in the end will increase the stress, is to deny the importance of the task (examination) that you must do. Statements such as "The examination is filled with trick questions anyway, so why

bother studying?" or "If I don't do well, I just wasn't lucky" are inappropriate and will not help you. You need to concentrate your efforts in proper study and positive thinking. The information presented in this chapter is generally applicable to paper-and-pencil examinations as well as computerized adaptive testing (CAT). If something is not relevant to CAT, a notation is made in the text.

Some of the characteristics frequently associated with test anxiety include[2]:

1. Feeling insecure about your performance
2. Worrying a great deal about things that are not under your control
3. Thinking about how much brighter or better others are
4. Thinking about what will happen if you fail
5. Feeling that you are not as prepared as you could or should be (assuming that you have prepared)
6. Worrying about not having enough time to finish the test
7. Feeling that you will be letting yourself or others down
8. Feeling that you could and should have done better

These eight feelings can be viewed as constituting four major symptoms of anxiety,[3] which can and must be handled to overcome the problem. Each of these four symptoms is discussed briefly in the following paragraphs.

Anxiety-Producing Mental Activities

Worrying about nonspecific problems or situations and fretting over everything that could go wrong is associated with this symptom. Self-criticism, self-blame, and general negative self-talk lead to low self-confidence and disorganized problem solving. Telling yourself that you cannot do something or that you are stupid leads to failure. Another trait associated with this symptom is false thinking about yourself and the world around you—the "everyone-is-so-much-smarter-than-I" syndrome.

Misdirected Attention

Instead of focusing on the task at hand, such as studying for or taking the examination, you focus on internal and external distractors. These could include watching other people study, looking at the clock, or daydreaming. If you focus on the wrong thing, you are less efficient and may become emotionally upset.

Physiological Distress

When you are anxious, your body reacts both physiologically and psychologically. Some of the physiological symptoms include sweating, increased heart rate, nervous stomach, and headache. If you focus significantly on the physiological symptoms, you will be less able to focus on your studies or the examination.

Inappropriate Behavior

This symptom is exhibited by avoiding the task that needs to be done (procrastination), withdrawing prematurely from the task, or doing something else when you should be focusing on the task at hand (e.g., talking to your roommate instead of studying). Other aspects of inappropriate behavior include rushing through the examination or study material without focusing on the information or, at the opposite extreme, being excessively compulsive and rereading everything more than is necessary. A final element is trying to push yourself to keep going when you are tense rather than taking time to relax.

Reducing Stress

To reduce stress to a manageable level, you need to determine what symptoms or behaviors you are exhibiting. One way to learn more about your individual expressions of stress is to find a comfortable, relaxing environment, close your eyes, and really imagine and concentrate on how you feel or what you do when you study. How are you going to feel when it is 1 week before the examination? When it is 1 day before the examination? When it is the day of the examination? When you are sitting in the room taking the examination? Try to think carefully about these events and how you *really* will feel. If you are honest in your evaluation of your feelings, you will be better able to change the way you handle stressful situations.

Another activity you can do to learn more about your own coping ability is to make notes of what you do while studying. Do you watch other people? Do you daydream? Do you begin to worry about the test? Do you give up studying because you think it will do no good? You will probably need to keep a log of your behaviors during several study periods so that you have a complete picture of your behaviors. After you have recorded all of your distractors, make a list of what you could do to reduce your level of anxiety. For instance, telling yourself that you can never learn the material is self-defeating; instead, remind yourself that you learned the material in the past and that you have done well in school. After all, you either have graduated or are ready to graduate, so you must have learned what is necessary to reach this point.

Another aid to learning more about yourself and your reaction to stress is to answer the following questions in terms of what *you* do or how *you* respond during periods of stress:

1. Do I bite my nails, fidget with my hair, or tap my fingers constantly?
2. Do I smoke or drink more frequently?
3. Do I tend to eat more or less or to eat less healthy foods?
4. Do I avoid doing what I should be doing, such as studying?
5. Do I feel as though there is too much to do in too little time?
6. Do I worry about everything—the examination, my health, my family, my work, and so on?
7. Do I seem to have more physical or health-related problems?
8. Do I become irritated or lose my temper more quickly over trivial matters?
9. Do I seem to have less energy or to want to sleep more?
10. Do I have trouble falling asleep or sleeping according to a normal schedule?
11. Am I more critical of myself, or do I think of myself as worthless?
12. Do I seem to forget more day-to-day activities or responsibilities, such as forgetting to shop for groceries, forgetting an appointment, or forgetting to return a phone call?
13. Do I have trouble relaxing and enjoying myself even when I am at a social event or with people I like?
14. Do I tend to daydream more?

Questions 1–3 may be viewed as bad habits that simply become more prevalent during times of stress or anxiety. The key to deciding whether any of these are major problems is to determine whether you are doing them *more than usual* during times of anxiety. If the answer is yes, they could negatively influence your effectiveness in preparing for and taking the examination. At the same time, if you try to be perfect and eliminate normal bad habits during a time of stress, you may actually increase your level of stress. Although it may not be necessary to eliminate bad habits at this time, you should keep them under control.

The other questions (4–14) focus more on symptoms of anxiety. If you responded "yes" to most of the questions, it is time to reevaluate your thoughts about yourself and the future examination. You need to focus less on what is going on around you or inside you and more on how to solve the problem that is causing the anxiety. Begin to view the examination as a problem to be solved or a challenge to be met. Do not view it as something that is a punishment or an imaginary catastrophic event.

Begin to view the test realistically. It is not a measure of your self-worth, your ability to succeed, or your future happiness. It is merely a measure of what you know, as well as your ability to take tests.

Develop a positive attitude toward the test. Eliminate the negative thoughts and feelings you have about it and do not think about how well you will or will not do.

Choose to take the test. The examination is not being forced on you; rather, you elected to take it. By viewing the examination as something you want to do, you are in control and the examination is no longer controlling you. Because you have chosen to take the examination, you must also choose to study for it.

Concentrate on what you can and must do *now*. Do not think about what you should have studied yesterday (the past) or what will happen when you take the exam (the future). Rather direct your attention on the present task of studying, and expend your energy on that.

As stated previously, some test anxiety is good for you. Too much, however, will hinder your performance, and you will not be able to demonstrate adequately the knowledge you actually have. Some ways test-anxious persons are helped are by[2]:

1. Learning to be less demanding of themselves
2. Revising their expectations about the consequence of failure and viewing the task as less alarming
3. Strengthening their study skills
4. Gaining more self-control over their worry and emotionality

If anxiety is handled in a positive manner, it can assist in "promoting survival, healthy adaptation and development. In its nonadaptive modes, it can promote incompetence and extreme and lasting misery."[2]

In any situation, if you convince yourself that you are going to fail, you will. Instead of being negative about yourself, trying to decide what others will think if you fail, or how poorly you might do on the examination, *think positively*. Negative statements made either to yourself or to others can significantly reduce the effectiveness of the studying you do. Think positively and you'll *feel* positive.

Read the examples of typical negative and positive statements shown in Table 2–1. Are you guilty of making any of the negative statements? If so, begin working at using statements in the positive column.

Avoid "why," "if only," and "what if" types of questions or statements; for example, "Why did I ever think I could be a nurse?," or "If only I had more time, I could do better," or "What if I don't do well on the examination?" These expressions tend to reinforce feelings of helplessness, frustration, and anger. Try to eliminate them from your internal thoughts and external statements.

Stress and anxiety can and will be reduced if you take *positive* action and think *positive* thoughts about yourself and your abilities. At the same time, recognize that you are going to worry about the examination. The statement "Don't worry" is useless advice because we all worry. You must, however, worry in a constructive manner and must have prepared for the examination.

Study Environment

Not only what you study but also the conditions under which you study are important in your ability to learn and remember. Both internal (daydreaming) and external (noise) distractors can lessen your ability to concentrate.

Think about where and how you typically study. Are you studying in an optimal place and manner? You want to be comfortable and relaxed while studying, yet at the same time you need to be able to focus all of your attention on the material you are reading and reviewing.

The following series of questions should assist you in your evaluation of whether the location and way in which you study are most conducive to learning.

1. When I begin studying, do I have all necessary books, paper, pencils, and other study materials with me so that I do not waste time finding them?
2. Do I schedule at least 1–2 hours at a time for studying?
3. Do I take short breaks (10–15 minutes) while studying for long periods of time and then return to work immediately?
4. Do I spread out my studying over a period of time rather than trying to do it all at the last minute?
5. If I study with friends, do they have good study habits?
6. Do I have a plan for studying and, if so, do I stick to it?
7. Do I feel rested when I study?

Table 2–1. **Changing Negative Self-Talk to Positive Self-Talk**	
Negative Statements	**Positive Statements**
"I have to get a perfect score."	"I want to do well, but I don't need to get every item right."
"I always get upset during a test."	"If I feel myself getting tense during the test, I know how to relax."
"I'm a failure because I didn't remember."	"Just because I forgot … doesn't mean I'm a failure; I remember lots of other material."
"If the test has questions on … topic, I'll fail."	"If the test has questions on … topic, I had better study it more."
"What if I fail the exam?"	"I don't expect to fail, but if I do, I'll just have to study harder and do better the next time."
"I'll let my family down if I don't pass this test."	"Sure, my family wants me to do well, but they'll still accept me if I don't pass."
"I'm too stupid to be a nurse."	"I made it through school and I can make it through the exam."
"The test is designed to trick candidates, so it doesn't matter."	"If I study, I can do well; it's my responsibility to prepare."
"I'll never be able to understand this material."	"Just relax and try rereading this section; I know I can figure it out."
"Thank heavens, I made it through this study session!"	"Wow, I really learned a lot while studying today. Hope tomorrow goes as well."
"I just know I'll be scared during the examination."	"I know I'll do well on the exam because I'm capable and I studied."
"Everyone expects me to do poorly, so why bother trying to do otherwise."	"I don't care what others think about my chance of passing the test; I know I can do it."
"I don't know why I have to take this test."	"I want to take this test simply because it will confirm that I really did learn while in school."

8. If I begin to feel tense or tired, do I stop studying for a while and try to relax?
9. If I begin daydreaming or worrying, do I take a few minutes' break to daydream or worry rather than let those activities interfere with my studying?
10. Do I concentrate on the material that I am studying rather than thinking about other things?
11. Have I included time in my schedule for social activities and exercise?
12. When I am finished studying for the day, do I feel I have accomplished something?
13. Am I able to remove myself mentally from the environment; that is, can I block out potential distractions?
14. Is the area in which I study relaxing and comfortable, but not so much so that I fall asleep?
15. Is the area in which I study quiet and basically free from interruptions?
16. Is my desk neat and well organized so that I have enough room to study effectively?
17. Is the lighting sufficient and nonglaring?
18. When it is time to study, do I do so immediately and eagerly?
19. Do I reward myself when I feel I have done an exceptionally good job of studying?

Each of these questions should have been answered "yes" if you are studying in an appropriate atmosphere and with the proper frame of mind. If there were some questions to which you answered "no," try to determine what you need to do to improve the conditions. Remember, how, when, and where you study do make a difference in your ability to learn.

Preparing For the NCLEX-PN

One of the first tasks for you to do is learn all you can about the actual test—how it is constructed, what type of questions are included, how long you have to complete the test, and so on. The information provided in Chapters 1 and 2 serves as a good starting point, but you should also read the material provided by the National Council of State Boards of Nursing (NCSBN) and ask your instructors about the test. The better informed you are about the examination, the better you can prepare in a positive manner. Computerized Adaptive Testing (CAT), the method of delivering NCLEX-PN examinations, uses computer technology and measurement theory. Beginning April 2005, examination items are primarily four-option and multiple-choice. Other types of formats include multiple-response, fill-in-the-blank, and hotspot. *Hotspot* is the term coined for charts, tables, or graphic images in which the test taker can select the correct response.

The suggestions in this chapter are provided so that you can learn to study aggressively and actively. Underlining or highlighting key words is a good start, but that is passive learning and is not as effective for long-term memory. You need to develop active learning skills to improve your chances for remembering the material.[4,5]

Relate the material you have just read to other information you have learned in the past. Does knowledge of something new relate to how you would handle a given situation? Is there a relationship between various facts you have learned? If so, what is that relationship? *Think, don't just memorize.*

Ask yourself questions about the material you have

read. Predict how the material might be worded in the examination.

Form study groups to review information and ask each other questions. You may wish to develop a list of questions during one study period and respond to them the next time. All members of the study group need to be actively involved in the process and willing to devote sufficient time for the group interaction to be effective.

Make notes of key concepts or facts that are important to remember. Also, take notes on areas in which you feel uncertain, and use these notes as a reminder that you need to continue learning about the topics.

Be interested in the material. Just because you want to be a practical nurse does not mean that everything you study will be personally interesting to you. However, as you prepare for the examination, you need to become interested in the total field so that you can learn better.

Use prepared test questions such as those in this book to help you study. Use the results of the tests to help you determine your own strengths and weaknesses. Take the tests more than once so that you can see improvement. Use other sources of test items to become more familiar with the different ways in which the same information can be presented.

Set specific goals for yourself. A goal of "needing to learn about nursing" is not much help. Rather, you need to establish a definite goal for each study period.

Establish a schedule for each day's studying and reviewing. Remain flexible, however, so that if you wish to go to a party or go out to dinner when you are supposed to be studying, you can do so without feeling guilty. This does not mean, however, that you forfeit that study time; rather you make it up later.

Write summaries of what you have read. Rephrase information so that you can better understand it. Restating information in your own words will help you remember it better.

If some information is not clear after reading it in one book, read another book to see if the material is explained any better. Do not forget to ask your instructors or peers for clarification.

Visualize the information that you have just read. Try to imagine how what you have read would actually look. Try to visualize a client with certain conditions or symptoms. What would you need to do?

Overlearn the material. Everyone forgets information, so you should not expect to remember everything you read. However, if you continue studying and learning material even after you think you have learned it, you will forget less.

At the end of each study period, take a few minutes to **outline the key material you just learned.** These outlines can then serve as your final review materials just before the examination. Some key elements of a good outline include:

1. Using underlining or symbols to identify key points
2. Using sufficient space to allow for clarification or expansion based on later studying
3. Recording all formulas, equations, and rules exactly
4. Writing legibly on one side of the paper
5. Writing your own ideas or questions as well as facts
6. Using your own words to help reinforce a concept
7. Using personal nursing care experiences to clarify points

Now that you have learned what you should be doing to become a more active learner, you need to put these activities

Table 2–2. **Study Approach Checklist**

	Yes	No

1. Did you note which material you were unsure of so that you can return to it later?
2. Did you look over the material before beginning to study it?
3. When you finished the initial reading, reciting, and reviewing, did you look over your notes and check your memory as to the major headings and subpoints under each heading?
4. Did you select what is important to be learned and determine your time frame for learning it?
5. Did you take brief notes as you reviewed?
6. Did you read the material and try to answer your own questions?
7. After reading the section or chapter, did you look away and try to recite the answers to questions and give examples of patients with similar problems?
8. Did you vary your speed of reading according to the difficulty and familiarity of the material and according to your purpose in reading?
9. Did you pause after reading each section to underline the important points and make marginal notes on the material about which you had questions?
10. Did you go back to the material that you were unsure of and review again?

into place. During the next few study periods, do not try to study any differently than you normally do. Instead, at the end of each study period, take the checklist test shown in Table 2–2. Use the questions to evaluate the ways in which you need to change your studying behavior.

Whenever you answered "no," keep those points in mind the next time you study. Do not feel frustrated if you find you have not included all of the steps in your studying; just keep trying to improve. The overused phrase "Rome wasn't built in a day" is applicable in this instance. It will take time and effort for you to learn how to study more effectively and actively.

How to Take an NCLEX Test

Multiple-Choice Questions

There is a right way and a wrong way to answer multiple-choice items. Although you have probably answered thousands of them during your course of study, you may find it advantageous to review the suggestions given in this section. Part of doing well on an examination is being "test wise"; that is, knowing how to figure out the correct answer even if you are not certain. You may have a wealth of knowledge and be one of the smartest in your class, but if you do not know how to respond to multiple-choice questions, you will be unable to prove this knowledge, and the new NCLEX test formats

pose additional challenges. For better or worse, part of the score you receive on any examination depends on your test-taking ability.

Use logic and common sense to figure out the correct response. The items are usually based on situations that a practical nurse entering the field would most likely encounter rather than exotic or unique situations.

Use cues in the stem and distractors to help you figure out the correct response.

Try to figure out the meaning of unfamiliar words in the stem in terms of the sentence context. You might also be able to figure out the meaning of words by dividing them into prefixes and suffixes that you know.

Read each question thoroughly but quickly. Do not keep reading the same question over and over. Select your response and move on. (In CAT, it is even more critical that you read each item thoroughly. Once you decide on an answer, you cannot change your mind later.)

Read all options before selecting the one you think is correct. A well-constructed test has four plausible responses, and it is your responsibility to select the *best*. Too often, candidates read the first and second options and decide that one of them is correct without reading the other options. Later they may discover that their choice was not really the best.

In the multiple-response item, there may be six plausible responses. It is your responsibility to select all the responses that are correct. There may be two to four correct responses out of the six plausible responses.

Eliminate the distractors that are obviously incorrect and then choose between or among the remaining ones.

Do not try to make an item any more difficult than it is. Do not read anything into the question and do not waste your time looking for "tricks" or hidden meanings. As a rule, the items are straightforward and basic.

Relate each option to the stem. Make sure that the answer you select fits the intent of the stem and is grammatically correct.

Focus on key words in the stem.

Select the option that is most inclusive. If two options are similar, but one contains more details, select the option that is more complete.

Break down complex stems into smaller, more manageable sections.

Make certain that the response you select is correct for each of the separate components.

Try answering the question before you have read the options given. This process will help you find the correct response and will also save you time even if the answer you give is not one of those provided. At least you will be thinking about what to look for.

Do not stop trying. Even if there are several items in a row that seem unfamiliar to you, do not start worrying about the examination as a whole. Just answer the items to the best of your ability and move forward.

Concentrate on one item at a time. Do not worry about how many more items you need to answer or how much time remains. Focus on the item that is before you.

Focus on whether the question is asking for a positive or negative response. Negative words (e.g., not, except) are usually emphasized in the stem to help you recognize that you must reverse your thought process.

If a question requires calculations, **talk yourself through each step of the process.** Double-check your computations to be certain you have not made some minor mistake. Generally, the options included in computational questions are based on mistakes typically made in calculation. This means you may find the answer as you worked the problem and still be wrong.

Try to relate a situation in the question to something with which you are familiar. Determine whether the same concepts would apply.

Reword a difficult question and see if that helps you better understand the intent of the item. If you are deciding between two reasonable answers, select the one that focuses on the client as being a worthy human being.

Look for the most common or typical response to the problem. The examination is designed for nurses entering the field; therefore, the test writers do not expect you to have knowledge that would normally be obtained from years of experience.

Never leave an item unanswered. There is no penalty for guessing, and you have a chance of getting the item correct by guessing. In CAT, you must answer all items presented before any other items are shown.

Use the drop-down calculator to answer the fill-in-the-blank questions. Questions that need to be calculated, such as drug dosages and parenteral formulas, are to be answered by using the drop-down calculator. You will need to know the drug dosages and formulas in order to answer these questions correctly.

If you must guess, do so logically. Eliminate the options that you know are wrong, and then see if there is any test construction flaw that might help you figure out the intended answer. Given the extensive editing done before assembling the NCLEX-PN, it is doubtful that these "errors" will be found, but you might as well look for them. Some of the more common test construction errors are:

Length: Select the longest response if all others are approximately equal.

Location: The correct response is more likely to be in the middle.

Grammar: Incorrect options may not grammatically fit the stem.

Language: Unusual or highly technical language typically indicates an incorrect option.

Qualification: If one option includes qualifiers such as "generally," "tends to," or "usually" and other options do not, select that option.

Generalizability: The correct option tends to have greater applicability or flexibility.

Specifics: Options that include "always" or "never" are typically not the correct answer.

Reread the question in its entirety as well as each option you select. Does your response still make sense? Usually your first response will be correct if you read the stem and all distractors carefully. There are instances, however, when you reread a question and decide that another option is better. If this is the case, then by all means change your answer. Do so only with sufficient reason and not just because you are uncertain. You need to read each item carefully as it is presented and respond accordingly.

Hotspot Questions

A hotspot question will have charts, tables, or graphic images for you to select the correct answer. You must use the computer mouse and direct the cursor to the correct "spot," thus answering the question. Hotspot questions are used to test knowledge of anatomy and physiology as well as skills questions. For example, where do you auscultate for heart sounds? Where do you give a child an intramuscular injection?

Study Schedule

The following schedule is provided to help you prepare for the NCLEX-PN without trying to learn and remember everything at the last minute. Keep in mind that cramming has no long-term benefit; you may remember the material for a few hours but not for the entire examination. At some point during your education, you probably stayed up all night studying for an examination, took the examination, and returned to your room and slept. How much of the material did you remember later that day? Probably not much. Therefore, if you want to do well on the examination, you will have to begin preparing early and *not* try to cram all the information into a few nights of studying.

2–3 Months Before the Examination

Although it may seem early to start preparing for the examination, it really is not. At this time, you should:

1. Begin organizing your textbooks and lecture notes meaningfully.
2. Begin noting areas about which you feel less comfortable.
3. Begin learning about the format (CAT) and content of the examination.
4. Take a practice test that includes items similar to those likely to be on the actual NCLEX-PN to see how well you do; assess your strengths and weaknesses.
5. Establish a study schedule that includes adequate time to prepare but also recognizes the need for flexibility (4–5 days per week, with 1–3 hours of study per day). Your schedule should be based on how well you did on the practice test, how confident you feel, and how many weeks are left before the examination.

4–8 Weeks Before the Examination

At this time, you should:

1. Begin reviewing areas of known weakness *first* so that you will have time to review them again before the examination.
2. Develop, organize, and maintain your own notes in each subject for a final review just before the examination.
3. Form a study group that meets at least weekly; prepare specific topics for discussion when the group meets.
4. Take at least one test a week to help you become more familiar with the types of questions that may be asked.
5. After several weeks of studying, take the original pretest to see how well you are doing, assess strengths and weaknesses again, and readjust your study schedule as necessary.

6. Develop your own situational questions as a technique for reviewing.
7. Maintain sufficient time for eating, sleeping, exercising, socializing, and working—do not become a study hermit.

1 Week Before the Examination

At this time, you should:
1. Begin a concentrated *review* of the material.
2. Take the pretest for the last time and evaluate your performance.
3. Recite key ideas to yourself; make sure all essential formulas or equations are memorized correctly.
4. Rest, eat well, and do not dwell on the test during the nonstudy times.
5. Make sure you have all documents required for admission to the examination. If you have any questions, call the Board of Nursing office or the agency that administers the examination.

1 Day Before the Examination

1. Do something you enjoy during the day; have a nice quiet dinner; and relax that evening by doing something pleasant that will keep your mind off the examination.
2. If you are with colleagues who are taking the test, refrain from discussing it.
3. If you feel the need to review your notes, do so once and then not again—do not keep returning to them.
4. Get sufficient sleep—you need to be both physically and mentally alert on the next day.
5. Double-check that you have all required documents and materials for the next day.

Actual Examination Administration

The examination day has finally arrived and, although you may be anxious or worried, you know how to maintain a helpful level of anxiety. Be confident as you start the day.
1. Get up early enough to have a good breakfast.
2. Wear comfortable clothes—preferably layered, so that you can be comfortable whether the room is warm or cool.
3. Make certain you have everything you need—admission card, identification, money for lunch or parking, and so on.
4. Arrive at the examination site *on time*. If you are driving, start at least 1/2–1 hour earlier than you think is necessary in case an unexpected problem occurs.

Most researchers have found that the greatest level of anxiety in a testing situation occurs while waiting for the test to begin or during the first few minutes of the examination. If you find this happening to you at the start of the test or at anytime during the test, some rapid relaxation may be helpful. You should use this technique as soon as you are aware of feelings of anxiety; if you wait, these feelings may become heightened and more difficult to allay.

One recommended procedure is as follows[3]:
1. Close your eyes. As you sit in your seat, tense all of your muscles. Really try to "scrunch up" as many muscles as you can.

2. Once you have tensed the muscles, take a deep breath (inhale through your nostrils) and hold your breath for a count of five, keeping your muscles tensed all of the time.
3. After counting to five, simultaneously exhale rapidly through your lips and quickly let go of your muscle tightness by silently telling yourself to *relax*.
4. With your eyes still closed, go as limp in the chair as you possibly can after relaxing.
5. Now with your muscles relaxed, take a second |deep breath through your nostrils. Hold your breath for a couple of seconds. Then *slowly* exhale through your lips.
6. As you exhale, repeat the word *"calm"* to yourself. You will probably repeat the word 7–10 times while slowly exhaling.
7. Repeat these steps once or twice to achieve greater relaxation. Each time through the steps will take about 30 seconds.

In addition to the foregoing relaxation technique, you should take a number of other steps to remain calm during the examination.
1. Once you are told to begin the test, jot down formulas or ideas that you think you might forget during the examination in the front of your booklet.
2. Develop an *assertive* yet realistic attitude. Approach the test determined that you will do your best, but also accept the limits of what you know. Use everything you know to do well, but do not blame yourself for what you do not know.
3. Remember the guidelines on how to take multiple-choice tests.
4. Do *not* spend too much time thinking about alternative responses, especially after you have selected the one you think is correct.
5. *Pay attention* to the test, not to yourself or others. Do not waste time worrying, doubting yourself, or wondering how others are doing. Do not worry about what you should have done; instead, pay attention to what you are doing now.
6. Do not let lapses of memory produce unhealthy anxiety or fear; such lapses are normal.
7. Do not waste time with emotional reactions to the questions.
8. *Remain confident* and resolve to work at top efficiency throughout the entire examination. At all times, remain positive and convinced that you will be successful on the examination.

REFERENCES

1. Fiore, N and Pescar, SC: Conquering Test Anxiety. Warner Books, New York, 1987.
2. Sarason, IG (ed): Test Anxiety: Theory, Research and Application. Laurence Erlbaum Associates, Hillsdale, NJ, 1980, pp 18, 12–113.
3. Ottens, AJ: Coping with Academic Anxiety, Revised Edition. Rosen Publishing Group, New York, 1991.
4. Sherman, TM and Wildman, TM: Proven Strategies for Successful Test Taking. Charles E Merrill, Columbus, OH, 1982.
5. Kesselman-Turkel, J and Peterson, F: Test Taking Strategies. University of Wisconsin Press, Madison, 2004.
6. NCLEX-PN Examination.Test Plan for the National Council Licensure Examination for Licensed Practical/Vocational Nurses, April 2005.

Clinical Specialties
Content Reviews
and Tests

CHAPTER 3

Maternity Nursing: Content Review and Test

Lizabeth L. Carlson, RN, DNS, BC
Larry D. Purnell, RN, PhD
Golden M. Tradewell, RN, PhD

The process of childbearing involves exciting changes in the life of a woman and her family. The changes in physical, emotional, and psychosocial factors have an enormous impact on the expectant family. Factors that affect successful adaptation to pregnancy include personal values, family member roles, social support factors, and cultural effects. Maternity nurses have both the opportunity and responsibility to help the expectant family make the necessary transitions to welcome their new baby into the family. The maternity nurse is responsible for incorporating the psychosocial, cultural, and physiological aspects of pregnancy in the educational, emotional, and physical needs of the childbearing woman and her family.

Antepartal Care

I. Conception
  A. Fertilization
    1. Conception occurs in the upper third of the fallopian tube when egg and sperm unite.
      a. Conception occurs approximately 14 days before the start of the next menstrual cycle.
        1) Each ovum has 23 chromosomes.
        2) Each sperm has 23 chromosomes.
        3) Each fertilized egg is called a *zygote*.
        4) Each zygote has a total of 46 chromosomes (23 from each parent).
          a) A female has two X chromosomes.
          b) A male has one X and one Y chromosome.
      b. The zygote moves from the fallopian tube to the uterus for implantation.
      c. The fertilized egg is called an *embryo* from implantation until the eighth week of gestation.
      d. From the eighth week of gestation until birth, the fertilized egg is called a *fetus*.

  B. Placenta
    1. Structure
      a. Made up of cotyledons
      b. Connects to the fetus via the umbilical cord
      c. Connected to the mother through adherence to the uterine wall
    2. Function
      a. Nutrient and waste exchange between maternal and fetal systems
      b. Gas (oxygen and carbon dioxide) exchange between maternal and fetal systems
      c. Production of pregnancy hormones
        1) Progesterone: stimulates placental growth, decreases uterine contractions, suppresses ovulation, maintains endometrium (decidua) throughout pregnancy
        2) Estrogen: stimulates enlargement of breasts and uterus; stimulates contractions
        3) Human placental lactogen (hPL): increases maternal metabolism; aids in preparing breasts for lactation
        4) Human chorionic gonadotropin (hCG): works to develop placenta until about 11 weeks' gestation
  C. Umbilical cord
    1. Structure
      a. Contains two arteries.
      b. Contains one vein.
      c. Arteries and vein are surrounded by Wharton's jelly (for protection).
    2. Function
      a. Attaches placenta to growing fetus at the umbilicus
      b. Carries nutrients, gases, and wastes between mother and fetus
  D. Amniotic membranes
    1. Structure

a. Thin membranous sac surrounding the fetus
b. Two layers
   1) Amnion
   2) Chorion
c. Filled with fluid
   1) Saline
   2) Alkaline
d. Fluid constantly replaced
2. Function
   a. Protects the fetus
   b. Allows free fetal movement
   c. Maintains a stable temperature
   d. Prevents amnion from adhering to the fetus
   e. Allows for fetal respiration
   f. Provides fluid for fetal swallowing
E. Maternal circulation
   1. Blood that is under pressure from the maternal heart is circulated to the aorta, common iliac vessels, hypogastric, uterine arteries through the uteroplacental shunt, to the cotyledons of the placenta. Three transfers take place:
      a. Oxygen: simple diffusion
      b. Glucose: facilitated diffusion
      c. Proteins: active transport
F. Fetal circulation
   1. Umbilical vein carries oxygen and nutrients to the fetus.
   2. Umbilical arteries carry carbon dioxide and waste from the fetus to the placenta.
   3. Ductus venosus bypasses digestive tract and liver; shunts blood directly to the inferior vena cava.
   4. Foramen ovale shunts blood from right to left atria bypassing lungs and ventricles.
   5. Ductus arteriosus shunts blood from pulmonary artery to aorta, bypassing the lungs.
G. Normal fetal heart rate: 110–160 bpm
H. Liver and lungs: little function in fetal life
   1. Liver is major source of oxyhemoglobin
   2. Fetus "practices" breathing amniotic fluid in and out (fetal respiration)
II. Disorders related to conception and implantation
   A. Abortion: termination of pregnancy before 20 weeks' gestation
      1. Types
         a. Spontaneous
            1) Threatened: possible loss of pregnancy evidenced by vaginal bleeding
            2) Incomplete: part but not all of pregnancy tissue expelled
            3) Habitual: spontaneous loss of three or more pregnancies
            4) Complete: all pregnancy tissue expelled
            5) Inevitable: cervical dilatation
         b. Induced
            1) Therapeutic: an abortion performed to save the woman's life
            2) Voluntary: occurs up to 24 weeks with medical intervention at the woman's request
            3) Criminal: an illegal termination of pregnancy
   B. Ectopic pregnancy: implantation of a fertilized ovum outside the uterus, usually in the fallopian tube
      1. Signs and symptoms

a. Sharp localized pain in the lower abdomen
b. Painless irregular vaginal bleeding
c. Unilateral shoulder pain
d. Syncope
e. Hypovolemic shock, pallor, anxiety, air hunger, increased thirst, palpitations
C. Hydatidiform mole: a disorder in placental development that causes the ovum to deteriorate and grapelike vesicles to form; may become malignant (choriocarcinoma), especially if a partial mole
   1. Signs and symptoms
      a. Vaginal bleeding around the 12th week of pregnancy
      b. Hyperemesis
      c. Larger fundal height than expected for dates
      d. Extremely high hCG levels
      e. No fetal heart tones
      f. Symptoms of pregnancy-induced hypertension (PIH) before 20 weeks of pregnancy
   2. Avoidance of pregnancy and follow-up for 1 year is essential to ensure hCG levels return to normal and to rule out malignancy
III. Therapeutic management; nursing interventions
   A. Data collection
      1. Physical
         a. Vaginal bleeding
            1) Amount
            2) Color
            3) Consistency
            4) Presence of clots
         b. Pain
            1) Type
               a) Sharp
               b) Crampy
               c) Dull
            2) Location
               a) Abdominal
               b) Pelvic
               c) Lower quadrants
               d) Shoulder
         c. Vital signs, especially blood pressure
         d. Tissue passed from vagina
         e. Level of consciousness
      2. Psychological
         a. Fear of death
         b. Anxiety
         c. Guilt
         d. Grief
         e. Disappointment
         f. Denial
         g. Uncooperative
      3. Laboratory tests
         a. hCG
            1) Lower for abortion and tubal pregnancies
            2) Elevated for hydatidiform mole
         b. Complete blood cell (CBC) count
            1) Values normally decreased during pregnancy
               a) Hemoglobin
               b) Hematocrit
            2) Values normally increased during pregnancy
               a) White blood cells
               b) Red blood cells

c. Other specialized evaluations
  1) Ultrasound
  2) Culdocentesis
  3) Pelvic exam
B. Medical and surgical intervention; planning and nursing implementation
  1. Provide information regarding treatment plan
  2. Prepare for surgery
    a. Dilatation and curettage
      1) Incomplete abortion
      2) Hydatidiform mole
    b. Laparoscopy
      1) Ectopic pregnancy
      2) Possible removal of tube/ovary or both
  3. Provide opportunity for support and counseling
  4. Prepare for recovery and self-care
  5. Nursing interventions
    a. Emphasize importance of bed rest
    b. Save all expelled tissue and clots
    c. Observe vaginal bleeding
      1) Count perineal pads
      2) Estimate blood loss with the centimeter/mililiter method (5-cm diameter on peripad equals approximately 10-mL blood loss)
      3) Monitor vital signs every 5 minutes to 4 hours, depending on the woman's condition
      4) Institute treatment for shock prn
      5) Observe for postsurgery hemorrhage or infection
    d. Drug therapies
      1) Oral contraceptives
        a) For 1 year post–hydatidiform mole
        b) For 3 months following ectopic pregnancy
      2) Anticancer drugs for hydatidiform mole
  6. Evaluation of nursing interventions
    a. The woman participates in decisions.
    b. The woman has normal vital signs according to her baseline and pain is controlled.
    c. The woman demonstrates physical and psychological recovery.
    d. The woman identifies support systems.
IV. Maternal adaptations to pregnancy
  A. Physiological
    1. Cardiovascular
      a. Pulse rate increases by 10 bpm.
      b. Blood volume increases by 50%.
      c. White blood cells (WBCs) increase to an average of 15,000 mm^3.
      d. Clotting factors increase.
      e. Systolic and diastolic blood pressures are lower by 5–10 mm Hg in the first and second trimesters; they return to prepregnant levels in the third trimester.
    2. Respiratory
      a. Rate does not change; depth becomes more shallow and diaphragmatic as the uterus enlarges.
      b. Oxygen consumption increases during the last half of pregnancy.
    3. Gastrointestinal
      a. Gums swell and bleed easily.

b. Nausea and vomiting common in the first trimester.
c. Delayed gastric emptying and decreased intestinal motility (caused by effects of progesterone).
d. Hemorrhoids and constipation common.
4. Urinary tract
  a. Frequency common in the first and third trimesters; caused by pressure from the uterus.
  b. Dilation of kidneys and ureters caused by progesterone.
  c. Enlarging uterus places pressure on the right ureter and the back flow of urine causes dilation of the right renal pelvis.
  d. Glycosuria is caused by increased glomerular filtration.
5. Reproductive
  a. Uterus
    1) Hypertrophy of myometrial cells results in uterine enlargement.
    2) Number of blood vessels to the uterus increase.
    3) Gentle, rhythmic contractions start in the first trimester (Braxton Hicks contractions).
  b. Cervix
    1) Goodell's sign: softening of the cervix
    2) Hegar's sign: softening of the lower uterine segment
    3) McDonald's sign: easy flexion of the uterus against the cervix
    4) Chadwick's sign: dark blue-purple coloration of the cervix (color change can extend to the vagina and labia)
    5) Development of a thick mucous plug
  c. Ovaries
    1) Cease egg production
    2) Produce corpus luteum (which produces progesterone to maintain the pregnancy) for first 12 weeks of pregnancy
  d. Vagina
    1) Increased vaginal secretions.
    2) May have color changes (Chadwick's sign).
  e. Breasts
    1) Increased size and tenderness.
    2) Nipples become more erectile.
    3) Areolas darken and enlarge.
    4) Montgomery's tubercules develop.
    5) Leakage of colostrum in third trimester.
6. Skin
  a. Darkening of areolas, nipples, vulva, and linea nigra.
  b. Mask of pregnancy (chloasma) may develop.
  c. Stretch marks (striae gravidarum) possible.
    1) Breasts
    2) Abdomen
    3) Hips
    4) Thighs
  d. Spider nevi may develop.
    1) Face
    2) Chest
    3) Arms
7. Skeletal

a. Relaxation of pelvic joints caused by influence of relaxin and progesterone
b. Postural changes (lordosis) as pregnancy advances

8. Metabolism
   a. Average desired weight gain: 25–35 pounds
   b. Increased water retention (caused by influence of estrogen)
   c. Physiological anemia caused by the increased volume of the blood plasma diluting the red blood cells (RBCs) (hemodilution)
   d. Increased iron demand

9. Psychological
   a. Accomplishment of developmental tasks depends on
      1) The woman's emotional make-up
      2) Her support systems
      3) Acceptance of the pregnancy
      4) Cultural beliefs
   b. Common responses
      1) Ambivalence in early pregnancy very common even with planned pregnancies
      2) Acceptance
         a) Happy
         b) Fewer physical discomforts
      3) Introversion
         a) A focus on self and the fetus
         b) Occurs in the second trimester
      4) Mood swings
         a) Common throughout pregnancy
         b) Caused by increased hormonal production
      5) Body image
         a) How the woman views herself
         b) Her perception of other's views (about her)

V. Care in the first trimester
   A. Data collection
      1. History: present obstetric (OB) experience
         a. Determine first day of last menstrual period (LMP).
         b. Assess for bleeding or cramping since LMP.
         c. Determine if this pregnancy was planned or unplanned.
      2. History: past OB experiences
         a. Number of pregnancies, abortions, stillbirths, premature births, and living children
         b. Difficulties with other pregnancies
         c. Blood type and Rh factor
      3. History: past medical
         a. Childhood diseases
         b. Any hospitalizations
         c. Serious illnesses
         d. Handicaps
      4. History: current medical
         a. Medications
         b. Usual weight and height
         c. Use of drugs, alcohol, tobacco
         d. Disease conditions or infections
      5. History: family
         a. Genetic diseases
         b. Chronic diseases
            1) Diabetes mellitus

2) Cardiovascular problems
3) Pulmonary diseases
4) PIH
5) Phenylketonuria (PKU)

   c. Multiple births

6. Physical
   a. Presumptive signs
      1) Amenorrhea
      2) Breast tenderness and enlargement
      3) Nausea and vomiting
      4) Urinary frequency
      5) Quickening
      6) Chloasma
      7) Linea nigra
   b. Probable signs
      1) Hegar's
      2) Goodell's
      3) Ballottement
      4) Chadwick's
      5) Enlargement of abdomen
      6) Changes in cervix and uterus
      7) Braxton Hicks contractions
   c. Positive (diagnostic) signs
      1) Fetal heartbeat heard
         a) By Doppler at 10–12 weeks
         b) By fetoscope at 18–20 weeks
      2) Ultrasound visualization of gestational sac, fetus, and fetal heartbeat
      3) Fetal movement felt by an experienced health-care provider
      4) Fetal heart rate (FHR) tracing (electrocardiogram [ECG])
      5) Uterine souffle

7. Psychological
   a. Emotional lability
   b. Disbelief or shock over pregnancy
   c. Physical symptoms possibly experienced by the male partner in addition to the expectant mother (couvade)
   d. Partner possibly protective
   e. How pregnancy viewed: as illness or as normal life process

B. Planning
   1. Provide education about pregnancy and safety.
   2. Promote maternal and fetal well-being.
   3. Assist with psychosocial adaptation.

C. Nursing implementation
   1. Obtain complete health history
      a. Gravidity (number of pregnancies)
         1) Primigravida: pregnant for first time
         2) Multigravida: pregnant for at least second time
      b. Parity: number of births past 20 weeks (alive or not)
         1) Nullipara: never delivered after 20 weeks
         2) Primipara: one birth after 20 weeks
         3) Multipara: several births after 20 weeks
   2. Calculate estimated date of delivery (EDD): Subtract 3 months from LMP and add 7 days
   3. Data collection
      a. Measure weight and height
      b. Assess blood pressure, pulse, and respirations

c. Palpate breasts
d. Assist with speculum exam
   1) Papanicolaou (Pap) smear
   2) Gonorrhea culture
e. Inspect abdomen by palpation and auscultation for FHR at 10–12 weeks.
f. Obtain urine specimen and check for sugar and protein.
g. Collect blood for syphilis (Venereal Disease Research Laboratory [VDRL]).
h. Collect blood for CBC, rubella, blood type, and Rh factor.
i. Provide nutritional information; encourage a nutritionally sound diet.

4. Provide education about:
a. Exercise: avoid
   1) High-impact aerobics and other exercise that increase the heart rate >120 bpm
   2) Saunas
   3) Hot tubs
b. Work: no heavy lifting (>10 lb)
c. Common discomforts
   1) Urinary frequency
   2) Breast tenderness
   3) Pelvic cramping (without vaginal bleeding)
   4) Backache
   5) Heartburn
   6) Mood swings
   7) Nausea and vomiting
   8) Constipation
   9) Broad ligament pain
d. Schedule for prenatal visits
e. Discuss childbirth education classes
f. Sexuality
g. Elimination of harmful substances
   1) Drugs (prescription, over-the-counter, street drugs)
   2) Tobacco
   3) Alcohol
   4) Caffeine
   5) Artificial sweeteners
h. Nausea: keep crackers at bedside
i. Danger signs and symptoms
   1) Sudden gush of fluid from vagina
   2) Severe headache, blurred vision, seeing spots before eyes
   3) Swelling of face, eyelids, hands, lower legs, feet
   4) Vaginal bleeding
   5) Fever and chills
   6) Lack of fetal movement
   7) Pain in abdomen or chest
   8) Scant or bloody urine
   9) Persistent vomiting
j. Testing
   1) Ultrasound
   2) Chorionic villus sampling (CVS)
   3) Amniocentesis

D. Evaluation of nursing intervention
1. Expectant woman participates in decisions.
2. Expectant woman verbalizes understanding of safety.

3. Expectant woman and her fetus maintain good health during the first 12 weeks.
4. Expectant woman asks questions about self-care.
5. Expectant woman voices acceptance of the pregnancy.

VI. Care in the second trimester
A. Data collection
1. Physical
   a. Weight gain 1 lb/week.
   b. Nausea and vomiting should cease.
   c. Gravid uterus moves upward and out of the pelvis; results in decreased urinary frequency.
   d. Quickening occurs (fetal movement 18–20 weeks).
   e. Blood pressure decreased compared with prepregnancy levels.
   f. FHR auscultated between 110 and 160 bpm.
   g. Fundus at umbilicus by 20 weeks.
2. Psychological
   a. Woman/family verbalizes feelings about pregnancy.
   b. Woman wears maternity clothes.
   c. Woman/family verbalizes changes they are making in planning for the new baby.
   d. Woman is reflective about maternal role.
B. Planning
1. Provide counseling about safety for mother and fetus.
2. Promote psychosocial adaptation by expectant woman.
   a. Therapeutic communication.
   b. Teaching.
      1) Family roles
      2) Fetal feedback (activity in response to a stimulus)
   c. Involve woman/family in childbirth education.
C. Nursing implementation
1. Document and report any abnormalities to the physician.
2. Listen to fetal heart tones, allowing woman and family to hear.
3. Determine fundal height.
4. Discuss common discomforts and treatment.
   a. Heartburn: benefits of eating small frequent meals, sitting up for 30 minutes after eating, avoiding fatty foods
   b. Varicose veins: elevation of legs, wearing support hose, avoid crossing legs
   c. Ankle edema: elevating legs, avoiding salty food, wearing support hose
   d. Hemorrhoids: advising patient to walk more, increase fiber in diet, take warm sitz baths
   e. Constipation: advising patient to walk more, increase fluids and fiber
   f. Backache: helpful to wear low-heeled shoes; use proper posture; perform pelvic-lift exercises
   g. Leg cramps: caused by calcium/phosphorus imbalance. Avoiding/limiting soft drinks containing phosphate, increasing calcium in diet, exercising leg to release cramp, dorsiflexion of foot
5. Review prenatal exercises.

D. Evaluation of nursing intervention
   1. Expectant woman verbalizes self-help therapies for common discomforts.
   2. Expectant woman verbalizes acknowledgement of the pregnancy.
   3. Expectant woman relates plans for incorporating the new baby into the family.
   4. Pregnancy proceeds normally during the fourth through the sixth months.

VII. Care in the third trimester
   A. Data collection
      1. Physical
         a. Weight gain approximately 16 lb by the beginning of the third trimester.
         b. FHR 110–160 bpm.
         c. Fetal activity monitored by expectant mother (kick count).
         d. Return of urinary frequency.
         e. No sugar or protein in urine.
         f. Slight edema in ankles; relieved by elevation.
         g. Determine growth by fundal height (each centimeter in height equals a week of pregnancy).
         h. Vaginal secretions clear; no bleeding.
         i. Blood pressure normally returns to prepregnancy levels (however, if 140 mm Hg systolic and/or 90 mm Hg diastolic, consider hypertension).
      2. Psychological
         a. Increased anxiety related to:
         b. Labor and birth
         c. Mutilation of her body
         d. Ability to cope
      3. Partner experiencing increased anxiety about:
         a. Healthy baby
         b. Safety of woman
         c. Preparation of home for baby
   B. Planning
      1. Involve couple in childbirth classes.
      2. Involve couple in parenting activities as preparation for baby.
      3. Provide opportunity for tour of the obstetric unit and hospital.
      4. Discuss fears and labor events.
      5. Provide support.
   C. Nursing implementation
      1. Document and report any abnormalities to the physician.
      2. Determine fundal height.
      3. Auscultate FHR.
      4. Discuss labor and delivery plan with the woman and her partner.
      5. Discuss:
         a. Signs of labor
         b. When to go to the hospital
         c. When to call the physician
         d. Possible sibling reactions
      6. Determine fetal presentation.
      7. Provide information about specialized tests.
         a. Ultrasound
         b. Amniocentesis for fetal maturity
            1) Lecithin/sphingomyelin (L/S) ratio
            2) Phosphatidylglycerol (PG)
            3) Creatinine

   c. Nonstress test
      1) Reactive: FHR accelerations with fetal movement last for 15 seconds at least 15 beats above the baseline; must occur at least twice in 20 minutes.
      2) Nonreactive: no FHR accelerations with fetal movement.
   d. Biophysical profile
      1) Includes nonstress testing
      2) Also sonogram to assess for
         a) Amniotic fluid volume
         b) Fetal tone
         c) Fetal respiration
         d) Gross body movement
      3) Scoring: 0–2 points for each parameter
         a) Score of 8–10 normal
         b) 6 points: suspected chronic asphyxia
         c) 4 points: nonreassuring
         d) 0–2 points: strong suspicion of chronic asphyxia
   e. Contraction stress test
      1) Oxytocin challenge test: use of oxytocin (Pitocin) to produce uterine contractions
      2) Nipple stimulation test: use of nipple self-stimulation to produce uterine contractions spontaneously
      3) Contraction stress test: performed when woman is already having uterine contractions
      4) Results
         a) Negative: no late decelerations with uterine contractions
         b) Positive: presence of two or more late decelerations with uterine contractions
         c) Equivocal: one late deceleration only, with uterine contractions; test must be repeated next day

D. Evaluation of nursing interventions
   1. Woman/couple attend childbirth classes and hospital tour.
   2. Woman aware of and reports fetal activity patterns.
   3. Couple expresses expectations of the birthing experience and parenthood.

Disorders/Complications of Pregnancy

I. Placental
   A. Placenta previa
      1. Types
         a. Complete: center of placenta completely covers cervical os
         b. Partial: a portion of placenta covers cervical os
         c. Marginal: lower edge of placenta lies on or near cervical os
      2. Data collection
         a. Physical
            1) Increased incidence with parity, multiple gestation, fetal defects, previous endometritis
            2) Painless, unexplained uterine bleeding or spotting, usually in third trimester

3) Intermittent gushes of blood

4) Profuse hemorrhage as cervix dilates

5) Fetal distress possibly present as late decelerations

  b. Psychological: apprehension about safety of self and fetus

3. Planning

  a. Maintain vital signs within normal limits.

  b. Monitor bleeding and fetal status.

  c. Provide support and information about condition.

4. Nursing implementation

  a. *No vaginal or rectal examination is permitted.*

  b. Do not give enemas or suppositories.

  c. Prepare for ultrasound of abdomen.

  d. Manage bleeding.

    1) Give nothing by mouth (NPO).

    2) Hydrate with intravenous (IV) fluids.

    3) Apply external fetal monitor.

    4) Perform pad count: weigh pads (1 g = 1 mL), or estimate vaginal bleeding with the centimeter/milliliter method hourly.

    5) Monitor vital signs.

    6) Obtain type and crossmatch for at least 2 units of blood.

    7) Have patient maintain bed rest.

    8) Prepare patient for cesarean delivery

      a) Get informed consent.

      b) Allow verbalization of feelings.

    9) Provide double setup for delivery if vaginal exam. performed (i.e., vaginal and cesarean instruments)

5. Evaluation of nursing interventions

  a. Woman prepared for cesarean if bleeding severe.

  b. Self-limited bleeding episodes do not endanger mother or fetus.

  c. Woman verbalizes anxiety, fear, and anger.

B. Abruptio placentae

1. Types

  a. Concealed: separation occurs centrally, causing uterus to fill with blood

  b. Marginal: separation occurs near edge, causing bright-red bleeding from the vagina

2. Data collection

  a. Physical

    1) Vaginal bleeding

      a) Scant

      b) Heavy

    2) Couvelaire uterus

      a) Tender

      b) Irritable contractions

      c) Rigidity

      d) Rising uterine baseline tone on fetal/contraction monitor

      e) Uneven tone

    3) Constant painful, low backache

    4) Abdominal pain constant or intermittent

    5) Maternal shock

    6) Low FHR with late decelerations

    7) Absent fetal heart tones

    8) Extreme fetal activity followed by inactivity

  b. Psychological

    1) Confusion due to shock or overwhelming pain

    2) Restlessness, weakness, uncooperative

3. Planning

  a. Monitor maternal vital signs closely

  b. Establish fetal well-being through electronic fetal monitoring (EFM).

  c. Reduce apprehension; explain procedures

4. Nursing implementation

  a. Treat shock

    1) Administer oxygen at 6–10 L/min by mask.

    2) Administer rapid infusion of IV fluids via large-bore IV catheter (16 gauge).

    3) Maintain patient in Trendelenburg's position.

    4) Assess vital signs every 5–10 minutes.

    5) Monitor intake and output (I&O).

    6) Use external fetal monitor for labor pattern and FHR.

  b. Remain at bedside.

  c. Prepare for emergency delivery.

  d. Prepare to transfuse.

  e. Monitor fibrinogen, prothrombin time (PT), partial thromboplastin time (PTT), platelets, hemoglobin (Hgb), and hematocrit (Hct).

5. Evaluation of nursing interventions

  a. Couple verbalizes understanding of treatment plan.

  b. Woman should be physically stable: normotensive with adequate Hgb and Hct.

  c. Woman verbalizes relief or gratitude, or both, once emergency over.

  d. Fetal status stabilizes.

C. Incompetent cervix: painless dilation of the cervix in the second trimester

1. Causes

  a. Previous surgical trauma (cone biopsy)

  b. Mechanical defect

2. Surgical treatment

  a. Cerclage

  b. McDonald's procedure

  c. Shirodkar's procedure

3. Data collection

  a. Physical

    1) Painless dilatation

    2) Presence of vaginal bleeding or bloody show

    3) Recurrent spontaneous second trimester abortions

    4) Fetal membranes visible with pelvic exam

  b. Psychological

    1) Discouragement about ability to deliver full-term infant

    2) Guilt about activity and sexual relations

    3) Anxiety about outcome

4. Planning

  a. Prepare for surgical procedure.

  b. Monitor for preterm labor.

  c. Provide opportunities for discussion of feelings.

  d. Teach woman warning signs of labor.

5. Nursing implementation

  a. Obtain history of other pregnancies.

b. Maintain bed rest.

c. Monitor FHR.

d. Prepare for surgery.

e. Observe for complications after surgery
   1) Spontaneous rupture of membranes
   2) Uterine contractions
   3) Signs of infection
   4) Vaginal bleeding

f. Discuss discharge teaching.
   1) Notify physician if cramping, bleeding, or gush of fluid present.
   2) Be aware of fetal activity.
   3) Notify physician if fever >100.4°F (38°C), chills, or dysuria present.

6. Evaluation of nursing interventions
   a. Woman voices understanding of the need for the procedure and what will be/was done.
   b. Labor delayed until 38–42 weeks' gestation.
   c. The woman verbalizes self-confidence regarding carrying a pregnancy to term.
   d. The woman lists signs and symptoms (S/S) of problems and agrees to notify the physician of the same.

D. Hyperemesis gravidarum: continuous episodes of vomiting due to hormones or stress or both
   1. Data collection
      a. Physical
         1) Weight loss
         2) Dehydration
         3) Epigastric pain
         4) Uncoordinated movements, jerking
         5) Electrolyte imbalance
      b. Psychological
         1) Excessive stress in the woman's/family's life
         2) Unplanned pregnancy
   2. Planning
      a. Establish normal fluid and electrolyte levels.
      b. Assist with coping strategies.
      c. Teach about nutrition.
      d. Provide therapy to stop vomiting and restore balance.
   3. Nursing implementation
      a. Administer IV fluids, vitamins, and antiemetics.
      b. Weigh daily.
      c. Observe vomitus for amount and consistency.
      d. Assess I&O every shift.
      e. Slowly introduce small, frequent meals high in complex carbohydrates.
      f. Obtain psychiatric consultation if needed.
   4. Evaluation of nursing interventions
      a. Attainment of adequate hydration, as evidenced by (AEB):
         1) Good skin turgor
         2) Moist mucous membranes
         3) Electrolytes within normal limits
         4) Urine output averaging at least 30 mL/hr
      b. Establish normal eating patterns.
      c. Promote woman's verbalization of ability to cope.

II. Preexisting conditions
   A. Cardiac
      1. Types

a. Mitral valve stenosis or prolapse common

b. Congestive heart failure from increased cardiac demands

2. Data collection
   a. Physical
      1) Pedal edema
      2) Generalized edema
      3) Moist cough
      4) Fatigue
      5) Tachycardia or irregular pulse
      6) Dyspnea on exertion
      7) Systolic murmurs
      8) Cyanosis of nailbeds and lips
   b. Psychological
      1) Anxiety about death of self or fetus
      2) Frustration over reduced activity
      3) Concern for other family members' functioning
      4) Family role changes

3. Planning
   a. Promote rest and relaxation; limit activity.
   b. Protect from infection.
   c. Promote acceptance of limitations and the condition.

4. Nursing implementation
   a. Prevent infection (prophylactic antibiotic therapy) early.
   b. Have patient avoid strenuous exercise.
   c. Provide frequent rest periods.
   d. Help patient/family identify acceptable methods of accomplishing tasks.
   e. Encourage woman/family to verbalize feelings.
   f. Prepare for vaginal delivery by assisting with administration of regional anesthesia and use of forceps.
   g. Help woman identify ways to avoid/deal with emotional stress.
   h. Administer medications:
      1) Digitalis
      2) Furosemide (Lasix)
      3) Penicillin
   i. Position patient for best circulatory perfusion (left lateral position).
   j. Administer oxygen at 6–10 L/min via mask.
   k. Fourth stage of labor most unstable due to rapid shifts in circulating blood volume.

5. Evaluation of nursing interventions
   a. Woman remains free of infection.
   b. Woman follows dietary and activity limitations.
   c. Woman's condition stable during labor and delivery.

B. Hypertension
   1. Essential
      a. Occurs in second trimester
      b. Permanent condition
      c. No preeclamptic symptoms
   2. Data collection
      a. Physical
         1) Blood pressure elevation above baseline or
         2) 140/90 mm Hg or greater
         3) Retinal changes

b. Psychological: may be depressed about permanent condition
3. Planning
   a. Monitor blood pressure frequently.
   b. Provide education about self-care.
   c. Assess fetal well-being.
4. Nursing implementation
   a. Monitor blood pressure every 2 weeks for first 24 weeks, and then weekly.
   b. Provide low-sodium diet information.
   c. Administer medications; teach self-administration.
      1) Diuretics
         a) Thiazides
         b) Furosemide
      2) Antihypertensives
         a) Calcium channel blockers
         b) Hydralazine
   d. Encourage frequent rest on left side.
   e. Avoid stress.
   f. Discuss disease and associated problems.
5. Evaluation of nursing interventions
   a. Woman remains normotensive.
   b. Woman demonstrates knowledge of treatment regimen.
   c. Pregnancy progresses without maternal/fetal complications.
C. PIH (toxemia)
1. Preeclampsia symptoms
   a. Edema
   b. Proteinuria
   c. Hyperreflexia
   d. Elevated blood pressure during pregnancy
2. Eclampsia symptoms
   a. Preeclampsia symptoms
   b. Severe frontal headache
   c. Visual changes
   d. Epigastric discomfort
   e. Convulsions
   f. Decreased urine output
3. Data collection
   a. Physical
      1) Edema in pretibial, facial, hand areas
      2) Proteinuria: 1+ to 4+
      3) Weight gain: 2 lb/week or more, or rapid increase
      4) Elevated blood pressure
         a) 140/90–160/110 mm Hg: preeclampsia
         b) 160/110 mm Hg: eclampsia
      5) Blurred vision, frontal headache
      6) Epigastric pain
      7) Hyperreflexia, twitching, convulsions
      8) Oliguria
   b. Psychological
      1) Anxiety about safety of self and fetus
      2) Frustration about activity restrictions and possible hospitalization
4. Planning
   a. Prevent progression to convulsions
   b. Promote fetal well-being
   c. Provide teaching about condition

5. Nursing implementation
   a. Assess blood pressure, urine for protein, edema, reflexes, and weight gain.
   b. Provide high-protein diet, no added salt.
   c. Encourage patient to rest on left side in quiet, shaded atmosphere.
   d. Teach S/S to report immediately.
   e. Teach self-administration of medications.
      1) Phenobarbital
      2) Hydralazine
      3) Magnesium gluconate
   f. Prevent convulsions.
      1) Obtain electrolyte, magnesium levels, and uric acid levels.
      2) Administer magnesium sulfate ($MgSO_4$).
         a) Loading dose IV piggyback
         b) Hourly maintenance dose of 1–2 g
         c) Never put $MgSO_4$ in the mainline IV infusion
         d) Administered by IV controller or pump
      3) Perform hourly assessment of output, respirations, reflexes, and proteinuria.
      4) Monitor vital signs every 15 minutes if woman is in labor.
      5) Have calcium gluconate available to reverse magnesium effects.
      6) Use fetal monitor to evaluate fetus and labor.
      7) Continue $MgSO_4$ administration for at least 24 hours after delivery.
6. Evaluation of nursing interventions
   a. Convulsions are avoided.
   b. Progress to delivery uncomplicated for mother and fetus.
   c. Woman/family verbalizes support and acceptable coping methods.
D. Diabetes mellitus
1. Types
   a. Gestational: carbohydrate intolerance during pregnancy
   b. Insulin-dependent: lack of insulin from pancreas requires external source; can be preexisting or develop in pregnancy
   c. Non–insulin dependent: partial insulin is secreted; requires diet control
2. Data collection
   a. Physical
      1) Hyperemesis during early pregnancy
      2) Sugar and ketones in urine
      3) Elevated results of fasting blood sugar (FBS), resting glucose level, and glucose tolerance test (GTT)
      4) Rapid weight gain
      5) Polyuria, polydipsia, polyphagia
      6) Previous large baby ≥4500 g
   b. Psychological
      1) Anxiety associated with fetal anomalies or death
      2) Stress in learning to cope with the disease
3. Planning
   a. Test regularly for glucose level.
   b. Periodic hemoglobin A1C (HgbA1c).
   c. Implement diet and medication if needed.

d. Provide teaching about disease and its effects on pregnancy.
e. Observe for signs of hypoglycemia or hyperglycemia.
f. Monitor fetal well-being.
4. Nursing implementation
 a. Obtain obstetric history.
 b. Test urine for sugar, protein, ketones, and bacteria.
 c. Assess for large size of fetus, FHR, weight gain, blood pressure, yeast infections, and polyhydramnois.
 d. Provide diet instruction.
 e. Instruct about insulin injections
  1) Blood sugar levels dictate dose.
  2) Use blood monitoring device before breakfast (fasting), 2 hours after each meal, and at bedtime.
  3) Synthetic (Humulin/Novulin) regular insulin is drug of choice.
  4) Synthetic Hagedorn (NPH) insulin may be used.
  5) No oral agents are permitted during pregnancy or lactation.
 f. Hypoglycemia and ketoacidosis require rapid intervention.
 g. Initiate and maintain fetal surveillance for fetal well-being.
  1) Fetal kick counts
  2) Nonstress test
  3) Biophysical profile
 h. Insulin needs increase during pregnancy; abruptly decrease after delivery.
 i. Encourage breast-feeding (decreases insulin requirements).
 j. Instruct woman to avoid use of oral contraceptives.
5. Evaluation of nursing interventions
 a. The woman will remain stable with normal blood sugar levels (60–110 mg/dL).
 b. The woman will verbalize her knowledge of reasons for fetal surveillance and blood glucose monitoring throughout her pregnancy.
 c. The woman will make decisions regarding her care whenever possible.
 d. The woman will comply with her diet and medication regimen.
E. Acquired immunodeficiency syndrome (AIDS) and human immunodeficiency virus (HIV)
 1. Acquired through blood contact (may be through vaginal or anal intercourse) with infected person (usually IV drug user, homosexual, or bisexual man), or through a blood transfusion, or from breast milk (newborns)
 2. Data collection
  a. Physical
   1) Detailed history of risk behaviors
   2) Night sweats
   3) Malaise
   4) Weight loss
   5) Fever or diarrhea or both
   6) Lymph node enlargements
   7) Kaposi's sarcoma (reddish purple lesions)
   8) *Pneumocystis carinii* pneumonia
  b. Psychological
   1) Anxiety about self and transmission to fetus
   2) Fear of worsening condition with pregnancy
 3. Planning
  a. Protect from opportunistic infection
  b. Prevent transmission to health-care workers
   1) Instruct about universal precautions
   2) Instruct health-care workers how the virus is and is not transmitted
   3) Administer combination therapy that includes ziduvodine (ZVD) during the third trimester and labor/delivery
  c. Provide counseling
 4. Nursing implementation
  a. Follow blood and body fluids precautions.
  b. Use aseptic technique to prevent infection.
  c. Test infant or cord blood for HIV antibodies.
  d. Teach woman about asepsis when handling the infant.
  e. Provide counseling about contraception and safe sex.
  f. Encourage bottle feeding.
 5. Evaluation of nursing interventions
  a. Woman verbalizes her feelings about prognosis of the disease for herself and her baby.
  b. Protection from infection should be maintained through universal precautions.
  c. Woman adheres to blood and body precautions in handling baby.
  d. Woman should not breast-feed her infant.

Intrapartal Care

I. Labor
 A. Premonitory signs
  1. Lightening: fetus settles into pelvis (drops)
  2. Bloody show: pink-tinged vaginal mucus
  3. Diarrhea
  4. Burst of energy
  5. Cervical softening (ripening)
  6. Spontaneous rupture of the amniotic membranes (bag of water)
  7. Braxton Hicks contractions become uncomfortable and frequent
 B. First stage (stage of dilation)
  1. Begins with labor contractions
   a. Come at regular intervals
   b. Increase in frequency and duration over time
   c. Are increased in intensity by walking
   d. Are typified by discomfort radiating from back to abdomen
  2. Ends with complete dilatation of cervix (10 cm)
  3. Latent phase (0–3 cm)
   a. Mild to moderate intensity of contractions
   b. Cervix dilates to 3 cm
   c. Contraction duration is short (15–30 seconds)
   d. Contraction frequency increased from 15 minutes apart to 3–5 minutes apart
   e. Mood of excitement

4. Active phase (4–7 cm)
   a. Moderate to strong intensity of contractions
   b. Cervix dilates to 7 cm
   c. Contraction duration is 45–60 seconds
   d. Contraction frequency 2–3.5 minutes
   e. Mood serious
5. Transition phase (7–10 cm)
   a. Strong intensity of contractions
   b. Cervix dilates to 10 cm
   c. Contraction duration 45–90 seconds
   d. Contraction frequency 1.5–2 minutes
   e. Mood of "losing control"
   f. Signs indicating that delivery (second stage) is impending: mustache of perspiration, bulging perineum, nausea and vomiting, anal dilation, increased restlessness, desire to push, desire to move bowels, cries of "my baby is coming"
C. Second stage: stage of expulsion
   1. Begins with complete cervical dilation
   2. Ends with birth of baby
   3. Includes a "bearing down," pushing effort
   4. Variable length of time ranging from one contraction to several hours
   5. Mood serious, with great energy expended
D. Third stage
   1. Begins with birth of baby
   2. Ends with delivery of placenta
   3. Lasts between 5 and 30 minutes
   4. Mood exhilarated
   5. Beginning of attachment
E. Fourth stage
   1. Begins with delivery of placenta
   2. Ends with stabilization of mother 1–4 hours after delivery
   3. Mood of exhilaration and/or exhaustion
   4. May be ravenously hungry
   5. Rest period
   6. Optimal time for interaction with baby
F. Mechanisms of descent (cardinal movements)
   1. Engagement: biparietal diameter of fetal head passes through midpelvis
   2. Descent: fetal head moves down into birth canal
   3. Flexion: fetal chin touching fetal chest
   4. Internal rotation: fetal head turns to pass ischial spines
   5. Extension: fetal head passes under symphysis pubis and raises chin off chest
   6. External rotation: turning of fetal head to allow shoulders to pass through the ischial spines
G. Physiological maternal response
   1. Cardiovascular
      a. Supine hypotension: caused by vena cava compression secondary to supine position
         1) Turn mother onto left side (left lateral position)
         2) Increase intravenous (IV) fluids
         3) Oxygen by face mask at 6–10 L/min.
         4) Monitor FHR
         5) Monitor maternal vital signs
      b. Systolic blood pressure rises during contractions

1) During labor, cardiac output increases (approximately 500 mL of blood that supplies the uterus is squeezed into the maternal circulation during contractions)
         2) Immediately after delivery, cardiac output surges
   2. Blood components
      a. WBCs increase up to 25,000/mm^3
      b. Increase in fibrinogen
   3. Respiratory
      a. Respiratory rate and depth increase during contractions
      b. Oxygen consumption doubles during second stage of labor
   4. Pain: variable
      a. First stage
         1) Felt in lower abdomen and back
         2) Caused by
            a) Hypoxia of uterine muscle tissue during contractions
            b) Cervical dilatation
            c) Stretching of cervix and lower uterine segment
      b. Second stage
         1) Felt in lower abdomen, thighs, and perineum
         2) Caused by
            a) Muscle hypoxia during uterine contractions
            b) Pressure and distention of vagina and perineum
      c. Third stage
         1) Caused by uterine contractions
         2) Caused by passage of the placenta
      d. Fourth stage
         1) Felt as
            a) Contractions
            b) Perineal pain
         2) Caused by
            a) Uterine involution
            b) Episiotomy repair
H. Fetal response
   1. FHR 110–160 bpm
      a. Early deceleration:
         1) A decrease in the FHR with contractions
            a) Generally starts before or at the peak of the contraction
            b) Ends with the end of the contractions
            c) Caused by fetal head compression during contractions and descent
            d) Reassuring pattern
      b. Variable deceleration
         1) Occurs at any time during the labor (not always associated with a contraction)
         2) Has an abrupt (sharp) onset and end
         3) Caused by umbilical cord compression
         4) Nonreassuring if:
            a) Deep
            b) Prolonged
            c) Repetitive
            d) Associated with decreased variability of the fetal heart tracing

c. Late deceleration
  1) Onset can occur at any time during the contraction
  2) Always continues after the end of the contraction
  3) Caused by uteroplacental insufficiency
  4) Nonreassuring pattern
d. Acceleration
  1) Short increase (8–15 beats) in heart rate in response to fetal movement or uterine contractions
  2) Reassuring pattern
e. Baseline variability
  1) Most important parameter to fetal well-being
  2) Indicates healthy fetal parasympathetic and sympathetic responses

II. Nursing care during first stage
  A. Data collection
    1. History
      a. Name and age
      b. Physician
      c. Gravida, para
      d. EDD
      e. Blood type, Rh factor
      f. Characteristics of contractions
      g. Status of the amniotic membranes
      h. Presence of bloody show
      i. Time of last meal
      j. Allergies
      k. Medications currently used
      l. History of substance use/abuse in pregnancy
      m. Labor and delivery plan
      n. Desires regarding infant feeding
    2. Physical
      a. Assess FHR
        1) Use Doppler, fetoscope, or electronic fetal monitor.
        2) FHR may not be heard during contractions and for 15–30 seconds afterward unless monitor is used.
        3) FHR can be heard between contractions.
        4) Normal range is 110–160 bpm.
      b. Evaluate FHR pattern
        1) Variability should fluctuate by 8–15 beats
          a) Beat-to-beat or short term: only seen with internal scalp electrode
          b) Long-term: 3–5 beat fluctuations per minute
          c) Monitor externally over 10 minutes
          d) Indicates whether fetus can tolerate stress of labor
        2) Accelerations
          a) Normal response to movement or other stimuli
          b) Indicates fetal well-being
          c) No intervention needed
        3) Early decelerations
          a) Indicates compression of fetal head against cervix
          b) Uniform shape
          c) Start and end with the contraction
          d) No intervention needed

        4) Late decelerations
          a) Indicate insufficient blood flow from placenta to fetus
          b) Smooth shape
          c) Can be 5- to 30-beat drop
          d) Usually start after peak of contraction
          e) End after contraction over by 5–60 seconds
          f) Indicate fetal distress
          g) Interventions
            i) Turn woman onto left side.
            ii) Start oxygen by mask at 6–10 L/min.
            iii) Increase IV fluids.
            iv) Turn off Pitocin if running.
            v) Notify physician.
        5) Variable decelerations
          a) Indicate umbilical cord compression, cord problems, and/or fetal disorders
          b) Irregular shape, usually in form of **V**, **W**, or **U**
          c) Can occur any time with or without contractions
          d) Interventions
            i) Change maternal position.
            ii) Start oxygen by mask at 6–10 L/min if severe.
            iii) Check for prolapsed cord.
            iv) Notify physician if persistent.
        6) Decreased variability
          a) Indicates:
            i) Fetal hypoxia
            ii) Medications for analgesia
            iii) Fetal sleep
          b) FHR fluctuations of ≤2 bpm
          c) May be ominous if persisting >30 minutes
          d) Interventions
            i) Turn woman onto left side.
            ii) Start oxygen by face mask at 6–10 L/min.
            iii) Notify physician.
        7) Tachycardia
          a) HR >160 bpm
          b) Indicates
            i) Fetal response to tocolytics
            ii) Maternal fever
            iii) Dehydration
            iv) Possible infection of amniotic sac
            v) Beginning fetal hypoxia
            vi) May be precursor to fetal distress
          c) Interventions
            i) Increase IV fluids.
            ii) Start oxygen face mask at 6–10 L/min.
            iii) Check maternal temperature.
            iv) Notify physician.
            v) Check vital signs.
            vi) Determine frequency, duration, and intensity of contractions by palpation or external monitor.
            vii) Examine for cervical dilation and effacement.

viii) Assess fetal presentation and station by Leopold's maneuvers and vaginal exam.

3. Psychosocial
   a. Assess anxiety level of woman and coach.
   b. Assess coping skills of woman and coach.
   c. Observe interactions between woman and coach.
   d. Assess support shown woman by coach.

B. Planning
   1. Provide explanation and honesty about maternal and fetal well-being in labor.
   2. Assist with self comfort measures in labor.
   3. Promote safety and familiarity with the area.
   4. Provide emotional support to the couple.

C. Nursing implementation
   1. Monitor vital signs (blood pressure, pulse, and respirations):
      a. Hourly in early labor
      b. Every 30 minutes in active labor
      c. Every 15 minutes in transition
      d. Every 15 minutes if blood pressure elevated or Pitocin infused
   2. Take oral temperature:
      a. Every 4 hours if membranes intact
      b. Every 2 hours if membranes ruptured
   3. Assess FHR:
      a. Every 30 minutes in latent stage
      b. Every 15 minutes in active stage
   4. Evaluate progress of labor:
      a. Dilatation, effacement, and descent
      b. Uterine contractions
         1) Every 30–60 minutes in latent stage
         2) Every 15 minutes in transition
   5. Support breathing patterns:
      a. Slow chest breathing
      b. Pant-blow
      c. Panting
   6. Provide comfort measures:
      a. Fluid or ice chips
      b. Massage and/or warm blankets to back
   7. Encourage ambulation.
   8. Encourage voiding every 1–2 hours.
   9. Change position frequently.
   10. Effleurage.
   11. Cool cloth to forehead and face.
   12. Administer analgesics as ordered/requested:
      a. Meperidine (Demerol)
      b. Butorphanol tartrate (Stadol)
      c. Pentazocine (Talwin)
      d. Morphine
   13. Assist with regional anesthesia:
      a. Give 500- to 1000-mL bolus of IV fluids unless woman has cardiac disease.
      b. Position with spine "curled" for administration of spinal/epidural.
      c. Teach woman sensations to expect, expected results, side effects.
      d. Monitor vital signs every 5 minutes for 30 minutes.
      e. Position woman off vena cava, using pillow (usually to left side).

f. Maintain IV fluids.
g. Provide emotional support.
14. Use electronic fetal monitor if:
   a. Abnormal FHR pattern
   b. Decreased fetal movement
   c. Meconium passage
   d. Small-for-dates or postdates fetus
   e. Maternal complications
   f. Pitocin use
   g. Vaginal bleeding
   h. Maternal fever or infection
15. Maintain hydration (administer IV fluids carefully—do not overload with fluid).
16. Watch for signs of fetal distress:
   a. Late decelerations
   b. Severe variable decelerations
   c. Loss of variability
   d. Lack of fetal activity
   e. Tachycardia
   f. Bradycardia (<110 bpm baseline)
   g. Meconium-stained fluid

D. Evaluation of nursing interventions
   1. Mother and fetus experience labor and delivery without complications.
   2. Couple verbalizes nurse's support during labor.
   3. Couple verbalizes feeling safe and secure in surroundings.

E. Woman verbalizes effectiveness of comfort measures used in labor.

III. Special procedures during labor
   A. Amniotomy: artificial rupture of membranes
      1. Purposes
         a. To stimulate labor
         b. To see color of amniotic fluid
         c. To enable application of internal monitor
      2. Disadvantages
         a. Commits woman to delivery
         b. Increased risk of infection
         c. Risk of prolapsed cord if fetal head not well applied to cervix
      3. Nursing interventions
         a. Auscultate FHR before and after procedure; record findings.
         b. Document color, consistency, and amount of fluid.
         c. Instruct woman regarding need for bed rest unless fetal head well engaged.
         d. Change linen frequently to keep woman dry.
   B. Application of electronic fetal monitor
      1. Purpose
         a. Continuous monitoring of FHR and contraction pattern to detect fetal distress
         b. Medical-legal record
      2. Ultrasound transducer (fetal)
         a. Requires belt and aquasonic jelly.
         b. Upper area of graph is FHR recording.
         c. Records FHR by sound waves.
         d. FHR can be heard through speaker on machine.
         e. FHR baseline, long-term variability, and decelerations can be determined.
      3. Toco transducer (uterine)
         a. Requires belt.

   b. Lower area of graph records contractions.
   c. Records contractions by pressure from the muscle tightening during a contraction.
      1) Contractions can still be palpated.
      2) Frequency and duration of contractions are recorded.
      3) Intensity cannot be determined without palpation because placement affects tracing on graph.
   4. Nursing interventions
      a. Explain procedure to couple.
      b. Demonstrate how to read contraction pattern and FHR.
      c. Chart important data on graph sheet.
      d. Assist physician with application of internal monitors.
      e. Readjust external monitor as needed to obtain a clear tracing.
      f. Save all tracings, properly labeled, for the medical record.
C. Induction of labor
   1. Purpose
      a. To artificially stimulate labor
      b. Medical intervention
         1) Postdate pregnancies
         2) PIH
         3) Diabetes mellitus
         4) Fetal death
         5) Premature rupture of membranes (PROM)
   2. Procedure
      a. Administration of IV oxytocin (Pitocin)
         1) Used IV piggyback.
         2) Always used with IV controller.
         3) Electronic fetal monitoring necessary.
         4) Monitor maternal blood pressure every 15 minutes.
      b. Risks
         1) Uterine hyperstimulation: not enough rest between contractions
         2) Tetanic uterine contractions: lasting >90 seconds
         3) Uterine rupture
         4) Increased blood pressure
         5) Risk of water intoxication if used in combination with 5% dextrose in water (D_5W) IV fluids
         6) Fetal distress related to uterine hyperstimulation
      c. Contraindications
         1) Previous classic cesarean incision
         2) Placenta previa or abruptio placentae
         3) Fetal distress
         4) Preterm fetus
   3. Nursing interventions
      a. Follow established protocols for initial dosage and incremental increases of Pitocin.
      b. Monitor vital signs and FHR at least every 15 minutes.
      c. Increase only after assessing FHR, blood pressure, and contractions.
      d. Do not increase once desired pattern achieved

(contractions 1–3 minutes apart, lasting 45–60 seconds).
   e. Discontinue immediately if fetal distress present, or if contractions <2 minutes apart or lasting >90 seconds—need at least 60 seconds of complete uterine relaxation for gas/waste exchange between woman and fetus.
      1) Turn patient on left side.
      2) Administer oxygen 6 L/min by face mask.
      3) Report to physician.
      4) Document.
D. Forceps or vacuum extraction delivery
   1. Purpose
      a. Assist with rotation and descent of presenting part.
      b. Provides help for exhausted woman.
      c. Provides help if regional anesthesia has blocked pushing urge.
      d. May decrease need for cesarean delivery.
   2. Complications
      a. Maternal
         1) Perineal tears
         2) Hematomas
         3) Vaginal lacerations
         4) Postpartum hemorrhage
      b. Newborn
         1) Facial bruising
         2) Facial nerve damage
         3) Forceps marks on cheeks or ears
         4) Severe edema of occiput (Chignon) possible with use of vacuum extractor
         5) Breast-feeding grasping ability difficulty
   3. Nursing interventions
      a. Explain procedure and feeling of pressure.
      b. Encourage woman to relax during application.
      c. Encourage woman to push with contractions.
      d. Examine newborn infant for injury.
E. Episiotomy: surgical incision of perineum
   1. Types
      a. Midline: straight toward rectum from vaginal orifice
      b. Mediolateral: cut angles from vaginal orifice to the right or left and down
   2. Purpose
      a. Increases size of outlet for birth
      b. Decreases length of pushing time
      c. Lessens trauma to the fetal head
   3. Nursing interventions
      a. Apply ice after delivery to reduce swelling in first 24 hours.
      b. Examine for bruising, swelling, hematoma, bleeding, and intact sutures.
      c. Teach proper hygiene.
      d. Use analgesics (as needed), warm packs, and/or sitz baths (after the first 24 hours) for pain.
F. Cesarean delivery: birth through an abdominal incision
   1. Indications
      a. Cephalopelvic disproportion (CPD)
      b. Fetal distress
      c. Dysfunctional labor

d. Failure of descent
e. Prolapsed cord
f. Placenta previa
g. Abruptio placentae
h. Active herpes
i. Breach presentation (in a primipara)
j. May be performed in women with HIV to prevent transmission to the fetus/newborn
2. Complications
   a. Infection
   b. Hemorrhage
   c. Maternal bladder injury
   d. Transient tachypnea (wet lung) of the newborn
3. Nursing interventions
   a. Obtain signature for consent.
   b. Explain procedure.
   c. Explain need for procedure.
   d. Obtain CBC and urinalysis (UA) if not already done.
   e. Ensure type and screen/cross done.
   f. Hydrate with IV fluids
   g. Explain cesarean prep procedures before carrying them out.
      1) Insert Foley catheter.
      2) Shave abdominal area.
      3) Reassure woman and significant other.
      4) Obtain FHR strip.
      5) Remove fetal monitor when ready to go to surgery.
   h. Recovery.
      1) Provide usual postpartum assessments.
      2) Check abdominal dressing for bleeding.
      3) Apply antiembolitic stockings.
      4) Have patient turn, cough, and deep breathe every 2 hours.
      5) Measure I&O every shift.
G. Vaginal birth after cesarean delivery
   1. Purpose: allow normal labor and delivery without surgical intervention in a woman who has had a previous cesarean delivery
   2. Advantages
      a. Fewer maternal and fetal complications
      b. Quicker maternal recovery
      c. Facilitates attachment process
   3. Disadvantages
      a. Increased risk of uterine rupture even with left sacrotransverse (LST) uterine incision
   4. Contraindications
      a. Cephalopelvic disproportion (CPD)
      b. Fetal distress
      c. Previous classic cesarean (longitudinal) scar on uterus
      d. Placenta previa
      e. Multiple gestation
   5. Nursing interventions
      a. Labor must be monitored closely.
      b. Check vital signs and FHR every 15 minutes.
      c. Watch for signs of uterine rupture.
         1) Loss of FHR
         2) Shearing pain followed by comfort
         3) Shock

4) Fetal parts easily palpated in the abdomen
5) Occult (in the abdomen) and vaginal bleeding
IV. Nursing care during second stage: delivery
   A. Data collection
      1. Physical
         a. Labor progress
            1) Complete dilatation and effacement
            2) Station of descent of presenting part
            3) Contractions 2–3 minutes apart, lasting 60–75 seconds, strong intensity
            4) Bloody show increases
            5) Urge to bear down
         b. Fetal status
         c. Maternal vital signs
      2. Psychological
         a. Willingness/eagerness to finish labor process
         b. Mood of intense concentration
         c. Coping skills may falter
   B. Planning
      1. Encourage effort of couple to deliver child.
      2. Support comfort measures.
      3. Monitor maternal and fetal status.
      4. Promote quiet, peaceful environment for delivery.
   C. Nursing implementation
      1. Monitor FHR every 5 minutes; document.
      2. Choose position for pushing that is comfortable and effective.
         a. Side-lying
         b. Squatting
         c. Hands-and-knees
         d. Semi-Fowler's
         e. Lithotomy
      3. Observe for impending birth.
         a. Strong urge to push continuously
         b. Perineal bulge
         c. Fetal hair or scalp
      4. Provide comfort measures.
      5. Prepare for delivery.
         a. Position instrument table
         b. Place warmer for baby
         c. Perform perineal scrub
         d. Assist physician
         e. Adjust mirror if woman desires to watch
         f. Record time and position of birth
   D. Evaluation of nursing implementation
      1. Woman's comfort maintained.
      2. Mother and fetus physiologically stable.
      3. Couple able to focus on delivery of baby.
      4. Atmosphere supportive of family/newborn interaction/attachment.
V. Nursing care during third stage: delivery of placenta
   A. Data collection
      1. Physical
         a. Contractions resume after birth of baby.
         b. Abdomen changes shape.
         c. Gush of blood from vagina.
         d. Cord lengthens.
         e. Placenta delivered 5–30 minutes after baby.
         f. Expulsion:

1) Schultze's placenta: shiny; fetal side first
2) Duncan's placenta: rough; red cotyledons appear first; associated with retained placental parts
g. After delivery of placenta:
1) Uterus remains firm.
2) Palpate two fingerbreadths below umbilicus.
3) Chills and shivering common.
4) Maternal blood pressure monitored every 15 minutes.
5) Neonate dried and placed in mother's arms and covered with a warm blanket:
  a) Dry newborn infant with warm blankets.
  b) Assign Apgar score (0–10 points):
    i) Color pink: 2 points
    ii) Heart rate >100: 2 points
    iii) Grimace or cry: 2 points
    iv) Muscle tone; motion: 2 points
    v) Respirations regular or crying present: 2 points
h. Examine newborn infant for:
1) Gross anomalies
2) Three-vessel cord
3) Clear lungs
4) Heart rate
5) Temperature
6) Color
7) Gestational age
8) Reflexes
2. Psychosocial
a. Readiness to interact with neonate
b. What is said about and to neonate
c. Need for support and praise after delivery
B. Planning
1. Promote stabilization of the newborn infant.
2. Provide opportunity for interaction with baby.
3. Monitor mother's and baby's statuses.
4. Provide comfort measures.
C. Nursing implementation
1. Record time of delivery of placenta and expulsion style.
2. Monitor maternal vital signs.
3. Complete neonatal assessment.
4. Provide neonatal care:
a. Warmth
b. Eye prophylaxis (delay up to 2 hours to promote eye contact and bonding)
c. Attachment process
5. Administer drugs as ordered to mother:
a. Oxytocins:
1) Pitocin
2) Methergine
3) Syntocinon
b. Analgesics
6. Massage uterus if required for uterine atony.
7. Assist physician.
D. Evaluation of nursing interventions
1. Newborn infant has stable vital signs.
2. Mother and newborn infant given the opportunity to interact.
3. Mother reports feeling comfortable.
4. Mother and newborn infant physically stable.

VI. Nursing care during the fourth stage
A. Data collection
1. Physical
a. Blood pressure and pulse return to prepregnant baseline measures.
b. Fundus is firm, midline, and at the umbilicus or 1–2 fingerbreadths below.
c. Lochia is red (rubra) and scant to moderate in amount.
d. No distended bladder.
e. Perineum is slightly swollen, with no bruising; sutures are intact.
f. Maternal exhaustion.
2. Psychosocial
a. Emotions possibly labile
b. Desire to interact with baby
B. Planning
1. Monitor vital signs, lochia, and uterine status.
2. Provide information on perineal and breast care.
3. Instruct woman to call for assistance getting up.
4. Measure first three voids:
a. Must be at least 100 mL each
b. If less than 100 mL, continue to measure until three voids of ≥100 mL each are obtained
5. Support maternal-infant attachment.
C. Nursing implementation
1. Palpate uterus for consistency and placement.
2. Observe lochia:
a. Color
b. Amount
c. Clots:
1) Number
2) Size
d. Odor
3. Check vital signs:
a. Every 15 minutes for 1 hour
b. Then every 30 minutes for 1 hour
c. Then hourly for 2 hours
4. Assist mother to empty bladder if full.
5. Massage uterus if not fully contracted (boggy).
6. Provide comfort measures:
a. Warm blanket
b. Ice pack to perineum
c. Change perineal pads prn and each time up to the bathroom
d. Shower or tub bath okay
e. Change linens as needed
f. Offer drink and/or food
g. Analgesics if needed
h. Bra for support
i. Breast binder if bottle feeding
D. Evaluation of nursing interventions
1. Mother's vital signs remain within normal limits (WNL) (based on the prepregnant baseline).
2. Fundus remains firmly contracted and at or just below the umbilicus.
3. Lochia remains scant to moderate.
4. Any clots are smaller than a half dollar.
5. Opportunity for family-newborn interaction provided.
6. Mother demonstrates perineal, breast care, and uterine massage.

Labor and Delivery Complications

I. Fetal death
  A. Caused by
    1. Chromosomal abnormality
    2. Spontaneous abortion
    3. Maternal or fetal illness
    4. Unrecognized fetal distress
  B. Data collection
    1. Physical
      a. Vaginal bleeding
      b. Uterine cramping
      c. Lack of fetal movement and FHR
      d. Fundal height small for dates
      e. Low weight gain
      f. Urine estriol level decreased
      g. Confirmation with abdominal or pelvic ultrasound necessary
    2. Psychological
      a. Stages of grieving:
        1) Shock (denial)
        2) Anger
        3) Guilt
        4) Acceptance
        5) May skip appointment(s) as means of denial
  C. Planning
    1. Provide information regarding delivery plan.
    2. Provide woman with emotional support; reassure her that she is not to blame.
    3. Discuss follow-up testing of woman or products of conception or both.
  D. Nursing implementation
    1. Obtain prenatal history to date.
    2. Review fetal activity with woman.
    3. Prepare for diagnostic tests to confirm fetal death.
    4. Clarify procedure for induction.
    5. Provide time alone for family with fetus.
    6. Assist in working through grief.
    7. Obtain consents for genetic testing, pathology, burial of fetus.
  E. Evaluation of nursing interventions
    1. Couple verbalizes understanding of procedure for delivery.
    2. Couple voices feelings.
    3. Woman demonstrates self-care after delivery.

II. Preterm labor: Uterine contractions that cause cervical dilation before 37 weeks' gestation
  A. Causes
    1. Preterm, PROM
    2. Infection
    3. Cocaine use
    4. Dehydration
    5. Fetal death
    6. Unknown
  B. Data collection
    1. Physical
      a. Spontaneous contractions
      b. Spontaneous rupture of membranes common
      c. Cervical dilation and thinning (effacement) with contractions
    2. Psychological
      a. Fear and anxiety
      b. Guilt feelings
  C. Planning
    1. Provide information about treatment.
    2. Administer medications to stop contractions (tocolytics).
    3. Promote verbalization of feelings.
  D. Nursing implementation
    1. Maintain woman at bed rest lying on left side.
    2. Oral or IV hydration.
    3. Assist with lab and ultrasound procedures.
    4. Assist with the initiation of tocolytic therapy to decrease or stop uterine contractions.
    5. Draw blood to assess:
      a. Electrolytes
      b. CBC
      c. Type and cross match before starting medication
    6. Apply external fetal monitor
    7. Monitor vital signs and breath sounds every 5–15 minutes
    8. Administer drugs:
      a. Always give as piggyback solution on a controller or pump.
      b. Observe for tachycardia, hypotension, and arrhythmias.
      c. Administer ritodrine, terbutaline, indomethacin, or magnesium sulfate by protocol.
      d. Monitor contraction pattern and FHR.
      e. Avoid narcotic administration.
      f. Administer steroids (betamethasone) if ordered:
        1) Helps mature fetal lungs.
        2) Use with caution with tocolytics, as pulmonary edema can occur.
    9. Alert nursery to prepare for preterm newborn.
  E. Evaluation of nursing interventions
    1. Uterine contractions slow to 0–4 per hour.
    2. Fetus and woman tolerate effects of therapy without serious side effects.
    3. Woman verbalizes concerns about self and fetus.
    4. Woman is able to verbalize:
      a. Warning signs of preterm labor
      b. Medication regimen
      c. Need for rest and limited activity
      d. When to call physician

III. Ineffective labor
  A. Hypotonic contractions: intensity of regular contractions decreases during active labor
  B. Hypertonic contractions (uterus does not rest sufficiently between contractions): contractions occur frequently, usually during latent phase
  C. Uncoordinated contractions (coupling): two pacing cells active
  D. Data collection
    1. Physical
      a. Cervical dilation slows or stops.
      b. Fetal descent slows or stops.
      c. Woman is exhausted and/or dehydrated.
      d. Extreme pain with hypertonic and uncoordinated contractions.
        1) Turn woman on her left side.
        2) IV hydration.

3) Observe for signs and symptoms of fetal distress.
4) Document.
5) Provide pain relief measures.

2. Psychological
   a. Feelings of discouragement
   b. Extreme fatigue
   c. Uncooperative

E. Planning
1. Hypertonic
   a. Assess progress of labor.
   b. Promote rest and relaxation.
   c. Administer analgesics, sedatives, tocolytics.
2. Hypertonic
   a. Assess progress of labor.
   b. Prepare for augmentation of labor with oxytocin.

F. Nursing implementation
1. Hypotonic
   a. Examine vaginally for:
      1) Descent
      2) Dilatation
      3) Effacement
      4) Position
   b. Assist with ultrasound or pelvimetry to rule out CPD.
   c. Hydrate woman vigorously.
   d. Promote rest and a quiet atmosphere.
   e. Sedate woman for sleep as ordered.
   f. Start IV oxytocin infusion:
      1) Give fluids as ordered except plain D_5W.
      2) Administer via IV piggyback on infusion controller or pump.
      3) Follow protocol.
2. Hypertonic
   a. Change woman's' position.
   b. Encourage woman to empty bladder.
   c. Teach and support relaxation techniques.
   d. Provide analgesia sedation.
   e. Monitor fetus closely.
   f. Use heavy sedation, tocolytics, or $MgSO_4$ to decrease uterine tone.

G. Evaluation of nursing interventions
1. Woman verbalizes understanding of and agrees with treatment plan.
2. Woman and fetus tolerate treatment without complications.
3. Woman reports comfort measures effective.

IV. Prolapsed cord
A. Types
1. Concealed: between presenting part and amnion
2. Palpable: protruding through the cervix or vagina or both

B. Data collection
1. Physical
   a. Umbilical cord seen or palpated
   b. FHR slow and irregular or absent
   c. Violent fetal activity followed by no activity
   d. Severe variable decelerations on the fetal monitor

e. Associated factors
   1) Breech or transverse presentation
   2) Multiple gestation
   3) Prematurity
   4) Polyhydramnios
2. Psychological
   a. Confusion and fear once woman realizes what has happened
   b. Anxiety over rapid intervention

C. Planning
1. Relieve pressure on the cord.
2. Monitor FHR constantly.
3. Provide for informed consent for emergency cesarean.
4. Offer emotional support.

D. Nursing implementation
1. Monitor FHR immediately after rupture of membranes.
2. Relieve cord compression immediately:
   a. Knee/chest position
   b. Trendelenburg's position
   c. Push the presenting part off the cord through the vagina with a sterile gloved hand:
      1) Do not try to push the cord back in.
      2) Do not remove hand until fetus is delivered.
      3) Administer oxygen at 10 L/min by face mask.
      4) Prepare for emergency cesarean delivery.
      5) Witness informed consent.
      6) Monitor FHR continuously.

E. Evaluation of nursing interventions
1. Infant born by cesarean section without S/S of hypoxia.
2. Couple verbalizes feelings of support after delivery.

V. Ruptured uterus: rupture due to
A. Uterine scars
B. Use of oxytocic drugs
C. Unknown cause
D. Data collection
1. Physical
   a. Pain
   b. Shearing or tearing
   c. Diffuse or local
   d. Severe
   e. Contractions cease; labor stops
   f. Loss of FHR or very low FHR (severe bradycardia)
   g. Abdominal rigidity
   h. Fetal parts palpated easily through abdomen
   i. Maternal shock
2. Psychological
   a. Anxiety, confusion
   b. Restless and combative even though weak

E. Planning
1. Initiate emergency care.
2. Deliver infant as soon as possible.
3. Maintain stable physiological status of mother.

F. Nursing implementation
1. Discontinue oxytocin if infusion is running.
2. Initiate treatment for shock:

a. Trendelenburg's position
b. Oxygen face mask at 10 L/min
c. Open IV fluids for rapid infusion
d. FHR monitoring
e. Transfusion preparation
f. Vital signs checked every 5–15 minutes
3. Prepare for emergency cesarean section with possible hysterectomy.
4. Inform family members.
G. Evaluation of nursing interactions
1. Infant born in stable condition, or successfully resuscitated.
2. Woman's uterus repairable, or hysterectomy performed without complications.
3. Woman's physiological status stable.
4. Couple verbalizes feelings of support.

Postpartum Complications

I. Hemorrhage
A. Early: loss >500 mL within 24 hours of delivery
B. Late: loss >500 mL after 24 hours postpartum
C. Data collection
1. Physical
a. Uterine atony
b. Lacerations of cervix, vagina, perineum
c. Retained placental parts
d. Overdistended uterus that will not clamp down
2. Psychological
a. Uncooperative because fundal massage painful
b. Confusion, restlessness
D. Planning
1. Assess abnormal bleeding.
2. Maintain vital signs.
3. Prevent shock.
E. Nursing implementation
1. Massage uterus.
2. Assess amount of bleeding (use centimeters/milliliter method).
3. Monitor vital signs (VSs) (increased heart rate is the first VS change, blood pressure the last VS to change).
4. Increase IV fluids.
5. Have woman empty bladder.
6. Administer oxytocic medication (Methergine).
7. Evaluate blood loss by Hgb and Hct.
8. Assist with transfusion prn.
9. Assist with dilatation and curettage (D&C) if required.
10. Treat shock.
F. Evaluation of nursing interventions
1. Woman's fundus firm, midline, and at appropriate level for postpartum day.
2. Vaginal bleeding scant to moderate.
3. Woman's vital signs remain WNL of prepregnant baseline.
4. Lab values stabilize WNL.
5. Woman verbalizes need to rest and drink fluids.
II. Infection: Any infection of reproductive system within 10 days of delivery, excluding the first 24 hours postpartum

A. Data collection
1. Physical
a. Fever >100.4°F (38°C) and chills
b. Urinary frequency, dysuria, inadequate emptying of bladder
c. Foul odor and greenish color to lochia
d. Abdominal tenderness, enlarged lymph nodes
e. Purulent drainage from incision(s)
f. Increased WBC count (>25,000 mm^3)
2. Psychological
a. Extreme fatigue
b. Distress over inability to be "back to normal"
c. Uncooperativeness
d. Anger
B. Planning
1. Promote proper hygiene after delivery.
2. Support woman in expression of feelings.
3. Administer medications.
C. Nursing implementation
1. Obtain cultures (blood, urine, cervical, incisional).
2. Evaluate area and amount of pain.
3. Evaluate lochia for color and odor.
4. Check vital signs every 2–4 hours.
5. Encourage use of sitz bath, K-pad hot pack, and warm compresses for pain relief.
6. Need for a private bathroom.
7. Offer reassurance.
8. Teach personal hygiene.
D. Evaluation of nursing interventions
1. Woman demonstrates personal hygiene care.
2. Woman verbalizes adequate pain relief.
3. Medication should be taken for full course.
III. Mastitis: inflammation of milk ducts in breasts 2–4 weeks postpartum
A. Data collection
1. Physical
a. Nipple cracks, fissures, bleeding
b. Hot, reddened area on breast
c. Fever and chills
d. Engorgement and pain
e. Causes:
1) Incomplete emptying during breast-feeding
2) Migration of bacteria through cracked nipples
2. Psychological
a. Feelings of inadequacy and guilt
b. Fatigue, depression
B. Planning
1. Promote breast hygiene.
2. Reassure woman about mothering skills.
C. Nursing implementation
1. Teach woman to take antibiotic and analgesic.
2. Complete emptying of breast essential (can continue to breast-feed, or use manual pump).
3. Warm compresses should be applied to area.
4. Bra should be worn day and night.
5. Reassure woman that normal lactation will return.
6. Reinforce breast hygiene care:
a. Wash with water only.

b. Apply breast milk to nipples and areola after feeding.
c. Expose nipples to air.
d. Change breast-feeding positions frequently:
    1) Cradle hold
    2) Football hold
    3) Side-lying hold
D. Evaluation of nursing interventions
    1. Decreased or absent signs and symptoms of infection.
    2. Breast-feeding continues.
    3. Woman verbalizes/demonstrates breast hygiene measures.

Postpartal Care

I. Immediate: during hospitalization
    A. Data collection
        1. Physical
            a. Temperature: first 24 hours normal up to 100.4°F (38°C)
            b. Pulse: bradycardia 50–70 common up to 10 days
            c. Blood pressure: should stay at prepregnant baseline
            d. Breasts
                1) Soft for up to 3 days, then may become engorged.
                2) Very firm and full when engorged.
                3) Nipples may become tender if breast-feeding.
            e. Abdomen
                1) Flabby and loose, with possible striae.
                2) There may be separation of rectus abdominis muscles, which may feel like a hernia.
            f. Gastrointestinal
                1) Extreme hunger and thirst
                2) Constipation common
                3) Hemorrhoids common
            g. Urinary
                1) Large urine output occurs over first 24 hours.
                2) Emptying bladder is sometimes difficult.
                    a) Swelling of perineum.
                    b) Nerve paralysis caused by pressure during delivery.
                    c) Woman should void within 6 hours after delivery.
            h. Uterus
                1) Fundus should be firm; if boggy, massage.
                2) Height is at level of umbilicus for a couple of days.
                3) Height decreases by one fingerbreadth per day.
                4) Uterus is not palpable above symphysis after ninth postpartum day.
                5) Lochia: discharge from uterus:
                    a) Rubra: blood, mucus, and decidua; red; first 2–3 days
                    b) Serosa: serous, watery; pink to brown; 3–10 days
                    c) Alba: leukocytes and cellular debris white; starts days 6–10, lasts 1–3 weeks
                    d) Foul odor indicative of infection
                    e) Commonly contains small clots (large clots should not be present)
                    f) Becomes heavier with activity and when getting out of bed after lying supine for a long period of time
        2. Psychological
            a. "Taking in" phase: first 24 hours
                1) Reflective of pregnancy, labor, delivery
                2) Dependent
                3) Sense of wonder about baby
            b. "Taking hold" phase: up to 2 weeks' postpartum
                1) Provides self-care
                2) Impatient with discomfort
                3) Independent
                4) Interested in baby; wants to learn
            c. "Letting go" phase: 3–4 weeks postpartum
                1) Feels loss of pregnancy
                2) Must view infant as separate person
                3) Emotional lability
                4) Exhaustion
    B. Planning
        1. Provide support and anticipatory guidance for parenting.
        2. Allow quiet time for parent-baby interaction.
        3. Instruct in self-care of perineum, breasts, bowels.
        4. Promote relaxing atmosphere.
    C. Nursing implementation
        1. Assess at least every 8 hours:
            a. Fundus
            b. Breasts
            c. Abdomen
            d. Perineum
            e. Calves (Homan's sign)
            f. Bowels
            g. Urinary function
            h. Vital signs (every 4 hours)
        2. Maintain bladder and bowel function:
            a. Measure urine to assess emptying.
            b. Implement nursing measures (running water, pouring warm water over perineum if unable to void).
            c. Catheterize woman as the last resort if unable to void.
            d. Insert Foley catheter if woman unable to void after third straight catheterization.
            e. Encourage intake of fluids (2000–3000 mL daily), especially water.
            f. Provide stool softener and suppositories as ordered.
            g. Encourage high fiber foods.
            h. Encourage natural laxative foods.
        3. Promote perineal healing:
            a. Ice pack, first 24 hours.
            b. Sitz baths, at least three per day after first 24 hours.
            c. Topical medications for pain and hemorrhoids.
            d. Teach importance of front-to-back wiping.

e. Perineal pads changed with each toileting: applied front to back.
f. Teach signs of infection and when to seek help.
g. Emphasize proper handwashing techniques.
h. Instruct in perineal lavage (pericare):
   1) Use plain warm tap water or warm tap water and a bactericidal.
   2) Apply stream of solution from front to back.
4. Encourage breast care:
   a. Bra should be worn all the time for support.
   b. Nipples should be washed with plain water only.
   c. Breasts should be massaged to promote the let-down reflex and/or relieve discomfort.
   d. Colostrum/breast milk should be applied to sore nipples. Hypoallergenic lanolin if woman prefers.
   e. Warm towels may be applied to breast for relief if engorged.
   f. Assist with breast-feeding.
   g. Apply breast binder if woman desires bottle feeding.
   h. Discuss signs and symptoms of mastitis.
5. Review postpartum exercises:
   a. Kegel's
   b. Modified situps
   c. Walking
6. Provide information about sexual relationships:
   a. Sex permitted when it feels comfortable (approximately 2 weeks' postpartum).
   b. CAN get pregnant, barrier method of contraception preferred (condoms, foams, creams, vaginal film, tabs, suppositories).
   c. May need lubricant until normal vaginal secretions return.
D. Evaluation of nursing interventions
   1. Parents given time to interact with baby.
   2. Woman verbalizes and demonstrates self-care methods.
   3. Anticipatory guidance regarding baby care discussed.
   4. Mother states she feels rested before discharge.
II. Hospital care of the newborn infant (term)
   A. Data collection
      1. Physical
         a. Vital signs
            1) Tympanic or axillary temperature 97.6°–98.8°F (36.4°–37.1°C)
            2) Apical pulse 110–160 bpm
            3) Respirations 30–60/min
         b. Measurements
            1) Length: average 19–20.5 inches
            2) Head circumference: average 33–35 cm (13–14 inches)
            3) Chest circumference: average 32 cm (12–13 inches)
            4) Average weight: 7–8 lb. (normal range: 2500–4500 g)
         c. Head
            1) Molded (caput succedaneum)

2) Fontanels (soft spots)
   a) Anterior: diamond-shaped
   b) Posterior: triangle-shaped
   c) Should be soft and flat
3) Face
   a) Puffy
   b) Round
4) Eyes
   a) Blue-gray
   b) Puffy
   c) Sclera white
5) Ears
   a) One-third above outer canthus of eye
   b) Flip back to position when folded over
6) Nose
   a) Pug
   b) Preferential nose breather
7) Mouth
   a) Hard and soft palates present and intact
   b) Sucking and rooting reflexes
   c) Symmetrical grimace
   d) Tongue smooth; should not protrude
d. Neck
   1) Short
   2) Skin folds present
e. Chest
   1) Symmetrical
   2) Possible breast engorgement
   3) Possible breast discharge
f. Abdomen
   1) Cylindrical shape
   2) Umbilical stump
   3) Bowel sounds present
   4) Femoral pulses present and equal
g. Genitalia
   1) Female
      a) Large labia minora
      b) White milky discharge (may be blood tinged)
      c) Majora covering minora when legs extended
   2) Male
      a) Small penis
      b) Urinary meatus in midline
      c) Foreskin cannot retract
      d) Testes descended
      e) Full rugae on scrotal sack
      f) Scrotum enlarged
   3) Urination within 24 hours
   4) Meconium stool within 24 hours
h. Back
   1) C shaped
   2) Dimples over sacrum
i. Extremities
   1) Short
   2) Symmetrical
   3) May have extra digits
j. Skin
   1) Milia: clogged glands on face
   2) Lanugo: fine, downy hair on body

3) Vernix caseosa: thick white substance found in creases
4) Acrocyanosis: bluish hands and feet
5) "Stork bites": flat, red birthmarks on eyes, forehead, neck; blanch with fingertip pressure
6) Newborn rash: red maculopapular lesions (erythema toxicum)

k. Sleep: periods of reactivity
1) First period of reactivity
a) First 1–2 hours after birth
b) Infant quiet and alert
c) Frequently sucks fingers/fist
d) Optimal time for breast-feeding and/or bonding
2) Period of quiet sleep
a) Period of 2–4 hours after birth
b) A period of very deep sleep, infant rarely moves
c) Respirations regular
3) Second period of reactivity
a) Occurs after period of quiet sleep
b) Awakens with increased secretions
c) Frequently chokes and gags, may aspirate if formula fed at this time

2. Psychological
a. Parents accept newborn infant and state that he or she is beautiful.
b. Parents hold infant close and speak to him or her.
c. Eye contact is established between newborn infant and parents.
d. Parents discuss infant's health.
e. Newborn infant is held during feedings.
f. Parents demonstrate tolerance of fussiness.

B. Planning
1. Monitor newborn infant's physical parameters.
2. Teach infant care to parents.
3. Encourage interaction with family.
4. Provide a safe environment for newborn infant.

C. Nursing implementation
1. Wear gloves for unwashed babies.
2. Admission data collection
a. Respiratory
1) Grunting
2) Nasal flaring
3) Sternal and intercostal retractions
4) Signs of distress
5) Tachypnea
6) Breath sounds:
a) May hear crackles; suction with bulb syringe.
b) Common for respiratory rate to be irregular.
b. Gestational age
c. Dextrostick for glucose
d. Blood type if mother O group or Rh negative
e. Eye prophylaxis
f. Vitamin K administered
g. Body temperature maintained
h. Identification bracelet checked

3. Ongoing care
a. Complete assessment every 8 hours and prn
b. Daily weight assessment
c. Infection precautions
1) Three-minute wash to elbow at beginning of shift.
2) Twenty-second wash between infants.
3) Keep infant's eyes free of discharge.
4) Apply triple dye or alcohol to umbilical cord stump.
5) Change diapers frequently.
6) Remove cord clamp after 24 hours if cord is dried.
d. Feeding
1) Breast at delivery or within first hour.
2) Glucose water at 4–6 hours for bottle-fed babies.
3) Breast-feeding or bottle-feeding on demand, at least every 4 hours.
4) Anticipate spitting-up mucus.
5) Assist with infant position for breast-feeding.
e. Elimination
1) Meconium: green or black first 24 hours
2) Transitional: green or brown
3) Then yellow
f. Circumcision
1) Observe for bleeding.
2) Apply petroleum jelly (Vaseline) or ointment if ordered.
3) Cleanse gently.
4) Document voiding after procedure.
5) Teach as needed regarding use of Plastibel clamp.

4. Discharge
a. Screen newborn infant.
1) PKU
2) Galactosemia
3) Hypothyroidism
4) Sickle cell depending on state law
b. Remove cord clamp.
c. Give instructions to parents:
1) What crying means
2) Methods to help with colic
3) How to suction baby
4) How to change diapers
5) How to take temperature
6) How to give bath
7) How to care for umbilical stump until healed
8) Discuss infant needs for feeding on demand
9) Positioning on the right side after feeding to promote gastric emptying
10) Positions for burping
11) Positioning the infant supine for sleeping (prevents sudden infant death syndrome [SIDS])
12) Follow-up care
13) Safety in the home
d. Complete birth certificate.

D. Evaluation of nursing interventions
1. Parents interacting appropriately with infant
2. Newborn infant eating and eliminating normally

a. Breast
  1) Nursing until at least one breast is completely soft and empty
  2) Has 6–10 wet diapers a day
  3) Stools: yellow soft, curdy, have a sharp odor
b. Bottle
  1) Takes 0.5–1.0 oz. at each feeding
  2) Minimal spitting up of formula
  3) Stools: yellow/brown, pasty, have an unpleasant odor
  4) Parents demonstrate infant care to nurse

Common Newborn Problems

I. Full-term infant
  A. Hypoglycemia: blood sugar <40 mg/dL
    1. Causes
      a. Infant stress from delivery
      b. Large infusion of D_5W to mother during labor
      c. Diabetic mother
      d. Hypertensive mother
      e. Infant large for gestational age (suspect maternal diabetes)
    2. Data collection
      a. Physical
        1) Jitteriness, twitching, jerking movements
        2) Poor, weak sucking reflex
        3) Skin cool, clammy
        4) Irregular respirations, possible respiratory distress
        5) Poor muscle tone
        6) Low blood sugar, low blood calcium
        7) Weak cry; may be high-pitched
      b. Psychological
        1) Parents anxious about physical condition of infant
        2) Guilt feelings if mother diabetic or hypertensive
    3. Planning
      a. Assess for signs of hypoglycemia.
      b. Stabilize and maintain normal blood sugar for infant.
      c. Discuss infant's condition with parents.
    4. Nursing implementation
      a. Monitor vital signs frequently.
      b. Obtain serum glucose level every 30 minutes as needed and before feedings.
      c. Administer 10%–15% glucose water by mouth (PO) or IV as ordered.
      d. Schedule frequent feedings to maintain blood sugar levels.
      e. May have to supplement breast-feeding first 48 hours.
      f. Maintain normal body temperature.
      g. Monitor I&O.
    5. Evaluation of nursing interventions
      a. Tremors cease.
      b. Parents verbalize questions/concerns about infant condition.

c. Hypoglycemia readily detected and treated rapidly.
d. Blood sugar levels stable by discharge.
  B. Respiratory distress
    1. Causes
      a. Fetal lung immaturity (lack of surfactant)
      b. Aspiration of fluid or meconium during labor and delivery
      c. "Wet lung" due to pulmonary fluid collection caused by absence of "thoracic squeeze"
        1) Usually in cesarean births
        2) Sometimes in precipitous vaginal births
      d. Pneumonia: infection of lungs
      e. Sepsis
    2. Data collection
      a. Physical
        1) Predisposing factors are low Apgar score, cesarean section, and bleeding.
        2) Hypothermia and hypotonia may be present.
        3) Skin may be mottled, pale, or cyanotic.
        4) Respirations
          a) Assessment of rate, rhythm, cyanosis, depth of respiration, type of retraction
          b) Grunting and wheezing
          c) Nasal flaring
          d) Tachypnea (respiratory rate 60 or greater)
          e) Diminished breath sounds
          f) Retractions
        5) Provisions for parent-infant interaction
      b. Psychosocial (parental)
        1) Anxiety presenting as anger, shock, and withdrawal
        2) Fear of having permanently disabled child
    3. Planning
      a. Assess if infant meets criteria for administration of surfactant.
      b. Assess infant's respiratory status frequently.
      c. Provide opportunity for parents to verbalize questions/concerns.
    4. Nursing implementation
      a. Ensure availability of surfactant.
      b. Administer antibiotics (intramuscular [IM] or IV).
      c. Administer IV fluids.
      d. Assess IV access site: umbilical or peripheral.
      e. Monitor respiratory function.
      f. Blood gases every 4 hours.
      g. Pulse oximetry.
      h. Oxygen via OxyHood or ventilator.
      i. Warm humidified air.
      j. Give bicarbonate if ordered to correct acidosis.
    5. Evaluation of nursing interventions
      a. Infant progresses to normal respiratory rate and pattern.
      b. Infant color is pink.
      c. Infant tissue perfusion adequate (capillary refill).
      d. Parents verbalize feelings.
      e. Parents state understanding of medical/nursing care of infant.

C. Hyperbilirubinemia
  1. Causes
     a. Physiological jaundice due to decreases in conjugation at 3–5 days of age
     b. ABO and Rh incompatibility caused by antigen and antibody breakdown of RBCs
     c. Breast milk, which produces a hormone that can delay excretion of bilirubin
     d. Bruises, cephalhematoma, and petechiae resulting from delivery
     e. Immature liver function
  2. Data collection
     a. Physical
        1) Lethargy, irritability
        2) Poor feeding and sucking ability
        3) Color ruddy to deep yellow
        4) Abdominal distention, bowel sounds present
        5) Dark urine
        6) Elevated total and direct bilirubin levels
     b. Psychological
        1) Parental anxiety and fear about having permanently disabled child (brain damage due to kernicterus)
        2) Guilt if dehydration occurs or phenol-containing agents used in cleaning bilirubin
  3. Planning
     a. Recognize jaundice.
        1) Tip of nose yellow
        2) Skin undertones yellow when blanched
        3) "Peach" coloring
        4) Sclera yellow
     b. Maintain good hydration of infant.
        1) Offer oral fluids every 2 hours (breast milk, water, formula).
        2) IV hydration in severe cases.
     c. Provide teaching and reassurance for parents.
  4. Nursing implementation
     a. Provide phototherapy treatment with fluorescent or natural (through the window) light.
     b. Undress infant with genitals only covered.
     c. Shield infant's eyes from lights with protective mask.
     d. Provide stable air temperature and monitor every 2 hours.
     e. Change infant's position every 2 hours.
     f. Monitor total and direct bilirubin every 6–8 hours.
     g. Cleanse skin with water after infant voids or has a bowel movement.
     h. Monitor I&O.
     i. Weigh infant every 12–24 hours.
     j. Encourage parents to visit nursery frequently.
     k. Provide auditory stimulation.
     l. Assist in providing exchange transfusion if needed:
        1) Obtain parental informed consent.
        2) Compare type and crossmatch for compatibility.
        3) Suction trachea if needed before starting.
        4) Place under radiant heater with easy access.
        5) Keep nothing by mouth (NPO) 3 hours before and during procedure.
        6) Restrain if necessary.
        7) Monitor vital signs every 5–15 minutes.
        8) Record amounts of blood withdrawn and replaced.
        9) Assess hydration.
        10) Watch for reaction to transfusion.
        11) Monitor blood glucose and calcium levels.
  5. Evaluation of nursing interventions
     a. Infant's jaundice resolves with bilirubin levels returning to normal.
     b. Parents demonstrate infant care skills.
     c. Parents consent to treatment plan.
D. Infection
  1. Caused by
     a. Prolonged labor
     b. PROM
     c. Maternal infection
     d. Multiple procedures on infant
  2. Data collection
     a. Physical
        1) Lethargy, irritability
        2) Abdominal distention
        3) Poor sucking and feeding
        4) Elevated WBC count ($>10,000/mm^3$)
        5) Hypothermia (infant is unable to maintain body temperature; most commonly seen in infection with β-streptococci) or hyperthermia (most commonly seen in *Escherichia coli* infections)
        6) Signs and symptoms
           a) Irregular respirations; sometimes periods of apnea
           b) Rapid respiratory rate
           c) "Grunting" with expiration
           d) Sternal, intercostal retractions
           e) Nasal flaring
     b. Psychological
        1) Parental anxiety related to infant's condition
        2) Guilt if mother had infection
  3. Planning
     a. Monitor for signs of infection.
     b. Provide education for parents about infant's condition.
     c. Provide parents opportunities to verbalize feelings.
  4. Nursing implementation
     a. Administer antibiotics as ordered.
     b. Maintain universal precautions.
     c. Obtain cultures (gastric, urine, blood, stool, cord).
     d. Provide oxygen; warmed and humidified, via hood or ventilator.
     e. Check temperature, pulse, and respirations every 2 hours.
     f. Weigh daily.

g. Monitor I&O.

h. Suction as needed.

i. Reposition every 2 hours.

j. Assess hydration:

    1) Fontanels

    2) Eyes

    3) Skin turgor

    4) Mucous membranes

k. Share infant's progress with parents.

5. Evaluation of nursing interventions

    a. No S/S of infection within 7–10 days.

    b. Parents verbalized feelings.

II. Preterm infant: delivered at <37 weeks' gestation

A. Data collection

  1. Physical

    a. Extremities thin

    b. Few creases on soles of feet

    c. Fine lanugo over body

    d. Respirations irregular; spells of apnea common

    e. Undescended testicles

    f. Protruding labia minora

    g. Hypothermia

    h. Skin parchmentlike, with many blood vessels visible

    i. Poor coordination of suck-and-swallow

    j. Sluggish peristalsis; infrequent stools

    k. Position with extremities extended (term infant has flexed extremities)

  2. Psychological

    a. Parental fear of attachment to fragile infant

    b. Parental grief: loss of perfect infant

    c. Parental depression caused by long-term care and financial cost required

    d. Parental anxiety over possibly harming the infant by touch

B. Planning

  1. Assess at frequent intervals.

  2. Avoid excess stimulation.

  3. Stabilize and maintain vital signs.

  4. Nutrition as ordered—likely to be parenteral at first.

  5. Promote normal growth and development.

  6. Encourage parent-infant interaction.

  7. Encourage "kangaroo care" (placing a diaper clad premature baby in an upright position on parent's bare chest).

C. Nursing implementation

  1. Provide developmental care

    a. Prepare warm, quiet environment.

    b. Block light and noise at night.

    c. Pacifier with gavage feedings and for nonnutritive sucking.

    d. Position with hands positioned to the midline to prevent shortening of the muscles between the shoulder blades.

    e. Kangaroo care per protocol.

  2. Monitor (axillary or tympanic) temperature every 2 hours.

  3. Take apical pulse and respirations every 2–4 hours.

  4. Maintain IV access and fluid balance.

  5. Administer medications IV.

  6. Handle infant very gently, turning every 2 hours.

  7. Monitor oxygenation (OxyHood or ventilator supplied).

  8. Coordinate lab, medical imaging, and pulmonary function studies.

  9. Maintain meticulous hygiene and universal precautions.

  10. Bathe head and diaper area as needed with small gentle strokes.

  11. Gavage feed every 2–3 hours when ordered; progress as ordered.

  12. Discuss infant's care with parents.

  13. Involve parents in infant care.

  14. Assist parents with expressing feelings.

  15. Help set realistic timeframe for hospitalization.

  16. Reinforce positive adaptive skills.

  17. Instruct mother in pumping and storing breast milk.

  18. Prepare parents for common problems of preterm infant:

    a. Jaundice

    b. Hypoglycemia

    c. Feeding difficulties

D. Evaluation of nursing interventions

  1. Frequent assessment facilitated early interventions.

  2. Parents verbalize feelings.

  3. Parents participate in infant care.

  4. Parents interact appropriately with infant:

    a. Touching

    b. Stroking

    c. Holding

    d. Feeding

  5. Infant condition stabilized.

  6. Infant gains weight appropriately.

  7. Parents demonstrate infant care skills.

Cultural Considerations

Pregnancy and childbearing are rich with cultural meaning, and good nursing care requires that nurses understand this fact. Table 3–1 presents cultural considerations regarding pregnancy and childbearing practices for a variety of the cultural and ethnic groups found in North America.

REFERENCES

Abrams, A: Clinical Drug Therapy: Implications for Nursing Practice, ed 5. JB Lippincott, Philadelphia, 1997.

Beare, PG: Davis's NCLEX-RN Review, ed 3. FA Davis, Philadelphia, 2001.

Burroughs, A and Leifer, G: Maternity Nursing: An Introductory Text, ed 8. WB Saunders, Philadelphia, 2000.

Fogel, A: Infancy: Infant, Family, and Society, ed 3. West Publishing, St. Paul, MN, 1997.

Martin, EJ (ed.): Intrapartum Management Modules: A Perinatal Education Program, ed 2. Williams & Wilkins, Philadelphia, 2002.

Mississippi State Board of Nursing: . Laws and Regulations, 2003. [Online] Available: http://www.msbn.state.ms.us/

Murray, S, McKinney, E, and Gorrie, T: Foundations of Maternal-Newborn Nursing, ed 3. WB Saunders, Philadelphia, 2002.

Oregon Board of Nursing: What Certified Nursing Assistants Need to Know, 2003. [Online] Available: http://www.osbn.state.or.us/

Table 3–1. Cultural Considerations in Pregnancy and Childbearing Practices

Cultural Group	Birth Control	Beliefs Affecting Pregnancy	Beliefs About Certain Foods	Postpartal Care	Newborn Care
African Americans	• Takes away their personal freedom • Viewed as African-American genocide • Opposes abortion • Uses rhythm method over birth control pills	• Family network guides practices • Do not take pictures, causes stillbirth • Taking a picture captures mother's soul • Do not reach over head, causes umbilical cord to wrap around fetus' head • Thought to be bad luck to purchase clothes for unborn child • Ways to induce labor are: taking a ride over a bumpy road, ingesting castor oil, eating a heavy meal, or sniffing pepper	• Geophagia, the eating of earth or clay • If food cravings not satisfied, child will be born with a birthmark of the food denied	• Mother at greater risk than the baby • Avoid cold air • Encouraged to get adequate rest	• Baby born with amniotic sac is believed to have special powers from God • Bellyband or coin placed on top of infant's umbilical area to prevent protruding
Amish	• Birth control interferes with God's will and must be avoided • May use rhythm method; occasional use of intrauterine devices	• Children are viewed as gifts from God • Women enjoy high status because of their childbearing role • Tend to have first child later than other cultures • Fewer teenage pregnancies • Lay midwives provide prenatal care • Prefer home births with midwives assisting • Have no major taboos for birthing • Laboring women seldom express discomfort • Some use herbal remedies to promote labor		• Mothers resume family role managing housework, cooking, and child care within a few days after childbirth • For a new mother, her mother comes to stay for several days to provide support and help with care of infant	• Older siblings are expected to help care for younger children and help learn newborn care • Day of celebration when newborn can be brought to church services
Appalachians	• Include: birth control pills, condoms, tubal ligation, and abortion if one chooses	• Taking laxative facilitates abortion • High number of teen pregnancies • To have healthy baby, mother must eat well and take care of themselves • Boys are carried higher and mother's belly appears pointy; girls are carried lower • Pictures cause stillbirths • Reaching over one's head can cause the cord to strangle the baby • Wearing an opal ring during pregnancy can cause harm to child • If mother experiences a tragedy, a congenital anomaly may occur • Childbearing is a family affair • Childbirth is believed to be a short, intense, natural process that will bring mother closer to earth and must be endured	• Eating strawberries or citrus fruits can cause birthmarks • If food cravings not satisfied, child will be born with a birthmark of the food denied	• Relatives and extended family members gather to assist the new mother	• Bands around the abdomen prevent umbilical hernias • An asafetida bag around the neck prevents or wards off contagious disease

	Fertility Control	Pregnancy/Birth	Food	Breast-feeding	Newborn Care
Arab Americans	• High fertility rates are favored • Procreation is viewed as the purpose of marriage and means of enhancing family strength • "Reversible" forms of birth control are undesirable, but not forbidden • "Irreversible" forms of birth control such as vasectomy and tubal ligations are unlawful • Unwanted pregnancies are aborted • Sterility in a woman could lead to rejection and divorce • Approved methods for treating infertility include: artificial insemination and in vitro fertilization • Pregnancy occurs at a younger age	• Preference for male offspring • Some women fast during religious holidays causing consequences • During labor, women openly express pain through facial expressions, verbalizations, and body movements • Few women smoke, drink alcohol, or gain too little weight	• Similar beliefs about food cravings as other cultures	• Breast-feeding often delayed until the second or third day after birth because mother needs rest • Nursing at birth causes "colic" pain for the mother • "Colostrum makes the baby dumb" • Special foods such as lentil soup to increase milk production and tea to flush and cleanse the body is given	• Care includes wrapping the stomach at birth to prevent cold or wind from entering the baby's body • Call to prayer is recited in the Muslim newborn's ear • Male circumcision is a religious requirement
Chinese Americans	• Intrauterine device used for birth control • Sterilization is common even though oral contraception is available • Contraception is free	• Pregnancy is seen as women's business • Women insist on female midwife or obstetrician • Unwilling to take iron because they believe that it makes the delivery more difficult	• Add more meat to their diets because their blood needs to be stronger for the fetus • Avoid shellfish during the first trimester because it causes allergies • Raw fruits and vegetables are avoided because they are considered "cold" food • Foods must be cooked and served warm • Eat five to six meals a day with high nutritional ingredients, including rice, soups, and seven to eight eggs • Brown sugar helps rebuild blood loss	• Women are encouraged to breast-feed • Drinking and touching cold water are taboo • Drinking rice wine increases the mother's breast milk production • Many do not expose themselves to the cold air and do not go outside or bathe for the first month postpartum because belief that cold air can enter the body and cause health problems	

(Continued on following page)

Table 3–1. Cultural Considerations in Pregnancy and Childbearing Practices *(Continued)*

Cultural Group	Birth Control	Beliefs Affecting Pregnancy	Beliefs About Certain Foods	Postpartal Care	Newborn Care
Cuban Americans	• Lowest reproductive rate in the developing world	• Women believe they are eating for two and end up gaining excessive weight • Wearing necklaces during pregnancy causes the umbilical cord to be wrapped around the baby's neck • Childbirth is a time of celebration • Vitamin preparations to promote healthy development of their children	• Believe that morning sickness is cured by eating excessive coffee grounds • Eating a lot of fruit ensures that the baby will be born with a smooth complexion	• Ambulation, exposure to cold, and bare feet place the mother at risk for infection • Family members and relatives care for the mother and baby for about 4 weeks postpartum • Many prefer breast-feeding over bottle feeding	• Infants are weaned from breast and introduced to solid food at a median age of 3 months • Prolonged breast-feeding may contribute to a deformity or asymmetry of the breasts
Filipino Americans	• In marriage, rhythm method only acceptable contraception • Female sterilization is common	• Culture is child centered • Pregnancy considered normal • It is a time when a woman can demand attention and pampering from her husband and family members • Many refuse to take vitamins because they are afraid that vitamins could deform the fetus • Women are protected from sudden fright or stress because of the belief that this may harm the developing fetus • Women prefer to have their mothers rather than their husbands in the delivery room • Many still prefer the squatting position for birthing	• Believes if the mother craves dark-skinned fruit or dark-colored food, the infant's skin will be dark	• Reasons for not breast-feeding include: insufficient milk, mother working, nipple and breast problems, and mother's poor health • Lactating mothers are encouraged to take plenty of hot soups to promote milk production • Exposure to cold is avoided • Showers are prohibited because they cause arthritis • Woman's mother gives a sponge bath with aromatic oils and herbs, followed by a full body massage, including the abdominal muscles	• Eighty percent are breast-fed with a median duration of 13 months • Supplementing breast-feeding with other liquids and foods occurs as early as 2 months
French Canadian	• Traditional trend was that marriage was necessary to have children • Current trend is that many couples are living together without marrying • High fertility rates • Birth control pill primary means for effective contraception • Tubal and vasectomy are the next most common methods of contraception	• Prenatal classes are well attended by both the mother and father • Alcohol and tobacco use are discouraged during pregnancy and lactation • Father participates fully in the delivery of the infant • Many women still deliver in a dorsal position • Use of analgesics, local anesthetics such as epidural is high • Very few practice natural childbirth • Washing a floor associated with the onset of labor and early or preterm deliveries • A full moon plays a role in the onset of labor once the full-term period has been reached • Belief that pregnant women who experience hyperglycemia give birth to boys and that lack of salt announces the birth of girls		• General hesitation to breast-feed relates to not having sufficient milk, experiencing sore nipples, losing breast firmness, and muscle wasting after the breast-feeding period • Maternity and paternity leaves are available and range from 6 to 20 weeks • Fathers often take a few days to a few weeks of leave to help the mother care for the new baby and other children	• Breast-feeding has regained importance

Group					
Iranian	• Immigrant families are child oriented • Young women are expected to remain virgins until they marry • Sexual activity by men outside of marriage is tolerated • Menstrual blood is believed to be ritually unclean and physically polluted to the body and must be discharged monthly • Contraception is rarely used • Current methods of birth control include: the pill, intrauterine devices, and natural methods • Infertility is blamed on the woman	• Women are expected to marry and bear sons as quickly as possible • Both daughters and sons stay at home until married • Woman's prestige is elevated, especially if she gives birth to a son • Heavy work is thought to cause a miscarriage • Sexual intercourse is allowed until the last month • Some request analgesia for pain	• Food cravings must be satisfied lest a miscarriage occur • Avoid fried foods and foods that cause gas • Fruits and vegetables are recommended with special attention to the balance of hot and cold foods	• Considerable support from female kin begins in the sixth month and continues until after the birth • Postpartum period is 30–40 days • Women are required to take a ritual bath after they stop bleeding, so they can resume normal religious activities • A ghorse kamar (a brown, flat disk of dried herbs) is mixed with eggs and placed on her lower back a few hours after bathing • New mothers avoid cold water for bathing, ablutions, or cleaning • Mothers of sons are considered to have hotter bodies, hotter milk, and hotter temperatures than mothers of girls • Mothers of girls are given a mixture of honey and other nutrients, an herbal extract called taranjebin, to raise their bodily heat to ensure that the next child is a boy	• Prolonged breast-feeding was used as a method of contraception • Baby boys are considered "hotter" than baby girls • Some families keep an infant home for the first 40 days • Baby is given a ritual bath between the 10th and 40th days
Irish Americans	• Some view sexual relationships as a "duty" • Acceptable methods are abstinence and the rhythm method	• Birth of a baby is a joyous occasion • Mother should not reach over her head during pregnancy because the umbilical cord may wrap around the baby's neck • If pregnant woman sees or experiences a tragedy during pregnancy, a congenital anomaly may occur • Plenty of rest, fresh air, and sunshine are important for maintaining the mother's health	• Not eating a well-balanced diet or not eating the right kind of food may cause the baby to be deformed • Eating a well-balanced diet during pregnancy and after delivery ensures a healthy baby and maintaining the mother's health		• Going to bed with wet hair or wet feet causes illness in the mother

(Continued on following page)

Table 3–1. Cultural Considerations in Pregnancy and Childbearing Practices *(Continued)*

Cultural Group	Birth Control	Beliefs Affecting Pregnancy	Beliefs About Certain Foods	Postpartal Care	Newborn Care
Italian	• Premarital sex and adultery are forbidden in first-generation Italians • Belief that a mother does not conceive while nursing • Sprinkling salt under and around the bed of a newly married couple is believed to make them fertile	• If a pregnant woman is not given the food she smells, the fetus moves and a miscarriage results • If she turns a certain way, the fetus does not develop normally • Woman should not reach over her head • Many fear hospitalization except for childbirth • Hospital delivery provides a means of avoiding the traditional sexual intercourse rites at the onset of labor	• Coffee spills result in the baby being born with a birthmark where the coffee was spilled • During pregnancy, sexual relations are abstained	• Woman is not allowed to wash her hair, take a shower, or resume her domestic chores for at least 2 or 3 weeks after birth so she can rest • Woman's mother and female family members tend to the chores and assist with the care of the newborn • New mothers are expected to breast-feed to restore the health of the reproductive organs and keep the mother and infant free of infections	
Japanese		• Pregnancy is highly valued as a woman's fulfillment of her destiny • Women enjoy attention and pampering • Keeping one's feet warm is said to promote uterine health • An obi (sash) obtained from a Shinto shrine may be wrapped around the abdomen for warmth and protection • Exercise classes are encouraged • Medical procedures, such as enemas and episiotomies, are routinely used to ease the baby's passage • Japanese midwives use perineal massage • Vaginal deliveries are usually performed without medication • To give into pain dishonors the husband's family • Mothers appreciate their babies if they suffer in childbirth	• Women are encouraged to eat full meals during labor so that they have energy for pushing	• Women return to their mother's home for the last 2 months or their pregnancy and through the first 2 months postpartum • Women may stay in the hospital up to 1 week while learning to breast-feed and attend daily mother-care classes • Rooming-in is thought to disrupt the mother's rest, so at feeding times the baby is brought to her or she goes to the nursery • Traditionally do not bathe, shower, or wash their hair for at least the first week • Since new mother stays with her mother, the new father may not see his baby until he comes to take the mother and baby back home • Maternal rest and relaxation are deemed essential for successful breast-feeding	• Loud noises, such as a train or a sewing machine, are thought to be bad for the baby • Unusual to see infants in public before the age of 3 months

Jewish	• Prevention of pregnancy implies deferring the commandment to be fruitful and multiply • Condom use is supported among liberal Jewish	• Children are considered a gift and duty • Families are encouraged to have at least 2 children • Couples who are unable to conceive should try all possible means to have children • When all natural attempts have been made, adoption may be pursued • Birth is determined when the head or "greater part" is born • During pregnancy, the fetus is merely part of the mother's body and has no independent identity • A Hasidic husband may not touch his wife during labor and may choose not to be present during delivery • Husband is not permitted to view his wife's genitals			• For male infants, circumcision is performed • Circumcision is both a medical procedure and a religious rite • If child is still in the hospital on the eighth day, it is important for the hospital to provide a room for a small private party to celebrate • At birth, a child is free of all sin • Failure to circumcise carries no eternal consequences should the child die
Korean	• Government promotes the concept of two children per household • Contraceptive devices are covered by the present national health insurance of Korea	• Mothers tend to view infants as passive and dependent and seek guidance from folklore and extended family • Pregnancy is a highly protected time for women • Both pregnancy and the postpartum period have been ritualized by the culture • Some wear tight abdominal binders toward the end of the pregnancy to increase the chances of having a small baby • Women commonly labor and deliver in the supine position	• Expectant mothers should avoid duck, chicken, fish with scales, squid, or crab because eating these foods may affect the child's appearance • Foods avoided include coffee, spicy foods, chicken and crab • Reason for not eating certain foods is that it might produce a skin disease on the infant and cause an unpleasant face	• Women are given seaweed soup, a rich source of iron, which is believed to increase lactation and promote healing of the mother • Bed rest is encouraged for 7–9 days • Women are encouraged to keep warm by avoiding showers, baths, and cold fluids or foods • Women are to protect their body from harmful strains and keep clean • Because pregnancy is a hot condition and heat is lost during delivery, women avoid cold foods and water after childbirth to prevent chronic illnesses such as arthritis • Herbal medicines are used to promote healing and health	• Baby should be wrapped in warm blankets to prevent harm from cold winds

(Continued on following page)

Table 3–1. **Cultural Considerations in Pregnancy and Childbearing Practices** (Continued)

Cultural Group	Birth Control	Beliefs Affecting Pregnancy	Beliefs About Certain Foods	Postpartal Care	Newborn Care
Mexican	• Men see a large number of children as proof of their virility • Acceptable methods are abstinence and the rhythm method • Some believe that prolonged breast-feeding is a method of birth control • Some use contraceptives, sterilization, or abortion for unwanted pregnancies	• With the extended family network and the woman's role of maintaining the health status of family members, many pregnant women seek family advice before seeking medical care • Many pregnant women sleep on their backs to protect the infant from harm, keep the vaginal canal well lubricated by having frequent intercourse to facilitate an easier birth, and keep active to ensure a smaller baby and to prevent a decrease in the amount of amniotic fluid • Pregnant women should not walk in the moonlight because it might cause a birth deformity • To prevent birth deformities, pregnant women may wear a safety pin, metal key, or some other metal object on their abdomen • Other beliefs include avoiding cold air, not reaching over the head to prevent the baby's cord from wrapping around its neck, and avoiding lunar eclipses because they may result in deformities • Father is not included in the delivery experience and should not see the mother or baby until after both have been cleaned and dressed • During labor, women may be very vocal and are taught to avoid breathing air in through the mouth because it can cause the uterus to rise up	• A woman is more likely to favor hot foods, which are believed to provide warmth for the fetus and enable the baby to be born into a warm and loving environment • Cold foods and environments are preferred during the menstrual cycle and in the immediate postdelivery period	• Immediately after birth, they may place their legs together to prevent air from entering the womb • Postpartum women refrain from bathing or hair washing up to 40 days • Women take sitz baths, wash their hair with a washcloth, and take sponge baths • Women wear a heavy cotton abdominal binder, cord, or girdle to prevent air from entering the uterus; covering one's ears, head, shoulders, and feet to prevent blindness, mastitis, frigidity, or sterility; and avoiding acidic foods to protect the baby from harm	• When baby is born, mother may place a belt around the umbilicus to prevent the naval from popping out when the child cries • Cutting the baby's nails in the first 3 months is thought to cause blindness and deafness
Navajo Indians	• Traditionally do not practice birth control, and thus, do not limit the size of their families	• Many women are reluctant to deliver their babies in a hospital setting • During labor process, the mother wears birthing necklaces made of juniper seeds and beads to assist with a safe birth. • Woven belts or sashes are used to help push the baby out • Taboo to buy clothes for baby before birth		• Immediately after birth, the placenta is buried as a symbol of the child being tied to the land • Sometimes the placenta is burned in a fire	• Twins are not looked on favorably and are frequently believed to be the work of a witch, in which case one of the babies must die • The baby is given a mixture with juniper bark to cleanse its insides and rid it of mucus • Ceremonial food of corn pollen and boiled water is given • Corn symbolizes healthy nutrients and an enduring nature

Polish		
• Pregnant women are expected to seek preventive health care, eat well, and get adequate rest to ensure a healthy pregnancy and baby • Many believe it is bad luck to have a "baby shower" • Birthing is done in a hospital	• Fertility practices are balanced between the needs of the family and the laws of the Church	• Women are expected to rest for the first few weeks after delivery • Breast-feeding is important

Puerto Rican		
• Pregnancy is a time of indulgence • Hygiene is highly valued during pregnancy, labor, and the postpartum period • Women are encouraged to rest, consume large quantities of food, and carefully watch what they eat • Strenuous physical activity and exercise are discouraged and lifting heavy objects is prohibited • Women are discouraged from consuming aspirin, Alka-Seltzer, and malt beverages because these substances are believed to cause abortions • Men are socialized to be tolerant, understanding, and patient regarding pregnant women and their preferences • Many women refrain from sexual intercourse after the first trimester to avoid hurting the fetus or causing preterm labor • During labor, women are loud and verbally expressive	• Women do not commonly use birth control methods such as foams, creams, and diaphragms • Sterilization choices were not made out of Puerto Rican women's free will, but in response to the social and political ideologies	• Receive help from their family and friends • First postpartum meal is homemade chicken soup to provide energy and strength • Women are encouraged to avoid exposure to wind and cold temperatures, not to lift heavy objects, and not to do housework for 40 days after delivery • Some do not wash their hair for 40 days after delivery • Mothers who breast-feed are encouraged to drink lots of fluids such as milk and chicken soup • If feeling weak or tired, they drink ponches, beverages consisting of milk or fresh juices mixed with a raw egg yolk and sugar • Hot foods such as chocolate beans, lentils, and coffee are discouraged because they are believed to cause stomach irritability, flatus, and colic for the mother and infant

(Continued on following page)

Table 3–1. Cultural Considerations in Pregnancy and Childbearing Practices *(Continued)*

Cultural Group	Birth Control	Beliefs Affecting Pregnancy	Beliefs About Certain Foods	Postpartal Care	Newborn Care
Vietnamese	• Abortions are commonly performed in the homeland because pregnancy outside of marriage is considered a disgrace to the family • Women often desire information on contraception, but are afraid to ask	• During the first trimester, the expectant mother is considered to be in a weak, cold, and antitonic state. In the second trimester, the pregnant woman is considered to be in a neutral state • During the third trimester, when the woman may feel hot and suffer from indigestion and constipation, cold foods are prescribed and hot foods are avoided or strictly limited • Gas producing foods are generally avoided throughout pregnancy • Women maintain physical activity to keep the fetus moving and to prevent edema, miscarriage, or premature delivery • Additional restrictive beliefs include avoiding heavy lifting and strenuous work, raising the arms above the head, which pulls on the placenta causing it to break, and sexual relations late in pregnancy, which may cause respiratory stress in the infant • Many consider it taboo for pregnant women to attend weddings or funerals • Once in labor, women try to maintain self-control and may ever smile continuously • Many prefer walking around during labor and squatting during the birth process • Because the head is considered sacred, neither that of the mother nor of the infant should be touched or stroked	• Food practices for a healthy pregnancy include noodles, sweets, sour foods, and fruit, but avoidance of fish, salty foods, and rice • Tonic foods include animal protein, fat, sugar, and carbohydrates; they are usually hot and sweet • Wind foods, often classified as cold, include leafy vegetables, fruits, beef, mutton, fowl, fish, and glutinous rice • Cold foods, including mung beans, green coconut, spinach, and melon, and antitonic foods, such as vinegar, pineapple, and lemon, are avoided during the first trimester	• To restore equilibrium and provide adequate warmth to the breast milk, women consume soups with chili peppers, salty fish and meat dishes, and wine seeped with herbs • Ritual cleansing of the mother does not involve actual bathing with water • Because body heat is lost during delivery, women avoid cold foods and beverages and increase consumption of hot foods to replace and strengthen their blood • Because water is cold, women traditionally do not fully bathe, shower, or wash their hair for a month after delivery • Women also avoid drafts and strenuous activity; wear warm clothing; stay in bed, indoors, or both for about a month; and avoid sexual intercourse for months • Some discard the colostrum and feed the baby rice paste or boiled sugar water for several days • After the milk comes in, both mother and infant benefit from the hot foods consumed by the mother for the first month	• Customary practices include clearing the neonate's throat using the finger, cutting the umbilical cord with a non-metal instrument, quickly burying the placenta to protect the infant's health • A newborn is often dressed in old clothes; it is considered taboo to praise the child lest jealous spirits steal the infant • The mother may be reluctant to cut the child's hair or nails for fear that this might cause illness • Maintained on a diet of milk for the first year, with the introduction of rice gruel at around 6 months • Little formal toilet training; the child usually learns by imitating an older child

Data from Purnell, LD, and Paulanka, BJ: Transcultural Health Care: A Culturally Competent Approach, 2nd ed. F.A. Davis, Philadelphia, 2003.

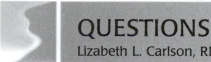

QUESTIONS
Lizabeth L. Carlson, RN, DNS, BC, and Golden M. Tradewell, RN, PhD

1. A client that is 6 months' pregnant comes to the clinic for a routine visit. She asks what she can do to relieve constipation. The nurse should teach the client that the most appropriate measures to alleviate this problem include which of the following recommendations?
   1. Take a mild laxative and use a Fleet enema as needed.
   2. Drink 8–10 cups of water and take a daily walk.
   3. Add more protein and fat to the daily diet.
   4. Drink hot coffee or tea each morning at breakfast.

2. A client at 26 weeks of gestation asks why she is having trouble with constipation during her pregnancy. Which of the following explanations by the nurse would be most accurate?
   1. The muscle movement of the intestines slows down, which causes dry, hard stools.
   2. The muscle movement of the intestines speeds up, which causes dry, hard stools.
   3. The intestines are compressed during pregnancy, which causes stool stasis.
   4. The intestines are expanded during pregnancy, which causes stool stasis.

3. A client was admitted to the obstetric unit on 9/10/02 with c/o labor. The nurse palpated regular uterine contractions every 5 minutes with moderate intensity. A sterile vaginal exam revealed a soft cervix that was 85% effaced and dilated to 2 cm. Which of the following admission information is most important in planning nursing care?
   1. The client's blood type and Rh were A+.
   2. The client's hemoglobin was 11 g/dL.
   3. The client's LMP was 2/15/02.
   4. The client's blood pressure was 100/64 mm Hg.

4. A 22-year-old client at 7 weeks' gestation attended the first trimester class on nutrition. Which of the following statements indicate a need for further teaching?
   1. "I should gain around 30 pounds by my due date."
   2. "Planning meals around the food pyramid guide is best."
   3. "Frozen foods are more nutritious than canned foods."
   4. "My cravings are probably caused by iron deficiency."

5. A client admitted to the obstetric unit with contractions every 8–10 minutes, with cervical effacement of 100%, and dilation of 3 cm. reported that she and her support person planned to use prepared childbirth techniques. The nurse would expect the couple to utilize which of the following pain relief methods during this phase of labor?
   1. Slow, deep breathing
   2. Rapid, shallow breathing
   3. Local anesthesia
   4. Narcotic analgesia

6. A 30-year-old gravida 5, para 4 (all female) client at 12 weeks' gestation asks the nurse, "Do you think I'm having a boy? If I don't have a boy this time, my husband will probably divorce me." Which of the following explanations by the nurse would be most accurate?
   1. "Girls probably run in your family, there's nothing you can do about it."
   2. "The heartbeat of the baby is fast, that means it's a boy."
   3. "The father's sperm determines if the baby is male or female"
   4. "Don't worry, you are carrying this baby low, that means it's a boy."

7. A client at term states, "I would like to breast-feed, but my mother-in-law told me my breasts are too small and I won't have enough milk for my baby." The best response by the nurse would be which of the following?
   1. "Your breasts are small, but if you don't produce enough milk, you can give the baby some formula."
   2. "The size of the breasts doesn't matter. All women have about the same amount of milk-producing tissue."
   3. "You will produce more milk if you use a breast pump and then give it to your baby in a bottle."
   4. "Milk production is increased by the hormone estrogen. You can ask your doctor for a prescription to take."

8. A 32-hour-old baby has yellowish skin undertones and a serum bilirubin level of 14 mg/100 mL. The blood type of the baby is B+. The mother's blood type is O+. The infant is being breast-fed. The nurse would include which of the following measures in her plan of care?
   1. No special measures are necessary; newborns normally get a little jaundiced.
   2. Tell the mother to stop breast-feeding and give the baby formula instead.
   3. Place the infant under the bililights and prepare for an exchange transfusion.
   4. Encourage the mother to increase the frequency of breast-feeding sessions.

9. A primiparous client at 18 weeks' gestation had an ultrasound examination done which showed the fetus in a breech position. The client asked the nurse, "Does this mean I will have to have a C-section?" Which of the following responses by the nurse would be most accurate?
   1. "If a first baby is breech, it must always be delivered by cesarean section."
   2. "The baby will have more room to turn as your delivery date nears."
   3. "You can probably deliver normally, most babies are born breech."
   4. "Many babies are breech at this stage of pregnancy, most turn by term."

10. A laboring client has been dilated 9–10 cm for 2 hours. The fetal head has remained at zero station for 45 minutes despite adequate pushing efforts by the client. A sterile vaginal exam reveals a position of occiput posterior. Which of the following actions by the nurse would be most appropriate?

   1. Assist the client to a hands and knees position.
   2. Assist the client to a supine position.
   3. Prepare the client for a forceps rotation.
   4. Prepare the client for a cesarean delivery.

11. A client with preterm contractions at 34 weeks' gestation has had an amniocentesis for fetal lung maturity. Which of the following laboratory tests should the nurse monitor?

   1. Human chorionic gonadotropin (hCG)
   2. Phosphatidylglycerol (PG)
   3. α-Fetoprotein (AFP)
   4. Partial thromboplastin time (PTT)

12. A client at 12 weeks' gestation has just been told that she is carrying dizygotic twins. She asks the nurse what the difference is between monozygotic and dizygotic twins. Which of the following explanations by the nurse would be most accurate?

   1. "Monozygotic twins come from two different eggs and sperm."
   2. "Dizygotic twins come from one fertilized egg that split."
   3. "Monozygotic twins come from one egg and two sperm."
   4. "Dizygotic twins come from two different eggs and sperm."

13. A 20-year-old client has come to the obstetric clinic because her menstrual period is 7 days late. She tells the nurse, "I'm sure I'm pregnant because my period is late and my breasts are tender." Which of the following responses by the nurse would be most accurate?

   1. "Missed menses and breast tenderness are positive signs of pregnancy."
   2. "Missed menses and breast tenderness are presumptive signs of pregnancy."
   3. "Missed menses and breast tenderness are probable signs of pregnancy."
   4. "Missed menses and breast tenderness are negative signs of pregnancy."

14. A client is seen in the emergency room at 16 weeks' gestation with pelvic cramping and bright red vaginal bleeding. Which of the following signs and symptoms should the nurse observe the client for?

   1. Increased temperature
   2. Increased pulse pressure
   3. Increasing heart rate
   4. Increased blood pressure

15. The anesthetist has just placed an epidural catheter dosed with bupivacaine hydrochloride (Marcaine) in a client at term in active labor. The nurse should observe the client for which of the following side effects?

   1. Hypotension
   2. Hypertension
   3. Hyperventilation
   4. Hypoventilation

16. A client at 12 weeks' gestation has a history of thromboembolitic disease. The client is placed on daily heparin therapy. The nurse should monitor the results of which of the following laboratory tests?

   1. Prothrombin time
   2. Partial thromboplastin time
   3. Bleeding time
   4. Clotting time

17. A postpartum client complains of sharp pain in the calf of her right leg when walking. The nurse notes that the leg has a circumscribed area of redness, warmth, and tenderness. Which of the following nursing actions is *most* appropriate in this client's nursing care?

   1. Instructing the client to massage the affected area to relieve the tenderness.
   2. Applying cold packs to the affected area to decrease inflammation.
   3. Encourage the client to ambulate to increase circulation.
   4. Elevating the affected extremity to promote venous blood flow.

18. A client has just started the third stage of labor. Which of the following nursing actions have priority at this time?

   1. Encouraging the client to push
   2. Administration of an oxytocic medication
   3. Physical assessment of the infant
   4. Promotion of the bonding process

19. A client who delivered 45 minutes ago comes into the transitional nursery to see her infant. She asks the nurse, "My baby's head is shaped like a cone! Will it stay like that?" Which of the following responses by the nurse is most accurate?

   1. "That is called a caput. It usually lasts for 3 or 4 days."
   2. "That is called molding. It usually lasts for a few days."
   3. "That is called a cephalhematoma. It usually lasts for a few weeks."
   4. "That is called a nevi. It usually lasts several months."

20. A 20-year-old primiparous client, who is breastfeeding, is preparing to be discharged home with her newborn son. The nurse has completed discharge instructions on newborn care. Which of the following statements by the client would indicate a need for further teaching?

   1. "I should clean the cord stump with alcohol or peroxide every day until it falls off."
   2. "If my baby has at least two wet diapers and one bowel movement a day, he is getting enough to eat."
   3. "I should dress my baby in clothing I would be comfortable in, plus a light blanket."
   4. "I should nurse my baby whenever he acts hungry and for as long as he wants to nurse."

21. The nurse is planning care for a client who had a spontaneous vaginal delivery with epidural anesthesia over an intact perineum. She is currently in the fourth stage of labor. Which of the following nursing goals would be *most* appropriate for this client?

1. The client will ambulate in the room without assistance.
2. The client will turn, cough, and deep breathe 10 times an hour.
3. The client's epsiotomy will remain clean, dry, and intact.
4. The client will maintain physiological homeostasis.

22. A client delivered a term infant 6 hours ago. Which of the following assessment findings indicate normal postpartum progression?

1. Firm fundus at the umbilicus and midline with moderate lochia rubra
2. Firm fundus 1–2 fingerbreadths above the umbilicus and midline with moderate lochia rubra
3. Firm fundus 1–2 fingerbreadths above the umbilicus and deviated to the right side with moderate lochia rubra
4. Firm fundus 3–4 fingerbreadths below the umbilicus and midline with moderate lochia rubra

23. A client is pregnant at 12 weeks' gestation. Which of the following laboratory tests would the nurse need to interpret that would indicate a need for change in the client's plan of care?

1. White blood count = 14 mm³
2. Hematocrit .= 32%
3. Hemoglobin = 10 g/dL
4. Serum glucose = 105 g/dL

24. A laboring client received epidural anesthesia with bupivacaine hydrochloride (Marcaine) for contraction pain 1 hour ago. Considering the effects of epidural anesthesia, which of the following nursing measures are important in her care?

1. Assessing the client hourly for respiratory depression
2. Assessing the client hourly for bladder distention
3. Assessing the client hourly for uterine atony
4. Assessing the client hourly for hypertension

25. A client arrived on the obstetric unit at term with mild irregular contractions. Findings from a sterile vaginal exam were as follow: cervical dilation of 3 cm, membranes were intact, and the presenting part at −1 station. An external fetal monitor was placed and the fetal heart tracing revealed a baseline of 130 with accelerations to the 150s during contractions. Which of the following nursing actions would be most appropriate considering the client's situation?

1. Prepare the client for an immediate operative delivery.
2. Turn the client to her left side and administer oxygen.
3. Notify the registered nurse to start an intravenous infusion stat.
4. Send the client home and encourage her to ambulate.

26. A 6-week postpartum client, who is breast-feeding, asks for information on birth control methods that do not affect breast milk production. Which of the following statements would indicate the client needs further instruction?

1. "Using condoms would be a good choice for me."
2. "I can use Depo-Provera and breast-feed without problems."
3. "Breast-feeding itself is effective at preventing pregnancy."
4. "I can use contraceptive foam for birth control."

27. An antepartum client at 16 weeks' gestation has tested positive for gonorrhea. All tests for other sexually transmitted infections were negative. Which of the following information is most important in planning her nursing care?

1. Client drug allergies
2. Fishy-smelling discharge
3. The presence of a chancre
4. The presence of vesicles

28. A non–insulin-dependent diabetic has just found out she is pregnant. She asks the clinic nurse what she should do to about her diabetes. The most appropriate response by the nurse would be which of the following?

1. "You can control your blood sugar with oral hypoglycemic agents."
2. "You can control your blood sugar with insulin injections."
3. "You can control your blood sugar with dietary changes."
4. "You can control your blood sugar by exercising more."

29. An insulin-dependent diabetic at 18 weeks' gestation has arrived for α-fetoprotein testing. She asks the nurse why this test is being performed. Which of the following explanations by the nurse would be most accurate?

1. "This test is to determine the sex of your baby."
2. "This test is for fetal lung maturity."
3. "This test is for neural tube defects."
4. "This test is to determine glycemic control."

30. A postpartum client had a spontaneous vaginal delivery 30 minutes ago. During the postpartum assessment, the nurse notes that there is constant trickling of bright red vaginal bleeding in the presence of a contracted uterus at midline. Which action by the nurse would be most appropriate in this situation?

1. Massage the fundus.
2. Call the health-care provider.
3. Have the client empty her bladder.
4. Increase the oxytocin (Pitocin) infusion.

31. The nurse enters the room of a breast-feeding client who delivered 3 hours ago and who is in tears. "I just don't know what I'm doing wrong!" she sobs "I can't get my baby to take the nipple!" Which of the following nursing diagnoses would be most appropriate in this case?

1. Altered parenting related to difficulty in breast-feeding
2. Altered comfort related to sore nipples

3. Altered bonding process related to maternal frustration
4. Knowledge deficit related to breast-feeding techniques

32. A client delivered her first infant 1 day ago at term. Which of the following actions by the nurse would most likely promote the attachment process?

1. Take pictures of the baby for the mother to see.
2. Tell the mother what her baby looks like.
3. Take the mother to the nursery window to see her baby.
4. Give the baby to his mother and point out his features.

33. A 20-year-old multipara at 18 weeks' gestation reports symptoms of thick white vaginal discharge and intense itching. A wet mount specimen reveals budding yeast cells with a diagnosis of *Candida albicans*. The client asks how to prevent future infections. Which of the following responses by the nurse is most accurate?

1. "Eat a serving of live culture yogurt daily."
2. "Douche after intercourse with vinegar and water."
3. "Douche with live culture yogurt daily."
4. "Take antibiotics as ordered until all are gone."

34. A 24-year-old primipara at 32 weeks' gestation comes into the clinic with complaints of nasal stuffiness, nosebleeds, and bilateral hearing loss. She asks why she is having these symptoms. Which of the following explanations by the nurse is most accurate?

1. "This sounds like a bad cold, you need to take a decongestant."
2. "These symptoms are common in pregnancy because pregnancy hormones cause increased blood flow, which causes head congestion."
3. "These are symptoms of a major problem. You need to be referred to a specialist."
4. "This sounds like a sinus infection. It is caused by exposure to allergens, such as cat dander or plant pollen. You need to take antibiotics and an antihistamine."

35. A client in the second trimester of pregnancy has blood drawn for routine 12-week lab work. Which of the following results would be considered normal for this stage of pregnancy?

1. Hemoglobin of 11 g/mL
2. Hemoglobin of 18 g/mL
3. Serum glucose of 80
4. Red blood cell count of 4

36. A nurse educator teaching a prenatal class asked for feedback from the class on the topic "Breast Changes During Pregnancy." Which of the following statements from one of the attendees would indicate further instruction is needed?

1. "My areolas will get smaller and lighter in color."
2. "My breasts will be tender and swollen."
3. "The nipples will get darker and more erect."
4. "My breasts will enlarge and may feel lumpy."

37. A 36-year-old professional woman who is pregnant for the first time at 10 weeks' gestation tells the nurse that her pregnancy was planned, but that "I'm feeling like maybe this wasn't such a good idea." Which of the following responses by the nurse would be most appropriate?

1. "These are unnatural feelings. You should be happy to be pregnant."
2. "Maybe you should consider abortion since you feel this way."
3. "Don't worry, you'll feel differently once the baby is born."
4. "Many women have mixed emotions when they are first pregnant."

38. A 20-year-old client came in for her first prenatal appointment at 10 weeks' gestation. Blood is drawn for routine prenatal screening. Which of the following laboratory results would indicate a risk to the fetus for erythroblastosis fetalis?

1. Low α-fetoprotein
2. B−, antibody+
3. L:S ratio of 2:1
4. O+, antibody−

39. A client is in active labor at term with cervical findings of 5 cm dilated, effacement of 90%, station −1. The FHR baseline is in the 120s with long-term variability. Three late decelerations were noted within the last hour with a quick return to the 150s and then baseline. Which of the following nursing actions would be most appropriate?

1. Position the client on her back so the monitor strip is more accurate.
2. Prepare for a stat cesarean section.
3. Turn the client to her left side.
4. Encourage the client to ambulate.

40. A client in the 26th week of gestation has been admitted to the obstetric unit with a diagnosis of pregnancy-induced hypertension. Which of the following symptoms would indicate worsening of the disease?

1. Epigastric discomfort
2. Blood pressure of 140/90 mm Hg
3. 2+ Deep tendon reflexes
4. 2+ Dependent edema

41. A client at 32 weeks' gestation was admitted to the obstetric ward 3 days ago with preterm labor. Oral terbutaline 2.5 mg every 3 hours was ordered. Which of the following nursing measures would have the highest priority in her antepartum care?

1. Check the pulse before each dose of terbutaline.
2. Maintain continuous fetal monitoring.
3. Place the client on strict bed rest.
4. Monitor closely for respiratory depression.

42. An Asian client in labor with her first child has a cervical dilation of 7 cm, effacement of 100%, and the presenting part is at 0 station. Contractions are every 3 minutes, strong in intensity, and lasting 90 seconds. The client smiles each time the nurse enters the room.

She stiffens her body during contractions, but does not otherwise indicate she is feeling any pain. She has not asked for any pain medication. Which of the following interpretations of the client's behavior would be most accurate?

1. The client is not experiencing acute pain.
2. The client is in control of her pain.
3. The client is demonstrating a moral value.
4. The client is demonstrating a cultural value.

43. A client who delivered a healthy term infant 1 day ago is talking on the telephone when the nurse enters her room to do her postpartum checks. Which response by the nurse would be most appropriate?

1. Instruct the client to hang up the phone immediately so she can be checked.
2. Ask the client if doing the check now or in a few minutes would be better.
3. Ask the client about her vaginal bleeding instead of doing a check.
4. Postpone the postpartum check until later in the shift.

44. A client at 28 weeks' gestation has been admitted to the obstetric unit for preeclampsia. Her blood pressures have been ranging from 140s/100s to 160s/110s. She has 3+ proteinuria and generalized edema, and has been complaining of a headache. Which care environment would be most appropriate for this client?

1. Semiprivate room, up ad lib, vital signs every shift with fetal heart tones, 2-g sodium diet
2. Private room, bedrest with bathroom privileges, vital signs with fetal heart tones every 4 hours, regular diet
3. Three-bed ward, ambulate three times a day, vital signs two times a day with fetal heart tones, low-protein diet
4. Labor room, strict bed rest, vital signs every 15 minutes with continuous fetal monitoring, nothing by mouth

45. A client at 24 weeks' gestation comes into the obstetric clinic for a routine visit and a CBC. Results of the CBC include a WBC of 10 mm³, RBCs of 5 mm³, hemoglobin 9 g/dL, and hematocrit 32 PCV%. The client asks what these results mean. Which of the following explanations by the nurse would be most accurate?

1. "Your lab results are normal for this stage of pregnancy."
2. "Your white count is high; you may have an infection."
3. "Your hemoglobin and hematocrit are on the low side of normal for pregnancy."
4. "Your hemoglobin and hematocrit are low. It looks like you are a little anemic."

46. A client with severe preeclampsia is being treated with intravenous magnesium sulfate. The nurse checks the deep tendon reflexes, which are absent. Which of the following nursing actions have priority?

1. Notify the registered nurse and continue to monitor the client.
2. Notify the registered nurse to decrease the rate of infusion.

3. Notify the registered nurse to increase the rate of infusion.
4. Notify the registered nurse to stop the infusion.

47. A 22-year-old nulliparous client at 16 weeks' gestation asks the nurse how she can help her husband to "get more excited about this pregnancy." Which of the following actions by the nurse would be most appropriate in assisting the father to attach to the fetus and validate the reality of the pregnancy?

1. Allow the father to listen to fetal heart tones.
2. Show the father a model of a fetus at the same developmental stage as his fetus.
3. Give the father a typed handout on fetal development.
4. Encourage the father to attend an ultrasound of his fetus.

48. A client at 36 weeks' gestation is admitted to the obstetric unit for severe PIH. The health-care provider performs an amniocentesis for fetal lung maturity to determine the risks of delivery. Which of the following nursing actions have priority after this procedure?

1. Monitor the puncture wound for S/S of infection.
2. Monitor fetal heart tones and for uterine contractions.
3. Explain the purpose of the procedure to the client.
4. Encourage the client to verbalize her concerns.

49. A client with PIH at 32 weeks' gestation has been admitted to the obstetric unit. The signs and symptoms she has been manifesting indicate mild PIH. The nurse should monitor which of the following laboratory tests that would signal progression of the disease?

1. Liver function tests
2. Serum glucose
3. Serum magnesium levels
4. Erythrocyte sedimentation rate

50. A 30-year-old client at term has had normal progression of her labor and is now completely dilated and pushing. The fetal presentation is vertex, with the presenting part OP (occiput posterior) and at 1+ station. For which of the following procedures would the nurse expect to prepare the client?

1. Assistance to a lithotomy position and pushing with the breath held
2. Simpson forceps rotation/delivery with a mediolateral episiotomy
3. Nurse-administered fundal pressure and midline episiotomy
4. Piper forceps rotation/delivery with a midline episiotomy

51. A 25-year-old client at term has been admitted to the labor and delivery unit for induction of labor. Sterile vaginal exam reveals cervical dilation of fingertip, effacement of 90%, and presenting part floating. Before the induction starts, the client calls the nurse and says "I felt a gush, I think my water broke." Which of the following nursing actions have the highest priority?

1. Check for cervical dilation.
2. Check maternal vital signs.

3. Check the fetal heart tones.
4. Check for vaginal bleeding.

52. A breast-feeding client is being discharged home with her 24-hour-old infant. Which of the following statements would indicate the client needs further instruction about nipple care?
    1. "I should clean my nipples with soap and water daily."
    2. "I should leave the flaps of my bra down between feedings."
    3. "I should run a little colostrum on my nipples after nursing."
    4. "I should change the position of the baby with each feeding."

53. A formula-feeding client has been discharged home with her term infant. She calls the nursery after 1 day at home. She is concerned because the infant is taking only 0.5 oz at each feeding. Which of the following explanations by the nurse would be most accurate?
    1. "The baby needs to take at least an ounce at each feeding no matter what you have to do to get it down."
    2. "Maybe the baby is allergic to that formula. You should switch to a soy formula."
    3. "If the baby is having at least four wet diapers a day, (s)he is getting enough."
    4. "One-half an ounce is all the stomach of a newborn can hold. The baby will take more in a few days."

54. A 16-year-old client in the 35th week of gestation has attended childbirth preparation classes at the local hospital. Which of the following statements made by the client to the nurse educator indicates a need for further instruction?
    1. "My boyfriend will be my coach and help me relax during contractions."
    2. "If I practice these techniques, I won't need any pain medication."
    3. "These techniques help control labor pain, but I can ask for pain meds if I need them."
    4. "I should practice Kegel exercises several times a day."

55. A newborn male infant was just delivered. Which of the following nursing actions has the highest priority?
    1. Completely dry the infant.
    2. Suction the nose and mouth.
    3. Put on ID bands.
    4. Check the heart rate.

56. A 24-year-old client delivered a term male infant 30 minutes ago over a midline episiotomy after normal progression of labor. Vital signs are currently stable. Oxytocin (Pitocin) 10 mg is infusing in 500 mL of D_5 lactated Ringer's solution at 125 mL/hr. The current postpartum check revealed firm fundus 1 fingerbreath below the umbilicus, moderate lochia rubra, and two nickel-sized clots were noted. The newborn is in the father's arms. The mother made the following statement to the nurse. "We were hoping for a little girl, but it's OK as long as the baby is healthy." Which of the following nursing diagnoses would be most appropriate for this situation?

1. Risk for injury related to uterine atony and hemorrhage
2. Altered family processes, potential for growth
3. Potential for infection related to altered skin integrity
4. Anxiety related to the new role of parenting

57. A primigravida with O− blood type and Rh factor has just delivered the placenta. She plans to bottle feed. Pitocin 20 units is added to 1000 mL of lactated Ringer's solution and hung. The client asks the nurse why she needs this medication. The most accurate explanation by the nurse would be which of the following?
    1. "This medication is to dry up your breast milk."
    2. "This medication will reduce blood clotting."
    3. "This medication is to prevent Rh antibodies from forming."
    4. "This medication is to make your uterus clamp down."

58. A client at 28 weeks' gestation admitted to the obstetric unit with symptoms of mild PIH complains of epigastric pain. Which of the following nursing actions would be most appropriate?
    1. Pad the siderails and position the client on her left side.
    2. Place the client on continuous fetal heart monitoring.
    3. Check the medication administration record to see when the client last received an antacid.
    4. Notify the registered nurse to start an intravenous line stat.

59. A client who has just found out she is pregnant tells the nurse, "I'm a vegan. What diet modifications should I follow?" The best reply by the nurse is which of the following responses?
    1. "You will have to eat meat during your pregnancy. Babies need complete proteins."
    2. "If you drink soymilk and combine grains and legumes, your protein intake will be sufficient."
    3. "You need to eat lots of dark yellow fruits and dark green leafy vegetables as protein substitutes."
    4. "You need to add cheese and eggs to your daily diet. These are high-quality protein sources."

60. A 14-year-old client at 24 weeks' gestation has come into the prenatal clinic for her first visit. She is underweight for her height and pregnancy stage. The nurse asked for a 24-hour diet recall which revealed a fast-food diet. Which of the following meal suggestions by the nurse would be both nutritious and acceptable to this client?
    1. Baked chicken, baked potato, broccoli, and milk
    2. Fried steak fingers, mashed potatoes, fried vegetable sticks, and iced tea
    3. Double cheese pizza with sweet peppers and ham and a strawberry milkshake
    4. Cheeseburger, french fries, fried apple pie, and a soft drink

61. A healthy term infant whose mother plans to breast-feed was admitted to the transitional nursery 30 min-

utes ago. The infant is under a radiant warmer. The nurse caring for the infant noted that she had an axillary temperature of 97°F (36.1°C), a respiratory rate of 60/min, and a heal stick glucose of 45 mg/dL. Which of the following actions by the nurse would be most appropriate?

1. Wrap the baby warmly, and take to the mother for breast-feeding.
2. Give the baby an oral glucose feeding of $D_{10}W$.
3. Increase the temperature setting on the radiant warmer.
4. Call the health-care provider for an order for a chest radiograph.

62. A cold-stressed infant was warmed to 99°F (37.2°C) (core temperature) over a period of 2 hours. The infant's temperature has been maintained within normal limits for the last 24 hours, and the infant has been breast-feeding well every 3–4 hours (per mother's report). The nurse should monitor which of the following laboratory results?

1. Serum calcium
2. Serum glucose
3. Serum sodium
4. Serum bilirubin

63. A 1-day-old infant has just been fed 0.5 oz of formula and burped. He is placed in his crib in the nursery. To prevent aspiration, in which position should the nurse place the infant?

1. Right lateral with the crib mattress flat
2. Left lateral with the crib mattress flat
3. Prone with the crib mattress flat
4. Prone with the foot of the crib mattress elevated

64. A pregestational diabetic client attending a prenatal class on breast-feeding reported to the nurse educator, "I want to breast-feed, but my friend told me that because I'm a diabetic, my milk will be too high in sugar and will make my baby diabetic also." Which of the following responses by the nurse would be most accurate?

1. "That information is correct. Diabetic women shouldn't breast-feed because of high sugar content in the breast milk."
2. "You should definitely breast-feed. It has major health advantages for you and your baby."
3. "You can breast-feed. The insulin you take will control sugar levels in your milk."
4. "Your breast milk won't have too much sugar in it, but you would have to add 500 calories to your diet. That is too many calories for a diabetic woman."

65. A routine postpartum assessment of a breast-feeding client reveals bilaterally reddened nipples. No cracking or blisters are noted. The client reported nipple soreness and asked what she could do to decrease the soreness. The best response by the nurse would be which of the following suggestions?

1. Limit nursing time to 5 minutes on each breast. Then increase nursing time by 1 minute at each subsequent feeding.

2. Dry the nipples with a soft cloth and then rub them with Massé cream after each feeding.
3. Make sure the infant's mouth is wide open before latching on, and that most of the areola is taken into the mouth.
4. Breast-feed only every other feeding to rest the nipples. Pump the breast milk into a bottle for other feedings.

66. A client at 8 weeks' gestation called the obstetric clinic at 10 AM to report streaking of blood on the toilet tissue when she used the bathroom that morning. She also reported having intercourse the night before. She denied any further bleeding or spotting. She asked, "What is causing this bleeding?" Which of the following responses by the nurse would be most accurate?

1. "You are probably having a miscarriage. You need to go to the emergency room right away."
2. "What you are experiencing is bleeding caused by implantation of the embryo. It is nothing to be concerned about."
3. "Some women continue to have a small period each month. Just take it easy during the time you would normally be having your period."
4. Penile penetration can cause slight bleeding. It is usually nothing to be concerned about, but call us if the bleeding gets heavier or if you start cramping."

67. A 26-year-old primigravida at 8 weeks' gestation is admitted to the obstetric unit for severe vomiting. She has been treated in the emergency room with IV fluids three times in the last week. She reports, "I can't keep anything down, even water." IV fluids are started and promethazine (Phenergan) 25 mg IM/PO every 4 hours is ordered. The client asks the nurse, "Why am I getting that medicine?" The most accurate reply by the nurse is which of the following answers?

1. "Hyperemesis is connected to emotional disorders. Phenergan reduces anxiety."
2. "Hyperemesis is caused by exhaustion. Phenergan will help you rest."
3. "Hyperemesis causes electrolyte imbalances. Phenergan is an electrolyte replacement."
4. "Hyperemesis is uncontrolled vomiting. Phenergan controls vomiting."

68. A client that just arrived on the obstetric unit for a nonstress test brought her clinic records with her. She looked at the records and asked the nurse the meaning of the following notation: G4 T2 P1 A0 L3. Which of the following explanations by the nurse would be most accurate?

1. "This means you have been scheduled for four prenatal visits—and you have been on time for two, canceled one, was a no-show for one, and was late for three."
2. "This means you have four children—two were born when they were due, one was early, and three were overdue."

3. "This means you have had four pregnancies—two babies were born when they were due, you had one baby born early, no miscarriages, and three living children."
4. "This means you have four children—two were born early, you miscarried one time, and three children were born when they were due."

69. A primigravida in the sixth week of gestation attended a prenatal class on self-care in the first trimester. In conversing with the nurse educator, she reviewed potential hazards to pregnancy. Which of the following statements would indicate a need for further teaching?

1. "I can clean out the cat box if I wear gloves."
2. "I shouldn't take any medicine without checking with my doctor first."
3. "It is better for me if I eat five small meals a day."
4. "I shouldn't use my hot tub while I'm pregnant."

70. A 15-year-old athlete, who weighs 110 lb and is 66 inches tall, is being seen in the obstetric/gynecologic clinic because her periods had stopped. She told the nurse she didn't understand why this had happened because she was a virgin. Which of the following explanations by the nurse would be most accurate?

1. "It could be caused by abnormal uterine tissue growth that causes scarring of the ovaries and stops ovulation."
2. "It could be caused by strenuous exercise that has resulted in low body fat percentage."
3. "It could be caused by monthly hormone changes that also cause headaches, irritability, and depression."
4. "It could be caused by a bacterial infection that has spread to the pelvic organs."

71. A client pregnant at 24 weeks" gestation had her hemoglobin checked at her routine prenatal visit. The hemoglobin level was 11 g/dL. She asked the nurse why the level was so low. The most accurate explanation by the nurse is which of the following statements?

1. "You are not getting enough iron in your diet."
2. "The hemoglobin is diluted by the fluid in your blood."
3. "The fetus is building up iron stores by taking it from you."
4. "During pregnancy, there is decreased production of red blood cells."

72. A client noticed that her health-care provider wrote "positive Chadwick's sign" on her prenatal record. She asked the nurse what this meant. The most accurate response by the nurse would be which of the following?

1. "It means your cervix is a bluish color."
2. "It means your cervix is getting softer."
3. "It means your uterus can flex against the cervix."
4. "It means your cervix is dilating."

73. A client at 20 weeks' gestation comes to the clinic for a routine prenatal visit. The nurse measures the fundal height and finds that it is at the umbilicus. The correct interpretation of this finding is which of the following?

1. The fundal height is lower than expected for gestational age.
2. The fundal height is higher than expected for gestational age.
3. The fundal height is appropriate for gestational age.
4. The fundal height is irrelevant to gestational age.

74. A client at 35 weeks' gestation is being seen at the obstetric clinic. Which of the following complaints by the client would require further nursing assessment?

1. Shortness of breath when doing housework
2. Swollen ankles at the end of the day
3. Sharp, intermittent groin pain
4. Increase in vaginal discharge

75. An Asian client delivered a term infant 2 hours ago. In teaching the client pericare, the nurse noted that she would not make eye contact. The correct interpretation of this behavior is which of the following?

1. The client is embarrassed.
2. The client does not understand English.
3. The client is excessively modest.
4. The client is demonstrating cultural beliefs.

76. A client in the first trimester of pregnancy is attending a prenatal class on nutrition for pregnancy. She tells the nurse educator that she is lactose intolerant and asks if there are any other food sources of calcium. The nurse should teach the client that her diet should include which of the following foods?

1. Sardines, peanuts, broccoli
2. Poultry, whole grains, tomatoes
3. Liver, dark yellow vegetables, green peppers
4. There are no food sources of calcium

77. A client at 28 weeks' gestation has gained 16 lb. She expresses concern to the nurse about her weight gain. Which of the following responses by the nurse is most appropriate?

1. "You have gained too much weight for this stage of pregnancy."
2. "You have not gained enough weight for this stage of pregnancy."
3. "Your weight gain is appropriate for this stage of pregnancy."
4. "Weight gain does not matter at this stage of pregnancy."

78. A client at 34 weeks' gestation is seen at the clinic for a nonstress test. She asks the nurse the purpose of the test. Which of the following explanations by the nurse would be most accurate?

1. "This test determines fetal well-being by assessing the fetal heart rate, body tone, and amniotic fluid."
2. "This test determines fetal well-being by assessing the response of the fetal heart rate to fetal movement."
3. "This test determines fetal well-being by assessing fetal movement several times each day."
4. "This test determines fetal well-being by assessing the response of the fetal heart rate to contractions."

79. A client at 41 weeks' gestation has undergone a non-stress test for fetal well-being. The results of the non-stress test were three fetal heart rate accelerations of 18 bpm that lasted for 15 seconds over a 15-minute period. The nurse knows these results would be considered to be which of the following?

1. Positive
2. Negative
3. Reactive
4. Nonreactive

80. A client at 18 weeks' gestation preparing to undergo amniocentesis for fetal anomalies made the following remark to the nurse, "My husband insisted that I have this test." Which of the following responses by the nurse would be most appropriate?

1. "Don't worry, everything will be fine."
2. "Make up your mind if you're having the test."
3. "I'll call the doctor to cancel the test"
4. "You seem to have some concerns about this test."

81. A client in active labor at term has been using prepared childbirth techniques effectively. She asks the nurse, "Why do contractions hurt so much?" The most accurate reply by the nurse is which of the following responses?

1. "It hurts because of stretching of uterine muscles."
2. "It hurts because of irritation to the nerves in the vagina."
3. "It hurts because the nerves in the uterus are inflamed."
4. "It hurts because of decreased oxygen to the uterine muscle."

82. A client at term has just been admitted to the obstetric unit in active labor. The admitting nurse noted the client had a prepregnancy history of IV drug use and is positive for herpes B virus (HBV+). Considering this client's history, which of the following substances would require the nurse to wear personal protective equipment?

1. All body fluids
2. Saliva
3. Feces
4. Amniotic fluid

83. A client at 24 weeks' gestation has gained 5 lb since becoming pregnant. The nursing diagnosis—alteration in nutrition; less than body requirements; related to diet choices inadequate to meet the nutrient requirements of pregnancy—was developed. Which of the following goals would be most appropriate for this client?

1. The client will develop a nutritious daily menu plan.
2. The client will gain 30 lb by term.
3. The client will take prenatal vitamins and iron daily.
4. The client will eliminate all snack foods.

84. The spouse of a laboring woman tells the nurse that he doesn't think he wants to be present for the birth of his child. "I feel like I should be there for my wife, but all that blood and everything is disgusting. Besides, new-born babies are ugly." Which of the following nursing diagnoses would be most appropriate for this situation?

1. Impaired parenting related to negative perceptions of childbirth and newborns
2. Role conflict related to unrealistic expectations of the childbearing process
3. Decisional conflict related to ambivalence toward the anticipated role in childbirth
4. Impaired family function related to father's nonsupportive attitude toward his wife

85. A client in early labor is complaining of back pain during contractions. Which of the following nursing interventions would be most effective for this type of pain?

1. Light massage over the abdomen
2. Massage of the upper back
3. Firm pressure over the sacrum
4. Encouraging pant/blow breathing

86. A client in the second trimester is seen in the obstetric clinic for a urinary tract infection (UTI). She asks the nurse what actions she can take to prevent recurrences. Which of the following responses by the nurse would be most accurate?

1. "Hold your urine for as long as you can before voiding."
2. "Empty your bladder before and after intercourse."
3. "Drink lots of cranberry juice to acidify your urine."
4. "Eat live culture yogurt every day to prevent infection."

87. A client dilated to 8 cm with the presenting part at 0 station and fetal heart rate ranging from 110–120 bpm is complaining of facial numbness and tingling of her hands and feet. Which of the following nursing interventions would be most appropriate for this situation?

1. Encourage deep breathing techniques.
2. Initiate oxygen therapy via face mask.
3. Turn the client to a lateral position.
4. Have the client blow into a paper bag.

88. A client attending a prenatal class on labor and delivery asks the nurse what factors can cause slowed or stopped descent of the presenting part during labor. Which of the following explanations by the nurse is most accurate?

1. "During labor, peristalsis decreases and slows fetal descent."
2. "If the uterus decreases in size during contractions, descent slows."
3. "If the urinary bladder is full, fetal descent is slowed."
4. "Ruptured membranes slow down descent of the fetus."

89. A client has been admitted to the obstetric unit for observation of labor. The admitting nurse auscultates fetal heart tones with a fetoscope for 1 minute. The fetal heart rate was 76 bpm. Which of the following nursing actions would be most appropriate?

1. Prepare for an emergency cesarean section.
2. Prepare to assist with internal fetal monitoring.

3. Report the finding to the registered nurse in charge.
4. Assess the maternal pulse.

90. A client who delivered a male infant 24 hours ago had her 2-year-old daughter in the room. The newborn was brought into the room. The 2-year-old girl turned her head away and stated, "I hate that baby, send him back." The mother asked the nurse to return the infant to the nursery. Which of the following nursing diagnoses would be most appropriate for this situation?

1. Altered parenting related to depression
2. Altered role performance related to postpartum psychosis
3. Low self-esteem related to lack of confidence in ability to care for two children
4. Altered family processes related to sibling rivalry

91. A breast-feeding client has put the infant to the breast for the first time. To facilitate latch-on, the nurse should teach the mother which of the following techniques?

1. Using a finger to depress the breast tissue so the infant can breathe while nursing
2. Placing the forefinger and middle fingers around the nipple in a "scissors" position
3. Ensuring that only the nipple is taken into the infant's mouth
4. Placing the infant in a "belly to belly" position with the mother

92. A new mother is preparing for discharge with her term male infant. In discussing infant safety concerns, which of the following statements by the client to the nurse would indicate a need for further instruction?

1. "We put the car seat in the back seat facing backwards."
2. "We bought a backpack to carry the baby in."
3. "We stripped my old crib and painted it with lead-free paint."
4. "We will put the baby to sleep on his back or side."

93. A 15-year-old client at 28 weeks' gestation tells the school nurse that she has decided to put her baby up for adoption. Which of the following responses by the nurse would be most appropriate?

1. Tell her it is too soon to make such an important decision.
2. Support her decision and acknowledge her maturity in making it.
3. Ask her if she is being pressured into making this decision.
4. Question her reasons for giving up her baby for adoption.

94. A primigravida at term is admitted to the obstetric unit in early labor. Contractions are every 5 minutes, moderate in intensity, and cervical changes are dilation at 4 cm, effacement at 100%, presenting part at –1 station. Which of the following changes would indicate the nurse would need to prepare for imminent delivery?

1. Cervical dilation of 8–9 cm, presenting part at 1+ station.
2. Client stating "I feel like I have to have a BM."

3. Contractions every 3 minutes, hard intensity.
4. The client vomits and states, "I can't do this anymore."

95. A client in preterm labor was treated with IV magnesium sulfate for 6 hours, and is now on SQ terbutaline. Intravenous hydration was given with several 500-mL boluses of crystalloid solution since admission. The IV is now infusing at 125 mL/hr. Which of the following symptoms would indicate the client has developed a fluid overload?

1. Pulse 120 bpm, heart palpitations
2. Intake of 3000 mL, output of 3500 mL
3. 2+ pedal edema
4. Fine crackles in the base of the lungs

96. A client who abused cocaine while pregnant is getting ready to be discharged home with her male infant. The infant has a rigid body posture and is difficult to console. The nurse discusses appropriate methods of play for the infant with the client. Which of the following nurse recommendations are appropriate for this situation?

1. "You need to get a musical mobile for his crib."
2. "A wind-up swing will quiet him when he cries."
3. "Tell your friends that rattles are a good toy for him."
4. "Get a tape player and play soft music in his room."

97. The transitional nursery nurse suspects that a newly delivered infant was born to a mother addicted to narcotics. Which of the following physical manifestations would the nurse expect to find in this newborn?

1. Rigid muscle tone, seizures, poor suck/swallow reflex
2. Flat midface, low-set ears, small for gestational age
3. Small for gestational age, decreased head circumference, developmental delays
4. Poor muscle tone, flat midface, epicanthal folds near the bridge of the face

98. A well-dressed client at 24 weeks' gestation presents to the emergency room with facial and abdominal bruises. She reported, "I walked into a door." Physical assessment reveals numerous bruises in various stages of healing. The nurse suspects intimate partner abuse. Which of the following nursing actions would be most appropriate in this situation?

1. Encourage the client to leave her partner.
2. Accept the story. Abuse does not occur in middle-class families
3. Refer the client to psychiatric counseling.
4. Ask the client, "Did someone hurt you?"

99. A client is admitted to the obstetric unit at 34 weeks' gestation with vaginal bleeding. Which of the following symptoms would indicate a placenta previa?

1. Decreased fundal height
2. Hard, boardlike abdomen
3. FHR rate of 180
4. Painless vaginal bleeding

100. A client whose newborn tested positive for PKU has received teaching from the nurse about the special dietary needs of her infant. Which of the following client statements indicate teaching has been effective?

1. "I'll continue breast-feeding."
2. "I'll have to change to regular formula."
3. "I'll have to use a soy formula."
4. "I'll have to get a low-phenylalanine formula."

101. A client at 32 weeks" gestation is admitted to the obstetric unit with a blood pressure of 142/90 mm Hg and 1+ proteinuria. No private rooms are available. Which room assignment should the charge nurse make?

1. A semiprivate room with a postpartum woman who delivered at term
2. A semiprivate room with a woman in preterm labor at 30 weeks' gestation
3. A semiprivate room with a woman with a placenta previa at 29 weeks' gestation
4. A semiprivate room with a woman with PIH at 36 weeks' gestation.

102. A client at 34 weeks' gestation with PIH complains of "heartburn." What nursing action has priority?

Answer:

_____

103. The nurse on the antepartum/postpartum unit has the following clients. Which client should she see first?

1. A G1P1 12 hours postpartum with an oral temp of 100.2°
2. G2P2 5 hours postpartum complaining of uterine contractions
3. A G1P1 48 hours postpartum complaining of profuse diaphoresis
4. A G2P2 24 hours postpartum complaining of right calf pain

104. A client who is 1 day postpartum has the following lab results. Which of the following lab values should be reported to the physician immediately?

1. Hemoglobin of 11 g/dL
2. WBC count of 15,000 mm³
3. Hematocrit of 18%
4. Serum glucose of 80 g/dL

105. You are caring for a client with intense contractions occurring every 2 minutes. She delivers less than 3 hours after her labor began. Based on your knowledge of the normal labor process, which of the following labor patterns did the client experience?

1. Hypotonic
2. Precipitous
3. Prolonged
4. Normal

106. Which of the following tasks are appropriate to be assigned to the licensed practical nurse (LPN) or a labor delivery room person (LDRP)? **Select all that apply.**

1. Admission assessment on a client with vaginal bleeding
2. Vital signs on a multiparous client who delivered 15 minutes ago
3. Assisting a 17-year-old primipara with breast-feeding
4. Giving ampicillin IV push to a postoperative cesarean client

107. A primipara at 32 weeks' gestation is seen in the obstetric/gynecologic clinic. Which of the following signs/symptoms should the nurse immediately report to the physician?

1. Puffy hands and face
2. Complaints of dyspnea
3. Pedal edema
4. Trace proteinuria

108. Which of the following tasks would be *inappropriate* for the LDRP charge nurse to assign to an LPN II? **Select all that apply.**

1. Managing the patient controlled analgesia (PCA) on a 1-day postoperative cesarean section client
2. Drawing a trough vancomycin level on a client 1 week postpartum with mastitis
3. Teaching a primipara who is 4 hours postpartum how to perform perineal care
4. Drawing routine admission labs on a client admitted to the observation room in early labor

109. The postpartum nurse is busy with a new admission. Which of the following assignments would be appropriate for the certified nursing assistant (CNA)? **Select all that apply.**

1. Hanging plain IV fluids on a laboring client
2. Assisting a client to the bathroom 2 hours after delivery
3. Taking vital signs on a client in the transition phase of labor
4. Inserting an in-and-out catheter on a postpartum client with urinary retention

110. While the postpartum nurse was in report, four of her clients called the nurses' station for assistance. Which client should the nurse see first?

1. A client with three nickel-sized clots on her perineal pad
2. A breast-feeding client who is complaining of uterine cramping
3. A client complaining of blood running down her legs upon standing
4. A client who had an epidural and is now complaining of a headache

111. The newborn nursery is filled to capacity. Which of the following infants should the nurse assess first?

1. A 1-hour-old female infant who is sucking her fist
2. A 2-day-old male infant who is crying loudly
3. A 3-day-old male infant 3 hours after circumcision
4. A 4-hour-female infant who is just waking up

112. The LDRP night shift staff is composed of a charge nurse, two LPNs, and one nursing assistant. Which of the following assignments is appropriate for the charge nurse to make to the nursing assistant? **Select all that apply.**

1. Total the intake and output on a postpartum client receiving IV fluids.
2. Vital signs on a 2-hour postpartum client.
3. Administration of ibuprofen (Tylenol) to a 2-day postpartum client with cramping
4. Monitoring a 6-hour postpartum client on IV magnesium sulfate
5. Setting up the room for delivery of a client dilated to 10 cm

113. The nurse assesses a multigravida who is 4 hours postpartum. She finds that the fundus is slightly boggy, 2 cm above the umbilicus, and deviated to the right side. The lochia is moderately heavy and bright red. Which of the following nursing interventions are appropriate? **Select all that apply.**

1. Massage the fundus.
2. Administer oral methylergonovine maleate (Methergine).
3. Check for a distended bladder.
4. Document these normal findings.
5. Assist the client up to void.

114. Which of the following clients should the labor nurse see first?

1. A primigravida on IV magnesium sulfate with deep tendon reflexes of 2+
2. A multigravida on PO terbutaline with a pulse rate of 110 bpm
3. A primigravida on IV oxytocin (Pitocin) with contractions every 3–4 minutes
4. A multigravida on PO methldopa (Aldomet) with a blood pressure of 142/86 mm Hg

115. A client is admitted to the obstetric unit who had her last menstrual period 10 weeks ago. She is currently complaining of sharp lower right-sided abdominal pain. Which of the following symptoms should be immediately reported to the registered nurse?

1. Presence of fetal heart tones
2. Right sided shoulder pain
3. Bright red vaginal bleeding
4. Severe uterine cramping

116. All of the beds in a 10-bed LDRP unit are full when one of the nurses assigned that day calls in sick. An LPN from the Medical/Surgical unit is pulled to postpartum. The charge nurse should assign her which of the following clients? **Select all that apply.**

1. A client at 32 weeks' gestation on oral terbutaline with four contractions/hour
2. A client 1 hour postpartum with a moderate amount of vaginal bleeding
3. A client 2 hours postpartum with complaints of intense perineal pain
4. A client at 36 week' gestation with a blood pressure of 145/90 mm Hg

117. Which of the following nursing task has priority for the nurse in the term nursery?

1. Preparing the circumcision equipment for a 2-day-old newborn male infant
2. Using a bulb syringe to suction a newborn who is gagging on formula
3. Performing the gestational age assessment on a 30-minute-old newborn female infant
4. Obtaining a heal stick blood sample on a 24-hour-old newborn for metabolic testing

118. The following newborns are in the term nursery. Which infant condition(s) should be reported immediately? **Select all that apply.**

1. A newborn at 12 hours of age with a direct bilirubin of 3 g/dL
2. A newborn at 24 hours of age with a positive direct Coombs' test
3. A newborn at 18 hours of age with peach-colored skin
4. A newborn at 24 hours of age with acrocyanosis

119. The charge nurse is making assignments on the LDRP unit. There are two LPNs and one nurse's aide assigned to work the unit today. Of the following clients, which would be the most appropriate for the charge nurse to assign to the LPNs?

Client A. A primipara needing assistance with first-time breast-feeding

Client B. A multipara complaining of a headache and epigastric discomfort

Client C. A primipara who is 2 days postop cesarean section

Client D. A multipara 4 hours after delivery of a 10-lb baby

Client E. A primipara receiving IV ampicllin for an infection due to β streptococci

Client F. A multipara postop cesarean section with a PCA pump

1. Assign the LPNs to clients A, B, and C.
2. Assign the LPNs to clients B, E, and F.
3. Assign the LPNs to clients A, C, and D.
4. Assign the LPNs to clients D, E, and F.

120. The newborn nursery is full at the beginning of the 3–11 shift. Which of the following infants should the nurse assess first?

1. A newborn with a positive Babinski's reflex
2. A newborn with circumoral cyanosis
3. A newborn with a negative Ortalini's sign
4. A newborn with talangiectatic nevi

121. A nurse who has worked on the LDRP for 6 weeks approaches the charge nurse after she has been given her assignment for the day. The nurse has received cross-training to all areas of the unit. Today, her assignment was to transition a newly born male infant. The nurse tells the charge nurse that she is uncomfortable caring for "such a tiny, new baby" and asks for an assignment change. What is the best response of the charge nurse?

1. "You have been cross-trained and all of our nurses have to care for each type of OB client. Your assignment will not change."
2. "If you are uncomfortable with your assignment, I will switch you to the postpartum clients."
3. "I will team you up with another nursery nurse so you can become more comfortable with newborn babies."
4. "I will not change your assignment. You will have to discuss this further with the shift supervisor."

122. What room assignment would be best for a primigravida with gestational diabetes who was admitted for glycemic control?

1. A private room near the nurses' station
2. Rooming with a client with a placenta previa
3. Rooming with a client with preterm labor
4. Rooming with a client with pregestational diabetes

123. A pregnant client has been receiving daily heparin injections for a history of deep venous thromboses during pregnancy. Which of the following laboratory test results should be immediately reported to the physician?

1. A PT of 16
2. A PTT of 22
3. An International Normalized Ratio (INR) of 2.5
4. A hemoglobin of 11

124. A charge nurse, two floor nurses, and two obstetric scrub technicians have been assigned to a 12-bed LDRP. Which of the following tasks are appropriate for the charge nurse to delegate to the scrub techs? **Select all that apply.**

1. Set up the delivery tables as needed.
2. Place labor clients on fetal heart monitors.
3. Obtain vital signs.
4. Conduct nonstress testing.
5. Obtain a nursing history.
6. Administer parenteral medications.

125. The oncoming nurse has just received report and is preparing to make her initial rounds. Which of the following postpartum clients should be seen first?

1. A primipara 6 hours postpartum saturating one peripad every 2 hours
2. A multigravida 1 hour postpartum with a constant trickle of vaginal bleeding
3. A primigravida 12 hours postpartum with the uterine fundus at the umbilicus
4. A multigravida 72 hours postpartum with a brownish pink lochia discharge

126. Ovulation usually occurs:

1. At varying, irregular intervals
2. Fourteen days before the end of the menstrual cycle
3. Two days after menstrual flow has ceased
4. When the ovary is stimulated by sexual intercourse

127. The sex of the developing fetus is externally identifiable at which trimester of gestation?

1. First trimester
2. Second trimester
3. Third trimester
4. Equally throughout the pregnancy

128. Heartburn during pregnancy is commonly attributed to the normal physiological changes of:

1. Increased output and work load of the heart
2. Increased peristalsis and increased gastric acidity
3. Increased peristalsis and decreased food intake
4. Decreased gastric motility with reflux of stomach contents

129. One of the main objectives of a childbirth preparation program is to:

1. Strengthen the couple's marital relationship
2. Enhance the pregnant woman's self-esteem
3. Provide practical tools for the labor process
4. Educate the mother about the changes in childbirth practices

130. The nurse explains to a woman that a diaphragm is an excellent method of contraception, provided she:

1. Does not use any contraceptive cream, jelly, or foam that might make it slip out of place
2. Removes it promptly following intercourse
3. Leaves it in place for 6–8 hours following intercourse
4. Inserts it at least 4–6 hours prior to intercourse to ensure a protective seal

131. The main purpose of relaxation during labor is to:

1. Allow the woman to conserve energy and allow the uterine muscles to work more efficiently
2. Promote resting and control
3. Replace unfavorable with controlled, favorable behaviors
4. Provide a quiet birthing environment

132. Vitamin K is administered to a newborn in order to:

1. Stimulate the growth of intestinal flora
2. Improve the conjugation of bilirubin
3. Prevent potential bleeding problems
4. Improve the production of RBCs

133. A neonate is delivered at 27 weeks' gestation weighing 1400 g. Based on this weight and gestational age, how would you classify this neonate?

1. Low birth weight
2. Small for gestational age
3. Large for gestational age
4. Preterm

134. The embryonic period of pregnancy is critical because:

1. Genetic information is duplicated at this time.
2. All organ systems are developed.
3. Urine is secreted by the kidneys.
4. Subcutaneous fat is deposited.

135. When conducting a urine pregnancy test, what specific hormone will produce a positive test for pregnancy?

1. Estrogen
2. Prolactin

3. α-Fetoprotein
4. Human chorionic gonadotropin

136. Chorioamnionitis is a maternal infection usually associated with:

1. Postterm deliveries
2. Maternal dehydration
3. Prolonged rupture of membranes
4. Maternal pyelonephritis

137. A positive Babinski's reflex in a newborn would indicate:

1. The infant has neurological dysfunction.
2. The infant has normal, intact neurological function.
3. The infant has experienced perinatal asphyxia.
4. The infant has experienced a spinal cord injury during the birthing process.

138. You are teaching a childbirth and parenting class to a group of expectant mothers. As you describe the different states of an infant, you tell the participants that the characteristics of the quiet alert state of an infant are:

1. Minimal body activity, widening of eyes, and a regular breathing pattern
2. Variable activity levels, heavy-lidded eyes, and an irregular breathing pattern
3. Nearly still body activity, no eye movements, and a smooth, regular breathing pattern
4. Minimal body activity, rapid eye movements, and an irregular breathing pattern

139. Molding of the fetal head during birth would result in:

1. Widely spaced suture lines
2. A collection of fluid across the scalp
3. Overriding suture lines or a small space between the cranial bones
4. Depressed fontanelles

140. To improve iron absorption, you should instruct your client at her prenatal visit to take the supplement:

1. At bedtime with citrus juice, and avoid coffee or tea
2. Between meals when her stomach is empty
3. When she takes her prenatal vitamins
4. Only when she does not eat foods rich in iron daily

141. *Effacement* is a term used to describe the process by which the cervix:

1. Opens to its widest diameter
2. Lengthens during a normal pregnancy
3. Becomes hypotonic to prepare for dilation
4. Softens and thins with contractions

142. A 21-year-old who is at 41 weeks' gestation is undergoing induction of labor with IV oxytocin. As the nurse monitoring this client, you should routinely assess for:

1. Uterine tetany
2. Deep tendon reflexes
3. Hyperglycemia
4. Tearing of the perineum

143. The client is recovering from a hysterectomy as a result of uncontrollable bleeding following placenta previa. One of the top-priority teaching needs prior to discharge would be:

1. Explanation of the rationale for the immediate onset of menopause
2. Explanation of resumption of a normal menstrual cycle
3. Discussion of the type of birth control most suited for posthysterectomy clients
4. Discussion of expected feelings of grief and loss

144. The nurse explains to the client that the most common side effect of the contraceptive Depo-Provera is:

1. Irregular and unpredictable menstrual bleeding
2. Weight loss
3. Hyperactivity
4. Hypertension

145. A major complication of eclampsia is:

1. Infection
2. Aspiration
3. Polyuria
4. Extremity injuries

146. The most common cause of early postpartal hemorrhage is:

1. Uterine atony
2. Retained placental fragments
3. Cervical lacerations
4. Infection

147. Magnesium sulfate ($MgSO_4$) is used in the treatment of preeclampsia to:

1. Prevent seizures
2. Decrease blood pressure
3. Increased urine output
4. Decrease edema

148. A client with three prior cesarean sections is in active labor and scheduled for a repeat cesarean delivery. The nurse's primary concern for the client would be:

1. Tetanic contractions
2. Precipitous labor
3. Uterine rupture
4. Abruptio placentae

149. Following an amniocentesis, the client should be monitored for an hour for:

1. Breast tenderness
2. Increased fetal activity
3. Temperature elevation
4. Rupture of membranes

150. A client reports a weight gain of 1 lb a week during her eighth month of pregnancy. Which of the following actions should be taken?

1. None because this is a normal weight increase
2. Make an appointment with the nutritionist
3. Suggest a weight-loss program
4. Check for proteinuria and hypertension

ANSWERS

1. **(2)** Integrated processes: nursing process — implementation; client need: physiological integrity; basic care and comfort; content area: maternity.

   RATIONALE

   (1) Laxatives and enemas stimulate the intestinal tract, but also can initiate uterine contractions. **(2)** Intestinal motility is slowed in pregnancy due to the influence of progesterone. Increasing fluid intake and exercise stimulates peristalsis. **(3)** High-fat and high-protein foods contribute to constipation. **(4)** Caffeine can cause tachycardia in the fetus and its use during pregnancy is discouraged.

2. **(1)** Integrated processes: nursing process — implementation; teaching/learning; client need: physiological integrity; physiological adaptation; content area: maternity.

   RATIONALE

   (1) Progesterone causes peristalsis to slow so more nutrients can be absorbed. **(2)** An increase in intestinal motility causes diarrhea. **(3)** Compression of the intestines during pregnancy does not contribute to constipation. **(4)** The intestines do not increase in diameter due to pregnancy.

3. **(3)** Integrated processes: nursing process — planning; client need: physiological integrity; reduction of risk potential; content area: maternity

   RATIONALE

   (1) Blood type A with Rh+ does not present any problems in patient care. Maternal blood type O and/or Rh− blood types can cause severe jaundice in the newborn due to maternal antibodies that destroy fetal red blood cells. **(2)** Red blood cells are diluted by the increase in plasma volume in pregnancy. A hemoglobin of 11 g/dL is physiological anemia, as opposed to true anemia. **(3)** Using Nagle's rule, an LMP of 2/15/97 would give an estimated date of delivery (EDD) of 11/29/97. This client is in preterm labor at 28 5/7 weeks' gestation. **(4)** During the first two trimesters of pregnancy, maternal blood pressure normally decreases by 5–10 mm Hg in both systolic and diastolic pressures. This decrease is due to peripheral vasodilatation caused by pregnancy hormones.

4. **(4)** Integrated processes: nursing process — data collection; teaching/learning; client need: physiological integrity; basic care and comfort; content area: maternity.

   RATIONALE

   (1) Appropriate weight gain for pregnancy is between 25 and 35 lb. **(2)** Intrauterine growth retardation can be caused by poor maternal diets. The U.S. Food and Drug Administration recommends following the food pyramid recommendations for improved dietary intake. **(3)** Canned foods lose some nutrients in processing. Foods that are frozen are processed less and more nutritious. **(4)** Pica is more related to cultural values and beliefs than to dietary deficiencies. Pica is more likely to cause iron deficiency than to be caused by it.

5. **(1)** Integrated processes: nursing process — planning; teaching/learning; client need: physiological integrity; basic care and comfort; content area: maternity

   RATIONALE

   (1) This client is in the early phase of labor; slow, deep breathing and relaxation techniques are usually effective in relieving contraction pain during this phase. **(2)** Rapid, shallow breathing, or hyperventilation, is inappropriate for any phase of labor. **(3)** local anesthesia is used for numbing of the perineum immediately before performance of an episiotomy and delivery of the fetus during the last phase of the first stage of labor. **(4)** Narcotic analgesia is not appropriate for use during early phases of labor. It can slow or stop labor if given before 5 cm dilation. In addition, minimizing use of narcotics is preferred when prepared childbirth techniques are used.

6. **(3)** Integrated processes: nursing process — implementation; teaching/learning; client need: physiological integrity; physiological adaptation; content area: maternity.

   RATIONALE

   (1) The sex chromosome of males is XY; the sex chromosome for females is XX. The mother contributes one X chromosome to the fetus, the father contributes either an X or a Y chromosome. **(2)** The heart rate of the fetus is neither faster nor slower according to fetal gender. The range for the fetal heart rate is 110–160 bpm regardless of gender. **(3)** Meiosis results in the X and Y chromosomes of the male splitting so that each sperm carries either an X or a Y chromosome, thus determining the gender of the fetus. **(4)** How a fetus is carried is related to maternal uterine and abdominal muscle tone. The gender of the fetus does not determine how high or low it is carried.

7. **(2)** Integrated processes: nursing process — implementation; teaching/learning; client need: psychosocial integrity; content area: maternity

   RATIONALE

   (1) The volume of breast milk produced is related to how often the breasts are emptied of milk. Formula supplementation decreases breast milk production since the infant nurses less often. **(2)** The amount of milk producing glandular tissue in all women is approximately the same. The size of large breasts is due to increased fatty tissue. **(3)** An infant is more efficient at emptying a breast than a breast pump. In addition, oral stimulation of the nipples by the infant stimulates the release of oxytocin, which triggers the let-down reflex. **(4)** Estrogen does not stimulate milk production. Oxytocin and prolactin are the hormones responsible for breast milk production and breast-feeding success.

8. **(4)** Integrated processes: nursing process — implementation; client need: physiological integrity; reduction of risk potential; content area: maternity

   RATIONALE

   (1) Bilirubin levels in excess of 12 mg/100 mL may indicate the presence of a pathological process. This jaundice is most likely due to an ABO incompatibility. **(2)** Breast-feeding jaundice occurs around the third day of age. Encouraging early and frequent feedings at the breast lowers neonatal bilirubin levels. **(3)** Light therapy requires an order from the physician. Exchange transfusions for ABO incompatibilities are seldom necessary. **(4)** Early and frequent breast-feeding tends to lower serum bilirubin levels.

9. **(4)** Integrated processes: nursing process — implementation; teaching/learning; client need: health promotion and maintenance; content area: maternity.

   RATIONALE

   (1) If the fetus remains in a breech position, external version may be attempted at approximately 37 weeks' gestation to change the position of the fetus. If version is unsuccessful in the nulliparous woman with a fetus in a breech position, cesarean delivery is *almost* always certain. (2) The uterus becomes more crowded, not less, as pregnancy progresses. (3) Few fetuses (3%–4%) are in a breech position by delivery; even fewer breech positions are delivered vaginally. (4) Approximately 96% of fetuses in a breech position will turn to a cephalic position by term.

10. **(1)** Integrated processes: nursing process — implementation; client need: physiological integrity; reduction of risk potential; content area: maternity

    RATIONALE

    (1) Maternal position changes such as sitting, kneeling, lateral, or hands and knees, can assist fetal head rotation to an occiput anterior position. (2) The gravid uterus compresses the pelvic blood vessels and compromises uteroplacental blood flow. This position not only has no effect on rotation of the fetal head, but can cause fetal compromise. (3) Use of forceps at zero station is considered to be a high forceps classification and is not acceptable practice according to the American College of Obstetricians and Gynecologists. (4) Cesarean delivery should be considered only if adequate pushing efforts of 2 or more hours do not result in descent of the fetal head.

11. **(2)** Integrated processes: nursing process — data collection; client need: physiological integrity; reduction of risk potential; content area: maternity.

    RATIONALE

    (1) hCG is a hormone produced by the placenta that stimulates the corpus luteum to persist and secrete estrogen and progesterone, which maintains the pregnancy for the first 20 weeks of gestation. It is found in maternal blood and urine. (2) PG is a major phospholipid of surfactant. The presence of PG in amniotic fluid indicates fetal lung maturity. (3) AFP is a plasma protein that is produced by the fetus. Abnormally high or low levels can indicate fetal anomalies. AFP levels are drawn from maternal blood. (4) PTT levels are drawn to determine if sodium warfarin levels are at a therapeutic level in women with thromboembolic disease.

12. **(4)** Integrated processes: nursing process — implementation; teaching/learning; client need: health promotion and maintenance; content area: maternity.

    RATIONALE

    (1) Monozygotic twins (identical twins) develop from one fertilized egg that splits into identical halves early in embryonic development. (2) Dizygotic twins develop from two different ova fertilized by two different sperm. (3) Once an egg has been penetrated by a single sperm, chemical changes take place that prevent multiple sperm fertilization. (4) See rationale 2.

13. **(2)** Integrated processes: nursing process — implementation; teaching/learning; client need: health promotion and maintenance; content area: maternity.

    RATIONALE

    (1) The only positive signs of pregnancy are auscultation of fetal heart tones, visualization of the fetus by ultrasound, and fetal movement felt by the health-care provider. (2) Presumptive signs of pregnancy are amenorrhea, fatigue, breast tenderness and enlargement, morning sickness, and quickening. (3) Probable signs of pregnancy are Hegar's sign, ballottement, positive pregnancy test, and Goodell's sign. (4) Amenorrhea and breast tenderness are presumptive signs of pregnancy.

14. **(3)** Integrated processes: nursing process — data collection; client need: physiological integrity; reduction of risk potential; content area: maternity.

    RATIONALE

    (1) Increased temperature may be a sign of infection; however, the risk of infection is greatest during the first 72 hours after spontaneous abortion or operative procedures. (2) The client is at risk for excess blood loss. The pulse pressure decreases with hemorrhage. (3) An increased pulse in the presence of visible bleeding indicates excessive blood loss. (4) Increased blood pressure at this stage of pregnancy would be a symptom of a hydatidiform mole.

15. **(1)** Integrated processes: nursing process — data collection; client need: physiological integrity; reduction of risk potential; content area: maternity

    RATIONALE

    (1) Hypotension is common with epidural anesthesia because the sympathetic nerves are also blocked by the medication, which results in vasodilation. (2) Hypertension is not a side effect of epidural anesthesia. (3) Hyperventilation is not a side effect of epidural anesthesia. A client is more likely to hyperventilate during painful contractions. Epidural anesthesia relieves contraction pain. (4) Hypoventilation is possible if epidural narcotics are used. An epidural narcotic (such as fentanyl) was not used in this case.

16. **(2)** Integrated processes: nursing process — data collection; client need: physiological integrity; reduction of risk potential; content area: maternity.

    RATIONALE

    (1) The PT is assessed to maintain correct dosages of warfarin (Coumadin). Coumadin crosses the placental barrier and is contraindicated in pregnancy. (2) The PTT is evaluated to determine the effectiveness of heparin therapy. (3) A bleeding time is obtained preoperatively to determine how quickly blood clots to maintain homeostasis. It is not routinely performed on pregnant women, and is unnecessary for a pregnant woman on heparin therapy. (4) A clotting time is a fictional test.

17. **(4)** Integrated processes: nursing process — implementation; client need: physiological integrity; basic care and comfort; content area: maternity

    RATIONALE

    (1) These are symptoms of thrombophlebitis; massage of the area can break the thrombus from the venous wall and cause an embolus. (2) Local application of heat is one of the treatments for superficial thrombosis. (3) The client with symptoms of thrombophlebitis should be placed on bed rest. (4) Administration of analgesics, local application of heat, bed rest for 5–7 days, and elevation of the affected extremity are often all that is needed to treat superficial thrombophlebitis.

18. **(3)** Integrated processes: nursing process — implementation; client need: physiological integrity; physiological adaptation; content area: maternity

    RATIONALE

    (1) The third stage of labor is the stage of delivery of the placenta. The placenta will spontaneously separate from the uterine wall and be expelled by uterine contractions. Maternal pushing is unnecessary. (2) Oxytocin should not be administered until after the placenta is delivered, which usually occurs 5–7 minutes after delivery of the infant. (3) The infant's physical condition is a priority at one and five minutes after delivery of the newborn. The physical assessment done at this time is known as Apgar scoring. (4) Initiation of the bonding process as soon as possible after birth is important, but the physical stability of the newborn is most important at this time.

19. **(2)** Integrated processes: nursing process — implementation; teaching/learning; client need: health promotion and maintenance; content area: maternity.
RATIONALE
(1) Caput succedaneum is an area of generalized edema of the scalp that was present at birth. **(2)** Molding is an overlapping of the skull bones at the occiput of the skull. The infant skull has a cone shaped appearance. **(3)** A cephalhematoma is a collection of blood between the skull bone and its periosteum. It is one-sided (does not cross suture lines), and appears within the first 2 days after delivery. **(4)** Nevi (also known as "stork bites") are pink areas on the upper eyelids, nose, upper lip, lower occiput, and the nape of the neck.

20. **(2)** Integrated processes: nursing process — data collection; teaching/learning; client need: health promotion and maintenance; content area: maternity.
RATIONALE
(1) The cord stump should be cleaned with the solution ordered by the health-care provider daily until it falls off. Cord care helps the cord to dry and prevents infection. **(2)** A breast-feeding infant should have at least six wet diapers daily. Adequate urinary output is a reliable indicator of adequate intake of breast milk. **(3)** The infant should be dressed as parents would dress themselves. Overdressing can cause prickly heat rash. Wrapping the infant in a light blanket maintains body temperature and makes the infant feel secure. **(4)** Breast milk is more completely and quickly digested than formula. Breast-fed infants should be fed on demand. It is important for the infant to completely empty the breast, so infant sucking time at the breast should also not be limited.

21. **(4)** Integrated processes: nursing process — planning; client need: physiological integrity; physiological adaptation; content area: maternity
RATIONALE
(1) The fourth stage of labor is the immediate (approximately 1 hour) postpartum period. Epidural anesthesia takes approximately an hour to wear off. The client will be unable to ambulate during this time. In addition, *all* postpartum clients should be assisted with ambulation the first few times out of bed. **(2)** Pulmonary hygiene is important in clients with a respiratory condition, or those who have undergone an operative procedure. The client doesn't have an episiotomy. **(3)** The most common complication of the fourth of labor is uterine atony and hemorrhage.

22. **(2)** Integrated processes: nursing process — data collection; client need: physiological integrity; physiological adaptation; content area: maternity
RATIONALE
(1) The fundal height is approximately 2 fingerbreadths below the umbilicus immediately after delivery. The fundal height increases to 1 fingerbreadth above the umbilicus within 12 hours. The fundal height will decrease approximately 1–2 fingerbreadths a day afterward. Lochia rubra will be present for 3–4 days after delivery. **(2)** Fundal height increases to 1 fingerbreadth above the umbilicus within 12 hours after delivery. **(3)** Fundal deviation to one side or the other indicates a full bladder and risk for hemorrhage. **(4)** The fundal height is 3–4 fingerbreadths below the umbilicus by the fourth to fifth postpartum day.

23. **(3)** Integrated processes: nursing process — data collection; client need: physiological integrity; reduction of risk potential; content area: maternity

RATIONALE
(1) White blood cell counts indicate the presence or absence of infection. The normal range for WBCs in pregnancy is 9–15 mm^3. There is no evidence of infection. **(2)** The normal hematocrit in pregnancy ranges from 32%–46%. **(3)** The normal hemoglobin in pregnancy ranges from 11–12 g/dL. This client is slightly anemic. **(4)** The normal serum glucose in pregnancy ranges from 65–110 g/dL.

24. **(2)** Integrated processes: nursing process — data collection; client need: physiological integrity; pharmacological therapies; content area: maternity.
RATIONALE
(1) Respiratory depression is associated with epidural narcotics. Marcaine is an anesthetic agent. **(2)** The woman may not sense the urge to void because of decreased sensation to the area. Pain caused by bladder distention can last for long periods of time. **(3)** Uterine atony is associated with administration of oxytoxic drugs. It is not an effect of epidural anesthesia. **(4)** Maternal hypertension is not an adverse effect of epidural anesthesia.

25. **(4)** Integrated processes: nursing process — implementation; client need: physiological integrity; physiological adaptation; content area: maternity
RATIONALE
(1) This is a reassuring fetal heart pattern; no immediate nursing actions other than comfort measures are necessary. **(2)** There is no fetal distress. **(3)** The client is in no need for fluid volume expansion; neither she nor the fetus is in distress. **(4)** This client is in very early labor. The fetal heart pattern is reassuring. Ambulation at home would stimulate labor and descent of the presenting part and decrease hospitalization time.

26. **(3)** Integrated processes: nursing process — data collection; teaching/learning; client need: health promotion and maintenance; content area: maternity.
RATIONALE
(1) Condoms are a mechanical barrier method of contraception with an effectiveness rate of 88%. Condom usage does not interfere with breast-feeding. **(2)** Depo-Provera is an injectable form of progestin with an effectiveness rate of 99.7%. Pregnancy is prevented for 3 months. It is safe for use during lactation once the milk supply is established. **(3)** High prolactin levels with exclusive breast-feeding can delay ovulation for up to 6 months. However, it is an unpredictable method of birth control. **(4)** The effectiveness of the contraceptive foams range from 72%–82%. It has no hormones to affect lactation, and is safe for use during the postpartum period.

27. **(1)** Integrated processes: nursing process — data collection; client need: safe, effective care environment; safety and infection control; content area: maternity
RATIONALE
(1) Gonorrhea is usually treated with penicillin. Drug allergies to penicillin are common and can result in an anaphylactic reaction. **(2)** A malodorous vaginal discharge is caused by *Gardnerella vaginalis*. **(3)** A chancre is seen with syphilis. **(4)** Vesicles are seen with herpes.

28. **(2)** Integrated processes: nursing process — implementation; teaching/learning; client need: physiological integrity; reduction of risk potential; content area: maternity
RATIONALE
(1) Oral hypoglycemic agents cross the placenta and can cause fetal anomalies. **(2)** Insulin does not cross the placenta and is safe for use in pregnancy. **(3)** Only gestational diabetes can be treated with diet during pregnancy. **(4)** Only gestational diabetes can be treated with exercise during pregnancy.

29. **(3)** Integrated processes: nursing process — implementation; teaching/learning; client need: health promotion and maintenance; content area: maternity.
    RATIONALE
    (1) Analysis of amniotic fluid from amniocentesis allows determination of fetal gender. **(2)** The presence of phosphatidylglycerol and the L/S ratio determine fetal lung maturity. It is obtained from amniotic fluid. **(3)** AFP is a maternal blood test that can detect neural tube defects (the most common anomaly) in fetuses of diabetic women. It can also indicate the presence of Down's syndrome. **(4)** Glycemic control is determined by hemoglobin A_{1C}, a maternal blood test.

30. **(2)** Integrated processes: nursing process — implementation; client need: physiological integrity; reduction of risk potential; content area: maternity
    RATIONALE
    (1) Uterine atony would reveal a constant trickle of bright red blood in the presence of a boggy uterus. **(2)** Excessive lochia in the presence of a contracted uterus suggests lacerations of the birth canal. The health-care provider must be notified so the laceration can be repaired. **(3)** Excessive bleeding caused by a full bladder would reveal a uterus that was high and deviated to one side. **(4)** Increasing the rate of an infusion of oxytocin would not correct the problem of a lacerated birth canal.

31. **(4)** Integrated processes: nursing process — data collection; client need: health promotion and maintenance; content area: maternity.
    RATIONALE
    (1) One session of breast-feeding problems does not result in altered parenting. **(2)** The difficulty is in infant latch-on, not sore nipples. **(3)** Success in breast-feeding has little to do with bonding/attachment. **(4)** Instruction and assistance from the nurse would most likely result in successful latch-on and breast-feeding.

32. **(4)** Integrated processes: nursing process — implementation; caring; client need: health promotion and maintenance; content area: maternity.
    RATIONALE
    (1) Giving the mother pictures of her baby is appropriate only when an infant is too ill for physical contact. **(2)** Descriptions of the infant do not replace physical contact between mother and baby. **(3)** Direct physical contact between mother and baby is most likely to promote attachment. **(4)** The combination of direct physical contact between mother and baby and discussion of the child's physical and personality attributes assists the mother in recognizing her infant as a distinct individual who is yet a part of her. This process is the beginnings of attachment.

33. **(1)** Integrated processes: nursing process — implementation; teaching/learning; client need: health promotion and maintenance; content area: maternity
    RATIONALE
    (1) Evidence indicates that ingestion of live-culture yogurt decreases the incidence of vaginal yeast infections. **(2)** Vinegar and water douches decrease vaginal pH and inhibit the growth of yeast cells. However, douching is not recommended in pregnancy. **(3)** Douching with live-culture yogurt decreases vaginal pH. However douching is not recommended in pregnancy. **(4)** All antimicrobials cross the placenta; many can cause fetal organ damage. In addition, antibiotic therapy can increase the incidence of vaginal yeast infections.

34. **(2)** Integrated processes: nursing process — implementation; teaching/learning; client need: physiological integrity; physiological adaptation; content area: maternity.

35. **(1)** Integrated processes: nursing process — data collection; client need: physiological integrity; physiological adaptation; content area: maternity
    RATIONALE
    (1) Increased estrogen levels cause congestion, swelling, and hyperemia of the capillaries in the upper respiratory tract. These symptoms will not be relieved by antihistamines. **(2)** The elevated levels of estrogen during pregnancy cause increased blood flow in the upper respiratory tract. Nasal stuffiness, ear aches, hearing loss, and nose bleeds are common. **(3)** Referral to a specialist is not necessary because these are normal pregnancy symptoms. **(4)** These are normal pregnancy symptoms. Many antibiotics cross the placenta and are contraindicated in pregnancy. Antihistamines are also generally not recommended in pregnancy.

35. **(1)** Integrated processes: nursing process — data collection; client need: physiological integrity; physiological adaptation; content area: maternity
    RATIONALE
    (1) Blood volume increases by 30%–50% in pregnancy. This causes hemodilution of red blood cells and physiological anemia. Normal hemoglobin levels in pregnancy range from 11–12 g/dL. **(2)** Plethora is not a normal finding in pregnancy. **(3)** Normal serum glucose in pregnancy is 65. **(4)** This is a normal red blood cell count for nonpregnant individuals. Normal RBCs in pregnancy range from 11–12.

36. **(1)** Integrated processes: nursing process — data collection; teaching/learning; client need: health promotion and maintenance; content area: maternity
    RATIONALE
    (1) Pregnancy causes the areolas to darken and enlarge. **(2)** Breast tenderness and swelling are almost universal findings in pregnancy. **(3)** Pregnancy causes darkening of the pigment in the nipples and causes them to become more erectile. **(4)** Breast enlargement is caused by the influence of progesterone and estrogen. Nodularity is caused by an increase in the size of the mammary glands during the second trimester.

37. **(4)** Integrated processes: nursing process — implementation; caring; client need: psychosocial integrity; content area: maternity
    RATIONALE
    (1) Ambivalent feelings about pregnancy are common in all women. In addition, this response is a block to therapeutic communication. The nurse is telling the client how she "should" feel. **(2)** Even women with a desired pregnancy have ambivalent feelings. Such feelings do not necessarily mean the woman desires an abortion. **(3)** "Mother love" does not necessarily appear right after birth, especially in a first pregnancy. It may take time for such feelings to grow. **(4)** Ambivalence is a normal response experienced by any individual preparing for a new role.

38. **(2)** Integrated processes: nursing process — data collection; client need: physiological integrity; reduction of risk potential; content area: maternity
    RATIONALE
    (1) AFP drawn in the second trimester around 18 weeks of gestation. Low AFP may indicate Down's syndrome. **(2)** Antibodies formed by a mother because of an ABO or Rh incompatibility cause erythroblastosis fetalis. Blood and Rh typing and antibody screening can alert the health-care provider to the possible development of this condition. **(3)** The L/S ratio is obtained from amniotic fluid analysis and indicates fetal lung maturity. **(4)** There is a possibility of ABO incompatibility that could result in erythroblastosis fetalis; however the antibody screen is negative.

39. **(3)** Integrated processes: nursing process — implementation; client need: physiological integrity; reduction of risk potential; content area: maternity

RATIONALE

(1) Compression of the major vessels of the pelvis occurs with a supine position. This will compromise placental perfusion and contribute to fetal distress. (2) Fetal reserves are still present as evidenced by long-term variability, "shoulders," and a return to baseline. An operative delivery is not yet required. (3) Late decelerations are caused by decreased uteroplacental perfusion. Positioning a woman on her left side promotes fetal well-being by increasing placental perfusion and subsequent fetal oxygenation. This position change may stop the late decelerations. (4) Ambulation will stimulate uterine contractions and promote fetal descent. Increased frequency and/or intensity of contractions will impair uterine perfusion.

40. (1) Integrated processes: nursing process — data collection; client need: physiological integrity; reduction of risk potential; content area: maternity

RATIONALE

(1) Epigastric pain/discomfort is a sign of impending seizure in the client with severe PIH. (2) A blood pressure reading of 140/90 mm Hg indicates hypertension. Hypertension is considered severe when diastolic blood pressures exceed 110 mm Hg. (3) Normal deep tendon reflexes are 2+. (4) Dependent edema is a normal finding of pregnancy. Edema of the hands or face or pitting edema indicate a worsening of the disease.

41. (1) Integrated processes: nursing process — implementation; client need: physiological integrity; pharmacological therapies; content area: maternity

RATIONALE

(1) Terbutaline can cause maternal tachycardia (>120 bpm). Maternal tachycardia can reduce cardiac output and oxygenation. The dosage may need to be reduced or discontinued if tachycardia occurs. (2) Continuous fetal monitoring is maintained during initial tocolysis and active labor. Fetal heart tones and fetal activity logs are more appropriate for determining fetal well-being at this stage of treatment. (3) Bed rest with bathroom privileges is the most common activity restriction for clients with preterm labor after initial stabilization. (4) Terbutaline is likely to cause hyperventilation. It does not cause respiratory depression.

42. (4) Integrated processes: nursing process — data collection; cultural awareness; client need: psychosocial integrity; content area: maternity

RATIONALE

(1) Absence of requests for pain medication and smiling do not mean a client is not experiencing pain. These responses may reflect personal or cultural values. (2) The progress of the client's labor and her tension may indicate the client needs help with pain control. (3) Moral values are related to an individual's sense of right and wrong. Pain control methods are not associated with morality. (4) Asian women usually value stoicism and maintaining harmonious relationships. It is incorrect to assume that pain relief is not needed because of these responses.

43. (2) Integrated processes: nursing process — implementation; caring; client need: safe, effective care environment; coordinated care; content area: maternity.

RATIONALE

(1) It is important to collaborate with postpartum clients. Postpartum checks can safely be deferred for a few minutes when a client is stable. (2) Allowing postpartum clients choices gives them more of a sense of autonomy. Obstetric nurses should foster independence as much as possible. (3) Important physical information can be missed if a thorough check is not done. A client may not know what constitutes normal lochia flow, cannot evaluate the episiotomy, and cannot describe the consistency of the fundus. (4) The nurse needs a baseline database in order to evaluate changes in the condition of the client later in the shift.

44. (2) Integrated processes: nursing process — planning; client need: safe, effective care environment; safety and infection control; content area: maternity

RATIONALE

(1) A semiprivate room would not afford the client the quiet environment she needs. Routine vital signs are not frequent enough to detect early changes in maternal or fetal condition. Salt restriction has no effect on the edema and is not necessary. (2) Loud noises and bright lights can trigger seizures in a preeclamptic client; these stimuli can be minimized in a private room. The client needs to rest as much as possible and avoid stress. Vital signs and fetal heart tones should be monitored a minimum of every 4 hours. There are no dietary restrictions for a client with PIH or preeclampsia. (3) This client needs to be in a quiet environment and on bed rest. The vital signs and fetal heart tones are not frequent enough to detect early changes in maternal or fetal condition. A low-protein diet is prescribed for clients with renal conditions. Pregnant clients need adequate amounts of protein to support the pregnancy. (4) Unless the condition of the client worsens, or she starts to labor, there is no reason for her to be in a labor room. Continuous fetal monitoring and vital signs every 15 minutes do not promote rest. NPO status is not necessary.

45. (4) Integrated processes: nursing process — implementation; teaching/learning; client need: physiological integrity; reduction of risk potential; content area: maternity.

RATIONALE

(1) Normal lab values for pregnancy are WBCs = 5,000–10,000, RBCs = 4.2–5.4, hemoglobin = 12–16, and hematocrit = 37–47. This client is anemic. (2) The WBC count is within the normal range for pregnancy. (3) The hemoglobin and hematocrit are below the normal ranges for pregnancy. (4) Most cases of iron deficiency develop after the 20th week of pregnancy because of expanding blood volume and fetal demands. Any hemoglobin value below 10 g/dL and/or hematocrit below 35 are considered to constitute a true anemia.

46. (4) Integrated processes: nursing process — implementation; client need: physiological integrity; reduction of risk potential; content area: maternity

RATIONALE

(1) Absence of deep tendon reflexes is an early indication of magnesium toxicity. The infusion should be stopped immediately. (2) Excessive magnesium depresses the entire central nervous system. Magnesium toxicity can culminate in respiratory arrest. (3) The infusion of magnesium should never exceed a rate of 150 mg/min. Administration of additional magnesium will make the condition worse. (4) Magnesium should be discontinued if the respiratory rate is 12 breaths/minute or if deep tendon reflexes are absent.

47. (4) Integrated processes: nursing process — implementation; client need: health promotion and maintenance; content area: maternity.

RATIONALE

(1) Listening to the fetal heart tones helps validate the reality of the pregnancy, but does not help; allowing the father to visualize the new family member best facilitates paternal/fetal attachment. (2) Fetal models are good teaching tools for explaining physical development and size of the fetus, but are not the best way of encouraging paternal attachment to the fetus. (3) Typed handouts are too abstract to be of help in encouraging paternal/fetal attachment. (4) Having a father present at the

ultrasound of his fetus promotes paternal/fetal bonding by allowing him to see the features of the fetus. This visualization makes the pregnancy and new role more real.

48. **(2)** Integrated processes: nursing process — implementation; client need: physiological integrity; reduction of risk potential; content area: maternity

    RATIONALE

    (1) Amniocentesis is performed under sterile conditions. In addition, signs and symptoms of infection usually take 12–24 hours to manifest after an invasive procedure. **(2)** Amniocentesis involves inserting a long needle through the uterus and into the amniotic sac. There is a risk for stimulation of uterine contractions and of fetal injury. **(3)** Informed consent is required before any invasive procedure. Explanations should take place prior to the procedure. **(4)** While encouraging a client to verbalize concerns is always a good nursing intervention, physical needs have priority over psychosocial needs in this instance.

49. **(1)** Integrated processes: nursing process — data collection; client need: physiological integrity; reduction of risk potential; content area: maternity

    RATIONALE

    (1) Liver function tests can indicate the development of HELLP (*hemolysis, elevated liver* enzymes, *low platelets*) syndrome. HELLP syndrome develops as PIH worsens. **(2)** Diabetics are at higher risk for developing PIH, but the serum glucose is not a diagnostic test for PIH. **(3)** Magnesium sulfate is administered to prevent convulsions in severe PIH (eclampsia). Magnesium levels indicate a therapeutic level of the medication. This client has mild PIH and is not on magnesium. **(4)** The erythrocyte sedimentation rate is not associated with PIH.

50. **(2)** Integrated processes: nursing process — planning; client need: safe, effective care environment; coordinated care; content area: maternity.

    RATIONALE

    (1) An OP position will result in prolonged pushing and maternal exhaustion because a larger diameter is presenting to the pelvis and birth canal. Fetal compromise can also result from prolonged pushing. **(2)** The OA position is desired for vaginal delivery. The occiput has the smallest fetal diameter, and passes through the birth canal easier. Forceps rotation is the quickest way of rotating the fetus to an OP position. Simpson forceps are most commonly used for vertex presentations. A mediolateral episiotomy gives the health-care provider more room for application of the forceps, with decreased risk of episiotomy extension into the anus. **(3)** In a face (OP) position, a midline episiotomy would very likely extend into the anus. Fundal pressure is always contraindicated because of the risk of uterine prolapse. Any assistive pressure by the nurse should be suprapubic. **(4)** Piper forceps are used in breech deliveries to deliver the after-coming head.

51. **(3)** Integrated processes: nursing process — implementation; client need: physiological integrity; reduction of risk potential; content area: maternity

    RATIONALE

    (1) A vaginal exam on a woman with ruptured membranes who is not in labor will increase the risk of infection. **(2)** Maternal vital signs are important to establish a baseline for comparison. However, they are not a priority at this time. **(3)** If the fetal presenting part is not well engaged prior to rupture of membranes, there is a high risk for a prolapsed fetal umbilical cord. A prolapsed cord can become trapped between the fetal presenting part and the maternal pelvis. The fetal oxygen supply will then be compromised. The presence of fetal heart tones can be a reassuring sign of adequate oxygenation to the fetus. **(4)** Vaginal

bleeding is a sign of either cervical dilation or of placenta previa, it is not associated with ruptured membranes unless the client is in active labor.

52. **(1)** Integrated processes: nursing process — data collection; teaching/learning; client need: health promotion and maintenance; content area: maternity.

    RATIONALE

    (1) Soap removes protective oils and dries out the nipples. This can lead to cracking, soreness, and infection. **(2)** Increased air circulation around the nipples prevents maceration. **(3)** Colostrum or breast milk contains healing properties such as lysozymes. **(4)** The area of the nipple directly in line with the infant's nose and chin is most stressed during feedings. Varying the position of the infant can prevent overstress of any one area.

53. **(4)** Integrated processes: nursing process — implementation; teaching/learning; client need: physiological integrity; physiological adaptation; content area: maternity

    RATIONALE

    (1) The stomach capacity of a newborn is approximately 15 mL. This lasts for the first few days of life. **(2)** Cow's milk allergy is manifested in a newborn by vomiting after each feeding. **(3)** A newborn infant should have six to ten wet diapers a day if the fluid intake is adequate. **(4)** The average capacity of a newborn's stomach increases to 75–90 mL by the age of 7 days.

54. **(2)** Integrated processes: nursing process — data collection; teaching/learning; client need: health promotion and maintenance; content area: maternity.

    RATIONALE

    (1) In the Lamaze method, the labor coach assists the woman by providing feedback during labor and helping her to relax. **(2)** Lamaze techniques are used to increase the ability of the woman to cope with pain though conditioning and relaxation. There are no promises that the methods will completely relieve pain. **(3)** Teachers of prepared childbirth recognize that labor is painful and do not promise that no other methods of pain control will be needed. Pain medications are always available for the laboring woman. **(4)** In the Lamaze method, women learn exercises to condition and tone muscles to prepare for childbirth. The exercises include the pelvic tilt, tailor sit, and Kegel exercises.

55. **(1)** Integrated processes: nursing process — implementation; client need: physiological integrity; reduction of risk potential; content area: maternity

    RATIONALE

    (1) Cold stress is extremely dangerous to the newborn. It increases oxygen demands and can cause hypoxia. Drying the infant decreases heat loss through evaporation. **(2)** The physician should suction the oropharynx of the infant while the head is on the perineum. Immediate suctioning after delivery can stimulate the vagus nerve and lower the infant's heart rate. **(3)** Placement of the ID bands can be done anytime after the infant is stabilized. **(4)** The heart rate should be checked at 1 minute after birth, after the infant is dried and warmed.

56. **(2)** Integrated processes: nursing process — data collection; client need: psychosocial integrity; content area: maternity.

    RATIONALE

    (1) There were normal findings on the postpartum assessment. In addition, actual problems have priority over those at risk. **(2)** This family has entered a new phase of development. The nurse needs to plan and implement measures to promote attachment so that the parents can start to assume their new roles. This is an actual problem. **(3)** There is a potential for infection of the episiotomy and IV sites; however actual problems have priority over potential ones. (4) There is no evidence of anxiety at this time. Altered family processes would be a more appropriate nursing diagnosis.

57. **(4)** Integrated processes: nursing process — implementation; teaching/learning; client need: physiological integrity; pharmacological therapies; content area: maternity

RATIONALE

(1) There are currently no approved drugs for lactation suppression. (2) Heparin is given to decrease blood-clotting ability. (3) Rh$_o$(D) immune globulin (RhoGAM) is given to prevent the formation of anti-Rh antibodies in Rh-negative women who deliver an Rh-positive infant. It is given within 72 hours of delivery. (4) Pitocin is an oxytocin that promotes firm contraction of the uterus after birth to control postpartum bleeding

58. **(1)** Integrated processes: nursing process — implementation; client need: safe effective care environment; safety and infection control; content area: maternity

RATIONALE

(1) Epigastric pain is caused by hepatic edema and hemorrhage in clients with PIH, and is a sign of impending seizures. (2) While fetal well-being is a concern, the priority is to ensure the safety of the mother. The fetal heart rate can be monitored after seizures have ceased if the fetus did not deliver during the seizures. (3) The epigastric area is located in the right upper quadrant of the abdominal area as opposed to "heartburn" or acid reflux, which is a burning sensation located just below the zyphoid process. (4) It is unlikely there will be time to start an IV before the onset of seizures. The client needs to be protected from injury first.

59. **(2)** Integrated processes: nursing process — implementation; self-care; client need: physiological integrity; basic care and comfort; content area: maternity.

RATIONALE

(1) Meat is not the only source of complete protein. (2) Soy is a good protein source. Combining legumes and grains results in proteins with all the essential amino acids. (3) Dark yellow fruits and dark green leafy vegetables are good sources of iron and vitamin C. They are not good sources of protein. (4) This client does not eat any animal product. This includes meats, eggs, and milk products.

60. **(3)** Integrated processes: nursing process — implementation; client need: physiological integrity; basic care and comfort; content area: maternity.

RATIONALE

(1) While this is a nutritionally well-balanced meal, it is likely too drastic a dietary change for this client. (2) Fried foods are occasionally okay, but this meal has too much fat. In addition, it is recommended that caffeine be avoided. (3) This diet is both nutritious and likely to be accepted by the client. The double-cheese pizza and milkshake help meet calcium and protein needs. Ham is usually the leanest meat available for pizza. The peppers are a good source of fiber and vitamin C. (4) This fast-food meal is likely to be highly acceptable to the client, but it is high in fat and nutrition poor.

61. **(1)** Integrated processes: nursing process — implementation; client need: physiological integrity; reduction of risk potential; content area: maternity

RATIONALE

(1) Cold stress increases an infant's need for oxygen and can upset the acid-base balance. The infant reacts by increasing its respiratory rate. The infant needs to be wrapped in double blankets and with a cap covering the head. Cold stress also increases the metabolic rate, and glucose stores are rapidly used up. A

protein feeding is preferred because it increases blood glucose levels and maintains them. (2) D$_{10}$W rapidly increases blood glucose levels, but does not sustain them. If glucose water is used, it should be followed with a protein feeding 1 hour later. In addition, the cause of the low glucose level is not addressed. (3) Too rapid warming can cause apnea. (4) The infant is not in respiratory distress. There are no retractions or grunting. The normal range for respirations in a newborn is 30–60 breaths/minute.

62. **(4)** Integrated processes: nursing process — data collection; client need: physiological integrity; reduction of risk potential; content area: maternity.

RATIONALE

(1) Hypocalcemia is strongly associated with newborns of diabetic mothers, perinatal asphyxia, trauma, low birth weight, and preterm birth. (2) Glucose levels normally fall in the newborn over the first few hours of life. Infants with risk factors (large or small for gestational age, low birth weight, ongoing cold stress, or neonatal asphyxia) may require frequent glucose monitoring for the first few hours of life. Feeding the infant treats hypoglycemia. (3) Water intoxication results in hyponatremia, and is associated with excessive feeding of water to infants. Diluting formula with water is another cause of water intoxication. This infant is breast-feeding and not at risk for hyponatremia. (4) Cold stress of the newborn can result in acidosis and raise the levels of free fatty acids. In the presence of acidosis, albumin binding of bilirubin is weakened and bilirubin is freed, resulting in hyperbilirubinemia.

63. **(1)** Integrated processes: nursing process — planning; client need: physiological integrity; reduction of risk potential; content area: maternity.

RATIONALE

(1) Turning the infant to the right side promotes emptying of the stomach into the small intestine. A side-lying position also facilitates drainage from the oropharynx. (2) The infant should be turned from one side to the other to help develop even contours of the head and to ease pressure on other parts of the body. The left lateral side, however, does not promote stomach emptying. (3) The prone position has been associated with an increased incidence of sudden infant death syndrome (SIDS). (4) The prone position has been associated with SIDS. Elevating the foot of the crib increases the risk of aspiration.

64. **(2)** Integrated processes: nursing process — implementation; teaching/learning; client need: health promotion and maintenance; content area: maternity.

RATIONALE

(1) Blood glucose levels do not affect the amount of lactose in breast milk. (2) Breast-feeding is encouraged in diabetic mothers because it decreases insulin requirements. In addition, breast-fed infants have a decreased risk of developing insulin diabetes than those who are formula fed. (3) Neither glucose nor insulin enters breast milk from the bloodstream of the lactating woman. (4) Adding calories for breast-feeding will not affect dietary control for the diabetic woman. The caloric demands of breast-feeding easily use up the extra 500 k/cal needed per day.

65. **(3)** Integrated processes: nursing process — implementation; teaching/learning; client need: physiological integrity; reduction of risk potential; content area: maternity

RATIONALE

(1) Limiting time at the breast does not prevent sore nipples, and can create a fussy, unsatisfied infant. The infant has to nurse at least 10 minutes to get the "hind milk," or the higher fat portion of breast milk. (2) Any technique that involves friction will

increase nipple soreness. Nipples should be air dried. Massé cream is made from lanolin and can create more problems if the woman is allergic to wool (a common allergy). **(3)** If the infant's mouth is open wide prior to latching on, it is more likely that most of the areola will be taken into the infant's mouth. When the infant is positioned with the nipple and most of the areola in his or her mouth, there should not be any tissue damage or pain. **(4)** Use of a breast pump contributes to nipple soreness because of to its mechanical action and friction.

66. **(4)** Integrated processes: nursing process — implementation; teaching/learning; client need: health promotion and maintenance; content area: maternity.

RATIONALE

(1) Signs of a miscarriage are bleeding with cramps, severe pain with or without vaginal bleeding, vaginal bleeding as heavy as menses, or light staining that continues for more than 3 days. **(2)** Implantation occurs from 7–10 days after conception. **(3)** Slight bleeding at the time a period would have been expected is common. No special precautions are necessary. **(4)** The cervix becomes very soft and vascular during pregnancy. Deep penetration of the penis may cause bleeding if the cervix is bumped.

67. **(4)** Integrated processes: nursing process — implementation; teaching/learning; client need: physiological integrity; pharmacological therapies; content area: maternity

RATIONALE

(1) Phenergan can decrease anxiety; however, it is no longer believed that women experiencing hyperemesis are attempting to "throw up" the pregnancy. **(2)** Phenergan can have the side effect of sleepiness; however, hyperemesis is not associated with maternal exhaustion. **(3)** Hyperemesis can cause fluid and electrolyte imbalances; however, phenergan is not an electrolyte solution. **(4)** Phenergan is used as an antiemetic in pregnancies in which nausea and vomiting are uncontrolled by other means.

68. **(3)** Integrated processes: nursing process — implementation; teaching/learning; client need: health promotion and maintenance; content area: maternity.

RATIONALE

(1) GTPAL stands for *gravida* (number of times pregnant, including the current pregnancy), *term* (number of babies delivered after 36 weeks' gestation), *preterm* (number of babies delivered before 36 weeks' gestation), *aborta* (number of pregnancies miscarried or therapeutically aborted), and *living* (number of living children). **(2)** The client has had four pregnancies, two were term deliveries, one preterm, no abortions, and three living. **(3)** See rationale 2. **(4)** See rationale 2.

69. **(1)** Integrated processes: nursing process — data collection; teaching/learning; client need: health promotion and maintenance; content area: maternity.

RATIONALE

(1) Cats can carry *Toxoplasma gondii* in their stools. This organism can cause fetal anomalies. It can be inhaled from litter box dust as well as be transferred on the hands. **(2)** Many medications, including over-the-counter (OTC) medicines, cross the placenta to the fetus. The greatest risk for teratogenic effects is during the first 12 weeks of gestation. **(3)** Gastrointestinal motility is decreased in pregnancy due to the influence of estrogen. The hormone hCG may also affect morning sickness. Pregnant women should avoid overloaded and/or empty stomachs. Five to six small meals a day accomplish this goal. **(4)** Any activity or condition that increases the body temperature to more than 102°F (38.8°C) for more than 10 minutes can cause fetal central nervous system damage.

70. **(2)** Integrated processes: nursing process — implementation; teaching/learning; client need: physiological integrity; physiological adaptation; content area: maternity.

RATIONALE

(1) Endometriosis is endometrial tissue that is found outside the uterus on other pelvic organs. This tissue bleeds at the time of the menses and causes scarring. This scarring can lead to infertility. Endometriosis does not cause cessation of menses. **(2)** Menstrual regularity requires maintenance of body weight and fat above a certain level. A woman who weighs less than 115 lb or who has lost 10 or more pounds through strenuous exercise often experiences cessation of menses. This condition is known as hypogonadotropic amenorrhea. **(3)** These are symptoms of premenstrual syndrome (PMS), which include edema, emotional instability, panic attacks, irritability, impaired ability to concentrate, headache, fatigue, and backache. The cause of PMS is unknown. PMS does not affect menses. **(4)** A generalized infection of the female pelvic organs (PID) is a significant cause of infertility and is commonly caused by sexually transmitted organisms. It causes severe lower abdominal pain and tenderness. Cessation of menses is not a symptom of PID.

71. **(2)** Integrated processes; nursing process — implementation; teaching/learning; client need: physiological integrity; physiological adaptation; content area: maternity.

RATIONALE

(1) Normal hemoglobin levels for pregnancy are 11–12 g/dL. If the hemoglobin level falls below 11, a true anemia is considered to exist. **(2)** Physiological anemia is the result of dilution of hemoglobin concentration by blood volume expansion. **(3)** The fetus does not rob the maternal body of iron. **(4)** Red blood cell production is increased during pregnancy.

72. **(1)** Integrated processes: nursing process — implementation; teaching/learning; client need: health promotion and maintenance; content area: maternity.

RATIONALE

(1) The increased vascularity of the cervix during pregnancy results in congestion of blood and a resulting bluish color. This is known as Chadwick's sign. **(2)** The cervix becomes softer as a result of pelvic vasocongestion. This is known as Goodell's sign. **(3)** Starting at about the sixth week of pregnancy, the lower uterine segment is so soft it can be compressed against the cervix. This is called McDonald's sign. **(4)** Dilation of the cervix occurs when uterine contractions thin and open the cervix. This is called cervical dilation.

73. **(3)** Integrated processes; nursing process — data collection; client need: physiological integrity; physiological adaptation; content area: maternity

RATIONALE

(1) Fundal height in centimeters is correlated to gestational age. The umbilicus is approximately 20 cm from the symphysis pubis. The fundal height is at the appropriate level for a gestational age of 20 weeks. **(2)** See rationale 1. **(3)** See rationale 1. **(4)** See rationale 1.

74. **(4)** Integrated processes: nursing process — data collection; client need: physiological integrity; reduction of risk potential; content area: maternity

RATIONALE

(1) Shortness of breath even at rest is a common complaint of late pregnancy. It is caused by abdominal organ pressure on the diaphragm. **(2)** Dependent edema is a common finding in pregnancy. **(3)** Sharp, intermittent groin pain is caused by stretching of the round ligaments as the uterus enlarges. **(4)** A change in vaginal discharge can indicate preterm labor or a vaginal infection. The health-care provider should be notified.

75. **(4)** Integrated processes: nursing process — data collection; cultural awareness; client need: psychosocial integrity; content area: maternity.

RATIONALE

(1) Making eye contact means different things in different cultures. It does not necessarily mean the client is embarrassed. **(2)** The lack of eye contact does not mean a lack of understanding. **(3)** Asian women are extremely modest. However, this modesty is not manifested in eye contact. **(4)** It is a sign of disrespect in the Asian culture to make eye contact with one considered to be in authority. This client is exhibiting a cultural belief.

76. **(1)** Integrated processes nursing process — implementation; teaching/learning; client need: health promotion and maintenance; content area: maternity.

RATIONALE

(1) Dietary calcium can be found in fish with the bones left in (i.e., sardines and salmon), legumes, nuts, dried fruits, and dark green leafy vegetables (except spinach or Swiss chard). **(2)** Poultry is a good source of protein, whole grains of fiber and phosphorus, and tomatoes of vitamin C. **(3)** Liver is high in iron and vitamin E, yellow vegetables contain riboflavin and vitamin A, and peppers are a good source of vitamin C. **(4)** See rationale 1.

77. **(3)** Integrated processes: nursing process — implementation; teaching/learning; client need: health promotion and maintenance; content area: maternity.

RATIONALE

(1) The recommended rate of gain is approximately 3.5 lb during the first 12 weeks of pregnancy and 0.8 lb each week thereafter. Total weight gained at 28 weeks' gestation should average between 16 and 20 lb. **(2)** For a woman of normal prepregnant weight, 16 lb is appropriate for this stage of pregnancy. **(3)** This weight gain is within the expected range for 28 weeks of gestation. **(4)** Weight gain in pregnancy, especially after the first trimester, is an important factor in fetal growth. Insufficient weight gain causes increased fetal mortality and morbidity, and excessive weight gain is associated with birth trauma and operative deliveries.

78. **(2)** Integrated processes: nursing process — implementation; teaching/learning; client need: physiological integrity; reduction of risk potential; content area: maternity

RATIONALE

(1) This response describes three of the five parameters of a biophysical profile. The other two parameters are fetal breathing and body movements. **(2)** A nonstress test evaluates the ability of the fetal heart to accelerate either spontaneously or in association with fetal movement. **(3)** A fetal kick count is a maternal assessment of the fetus. Fetal movement is associated with fetal condition. **(4)** A contraction stress test is another method of evaluating fetal well-being. Uterine contractions are initiated with either nipple stimulation or IV administration of Pitocin. The fetal response on an external monitor strip is then evaluated once three contractions are obtained in 10 minutes. The test indicates how well a fetus will tolerate labor.

79. **(3)** Integrated processes: nursing process — evaluation; client need: health promotion and maintenance; content area: maternity.

RATIONALE

(1) Nonstress test results are either reactive or nonreactive. Contraction stress tests are either positive or negative. **(2)** See

rationale 1. **(3)** A reactive nonstress test is normal (reactive) when there are two or more fetal heart rate accelerations of at least 15 bpm with a duration of at least 15 seconds in a 20-minute period. **(4)** A nonreactive nonstress test would be less than two fetal heart rate accelerations, or there was an increase of less than 15 seconds in the two accelerations, or the duration of the accelerations lasted less than 15 seconds, or the accelerations did not occur within a 20-minute time period.

80. **(4)** Integrated processes: nursing process — implementation; teaching/learning; client need: psychosocial integrity; content area: maternity.

RATIONALE

(1) False reassurances are a block to communication. **(2)** Impatience is a block to communication. **(3)** The client has not indicated that she wishes to have the test canceled. This is also a block to communication. **(4)** Open-ended comments or questions that reflect the meaning of the statement by the client are most likely to lead to therapeutic communication.

81. **(4)** Integrated processes: nursing process — implementation; teaching/learning; client need: health promotion and maintenance; content area: maternity.

RATIONALE

(1) Uterine muscle contracts during labor. **(2)** There are few nerve endings in the vaginal walls. **(3)** Nerve inflammation is painful, but it does not cause contraction pain. **(4)** When the uterus contracts, blood flow is reduced to uterine muscle, resulting in ischemia and pain.

82. **(4)** Integrated processes: nursing process — planning; client need: safe, effective care environment; safety and infection control; content area: maternity

RATIONALE

(1) Universal Precautions do not always apply to certain body fluids. Body fluids such as feces, nasal secretion, saliva, sputum, and sweat do not require the use of personal protective equipment unless they are visibly contaminated with blood. **(2)** Universal Precautions do not apply to saliva except in dental settings. **(3)** Universal Precautions do not apply to feces unless they are contaminated with visible blood. **(4)** Universal Precautions apply to blood, amniotic fluids, pericardial fluid, peritoneal fluid, pleural fluid, synovial fluid, cerebrospinal fluid, semen, vaginal secretions, and any body fluid visibly contaminated with blood.

83. **(1)** Integrated processes: nursing process — planning; client need: physiological integrity; basic care and comfort; content area: maternity.

RATIONALE

(1) Involving the client in developing menus that incorporate her food preferences will result in better adherence to a nutritional plan. **(2)** Weight gain is important in pregnancy, but the nutrient value of the calories ingested is even more important. **(3)** Dietary sources of nutrients are preferable to supplements because they are absorbed better. In addition, foods often have other beneficial nutrients that are not contained in vitamin and mineral supplements. **(4)** It is unrealistic to expect elimination of all snack foods. This goal will almost assure nonadherence to a nutritional plan.

84. **(3)** Integrated processes: nursing process — planning; communication and documentation; client need: psychological integrity; content area: maternity.

RATIONALE

(1) Perceptions of the childbirth process do not impact parenting abilities. **(2)** These are not unrealistic expectations. **(3)**

Ambivalence is manifested by mixed emotions about an event impacting one's life. This father feels he "should" be present for the birth, but is uncertain about the process. Ambivalent feelings are common during pregnancy and childbirth for both mother and father. **(4)** Factors that interfere with family function are low socioeconomic status, inadequate family support, the birth of a special needs child, unhealthy habits, and the inability to make mature decisions.

85. **(3)** Integrated processes: nursing process — implementation; client need: physiological integrity; basic care and comfort; content area: maternity

    RATIONALE
    Effleurage is massage of the abdomen performed during contractions. Light-pressure effleurage stimulates small-diameter nerve fibers and may actually increase pain. **(2)** Massage of the shoulders may help women relax that area; however, this pain is in the lower back. **(3)** Firm sacral pressure is effective when a woman is experiencing most of the contraction pain in her back. This technique can be combined with thermal stimulation to increase effectiveness. **(4)** Patterned paced breathing is used when slow-paced and modified-paced breathing are no longer effective. It is commonly used during transition (8- to 10- cm dilation).

86. **(2)** Integrated processes: nursing process — implementation; teaching/learning; client need: health promotion and maintenance; content area: maternity.

    RATIONALE
    (1) The bladder should be emptied frequently to prevent urine stasis and growth of bacteria. **(2)** Emptying the bladder before and after intercourse helps wash out any microorganisms that may be introduced onto the urinary meatus/urethra. **(3)** Cranberry juice does not acidify the urine; it prevents adherence of bacteria to the bladder wall. **(4)** Ingestion of live-culture yogurt helps prevent vaginal yeast infections, not bladder infections.

87. **(4)** Integrated processes: nursing process — implementation; client need: physiological integrity; reduction of risk potential; content area: maternity

    RATIONALE
    (1) The client is hyperventilating during an extremely difficult period of labor. The maternal focus is inward. Deep breathing will not reverse the effects of hyperventilation rapidly enough to reverse the respiratory alkalosis this client is developing. **(2)** The client has already blown off too much carbon dioxide. **(3)** A position change to lateral is done to increase uteroplacental oxygenation. The fetus is not in distress. **(4)** Rapid, deep respirations cause the laboring woman to lose carbon dioxide during exhalation and causing respiratory alkalosis. Rebreathing exhaled carbon dioxide in the paper bag will help reverse this condition.

88. **(3)** Integrated processes: nursing process — implementation; teaching/learning; client need: health promotion and maintenance; content area: maternity.

    RATIONALE
    (1) Slowed peristalsis can cause vomiting during labor and a higher risk for aspiration of gastric contents. It does not affect fetal descent. **(2)** The uterine muscle shortens during labor contractions. This results in decreased uterine size, which facilitates fetal descent. **(3)** A full urinary bladder inhibits fetal descent because it occupies space in the pelvic cavity. **(4)** Ruptured membranes decrease the duration of labor by an average of 30 minutes.

89. **(4)** Integrated processes: nursing process — planning; client need: physiological integrity; reduction of risk potential; content area: maternity

RATIONALE
(1) Auscultation of a FHR of less than 100 does not indicate operative delivery. If fetal bradycardia is verified, then noninvasive measures should be attempted first and their effectiveness evaluated. **(2)** Internal fetal monitoring is an invasive procedure that requires rupture of membranes. In the absence of verified fetal bradycardia, this intervention is not warranted. **(3)** Fetal bradycardia should be verified before any other action is taken. **(4)** The fetoscope may be placed over the placental or uterine blood vessels and may reflect the maternal pulse rather than fetal bradycardia.

90. **(4)** Integrated processes: nursing process — planning; client need: psychological integrity; content area: maternity.

    RATIONALE
    (1) Postpartum depression is characterized by the woman showing less interest in her surroundings and a loss of usual emotional responses toward her family. She is unable to feel pleasure in her new baby, and often has strong feelings of guilt and shame. **(2)** Postpartum psychosis is characterized by tearfulness, guilt feelings, sleep and appetite disturbances, and thoughts of harming the infant or self. **(3)** There is no evidence that this client has low self-esteem or is feeling unable to care for both of her children. **(4)** Sibling rivalry is characterized by the older child experiencing feelings of jealously and fear that he or she will be replaced in the parent's affections by the newcomer. Parental reassurance of love and time spent alone with the older child can help him or her cope with these feelings.

91. **(4)** Integrated processes: nursing process — implementation; teaching/learning; client need: health promotion and maintenance; content area: maternity.

    RATIONALE
    (1) Infants' noses are made so they can breathe while nursing. Depressing breast tissue at the nose can pull the nipple and areola out of the correct position in the infant's mouth. **(2)** Using the "scissors" position of the fingers can prevent the infant from taking in enough of the areola for effective breast-feeding. **(3)** The lactiferous ducts are found underneath the areola. Proper latch-on includes the nipple and as much of the areola as can be gotten into the infant's mouth. **(4)** Positioning the infant at nipple level prevents nipple trauma. Keeping the body of the infant in a straight line with the head allows the infant to swallow while nursing.

92. **(2)** Integrated processes: nursing process — data collection; teaching/learning; client need: health promotion and maintenance; content area: maternity.

    RATIONALE
    (1) The back seat is the safest place in a car. The car seat should face the back of the car until the infant weighs at least 20 lb. **(2)** Backpacks should only be used for infants old enough to hold his or her head up well alone. **(3)** An infant may chew the crib during teething. Lead paint causes brain damage. **(4)** SIDS is associated with the prone position in young infants.

93. **(2)** Integrated processes: nursing process — implementation; caring; client need: physiological integrity; physiological adaptation; content area: maternity

    RATIONALE
    (1) An adolescent who becomes pregnant must decide what course of action she is going to take. Putting up a child for adoption can be a painful process. Making a decision earlier in the pregnancy allows painful feelings to be resolved before the birth of the baby. **(2)** The autonomous decision by an adolescent to give up her baby for adoption can be considered an important step toward maturity. **(3)** Teenagers who place their infant for adoption because of external pressure frequently feel anger at

those who placed the pressure upon them. (4) The choice of adoption leaves the teenager with mixed messages from society regarding her pregnancy. She needs affirmation that this decision is a significant event and help in dealing with her feelings.

94. **(2)** Integrated processes: nursing process — data collection; client need: health promotion and maintenance; content area: maternity.

RATIONALE

(1) These are the findings of transition, which is cervical dilation from 8–10 cm. Delivery will take place in approximately 2 hours. (2) Pressure of the presenting part as it progresses through the birth stimulates the sensation of needing to have a bowel movement. A vaginal exam needs to be done stat, as delivery may occur very quickly. (3) Contractions can increase in frequency and intensity without much change in the cervix. A judgment about delivery cannot be made from this information. (4) Vomiting and a sense of "having enough" are signs of transition.

95. **(4)** Integrated processes: nursing process — data collection; client need: physiological integrity; pharmacological therapies; content area: maternity

RATIONALE

(1) A pulse rate up to 120 and palpitations are normal side effects of terbutaline. (2) This output exceeds the intake, which decreases the risk of fluid overload. (3) Pedal edema is not uncommon in pregnant women; 3+ edema could indicate PIH, not pulmonary edema. (4) Fluid overload would result in pulmonary edema. The lower bases of the lungs are the first to fill with fluid.

96. **(4)** Integrated processes: nursing process — implementation; teaching/learning; client need: health promotion and maintenance; content area: maternity.

RATIONALE

(1) Visual and auditory stimulation should not be presented to the infant at the same time. Drug-exposed infants are easily stressed. (2) Wind-up swings make a clicking noise and also stimulate the visual system. (3) Rattles are both visual and auditory stimulations. (4) Drug-exposed infants need physical contact and soft auditory stimulation.

97. **(1)** Integrated processes: nursing process — data collection; client need: physiological integrity; physiological adaptation; content area: maternity.

RATIONALE

(1) Hypertonicity and poor coordination of the suck and swallow reflexes are characteristic of the narcotic-exposed infant. Seizures may also be present. (2) These are the typical features of the baby with fetal alcohol syndrome. (3) These are the typical features of the tobacco-exposed newborn. (4) These are the typical features of Down's syndrome.

98. **(4)** Integrated processes: nursing process — implementation; teaching/learning; client need: psychosocial integrity; content area: maternity.

RATIONALE

(1) Many women fear that disclosure of abuse will result in being told she must leave her partner in order to receive treatment. Women who are pregnant or with a newborn are least likely to leave a relationship. (2) One in three women is a victim of partner abuse regardless of socioeconomic status. (3) The client does not have a psychiatric problem. What is needed is sensitivity, acceptance, and guidance on where she can receive help once she is ready. (4) The most significant intervention for partner abuse is being asked about being hurt or frightened by a partner. Studies show that victims of partner abuse frequently go to a health-care provider with obvious injuries and wait for

the provider to ask about them because they were too ashamed to volunteer the information.

99. **(4)** Integrated processes: nursing process — data collection; client need: physiological integrity; reduction of risk potential; content area: maternity

RATIONALE

(1) Decreased fundal height is associated with "lightening" or engagement of the fetal presenting part in the pelvis. (2) Abruptio placentae is the separation of the placenta from the uterine wall. If the separation is in the middle of the placenta, bleeding is concealed. (3) Fetal tachycardia can occur with tocolysis or maternal infection. (4) Painless, bright red vaginal bleeding is symptomatic of placenta previa.

100. **(4)** Integrated processes: nursing process — evaluation; teaching/learning; client need: health promotion and maintenance; content area: maternity.

RATIONALE

(1) Breast milk contains the amino acid phenylalanine, which cannot be metabolized by the infant with PKU. Moderate to high levels of phenylalanine can result in mental retardation. (2) Formula is modified cow's milk which contains phenylalanine. (3) Soy milk contains phenylalanine. (4) PKU is treated with a special low-phenylalanine diet. A special formula is used for infants.

101. **(4)** Integrated processes: nursing process — planning; communication and documentation; client need: physiological integrity; reduction of risk potential; content area: maternity

RATIONALE

(1) The client in room A with the term newborn will likely have a great deal of activity in her room. This client has symptoms of preeclampsia and should either be in a private room or in a quiet, darkened room to minimize stimuli that could trigger seizures. (2) and (3) are incorrect because they are likely to need bright lights and activity in their rooms if their conditions worsen. (4) A roommate requiring a similar environment would be most appropriate when there are no private rooms available.

102. **(Check her blood pressure)** Integrated processes: nursing process — implementation; client need: health promotion and maintenance; content area: maternity.

RATIONALE

Epigastric discomfort is commonly described as "heartburn" by pregnant clients; and epigastric discomfort is a symptom of impending rupture of the liver capsule and seizures associated with worsening PIH and eclampsia.

103. **(4)** Integrated processes: nursing process — planning; client need: physiological integrity; reduction of risk potential; content area: maternity

RATIONALE

(1) A temperature of 100.1°F (37.7°C) within the first 24 hours postpartum is common because of the dehydrating effects of labor and delivery. (2) and (3) are incorrect because these are normal findings postpartum. (4) Postpartum clients are at high risk for DVTs because of the hypercoaguable state of pregnancy that still exists and the dehydration caused by labor. Right calf pain is a common symptom of a DVT.

104. **(3)** Integrated processes: nursing process — data collection; client need: physiological integrity; reduction of risk potential; content area: maternity.

RATIONALE

(1) A hemoglobin of 11 g/dL is considered to be normal for pregnancy and postpartum. (2) It is not unusual for a post-

partum woman to have a WBC up to 25000 mm³ without infection because of the healing process of the reproductive system. **(3)** A hematocrit in postpartum women can drop as low as 20% and not require transfusion in the absence of symptoms of hypovolemia. A hematocrit of 18% and lower should be reported even in the absence of dizziness, light-headedness, shortness of breath with exertion, and syncope. **(4)** A serum glucose of 89 g/dL is within the normal range of glycemic control.

105. **(2)** Integrated processes: nursing process — data collection; client need: physiological integrity; physiological adaptation; content area: maternity

RATIONALE
(1) Hypotonic contractions are weak and infrequent, and usually are not effective in progressing labor. **(2)** The definition of precipitous labor is labor lasting less than 3 hours from the beginning of labor to delivery. This type of labor is characterized by frequent, intense contractions and rapid progression through the phases and stages of labor. **(3)** Prolonged labor is defined as labor that exceeds the normal. **(4)** Normal labor lasts about 8–12 hours, with less than 3 hours being the definition of precipitous labor.

106. **(2 and 3)** Integrated processes: nursing process — planning; communication and documentation; client need: safe, effective care environment; coordinated care; content area: maternity.

RATIONALE
(1) This is a high-risk client who requires nursing care by a more advanced practitioner. In addition, it is outside the scope of an LPN to perform admission assessments. **(2)** LPNs may assess vital signs. **(3)** LPNs may assist clients with feeding their infants. **(4)** LPNs may not give IV push medications even if they have completed the criteria for an expanded role.

107. **(1)** Integrated processes: nursing process — data collection; client need: health promotion and maintenance; content area: maternity.

RATIONALE
(1) Facial and upper extremity edema can be a sign of preeclampsia, which can endanger both the mother and fetus. **(2), (3),** and **(4)** Dyspnea, pedal edema and trace proteinurea are benign common complaints in the third trimester of pregnancy.

108. **(1)** Integrated processes: nursing process — planning; communication and documentation; client need: safe, effective care environment; coordinated care; content area: maternity.

RATIONALE
(1) Management of a PCA is outside the scope of practice for LPNs regardless of extra education and training. **(2)** and **(4)** LPN IIs may perform venipunctures and draw blood. **(3)** Client teaching is an appropriate task for LPNs.

109. **(2, 3, and 4)** Integrated processes: nursing process — planning; communication and documentation; client need: safe, effective care environment; coordinated care; content area: maternity

RATIONALE
(1) Nursing assistants may not hang IV fluids. **(2)** Nursing assistants may assist clients with activities of daily living, including toileting. **(3)** Nursing assistants are qualified to take and report vital signs. **(4)** A nursing assistant may insert a straight urinary catheter under the direction of a licensed nurse.

110. **(4)** Integrated processes: nursing process — planning; client need: safe effective care environment; coordinated care; content area: maternity

RATIONALE
(1) Clots smaller in size than a silver dollar are normal findings postpartum. **(2)** This is a normal finding. Breast-feeding causes the release of endogenous oxytocin from the pituitary, which causes the uterus to contract. **(3)** The blood pools in the vagina while a client is lying prone and the peripad cannot contain it all when the client stands. This results in a "gush" of blood that can run down the legs. **(4)** A postepidural headache can be an indication of inadvertent puncture of the dural membrane. This client will need to be positioned prone, push fluids, and given caffeine, and may need a blood patch to seal the dural leak.

111. **(4)** Integrated processes: nursing process — planning; safe effective care environment; coordinated care; content area: maternity

RATIONALE
(1) This infant is in the first period of reactivity; infants during this period are frequently quiet and alert and sucking their fists or fingers. **(2)** Loud cries should always be investigated, but there is no other indicator that this infant is in physiological distress. **(3)** The risk of bleeding is greatest during the first hour after a circumcision. **(4)** The second period of reactivity, which occurs after the period of deep sleep approximately 3–5 hours after delivery, is the most unstable for the newborn. This is when they are most likely to bring up and gag on mucus and may aspirate.

112. **(1, 2, and 5)** Integrated processes: nursing process — planning; communication and documentation; client need: safe, effective care environment; coordinated care; content area: maternity

RATIONALE
(1) A nursing assistant has the education and training to accurately total I&O. **(2)** Nursing assistants are qualified to take vital signs. **(3)** Nursing assistants may not administer medication in an acute care setting. **(4)** A client on IV magnesium sulfate is high risk and may not be monitored by a nursing assistant. **5.** Setting up the room for a delivery is an appropriate task for a nursing assistant.

113. **(3 and 5)** Integrated processes: nursing process — implementation; client need: safe effective care environment; coordinated care; content area: maternity

RATIONALE
(1) A boggy fundus should be massaged until firm if it is caused by hypotonicity. However, the assessment findings also state that the fundus is high and deviated to the side. This indicates that a full bladder is pushing the uterus upward and preventing its full contraction. **(2)** Methergine is indicated with persistent heavy vaginal bleeding that is refractory to nursing measures such as massaging the fundus, checking for a full bladder, and assisting the client up to void. **(3)** A full bladder pushes the uterus upward and to the side (usually the right side). It also prevents the uterus from contracting down and achieving homeostasis. **(4)** These findings should be documented after the client is assisted to empty her bladder and her fundus and lochia flow reassessed. **5.** Once the bladder is empty, the fundus will contract adequately and return to its expected normal location below the umbilicus and in the midline.

114. **(2)** Integrated processes: nursing process — planning; client need: safe, effective care environment; coordinated care; content area: maternity

RATIONALE

(1) A finding of 2+ DTRs is normal. (2) Terbutaline causes fetal and maternal tachycardia. However, a maternal heart rate <120 is considered safe. (3) The desired contraction pattern for a client on Pitocin is three in 10 minutes. (4) A systolic blood pressure of >140 mm Hg or a diastolic BP of >90 mm Hg indicates hypertension. This client is already on methyldopa (Aldomet), which is an antihypertension medication. Her hypertension is worsening and may compromise fetal well-being.

115. **(2)** Integrated processes: nursing process — data collection; communication and documentation; client need: physiological integrity; reduction of risk potential; content area: maternity

RATIONALE

(1) Fetal heart tones cannot be auscultated until at least 12 weeks' gestation. (2) Right-sided shoulder pain is referred pain caused by pressure on the diaphragm due to blood spilling into the abdominal cavity from a ruptured ectopic pregnancy. This client is at high risk for hemorrhage. (3) Bright red vaginal bleeding is an indicator of threatened abortion. (4) Severe uterine cramping is a sign of threatened abortion.

116. **(1 and 2)** Integrated processes: nursing process — planning; communication and documentation; client need: safe effective care environment; coordinated care; content area: maternity

RATIONALE

(1) Client A is at lowest risk for complications. She is having infrequent contractions and is not at high risk for preterm delivery. She is also receiving an oral tocolytic (terbutaline) to treat her preterm labor. (2) Moderate vaginal bleeding is a normal finding immediately postpartum. (3) Intense perineal pain is a symptom of a genital tract hematoma. A client can lose 500 mL of blood into the perineal tissues in a very short period of time. Immediate intervention is needed for this client. (4) A systolic blood pressure greater then 140 mm Hg indicates the complication of PIH.

117. **(2)** Integrated processes: nursing process — planning; client need: safe, effective care environment; coordinated care; content area: maternity.

RATIONALE

(1) This is not an emergent situation. The infant who is gagging has priority. (2) Remember the ABCs of Airway, Breathing, and Circulation. This infant is at high risk for aspiration, which will occlude his airway. (3) Performing a gestational age assessment is outside the scope of practice of an LPN. (4) LPN can perform laboratory procedures on clients; however, this test can be safely delayed to 48–72 hours.

118. **(1, 2 and 3)** Integrated processes: nursing process — planning; client need: safe, effective care environment; coordinated care; content area: maternity

RATIONALE

Answers (1), (2), and (3) are all abnormal findings that indicate pathologic jaundice and risk for brain damage. (4) Acrocyanosis is a bluish discoloration of the hands and feet. This is a normal finding in stable, healthy newborn infants because of their poor circulation to the extremities.

119. **(3)** Integrated processes: nursing process — planning; communication and documentation; client need: safe, effective care environment; coordinated care; content area: maternity

RATIONALE

(1) Client B is exhibiting symptoms of postpartum-onset PIH, which places her into a higher risk category. (2) LPN IIs are qualified to hang plain IV fluids. Client E is receiving an IV antibiotic. (3) These are stable clients whose care is within the scope of practice of an LPN. (4) Client F has an IV narcotic infusing.

120. **(3)** Integrated processes: nursing process — planning; client need: physiological integrity; reduction of risk potential; content area: maternity

RATIONALE

(1) This is a normal newborn finding. Absence of the Babinski's reflex is abnormal. (2) Circumoral cyanosis is bluish discoloration of and around the lips. It is an indicator of a cyanotic heart defect. Answer 1 is incorrect because absence of the Babinski's reflex is abnormal. (3) A negative Ortalini's sign indicates normal hip structure. A positive Ortalini's sign is an indicator of congenital hip dislocation. (4) The common term for this type of nevi is "stork bite," which is a normal newborn finding.

121. **(3)** Integrated processes: nursing process — planning; communication and documentation; client need: safe, effective care environment; coordinated care; content area: maternity

RATIONALE

(1, 2, and 4). The nurse has been cross-trained to L and D and the nursery, and this implies that her job description requires her to care for all of these types of clients. She can request additional training and support, but cannot refuse her assignment unless client safety will be compromised. The best answer is (3), because this both recognizes the nurse's concern and promotes the efficient management of the unit.

122. **(4)** Integrated processes: nursing process — planning; client need: psychosocial integrity; content area: maternity.

RATIONALE

(1) This client needs teaching regarding diet and exercise and monitoring of her blood glucose levels. She does not have a risk condition that requires the close observation a room near the nurses" station would have. (2) A client with a placenta previa can have unpredictable episodes of bright red bleeding that may compromise the health of both her and her fetus. This can result in sudden and intense activity in the room. (3) A client in preterm labor requires close observation and frequent monitoring. This could result in an environment that is not conducive to rest and calm. (4) Placing clients with similar diagnoses together can result in information sharing and emotional support between the two women because of their similar needs and goals for a health pregnancy.

123. **(2)** Integrated processes: nursing process — implementation; communication and documentation; client need: safe, effective care environment; coordinated care; content area: maternity

RATIONALE

(1) The PT monitors the efficacy of Coumadin. This level is nontherapeutic, however, Coumadin is not used in pregnancy because it crosses the placenta and may have teratogenic effects. (2) The test that monitors the efficacy of heparin is the PTT. This level is not therapeutic and will not prevent blood clots. The therapeutic range for a PTT is 27–31. (3) Even though the INR level of 2.5 is therapeutic, this test also measures the effectiveness of Coumadin, which is not used in pregnancy because of possible teratogenic effects. (4) A hemoglobin level of 11 is considered adequate in pregnancy.

124. **(4, 5, and 6)** Integrated processes: nursing process — planning; communication and documentation; client need: safe, effective care environment; coordinated care; content area: maternity

RATIONALE

(1, 2, and 3) These tasks are within the scope of practice for OB scrub techs. **(4, 5 and 6)** Only LPNs or RNs can perform these tasks.

125. **(2)** Integrated processes: nursing process — planning; client need: safe effective care environment; coordinated care; content area: maternity

RATIONALE

(1) This is within a normal lochial flow. Saturating more than one peripad in 1 hour is considered hemorrhage. **(2)** A continuous trickle of lochia is abnormal and a sign of an unrepaired genital tract laceration. This client can lose a large amount of blood in a short period of time. Surgical repair is indicated. **(3)** The fundus is between the umbilicus and pubis the first 12 hours after delivery. It then rises to 1–2 cm above the umbilicus and then descends 1–2 cm every 24 hours afterward. This uterus is going through the normal process of involution. **(4)** This is a normal finding for a 3-day postpartum client. Lochia serosa is seen approximately 72 hours after delivery. It is brown-pink in color.

126. **(2)** Integrated processes: nursing process — data collection; client need: health promotion and maintenance; content area: maternity.

RATIONALE

(1) Ovulation may vary for some individuals; however, the term *cycle*, referring to the menstrual cycle, implies regularity and predictability. Generally speaking, each woman's body establishes a routine reproductive cycle with ovulation occurring at a regular interval for her. **(2)** Ovulation generally occurs at the end of the proliferative phase, beginning the secretory phase of the menstrual cycle. This usually occurs approximately the 14th day of the cycle based on a 28-day menstrual cycle. **(3)** Ovulation does not occur until the estrogen and progesterone levels have risen and the endometrium has begun to prepare for implantation of the fertilized ova. **(4)** Intercourse does not play a part in the stimulation or maturation of the ovum.

127. **(2)** Integrated processes: nursing process — data collection; client need: health promotion and maintenance; content area: maternity.

RATIONALE

(1) At conception, chromosomal or genetic sex is determined. During the first month, primordial germ cells are internally visible. **(2)** External genitalia are not well developed and identifiable until after the ninth week. **(3)** By the 20th week, the external genitalia are well defined, although they continue to refine until close to term. **(4)** The seventh month finds the fetal external genitalia continuing to be more clearly defined. The sexual characteristics of the external genitalia are easily distinguished at this time.

128. **(4)** Integrated processes: nursing process — data collection; client need: health promotion and maintenance; content area: maternity.

RATIONALE

(1) The cardiac output and workload of the heart are not related to the incidence of heartburn during pregnancy. **(2)** Although gastric acidity does change during pregnancy, peristalsis decreases rather than increases. **(3)** Peristalsis decreases during pregnancy by about 50%. **(4)** The common complaint of heartburn in pregnancy is a result of the diminished gastric emptying time and acid reflux into the esophagus.

129. **(3)** Integrated processes: nursing process — planning; client need: health promotion and maintenance; content area: maternity.

RATIONALE

(1) Many expectant mothers may not have a supportive partner; therefore, this is not the purpose of childbirth preparation programs. **(2)** Although childbirth education may increase a woman's self-esteem, this is not the primary purpose of the program. **(3)** Educating the mother in order to provide her with practical tools that will equip her to cope effectively with the stress brought about by the last weeks of pregnancy, the birth of her baby, and the early postpartal period are the main objectives in childbirth programs. **(4)** Many childbirth preparation classes do include this type of information; however, it is not the primary focus of the class.

130. **(3)** Integrated processes: nursing process — implementation; teaching/learning; client need: health promotion and maintenance; content area: maternity.

RATIONALE

(1) A diaphragm, which is a curved rubber dome enclosed by a flexible metal ring, is used as a mechanical barrier for contraception. Spermicidal cream or jelly is placed in the cup portion and on the rim of the diaphragm before insertion. **(2)** The diaphragm should be left covering the cervix at least 6 hours, but no longer than 24 hours following intercourse. **(3)** The diaphragm should be left covering the cervix at least 6 hours, but no longer than 24 hours following intercourse. **(4)** It is effective for contraception as soon as it is in place. It should be placed just prior to intercourse.

131. **(1)** Integrated processes: nursing process — data collection; client need: health promotion and maintenance; content area: maternity.

RATIONALE

(1) The applications of skills of controlled relaxation helps a woman withstand the stress of labor. It teaches her body awareness, improves her ability to conserve energy between contractions, and provides relaxation of the uterine muscles. This improves the work of each contraction to more effectively move the fetus through the birth canal. **(2)** Movement of the infant through the birth canal is an important reason for relaxation. **(3)** Although this is a hoped-for result of remaining relaxed, it is not the main focus. **(4)** A quiet environment is ideal and may be a factor that will assist the mother to be more in control and relaxed.

132. **(3)** Integrated processes: nursing process — implementation; client need: physiological integrity; reduction of risk potential; content area: maternity.

RATIONALE

(1) Vitamin K does not increase the growth of the intestinal flora. **(2)** Vitamin K does not improve the conjugation of bilirubin. **(3)** Hemorrhagic disease of the newborn results from a deficiency of prothrombin and other clotting factors. Vitamin K, which is produced in the bowel, is low in the newborn due to the decreased bacterial flora. **(4)** Healthy full-term infants have sufficient iron stores for synthesis of red blood cells until the third or fourth month after birth.

133. **(4)** Integrated processes: nursing process — data collection; client need: health promotion and maintenance; content area: maternity.

RATIONALE

(1) An infant of less than 37 weeks' gestation is considered preterm. (2) In order to determine whether an infant is small or large for gestational age, the length and weight is required for calculation. (3) In order to determine whether an infant is small or large for gestational age, the length and weight are required for calculation. (4) An infant of less than 37 weeks' gestation is considered preterm.

134. **(2)** Integrated processes: nursing process — data collection; client need: health promotion and maintenance; content area: maternity.

RATIONALE

(1) Duplication of genetic material occurs during the preembryonic period (weeks 1–3) following conception. (2) Weeks 4–8, known as the embryonic period, is the period when organogenesis occurs. During this period of growth and development, the greatest potential for major congenital malformation exists. (3) Kidneys do not secrete urine until weeks 13–16 of gestation. (4) Subcutaneous fat is not deposited until the final week prior to delivery at term.

135. **(4)** Integrated processes: nursing process — data collection; client need: health promotion and maintenance; content area: maternity.

RATIONALE

(1) Although estrogen levels do change during pregnancy, it is not used as the main hormone of evaluation in pregnancy tests. (2) Maternal serum levels of prolactin rise throughout pregnancy in preparation for breast-feeding, but there is no evidence of increased urine levels that could be used to determine pregnancy. (3) AFP is the major protein in the serum of the embryo produced initially by the yolk sac. It is not the hormone used to detect pregnancy. (4) Human chorionic gonadotropin is the biochemical basis for pregnancy tests. Levels increase rapidly following conception, peaking at about 8 weeks and gradually decreasing to low levels at about 16 weeks.

136. **(3)** Integrated processes: nursing process — data collection; client need: physiological integrity; physiological adaptation; content area: maternity.

RATIONALE

(1) Postterm deliveries have not been shown to increase the incidence of chorioamnionitis unless there has been prolonged rupture of membranes. (2) Maternal dehydration is not related to chorioamnionitis. (3) Chorioamnionitis, an inflammation of the amnion and chorion, is generally associated with premature or prolonged rupture of membranes. (4) Pyelonephritis, a kidney infection that develops as a result of an untreated urinary tract infection, is the most common nonobstetrical cause for hospitalization during pregnancy.

137. **(2)** Integrated processes: nursing process — data collection; client need: health promotion and maintenance; content area: maternity.

RATIONALE

(1) The absence of the Babinski's reflex in a newborn would indicate neurological dysfunction. (2) A positive Babinski's reflex in a newborn indicates a normal, intact neurological function. This reflex disappears before 2 years of age. (3) The absence of a palmar grasp reflex indicates an infant has suffered hypotonia or perinatal asphyxia. (4) The absence of a plantar grasp reflex indicates an infant has hypotonia or spinal cord injuries.

138. **(1)** Integrated processes: nursing process — implementation; teaching/learning; client need: health promotion and maintenance; content area: maternity.

RATIONALE

(1) This is a correct description of a quiet alert state in an infant. Infants react to sensory stimuli because this is the most optimum state of arousal. (2) This describes an infant in a drowsy awake state. (3) This describes an infant in a deep sleep state. (4) This describes an infant in a light sleep state.

139. **(3)** Integrated processes: nursing process — data collection; client need: health promotion and maintenance; content area: maternity.

RATIONALE

(1) Widely spaced suture lines in a newborn may be indicative of hydrocephaly. (2) A collection of fluid across the scalp is called caput succedaneum. (3) Molding is a normal process during delivery as a result of the pressure on the fetal head. The cranial bones are not fused, allowing the movement necessary for the fetal head to pass through the birth canal. (4) Depressed fontanelles indicate dehydration.

140. **(1)** Integrated processes: nursing process — implementation; teaching/learning; client need: health promotion and maintenance; content area: maternity.

RATIONALE

(1) Absorption of iron is best when the supplement is taken at bedtime with a citrus juice. Coffee, tea, milk, and calcium supplements decrease absorption of iron. (2) Taking an iron supplement between meals on an empty stomach will likely cause gastrointestinal upset. (3) Taking a prenatal vitamin that has calcium will decrease the absorption of iron. (4) Iron absorption from the diet does increase during pregnancy; however, it is impossible for a client to meet her iron requirements from food intake without overeating.

141. **(4)** Integrated processes: nursing process — data collection; client need: health promotion and maintenance; content area: maternity.

RATIONALE

(1) Opening of the cervix is called dilation. (2) The cervix does not lengthen during pregnancy. (3) *Hypotonic* is not a term used to describe the cervix. (4) Effective contractions lead to cervical changes. The cervix softens and thins with each contraction, drawing slowly and progressively up into the lower uterine segment.

142. **(1)** Integrated processes: nursing process — data collection; client need: physiological integrity; pharmacological therapies; content area: maternity

RATIONALE

(1) One main adverse reaction to oxytocin is uterine tetany. (2) It is not necessary to monitor deep tendon reflexes when a patient is receiving oxytocin. (3) Hyperglycemia is not a side effect of oxytocin. (4) Tearing of the perineum is not a side effect of oxytocin.

143. **(4)** Integrated processes: nursing process — implementation; teaching/learning; client need: psychosocial integrity; content area: maternity.

RATIONALE

(1) Since only the uterus is removed during a hysterectomy and not the ovaries, the secretion of ovarian hormones is not affected and, consequently, menopause does not occur as a result. (2) With removal of the uterus, menstruation does not occur. (3) The posthysterectomy client no longer needs birth control. (4) Feelings of grief and loss may result following an

unplanned hysterectomy. Clients should be taught their feelings of loss or depression are normal and be provided with emotional support.

144. **(1)** Integrated processes: nursing process — implementation; teaching/learning; client need: physiological integrity; pharmacological therapies; content area: maternity

    RATIONALE

    (1) Depo-Provera prevents the regular release of ova, inhibiting normal changes in the endometrial lining of the uterus. **(2)** Women report weight gain more often than weight loss. **(3)** Women experience fatigue rather than increased metabolic activity. **(4)** Hypertension is not a side effect of Depo-Provera.

145. **(2)** Integrated processes: nursing process — data collection; client need: physiological integrity; physiological adaptation; content area: maternity

    RATIONALE

    (1) Infection is not associated with eclampsia. **(2)** Eclampsia is characterized by seizure activity, which often results in aspiration as a major complication. **(3)** Renal perfusion is decreased with eclampsia-induced hypertension, resulting in decreased urine output. **(4)** Extremity injuries may occur with seizure activity, but are not considered a major complication.

146. **(1)** Integrated processes: nursing process — data collection; client need: physiological integrity; physiological adaptation; content area: maternity.

    RATIONALE

    (1) Uterine atony, failure of the uterine muscle to contract firmly, occurs in 75%–85% of postpartum clients. **(2)** Retained placental fragments commonly cause late postpartal hemorrhage. **(3)** Cervical lacerations, seen less often, are characterized by slow, continuous bleeding with a contracted uterus. **(4)** Only 6% of postpartum women have a postpartal infection and is usually not associated with postpartal hemorrhage.

147. **(1)** Integrated processes: nursing process — implementation; client need: physiological integrity; pharmacological therapies; content area: maternity.

RATIONALE

(1) Magnesium sulfate prevents seizure by blocking neuromuscular transmission. **(2)** Magnesium sulfate may drop blood pressure as a result of the relaxation of smooth muscle, but it is not used as a hypertensive agent. **(3)** Magnesium sulfate treatment may cause a decrease in urine output because of the toxic effect it has on the kidneys. **(4)** The purpose of using magnesium sulfate is to prevent seizures.

148. **(3)** Integrated processes: nursing process — planning; client need: physiological integrity; reduction of risk potential; content area: maternity.

    RATIONALE

    (1) Tetanic contractions are not associated with repeat cesarean delivery. **(2)** Precipitous labor is not associated with repeat cesarean delivery. **(3)** Uterine rupture along the previous scar is a primary concern for clients who previously have had cesarean deliveries. **(4)** Abruptio placentae is not associated with repeat cesarean delivery.

149. **(4)** Integrated processes: nursing process — evaluation; client need: physiological integrity; reduction of risk potential; content area: maternity

    RATIONALE

    (1) Breast tenderness is not associated with an amniocentesis. **(2)** Increased fetal activity may occur with an amniocentesis, but does not present a problem. **(3)** Signs of infection would not be evident in the first hour after the procedure. **(4)** Rupture of the membranes is a potential complication of amniocentesis.

150. **(1)** Integrated processes: nursing process — evaluation; client need: health promotion and maintenance; content area: maternity.

    RATIONALE

    (1) This weight gain is normal during the third trimester. **(2)** An appointment with a nutritionist is not necessary since this weight gain is normal during the third trimester. **(3)** A weight gain of 1 lb is normal during the third trimester. **(4)** It is not necessary to check for proteinuria and hypertension because of a 1-lb weight gain.

CHAPTER 4

Pediatric Nursing: Content Review and Test

Nora F. Steele, RN.C, DNS, PNP
Susan I. Ray, RN, MS
Larry D. Purnell, RN, PhD

The Ill or Hospitalized Child

Nursing Care of the Ill Child

Meaning of Illness to Child

I. Infant
   A. Change in familiar routine and own bedroom
   B. Separation from favorite toy or blanket
II. Toddler
   A. Fear of separation, being left alone; separation anxiety highest in this age group
   B. Blames self for illness
III. Preschool
   A. Fear of being hurt or fear of mutilation
   B. Afraid of pain and bleeding
   C. Separation anxiety less than for toddler
   D. Often considers illness punishment for wrongdoing
IV. School-age
   A. Fear of physical nature of illness
   B. Concern regarding separation from peers and ability to maintain position in group
   C. Thinks there is an external cause for illness, although located in body
V. Adolescent
   A. Anxiety regarding loss of independence, control, identity
   B. Concern about privacy
   C. Able to explain illness

Response to Separation

I. Greatest impact between ages 1 and 3 years
II. Three phases identified:
   A. Protest: cries for parents; refuses attention of anyone else
   B. Despair: ceases crying; shows evidence of depression; "settles in"
   C. Detachment (denial): superficially appears to adjust; ignores parent in effort to escape emotional pain

Signs and Symptoms of Separation Anxiety

I. Protest: lasts from hours to days
   A. Cries and screams
   B. Searches with eyes for parent
   C. Clings to parent when present
   D. Avoids and rejects contact with strangers
   E. Verbally and physically attacks strangers
   F. Attempts physically to prevent parent from leaving
II. Despair: length of time variable
   A. Inactive
   B. Withdrawn
   C. Depressed, sad
   D. Uninterested in environment
   E. Noncommunicative
   F. Regresses to earlier behaviors (e.g., thumb sucking, bed-wetting, use of bottle)
   G. Often refuses to eat
III. Detachment: rarely seen
   A. Shows increased interest in surroundings
   B. Interacts with strangers or familiar caregivers
   C. Forms new but superficial relationships
   D. Appears happy
   E. Shows only passive or superficial interest in parents

Response to Pain

I. Young infant (0–1 years old)
   A. Generalized body response: sometimes local reflex withdrawal on stimulation
   B. Movements may be increased: squirming, jerking, and flailing
   C. Crying becoming more intense
   D. Facial expression reflecting pain

E. Skin changes: pale or flushed

F. Vital sign (VS) fluctuations

G. Irregular eating and sleeping patterns

II. Older infant or toddler (1–3 years old)

  A. Localized body response: deliberate withdrawal on stimulation

  B. Loud crying

  C. Facial expression reflects pain

  D. Physical resistance; attempt to push stimulus away when applied

III. Young child or preschooler (3–6 years old)

  A. Loud crying, screaming

  B. Verbal expressions

  C. Thrashing of extremities

  D. Physical resistance before and during application of stimulus

  E. Requires physical restraint for painful procedures

  F. Clings to parent; solicits emotional support

  G. Restless and irritable with continuing pain

  H. May see these behaviors if child anticipates painful experience

IV. School-age child (6–11 years old)

  A. Same behaviors observed in young child

  B. Stalling behavior in anticipation of painful procedure

  C. Muscular rigidity in anticipation

V. Adolescent (12–18 years old)

  A. Less vocal protest and motor activity

  B. More verbal complaints such as "It hurts"

  C. Increased muscle tension and body control

Fear and Anxiety Reduction

Reducing Response of Fear From Separation, Anxiety, and Pain

I. Infants

  A. Promote interaction between infant and primary caregiver.

  B. Role-model comfort activities such as cuddling and talking to infant.

  C. Provide appropriate activities and toys for age, such as swing, bath toys, mobiles.

  D. Be calm and gentle during procedures.

  E. Allow caregivers time to comfort infant after procedure.

  F. Provide consistent staff.

  G. Avoid performing procedures in crib.

II. Toddler

  A. Promote visitation from primary caregiver.

  B. Provide consistent staff.

  C. Play games of disappearance such as hide-and-seek, peek-a-boo.

  D. Encourage parents to bring items from home, such as toy, blanket, pictures, and tape recording of bedtime story.

  E. Discourage parental departure when child is asleep.

  F. Comfort and cuddle child when crying.

  G. Continue home habits such as bottle, pacifier, potty chair if trained, diapers if not.

  H. Explain unpleasant procedures to child just before procedure. Be honest.

I. Provide distraction: blowing bubbles, kaleidoscope, and pop-up toys.

J. Allow child to play with hospital supplies and equipment that are safe for age: bandages, tongue blade, and stethoscope.

K. Avoid performing painful procedures in crib or bed.

III. Preschool child

  A. Prepare child for hospitalization.

  B. Reassure child that he or she is not responsible for the hospitalization.

  C. When parents or primary caregivers leave, they should relate their return to time frame the child can understand, such as breakfast, lunch, dinner, bedtime. Do not give false return times.

  D. Prepare child for procedures by explaining or illustrating the body part that will be involved and what the part will look like after the procedure.

  E. Answer child's questions in age-appropriate terms.

  F. Allow child to play with hospital supplies and equipment that are safe for age.

IV. School-age child

  A. Encourage parents or primary caregiver to avoid extended absences from hospitalized child.

  B. Allow child to talk and ask questions. Listen and respond to questions.

  C. Promote play through competitive table games.

  D. Be familiar with child's home routine and incorporate it into hospital routine as much as possible.

  E. Provide positive reinforcement for behavior. Avoid negative feedback.

  F. Encourage continuation of school work if child's condition permits.

  G. Provide a familiar face (consistent nurse) during procedures when possible.

  H. Allow children to express feelings regarding procedure through drawing and talking or acting-out procedure with doll or stuffed animal.

V. Adolescent

  A. Allow adolescent to participate in decisions related to treatment and care. Give information on the rules and policies of the hospital unit.

  B. Promote support and visitation from peers and family.

  C. Promote positive perception of illness.

  D. Explain procedures and what can be expected after a procedure. Allow a question-and-answer period. Be honest.

  E. Provide privacy as much as possible.

Nursing Care of the Hospitalized Child

Data Collection

I. Assist in obtaining health history and history of hospitalization.

II. Assist with diagnostic procedures.

Planning

I. Safe, effective care environment

  A. Reduce or eliminate environmental hazards.

  B. Transport, restrain, and position child safely.

  C. Ensure safety during procedures, including surgery.

II. Physiological integrity
  A. Carry out procedures with minimum distress to child.
  B. Prevent or minimize bodily injury or pain or both.
III. Psychosocial integrity
  A. Prevent or minimize effects of separation.
  B. Support and educate child and family.
  C. Help child to maintain control.
  D. Prepare child and family for procedures, surgery as needed.
  E. Use play as diversion and for stress reduction.
IV. Health promotion and maintenance
  A. Promote optimum health.
  B. Promote nutrition and hydration.
  C. Prepare family for home care.

Implementation

I. Keep harmful items out of reach of child.
II. Keep side rails up for infants and young children.
III. Allow freedom on unit within defined and enforced limits.
IV. Restrain child if necessary for safety, but limit use of restraints.
V. Explain hospital routines, items, procedures, and events in language appropriate for child's age.
VI. Use terms familiar to the child (e.g., those for bodily functions).
VII. Maintain a routine similar to that of child at home whenever possible.
VIII. Provide consistency of personnel as much as possible.
IX. Promote family interaction; encourage child and family contact and rooming-in whenever possible.
X. Allow parents to participate in care.
XI. Maintain contact with family: talk to child about home.
XII. Allow sibling visitation if possible.
XIII. Provide an atmosphere that allows free expression of feelings.
XIV. Allow child choices whenever possible.
XV. Explain procedures to the child, what child will experience, and what he or she can do to help: explain at the child's level of understanding; relate unfamiliar things and events to those familiar to the child; clarify terms; explain just before performing procedure.
XVI. Convey an attitude of confidence and indicate that cooperation is expected.
XVII. Allow child to see and handle strange and potentially frightening items, if possible.
XVIII. Be honest with child.
XIX. Be consistent in behaviors toward child.
XX. Communicate disapproval of undesired behavior—not disapproval of child.
XXI. Accept regressive behaviors.
XXII. Praise child for cooperation.
XXIII. Allow ample time for play.
XXIV. Encourage play activities and diversions appropriate to child's age, condition, and interests.
XXV. Use play as a way of explaining procedures.
XXVI. Encourage interaction with other children, when appropriate.
XXVII. Help family support child and refer to agencies providing family support.
XXVIII. Use services as available in neighborhood or region (e.g., Cystic Fibrosis Foundation, Easter Seals, Spina Bifida Association, American Cancer Society).
XXIX. Refer for home health nursing as indicated with discharge planning.

Evaluation

I. Child has consistent caregivers.
II. Child exhibits no evidence of discomfort.
III. Child verbalizes or plays out feelings and concerns.
IV. Child discusses home and family.
V. Child exhibits an understanding of information presented.
VI. Child cooperates in care and participates in care activities.
VII. Parents visit frequently or constantly.
VIII. Parents cooperate in care.
IX. Family demonstrates an understanding of child's behavior and becomes familiar with therapies.
X. Family demonstrates the ability to provide home care.
XI. Family demonstrates an understanding of the child's behavior.
XII. Family uses community resources appropriately.

Nursing Care of the Chronically Ill or Disabled Child

Data Collection

I. Observe for signs of suspected or determined diagnosis.
II. Assist with diagnostic procedures.
III. Be alert for evidence of overprotection or neglect.
IV. Determine family routines and abilities related to special care needs at home.

Planning

See also Nursing Care of the Ill Child.
  I. Safe, effective care environment
    A. Promote safe environment according to needs of individual child.
  II. Physiological integrity
    A. Follow plan of care.
    B. Prevent complications.
  III. Psychosocial integrity
    A. Teach child and family as needed.
    B. Prepare child and family for procedures, surgery as needed.
  IV. Health promotion and maintenance
    A. Promote optimum health.
    B. Prepare family for home care.

Implementation

  I. Support child and family at time of diagnosis.
    A. Project an attitude that shows acceptance of child and family.
    B. Allow expression of feelings and concerns.

II. Explain or reinforce explanation of condition or disease and treatment.
III. Help family develop a thorough plan of care.
IV. Encourage participation in care of hospitalized child.
V. Be available to family as listener or a resource.
VI. Encourage social activity for both child and family.
VII. Emphasize child's abilities.
VIII. Assist with improving appearance and grooming.
IX. Encourage self-care appropriate to capabilities and as much independence as condition allows.
X. Teach family skills and procedures needed for home care.
XI. Encourage sibling participation when possible.

Evaluation

I. Child exhibits no evidence of overprotection or neglect.
II. Child appears clean, well groomed, and attractively dressed.
III. Child and family (when appropriate) demonstrate an understanding of the disease or condition and the ability to provide home care.
IV. Child and family verbalize feelings and concerns.
V. Child and family develop realistic short- and long-term plans.
VI. Child and family comply with plan of care.
VII. Family displays an attitude of confidence in ability to cope.

Newborn Disorders

The Preterm Infant

Description

Infant born before completion of 37 weeks' gestation, regardless of birth weight.
I. Low-birth-weight infant: infant whose birth weight is <2500 g regardless of gestational age
II. Very-low-birth-weight infant: infant whose birth weight is <1500 g.
III. Small-for-date or small-for-gestational-age infant: infant whose rate of intrauterine growth was slowed and who was delivered at or later than term; the infant's birth weight falls below the 10th percentile on intrauterine growth curves
IV. Intrauterine growth retardation: infant whose prenatal growth is retarded or below 10th percentile on standardized growth curves

Pathophysiology

I. Factors related to prematurity (more than one often involved)
   A. Multiple pregnancies
   B. Maternal disease
   C. Heavy smoking
   D. Poor maternal nutrition
   E. Teenage pregnancy
   F. Illegal drug use or abuse
   G. Low income or socioeconomic status
II. Intensive care nursery necessary

Signs and Symptoms

I. Very small, wrinkled
II. Skin: red to pink with visible veins
III. Fine, feathery hair; lanugo on back and face
IV. Little or no evidence of fat
V. Head large in relation to body
VI. Limbs extended
VII. Lax, easily manipulated joints
VIII. Absent, weak, or ineffectual grasping, sucking, and swallowing reflexes
IX. Inability to maintain body temperature
X. Small thorax
XI. Breathing irregular
XIII. Bottom of feet smooth: absence of creases
XIV. Undescended testes in male infant

Therapeutic Management

I. Determination by status of infant, especially in relation to:
   A. Respiratory support
   B. Body temperature regulation
   C. Ability to suck
   D. Susceptibility to infection
   E. Activity intolerance
II. Prevention of complications

Nursing Care

DATA COLLECTION

I. Perform routine newborn assessment.
II. Assist with diagnostic procedures.
III. Perform ongoing systematic assessment of functioning:
   A. Weigh twice daily.
   B. Provide respiratory assessment:
      1. Rate and regularity
      2. Presence of retractions, nasal flaring
      3. Breath sounds, secretions
   C. Assess cardiovascular system:
      1. Heart rate, rhythm
      2. Heart sounds, including suspected murmurs
   D. Make gastrointestinal (GI) assessment:
      1. Feeding behavior
      2. Regurgitation or emesis
      3. Stool patterns: color, amount, odor, consistency
      4. Abdominal distention
      5. Bowel sounds
   E. Make genitourinary assessment:
      1. Abnormalities, if any
      2. Urinary output: amount, color, consistency
      3. Hydration
   F. Assess neurological and musculoskeletal systems:
      1. Movements: random, jittery, twitching, spontaneous, elicited
      2. Position at rest
      3. Changes in head circumference
      4. Reflexes: level of response
   G. Assess temperature:
      1. Axillary
      2. Rectal

H. Assess skin:
1. Color: cyanosis or jaundice
2. Discolored areas
3. Texture, turgor, characteristics (dry, flaky, peeling)
4. Skin lesion, rash

PLANNING

I. Safe, effective care environment
   A. See Hospital Care of the Newborn Infant under Postpartal Care in Chapter 3
   B. Provide external warmth.
   C. Protect from infection.
II. Physiological integrity
   A. Facilitate respiratory efforts.
   B. Conserve energy.
   C. Prevent complications.
III. Psychosocial integrity
   A. Promote parent-infant relationships.
   B. Support and educate family.
   C. Prepare family for procedures.
IV. Health promotion and maintenance
   A. Promote optimum health.
   B. Achieve and maintain optimum hydration and nutrition.
   C. Prepare family for home care.

IMPLEMENTATION

I. Position for maximum respiration: head of crib slightly elevated.
II. Provide supplemental oxygen.
III. Provide external warmth according to infant's condition and tolerance:
   A. Keep well wrapped if placed in open crib.
   B. Use Isolette.
   C. Use overhead warming unit.
   D. Position away from windows or drafts to prevent heat loss.
   E. Provide humidified atmosphere to reduce evaporative heat loss.
   F. Provide infant with knitted cap.
IV. Reduce energy expenditure.
   A. Ease respiratory effort.
   B. Maintain neutral thermal environment.
   C. Implement gavage feeding if infant becomes tired with conventional feeding methods to promote growth and conserve energy.
   D. Organize nursing activities and assessments to minimize disturbance.
   E. Promote rest: reduce environmental distractions (e.g., dim lights or cover crib with blanket, eliminate or reduce noise).
V. Implement institutional policies to prevent spread of infection; teach precautions to family.
VI. Provide nutrition:
   A. Nipple-feed with soft nipple that supplies nourishment without exertion (expressed mother's milk, banked breast milk, special formula).
   B. Assist with breast-feeding (with families who indicate desire).
   C. Gavage-feed.

VII. Prevent skin breakdown.
   A. Clean with clear water or mild, nonalkaline cleanser two to three times a week.
   B. Avoid damage to delicate skin (e.g., removing tape, careful use of scissors for removal of bandages).
   C. Change position of infant every 1–2 hours.
VIII. Encourage family to become involved in infant's care.
IX. Teach family skills needed for home care.

EVALUATION

I. Infant's breathing is regular, unlabored, and within normal limits.
II. Infant's temperature remains within desirable limits (97.7°F [36.5°C]).
III. Infant exhibits no evidence of dehydration.
IV. Infant consumes appropriate amount of nourishment without difficulty.
V. Infant exhibits a steady weight gain.
VI. Infant remains free of complications.
VII. Infant responds to appropriate stimuli.
VIII. Family becomes involved in infant's care.
IX. Family demonstrates an understanding of the condition and the ability to provide home care.

Hyperbilirubinemia

Description

Hyperbilirubinemia is excessive accumulation of bilirubin in the blood.

Classification

I. Pathological
   A. Before 24 hours of age
   B. With Rh-negative mother
II. Physiological
   A. After 24 hours of age
   B. With a bilirubin level of <12 normal (reference value) for full-term infant 2–5 days old; preterm level <16

Pathophysiology

I. Breakdown of red blood cells (RBCs)
II. Increased levels of bilirubin in the blood
III. Associated with breastfeeding
   A. Cause: unknown
   B. Early: 3–4 days of age
   C. Late: 4–5 days of age

Signs and Symptoms

I. Jaundice: yellowish discoloration of skin
   A. Bright yellow or orange
   B. Greenish, muddy yellow

Therapeutic Management

I. Observe closely for increase in jaundice.
II. Remove excess bilirubin.
   A. Phototherapy to alter bilirubin into a more soluble form
   B. Exchange transfusion

C. Prevention of blood incompatibility by administration of Rh_o immune globulin to all unsensitized Rh-negative mothers after delivery

Nursing Care

DATA COLLECTION

I. Perform routine assessment.
II. Assist with diagnostic procedures: serum bilirubin levels, Coombs' test (infants of Rh-negative mothers).

PLANNING

I. Safe, effective care environment (see Hospital Care of the Newborn Infant under Postpartal Care in Chap. 3)
II. Physiological integrity
  A. Assist with measures to reduce serum bilirubin levels.
  B. Prevent complications from therapy.
III. Psychosocial integrity
  A. Support and educate family.
IV. Health promotion and maintenance
  A. Promote optimum health.
  B. Prepare family for home care.

IMPLEMENTATION

I. Explain or reinforce explanation of condition and therapies.
II. Place infant under fluorescent light.
III. Turn frequently to expose all body surface areas to light.
IV. Shield infant's eyes with opaque mask of proper size.
  A. Close eyes before application.
  B. Position to prevent occlusion of nares.
  C. Assess several times per day for evidence of discharge, excessive pressures on lids, corneal irritation.
V. Avoid oily lubricants or lotions on skin.
VI. Promote adequate fluid intake.
VII. Observe for evidence of dehydration and drying skin.
VIII. Assist with exchange transfusion.
  A. Use sterile technique.
  B. Assist with procedure.
  C. Keep accurate records of blood volumes exchanged.
  D. Monitor infant's condition: VSs, temperature.

EVALUATION

I. Infant exhibits no evidence of jaundice.
II. Infant's serum bilirubin is within normal limits.
III. Infant remains well hydrated and free of complications.
IV. Family demonstrates an understanding of the condition.
V. Family demonstrates the ability to care for child.

Respiratory Distress Syndrome (Hyaline Membrane Disease)

Description

Respiratory distress syndrome is a dysfunction in newborns, primarily related to developmental delay in lung maturation.

Pathophysiology

I. Decreased surfactant production
II. Diminished oxygen to tissues and inability to excrete excess carbon dioxide

III. With each breath, increased energy expenditure to reinflate
IV. Decreased lung expansion, with fewer inflated alveoli

Signs and Symptoms

I. Dyspnea
II. Tachypnea (up to 80–120 breaths/min)
III. Pronounced retractions
IV. Audible expiratory grunt
V. Flaring of external nares
VI. Cyanosis

Therapeutic Management

I. Provide oxygen.
  A. Increased oxygen concentration provided in Isolette or by oxygen hood
  B. Assisted ventilation instituted: continuous positive airway pressure (CPAP)
II. Maintain acid-base status.
III. Maintain thermal environment to conserve energy and oxygen use.
IV. Conserve energy by minimal handling and use of gavage feeding.

Nursing Care

DATA COLLECTION

I. Perform routine assessment of premature infant.
II. Perform thorough respiratory assessment.
  A. Determine respiratory rate and regularity.
  B. Describe retractions and nasal flaring.
  C. Describe breath sounds: wet diminished sounds, areas of absence of sound, grunting.
  D. Describe secretions.
  E. Determine whether suctioning is needed.
  F. Describe cry.
  G. Describe oxygen and method of delivery; if infant is intubated, describe size of tube, type of ventilator, and settings.
III. Assist with diagnostic procedures: x-ray, blood gas measurements.

PLANNING

I. Safe, effective care environment
  A. Protect from injury and infection.
  B. Provide warmth.
II. Physiological integrity
  A. Promote respiratory effort.
  B. Conserve energy.
  C. Prepare family for procedures.
III. Psychosocial integrity
  A. See Hospital Care of the Newborn Infant under Postpartal Care in Chapter 3.
  B. Support and educate family.
  C. Prepare family for procedures.
IV. Health promotion and maintenance
  A. Promote optimum health.
  B. Achieve and maintain optimum hydration and nutrition.
  C. Prepare family for home care.

IMPLEMENTATION

I. Place infant in Isolette or crib with overhead warmer.
II. Maintain a thermal environment.
III. Maintain oxygen as prescribed.
IV. Remove secretions from airway as needed.
V. Monitor oxygen administration, including ventilator if used.
VI. Provide nutrition by one of the following:
   A. Gavage feed to conserve energy and provide sufficient calories.
   B. Nipple feed with soft nipple, allowing sufficient time for rest.
VII. Employ careful skin care to prevent breakdown or injury.
VIII. Teach family skills needed for home care.

EVALUATION

I. Infant breathes without effort.
II. Infant maintains optimum blood gas measurements without ventilatory assistance.
III. Infant remains free of complications.
IV. Family demonstrates an understanding of the condition and the ability to provide home care.

Neonatal Sepsis (Septicemia)

Description

Neonatal sepsis is generalized bacterial disease in the bloodstream.

Pathophysiology

I. Acquired
II. Prenatal: infected amniotic fluid, across placenta from maternal bloodstream
III. Birth: contact with maternal tissues
IV. Postnatal: cross-contamination from other infants, personnel, or objects in environment
V. Occurs more frequently in high-risk infants: preterm infants and those born after a difficult or traumatic delivery

Signs and Symptoms

I. Respiratory distress
   A. Apnea
   B. Irregular, grunting respirations
   C. Retractions
II. Gastric distress
   A. Vomiting
   B. Diarrhea
   C. Abdominal distention
   D. Absent stools (from paralytic ileus)
   E. Poor sucking and feeding
III. Skin manifestations
   A. Cyanosis
   B. Pallor
   C. Jaundice
IV. Central nervous system (CNS) involvement
   A. Irritability
   B. Apathy
   C. Seizures
V. Temperature instability

Therapeutic Management

I. Administration of antibiotics
II. Oxygen administration
III. Careful regulation of fluid and electrolytes

Nursing Care

DATA COLLECTION

I. Perform routine physical assessment.
II. Assist with diagnostic procedures: cultures of blood, spinal fluid, urine, stool, and any skin lesion examinations.
III. Observe for side effects of antibiotics.

PLANNING

I. Safe, effective care environment
   A. See Hospital Care of the Newborn Infant under Postpartal Care in Chapter 3.
   B. Prevent spread of infection.
II. Physiological integrity
   A. Help to eradicate organisms.
   B. Prevent complications.
III. Psychosocial integrity
   A. Support family.
IV. Health promotion and maintenance
   A. Promote optimum health.
   B. Achieve and maintain optimum hydration and nutrition.

IMPLEMENTATION

I. Provide external warmth (see Nursing Care under The Preterm Infant).
II. Reduce energy expenditure (see Nursing Care under The Preterm Infant).
III. Maintain and implement institutional policies to prevent spread of infection.
IV. Monitor intravenous (IV) infusion.
V. Administer antibiotics as prescribed.
VI. Explain or reinforce explanation of condition and therapies.
VII. Teach family skills needed for home care.

EVALUATION

I. Infant exhibits no evidence of infection.
II. Infant remains free of complications.
III. Family demonstrates an understanding of the condition and the ability to provide home care.

Respiratory Disorders

Croup (Laryngotracheobronchitis)

Description

Croup is an inflammation of the larynx, trachea, and bronchi.

Pathophysiology

I. Narrowing of the air passages produced by edema of respiratory mucosa, causing variable degrees of airway obstruction

II. Condition usually follows 1- to 3-day cold
III. Most common in children aged 3 months to 3 years
IV. Usually viral in origin

Signs and Symptoms

I. Restlessness
II. Hoarseness
III. "Brassy" or "barking" cough
IV. Inspiratory stridor
V. Respiratory distress
VI. Fever: low grade
VII. Condition usually occurs suddenly during night

Therapeutic Management

I. Mild disease; can be treated at home
  A. Careful observation for symptoms of respiratory obstruction
  B. Bed rest
  C. Cool, humidified environment
  D. Encouragement of fluid intake
  E. Temperature reduction (if elevated)
II. Severe disease; hospitalization
  A. As previously listed
  B. High-humidity environment
  C. Oxygen
  D. IV fluids
  E. Corticosteroid therapy
  F. Epinephrine for transient relief
  G. Availability of endotracheal intubation equipment

Nursing Care

DATA COLLECTION

I. Perform routine physical assessment.
II. Perform in-depth assessment for:
  A. Rate, depth, and rhythm of respirations
  B. Presence of flaring nares, grunting, and retractions
  C. Pallor, cyanosis
  D. Dyspnea
  E. Stridor
  F. Type, frequency, and intensity of cough
  G. Sputum
  H. Oxygen saturation
III. Assist with diagnostic procedures: chest radiograph, serum electrolytes, blood gas measurements, pH.

PLANNING

I. Safe, effective care environment
  A. See Nursing Care of the Ill Child.
  B. Prevent spread of infection.
II. Physiological integrity
  A. Assist respiratory efforts.
  B. Promote rest.
  C. Promote comfort.
  D. Reduce temperature (for significant elevation).
III. Psychosocial integrity
  A. Support child and family.
IV. Health promotion and maintenance
  A. Prevent dehydration.
  B. Provide nourishment.
  C. Prevent complications.
  D. Prepare family for home care.

IMPLEMENTATION

I. Administer humidified oxygen as prescribed (mist tent, nasal).
II. Position for optimum breathing with head of bed elevated.
III. Monitor respiratory status regularly.
IV. Administer nose drops and suction nasal passages to facilitate breathing.
V. Administer medication as prescribed.
VI. Support child and family (see Nursing Care of the Ill Child or Nursing Care of the Hospitalized Child).
VII. Encourage presence of family.
VIII. Provide constant attendance during acute illness.
IX. Encourage intake of cool fluids such as fruit juices, soft drinks, and gelatin.
X. Monitor parenteral fluid administration, if prescribed.
XI. Have emergency endotracheal or tracheostomy equipment available.
XII. Implement measures to prevent spread of infection to others.
XIII. Administer antibiotics as prescribed.
XIV. Administer chest physiotherapy, if prescribed.
XV. Teach family procedures needed for home care, including expected results of medication and their possible side effects.

EVALUATION

I. Child remains free of respiratory distress.
II. Child rests comfortably and plays quietly.
III. Child demonstrates adequate nutrition.
IV. Child and family comply with therapeutic regimen.

Epiglottitis

Description

Epiglottitis is an inflammation of the glottitis.

Pathophysiology

I. Edema of tissues above the vocal cords (supraglottic swelling)
II. Narrowing of airway inlet that can result in total obstruction
III. Usually caused by *Haemophilus influenzae* type B
IV. Most common in children 2–5 years old
V. Possible precursor: sore throat

Signs and Symptoms

I. Abrupt onset
II. Rapid progression to severe respiratory distress
III. Elevated temperature
IV. Toxic appearance
V. Characteristic posture with client insisting on sitting upright, leaning forward with chin thrust out, mouth open, and tongue protruding
VI. Irritability
VII. Anxious, apprehensive, frightened expression

VIII. Thick, muffled voice and "croaking, froglike" sound on inspiration
IX. Red, inflamed throat with distinctive large, cherry-red edematous epiglottitis (seldom observed except by qualified examiner, as described earlier)
X. Predictive symptoms: absence of spontaneous cough, drooling, and agitation.

Therapeutic Management

I. Throat examined with extreme care and where facilities are available for emergency endotracheal intubation or tracheostomy
II. Antibiotics to eradicate organisms
III. Corticosteroids to reduce edema

Nursing Care

DATA COLLECTION

I. Assessment is same as for laryngotracheobronchitis.
II. Perform routine physical assessment.
III. Collect data for:
   A. Rate, depth, and rhythm of respirations
   B. Presence of flaring nares, grunting, and retractions
   C. Pallor, cyanosis
   D. Dyspnea
   E. Stridor
   F. Type, frequency, and intensity of cough
   G. Sputum
   H. Oxygen saturation
IV. Assist with diagnostic procedures: chest radiograph, serum electrolytes, blood gas measurements, pH.

PLANNING

I. Prevention of respiratory obstruction
II. Safe, effective care environment
   A. See Nursing Care of the Ill Child.
   B. Prevent spread of infection.
III. Physiological integrity
   A. Assist respiratory efforts.
   B. Promote rest.
   C. Promote comfort.
   D. Reduce temperature (significant elevation).
IV. Psychosocial integrity
   A. Support child and family.
V. Health promotion and maintenance
   A. Prevent dehydration.
   B. Provide nourishment.
   C. Prevent complications.
   D. Prepare family for home care.

IMPLEMENTATION

I. Refer to physician immediately.
II. Administer humidified oxygen as prescribed (mist tent, nasal).
III. Position for optimum breathing with head of bed elevated.
IV. Monitor respiratory status regularly.
V. Administer nose drops and suction nasal passages to facilitate breathing.
VI. Administer medication as prescribed.

VII. Support child and family (see Nursing Care of the Ill Child or Nursing Care of the Hospitalized Child).
VIII. Encourage presence of family.
IX. Provide constant attendance during acute illness.
X. Encourage intake of cool fluids such as fruit juices, soft drinks, and gelatin.
XI. Monitor parenteral fluid administration, if prescribed.
XII. Have emergency endotracheal or tracheostomy equipment available.
XIII. Implement measures to prevent spread of infection to others.
XIV. Administer antibiotics and corticosteroids as prescribed.
XV. Administer chest physiotherapy, if prescribed.
XVI. Teach family procedures needed for care, including expected results of medication and their possible side effects.

EVALUATION

I. Child remains free of respiratory distress.
II. Child rests comfortably and plays quietly.
III. Child has adequate nutritional intake.
IV. Child and family comply with therapeutic regimen.

Pneumonia

Description

Inflammation in the lungs resulting in the alveoli becoming filled with exudate. It can be primary illness or secondary to another infection or surgery.

Pathophysiology

Cause of the pneumonia is usually viral in children but can be from bacteria, mycoplasma, or aspiration. Less often caused by histomycosis, coccidioidomycosis, or fungi.

Signs and Symptoms

I. Dry cough, progressing to productive cough.
II. Fever (103–104°F [39.3–40.0°C]).
III. Shallow, rapid respirations.
IV. Sternal retractions and nasal flaring can occur.
V. Listlessness.
VI. Poor appetite.
VII. Preference for positioning on affected side.
VIII. Onset could be sudden or preceded by upper respiratory infection (URI).

Therapeutic Management

I. Chest radiographs to confirm diagnosis.
II. Elevated white blood cell (WBC) count.
III. Cultures from sputum, nose, and throat may be taken.
IV. Bacterial pneumonia is treated with antibiotics.
V. Viral pneumonia treatment is supportive; if respiratory syncytial virus is present, may treat with riboviran via inhalation.
VI. Antipyretics for fever.
VII. Oxygen for cyanosis and dyspnea.
VIII. Oxygen administration with cool mist, chest physiotherapy, and postural drainage in some cases.

Nursing Care

DATA COLLECTION

I. Perform routine physical assessment.
II. Collect data for:
  A. Rate, depth, and rhythm of respirations.
  B. Presence of nasal flaring, grunting, and retractions.
  C. Pallor, cyanosis.
  D. Dyspnea.
  E. Stridor.
  F. Cough, nonproductive or productive. Note characteristics of productive cough.
  G. Oxygen saturation.
  H. Alertness of child.
  I. Vital signs.
  J. Fluid status.

PLANNING

I. Safe, effective care environment
  A. Avoid exposure to infectious agents.
  B. Provide environment appropriate for age.
  C. Routine safety precautions with oxygen.
II. Physiological integrity
  A. Relieve symptoms.
  B. Adhere to therapeutic regimen.
III. Psychosocial integrity
  A. Promote growth and development.
  B. Promote family involvement.
IV. Health promotion and maintenance
  A. Maintain optimum health, good nutrition, and adequate rest.
  B. Prepare child and family for home care.
  C. Promote self-care management.

IMPLEMENTATION

I. Position for optimum ventilation.
II. Provide humidified oxygen as prescribed.
III. Administer antipyretics for fever.
IV. Administer medications as ordered.
V. Assist in chest physiotherapy and postural drainage.
VI. Monitor intake and output (I&O); prevent dehydration through adequate hydration.

EVALUATION

I. Child exhibits normal respiratory rate, rhythm, and quality.
II. Child exhibits appropriate nutritional intake for age.
III. Child and family adhere to prescribed regimen.

Tonsillitis

Description

Tonsillitis is an inflammation of the tonsillar structures in the oropharynx.

Pathophysiology

I. Bacterial or viral invasion of tonsillar tissues with inflammation, swelling, and erythema (sometimes exudate)
II. Usually occurs in association with pharyngitis
III. Tonsillar enlargement, which causes discomfort and difficulty in swallowing

Signs and Symptoms

I. Difficulty swallowing and breathing
II. Nasal, muffled voice
III. Persistent cough common
IV. Condition often associated with otitis media and hearing difficulty
V. Enlargement of tonsils causing discomfort and difficulty in swallowing
VI. Elevated body temperature possible

Therapeutic Management

I. Medical
  A. Symptomatic treatment
  B. Antibiotics (for throat culture positive for group A β-hemolytic streptococcus)
II. Surgical
  A. Tonsillectomy (removal of the palatine tonsils)
  B. Usually with adenoidectomy (removal of adenoids)

Nursing Care (Tonsillectomy)

DATA COLLECTION

I. Preoperatively
  A. Perform routine assessment.
  B. Assist with diagnostic procedures: bleeding and clotting times.
  C. Prepare child in advance for procedure using simple explanation of procedure. Include what child can expect when he or she awakes.
II. Postoperatively
  A. Take pulse and respirations frequently.
  B. Observe for signs of bleeding:
    1. Rapid pulse
    2. Restlessness
    3. Frequent swallowing, clearing of throat
    4. Nausea and vomiting
  C. Inspect throat for evidence of oozing or hemorrhage.
  D. Inspect vomitus for evidence of fresh bleeding.

PLANNING

I. Safe, effective care environment
  A. See Nursing Care of the Ill Child.
II. Physiological integrity
  A. Promote hydration and nutrition.
  B. Relieve discomfort.
  C. Facilitate drainage.
  D. Prevent complications.
III. Psychosocial integrity
  A. Support child and family.
IV. Health promotion and maintenance
  A. Prepare family for home care.

IMPLEMENTATION

I. Offer cool fluids and liquid diet when child is fully alert and there is no evidence of bleeding.
II. Apply ice collar.
III. Offer soft diet after 24 hours; then advance to regular diet for age. Avoid red or brown popsicles to distinguish any bleeding.

IV. Administer analgesics the first 24 hours for discomfort and then as needed for discomfort.
V. Position on side or stomach while child is sleeping and when he or she is awake.
VI. Discourage child from swallowing mucous secretions.
VII. Discourage child from coughing frequently, clearing throat, or blowing nose.
VIII. Avoid acidic fluids or foods (e.g., orange or tomato juice) until healing takes place; do not use straw.
IX. Reassure child and family about what to expect (e.g., expectoration of blood-tinged mucus, temporary alteration in voice).
X. Support child and family.
XI. Teach skills needed for home care.

EVALUATION

I. Child recovers from surgery uneventfully:
A. No evidence of bleeding
B. No difficulty with nutritional intake

Acute Otitis Media

Description

Acute otitis media is an infection of the middle ear.

Pathophysiology

I. Usually following an upper respiratory infection
II. Primarily the result of a blocked eustachian tube
III. Impaired drainage, which prevents normal drainage of middle-ear secretions
IV. Rapid growth of organisms in this warm, fertile environment
V. Usual causes: *Streptococcus pneumoniae, Haemophilus influenzae,* and *Moraxella catarrhalis*

Signs and Symptoms

I. General
A. Earache
B. Fever
C. Possible purulent drainage
D. Loss of appetite
E. Irritability
F. Complaints of pain (older children)
G. Evidence of hearing loss in affected ear
II. In infants
A. Crying
B. Restless and difficult to comfort
C. Rolling of head from side to side
D. Tendency to rub, hold, or pull affected ear
III. Otoscopic examination reveals:
A. Bright-red or opaque, bulging or retracting tympanic membrane with diminished mobility
B. Possibly no visible bony landmarks or light reflex

Therapeutic Management

I. Medical
A. Antibiotics to eradicate organisms
B. Analgesics to control discomfort
C. Acetaminophen for high fever
D. Decongestants (of questionable value)
II. Surgical
A. May require myringotomy (surgical incision of eardrum)

Nursing Care

DATA COLLECTION

I. Perform routine assessment.
II. Assess for evidence of generalized infection.
III. Examine external auditory canal for evidence of inflammation.
IV. Assess child for evidence of hearing loss in affected ear.
V. Perform or assist with diagnostic procedures: audiography, tympanometry, pneumatic otoscopy, acoustic reflectometry.

PLANNING

I. Safe, effective care environment
A. See Nursing Care of the Ill Child.
II. Physiological integrity
A. Assist in eradication of organism.
B. Relieve discomfort.
III. Psychosocial integrity
A. Support child and family.
B. See Nursing Care of the Ill Child.
IV. Health promotion and maintenance
A. Prevent complications.
B. Prepare family for home care.

IMPLEMENTATION

I. Administer antibiotics as prescribed.
II. Administer analgesics as prescribed.
III. Administer decongestants, if prescribed.
IV. Apply local heat; have child lie (affected ear down) on a heating pad wrapped in a towel.
V. Cleanse external ear with sterile cotton swabs or pledgets soaked in saline; then keep ear dry to prevent excoriation.
VI. Cleanse any drainage from ear and keep area dry to prevent excoriation.
VII. Encourage fluid intake.
VIII. Prepare family for surgical intervention, if appropriate:
A. Myringotomy
B. Placement of pressure-equalizing tubes
IX. Emphasize the importance of following a full course of antibiotics.
X. Emphasize the importance of follow-up care.
XI. Teach primary caregiver measures to reduce occurrence of otitis media.
XII. Teach family skills needed for home care, including expected results of medications and their possible side effects.

EVALUATION

I. Child appears comfortable.
II. Child's ear canal and surrounding skin are free of drainage and irritation.
III. Child remains free of complications.
IV. Family complies with therapeutic regimen.

Bronchial Asthma

Description

Bronchial asthma is a lower-airway disorder characterized by smooth muscle constriction (bronchospasm), increased thick mucous secretions, and mucosal edema—usually in response to an allergen.

Pathophysiology

I. Symptoms possibly precipitated by allergic response to an allergen (pollens, dust, animal dander), exercise, certain foods, smoke or other irritants, rapid changes in environmental temperature, upper respiratory infection, or emotional stress
II. Bronchospasm
III. Increased mucous secretion
IV. Edema
V. Reduced diameter of air passage

Signs and Symptoms

I. Hacking, paroxysmal, irritative, nonproductive cough
II. Shortness of breath; flaring nares
III. Elevated pulse
IV. Prolonged expiratory phase of respiration
V. Audible wheeze
VI. Restlessness and apprehension accompanied by an anxious facial expression
VII. In children, speaking with short, panting, broken phrases common
VIII. In older children sitting upright, hunched over, with hands on bed or chair and arms braced common
IX. Chest auscultation revealing coarse, loud breath sounds; sonorous rales; coarse rhonchi; and generalized expiratory wheezing, which becomes increasingly high pitched
X. With repeated episodes, common for children to develop barrel chest, elevated shoulder, and use of accessory muscles of respiration

Therapeutic Management

I. Eliminate or avoid proved or suspected irritants and allergens.
II. Prevent attacks: avoid precipitating factors; administer cromolyn sodium.
III. Relieve or minimize symptoms:
    A. Bronchodilators to relax bronchiole musculature
       1. Rapid-acting β-adrenergic agonists and methylxanthines
    B. Corticosteroids to reduce edema
IV. Treat acute attacks promptly.
V. Educate child and family regarding short- and long-range management.

STATUS ASTHMATICUS

I. Hospitalization with intensive nursing care
II. IV fluids
III. Continuous respiratory and cardiac monitoring
IV. Bronchodilators

A. Short, rapid-acting sympathomimetics: epinephrine (Sus-Phrine), terbutaline
V. Corticosteroids
VI. Humidified oxygen therapy

Nursing Care

DATA COLLECTION

I. See Assessment under Respiratory Distress Syndrome.
II. Obtain history to determine possible precipitating factors.
III. Gather data on environment for presence of possible allergens.
IV. Assist with diagnostic procedures: chest radiograph, sputum examination, immunologic blood tests, skin tests, pulmonary function tests, challenge tests.
V. Assess family interpersonal relationships for evidence of dissension, overprotection, or manipulation.
VI. Provide acute care:
    A. Monitor IV fluids and output.
    B. Monitor VSs frequently.

PLANNING

I. Safe, effective care environment
   A. Remove allergenic materials from environment.
   B. Avoid exposure to infection.
   C. Prevent situations that precipitate an attack (e.g., extremes of weather; air pollutants, especially smoke; and infections).
II. Physiological integrity
   A. Relieve symptoms (e.g., bronchospasm).
   B. Adhere to therapeutic regimen (e.g., medications, breathing exercises).
III. Psychosocial integrity
   A. Promote normal activities.
   B. Discourage overprotection by family.
   C. Promote short- and long-term adaptation to the disease.
IV. Health promotion and maintenance
   A. Maintain optimum health with good nutrition, adequate rest, and appropriate exercise.
   B. Avoid exposure to infections.
   C. Manage minor illnesses at onset.
   D. Prepare child and family for home care.
   E. Promote self-care management.

IMPLEMENTATION

I. Acute attack
   A. Administer bronchodilators, corticosteroids, and antibiotics as prescribed.
   B. Position in high-Fowler's position for optimum ventilation.
   C. Provide humidified oxygen as prescribed.
   D. Administer mucolytic agents as prescribed.
II. Long-term supervision and support
   A. Teach preventive management, avoidance of precipitating factors, appropriate exercise, sound health maintenance.
   B. Explain expected results of medications and their possible side effects.

EVALUATION

I. Child exhibits normal respiratory rate, rhythm, and quality.
II. Child engages in activities appropriate to age and interests.
III. Child and family comply with therapeutic regimen.
IV. Child and family maintain optimum health practices.
V. Child and family cope with life stresses appropriately.

Cystic Fibrosis

Description

Cystic fibrosis is a multisystem disorder primarily affecting the exocrine (mucus-producing) glands.

Pathophysiology

I. Instead of thin, freely flowing secretions, mucous glands produce a thick mucus.
II. Mucus accumulates, dilating and eventually obstructing small ducts and passages.
III. Pancreatic ducts become blocked:
   A. Prevents enzymes from reaching the duodenum
   B. Results in marked impairment in the digestion and absorption of nutrients
   C. Also results in cystic dilatation, degeneration, and eventual fibrosis of the acini (small gland lobes)
IV. Respiratory tract bronchioles and bronchi become blocked:
   A. Manifests as patchy atelectasis and hyperinflation
V. Males usually do not produce sperm.
VI. Sweat glands fail to reabsorb sodium.
VII. Abnormally high levels of sodium and chloride are present in the sweat.
VIII. Sodium depletion may occur.
IX. Disease is inherited as an autosomal recessive trait.

Signs and Symptoms

I. Meconium ileus in newborn period (earliest sign)
   A. Abdominal distention
   B. Vomiting
   C. Failure to pass stools
II. Gastrointestinal
   A. Large, bulky, loose, frothy, extremely foul-smelling stools
   B. Weight loss
   C. Marked tissue wasting
   D. Failure to grow
   E. Abdominal distention
   F. Thin extremities
   G. Decreased or absent pancreatic enzymes, especially trypsin, in stools
III. Pulmonary
   A. Frequent upper respiratory infections
   B. Chronic cough, which becomes paroxysmal
   C. Thick, tenacious mucus
   D. Eventual barrel chest, dyspnea, clubbing of fingers and toes
   E. Radiographic evidence of patchy areas of atelectasis and obstructive emphysema

IV. Biochemical
   A. Diagnosis by sweat chloride concentrations >60 mEq/L
   B. Salty taste to sweat (often reported by parents)
V. Delayed puberty

Therapeutic Management

I. Remove obstruction (meconium ileus).
II. Facilitate lung clearance.
III. Prevent and treat pulmonary infections.
IV. Replace pancreatic enzymes.
V. Facilitate growth.
VI. Prevent complications.

Nursing Care

DATA COLLECTION

I. See Data Collection under Respiratory Distress Syndrome.
II. See Data Collection under The Preterm Infant.
III. Perform or assist with diagnostic tests: chest radiograph, sweat electrolytes, pulmonary function, tests for pancreatic enzymes, fat-absorption tests.
IV. Assess family's interpersonal relationships with child and response to the disease.

PLANNING

I. Safe, effective care environment
   A. See Nursing Care of the Ill Child.
   B. Avoid exposure to infections.
II. Physiological integrity
   A. Improve breathing.
   B. Facilitate bronchial clearance.
   C. Promote growth.
III. Psychosocial integrity
   A. Explore feelings regarding an inherited disease.
   B. Explore family's feelings regarding a child with a potentially terminal illness.
   C. Encourage genetic counseling.
   D. Provide long-term support and follow-up care.
IV. Health promotion and maintenance
   A. Maintain optimum health.
   B. Prevent complications.
   C. Prepare family for home care.
   D. Encourage as normal a lifestyle as possible.

IMPLEMENTATION

I. Assist with diagnostic procedures (perform sweat chloride test as prescribed).
II. Provide and/or supervise respiratory therapy as prescribed:
   A. Nebulization
   B. Chest physiotherapy
   C. Breathing exercises
III. Administer antibiotics, mucolytics, and expectorants as prescribed.
IV. Provide nutritious and attractive meals and snacks. Diet should have increased protein and moderate amount of fat.
V. Encourage extra intake of fluids.

VI. Monitor IV infusion, if prescribed.
VII. Administer pancreatic enzymes as prescribed.
VIII. Provide conscientious skin care (salt accumulation may be irritating).
IX. Implement and maintain appropriate infection-control measures.
X. Teach family administration of medications, including expected results and possible side effects.
XI. Teach family about use of equipment and about respiratory management.
XII. Promote compliance with prescribed therapies.
XIII. Encourage and promote self-care.
XIV. Promote as normal a lifestyle as possible (e.g., engaging in activities within capabilities, attending school, developing peer relationships).
XV. Support child and family.
XVI. Refer to genetic counseling services.

EVALUATION

I. Child breathes easily.
II. Child manages bronchial secretions with minimal stress.
III. Child appears well nourished and gains weight appropriate for developmental stage.
IV. Child remains free of complications, especially upper respiratory tract infections (URIs).
V. Child engages in activities appropriate to developmental level, capabilities, and interests.
VI. Family complies with therapeutic regimen.
VII. Family seeks appropriate counseling.

Gastrointestinal Disorders

Cleft Lip and/or Cleft Palate

Description

Cleft lip is a congenital malformation consisting of one or more clefts in the upper lip. Cleft palate is a congenital defect consisting of a fissure in the midline of the palate.

Pathophysiology

I. Cleft lip: failure of the maxillary and median nasal processes to fuse during prenatal development
   A. May range from a notch in the vermilion border of lip to complete separation extending to the floor of the nose
II. Cleft palate: failure of the two sides of the palate to fuse during prenatal development
   A. May occur as an isolated defect or in association with cleft lip

Signs and Symptoms

These defects are readily apparent at birth.

Therapeutic Management

I. Surgically close the defects at the optimum age.
II. Prevent complications.

III. Facilitate normal growth and development of the child.
IV. Rehabilitate for optimum speech and hearing within limitation of residual impairment, if any.

Nursing Care

DATA COLLECTION

I. Assess for palatal defects by placing examining fingers directly on palate.
II. Assess infant's or child's ability to suck and take nourishment.
III. Assess nutritional status of the child.

PLANNING

I. Safe, effective care environment
   A. See Hospital Care of the Newborn Infant under Postpartal Care in Chapter 3.
   B. Provide an environment appropriate for age.
   C. Promote the involvement of the primary caregiver.
II. Physiological integrity
   A. Facilitate healing of operative site.
   B. Prevent complications.
   C. Facilitate nutritional intake.
III. Psychosocial integrity
   A. Facilitate family's adjustment to a child with a facial defect.
   B. Promote normal lifestyle for child.
IV. Health promotion and maintenance
   A. Implement a feeding method appropriate to extent of the defect, parental preference, and ease of management.
   B. Prepare family for home care.

IMPLEMENTATION

I. Use special nipple or appliance when feeding (e.g., lamb's nipple, flanged nipple, gravity-flow nipple, rubber-tipped syringe, or specially designed feeding appliance); modify standard nipple with small single slit or cross-cut at end.
II. Feed with infant's head held upright to prevent aspiration.
III. Provide soft diet postoperatively for older children until healing takes place.
IV. Breast-feeding mothers are taught positioning of infant as for formula feeding and placing nipple well back in the infant's mouth for more efficient compression.
V. Bubble (burp) frequently during feeding.
VI. Convey an attitude of acceptance of infant and family; indicate by behavior that infant is a valuable human being.
VII. Protect operative site (cleft lip):
   A. Avoid positioning on stomach.
   B. Apply elbow restraints.
   C. Maintain metal appliance (if applied in the operating room).
   D. Cleanse operative site, as prescribed, after feeding and as indicated.
   E. Prevent excessive crying.
VIII. Protect operative site (cleft palate):
   A. Avoid placing objects in child's mouth (e.g., stan-

dard spoon: use only wide-bowled spoon, tongue depressor, thermometer).
  B. Restrain arms.
IX. Support and educate family regarding home care.
X. Teach family to observe for signs of speech or hearing impairment.

EVALUATION

I. Infant takes feedings well and displays appropriate weight gain.
II. Surgical site remains clean and free of trauma and infection.
III. Child develops normal patterns of speech articulation and intonation.
IV. Child hears without difficulty.
V. Family uses community resources appropriately.
VI. Family exhibits evidence that the child is an accepted and loved member of the household.

Tracheoesophageal Fistula, Esophageal Atresia

Description

Tracheoesophageal fistula is a congenital malformation resulting from failure of the esophagus to develop a continuous passage; the esophagus may or may not form a connection to the trachea.

PATHOPHYSIOLOGY

The anomaly appears in one of the following ways:
I. Proximal esophageal segment terminating in a blind pouch; distal segment connected to the trachea or primary bronchus by a short fistula at or near the bifurcation (most common anomaly)
II. Blind pouches at end of the proximal and the distal esophagus, which are widely separated and have no communication to the trachea
III. Otherwise normal trachea and esophagus connected by a common fistula
IV. Fistula from the trachea to the upper esophageal segment or to both the upper and lower segments (rare)

Signs and Symptoms

I. Excessive salivation and drooling
II. Coughing
III. Choking
IV. Cyanosis
V. Cessation of breathing possible
VI. Possibility of catheter gently passed into the esophagus meeting with resistance if the lumen is blocked
VII. Diagnosis established by radiographic demonstration of anomaly

Therapeutic Management

I. Patent airway
II. Prevention of pneumonia
  A. Feed by gastrostomy.
  B. Drain oral secretions via tube inserted into proximal blind pouch or cervical esophagostomy.

III. Surgical repair of defect (time of repair depends on the type of defect and condition of the infant)

Nursing Care

DATA COLLECTION

I. Perform routine assessment. (Does mother have a history of polyhydramnios?)
II. Observe for evidence of anomaly, primarily the three Cs: coughing, choking, and cyanosis (especially following ingestion of fluid). Also excessive salivation.
III. Assist with diagnostic procedures: gastric lavage, chest radiograph.

PLANNING

I. Safe, effective care environment
  A. Prevent complications.
  B. Provide safe environment according to the needs of the child.
II. Physiological integrity
  A. Prevent aspiration of fluid and secretions into trachea.
  B. Feed via gastrostomy as prescribed.
  C. Provide conscientious postoperative care at time of surgical correction.
III. Psychosocial integrity
  A. Meet oral needs of infant.
  B. Facilitate family's adjustment to an infant with a physical defect.
IV. Health promotion and maintenance
  A. Provide health supervision as appropriate.
  B. Prepare family for home care.

IMPLEMENTATION

I. Recognize defect as soon after birth as evident.
II. Position for optimum drainage of secretions—usually supine, with head elevated at least 30 degrees.
III. Suction oropharynx as needed.
IV. Aspirate secretions from proximal blind pouch manually or by intermittent or continuous suction.
V. Feed prescribed formula via gastrostomy tube.
VI. Provide for infant's sucking needs with pacifier, especially during gastrostomy feedings.
VII. Observe postoperatively for ability to swallow without choking and for satisfactory eating behavior.
VIII. Prepare family for appearance of child (e.g., presence of chest tubes).
IX. Assist family in coping with the infant's needs and therapies.
X. Provide for maternal and infant bonding.
XI. Teach family skills needed for home care.

EVALUATION

I. Infant remains free of respiratory distress.
II. Infant's lungs remain clear.
III. Infant retains feedings and exhibits appropriate weight gain.
IV. Family exhibits appropriate behavior with infant.
V. Family demonstrates an understanding of the condition and the ability to provide home care.

Pyloric Stenosis

Description

Pyloric stenosis is a narrowing of the opening at exit of the stomach.

Pathophysiology

I. Enlargement (hypertrophy) of the pyloric musculature causing obstruction at the stomach exit (may be genetic)

Signs and Symptoms

I. Vomiting
  A. Is forceful to projectile
  B. Occurs shortly after a feeding
  C. May follow each meal or appear intermittently
II. Infant hungry and irritable; accepts second feeding after vomiting
III. No evidence of pain or discomfort
IV. Weight loss
V. Signs of dehydration
VI. Hard, olive-shaped tumor possibly palpable

Therapeutic Management

I. Correct any dehydration and electrolyte imbalance.
II. Provide surgical relief of obstruction by pyloromyotomy (Fredet-Ramstedt procedure).

Nursing Care

DATA COLLECTION

I. Perform routine assessment.
II. Observe infant's eating behaviors, especially vomiting pattern.
III. Assess for dehydration. Monitor electrolytes.
IV. Assist with diagnostic procedures: upper GI series, ultrasound, laboratory assessment of electrolyte status.

PLANNING

I. Safe, effective care environment
  A. See Nursing Care of the Ill Child.
  B. Promote an environment that is appropriate for the age of the child.
II. Physiological integrity
  A. Provide nutrition.
  B. Prevent vomiting.
  C. Prevent complications.
III. Psychosocial integrity
  A. Meet infant's sucking needs.
  B. Support family and prepare for surgery.
  C. Promote healthy parent-child relationships.
IV. Health promotion and maintenance
  A. Provide health supervision.
  B. Prepare family for home care.

IMPLEMENTATION

I. Obtain baseline weight and monitor daily.
II. Monitor IV infusion as prescribed.
III. Monitor I&O.
IV. Monitor electrolytes.
V. Monitor nasogastric suction, if present.
VI. If feeding, minimize vomiting by:
  A. Feeding slowly
  B. Holding infant in semiupright position
  C. Bubbling frequently (before, during, and after feeding)
  D. Placing on right side after feeding
  E. Handling minimally after feeding
VII. Teach family skills needed for home care.

EVALUATION

I. Infant takes and retains feedings.
II. Infant exhibits a satisfactory weight gain.
III. Parents demonstrate an understanding of the condition and the ability to provide home care.

Imperforate Anus

Description

Imperforate anus is a congenital malformation in which the rectum has no outside opening.

Pathophysiology

I. Rectum ends as a closed or blind pouch.
II. End may connect to the vagina by a fistula.

Signs and Symptoms

I. Absence of an anus; dimple present
II. Failure to pass meconium stool
III. Passage of stool through inappropriate opening

Therapeutic Management

I. Perform surgery to construct opening.
II. Sometimes a temporary colostomy may be necessary.
III. In vaginal fistula, surgery may be delayed 4–6 months.

Nursing Care

DATA COLLECTION

I. Perform routine assessment.
II. Observe for meconium stool.
III. Assist with diagnostic procedures: endoscopy, radiography, renal ultrasound.

PLANNING

I. Safe, effective care environment
  A. See Hospital Care of the Newborn Infant under Postpartal Care in Chapter 3.
  B. Promote environment appropriate for age.
II. Physiological integrity
  A. Promote wound healing.
  B. Promote normal bowel function.
  C. Prevent infection and trauma.
III. Psychosocial integrity
  A. See Hospital Care of the Newborn Infant under Postpartal Care in Chapter 3.

B. Support family.

C. Prepare family for surgical procedure.

D. Promote involvement of primary caregiver in the care.

IV. Health promotion and maintenance

A. Provide appropriate hydration and nutrition.

B. Prepare family for home care.

IMPLEMENTATION

I. Avoid taking temperature rectally.

II. Monitor IV fluids as prescribed.

III. Monitor I&O; weigh daily.

IV. Maintain nasogastric suction, if prescribed.

V. Offer pacifier to satisfy nonnutritive sucking needs.

VI. Observe stool pattern.

VII. Support family and teach skills needed for home care.

EVALUATION

I. Infant is well hydrated and well nourished.

II. Infant displays normal stool pattern.

III. Operative site remains free of infection.

IV. Family demonstrates an understanding of the condition and the ability to provide home care.

Hirschsprung's Disease (Megacolon)

Description

Hirschsprung's disease is a lack of normal peristalsis.

Pathophysiology

I. Lack of peristaltic movements due to absence of autonomic parasympathetic ganglion cells

II. Retention of stool

III. Distention of the bowel

Signs and Symptoms

I. Absence or small amount of stool in the newborn period

II. Anorexia

III. Abdominal distention and vomiting

IV. Constipation

V. Ribbon-like stool

VI. Inadequate weight gain in infancy

Therapeutic Management

I. Temporary colostomy

II. Bowel reconstruction (usually at 1 year of age)

Nursing Care (Operative)

DATA COLLECTION

I. Perform routine assessment.

II. Observe bowel pattern.

III. Assess general hydration and nutritional status.

IV. Assist with diagnostic procedures: radiography, rectal biopsy, anorectal manometry.

PLANNING

I. Safe, effective care environment

A. See Nursing Care of the Ill Child.

II. Physiological integrity

A. Provide nutrition and hydration.

B. Facilitate bowel movements.

III. Psychosocial integrity

A. Foster healthy parent-child relationships.

B. Prepare child and family for surgical procedure and postoperative colostomy care.

IV. Health promotion and maintenance

A. Prevent complications.

B. Prepare family for home care, including postoperative colostomy care.

IMPLEMENTATION

I. Preoperative

A. Maintain nasogastric suction.

B. Keep client on nothing by mouth (NPO) regimen.

C. Monitor IV therapy.

D. Administer enemas and laxatives as prescribed.

E. Administer antibiotics as prescribed.

II. Postoperative

A. Maintain nasogastric suction.

B. Avoid rectal temperatures.

C. Monitor IV therapy.

D. Provide colostomy care as prescribed.

E. Provide diet as prescribed.

F. Support family and teach colostomy or wound care or both as indicated.

EVALUATION

I. Child exhibits a normal bowel elimination pattern.

II. Child remains well nourished and well hydrated.

III. Child exhibits no evidence of infection.

IV. Family demonstrates an understanding of the disease and the ability to provide home care.

Celiac Disease

Description

Celiac disease is a malabsorption disease characterized by hypersensitivity to gluten.

Pathophysiology

I. Inability to digest wheat, barley, rye, and oats (gluten)

II. Accumulation of toxic substances in the gut

III. Inflammation and ulceration of intestinal mucosa

Signs and Symptoms

I. Age of onset: 1–5 years

II. Failure to thrive: malnutrition and hypocalcemia

III. Muscle wasting, especially of buttocks and extremities

IV. Diarrhea, acute or insidious; stools often pale and watery with odor

V. Some cases of vomiting and constipation

VI. Anemia; easy bruising and bleeding

VII. Irritability, uncooperativeness, apathy
VIII. Celiac crisis
    A. Precipitated by infection
    B. Prolonged fluid and electrolyte depletion
    C. Emotional disturbance

Therapeutic Management

    I. Dietary elimination of wheat, barley, rye, and oats
   II. Supplemental vitamins and minerals

Nursing Care

DATA COLLECTION

    I. Perform routine assessment.
   II. Pay particular attention to bowel elimination patterns, amount, color, and character.
  III. Assist with diagnostic procedures (such as stool collection, intestinal biopsy, gluten challenge).

PLANNING

    I. Safe, effective care environment
    A. See Nursing Care of the Ill Child.
    B. Promote an appropriate environment for age.
   II. Physiological integrity
    A. Implement and maintain gluten-free diet.
  III. Psychosocial integrity
    A. See Nursing Care of the Ill Child.
    B. Promote healthy parent-child relationship.
    C. Promote normal lifestyle and peer relationships.
  IV. Health promotion and maintenance
    A. Promote good health practices.
    B. Prepare family for home care.

IMPLEMENTATION

    I. Provide special gluten-free diet: eliminate barley, wheat, oats, and rye.
   II. Substitute offending grains with other grains: corn, rice, or soybean.
  III. Administer vitamin and mineral supplements as prescribed.
  IV. Teach family about the disease and its management.
   V. Teach family diet planning:
    A. Appropriate grain products
    B. Reading food labels for hidden presence of gluten, including gravies, hydrogenated vegetable protein, and vegetable protein added
    C. Introducing recipes that promote adherence to diet
  VI. Teach family signs of celiac crisis.
 VII. Reinforce explanations of the disease and therapies.
VIII. Encourage child to assume responsibility for diet adherence as early as possible.
  IX. Stress that gluten restriction is usually a lifelong necessity.

EVALUATION

    I. Child achieves age-appropriate weight and height.
   II. Child engages in activities appropriate to age.
  III. Family complies with prescribed diet.

Intussusception

Description

Intussusception is telescoping of a portion of the intestine into an adjacent portion.

Pathophysiology

    I. Most common site for telescoping is the ileocecal valve.
   II. Stopping passage of intestinal contents beyond the defect.
  III. Inflammation, edema, and decreased blood flow.
  IV. Stool contains primarily blood and mucus: the characteristic "currant-jelly" stool.
   V. Condition usually affects male infants between 3 and 6 months old.

Signs and Symptoms

    I. Sudden, intermittent, severe abdominal pain.
    A. Child screams and draws knees up to chest.
    B. Child appears comfortable between pain episodes.
   II. Vomitus is bile stained or contains stool.
  III. Loose, scant stools.
  IV. Passage of red currant-jelly–like stools, usually 12 hours after the onset of pain.
   V. Tender, distended, boardlike abdomen.

Therapeutic Management

    I. Nonsurgical: reduction by barium enema
   II. Surgical: reduction or resection

Nursing Care

DATA COLLECTION

    I. Perform routine assessment.
   II. Listen carefully to family's description of symptoms.
  III. Assess vomitus.
  IV. Assess stools.
   V. Assess patterns of pain and relief.
  VI. Assist with diagnostic procedure: radiography.

PLANNING

    I. Safe, effective care environment
    A. See Nursing Care of the Ill Child.
   II. Physiological integrity
    A. Prepare child for emergency therapeutic procedures.
    B. Observe child for complications (e.g., fever, dehydration, peritonitis).
  III. Psychosocial integrity
    A. Support child and family.
    B. Prepare child and family for procedures.
  IV. Health promotion and maintenance
    A. Promote and maintain optimum hydration and nutrition.
    B. Promote elimination.
    C. Prepare family for home care.

IMPLEMENTATION

    I. Monitor stooling pattern.
   II. Monitor vital signs and IV infusion.
  III. Maintain nasogastric suction, if used.

EVALUATION

I. Child exhibits normal stooling pattern.
II. Child is free of discomfort.
III. Family demonstrates an understanding of the condition and the ability to provide home care.

Diarrhea

Description

I. A noticeable or sudden increase in the number of or change in consistency of stools
II. Watery stools

Pathophysiology

I. Infection
II. Malabsorption syndromes
III. Loss of fluid and electrolytes

Signs and Symptoms

I. Mild diarrhea: few loose stools daily but no other symptoms
II. Moderate diarrhea: several loose or watery stools daily
III. Severe diarrhea: numerous stools to continuous stooling
IV. Accompanying signs
   A. Weight loss
   B. Dry skin and mucous membranes
   C. Decreased urine

Therapeutic Management

I. IV fluid therapy
II. Correction of electrolyte and acid-base imbalances
III. Elimination and/or correction of cause of diarrhea
IV. Prevention of spread of infection
V. Prevention of complications

Nursing Care

DATA COLLECTION

I. Perform routine assessment.
II. Observe stool pattern and consistency.
III. Assess (on admission and throughout care) weight and state of hydration.
IV. Assist with diagnostic procedures: laboratory tests of fluid and electrolyte status, acid-base balance; stool examination.
V. Test stools for pH, glucose, and blood, if prescribed.

PLANNING

I. Safe, effective care environment
   A. See Nursing Care of the Hospitalized Child.
   B. Prevent spread of diarrhea to others.
II. Physiological integrity
   A. Promote rehydration and maintain adequate hydration.
   B. Reestablish nutrition appropriate to age and condition.
   C. Prevent complications.

III. Psychosocial integrity
   A. See Nursing Care of the Hospitalized Child.
   B. Support and educate child and family.
   C. Prepare child and family for procedures.
IV. Health promotion and maintenance
   A. Promote optimum health.
   B. Prepare family for home care.

IMPLEMENTATION

I. Monitor IV fluid administration, if prescribed.
II. Feed oral rehydration fluids as prescribed.
III. Gradually reintroduce diet for age as indicated.
IV. Implement appropriate isolation precautions. Instruct family and others in their use.
V. Record color, consistency, and appearance of stool.
VI. Keep accurate I&O records.
VII. Measure and record weight.
VIII. Avoid rectal temperature measurements.
IX. Provide skin care, especially of anal, perineal, and buttock areas.
X. Provide for sucking needs with pacifier if NPO or if receiving limited oral fluids.
XI. Promote parent-child interaction.
XII. Teach family skills and procedures needed for home care.

EVALUATION

I. Child takes and retains prescribed oral fluids.
II. Child exhibits evidence of good hydration and satisfactory weight for age.
III. VSs remain within normal range for age.
IV. Child consumes adequate diet for age.
V. Child's skin exhibits no evidence of discoloration or irritation.
VI. Mucous membranes remain moist and clean.
VII. Family demonstrates an understanding of the condition and the ability to provide home care.

Pinworms

Description

Pinworms are an intestinal infestation with *Enterobius vermicularis,* the common pinworm.

Pathophysiology

I. Infection begins when eggs are inhaled or swallowed.
II. Eggs hatch in intestine and mature.
III. Female worms proceed to anal area and lay eggs.
IV. Movement of worms on skin and mucous membrane surfaces causes intense itching.
V. Eggs are deposited on hands and under fingernails during scratching, and child puts fingers in mouth, causing reinfection.

Signs and Symptoms

I. Intense perianal itching
II. Evidence of itching in young children
   A. General restlessness and irritability
   B. Sleep disturbances
   C. Bed-wetting

Therapeutic Management

I. Administration of mebendazole (Vermox) or pyrantel pamoate (Antiminth)

Nursing Care

DATA COLLECTION

I. Perform routine assessment.
II. Assist with diagnostic procedures: identify parasite. Specimens must be sent to laboratory while still warm.

PLANNING

I. Safe, effective care environment
   A. Prevent spread of infestation.
II. Physiological integrity
   A. Help to eradicate organisms.
III. Psychosocial integrity
   A. Support and educate child and family.
   B. Prepare child and family for collection of specimens and administration of medication.
IV. Health promotion and maintenance
   A. Promote optimum health.

IMPLEMENTATION

I. Explain or reinforce explanation of condition and therapies.
II. Collect specimens for examination.
   A. Construct loop of transparent tape, sticky side out, and place around the end of a tongue depressor.
   B. Apply to perianal region in morning as soon as child awakens and before a bowel movement or bath.
   C. Place in jar or plastic bag loosely.
III. Teach family to administer medication: single dose, followed in 2 weeks by second dose.
IV. Teach child and family preventive measures:
   A. Wash hands after toileting and before eating.
   B. Keep child's fingernails short.
   C. Bathe or shower daily.
   D. Discourage child from biting nails, placing fingers in mouth, and scratching anal area.
   E. Wash linen in hot water.
   F. Sanitize linen, underpants, and diapers in hot water.
V. Prevent spread by keeping toys separate and avoid shaking linen.

EVALUATION

I. Child exhibits no evidence of infestation.
II. Family demonstrates an understanding of the condition and the ability to perform home care.
III. Others exhibit no evidence of infestation.

Cardiovascular Disorders

Congenital Heart Disease

Description

Congenital heart disease is a defect in the heart resulting from developmental arrest or deviation during the prenatal period.

Pathophysiology

I. Acyanotic defects
   A. A narrowing of the pulmonary artery
   B. An opening that moves arterial blood into the venous system (left to right shunting)
II. Cyanotic defects
   A. Unoxygenated blood mixed with oxygenated blood in the systemic circulation
   B. Usually right-to-left shunting of blood through an abnormal opening and/or vessel configuration
III. Characteristics of major acyanotic defects
   A. Patent ductus arteriosus: failure of fetal ductus arteriosus to close completely after birth, increasing pulmonary circulation
   B. Coarctation of aorta: narrowing of the aorta, causing decreased circulation
   C. Atrial septal defect: abnormal opening between the right and left atria
   D. Ventricular septal defect: abnormal opening between the right and left ventricles (defect can vary in size from pinhole to complete absence of septum)
   E. Pulmonary stenosis: narrowing or stricture at the entrance to the pulmonary artery
   F. Aortic stenosis: narrowing or stricture of the aortic valve or the entrance to the aorta
IV. Characteristics of major cyanotic defects
   A. Tetralogy of Fallot: classic form consists of four defects:
      1. Ventricular septal defect
      2. Pulmonic stenosis
      3. Overriding aorta
      4. Right ventricular hypertrophy
   B. Transposition of the great vessels (arteries) (pulmonary artery leaves the left ventricle and the aorta exits from the right ventricle, with no blood flow between systemic and pulmonary circulations)

Signs and Symptoms

I. Infants
   A. Generalized cyanosis
   B. Cyanosis during exertion, especially crying, feeding, straining
   C. Dyspnea, especially following physical effort
   D. Fatigue (with eating)
   E. Failure to thrive
   F. Tachypnea
II. Older children
   A. Small for age
   B. Delicate, frail body
   C. Fatigue
   D. Dyspnea with exercise
   E. Clubbed fingers (cyanotic defects)
   F. Squatting for relief of dyspnea (cyanotic defects)
III. Other possible observations
   A. Bounding pulse
   B. Murmur
   C. Thrill
   D. Tachycardia
   E. Difference in pulse between upper and lower extremities (coarctation of the aorta)

Therapeutic Management

I. Medical
   A. Improve circulatory effort:
      1. Digitalis administration
   B. Remove and prevent excess fluid retention:
      1. Low-sodium diet (formula)
      2. Diuretic administration
   C. Prevent complications:
      1. Supplemental vitamin administration
      2. Supplemental iron administration
      3. Potassium chloride administration
II. Surgical
   A. Cardiac catheterization to establish diagnosis
   B. Surgical correction appropriate to the specific defect
   C. Relief of symptoms until surgical correction can be accomplished

Nursing Care

DATA COLLECTION

I. Perform routine assessment, with particular attention to the following:
   A. Assess rate and quality of pulses.
   B. Measure blood pressure.
   C. Observe for cyanosis, dyspnea, and clubbing of fingers.
   D. Listen for murmurs.
II. Take careful health history, especially relative to:
   A. Weight gain
   B. Feeding behavior
   C. Exercise intolerance
   D. Frequency of infection
   E. Unusual posturing (squatting, assuming knee-chest position)
III. Assist with diagnostic procedures: electrocardiography (ECG), radiography, sonography, echocardiography, cardiac catheterization.

PLANNING

I. Safe, effective care environment
   A. See Nursing Care of the Ill Child.
   B. Promote environment appropriate for age.
II. Physiological integrity
   A. Decrease energy output.
   B. Improve circulatory effort.
   C. Prevent complications (e.g., excess fluid retention, congestive heart failure [CHF], URI).
III. Psychosocial integrity
   A. See Nursing Care of the Ill Child.
   B. Assist child and family to cope with the condition.
   C. Support and educate child and family.
   D. Prepare child and family for procedures or surgery.
   E. Promote as normal a lifestyle as possible.
IV. Health promotion and maintenance
   A. Promote optimum health.
   B. Maintain optimum fluid and nutrition.
   C. Prepare family for home care.

IMPLEMENTATION

I. Limit physical activity.
II. Feed slowly.
III. Allow for frequent rest periods; schedule nursing activities to minimize disturbance of rest.
IV. Help child and family select activities appropriate to the condition.
V. Monitor I&O.
VI. Avoid extremes of temperature.
VII. Administer drugs as prescribed: digoxin (Lanoxin), iron preparation, diuretic, potassium chloride.
VIII. Administer oxygen as prescribed.
IX. Administer oral and IV fluids as prescribed.
X. Feed low-salt formula, if prescribed.
XI. Protect child from contact with persons with infections.
XII. Explain or reinforce explanation of condition and therapies.
XIII. Teach family skills and procedures needed for home care, including expected results of medications and their possible side effects.
XIV. See Nursing Care of the Ill Child.

EVALUATION

I. Child rests quietly and breathes easily.
II. Child's VSs are within acceptable limits.
III. Child consumes enough fluid and food for age.
IV. Child achieves normal growth for age.
V. Child exhibits no evidence of infection.
VI. Family demonstrates an understanding of the condition and therapies and the ability to provide home care.

Rheumatic Fever

Description

Rheumatic fever is an inflammatory disease affecting the heart, joints, central nervous system (CNS), and subcutaneous tissue.

Pathophysiology

I. Occurs after an infection with group A β-hemolytic streptococcus
II. Believed to occur as an autoimmune response
III. Characterized by inflammatory reaction of heart, joints, and skin
IV. Characterized by edema of involved tissues

Signs and Symptoms

I. Diagnosis based on Jones' criteria
II. Major manifestations
   A. Carditis: tachycardia, cardiomegaly, murmur
   B. Polyarthritis: migratory swollen, hot, red, painful joints
   C. Chorea: sudden aimless, irregular movements of extremities, involuntary facial grimaces, speech disturbances
   D. Subcutaneous nodes: nontender swelling located over bony parts
   E. Erythema marginatum: transitory, nonitching rash
III. Minor manifestations
   A. Fever: low-grade
   B. Arthralgia without arthritic changes
   C. History of previous rheumatic fever or rheumatic heart disease
   D. Increased erythrocyte sedimentation rate (ESR)

E. C-reactive protein (CRP)
F. Leukocytosis
G. Anemia
H. Prolonged PR interval on electrocardiogram (ECG)
I. Elevated antistreptolysin-O titer

Therapeutic Management

I. Treatment of group A β-hemolytic streptococci with penicillin
II. Prevention of permanent cardiac damage
   A. Bed rest during acute phase
   B. Corticosteroids to decrease inflammation
III. Supportive care for other symptoms
   A. Anti-inflammatory agents to suppress joint inflammation
   B. Mild sedation to decrease anxiety and restlessness caused by chorea
   C. Acetaminophen to relieve discomfort
IV. Prevention of further infections with long-term penicillin

Nursing Care

DATA COLLECTION

I. Perform routine assessment.
II. Take history of infections in the last 2 weeks.
III. Assist with diagnostic procedures: ECG, laboratory tests.

PLANNING

I. Safe, effective care environment
   A. See Nursing Care of the Ill Child.
   B. Provide appropriate environment for age.
II. Physiological integrity
   A. Help to eradicate organism.
   B. Alleviate symptoms.
   C. Prevent complications.
III. Psychosocial integrity
   A. See Nursing Care of the Ill Child.
   B. Support and educate child and family.
   C. Prepare child and family for procedures, surgery as needed.
   D. Promote child and primary caregiver interaction.
IV. Health promotion and maintenance
   A. Maintain and promote optimum health.
   B. Prepare family for home care.

IMPLEMENTATION

I. Administer penicillin or other antibiotic as prescribed.
II. Administer corticosteroids, anti-inflammatory drugs, analgesics, and sedatives as prescribed.
III. Help family cope with child's enforced limited activity, if prescribed.
IV. Teach family skills and procedures needed for home care, including expected results of medications and their possible side effects.
V. Teach the importance of long-term penicillin therapy.

EVALUATION

I. Child exhibits no evidence of cardiac problems.
II. Child exhibits no rash or swollen nodes and moves joints without pain.
III. Child displays no evidence of streptococcal infection.
IV. Child is able to exercise without fatigue.

Kawasaki Disease

Description

Kawasaki disease (KD) is a systemic vasculitis that usually affects children younger than 5 years of age. The cause is unknown.

Pathophysiology

I. Inflammation develops in small vessels (capillaries, venules, arterioles), progressing to medium-size blood vessels.
II. Pericarditis
III. Aneurysms may develop because of damage to vascular wall.
IV. Vessel walls can be damaged, resulting in scarring, calcification, and stenosis.
V. Thrombus formation can occur.

Signs and Symptoms

I. Acute phase
   A. Irritable, inconsolable child with high fever unresponsive to antipyretics.
   B. Conjunctiva becomes reddened and eyes are dry.
   C. Inflammation of pharynx and oral mucosa.
   D. Strawberry tongue with dryness of lips.
   E. Rash is variable, often affecting perineum.
   F. Lymphadenopathy.
   G. Edematous extremities with erythema of palms of hands and soles of feet.
   H. Decrease in left ventricle function, and ECG changes associated with myositis.
   I. Symptoms of congested heart failure.
II. Subacute phase
   A. Fever subsided, but irritability present.
   B. Clinical symptoms resolving.
   C. Changes in echocardiogram.
   D. Periungual desquamation.
   E. Arthritis can persist into this phase.
   F. Chances of thrombocytosis increase.
   G. Cardiac involvement indicating myocardial infarction (abdominal pain, vomiting, restlessness, inconsolable crying, pallor, and shock).
III. Convalescent phase
   A. Clinical symptoms subsided.
   B. Sedimentation rate increases.
   C. Thrombocytosis may be apparent, and coronary complications are still of concern.
   D. Arthritis can still be present.

Therapeutic Management

I. High dose of IV gamma globulin
II. Salicylate therapy
III. Coumadin when large aneurysms are present.

Nursing Care

DATA COLLECTION

I. Perform routine assessment.
II. Monitor cardiac status (CHF, tachycardia, and respiratory distress).

III. I&O with daily weights. Watch for dehydration.
IV. Assist with ECG and echocardiogram.

PLANNING

I. Safe, effective care environment
   A. Provide environment appropriate for age.
   B. Provide environment for convalescence.
II. Physiological integrity
   A. Promote hydration status.
   B. Prevent complications (CHF, respiratory distress, dehydration, myocardial infarction).
III. Psychosocial integrity
   A. Promote child-parent bonding.
   B. Support and educate the family.
   C. Prepare the child and family for procedures.
IV. Health promotion and maintenance
   A. Promote optimum health.
   B. Prepare family for home care.

IMPLEMENTATION

I. Monitor cardiac status.
II. Monitor I&O along with daily weights.
III. Monitor IV fluids carefully because of the increased chances of CHF.
IV. Monitor infusion of gamma globulin.
V. Advise to dress in cool, loose clothing.
VI. Administer acetaminophen for fever.
VII. Provide good oral hygiene with lubricant for lips.
VIII. Perform range-of-motion (ROM) exercises to prevent stiffness of joints with arthritis. Bath time is an appropriate time for this.
IX. Provide quiet environment to help console child.
X. Teach family skills needed for home care.

EVALUATION

II. Family understands signs and symptoms that require medical attention.
III. Family demonstrates an understanding of the disease and the ability to provide home care.

Hematopoietic Disorders

Leukemia

Description

Leukemia is cancer of the blood-forming tissues.

Pathophysiology

I. Abnormal increase of immature WBCs prevents production and development of normal blood cells in bone marrow.
II. Abnormal WBCs invade tissue and cause symptoms.
III. Symptoms depend on the area of the body invaded by leukemia cells.

Signs and Symptoms

I. Pallor, easy fatigability
II. Susceptibility to infections
III. Easy bruising and bleeding
IV. Bone pain and fractures
V. Enlarged liver, spleen, lymph glands
VI. Headache
VII. Nausea and vomiting
VIII. Irritability
IX. Anorexia and weight loss

Therapeutic Management

I. Achieve and maintain remission.
II. Administer antimetabolites and immunosuppressants.
III. Prevent complications of chemotherapy.
   A. Prevent infection with protective isolation or other appropriate precautions.
IV. Replace blood elements.
V. Relieve pain.

Nursing Care

DATA COLLECTION

I. Perform routine assessment.
II. Assist with diagnostic tests (e.g., blood counts, lumbar puncture, bone marrow aspiration, biopsy).
III. Observe for signs of complications (e.g., bleeding, ulceration, CNS symptoms).
IV. Assess family's coping capabilities and support systems.

PLANNING

I. Safe, effective care environment
   A. See Nursing Care of the Ill Child.
   B. Prevent transfer of infection to the child.
   C. Prevent trauma that might cause bleeding.
II. Physiological integrity
   A. Help to achieve a remission.
   B. Relieve pain.
   C. Alleviate symptoms.
III. Psychosocial integrity
   A. See Nursing Care of the Ill Child.
   B. Educate child and family.
   C. Help child and family to cope with effects of the disease and its therapies.
   D. Prepare child and family for procedures and therapies.
IV. Health promotion and maintenance
   A. Promote optimum health.
   B. Achieve and maintain optimum fluid and nutrition.
   C. Prepare family for home care.

IMPLEMENTATION

I. Implement and maintain protective isolation.
II. Administer antimetabolites and immunosuppressive agents as prescribed.
III. Administer blood products as prescribed.
IV. Administer analgesics as prescribed.
V. Provide frequent oral hygiene with soft toothbrushes or swabs.
VI. Use minimal and gentle physical manipulation.
VII. Avoid taking rectal temperatures.
VIII. Administer antiemetic for nausea as prescribed.
IX. Provide meticulous, nontraumatic skin care.
X. Change position frequently.
XI. Promote rest; encourage frequent rest periods.
XII. Stimulate appetite with attractive meals and foods of child's choice; provide nutritious supplements.

XIII. Encourage family to be with the child at meal times.
XIV. Teach family skills and procedures needed for home care.

EVALUATION

I. Child attains and maintains a remission.
II. Child appears comfortable and verbalizes no complaints of pain.
III. Child eats an adequate amount of appropriate foods.
IV. Child exhibits no evidence of infection, bleeding, or other complications.
V. Child appears rested and engages in appropriate activities.
VI. Child and family cope with effects of therapies.
VII. Family demonstrates an understanding of the disease, the consequences of therapies, and the ability to provide home care.

Sickle Cell Disease

Description

Sickle cell disease is a genetically transmitted disease in which normal adult hemoglobin (HbA) is partly or completely replaced by hemoglobin S (HbS).

Pathophysiology

I. HbS transmitted as an autosomal dominant gene but displaying an autosomal recessive inheritance pattern
II. Disease occurring primarily in blacks or persons of Mediterranean ancestry
III. Rigid crescent or sickle shape assumed by RBCs when oxygen released to tissues (HbS has decreased oxygen-carrying capacity and short life span or increased destruction rate)

Signs and Symptoms

I. Growth retardation and delayed puberty
II. Chronic anemia
III. Marked susceptibility to infection
IV. Vaso-occlusive crisis (sickle cell crisis)
  A. Pain in involved areas
  B. Extremities: painful swelling of hands, feet, joints; ulceration
  C. Abdomen: severe abdominal pain
  D. Chest: pain, pulmonary disease
  E. Liver: jaundice, hepatomegaly
  F. Kidney: hematuria
V. Laboratory evidence of disease
  A. Presence of HbS in blood
  B. Hemoglobin electrophoresis identifies type and extent of abnormal hemoglobin

Therapeutic Management

I. Identify presence of HbS.
II. Prevent sickling phenomenon: promote adequate oxygenation and maintain hemodilution.
III. Treat sickle cell crisis:

A. Bed rest to minimize oxygen use
B. Oral or IV fluids
C. Electrolyte replacement
D. Administration of analgesics for pain relief
E. Blood replacement for anemia; exchange transfusion in selected cases
F. Antibiotics to treat existing infections
G. Short-term oxygen therapy for severe anoxia
IV. Perform splenectomy for recurrent pooling of blood in the organ (sequestration).

Nursing Care

DATA COLLECTION

I. Perform routine assessment.
II. Assist with screening or diagnostic tests or both: Sickledex, electrophoresis, blood count.
III. Assist in diagnostic testing to assess effects of complications: radiography, tomography, renal function tests, liver function tests.

PLANNING

I. Safe, effective care environment
  A. See Nursing Care of the Ill Child.
II. Physiological integrity
  A. Relieve pain (crisis).
  B. Promote adequate fluid intake.
  C. Prevent complications.
III. Psychosocial integrity
  A. See Nursing Care of the Ill Child.
  B. Support and educate child and family.
  C. Prepare child and family for procedures, surgery as needed.
IV. Health promotion and maintenance
  A. Prevent sickling crisis.
  B. Promote optimum health.
  C. Prepare family for home care.

IMPLEMENTATION

I. Administer oxygen, if ordered.
II. Administer analgesics as prescribed for pain.
III. Provide warmth to affected areas.
IV. Encourage ample oral fluids; force fluids, if needed; monitor IV infusion, if present.
V. Teach family skills and procedures needed for home care.
VI. Emphasize need for medical attention for infections.

EVALUATION

I. Child does not suffer a sickle cell crisis (i.e., should be free of pain or other symptoms).
II. Child is well hydrated.
III. Child exhibits no evidence of infection.
IV. Family demonstrates an understanding of the disease and the ability to provide home care.
V. Family seeks genetic counseling.

Hemophilia

Description

Hemophilia comprises a group of bleeding disorders in which one of the factors needed for clotting of blood is deficient.

I. Hemophilia A: deficiency of factor VIII (antihemophilic factor; antihemophilic globulin)
II. Hemophilia B (Christmas disease): deficiency of factor IX

Pathophysiology

I. Transmitted by X-linked recessive inheritance pattern
II. Inability of blood to clot
III. Bleeding into tissues possible anywhere

Signs and Symptoms

I. Prolonged bleeding anywhere from or in the body
II. Prolonged bleeding from trauma (e.g., umbilical cord, circumcision, cuts, loss of teeth, nosebleed, injection, surgery)
III. Excessive bruising, even from slight injury

Therapeutic Management

I. Replace missing blood factor with one of the following:
   A. Factor VIII concentrate
   B. Cryoprecipitate
   C. Fresh frozen plasma
II. Prevent chronic crippling effects of joint bleeding:
   A. Corticosteroids or nonsteroid anti-inflammatory agents (or both), to reduce inflammation
   B. Cold compresses applied to joint
III. Administer ibuprofen for discomfort as prescribed.
IV. Identify persons at risk for the disorder.

Nursing Care

DATA COLLECTION

I. Perform routine assessment.
II. Take careful histories:
   A. Health history for evidence of previous bleeding episodes, and present problem
   B. Family history for evidence of other affected members

PLANNING

I. Safe, effective care environment
   A. See Nursing Care of the Ill Child.
   B. Prevent trauma.
II. Physiological integrity
   A. Relieve discomfort.
   B. Prevent and control bleeding episodes.
   C. Prevent crippling effects of bleeding into joints.
III. Psychosocial integrity
   A. See Nursing Care of the Ill Child.
   B. Support and educate child and family.
   C. Prepare child and family for procedures, surgery as needed.
IV. Health promotion and maintenance
   A. Maintain and promote optimum health.
   B. Prepare family for home care.
   C. Promote self-management of therapies.

IMPLEMENTATION

I. Administer clotting factor as prescribed.
II. Administer ibuprofen as prescribed for pain.
III. Prevent trauma.

A. Prevent falling and impact injuries.
B. Alter environment to reduce injury, especially in toddlers (carpeted floors, padded furniture).
C. Encourage use of soft toothbrush.
IV. Control or decrease local bleeding.
   A. Immobilize and elevate affected part.
   B. Apply pressure for 10–15 minutes.
   C. Apply cold to promote vasoconstriction.
V. Prevent crippling effects.
   A. Apply splints as prescribed.
   B. Encourage or perform passive ROM exercises.
VI. Teach family (including the child) skills and procedures needed for home care, especially administration of clotting factor.
VII. Encourage child to assume responsibility for own care.

EVALUATION

I. Child exhibits no evidence of bleeding.
II. Child exhibits no evidence of tissue damage.
III. Family demonstrates an understanding of the disease and the ability to provide home care.
IV. Family seeks genetic counseling.

Idiopathic Thrombocytopenic Purpura

Description

Idiopathic thrombocytopenic purpura (ITP) is an acquired hemorrhagic disorder characterized by a marked decrease in the number of platelets.

Pathophysiology

I. Involves excessive destruction of platelets
II. Interferes with blood clotting
III. Causes easy bleeding, particularly noted beneath the skin

Signs and Symptoms

I. Occurs in children 2–8 years of age
II. Most commonly seen after upper respiratory infections or childhood communicable diseases
III. Makes child prone to easy bruising: evidenced as petechiae, ecchymoses
IV. Results in bleeding from mucous membranes
   A. Epistaxis
   B. Bleeding gums
   C. Hematuria
   D. Hematemesis

Therapeutic Management

I. Restriction of child's activity at onset and if bleeding is active
II. Administration of corticosteroids for children at highest risk for serious bleeding
III. Administration of packed red cells for blood loss
IV. Administration of gamma globulin to increase platelet count (in chronic ITP)
V. Splenectomy in selected cases

Nursing Care

DATA COLLECTION

I. Perform routine assessment.
II. Assist with diagnostic tests.

PLANNING

I. Safe, effective care environment
   A. See Nursing Care of the Ill Child.
II. Physiological integrity
   A. Prevent and/or control bleeding.
   B. Prevent complications.
III. Psychosocial integrity
   A. See Nursing Care of the Ill Child.
   B. Support and educate child and family.
   C. Prepare child and family for procedures, surgery as needed.
IV. Health promotion and maintenance
   A. Promote optimum health.
   B. Prepare family for home care.

IMPLEMENTATION

I. Administer corticosteroids as prescribed.
II. Implement measures to prevent bleeding (see Hemophilia).
III. Administer nonsalicylate preparations for discomfort.
IV. Teach family skills and procedures needed for home care.

EVALUATION

I. Child exhibits no evidence of bleeding.
II. Family demonstrates an understanding of the condition and the ability to provide home care.

Endocrine Disorders

Diabetes Mellitus

Description

Diabetes mellitus is a disease of metabolism characterized by a deficiency of the hormone insulin.
   I. Insulin-dependent diabetes mellitus or type I diabetes: onset typically in childhood and adolescence
   II. Maturity-onset diabetes of youth or type II diabetes: decrease in the amount of needed insulin

Pathophysiology

I. Inadequate insulin for metabolism of carbohydrates, fats, and proteins
II. Inadequate glucose to fuel body needs; proteins and fats broken down
III. Blood glucose concentration increased, spilling over in urine
IV. Increased fluid and electrolytes lost in diuresis

Signs and Symptoms

I. Three "polys"
   A. Polyphagia
   B. Polyuria
   C. Polydipsia
II. Weight loss
III. Fatigue
IV. Hyperglycemia
V. Possible diabetic ketoacidosis
   A. Ketones as well as glucose in urine
   B. Dehydration
   C. Vomiting
   D. Electrolyte imbalance
   E. Metabolic acidosis
   F. Abdominal pain
   G. Fruity acetone breath
   H. Drowsiness progressing to coma

Therapeutic Management

I. Insulin replacement
II. Exercise
III. Nutritional intake that:
   A. Provides sufficient calories to balance daily expenditure of energy
   B. Satisfies requirements for growth and development
   C. Contains no concentrated sugars
IV. Management of hypoglycemia, illness, ketoacidosis
V. Promotion of adherence to regimen and self-management of disease

Nursing Care

DATA COLLECTION

I. Perform routine assessment.
II. Assist with diagnostic tests (e.g., fasting blood sugar, chemical strips, ketones, glucose tolerance).

PLANNING

I. Safe, effective care environment
   A. See Nursing Care of the Ill Child.
   B. Monitor blood sugar regularly.
II. Physiological integrity
   A. Promote regular monitoring of blood sugar and insulin intake.
   B. Promote careful balancing of nutrition and exercise.
   C. Prevent complications.
III. Psychosocial integrity
   A. Support and educate family and child.
   B. Encourage regular activities to prevent child from becoming emotionally crippled.
IV. Health promotion and maintenance
   A. Promote optimum health.
   B. Prepare family for home care.

IMPLEMENTATION

I. Monitor blood sugar regularly.
II. Keep accurate records of food intake and exercise.
III. Monitor for signs of hypoglycemia and hyperglycemia.
IV. Administer insulin as prescribed.
V. Teach family and child to check blood sugar and monitor food intake and exercise.
VI. Teach family and child to give injections.

VII. Teach family and child to regulate insulin intake according to food intake and exercise.

EVALUATION

I. Child has no episodes of hyperglycemia or hypoglycemia.
II. Child participates in normal childhood activities.
III. Family and child demonstrate ability to prepare medications and to give injections safely.
IV. Family and child demonstrate the ability to regulate diet.
V. Family and child demonstrate ability to modify insulin intake to match food and exercise.

Hypothyroidism (Congenital)

Description

Congenital hypothyroidism is a deficiency in secretion of thyroid hormones.

Pathophysiology

I. Deficiency of thyroid hormones causing retardation in growth and development

Signs and Symptoms

I. Infancy
   A. Cool, dry, mottled skin
   B. Coarse, sparse hair
   C. Enlarged tongue
   D. Hoarse cry
   E. Diminished activity
   F. Difficulty feeding
II. Childhood
   A. Continuous constipation
   B. Growth retardation
   C. Mental retardation

Therapeutic Management

I. Administer thyroid hormone.

Nursing Care

DATA COLLECTION

I. Perform routine assessment.
II. Assist with diagnostic procedures: thyroid hormone tests.

PLANNING

I. Safe, effective care environment
   A. See Nursing Care of the Ill Child.
II. Physiological integrity
   A. Prevent complications.
III. Psychosocial integrity
   A. See Nursing Care of the Ill Child.
   B. Support and educate child and family.
   C. Prepare child and family for procedures or surgery, if needed.

IV. Health promotion and maintenance
   A. Promote optimum health.
   B. Prepare family for home care.

IMPLEMENTATION

I. Explain or reinforce explanation of disease and therapies.
II. Teach family administration of thyroid hormone.

EVALUATION

I. Child displays normal growth and development.
II. Family demonstrates an understanding of the disease and the ability to provide home care.

Genitourinary Disorders

Urinary Tract Infection

Description

Urinary tract infection is an infection of any portion of the urinary tract and includes urethritis, cystitis, ureteritis, pyelonephritis.

Pathophysiology

I. Bacterial invasion of urinary structures, usually confined to the bladder but possibly ascending to upper collecting system and kidney, where it produces inflammatory changes, with scarring and loss of renal tissue

Signs and Symptoms

I. Children <2 years old
   A. Fever of abrupt onset
   B. Poor feeding
   C. Vomiting
   D. Diarrhea
   E. Abdominal distention
   F. Frequent or infrequent voiding
   G. Constant squirming
   H. Strong-smelling urine
   I. Diaper rash
II. Children >2 years old
   A. Bed-wetting
   B. Daytime incontinence (toilet-trained child)
   C. Fever and chills
   D. Strong or foul-smelling urine
   E. Increased frequency of urination
   F. Localized sharp or dull pain
   G. Urgency
   H. Abdominal pain
   I. Flank pain
   J. Bloody urine
   K. Vomiting (in preschool children)

Therapeutic Management

I. Treat with antibacterial preparations (systemic penicillins, sulfonamides).
II. Detect or correct anatomic abnormalities.

III. Prevent recurrences.
IV. Preserve renal function.

Nursing Care

DATA COLLECTION

I. Perform routine assessment.
II. Observe elimination behaviors, including amount and character of urine output.
III. Assist with diagnostic procedures: urinalysis, IV pyelography, cystoscopy, cystourethrography, ultrasonography.

PLANNING

I. Safe, effective care environment
  A. See Nursing Care of the Ill Child.
II. Physiological integrity
  A. Help to eradicate organisms.
  B. Prevent complications.
III. Psychosocial integrity
  A. See Nursing Care of the Ill Child.
  B. Support and educate child and family.
  C. Prepare child and family for procedures.
IV. Health promotion and maintenance
  A. Promote optimum health.
  B. Achieve and maintain optimum hydration.
  C. Prevent recurrence.
  D. Prepare family for home care.

IMPLEMENTATION

I. Administer antibacterial medications as prescribed.
II. Teach child and family preventive hygiene habits (e.g., wipe genitals from front to back, avoid tight-fitting clothing in genital area).
III. Encourage adequate fluid intake.
IV. Explain procedures needed for diagnosis and evaluation.
V. Teach family skills and procedures needed for home care, including expected results of medication and possible side effects.

EVALUATION

I. Child exhibits no evidence of infection.
II. Child and family demonstrate good hygienic practices.
III. Family demonstrates an understanding of the disease and the ability to provide home care.

Nephrotic Syndrome

Description

Nephrotic syndrome is a chronic renal disease.

Pathophysiology

I. Protein leakage into urine (proteinuria)
II. Fluid accumulation in tissues
III. Reduced renal blood flow

Signs and Symptoms

I. Weight gain
II. Edema

  A. Puffiness around eyes
  B. Abdominal swelling
III. Diarrhea
IV. Anorexia
V. Normal or slightly decreased blood pressure
VI. Increased susceptibility to infection
VII. Easy fatigability
VIII. Urine
  A. Decreased
  B. Frothy
  C. Darkly opalescent

Therapeutic Management

I. Activity as tolerated
II. Salt restriction (during edematous stage)
III. Fluid restriction, if severe edema present
IV. Corticosteroids (prednisone)
V. Immunosuppressive agents in severe cases (cyclophosphamide)
VI. Prevention of infection with prophylactic antibiotics (sometimes)

Nursing Care

DATA COLLECTION

I. Perform routine assessment.
II. Observe amount and character of urine.
III. Assess edema: measure I&O, specific gravity of urine; weight; abdominal girth.
IV. Assess pulse and blood pressure.
V. Assist with diagnostic procedures: urinalysis, serum protein measurements, renal biopsy (sometimes).

PLANNING

I. Safe, effective care environment
  A. See Nursing Care of the Ill Child.
  B. Prevent infection.
II. Physiological integrity
  A. Decrease urinary protein output.
  B. Prevent complications.
  C. Conserve energy.
III. Psychosocial integrity
  A. See Nursing Care of the Ill Child.
  B. Support and educate child and family.
  C. Prepare child and family for procedures, surgery as needed.
IV. Health promotion and maintenance
  A. Promote optimum health.
  B. Achieve and maintain optimum fluid and nutrition.
  C. Prepare family for home care.

IMPLEMENTATION

I. Practice careful medical asepsis.
II. Avoid contact with infected persons or items.
III. Administer corticosteroids, immunosuppressive agents, and antibiotics as prescribed.
IV. Administer drugs orally or IV, but never intramuscularly or subcutaneously.
V. Provide good skin care, especially in skinfolds of edematous areas (powder).

VI. Change child's position frequently.
VII. Promote quiet activities.
VIII. Provide high-protein diet, appropriate for age, and snacks to encourage eating.
    A. Use no added salt and discourage salty foods (e.g., potato chips).
    B. Fluids may be restricted to control edema.
IX. Weigh daily, with same clothes and at same time of day.
X. Accurately record I&O.
XI. Teach family skills and procedures needed for home care, including expected results of medication and possible side effects.

EVALUATION

I. Child exhibits no evidence of edema.
II. Child achieves normal urinary output.
III. Child exhibits no evidence of infection or skin breakdown.
IV. Child engages in activities appropriate to age and condition.
V. Family demonstrates an understanding of the disease and the ability to provide home care.

Acute Poststreptococcal Glomerulonephritis

Description

Acute poststreptococcal glomerulonephritis is an inflammation of the renal glomeruli after a streptococcal infection.

Pathophysiology

I. Reaction of renal tissues to group A β-hemolytic streptococci
II. Retention of water and sodium

Signs and Symptoms

I. Edema, especially periorbital
II. Anorexia
III. Hematuria
IV. Pallor
V. Irritability
VI. Lethargy
VII. Ill appearance
VIII. Headache
IX. Abdominal or flank pain
X. Dysuria
XI. Vomiting
XII. Mild to moderately elevated blood pressure
XIII. Urine
    A. Severely reduced volume
    B. Cloudy appearance
    C. Smoky brown color
XIV. Hematological tests
    A. Elevated antistreptolysin-O titer, ESR, CRP

Therapeutic Management

I. Restricted activity during acute phase
II. Regular diet with sodium restricted according to severity of symptoms
III. Dietary potassium restricted during periods of decreased urinary output
IV. Antibiotics
V. Antihypertensives

Nursing Care

DATA COLLECTION

I. Perform routine assessment.
II. Take health history for evidence of recent streptococcal infection.
III. Monitor vital signs and weight.
IV. Assess for signs of cerebral edema.
V. Carefully measure I&O.
VI. Observe character of urine.
VII. Assist with diagnostic procedures: urinalysis, blood count, throat culture, serological tests (e.g., ESR, CRP), streptozyme titer test, and antistreptolysin titer test.

PLANNING

I. Safe, effective care environment
    A. See Nursing Care of the Ill Child.
    B. Promote rest.
II. Physiological integrity
    A. Provide appropriate diet and promote appetite.
    B. Prevent and observe for complications.
III. Psychosocial integrity
    A. See Nursing Care of the Ill Child.
    B. Support and educate child and family.
    C. Prepare child and family for procedures, surgery as needed.
IV. Health promotion and maintenance
    A. Promote optimum health.
    B. Prepare family for home care.

IMPLEMENTATION

I. Encourage frequent rest periods.
II. Provide and encourage quiet activities.
III. Administer antibiotics and antihypertensives as prescribed.
IV. Use no added salt at meals; discourage highly salted foods (e.g., potato chips, salted nuts).
V. Provide low-potassium diet, if prescribed.
VI. Separate from other children with infections.
VII. Teach home care, including expected results of medication and possible side effects.

EVALUATION

I. Child plays quietly and rests as needed.
II. Child eats appropriate diet.
III. Child remains free of complications.
IV. Family demonstrates an understanding of the condition and the ability to provide home care.

Cryptorchism

Description

Cryptorchism is a failure of one or both testes to descend normally into the scrotum.

Pathophysiology

I. Descent can be arrested at any point along the inguinal canal.
II. Condition is usually unilateral and associated with inguinal hernia.
III. Usual course is spontaneous descent within a year.

Signs and Symptoms

I. Rarely a cause of discomfort
II. Empty scrotum: unilateral or bilateral
III. Testes palpable if within the inguinal canal

Therapeutic Management

I. Medical: human gonadotropin administration after 1 year of age
II. Surgical: orchiopexy before 3 years of age

Nursing Care

DATA COLLECTION

I. Perform routine assessment.

PLANNING

I. Safe, effective care environment
   A. See Nursing Care of the Ill Child.
II. Physiological integrity
   A. Prevent complications.
III. Psychosocial integrity
   A. See Nursing Care of the Ill Child.
   B. Promote a positive body image.
   C. Support and educate child and family.
   D. Prepare child and family for surgery.
IV. Health promotion and maintenance
   A. Promote optimum health.
   B. Prepare family for home care.

IMPLEMENTATION

I. Provide clean wound care.
II. Present positive feedback to child and family.
III. Teach family skills and procedures needed for home care.

EVALUATION

I. Family seeks early evaluation and therapy.
II. Family demonstrates an understanding of the condition and the ability to provide home care.
III. Child exhibits no evidence of infection.
IV. Child displays a positive body image.

Wilms' Tumor

Description

Wilms' tumor is a malignant neoplasm of the kidney.

Pathophysiology

I. Develops from abnormal embryonic tissue usually by age 3 years

II. Starts in renal capsule and grows into the surrounding tissues

Signs and Symptoms

I. Abdomen that becomes large
II. Firm, nontender abdominal mass
III. Symptoms related to pressure of tumor on tissues
   A. Constipation
   B. Vomiting
   C. Difficult breathing

Therapeutic Management

I. Surgical removal of tumor
II. Chemotherapy and sometimes radiation to treat disease and to minimize metastasis

Nursing Care

DATA COLLECTION

I. Perform routine assessment.
II. Assist with diagnostic procedures (e.g., tomography, IV pyelography, ultrasound, biochemical and hematological studies, urinalysis).

PLANNING

I. Safe, effective care environment
   A. See Nursing Care of the Ill Child.
   B. Avoid touching abdomen and tumor before surgery.
II. Physiological integrity
   A. Prevent complications.
   B. Assist with chemotherapy and radiation.
III. Psychosocial integrity
   A. See Nursing Care of the Ill Child.
   B. Support and educate child and family.
   C. Prepare child and family for procedures, surgery as needed.
IV. Health promotion and maintenance
   A. Promote optimum health.

IMPLEMENTATION

I. Avoid palpating abdomen after diagnosis is suspected or confirmed.
II. Administer antimetabolites as prescribed.
III. Provide support to family and encourage expression of feelings regarding a child with a life-threatening disorder.
IV. Educate family regarding observations for symptoms of side effects of chemotherapy or radiotherapy.
V. Teach family skills and procedures needed for home care.

EVALUATION

I. Child displays no ill effects of therapies.
II. Child does not exhibit signs of metastasis.
III. Caregiver ensures that child has uneventful recovery from surgery.
IV. Family members express their feelings and concerns.
V. Family demonstrates an understanding of the condition and the ability to provide home care.

Neurological Disorders

Myelomeningocele (Infant)

Description

I. Spina bifida: defect in closure of vertebral column, with varying degrees of tissue protrusion through vertebral opening
II. Spina bifida occulta: failure of complete closure of the vertebral column with no outpouching
III. Meningocele: hernial protrusion of saclike cyst of meninges containing spinal fluid
IV. Myelomeningocele: hernial protrusion of a saclike cyst containing meninges, spinal fluid, and a portion of the spinal cord with its nerves

Pathophysiology

I. Degree of neurological damage dependent on extent and location of the outpouching.
II. Sensory disturbances match the motor dysfunction (see Signs and Symptoms).

Signs and Symptoms

I. Hernia evident with myelomeningocele and meningocele
II. If lesion is high, severe paralysis
III. If lesion is low, in sacral spine only, minimal weakness of legs
IV. Incontinence
V. Lack of bowel control
VI. Loss of feeling below the lesion

Therapeutic Management

I. Surgically cover skin and close lesion.
II. Treat complications: infections, hydrocephalus, renal problems.
III. Correct any associated orthopedic deformities.
IV. Provide mobility.

Nursing Care

DATA COLLECTION

I. Perform routine assessment.
II. Assess neurological status.
III. Assist with diagnostic procedures: transillumination, radiography.
IV. Observe pressure areas for signs of skin breakdown.
V. Assess for evidence of complications (e.g., enlarging head, dislocated hip, meningitis).

PLANNING

I. Safe, effective care environment
   A. See Nursing Care of the Ill Child.
II. Physiological integrity
   A. Prevent injury to the sac (preoperative).
   B. Prevent complications.
III. Psychosocial integrity
   A. See Nursing Care of the Ill Child.
   B. Support and educate child and family.

   C. Prepare child and family for procedures, surgery as needed.
IV. Health promotion and maintenance
   A. Promote optimum health.
   B. Achieve and maintain optimum fluid and nutrition.
   C. Prepare family for home care.

IMPLEMENTATION

I. Apply sterile, moist dressing over sac and moisten with saline or antimicrobial solution as prescribed.
II. Use care in cleaning soiled sac.
III. Position infant on stomach or side.
IV. Place infant on fleece pad to reduce pressure on knees and ankles.
V. Maintain legs in abduction with pad between knees and roll beneath ankles.
VI. Avoid diapering; place infant on diaper or pad and change as needed.
VII. Employ meticulous skin care, especially in genital area, because of leaking urine and stool.
VIII. Provide gentle range of motion (ROM) exercises to paralyzed extremities as prescribed.
IX. Observe sac for any change in size.
X. Observe for any leaking fluid.
XI. Teach family skills needed for home care, including signs of increased intracranial pressure (hydrocephalus is frequent complication of myelomeningocele).

EVALUATION

I. Infant's skin remains clean and intact, with no evidence of infection or breakdown.
II. Infant exhibits no evidence of infection.
III. Signs of complications are detected early and appropriate interventions implemented.
IV. Family demonstrates an understanding of the condition and the ability to provide home care.

Hydrocephalus

Description

Hydrocephalus is a condition caused by an increase in the amount of cerebrospinal fluid (CSF) within the cranium.

I. Communicating: CSF flows freely through the ventricular system to the subarachnoid space.
II. Noncommunicating: flow of CSF in the ventricular system is obstructed.

Pathophysiology

I. Increased accumulation of CSF in the ventricles
II. Ventricles enlarging
III. Pressure on the brain against the skull
IV. Damage to brain tissue

Signs and Symptoms

I. Infancy
   A. Irritability and vomiting
   B. Bulging fontanels
   C. Crying when picked up; yawning, quiet when set down

D. Display of changes in level of consciousness possible
E. Feeding difficulties
F. Brief, shrill, high-pitched cry
II. Early infancy
   A. Abnormal rapid head growth
   B. Bulging, tense, nonpulsating fontanels
   C. Separated cranial sutures
   D. High-pitched cry
III. Later infancy
   A. Enlarging frontal bones ("bossing")
   B. Depressed eyes
   C. Sclera visible above iris ("setting sun" sign)
IV. Childhood
   A. Headache
   B. Deviation of the eyes
   C. Irritability
   D. Lethargy
   E. Apathy
   F. Confusion

Therapeutic Management

I. Surgical
   A. Remove obstruction (e.g., tumor, cyst).
   B. Relieve intracranial pressure via ventricular tap during preoperative period.
   C. Shunt CSF from ventricle to extracranial compartment (usually the peritoneum), to relieve intracranial pressure.
   D. Revise shunt as needed during growth.
II. Medical
   A. Treat complications (infection, shunt malfunction).

Nursing Care

DATA COLLECTION

I. Perform routine assessment.
II. Measure head circumference routinely.
III. Perform neurological examination; observe for signs of increasing intracranial pressure.
IV. Observe for signs of infection preoperatively and postoperatively.
V. Assist with diagnostic procedures: echoencephalography, tomography.

PLANNING

I. Safe, effective care environment
   A. See Nursing Care of the Ill Child.
II. Physiological integrity
   A. Prevent complications of the disorder or the corrective surgery.
III. Psychosocial integrity
   A. See Nursing Care of the Ill Child.
   B. Support and educate child and family.
   C. Prepare child and family for procedures, surgery as needed.
IV. Health promotion and maintenance
   A. Promote optimum health.
   B. Prepare family for home care.

IMPLEMENTATION

I. Preoperatively, support head to prevent strain on neck; turn frequently to avoid pressure injury.

II. Position on back or on operated side to prevent pressure on shunt valve.
III. Keep flat to prevent too-rapid reduction of intracranial fluid, if ordered.
IV. Place on sheepskin.
V. Pump valve mechanism as prescribed.
VI. Monitor I&O, including IV infusion, to prevent fluid overload.
VII. Check pupil equality.
VIII. Measure head circumference daily.
IX. Teach family skills needed for home care.

EVALUATION

I. Child exhibits no evidence of infection or increased intracranial pressure.
II. Family demonstrates understanding of the condition and the ability to provide home care.

Bacterial Meningitis

Description

Bacterial meningitis is an infection of the meninges.

Pathophysiology

I. Usual organisms: *Haemophilus influenzae* (type B), *Streptococcus pneumoniae,* meningococci
II. Most commonly a result of infection elsewhere in the body

Signs and Symptoms

I. Fever
II. Vomiting
III. Irritability
IV. Seizures
V. Rigidity of neck, possibly progressing to opisthotonos
VI. Infants and young children
   A. Bulging fontanel (infants)
VII. Children and adolescents
   A. Headache
   B. Changes in ability to feel sensations
   C. Positive Kernig's and Brudzinski's signs
   D. Possible development of delirium, coma

Therapeutic Management

I. Prevent spread of infection.
II. Administer antimicrobials.
III. Maintain optimum fluids.
IV. Maintain breathing.
V. Reduce intracranial pressure.
VI. Manage shock.
VII. Control seizure.
VIII. Control extremes of body temperature.
IX. Treat complications.

Nursing Care

DATA COLLECTION

I. Perform routine assessment.
II. Perform regular neurological assessment.

III. Observe for signs of increased intracranial pressure, shock, respiratory distress.
IV. Assist with diagnostic procedures: lumbar puncture, cultures (CSF, blood), complete blood count (CBC), other laboratory tests.

PLANNING

I. Safe, effective care environment
   A. See Nursing Care of the Ill Child.
   B. Prevent or reduce environmental stimulation.
   C. Prevent transmission of disease to others.
II. Physiological integrity
   A. Help to treat organisms.
   B. Prevent complications.
III. Psychosocial integrity
   A. See Nursing Care of the Ill Child.
   B. Support and educate child and family.
   C. Prepare child and family for procedures, surgery as needed.
IV. Health promotion and maintenance
   A. Promote optimum health.
   B. Achieve and maintain optimum hydration and nutrition.
   C. Prepare family for home care.

IMPLEMENTATION

I. Implement appropriate isolation precautions and maintain as needed.
II. Teach family proper protective procedures.
III. Administer antimicrobials as prescribed.
IV. Monitor and maintain IV infusion.
V. Keep environmental stimuli at minimum (e.g., quiet, dimly lit room); avoid noisy activities and excessive handling of child.
VI. Implement seizure precautions.
VII. Position for comfort: head of bed slightly elevated, side-lying position; no pillow to reduce neck stretching.
VIII. Observe and record any seizure activity.
IX. Administer anticonvulsive medication, if ordered.
X. Teach family skills needed for home care, including expected results of medication and possible side effects.

EVALUATION

I. Child appears comfortable and alert and interacts with family.
II. Child remains free of seizures.
III. Signs of complications are detected early and appropriate interventions implemented.
IV. Family demonstrates an understanding of the disease and the ability to provide home care.
V. Others remain free of infection.

Epilepsy (Generalized, Tonic-Clonic, Grand Mal Seizures)

Description

Epilepsy consists of recurrent convulsive seizures of unknown cause.
I. Petit mal seizure (also known as absence seizure)
   A. Moments of blank staring
   B. Breaks in speech and thinking
   C. Minor tremors
   D. No loss of consciousness

II. Grand mal seizure
   A. Involuntary muscular contractions of the large muscles (tonic-clonic type)

Pathophysiology

I. Spontaneous electric discharge.
II. Partial seizures: discharges limited to a more or less specific region of the cerebral cortex.
III. Generalized seizures: discharges arise in the brain and involve both hemispheres of brain.

Signs and Symptoms

I. Absence seizures
   A. Brief loss of consciousness
   B. Abrupt onset; 20 or more attacks per day
   C. Minor tremors
   D. Often mistaken for inattentiveness or daydreaming
II. Tonic-clonic seizures
   A. Occurrence without warning
   B. Tonic phase lasting about 10–20 seconds
      1. Immediate loss of consciousness
      2. Falling to floor, if standing
      3. Eyes rolling upward
      4. Stiffening in generalized, symmetrical tonic contraction of entire body
      5. Arms usually flexed
      6. Legs, head, and neck extended
      7. Increased salivation
      8. Possibly a peculiar piercing cry
      9. Apneic, possibly becoming cyanotic
   C. Clonic phase lasting about 30 seconds
      1. Violent jerking movements as the trunk and extremities undergo rhythmic contraction and relaxation
      2. Foaming at the mouth possible
      3. Incontinence of urine and feces possible
   D. As attack ends, movements becoming less intense, occurring at longer intervals, then ceasing entirely

Therapeutic Management

I. Control seizures or reduce their frequency with anticonvulsants.
II. Discover and correct cause when possible.
III. Promote as normal a lifestyle as possible.

Nursing Care

DATA COLLECTION

I. Perform routine assessment.
II. Take family history for evidence of seizures.
III. Take careful history of the seizure:
   A. Age at onset of seizures
   B. Time of day when seizures occur
   C. Detailed description of seizure
   D. Any factors causing seizure: environmental, physical
   E. Sensory warning associated with seizure (aura)
   F. Length and progression of seizure
   G. Feelings and behavior after seizure
IV. Observe seizure:
   A. Behavior at onset of seizure

1. Change in facial expression
2. Cry or other sound
3. Involuntary movements
4. Random activity
5. Position of head, body, extremities
6. Time of onset
   B. Movement
   1. Change of position, if any
   2. Description of place movement began
   3. Tonic phase: length, parts of body involved
   4. Clonic phase: twitching or jerking, parts of body involved, sequence of parts involved, any change in movements
   5. Face
      a. Color change: pallor, cyanosis, flushing
      b. Perspiration
      c. Mouth position, teeth clenching, frothing, tongue biting
   6. Eyes
      a. Position: straight ahead, deviation
      b. Pupils (if able to assess): change in size, equality
   7. Respiratory effort
      a. Presence and length of apnea
      b. Any cyanosis
   8. Other: involuntary urination or defecation
   C. Behavior after seizure
   1. State of consciousness
   2. Orientation
   3. Motor ability
   4. Speech
   5. Sensations
V. Assist with diagnostic procedures: electroencephalogram (EEG), skull radiograph, tomography, blood studies.

PLANNING

I. Safe, effective care environment
   A. See Nursing Care of the Ill Child.
   B. Prevent injury to child during seizure.
   C. Provide an environment with seizure precautions.
II. Physiological integrity
   A. Prevent seizures if possible.
III. Psychosocial integrity
   A. See Nursing Care of the Ill Child.
   B. Support child and family.
   C. Educate child and family.
   D. Prepare child and family for procedures.
   E. Promote positive self-image in child.
IV. Health promotion and maintenance
   A. Promote optimum health.
   B. Prepare family for home care.

IMPLEMENTATION

I. Administer anticonvulsants as prescribed.
II. Protect child from injury during seizure:
   A. Do not attempt to restrain child or use force.
   B. If child is standing or sitting, ease child down to prevent falling.
   C. Avoid placing anything in child's mouth.
   D. Loosen restrictive clothing.
   E. Prevent child from hitting hard or sharp objects during uncontrolled movements.

F. Move furniture or other objects out of way.
G. Do not attempt to move child unless he or she is in danger.
III. Promote use of protective helmet for child subject to frequent seizures.
IV. Maintain side rails on bed.
V. Pad bumpers or add padding to the side rail.
VI. Discourage a child subject to daily seizures from engaging in activities in which injury might occur.
VII. Provide comfort after seizure as the child may feel tired and sore.
VIII. Help child and family deal with problems related to the disorder.
IX. Emphasize need for adherence to medical regimen.
X. Help child and family determine activities appropriate to child's condition, interests, and developmental level: avoid contact sports, climbing trees, or apparatus from which child might fall.
XI. Teach family skills needed for home care, including expected results of medication and possible side effects.

EVALUATION

I. Child remains seizure free.
II. Child exhibits no evidence of physical injury.
III. Child expresses feelings and concerns regarding his or her disease and its ramifications.
IV. Family follows instructions.
V. Family treats child as any other child in the family.
VI. Family demonstrates an understanding of the disease and the ability to provide home care.

Musculoskeletal Disorders

Clubfoot

Description

Clubfoot is a deformity in which the foot is twisted out of its normal shape or position.
   I. Talipes: deformity involving the heel
   II. Pes: deformity involving the foot

Pathophysiology

I. Cause unknown
II. Some distortions caused by prenatal positioning, not structural problem

Signs and Symptoms

I. Some positional deformities are:
   A. Inversion, or bending inward
   B. Eversion, or bending outward
   C. Plantar flexion (in which toes are lower than heel)
   D. Dorsiflexion (in which toes are higher than heel)
II. Most common deformity is:
   A. Talipes equinovarus: foot points downward and inward in various degrees of deformity

Therapeutic Management

I. Correct deformity by application of successive casts or by surgery.

II. Maintain correction until normal muscle balance is attained.

III. Observe as a follow-up to prevent possible recurrence.

Nursing Care

DATA COLLECTION

I. Perform routine assessment.

PLANNING

I. Safe, effective care environment
   A. See Nursing Care of the Ill Child.
   B. Promote safety for age.

II. Physiological integrity
   A. Promote correction of deformity.
   B. Prevent complications.

III. Psychosocial integrity
   A. See Nursing Care of the Ill Child.
   B. Support family.
   C. Prepare family for casting.

IV. Health promotion and maintenance
   A. Promote optimum health.
   B. Prepare family for home care.

IMPLEMENTATION

I. Implement cast care.

II. Implement stretching or strapping as directed.

III. Teach family skills needed for home care.

EVALUATION

I. Cast remains clean and intact.

II. Family is able to do stretching exercises or to handle straps if that method is prescribed.

Congenital Hip Dysplasia

Description

Congenital hip dysplasia is imperfect development of the hip or dislocation of the hip.

Pathophysiology

I. Subluxation: incomplete dislocation of hip
   A. Femoral head staying in contact with acetabulum
   B. Relaxed ligaments

II. Dislocation
   A. Femoral head out of contact with acetabulum
   B. Displacement posteriorly and superiorly over the rim
   C. Click heard as femur slips out of acetabulum

Signs and Symptoms

I. Infant
   A. Shortening of limb on affected side
   B. Restricted movement of hip on affected side
   C. Unequal thigh folds

Therapeutic Management

Varies with age of child and extent of dislocation

I. 0–6 months old
   A. Application of external device (Pavlik harness) that maintains femur centered in the acetabulum in the attitude of flexion

II. 6–18 months
   A. Traction followed by plaster cast immobilization

III. Older child (18 months old)
   A. Surgical reduction

Nursing Care

DATA COLLECTION

I. Perform routine assessment.

II. Assess corrective device for proper application and/or maintenance.

III. Assist with diagnostic procedures: radiography, sonography.

PLANNING

I. Safe, effective care environment
   A. See Nursing Care of the Ill Child.
   B. Promote an appropriate environment for age.

II. Physiological integrity
   A. Maintain correct position of hip in acetabulum.
   B. Prevent complications related to wearing corrective device.

III. Psychosocial integrity
   A. See Nursing Care of the Ill Child.
   B. Support and educate child and family.
   C. Prepare child and family for procedures, surgery as needed.

IV. Health promotion and maintenance
   A. Promote optimum health.
   B. Prepare family for home care.

IMPLEMENTATION

I. Teach family the purpose, function, application, and maintenance of the Pavlik harness, cast, or traction.

II. Help family to adapt routine nurturing activities and equipment to accommodate corrective device or cast: feeding, sleeping, playing, safety measures (e.g., car seat).

III. Avoid lifting child by legs to diaper.

EVALUATION

I. Child is properly maintained in corrective device.

II. Child engages in activities appropriate to age or plays as much as possible.

III. Family demonstrates understanding of the condition and its therapy and the ability to provide home care.

Coxa Plana (Legg-Calvé-Perthes Disease)

Description

Coxa plana is a progressive destruction of the femoral head, producing varying degrees of deformity.

Pathophysiology

I. Lack of circulation to the femoral head

II. Degeneration by bone absorption

III. Regeneration of the bone

IV. Process taking about 4 years

Signs and Symptoms

I. Limp on affected side
II. Pain: soreness or aching
   A. In hip, entire length of thigh, or knee
   B. Worse on rising or at end of a long day
   C. Tenderness over hip capsule
III. Joint dysfunction and limited ROM
IV. Stiffness
V. External hip rotation (late sign)

Therapeutic Management

I. Rest, initially, to reduce inflammation and restore motion
II. Traction to stretch tight adductor muscles (sometimes)
III. Containment of femoral head in acetabulum by non–weight-bearing device (abduction brace, leg cast, leather harness)
IV. Surgical correction (sometimes)

Nursing Care

DATA COLLECTION

I. Perform routine assessment.
II. Assess corrective device for proper application and signs of irritation.
III. Assist with diagnostic procedure: radiography.

PLANNING

I. Safe, effective care environment
   A. Alter physical environment as necessary to accommodate corrective device.
II. Physiological integrity
   A. Maintain corrective device.
   B. Prevent complications.
III. Psychosocial integrity
   A. Support and educate child and family.
   B. Prepare child and family for procedures.
IV. Health promotion and maintenance
   A. Promote optimum health.
   B. Prepare family for home care.

IMPLEMENTATION

I. Encourage child to maintain usual activities within limitations imposed by the disease and its therapy.
II. Teach family purpose, function, application, and maintenance of corrective device.

EVALUATION

I. Child engages in usual activities.
II. Family complies with therapeutic regimen.
III. Family demonstrates an understanding of the disease and the ability to provide home care.

Scoliosis

Description

Scoliosis is lateral curative of the spine. Usually consists of two curves: the original curve and a compensatory curve in the opposite direction.

I. Functional: caused by another deformity (e.g., unequal leg length)
II. Structural: caused by changes in the spine and its supporting structures

Pathophysiology

I. Structural scoliosis
   A. Spinal and support structure changes
   B. Loss of flexibility

Signs and Symptoms

I. Undressed subject viewed from back:
   A. Primary curvature with a compensatory curvature that places head in alignment
   B. Head and hips out of alignment
   C. Rib hump and asymmetry when child bends forward from waist
II. Dressed subject
   A. In girls wearing dresses, hems that do not hang straight

Therapeutic Management

I. Spinal strengthening and realignment
   A. Medical
      1. External bracing (Milwaukee)
      2. Casting
      3. Skeletal traction techniques
         a. Halo: femoral
         b. Halo: pelvic
      4. Electrical stimulation
   B. Surgical: internal fixation
      1. Harrington rod
      2. Spinal fusion

Nursing Care

DATA COLLECTION

I. Perform routine assessment.
II. Inspect corrective appliance and skin regularly for possible problems (e.g., skin irritation), and assess for correct application and fit.
III. Assist with diagnostic procedure: radiography.

PLANNING

I. Safe, effective care environment
   A. Prevent injury.
II. Physiological integrity
   A. Nonsurgical treatment: Maintain prescribed appliance.
   B. Surgical treatment: Provide competent postoperative care.
   C. Prevent complications.
III. Psychosocial integrity
   A. Prepare child and family for long-term therapy.
   B. Support and educate child and family.
   C. Prepare child and family for procedures, surgery as needed.
   D. Help child adjust to appliance.
   E. Promote a positive self-image.

IV. Health promotion and maintenance
   A. Promote optimum health.
   B. Prepare child and family for home care.

IMPLEMENTATION

I. Explain or reinforce explanation of condition, including:
   A. How appliance corrects defect
   B. Reason for lengthy treatment
   C. Anticipated results of therapy
   D. How client can help achieve desired goals
   E. Maintenance of therapeutic devices
II. Help child adjust to restricted movement.
III. Provide guidance regarding selection of appropriate exercises and anticipated problems (e.g., selection of clothing, reactions of peers).
IV. Discuss freedoms and restraints imposed by brace or rod.
V. Encourage independence and self-care when appropriate.
VI. Emphasize positive long-term outcome.
VII. Provide feedback and praise for positive behavior and compliance.

EVALUATION

I. Child engages in activities appropriate to age and capabilities.
II. Child displays evidence of positive self-image.
III. Child and family comply with therapeutic regimen.
IV. Child and family demonstrate an understanding of the condition and the ability to provide home care.

Fractures

Description

Fractures are traumatic injuries to bone in which the bone is broken.

Pathophysiology

I. Complete: bone fragments separated
II. Incomplete: bone fragments attached
III. Simple, or closed: no break in skin
IV. Open, or compound: bone protruding through break in skin
V. Greenstick: incomplete fracture because soft bone bends
VI. Comminuted: multiple breaks in one spot
VII. In children, at fracture site the periosteum remains intact and remarkably stable

Signs and Symptoms

I. Pain or tenderness at site of break
II. Generalized swelling
III. Diminished functional use of affected part
IV. Possible bruising, severe muscular rigidity
V. Because of attached periosteum at fracture site, child possibly able to use affected part

Therapeutic Management

I. Reduce fracture; regain alignment of bony fragments.
   A. Closed or open reduction

II. Retain alignment and length of part through immobilization.
III. Restore function of injured parts.

Nursing Care

DATA COLLECTION

I. Perform routine assessment.
II. Obtain history of trauma.
III. Assist with diagnostic procedure: x-ray.
IV. Assess casted extremity regularly for pain, swelling, discoloration (pallor or cyanosis), ability to move part, paresthesia, pulse, odor.
V. Assess extremity in traction for maintenance of desired pull, body alignment, correct functioning of apparatus.
VI. For open reduction, assess bleeding over operative site; outline edges of stain to assess increase.

PLANNING

I. Safe, effective care environment
   A. See Nursing Care of the Ill Child.
   B. Prevent injury.
   C. Provide an environment that facilitates healing.
II. Physiological integrity
   A. Maintain bone immobility.
   B. Promote bone healing.
   C. Prevent complications.
III. Psychosocial integrity
   A. See Nursing Care of the Ill Child.
   B. Support and educate child and family.
   C. Prepare child and family for procedures.
IV. Health promotion and maintenance
   A. Prepare family for home care.

IMPLEMENTATION

I. Keep casted extremity elevated on pillows or other support for first day, or as directed.
II. Apply "petaling" moleskin to rough edges of cast.
III. Maintain integrity of cast; keep clean and dry, avoiding damage to cast.
IV. Prevent child from placing crumbs or small items inside cast.
V. For open reduction, administer pain medication as needed.
VI. Teach crutch walking to child with lower-extremity injury.
VII. Teach family skills needed for home care: care of cast, signs of complications.

EVALUATION

I. Cast remains dry and intact.
II. Child exhibits no evidence of circulatory or neurological impairment.
III. Family demonstrates an understanding of the condition and the ability to provide home care.

Cerebral Palsy

Description

Cerebral palsy is impaired muscular control resulting from brain injury or occurring during a period of early brain growth.

Pathophysiology

I. Injury to the brain from pressure or oxygen deprivation before birth
II. Infection or toxicity after birth

Signs and Symptoms

I. Disorder of motor development
II. Possibly abnormal motor performance—slight to severe impairment
   A. Inability to stand or sit
   B. Increased stiffness of muscles
   C. Difficulty in chewing and swallowing
   D. Drooling and impaired speech articulation
   E. Spastic movements—especially scissors gait
   F. Nonspastic: athetoid or atoxic
   G. Seizures
   H. Constipation
   I. Respiratory problems
   J. Orthopedic complications
   K. Dental problems
III. Behavior problems
IV. Vision and hearing problems
V. Learning disabilities
VI. Attention-deficit hyperactivity disorder

Therapeutic Management

I. Establish movement, communication, and self-help with braces, mobilizing devices, speech therapy.
II. Gain optimum appearance and use of motor abilities:
   A. Skeletal muscle relaxants (some older children)
   B. Antianxiety agents to relieve excessive motion
   C. Anticonvulsants for seizures
   D. Dextroamphetamine or methylphenidate (Ritalin) for hyperactivity
III. Correct any associated defects with orthopedic surgery when possible.
IV. Provide educational opportunities adapted to the individual child's needs and capabilities.

Nursing Care

DATA COLLECTION

I. Perform routine assessment.
II. Obtain history of child's behavior and attainment of developmental milestones.
III. Assist with diagnostic procedures: EEG, tomography, screening for metabolic defects, serum electrolytes.

PLANNING

I. Safe, effective care environment
   A. Help modify environment to conform to needs of child.
   B. Promote age-appropriate safety precautions.
II. Physiological integrity
   A. Promote relaxation.
   B. Establish movement and communication.
   C. Prevent complications.

D. Promote adequate nutritional intake for age.
   E. Promote normal elimination.
III. Psychosocial integrity
   A. Assist with educational program.
   B. Promote positive self-image.
IV. Health promotion and maintenance
   A. Promote optimum health.
   B. Support family in its efforts to meet the needs of the child.

IMPLEMENTATION

I. Provide safe environment with padded furniture, side rails on beds, and sturdy furniture that does not slip; avoid scatter rugs and polished floors.
II. Restrain child when in chair or wheelchair.
III. Provide helmet for child who is prone to falls.
IV. Apply and correctly use braces.
V. Carry out and teach family to perform stretching exercises.
VI. Encourage sitting, crawling, and walking at appropriate ages.
VII. Use play that encourages desired behavior.
VIII. Use special devices that allow child independent motion.
IX. Maintain a well-regulated schedule that allows for adequate rest and sleep.
X. Help family modify equipment and activities to meet needs of child.
XI. Provide extra calories to meet extra energy demands of increased muscle activity.
XII. Encourage child to assist in care.
XIII. Enlist efforts of speech therapist.
XIV. Employ nonverbal communication methods.
XV. Promote and assist bowel elimination.
XVI. Teach family skills needed for care, including expected results of medication and possible side effects.
XVII. See Nursing Care of the Chronically Ill or Disabled Child.

EVALUATION

I. Child is sufficiently rested.
II. Child eats a balanced diet with sufficient calories for needs.
III. Child has normal bowel elimination.
IV. Child is able to communicate his or her needs to caregivers.
V. Family provides a safe environment for the child.
VI. Family demonstrates an understanding of the condition and the ability to provide home care.

Juvenile Rheumatoid Arthritis

Description

Juvenile rheumatoid arthritis is an inflammatory disease of the joints and connective tissues.

Pathophysiology

I. Similar to adult arthritis
II. Chronic inflammation of the joints

III. Joint swelling
IV. Limited motion caused by muscle spasm and inflammation
V. Eventual erosion, destruction, and fibrosis of articular cartilage

Signs and Symptoms

I. Joint characteristics
   A. Stiffness and swelling
   B. Tenderness
   C. Possibly painful to touch or relatively painless
   D. Warm to touch (seldom red)
   E. Loss of motion
   F. Characteristic morning stiffness or "gelling" on arising in the morning or after inactivity
II. Systemic
   A. Fever, higher in evening
   B. Enlarged liver, spleen, and lymph nodes
   C. Anemia
   D. Pallor
   E. Rash
   F. Pericarditis, myocarditis, and uveitis
   G. Aggravated by stress and fatigue

Therapeutic Management

I. Suppress inflammatory process with:
   A. Nonsteroidal anti-inflammatory drugs
   B. Cytotoxic drugs
   C. Corticosteroids
II. Preserve function or prevent deformity (or both) with physical therapy, occupational therapy, splinting, and positioning.
III. Reduce pain with analgesia and heat application.

Nursing Care

DATA COLLECTION

I. Perform routine assessment.
II. Observe for joint discomfort and movement.
III. Assist with diagnostic tests: radiography, WBC count, rheumatoid factors, ESR, antinuclear antibodies; result of latex fixation test to detect disease in adults is negative in most children.

PLANNING

I. Safe, effective care environment
   A. See Nursing Care of the Ill Child.
   B. Modify environment as needed to facilitate child's mobility.
   C. Promote safe environment appropriate for age.
II. Physiological integrity
   A. Relieve discomfort.
   B. Prevent physical deformity and preserve joint function.
   C. Promote positive self-image and good self-esteem.
III. Psychosocial integrity
   A. See Nursing Care of the Ill Child.
IV. Health promotion and maintenance
   A. Promote good health practices.

   B. Promote self-care.
   C. Prepare family for home care.

IMPLEMENTATION

I. Administer anti-inflammatory preparations as prescribed.
II. Carry out or assist with physical therapy plan.
III. Provide heat to affected joints via bath, hot compresses, paraffin baths.
IV. Carry out ROM activities in appropriate locations (e.g., bath, pool, playroom).
V. Encourage activity appropriate to capabilities.
VI. Apply splints and support equipment (e.g., bolsters, sandbags, pillows) as prescribed.
VII. Help modify environment for safety and utensils to facilitate self-help.
VIII. Use child's natural affinity for play to encourage motion and activity.
IX. Teach family skills needed for home care:
   A. Administration of medications, including possible side effects
   B. Purpose and correct application of splints or appliances
   C. Modification of environment, clothing, and utensils to facilitate self-help

EVALUATION

I. Child moves with minimal or no discomfort.
II. Child engages in suitable play and self-help activities.
III. Child and family demonstrate an understanding of the disease and therapies and the ability to provide home care.

Cognitive and Sensory Disorders

Strabismus and Amblyopia

Description

Strabismus and amblyopia are disorders of vision: respectively, a malalignment of the eyes and a weakness of eye muscle.

Pathophysiology

I. Image viewed does not fall on corresponding parts of retina in both eyes.
II. Double vision (diplopia) occurs.
III. Child suppresses image in deviating eye to avoid double vision.
IV. Disuse causes impaired vision in involved eye.

Signs and Symptoms

I. Deviation apparent on inspection
II. Squinting in attempt to produce clearer vision

Therapeutic Management

I. Uninvolved-eye patching to force child to use and strengthen involved eye

II. Corrective lenses to help focus object on retina
III. Surgical correction

Nursing Care

DATA COLLECTION

I. Perform routine assessment.
II. Assist with diagnostic procedure: ophthalmologic examination.

PLANNING

I. Safe, effective care environment
  A. Provide safe environment for child with both eyes patched.
II. Physiological integrity
  A. Provide postoperative care after surgical correction.
  B. Promote compliance in nonsurgical therapies.
III. Psychosocial integrity
  A. Support and educate child and family.
  B. Prepare child and family for procedures, surgery as needed.
IV. Health promotion and maintenance
  A. Promote optimum health.

IMPLEMENTATION

I. Implement safety precautions as for blind adult.
II. Provide safe postoperative care.
III. Apply sterile dressing changes.
IV. Teach child and family proper use of patching or glasses.

EVALUATION

I. Child exhibits desired oculomotor movements and eye alignment.
II. Child and family comply with therapeutic regimen.
III. Family demonstrates an understanding of the condition and the ability to provide home care.

Mental Retardation

Description

Mental retardation is defined as significantly subaverage general intellectual functioning: an IQ of 70 or below on an individually administered IQ test.

Pathophysiology

I. Inherited disease (e.g., phenylketonuria, galactosemia)
II. Infection (e.g., rubella)
III. Drugs (e.g., excessive alcohol, chronic lead ingestion)
IV. Down's syndrome
V. Congenital malformations (e.g., microcephaly, hydrocephaly)
VI. Birth injuries
VII. Inadequate nutrition
VIII. Failure to thrive

Signs and Symptoms

I. Motor delay
II. Intellectual delay: slower than normal rate of learning new skills

A. Basic patterns of development maintained
B. Time scale prolonged
III. Delayed vision and hearing development
IV. Delayed language
V. Neurobehavioral disturbances

Therapeutic Management

I. Infant stimulation
II. Special education
III. Appropriate protective care (home, institution)
IV. General health supervision
V. Correction of associated anomalies (e.g., heart defects, facial defects, impaired mobility)

Nursing Care

DATA COLLECTION

I. Perform routine assessment.
II. Obtain history of possible etiologic factors.
III. Obtain developmental history.
IV. Perform or assist with diagnostic procedures: developmental screening tests, IQ test, specific diagnostic tests (e.g., chromosomal analysis, metabolic studies).

PLANNING

I. Safe, effective care environment
  A. Ensure protected environment.
  B. Ensure safety for age.
II. Physiological integrity
  A. Promote development.
III. Psychosocial integrity
  A. Support and educate family.
  B. Promote acceptance by family.
  C. Promote special education for the child.
  D. Promote positive self-esteem in child and family.
IV. Health promotion and maintenance
  A. Promote optimum health.
  B. Help family adjust to future care.

IMPLEMENTATION

I. Help family to identify both short- and long-term goals.
II. Teach family skills needed for home care:
  A. Set realistic goals for child to learn new activities.
  B. Promote self-help skills and independence.
  C. Provide play materials that stimulate development and promote self-help.
  D. Promote development of interpersonal skills.
III. Help family to investigate and obtain special help for the child:
  A. Infant stimulation programs
  B. Special education
  C. Appropriate institutional care
IV. Help to identify activities that promote self-esteem.

EVALUATION

I. Child attains developmental milestones commensurate with cognitive level.
II. Child develops optimum self-help within the limits of his or her capabilities.
III. Family demonstrates an understanding of the condition and the ability to provide home care.

Down's Syndrome

Description

Down's syndrome, also called trisomy 21, is a genetic disorder characterized by varying degrees of mental retardation and multiple defects.

Pathophysiology

I. Increased incidence in children whose mothers were >35 years of age at the time of birth
II. In 92%–95% of the cases, attributed to an extra chromosome 21

Signs and Symptoms

I. Physical characteristics
  A. Small rounded skull with a flattened appearance
  B. Inner epicanthal folds and eyes slant upward and outward
  C. Small nose with depressed bridge ("saddle nose")
  D. Protruding tongue
  E. Short hands and fingers
  F. Floppy infant
  G. Simian line (transverse palmar crease)
II. Associated characteristics
  A. Cardiac anomalies (most common congenital defects)
  B. Delayed eruption of teeth
  C. Fissured tongue
  D. High susceptibility to upper respiratory illness (URI)
  E. Umbilical hernia
  F. Affectionate, placid personality

Therapeutic Management

I. See Mental Retardation.
II. Correct physical defects.
III. Treat infections.

Nursing Care

DATA COLLECTION

I. Perform routine assessment.
II. Assist with diagnostic procedures: chromosome analysis, tests to diagnose suspected anomalies.

PLANNING

I. Safe, effective care environment
  A. See Mental Retardation.
  B. Prevent infection.
II. Physiological integrity
  A. See Mental Retardation.
III. Psychosocial integrity
  A. See Mental Retardation.
IV. Health promotion and maintenance
  A. See Mental Retardation.
  B. Prevent infections.
  C. Prevent additional children with Down's syndrome.

IMPLEMENTATION

I. See Mental Retardation.
II. Avoid exposure to persons with URIs.

III. Encourage genetic counseling when disorder is caused by a translocation.
IV. Prenatal: Encourage amniocentesis for pregnant women >35 years of age.
V. Encourage exercise (e.g., Special Olympics).

EVALUATION

I. See Mental Retardation.
II. Child exhibits no evidence of infection.

Skin Disorders

Scabies

Description

Scabies is a superficial infestation produced by the scabies mite, *Sarcoptes scabiei*.

Pathophysiology

I. Impregnated female mite burrows under the skin and lays eggs.
II. Child is sensitized to mite.
III. Inflammatory response occurs 30–60 days after initial contact. If child is sensitized to mite, inflammatory response occurs in 48 hours.

Signs and Symptoms

I. Itching
II. Lesions: minute grayish brown, threadlike lesion (burrow) with black dot at end
III. Distribution: primarily between fingers and toes, and in axillae, groin, and abdominal areas

Therapeutic Management

I. Treat mite with scabicide, usually 1% lindane (Kwell).
II. Relieve itching with soothing ointments or lotions.

Nursing Care

DATA COLLECTION

I. Perform routine assessment.
II. Assist with diagnostic procedure: skin scrapings observed under microscope for evidence of mite.

PLANNING

I. Safe, effective care environment
  A. Prevent spread of mite to others.
II. Physiological integrity
  A. Eliminate scabies mite.
  B. Relieve discomfort.
  C. Prevent or minimize scratching.
III. Psychosocial integrity
  A. Support and educate child and family.
IV. Health promotion and maintenance
  A. Promote optimum health.

IMPLEMENTATION

I. Explain or reinforce explanation of condition and therapies.

II. Teach family application of scabicide; follow directions accurately:
   A. Apply on cool, dry skin (not after a bath).
   B. Leave on for prescribed time.
   C. Treat all members of household.
III. Apply lotion or ointment to affected areas.
IV. Employ methods to prevent scratching.
   A. Keep fingernails short and clean.
   B. Keep child in T-shirt or other soft clothing to cover itching area.
   C. Wrap hands in soft cotton gloves or stockings, if needed; pin gloves to shirt sleeves.

EVALUATION

I. Child's skin remains clean and dry with no evidence of scratching.
II. Child rests and plays with no evidence of discomfort.
III. Child and family exhibit no evidence of infestation.
IV. Family demonstrates an understanding of the condition and the ability to provide home care.

Pediculosis Capitis

Description

Pediculosis capitis is an infestation of the head by *Pediculus humanus capitis* (head louse).

Pathophysiology

I. Female louse lays eggs at night on a hair shaft close to junction with skin.
II. Eggs hatch in approximately 7–10 days.
III. Crawling insect and insect saliva on skin produce itching and irritation.

Signs and Symptoms

I. Itching.
II. Nits and nit cases observable on hair shaft.
III. Distribution: usually found in hair at occipital area, nape of neck, behind ears. Has been found in eyebrows and eyelashes.

Therapeutic Management

I. Elimination of lice and nits with pediculocidal shampoos (Kwell, RID, Nix)
II. Manual removal of nit cases

Nursing Care

DATA COLLECTION

I. Perform routine assessment.
II. Inspect scalp for evidence of nits or nit cases at base of hair shaft:
   A. Systematically spread hair with two tongue depressors or popsicle sticks.
   B. Observe for:
      1. Any movement that indicates a louse
      2. Nits (whitish oval specks adhering to hair shaft)
      3. Empty nit cases (translucent oval specks)

C. Condition is distinguished from dandruff by adherent nature; dandruff falls off hair readily.

PLANNING

I. Safe, effective care environment
   A. Prevent spread to others.
II. Physiological integrity
   A. Eliminate lice and nits.
III. Psychosocial integrity
   A. Support and educate child and family.
IV. Health promotion and maintenance
   A. Promote optimum health.

IMPLEMENTATION

I. Caution children against sharing combs, hats, caps, scarves, coats, and other items used on or near the hair.
II. Reassure family that anyone can get pediculosis, regardless of age, cleanliness, or socioeconomic level.
III. Teach family application of shampoo:
   A. Follow directions described on label of pediculocide:
      1. Read directions several times in quiet environment before application.
   B. Make child as comfortable as possible.
   C. Avoid getting preparation in eyes.
      1. If irritation occurs, flush well with tepid water.
   D. Remove nits with tweezers or between the fingernails.
IV. Launder washable items of clothing and linens in hot water and dry in dryer.
V. Soak combs, brushes, and so on, in pediculocide or lotion and very hot water for 5–10 minutes.
VI. Vacuum mattresses and upholstered furniture carefully.
VII. Support child to prevent feelings of shame or embarrassment.
VIII. Caution family against cutting child's hair or shaving head.

EVALUATION

I. Child and family exhibit no evidence of reinfestation.
II. Family demonstrates an understanding of the condition and the ability to provide home care.

Dermatophytosis (Ringworm)

Description

Infections are caused by a group of closely related fungi.
I. Tinea capitis: ringworm of the scalp
II. Tinea corporis: ringworm of the body
III. Tinea pedis: athlete's foot

Pathophysiology

I. Fungus that invades the skin
II. Production of an enzyme that causes hair to break off at roots

Signs and Symptoms

I. Tinea capitis
   A. Scaly, round patches

B. Patch, scaling areas of baldness
C. Itching
II. Tinea corporis
  A. Round or oval red scaling patches that spread outward and heal centrally
III. Tinea pedis
  A. Most frequent in adolescents; rare in young children
  B. Blisters and fissuring between toes
  C. Patches with pinhead-sized vesicles on plantar surface
  D. Itching

Therapeutic Management

I. Eliminate fungus.
  A. Administration of oral griseofulvin
  B. Topical applications of antifungal preparations

Nursing Care

DATA COLLECTION

I. Perform routine assessment.
II. Assist with diagnostic procedure: direct microscopic examination of scales from skin scrapings.

PLANNING

I. Safe, effective care environment
  A. Prevent spread to others.
II. Physiological integrity
  A. Help eliminate fungus.
III. Psychosocial integrity
  A. Support and educate child and family.
IV. Health promotion and maintenance
  A. Promote optimum health.
  B. Prepare family for home care.

IMPLEMENTATION

I. Suggest examination of animals in child's environment for evidence of infection (tinea corporis).
II. Teach family how to administer oral medication and apply topical ointments.
III. Teach family desired effects of medications and possible side effects.
IV. Teach family to improve the ventilation of the feet.

EVALUATION

I. Child exhibits no evidence of infection.
II. Family complies with therapeutic regimen.
III. Family demonstrates an understanding of the condition and the ability to provide home care.

Diaper Dermatitis

Description

Diaper dermatitis is an acute inflammatory disorder caused directly or indirectly by the wearing of diapers.

Pathophysiology; SIGNS AND SYMPTOMS

I. Various types of lesions observed, depending on cause of irritation and inflammation
II. Primary causes

  A. Allergy
  B. Poorly washed diapers
  C. Infrequent diaper change
  D. Ammonia formation from urine

Therapeutic Management

I. Promote skin healing.
II. Apply corticosteroids for stubborn inflammations.
III. Apply antifungal ointments or powders for candidiasis.
IV. Prevent recurrence.

Nursing Care

DATA COLLECTION

I. Perform routine assessment.

PLANNING

I. Safe, effective care environment
  A. Promote cleanliness.
II. Physiological integrity
  A. Minimize skin wetness.
  B. Promote normal skin pH.
  C. Prevent secondary infection.
III. Psychosocial integrity
  A. Support and educate family.
IV. Health promotion and maintenance
  A. Promote optimum health.

IMPLEMENTATION

I. Change diaper as soon as wet; change at least once during night.
II. Clean, rinse, and dry area before diapering.
III. Apply ointment (petrolatum, zinc oxide) over clean, dry, *noninflamed* skin to prevent moistness from reaching skin.
IV. Encourage use of diapers that reduce wetness next to skin (e.g., those with absorbent gel).
V. Avoid diaper covering (plastic pants, some elasticized disposable diapers).
VI. Teach diaper care to families who prefer cloth diapers.
  A. Encourage commercial diaper laundries.
  B. Home care: Soak diapers in quaternary ammonium compound:
    1. Wash in hot water with simple laundry soap (e.g., Ivory).
    2. Run through rinse cycle twice.
    3. A dryer enhances softness.
VII. Teach families application of any prescribed medication.

EVALUATION

I. Child remains free of dermatitis in the diaper area.
II. Family demonstrates an understanding of the condition, treatment, and prevention and the ability to provide home care.

Atopic Dermatitis (Eczema)

Description

Atopic dermatitis is a superficial inflammatory process involving primarily the skin.

Pathophysiology

I. Affected individuals have a lower threshold for itching.
II. Characteristic lesions appear after irritation (scratching, rubbing).
III. Appearance and distribution of lesions vary with age of child.
IV. Frequently a family history of sensitivity exists.

Signs and Symptoms

I. Intense itching
II. Unaffected skin dry and rough
III. Infantile form
   A. Generalized distribution, especially cheeks, scalp, trunk, extremities
   B. Erythema
   C. Vesicles and papules
   D. Weeping and oozing
   E. Crusting and scaling

Therapeutic Management

I. Prevent itching with antihistamines, mild baths, detergents, and soaps.
II. Hydrate the skin with emollients and limit bathing.
III. Reduce inflammation with topical corticosteroids.
IV. Prevent or control secondary infection.
V. Modify diet, if indicated.

Nursing Care

DATA COLLECTION

I. Perform routine assessment.
II. Assist with elimination diet, if indicated.

PLANNING

I. Safe, effective care environment
   A. Protect from known irritants.
II. Physiological integrity
   A. Prevent or minimize scratching.
   B. Prevent complications.
III. Psychosocial integrity
   A. Support and educate child and family.
IV. Health promotion and maintenance
   A. Promote optimum health.

IMPLEMENTATION

I. Keep fingernails and toenails short and clean.
II. Wrap hands in soft cotton gloves or stockings and pin gloves to shirt sleeves as needed to prevent scratching.
III. Avoid overheating child.
IV. Provide soothing and emollient tepid water baths or compresses as prescribed.
V. Administer antihistamines, sedatives, topical corticosteroids, and/or antibiotics as prescribed.
VI. Teach family diet planning (if food sensitivity is implicated).
VII. Teach family skills needed for care, including expected results of medications and their possible side effects.
VIII. Provide psychological and supportive care to promote a positive self-image.

IX. Teach parents to keep child protected from people who have infections.

EVALUATION

I. Child's skin remains intact without redness.
II. Child exhibits no evidence of secondary infection or trauma.
III. Family demonstrates an understanding of the condition and the ability to provide care.

Seborrheic Dermatitis

Description

Seborrheic dermatitis is a chronic, recurrent inflammatory condition of the skin.

Pathophysiology

I. Occurs most commonly on scalp ("cradle cap"), eyebrows, external ear canal (otitis externa), inguinal region
II. Related to excessive secretion from sebaceous glands
III. Cause unknown

Signs and Symptoms

I. Characteristic thick, adherent, yellowish, scaly, oily patches
II. May or may not include mild itching

Therapeutic Management

I. Symptomatic treatment
II. Corticosteroid ointment for persistent rash
III. Antibiotics for infected rash

Nursing Care

DATA COLLECTION

I. Perform routine assessment.

PLANNING

I. Safe, effective care environment
   A. Maintain cleanliness.
II. Physiological integrity
   A. Remove lesions.
   B. Prevent complications.
III. Psychosocial integrity
   A. Support and educate family.
IV. Health promotion and maintenance
   A. Promote optimum health.
   B. Prepare family for home care.

IMPLEMENTATION

I. Clean scalp (or other affected area).
II. Shampoo three to four times weekly with mild soap or shampoo.
III. Apply oil to lesion; massage into scalp; allow to penetrate and soften crusts; thoroughly wash out.
IV. Remove loosened crusts from hair strands with fine-toothed comb.
V. Apply any prescribed topical preparation.

VI. Explain or reinforce explanation of condition and therapies, especially regarding fear of damaging infant's soft spot.
VII. Teach family skills needed for care.

EVALUATION

I. Child's skin remains free of lesions.
II. Family demonstrates an understanding of the condition and the ability to provide care.

Acne Vulgaris

Description

Acne vulgaris is an inflammatory disease of the skin.

Pathophysiology; Signs and Symptoms

I. Hormones and bacteria, among other factors, have been implicated in production of lesions.
II. Distribution: face, neck, shoulders, back, and upper chest
III. Noninflamed lesions: comedones
   A. Compact masses of keratin, lipids, fatty acids, and bacteria
   B. Dilated follicular duct, which may be closed (whitehead) or open (blackhead); open lesions discolored as fatty acids oxidized by air
IV. Inflamed lesions
   A. Dilated follicular wall rupturing to produce papules, pustules, nodules, and cysts
   B. Description and possibility of scarring.
V. Lesions potentially complicated by secondary infection by *Staphylococcus albus*

Therapeutic Management

I. Prevent or reduce formation of new lesions with topical applications of retinoic acid, benzoyl peroxide, or a combination of these.
II. Reduce lesion formation in older adolescent females with cyclic estrogen-progesterone therapy.
III. Reduce inflammatory process and scarring with antibiotics and intralesional steroids.

Nursing Care

DATA COLLECTION

I. Perform routine assessment.

PLANNING

I. Safe, effective care environment
   A. Promote cleanliness.
II. Physiological integrity
   A. Remove comedones.
   B. Reduce number of lesions.
   C. Prevent inflammation and scarring.
   D. Prevent secondary infection.
III. Psychosocial integrity
   A. Support and educate child and family.
   B. Prepare child and family for procedures.
   C. Promote a positive self-image.

IV. Health promotion and maintenance
   A. Promote optimum health.
   B. Prepare child and family for home care.

IMPLEMENTATION

I. Encourage child to assume responsibility for own care.
II. Teach child how to carry out prescribed regimen:
   A. Skin cleansing and hair shampooing
   B. Application of topical preparations
   C. Administration of prescribed medications, including desired effects and possible side effects
III. Teach measures to reduce lesion formation:
   A. Hair styling (off forehead)
   B. Selection and application of makeup (water-based preparations)
   C. Avoidance of excessive scrubbing or pinching, squeezing, or otherwise manipulating lesions
   D. Avoidance of oily substances
IV. Caution against self-medication with over-the-counter preparations.
V. Emphasize importance of clean skin, hair, hands, and implements coming in contact with lesions.
VI. Dispel myths related to cause and treatment of acne.
VII. Allow child to express feelings.
VIII. Provide positive reinforcement for compliance.
IX. Emphasize improved appearance, self-limited nature of disorder.
X. Caution family against nagging or blaming or both.

EVALUATION

I. Child assumes responsibility for care.
II. Acne lesions diminish in number and severity.
III. Acne lesions do not become secondarily infected.
IV. Family displays a supportive attitude.
V. Child and family comply with therapeutic regimen.
VI. Child and family demonstrate an understanding of the condition and the ability to provide home care.

Impetigo Contagiosa

Description

Impetigo contagiosa is a superficial bacterial infection of the skin.

Pathophysiology

I. Caused by staphylococci, streptococci, or both
II. Begins as discolored spots
III. Followed by appearance of vesicles or bullae
IV. Rupture of vesicles or bullae, leaving superficial, moist erosion
V. Spread of germ-laden fluid to surrounding skin
VI. Drying of exudate forms heavy, honey-colored crusts and scabs
VII. Tends to spread outwardly

Signs and Symptoms

I. Vesicles, bullae, and weeping crusts as just described
II. Most often observed on face, hands, or perineum
III. Pruritus common

Therapeutic Management

I. Topical application of bactericidal ointment
II. Systemic administration of antibiotics in severe cases

Nursing Care

DATA COLLECTION

I. Describe lesion accurately; examine skin for evidence of spread to other areas.
II. Assist with diagnostic procedures: exudate culture.

PLANNING

I. Safe, effective care environment
  A. Prevent spread of infection.
II. Physiological integrity
  A. Help to eliminate lesions.
  B. Prevent complications.
III. Psychosocial integrity
  A. Support and educate child and family.
IV. Health promotion and maintenance
  A. Promote optimum health.
  B. Prepare family for home care.

IMPLEMENTATION

I. Practice and teach child and family careful handwashing.
II. Caution child against touching lesions to prevent spread.
III. Treat lesions:
  A. Soak crusts with warm-water compresses.
  B. Carefully remove crusts.
  C. Apply antibiotic ointment to affected areas.
IV. Administer antibiotics, if prescribed.
V. Teach family management of lesions and administration of medications.

EVALUATION

I. Child's skin remains free of lesions.
II. Family demonstrates an understanding of the disease and the ability to provide home care.
III. Others do not contract disease.

Thermal Burns

Description

A thermal burn is an injury to tissues caused by application of excessive heat to skin.

Pathophysiology

I. Physiological response directly related to amount of tissue destroyed
II. Extent of injury: expressed as percentage of body surface area involved; varies according to size of child
III. Depth of injury
  A. Superficial (first-degree): involves epidermis; heals without scarring
  B. Partial-thickness (second-degree): involves epidermis and variable portion of dermis (superficial or deep)
    1. Superficial: heals uneventfully
    2. Deep: may convert to full-thickness injury
  C. Full-thickness (third-degree): involves all layers of the skin
    1. Usually combined with extensive partial-thickness damage
    2. Scarring
  D. Full-thickness (fourth-degree): involves all layers of skin, subcutaneous tissue, and muscle
IV. Severity of injury
  A. Minor burns
    1. Partial-thickness burns over <15% of body surface
    2. Full-thickness burns over <2% of body surface
  B. Moderate burns
    1. Partial-thickness burns over <15%–25% of body surface
    2. Full-thickness burns over <10% of body surface, except in small children or when burns involve critical areas (e.g., face, hands, feet, genitalia)
  C. Severe burns
    1. Burns complicated by respiratory tract injury
    2. Partial-thickness burns over 25% or more of body surface
    3. Burns of face, hands, feet, or genitalia
    4. Full-thickness burns over 10% or more of body surface
    5. Any child <2 years of age, unless burn is very small and very superficial
    6. Electrical burns that penetrate
    7. Deep chemical burns
    8. Burns complicated by fractures or soft-tissue injury
    9. Burns complicated by concurrent illness (e.g., obesity, diabetes, epilepsy, cardiac or renal disorders)
V. Local responses
  A. Edema formation
  B. Fluid electrolyte and protein loss
  C. Circulatory stasis
VI. Systemic responses
  A. Circulatory
  B. Anemia from heat-damaged RBCs at burn site
VII. Healing
  A. Superficial burns: damaged epithelium peeling off in small scales or sheets, in 5–10 days, leaving no scarring
  B. Partial-thickness burns: crust forming in 3–5 days; healing occurring from underneath
  C. Deep dermal burns (deep partial-thickness, full-thickness burns): healing slow; thin epithelial covering forming in 25–35 days; scarring common
VIII. Systemic effects of severe burns
  A. Asphyxia from irritation and edema of lungs and respiratory passages
  B. Shock from fluid and protein loss from denuded skin, edema from increased capillary permeability and vasodilation at burn site, diminished intravascular colloidal osmotic pressure (greatest hazard first 48–72 hours)
  C. Renal shutdown from shock

Signs and Symptoms

I. Superficial (first-degree) burns
   A. Dry, red surface
   B. Blanches on pressure, then refills
   C. Painful
II. Partial-thickness (second-degree) burns
   A. Blistered, moist
   B. Mottled pink or red
   C. Red; blanches on pressure, then refills
   D. Very painful
III. Full-thickness (third-degree) burns
   A. Tough, leathery
   B. Dull, dry surface
   C. Brown, tan, red, or black
   D. Does not blanch on pressure
   E. Little pain, but surrounded by painful partial-thickness burns

Therapeutic Management

I. Minor burns
   A. Cleanse and debride wound.
   B. Cover with dry or medicated dressing.
II. Major burns: general care
   A. Hospitalize client.
   B. Establish adequate airway.
   C. Replace and maintain IV fluids and electrolytes.
   D. Feed a high-calorie, increased-protein diet or regular diet.
   E. Administer morphine sulfate for pain on scheduled basis.
   F. Administer zinc and vitamin A preparations to promote epithelial growth.
   G. Use prophylactic antibiotics (controversial).
   H. Administer tetanus toxoid (based on immunization history).
III. Wound management
   A. Debridement of devitalized tissue: hydrotherapy
   B. Topical antimicrobial therapy
   C. Cover: temporary dressing (gauze, biological, synthetic, allograft, and autographs)
   D. Graft
      1. Permanent cover (partial-thickness, full-thickness burns)
      2. Full-cover, postage-stamp, mesh, lace, or slit
   E. Primary excision
IV. Prevention of deformity using splinting and compression garments

Nursing Care

DATA COLLECTION

I. Assess respiratory status.
II. Help to assess burn injury.
III. Obtain a history of burn injury—especially time of injury, nature of burning agent, duration of contact, whether in enclosed area, any medication given.
IV. Obtain pertinent history—especially preburn weight, preexisting illness, allergies.
V. Assess pain.

VI. Check eyes for evidence of injury or irritation.
VII. Observe for signs of respiratory distress.
VIII. Check nasopharynx for edema or redness.
IX. Monitor vital signs frequently.
X. Weigh on admission and daily, or as prescribed.
XI. Measure I&O.
XII. Assess circulation to areas peripheral or distal to burns.
XIII. Assess level of consciousness.
XIV. Observe for signs of altered behavior.
XV. Observe for signs of impending overhydration.
XVI. Observe wound for evidence of healing, stability of temporary cover or graft, and infection.
XVII. Assist with diagnostic tests: CBC, urinalysis, wound cultures, hematocrit.

PLANNING

I. Safe, effective care environment
   A. See Nursing Care of the Ill Child.
   B. Prevent heat loss.
   C. Prevent infection and trauma.
II. Physiological integrity
   A. Relieve pain.
   B. Facilitate wound healing.
   C. Preserve graft site.
   D. Provide nutrition.
   E. Prevent complications.
III. Psychosocial integrity
   A. See Nursing Care of the Ill Child.
   B. Promote positive self-image.
IV. Health promotion and maintenance
   A. Promote optimum health.
   B. Prepare family for home care.

IMPLEMENTATION

I. Place in protective environment according to unit policy:
   A. Prevent contact with infected persons or objects.
   B. Administer good oral hygiene.
II. Maintain environmental temperature to prevent heat loss or place under heat source.
III. Administer analgesics for pain as prescribed.
IV. Administer antibiotics as prescribed.
V. Administer tetanus toxoid (or antitoxin), if prescribed.
VI. Maintain meticulous medical and surgical asepsis.
VII. Carry out wound care as prescribed.
   A. Avoid injury to crusts and eschar.
   B. Keep child from scratching and picking at wound.
   C. Provide distraction (young child) and reasoning (older child).
   D. Restrain infant or younger child as needed.
   E. Position for minimal disturbance of grafted area.
VIII. Provide highly nutritious meals and snacks.
   A. Provide extra calories and protein.
   B. Promote appetite by providing attractive meals, preferred foods, and companionship during meals.
   C. Encourage self-help.
   D. Encourage oral feedings, but feed via other means, if necessary: nasogastric tube.
   E. Administer supplementary vitamins and minerals as prescribed.

IX. Administer antacids as prescribed.
X. Carry out active or passive ROM exercises.
XI. Encourage mobility of affected (if it does not disturb graft) and unaffected areas.
XII. Ambulate as soon as feasible.
XIII. Encourage and promote self-help activities appropriate to abilities and developmental level.
XIV. Position in functional attitude for minimum deformity.
XV. Apply splints as ordered and designed.
XVI. Wrap healing tissue with elastic bandage or dress in elastic garments as ordered.
XVII. Convey a positive attitude to child.
XVIII. Provide reinforcement for positive aspects of appearance and capabilities.
XIX. Explore child's feeling regarding altered physical appearance.
  A. Discuss aids that hide any disfigurement.
XX. Promote positive thinking in child.
XXI. Encourage continuing schooling.
XXII. Encourage peer contact.
XXIII. Help family members to set realistic goals for themselves and the child.
XXIV. Teach family skills needed for home care, including wound care, rehabilitation, diet planning, administration of medication (if needed), and diet supplements.

EVALUATION

I. Child exhibits little or no evidence of pain.
II. Child's wound heals with minimal disfigurement.
III. Child recovers uneventfully.
IV. Child exhibits a positive body image.
V. Child and family comply with rehabilitative efforts.

Communicable Diseases

Chickenpox

Description

Chickenpox is a disease characterized by crops of itching, vesicular skin eruptions, with few systemic symptoms.

Pathophysiology

I. Highly contagious infection with varicella-zoster virus
II. Source of infection: respiratory tract secretions
III. Transmission by direct contact, droplet spread, and contaminated objects
IV. Incubation period: usually 13–17 days
V. Period of communicability: Probably 1 day before eruption of lesions to 6 days after vesicles erupt when crust begins to form.

Signs and Symptoms

I. Slight fever
II. Malaise
III. Anorexia
IV. Highly itchy rash
  A. Lesions: papules, vesicles, and crusts present in varying degrees at any time
  B. Distribution: torso, spreading to face and extremities

Therapeutic Management

I. Symptomatic
II. Aspirin administration contraindicated because of association with Reye's syndrome

Nursing Care

DATA COLLECTION

I. Perform routine assessment.
II. Pay particular attention to type and configuration of lesions.

PLANNING

I. Safe, effective care environment
  A. See Nursing Care of the Ill Child.
  B. Prevent spread of infection to other children.
II. Physiological integrity
  A. Prevent development of secondary infection of lesions.
III. Psychosocial integrity
  A. See Nursing Care of the Ill Child.
  B. Reduce scarring.
IV. Health promotion and maintenance
  A. Promote optimum health.

IMPLEMENTATION

I. Isolate infected child and his or her secretions from others.
II. Implement hospital policy for hospitalized child.
III. Administer soothing lotion (e.g., calamine) to itchy areas.
IV. Prevent scratching:
  A. Keep skin clean.
  B. Keep child's fingernails short.
  C. Apply mittens or elbow restraints, if necessary.
  D. Explain the danger of secondary infection and scarring to older children.
  E. Suggest applying pressure to areas to relieve discomfort.
V. Keep child occupied with diversional activities.
VI. Teach family skills needed for home care, including preventing spread of infection

EVALUATION

I. Child recovers uneventfully, with minimal or no scarring.
II. Others remain free of infection.

Diphtheria

Description

Diphtheria is an infectious disease characterized by respiratory infection and membrane on the pharynx.

Pathophysiology

I. Infection with the bacterium *Corynebacterium diphtheriae*.
II. Toxins produced may affect nervous system and heart.
III. Sources of infection: nasopharyngeal secretions, skin, eye, and lesions of affected person.

IV. Incubation period: 2–5 days or longer.
V. Period of communicability: until bacilli are no longer present—usually 2 weeks, but can extend to 4 weeks.

Signs and Symptoms

I. Nasal: resembles common cold
II. Pharyngeal
   A. Anorexia
   B. Malaise
   C. Fever
   D. Smooth, adherent white or gray membrane on mucous membrane
III. Laryngeal
   A. Fever
   B. Hoarseness
   C. Cough
   D. Signs of airway obstruction possible

Therapeutic Management

I. Administer antitoxin.
II. Administer antibiotics.
III. Allow complete bed rest.
IV. Perform tracheostomy or intubation for airway obstruction.
V. Provide symptomatic treatment of shock.
VI. Treat infected contacts and carriers.

Nursing Care

DATA COLLECTION

I. Perform routine assessment.
II. Observe for evidence of respiratory obstruction.
III. Assist with diagnostic procedures: nose and throat culture, sensitivity testing.

PLANNING

I. Safe, effective care environment
   A. See Nursing Care of the Ill Child.
   B. Prevent spread of infection.
II. Physiological integrity
   A. Help to eradicate organisms.
   B. Prevent complications.
III. Psychosocial integrity
   A. See Nursing Care of the Ill Child.
IV. Health promotion and maintenance
   A. Promote optimum health.
   B. Immunize susceptible individuals.

IMPLEMENTATION

I. Maintain strict isolation according to hospital policy and strict bedrest.
II. Immunize susceptible individuals.
III. Administer antibiotics and antitoxin as prescribed.
   A. Participate in sensitivity testing; have emergency equipment (tracheostomy set, epinephrine) readily available in the event of a reaction.
IV. Provide total care to promote rest and prevent cardiac complications.
V. Administer oxygen, humidity, and so on, as prescribed.

VI. Teach family skills needed for home care, including preventing spread of infection.

EVALUATION

I. Child recovers uneventfully.
II. Child remains free of complications.
III. Others remain free of infection.

Infectious Mononucleosis

Description

Infectious mononucleosis is an acute, self-limiting, contagious disease presumed to be of viral origin.

Pathophysiology

I. Mildly contagious disease caused by Epstein-Barr virus
II. Source: oral secretions
III. Transmitted by direct intimate contact with oral secretions
IV. Incubation period approximately 2–8 weeks

Signs and Symptoms

I. Headache
II. Malaise
III. Fatigue
IV. Fever
V. Loss of appetite
VI. Enlarged lymph nodes
VII. Enlarged spleen
VIII. Some liver involvement with jaundice

Therapeutic Management

I. Supportive treatment:
   A. Analgesic (acetaminophen) for headache, fever, malaise
   B. Gargles, hot drinks, analgesic lozenges for sore throat
II. Bed rest for fatigue.
III. Regulate activities according to tolerance.

Nursing Care

DATA COLLECTION

I. Perform routine assessment.
II. Assist with diagnostic procedures: CBC, heterophil antibody test, enzyme immunoassay test, Monospot.

PLANNING

I. Safe, effective care environment
   A. See Nursing Care of the Ill Child.
II. Physiological integrity
   A. Provide comfort.
   B. Prevent secondary infection.
III. Psychosocial integrity
   A. See Nursing Care of the Ill Child.
   B. Support and educate child and family.
IV. Health promotion and maintenance
   A. Promote optimum health.
   B. Prepare family for home care.

IMPLEMENTATION

I. Provide comfort measures (e.g., analgesics, gargles).
II. Help child and family to determine appropriate activities according to symptoms and interests.
III. Allow child to express feelings of depression and resentment related to lengthy convalescence, fatigue, and restriction of activities.

EVALUATION

I. Child verbalizes feelings and concerns.
II. Child and family comply with therapeutic regimen.
III. Family demonstrates an understanding of the disease and the ability to provide home care.

Measles (Rubeola)

Description

Measles is an acute, highly contagious disease involving the respiratory tract and characterized by a blotchy, macular rash.

Pathophysiology

I. Highly contagious infection with the measles virus
II. Source of infection: respiratory tract secretions
III. Transmission by direct contact with infectious droplets
IV. Incubation period: 10–20 days; 14 days to appearance of rash
V. Period of communicability: from 4 days before to 5 days after appearance of rash
VI. Complications: otitis media, bronchopneumonia, or encephalitis

Signs and Symptoms

I. Onset
  A. Fever and malaise
  B. Cough, conjunctivitis, runny nose
  C. Small, irregular red (Koplik's) spots on mucous membrane of mouth
II. Rash: appears 3–4 days after onset
  A. Begins as red, round, raised rash on face
  B. Gradually spreads downward
III. Photophobia (often)
IV. Anorexia
V. Enlarged lymph nodes

Therapeutic Management

I. Supportive
II. Acetaminophen for fever and discomfort
III. Prophylactic antibiotics

Nursing Care

DATA COLLECTION

I. Perform routine assessment.

PLANNING

I. Safe, effective care environment
  A. See Nursing Care of the Ill Child.

  B. Reduce irritating environmental stimuli.
  C. Prevent spread of infection to others.
II. Physiological integrity
  A. Promote comfort.
  B. Prevent complications.
III. Psychosocial integrity
  A. See Nursing Care of the Ill Child.
IV. Health promotion and maintenance
  A. Promote optimum health.
  B. Prepare family for home care.

IMPLEMENTATION

I. Isolate as appropriate and according to hospital policy.
II. Immunize susceptible individuals.
III. Maintain bed rest and provide quiet activity.
IV. Dim light in room if child is photophobic.
V. Administer acetaminophen as prescribed.
VI. Avoid chilling.
VII. Cleanse eyelids with warm saline to remove secretions and crusts.
VIII. Teach family skills needed for home care, including preventing spread of infection.

EVALUATION

I. Child exhibits no evidence of discomfort.
II. Child recovers uneventfully.
III. Child remains free of complications.
IV. Others do not contract the disease.

Mumps

Description

Mumps is an acute infectious disease characterized by swelling of the parotid glands.

Pathophysiology

I. Highly contagious infection with paramyxovirus
II. Sources of infection: direct contact and droplet
III. Incubation period: 14–21 days
IV. Period of communicability: immediately before and after swelling begins.
V. Unilateral or bilateral involvement of the parotid glands chiefly
VI. Frequently extends to include testes in adult men

Signs and Symptoms

I. Onset: 24 hours
  A. Fever
  B. Headache
  C. Malaise
  D. Anorexia
II. Parotid gland enlarging to maximum size in 1–3 days
III. Accompanied by pain and tenderness

Therapeutic Management

I. Primarily supportive
II. Respiratory isolation advised

Nursing Care

DATA COLLECTION

I. Perform routine assessment.
II. Assist with diagnostic tests: culture from throat washings, urine, or spinal fluid; viral studies.

PLANNING

I. Safe, effective care environment
   A. See Nursing Care of the Ill Child.
   B. Prevent spread of infection.
II. Physiological integrity
   A. Promote comfort.
   B. Prevent complications.
III. Psychosocial integrity
   A. See Nursing Care of the Ill Child.
IV. Health promotion and maintenance
   A. Promote optimum health.
   B. Prepare family for home care.

IMPLEMENTATION

I. Use respiratory isolation precautions during hospitalization.
II. Avoid contact with individuals who have not had mumps.
III. Offer easily swallowed bland foods.
IV. Administer analgesics for discomfort as prescribed.
V. Apply warm or cool compresses to area of neck swelling.
VI. Encourage quiet play and nonstrenuous activity.
VII. Teach family skills needed for home care, including preventing spread of infection.

EVALUATION

I. Child recovers uneventfully.
II. Child remains free of complications.
III. Others do not contract the disease.

Pertussis (Whooping Cough)

Description

Pertussis is an acute, highly contagious respiratory disease characterized by a paroxysmal cough that ends with a loud "whooping" inspiration.

Pathophysiology

I. Highly contagious infection with the bacillus *Bordetella pertussis*
II. Source of infection: respiratory tract
III. Transmission by direct contact, droplet spread, freshly contaminated articles
IV. Incubation period: 3–21 days; usually 10 days
V. Period of communicability: highest during runny nose stage; risk diminishing rapidly but lasting up to 3 weeks

Signs and Symptoms

I. Catarrhal stage
   A. Runny nose
   B. Sneezing
   C. Teary eyes
   D. Cough
   E. Low-grade fever
II. Paroxysmal stage
   A. Frequent attacks
   B. Cough becoming paroxysmal after 1–2 weeks
      1. Series of short, rapid bursts during exhalation
      2. Followed by characteristic "whoop"
   C. Large amounts of mucus being expelled during or after paroxysm
   D. Vomiting frequently after coughing attacks

Therapeutic Management

I. Hospitalization of infants and children with potentially severe disease
II. Supportive care
III. Antimicrobials

Nursing Care

DATA COLLECTION

I. Perform routine assessment.
II. Observe coughing.
III. Observe for signs of airway obstruction.
IV. Assist with diagnostic procedures: throat culture, WBC, direct immunofluorescence to nasal secretions.

PLANNING

I. Safe, effective care environment
   A. See Nursing Care of the Ill Child.
   B. Reduce or eliminate factors that cause coughing.
   C. Prevent spread of infection.
II. Physiological integrity
   A. Reduce coughing.
   B. Ease upper respiratory symptoms.
III. Psychosocial integrity
   A. See Nursing Care of the Ill Child.
   B. Reassure child and family during coughing episodes.
IV. Health promotion and maintenance
   A. Promote optimum health.
   B. Prepare family for home care.

IMPLEMENTATION

I. Isolate hospitalized child according to hospital policy.
II. Avoid contact with nonimmunized children.
III. Immunize susceptible individuals.
IV. Administer antibiotics as prescribed.
V. Reduce factors that cause coughing:
   A. Keep room well ventilated.
   B. Keep environment smoke and dust free.
   C. Avoid extremes of temperature or chilling.
   D. Keep child playing quietly.
VI. Provide comfort measures to prevent distress.
VII. Maintain child in mist tent with high humidity.
VIII. Encourage fluid intake.
IX. Refeed if child vomits.
X. Teach family skills needed for home care, including preventing spread of infection.

EVALUATION

I. Child exhibits minimal coughing.
II. Child recovers uneventfully.
III. Child remains free of complications.
IV. Others remain free of infection.

Rubella (German Measles)

Description

Rubella is a mild contagious disease characterized by red, raised rash; swollen lymph nodes; and slight fever.

Pathophysiology

I. Contagious infection with rubella virus
II. Source of infection: nasogastric secretions
III. Transmission by direct contact
IV. Incubation period: 14–21 days; usually 16–18 days
V. Period of communicability: 7 days before to 5 days after appearance of rash

Signs and Symptoms

I. Postnatal
   A. Low-grade fever, malaise, headache
   B. Swollen lymph nodes
   C. Rash
      1. Pinkish-red, round, raised
      2. On face initially
      3. Spreading downward to neck, trunk, and extremities
      4. Disappearing in 3 days in same order as it began
II. Congenital rubella syndrome
   A. Various deformities in infant if contracted during the first trimester of pregnancy
   B. Growth retardation of infant

Therapeutic Management

I. Supportive care

Nursing Care

DATA COLLECTION

I. Perform routine assessment.
II. Assist with diagnostic tests: serological tests; throat, blood, urine, or spinal fluid culture; specific IgM antibody titer.

PLANNING

I. Safe, effective care environment
   A. See Nursing Care of the Ill Child.
   B. Prevent spread of disease.
   C. Prevent prenatal disease.
II. Physiological integrity
   A. Provide comfort measures.
III. Psychosocial integrity
   A. See Nursing Care of the Ill Child.
IV. Health promotion and maintenance
   A. Promote optimum health.
   B. Prepare family for home care.

IMPLEMENTATION

I. Immunize susceptible individuals.
II. Prevent contact with pregnant women.
III. Administer acetaminophen for discomfort.
IV. Teach family skills needed for home care, including preventing spread of infection.

EVALUATION

I. Child recovers uneventfully.
II. Child remains free of complications.
III. Others do not contract the disease.

Streptococcal Infection (Scarlet Fever)

Description

Streptococcal infection, or scarlet fever, is an acute infectious disease of childhood characterized by sore throat, fever, enlarged lymph nodes, and rash.

Pathophysiology

I. Contagious infection with group A β-hemolytic streptococci
II. Source of infection: nasopharyngeal secretions
III. Transmission by direct contact or droplet spread, freshly contaminated articles
IV. Incubation period: 2–4 days
V. Period of communicability: 7 days before to about 5 days after appearance of rash
VI. Complications: otitis media, tonsillar abscess, sinusitis, rheumatic fever, nephritis, or carditis

Signs and Symptoms

I. Onset
   A. Abrupt high fever
   B. Pulse increased out of proportion to fever
   C. Chills, malaise, headache
   D. Vomiting, abdominal pain
II. Sore throat
   A. Tonsils: red, enlarged
   B. Tongue: red, swollen, coated with white ("red strawberry tongue")
III. Skin
   A. Red, pinhead-sized rash (occurs in 12–36 hours)
   B. Rash generalized, seldom seen on face
   C. Face flushed
   D. Desquamation begins at end of first week; usually complete by 3 weeks

Therapeutic Management

I. Full course of penicillin
II. Supportive measures during fever phase

Nursing Care

DATA COLLECTION

I. Perform routine assessment.
II. Assist with diagnostic test: throat culture.

PLANNING

I. Safe, effective care environment
   A. See Nursing Care of the Ill Child.
   B. Prevent spread of infection.
II. Physiological integrity
   A. Promote comfort.
   B. Prevent complications.
III. Psychosocial integrity
   A. See Nursing Care of the Ill Child.
IV. Health promotion and maintenance
   A. Promote optimum health.
   B. Prepare family for home care.

IMPLEMENTATION

I. Administer penicillin as prescribed.
II. Promote bed rest during fever phase.
III. Administer acetaminophen for sore throat.
IV. Emphasize importance of adherence to penicillin regimen.
V. Teach family skills needed for home care, including preventing spread of infection.

EVALUATION

I. Child recovers uneventfully.
II. Child remains free of complications.
III. Others do not contract the disease.

Childhood Immunizations

Description

I. Most effective way to prevent many communicable childhood illnesses from developing.
II. The American Academy of Pediatrics and the Centers for Disease Control have established guidelines for routine administration of currently licensed immunizations which are revised with the development of new vaccines, scientific knowledge, and changes in disease patterns.
III. The recommended schedule for all babies regardless of birth weight or gestational age starts at birth with the hepatitis B immunization in the United States.
IV. Subsequent immunizations for diphtheria, tetanus, pertussis, *Haemophilus influenzae* type B (Hib), poliomyelitis (IPV), pneumonococcus (PCV), measles, mumps, rubella, and varicella follow at regular intervals.
V. Immunizations are referred to by the names of the disease they mimic.
VI. Immunizations against influenza, hepatatis A, cytomegalovirus (CMV), herpes simplex virus, human immunodeficiency virus (HIV/AIDS), malaria, meningococcus, rabies, pneumococcus, and streptococcus among others are in various stages of development and may be recommended for specific at risk populations.

Pathophysiology

I. Vaccinations work by prompting the body to develop an antibody to fight the disease. See Communicable Diseases for information about several diseases preventable through vaccination.

2003 Recommended Immunization Schedule*	
Age	**Vaccination**
Birth	HepB #1
2 months	HepB #2, DTaP, Hib, IPV, PCV
4 months	DTaP, Hib, IPV, PCV
6 months	HepB #3, DTaP, Hib, IPV, PCV
12 months	MMR #1, Varicella, PCV
15 months	DTaP
4–6 years	DTaP, IPV, MMR#2
11–12 years	Td

*Adapted from www.cdc.gov/nip/acip

II. Full-term babies are born with some antibodies from their mother but over time these antibodies disappear.
III. Vaccinations stimulate the body's immune system to make its own antibodies.
IV. More than one dose of a vaccine may be required to develop immunity. Recommended timing for subsequent doses varies for each vaccine. Boosters may be necessary to maintain immunity.
V. Side effects of vaccines include tenderness, redness, hardness, or swelling at the injection (shot)] site; irritability, fatigue, malaise, or nausea.
VI. Immunizations are extremely safe and there are ongoing efforts to make them safer.
VII. True contraindications to vaccinations are moderate or severe illness or previous anaphylactic reaction to a vaccine or any vaccine component.
VII. Vaccines must be stored and handled properly.
VIII. Consult the National Immunization Program for detailed information about vaccines, including timing, precautions, and contraindications at www.cdc.gov/nip/acip.

Nursing Care

DATA COLLECTION

I. Assess immunization status at each health encounter; e.g., office visit, emergency room visit.
II. Determine family's knowledge and beliefs about immunizations.

PLANNING

I. Safe, effective care environment.
   A. Include pain reduction strategies. See Fear and Anxiety Reduction.
   B. Recommend use of acetaminophen at time of vaccine and every 4–6 hours for 1 day with diphtheria-tetanus-pertussis (DTaP), measles-mumps-rubella (MMR), and varicella vaccines to decrease side effects.
   C. Consult appropriate schedule for vaccine administration; e.g., catch-up schedule if child not immunized in first year of life.
II. Physiologic integrity.
   A. Follow manufacturer's recommendations for preparation of individual vaccinations.

B. Note identifying information about vaccine; e.g., manufacturer and lot numbers and expiration date, before administering any injection.

C. Rotate injection sites giving separate injections in different sites.

III. Psychosocial integrity.

   A. Prepare child and family for procedure(s).

   B. Use combined vaccines as much as possible to decrease the number of injections.

IV. Health promotion and maintenance.

   A. Provide parents with complete vaccination information at any opportunity.

   B. Prepare family for home care.

   C. Minimize barriers to immunization; e.g., long waiting lines and limited hours.

IMPLEMENTATION

I. Choose needle to deposit antigen deep in vastus lateralis or ventrogluteal muscle (1 inch in infants). Deltoid may be used after 18 months of age

II. Provide parents or guardians with information about the risks of the disease and of the vaccine, an opportunity to ask questions, and obtain signed informed consent forms for immunizations.

III. Report any vaccine reaction.

IV. Document information about vaccine for medical and family records; e.g., manufacturer and lot numbers, date, and injection site.

EVALUATION

I. Child's immunization status remains current.

II. Family keeps the immunization record.

III. Child remains free of complications

Psychosocial Disorders

Failure to Thrive

Description

Failure to thrive (FTT) is a deviation from the established growth pattern in child <3 years of age.

I. Organic FTT: growth failure due to major illness

II. Nonorganic FTT: presence of growth retardation in the absence of organic dysfunction

Pathophysiology

I. Organic FTT causes: principally neurological, GI, or endocrine dysfunction

II. Nonorganic FTT causes: neglect, poverty

Signs and Symptoms

I. Growth failure

   A. Weight 20% or more below the ideal weight for an infant's height

II. Nonorganic

   A. Apathy

   B. Withdrawal behavior

   C. Feeding or eating dysfunction

D. No fear of strangers (at age when stranger anxiety expected)

E. Avoidance of eye contact

F. Wide-eyed gaze, continual scan of the environment

G. Muscles stiff and unyielding or flaccid and unresponsive

H. Minimum amount of smiling

Therapeutic Management

I. Organic: determination and treatment of cause

II. Nonorganic: hospitalization for feeding trial and observation

   A. Home treatment

      1. Implement feeding program.

      2. Provide infant stimulation program.

      3. Refer to community resources that provide services to reduce family stress.

      4. Provide mental health services (individual or group).

      5. Perform conscientious medical follow-up.

   B. Recommendation of termination of parental rights, if necessary

Nursing Care

DATA COLLECTION

I. Perform routine assessment.

II. Assess feeding behaviors, parent-child interaction.

III. Obtain detailed history.

IV. Assist with diagnostic procedures.

PLANNING

I. Safe, effective care environment

   A. See Nursing Care of the Ill Child.

   B. Provide a nurturing environment for child.

   C. Promote trusting environment between caregiver and child.

II. Physiological integrity

   A. Plan feeding program that encourages an adequate caloric intake.

   B. Implement care plan for specific organic disorder (if identified).

III. Psychosocial integrity

   A. See Nursing Care of the Ill Child.

   B. Promote a trusting relationship.

   C. Provide appropriate infant stimulation.

   D. Provide nurturing environment for family.

   E. Foster parental self-esteem.

IV. Health promotion and maintenance

   A. Promote optimum health.

   B. Achieve and maintain optimum nutrition.

   C. Prepare family for home care.

IMPLEMENTATION

I. Maintain structured routine in care.

II. Provide continuity of nursing personnel for care.

III. Implement feeding program:

   A. Provide unlimited feeding of diet for age.

   B. Avoid interruptions of feedings (e.g., laboratory studies, radiology, examinations).

C. Remain calm and relaxed during feeding.

D. Follow child's rhythm during feeding.

E. Continue feeding even when child tries to refuse food.

IV. Provide eye contact during care.

V. Praise child for desired behavior.

VI. Provide sensory stimulation—tactile, visual, and auditory—appropriate to child's developmental level.

VII. Provide nurturing environment for family.

VIII. Teach family about child's physical care, developmental skills, and emotional needs.

IX. Serve as role model in child's care.

X. Afford family the opportunity to discuss feelings and concerns.

XI. Provide emotional nurturance without encouraging dependency.

XII. Build family's self-esteem with praise for positive behaviors and achievements.

XIII. Teach skills needed for home care:

A. Continue teaching skills needed for care.

B. Provide for continued infant stimulation program.

C. Provide for a consistent contact system.

D. Refer to community resources that provide ongoing care and services to reduce family stress.

EVALUATION

I. Infant attains and maintains desired weight.

II. Infant accomplishes expected developmental tasks.

III. Family demonstrates an understanding of the condition and the ability to provide home care.

IV. Family demonstrates nurturing behaviors toward infant.

Child Maltreatment

Description

Child maltreatment is intentional physical abuse or neglect, emotional abuse, or sexual abuse of children.

Pathophysiology

I. Possible characteristics of child

A. Viewed as difficult or different

B. Child reminds caregiver of an unliked person in life

C. Often born prematurely

D. Born to unmarried parents or from an unwanted pregnancy

E. Seriously or chronically ill

II. Possible parental characteristics

A. Victim of abuse as a child

B. Emotionally immature

C. Violent behavior

D. Low self-esteem

E. Inadequate understanding of normal growth and development; expectations beyond capabilities of the child

F. Role reversal: parent expects child to be nurturer

G. Living in social isolation

H. Not seeking support or assistance from others

III. Situational characteristics

A. Environment of chronic stress: interpersonal relationships, financial, unemployment, alcoholism, drug addiction, poor housing

B. Lack of adequate support systems

Signs and Symptoms

I. Physical evidence of abuse or neglect or both

A. Soft-tissue injuries: abrasions, lacerations, bruises

B. Traumatic bruises in varying stages of healing

C. Burns, especially symmetrical burns of buttocks, genitalia, legs, or hands; round "dug-out" craters (cigarette burns)

D. Bites, hair loss

E. Fractures

F. Drug intoxication

II. Neglect

A. Evidence of noncare: dirty, ill-fed, and ill-clothed

B. Evidence of lack of stimulation

C. FTT

D. Medical neglect

III. Emotional abuse: extremely varied; difficult to define and identify

A. Self-destructive behavior

B. Antisocial behavior

C. Child humiliated, labeled, put down

D. Child as family scapegoat

E. Family with unrealistic expectations of child

F. Suicide attempts

IV. Sexual abuse

A. Injuries in genital area

B. Torn, stained, or bloody underclothing

Therapeutic Management

I. Protect from further abuse.

II. Treat injuries.

III. Provide nurturing environment.

Nursing Care

DATA COLLECTION

I. Perform routine assessment.

II. Describe any physical injury.

III. Observe parent-child interaction.

IV. Identify family strengths and possible support systems.

V. Assist with diagnostic procedures.

PLANNING

I. Safe, effective care environment

A. Remove child from abusive situation.

II. Physiological integrity

A. Promote healing of physical injuries.

B. Prevent complications.

III. Psychosocial integrity

A. See Nursing Care of the Ill Child.

B. Promote nonthreatening, nurturing environment.

C. Support and educate family.

IV. Health promotion and maintenance

A. Promote optimum health.

B. Prepare family for home care.

IMPLEMENTATION

I. Establish protective measures for child as indicated.
II. Report suspected abuse to proper authorities.
III. Keep factual, objective records.
IV. Teach family about normal growth and developmental patterns and appropriate expectations for age.
V. Help family accept its parenting role.
VI. Provide anticipatory guidance.
VII. Refer to community resources that provide services to reduce family stresses.
VIII. Reinforce family strengths.

EVALUATION

I. Child remains free of injury.
II. Child exhibits appropriate behavior for developmental level.
III. Child exhibits minimal or no evidence of distress.
IV. Child accepts foster family, when necessary.
V. Family demonstrates an understanding of the condition and the ability to provide safe home care.

Poisoning

General Concepts of Poisoning

Description

Poisoning consists of eating, drinking, or inhaling toxic amounts of drugs, household products, or any item.

Pathophysiology

I. Depends on poison

Signs and Symptoms

I. Increased respirations
II. Severe acidosis
III. Electrolyte imbalance
IV. Restlessness
V. Thirst
VI. Fever
VII. Sweating
VIII. Oliguria
IX. Tinnitus
X. Tremors
XI. Convulsions
XII. Coma

Therapeutic Management

I. Identify toxic substance and antidote.
II. Stabilize cardiovascular and respiratory systems.
III. Remove remaining poison from body.
IV. Increase excretion of toxin.
V. Prevent and/or correct effects of absorbed toxin.
VI. Prevent complications.

Nursing Care

Data Collection
I. Acquire careful and detailed history regarding what, when, and how much of toxic substance has entered the body.
II. Collect assessment data on area exposed to poison and VSs.
III. Assist with diagnostic procedures: blood and urine examination for presence of specific substances.
IV. Save all evidence of poison (container, plant, vomitus, urine).
V. Observe client for latent symptoms of poisoning.

PLANNING

I. Safe, effective care environment
   A. Protect from injury.
II. Physiological integrity
   A. Dilute poisonous substance.
   B. Remove substance from stomach.
   C. Prevent aspiration of vomitus.
   D. Absorb remaining substance.
   E. Prevent complications.
III. Psychosocial integrity:
   A. Support and educate child and family.
   B. Prepare child and family for procedures.
IV. Health promotion and maintenance
   A. Prevent recurrence.
   B. Prepare family for home care.

IMPLEMENTATION

I. Contact physician for immediate advice regarding treatment, local poison control center, or emergency facility.
II. Implement measures to eliminate or reduce effects of poison.
III. Ingested poison:
   A. Remove pills, plant parts, or other materials from mouth.
   B. Administer water to dilute substance unless contraindicated.
   C. Administer ipecac syrup to induce vomiting (unless client swallowed hydrocarbons or corrosives or is comatose).
   D. Position to prevent aspiration.
   E. Prepare for and assist with gastric lavage, if prescribed.
   F. Administer activated charcoal after vomiting has occurred, to absorb remaining poison, following hospital protocol.
IV. Carry out orders for management of specific poisons (e.g., IV infusion, artificial ventilation), and administer specific antidotes (e.g., chelating agents, antivenom) and anticonvulsants.
V. Provide comfort and reassurance to child and family.
VI. Teach poison prevention.

EVALUATION

I. Child eliminates poison from body.
II. Child remains free of complications.
III. Child does not have a repeated episode of poisoning.
IV. Family demonstrates an understanding of the condition and the ability to provide a child safe home environment.

Cultural Considerations

Table 4–1 describes the roles that children and adolescents play in a variety of cultural groups found in the United States. An understanding of cultural factors is important to the delivery of quality nursing care.

Table 4–1. Cultural Roles for Children and Adolescents

Cultural Group	Roles for Children	Roles for Adolescents
African American Heritage	• Parents value self-reliance and education for their children • Respectfulness, obedience, conformity to parent-defined rules, and good behavior are stressed for children	• Adolescents are assigned household chores as part of their family responsibility or seek employment for pay when they are old enough, thus learning "survival skills" • Has been a drop in teenage pregnancy • Teenage mother is expected to assume primary responsibilities for her child where the extended family becomes a strong support system
Amish Heritage	• Before and during elementary school years, parents are more directive as they guide and train their children to assume responsibility, productive roles in Amish society	• Young people over age 16 may be encouraged to work away from home to gain experience, but their wages are still sent home to the parental household • Some experimentation with non-Amish dress and behavior among Amish teenagers is tolerated during this period of relative leniency • Expectation is that an adult decision to be baptized before marriage will call the young people back to the discipline of the church, as they take on full adult roles
Appalachian Heritage	• Children are accepted regardless of their negative behaviors in school or with authority figures • Permissive behavior at home is unacceptable, and hands-on physical punishment, to a degree that some perceive as abuse, is common • For children who have problems with school performance, the most effective approach for increasing performance is to provide individualized attention rather than group support or attention	• As children progress into their teens, mischievous behavior is accepted but not condoned • Continuing formal education may not be stressed because many teens are expected to get a job to help support the family • Not uncommon for teenagers to marry by the age of 15 and some as early as 13. • Children, single or married, may return to their parents' home, where they are readily accepted whenever the need arises
Arab Heritage	• Children are dearly loved, indulged, and included in all family activities • A child's character and successes (or failures) in life are attributed to upbringing and parental influence • Children are expected to behave in an honorable manner and not bring shame to the family • Children are raised to not question elders and to be obedient to older brothers and sisters • Children are made to feel ashamed because others have seen them misbehave, rather than to experience guilt arising from self-criticism and inward regret	• Adolescents are expected to remain enmeshed in the family system • Adolescents are pressed to succeed academically; in part because of the connections between professional careers and social status • Conversely, behaviors that would bring family dishonor, such as academic failure, sexual activity, illicit drug use, and juvenile delinquency, are avoided • Girls are expected to maintain chastity and decency
Chinese Heritage	• Children are well dressed and kept clean and well fed • Child is protected and independence is not fostered • Children usually depend on the family for everything • Children feel a lot of pressure to succeed to help improve the future of the family and the country • Most children value studying over playing and peer relationships • In rural areas, male children are more valued than female children because they continue the family line and provide labor • In urban areas, female children are valued as highly as male children • Children today are becoming more outspoken as they read more and watch more television and movies	• Few teens earn money because they are expected to study hard and to help the family with daily chores rather than to seek employment • Most adolescents value studying over playing and peer relationships • Adolescents are expected to determine who they are and where they want to end up in life • Teens value a strong and happy family life, and seldom do things that jeopardize that unanimity • Adolescents question affairs of life and make great efforts to see at least two sides of every issue. • They enjoy exploring different views with their peers and try to explore them with their parents

(Continued on following page)

Table 4–1. **Cultural Roles for Children and Adolescents** *(Continued)*		
Cultural Group	**Roles for Children**	**Roles for Adolescents**
	• Children are expected to help their parents in the home • Boys and girls play together when they are young, but as they get older, this changes because their roles, and the corresponding expectations, are predetermined by Chinese society • Boys are more active, and take pride in physical fitness • Girls are not nearly as interested in fitness as boys, and often enjoy reading, art, and music	• Teenage pregnancy is not common among Chinese, but it is increasing among Chinese Americans • Young men and women enter the workforce immediately after high school if they are unable to continue their education • Many continue to live with their parents and contribute to the family even after marriage and the birth of a child
Cuban Heritage	• Children study, respect their parents, and follow the straight and narrow • A boy is expected to learn a trade or prepare himself for work • A girl is expected "to keep herself honorable while single" and to prepare herself for marriage • Girls are instructed to avoid the opposite sex and not to go out without "ample protection"	• When a daughter reaches 15, a birthday party is typically held to celebrate this rite of passage • This rite of passage is indicative of the young woman's readiness for courting by a boyfriend • Adolescents may undergo an identity crisis, not knowing whether they are fully Cuban or American • One area of conflict is the Cuban practice of chaperoning unmarried couples when they go dating
Filipino Heritage	• Childhood socialization to the mechanism of shame reinforces the value of *utang na loob,* a personal sense of indebtedness and loyalty to kin, and generational respect • Children learn early to behave differently toward insiders and outsiders	• Dating at an early age is discouraged for young daughters who are advised that a short courtship period may suggest that they are "easy to get" • Young men with sincere intent must strive to get on the good side of the family and have patience with a long courtship • Open demonstrations of affection with sexual undertones are to be avoided by the young couple • Traditional families desire that their daughters remain chaste before marriage • Pregnancy out of wedlock brings shame to the whole family • High school students admitted that they were taught that all problems should be kept within the family, and that talking to outsiders such as friends, teachers, or counselors would bring shame to the family
Iranian Heritage	• Children in rural Iran are just as responsible for the family economy as adults • Children are expected to be loyal to their families and behave respectfully toward their elders • Manners are considered important even outside the home, where children are expected to be clean and well behaved and to refrain from rowdiness • Children are taught at an early age to avoid eating if no one else has yet been served at a meal, and never to speak rudely to elders	• Girls are expected to behave and dress more modestly than boys, especially as they approach adolescence • Young women are expected to remain virgins until they marry, but sexual activity by men outside marriage is tolerated • Dating is not allowed in the most traditional families • Adolescents behave more respectfully toward family members, particularly the elderly and other highly respected individuals • The fear of shaming the family and losing face in public act as a strong social constraint • Adolescents are often caught in a dilemma, pulled between their parents' attempts to maintain control and instill Iranian heritage and values, and their own desire to be like their American peers

(Continued on following page)

Cultural Group	Roles for Children	Roles for Adolescents
Irish Heritage	• Boys are allowed and expected to be more aggressive than girls, who are raised to be respectable, responsible, and resilient • Children are expected to have self-restraint, self-discipline, respect, and obedience for their parents and elders	• Adolescents are expected to obey and show respect for their parents as well as church and community figures • Peer group pressures at school may have a significant influence and are often incongruent with the belief systems of Irish Americans, resulting in the family relationships with teenagers containing mixed motivations of love and hatred
Japanese Heritage	• Customary for a mother to sleep with the youngest child until that child is 10 years old or older • When a new baby is born, the older sibling may sleep with the father or a grandparent • The primacy of the mother-son relationship and the absence of the fathers contribute to the known problem of mother-son incest • Japanese men are presumed to be incapable of managing day-to-day matters. • Young Japanese children, especially sons, are quite indulged by Western standards • Children are socialized to study hard, make their best effort, and be good group members • They are taught to take care of each other, and girls are taught to take care of boys • Children who are bullied by schoolmates typically have different looks, interests, or family structures	• Adolescents in Japan have their rebellions; e.g., rock music and pornography allow escape from social restrictions as well as smoking • Once young people graduate from high school, they may express themselves through their clothing, hair, and makeup • Teens and college students in Japan generally do not date • 40% of Japanese high school seniors have had sexual intercourse; 1% of Japanese girls have had abortions by their late teens • Other health concerns among young people include the pressure to conform within a peer group and to perform well in school, known factors in depression and suicide risk • After graduation from high school or college, young adults are traditionally expected to be employed through their network of school contacts or family friends • Young women typically live with their parents, while young men are likely to live in company housing until marriage
Jewish Heritage	• Children are the most valued treasure of the Jewish people • They are considered a blessing and are to be treated with respect and provided with love • Children typically attend Hebrew school at least two afternoons a week after public school throughout the school year • Children play an active role in most holiday celebrations and services • Children should be forever grateful to their parents for giving them the gift of life	• In Judaism, the age of majority is 13 years for a boy and 12 for a girl • At this age, teens are deemed capable of differentiating right from wrong and capable of committing themselves to performing the commandments • Recognition of adulthood occurs during a religious ceremony • Because the sons and daughters are still teenagers living at home, it is recognized that they are still the responsibility of their parents
Korean Heritage	• Children over the age of 5 are expected to be well behaved because the whole family is disgraced if a child behaves in an embarrassing manner • Most children are not encouraged to state their opinions • Future of Korean students is determined by their teachers' recommendations, and this pressure can be extremely intense for students who are not doing well • A student rarely questions a teachers' authority • Girls in elementary school are given a class regarding their menstrual cycle, but no information is given regarding sexual relations • Information about sexual relations is exchanged by word of mouth from friend to friend as the students piece details together	• The pressure of doing well in school and attending a university of high quality leaves adolescents little room for social interactions • Students frequently attend study groups after school or special tutoring sessions paid for by their families in preparation for examinations to enter a university • Dating is uncommon among high school students • Group outings are common for meeting the opposite sex • Neither the school system nor the family assumes responsibility for sex education
Mexican Heritage	• Children are highly valued because they ensure the continuation of the family and cultural values • They are closely protected and not encouraged to leave home	

(Continued on following page)

Table 4–1. **Cultural Roles for Children and Adolescents** (Continued)		
Cultural Group	**Roles for Children**	**Roles for Adolescents**
	• Each child must have godparents in case something interferes with the parents' ability to fulfill their child-rearing responsibilities • Children are taught at an early age to respect parents and older family members, especially grandparents	
Navajo Indians	• Children are looked on with joy and proudly welcomed into the family • Even though children may be named at birth, their names are not revealed until their first laugh, when they are considered officially to have a soul and self-identity • Children are frequently allowed to make decisions that other cultures might consider irresponsible • Children who do not listen to their parents or elders accept the consequences regardless of their age • Navajo children are usually shy and wary of strangers	• An important ritual in Navajo society for teenage girls is the onset of menarche, which is celebrated with special foods that symbolize passage into adulthood • Men are usually excluded from this celebration, with only aunts and grandmothers participating • Older children may be more comfortable with physical closeness rather than actual contact • Older children are taught to be stoic and uncomplaining
Polish Heritage	• The most valued behavior among children is obedience • Children are disciplined not to feel helpless, fragile, or dependent • Taboo child behaviors include anything that undermines parental authority	
Puerto Rican Heritage	• From childhood through adolescence, children are socialized to have respect for adults, especially the elderly • Many families believe that a healthy child is one who is overweight and has red cheeks • Many socialize male children to be powerful and strong • Female children are socialized with a focus on home economics, family dynamics, and motherhood, which places women in a powerful social status • Most families expect their children to stay home until they get married or pursue a college education • Children are expected to follow family traditions and rules	• Teen pregnancy, substance abuse, delinquent behaviors, and depression have been associated with the conflict between Puerto Rican and U.S. cultural values • The value placed on motherhood may be a precursor to teenage pregnancy among adolescents who are seeking power, support, and cultural recognition • Adolescent girls are socialized to be modest, sexually ingenuous, respectful, and subservient to men • Many mothers use threats of punishment, guilt, and discipline, which can create stress and difficulties for adolescents as they struggle with the more permissive cultural patterns in the U.S.
Vietnamese Heritage	• Children are expected to be obedient and devoted to their parents • Children are obliged to do everything possible to please their parents while they are alive and to worship their memory after death • Children are prized and valued because they carry the family lineage • For the first 2 years, their mothers primarily care for them	• Young people are expected to continue to respect their elders and to avoid behavior that might dishonor the family • Parents show relative approval for adolescent freedom of choice regarding dating, marriage, and career choices • Most adolescents have the same pressures and concerns as the U.S. youths

Data from Purnell, LD, and Paulanka, BJ: Transcultural Health Care: A Culturally Competent Approach, ed 2. Phialdelphia, F.A. Davis, 2003.

QUESTIONS

Nora F. Steele, RN.C, DNS, PNP, Susan I. Ray, RN, MS and Golden M. Tradewell, RN, PhD

1. A baby born today at 38 weeks' gestation weighs 5 lb 2 oz (2335 g). The nurse would describe the baby as:

1. A normal newborn
2. Chronically ill
3. Low birth weight
4. Very low birth weight

2. A baby is a low-birth-weight infant born at 36 weeks' gestation. The nurse planning care for this infant would focus on:

1. Conservation of energy and warmth
2. Bathing infant every shift in warm water
3. Prevention of cradle cap by daily shampooing
4. Stimulation of senses

3. The nurse knows that pain responses in a low-birth-weight neonate:

1. Are easy to assess in neonates
2. Do not exist because of an immature neurological system
3. Produce crying and flexing of extremities
4. Require special equipment to assess

4. In a neonate at 36 weeks' gestation, the nurse would anticipate implementation of nursing care for which disorder?

1. Acne
2. Chickenpox
3. Jaundice
4. Scoliosis

5. The nurse would clean a neonate with clear water or mild nonalkaline cleanser two or three times per week because:

1. Cleaning stimulates circulation.
2. Growth of bacteria is minimized.
3. Oils provide nourishment to tissues.
4. Regular cleansing prevents irritation.

6. If a neonate develops respiratory distress syndrome, the nurse should include as an evaluation outcome:

1. Neonate breathes without effort.
2. Neonate recovers from surgery uneventfully.
3. Family seeks genetic counseling.
4. Others do not contract disease.

7. A 2-year-old infant is diagnosed with severe croup (laryngotracheobronchitis). The nurse caring for this child identifies essential therapeutic measures as being hospitalization and:

1. Corticosteroids
2. Cool humidification
3. Intubation
4. Whirlpool baths

8. The nurse is planning for an admission of a preschooler. The nurse knows that a preschooler thinks about illness in terms of:

1. Concerns about privacy
2. External causes for body illnesses
3. Punishment for wrongdoing
4. Separation from a favorite toy or blanket

9. A 3-year-old child is being admitted to the pediatric unit. Phases of separation anxiety that the nurse would observe for are:

1. Crying, withdrawal, and attachment
2. Depression, detachment, and acceptance
3. Protest, despair, and acceptance
4. Protest, despair, and detachment

10. When providing care for a toddler, the nurse knows that the following nursing measures would promote hospital adjustment. (**Select all that apply.**)

1. Allow the toddler to imitate medical procedures.
2. Discourage parental departure when child is sleeping.
3. Institute visitation provisions for siblings.
4. Minimize parental involvement in care.
5. Provide detailed, professional explanations of routines.
6. Use side rails when child is sleeping.

11. A toddler is in respiratory distress, but he refuses to stay in his mist tent. The mother wants you to help. The best intervention by the nurse would be to:

1. Give the child a favorite toy to play with under the tent.
2. Have the mother read to the child as she sits under the tent with him.
3. Administer strong sedation to put the child to sleep.
4. Tell the child that the tent is a spaceship that will take off if he cries.

12. A school-age child is being discharged home from the hospital after being treated for respiratory distress from an asthma attack. Criteria for evaluating nursing care would include outcome objectives such as:

1. Family instead of nursing staff assumes all care.
2. Family demonstrates ability to provide home care.
3. Child accepts all care without responding.
4. Child rejects family as providers of care.

13. The mother of a female toddler tells you that her child has been attending day care for 3 weeks. Today, when she picked up the child, she noticed that the toddler had been scratching her chest, which had red bumps on it. The nurse would suspect which condition?

1. Chickenpox
2. Diphtheria

3. Measles
4. Mumps

14. Which of the following would be the most important nursing intervention for a child with chicken-pox?
    1. Administering aspirin to control elevated temperature
    2. Avoiding the use of calamine lotion because of chances of secondary infection
    3. Keeping the child's fingernails short
    4. Encouraging siblings to visit to prevent isolation and promote adaptation to illness

15. An infant is admitted to the pediatric unit with a diagnosis of failure to thrive (FTT). The infant is apathetic and withdrawn, avoids eye-to-eye contact with a wide-eyed gaze, and continually watches the environment. On the basis of the signs and symptoms, the nurse would suspect the infant of presenting with:
    1. Endocrine dysfunction
    2. Gastrointestinal dysfunction
    3. Neurological dysfunction
    4. Nonorganic FTT

16. When a nurse observes signs and symptoms of child neglect, appropriate action includes which of the following?
    1. Ensure involvement of a variety of caregivers.
    2. Oppose parental decision making.
    3. Promote a trusting relationship.
    4. Provide extra stimulation.

17. The nurse would consider which objective appropriate to evaluate the outcome of care for an infant with nonorganic FTT?
    1. Family demonstrates dependence on nursing staff for care.
    2. Family demonstrates nurturing behaviors toward infant.
    3. Infant maintains admission weight.
    4. Infant makes slow progress toward developmental milestones.

18. A 4-year-old child has swallowed the contents of one bottle of baby aspirin. The physician has ordered administration of ipecac. The clinic nurse understands that the rationale for this medication is to:
    1. Absorb remaining substance.
    2. Dilute poisonous substance.
    3. Prevent aspiration of vomitus.
    4. Remove substance from stomach.

19. A 6-year-old child is admitted to the pediatric unit with partial- and full-thickness third-degree burns. From this information, the nurse can plan burn care that affects:
    1. Dermis only
    2. Epidermis only
    3. All layers of skin
    4. All layers of skin, subcutaneous tissues, and muscle

20. Nursing care for a child with a third-degree burn on the body would focus on:
    1. Encouraging mobility
    2. Helping child to scratch wound
    3. Limiting fluid intake
    4. Removing crusts and eschar

21. Morphine sulfate is prescribed every 4 hours for a burned school-age child. When the nurse arrives to give the medicine, the child's eyes are closed and the child appears to be sleeping. The most appropriate initial response by the nurse is to:
    1. Assess nonverbal pain cues.
    2. Give the shot quickly and leave.
    3. Leave and go back in 30 minutes.
    4. Report the problem to the doctor.

22. You are the nurse who takes a burned client to the playroom for the first time. The client has bandages on both arms. The other children are playing and ignore the client. Your response should be to:
    1. Act as a role model, bringing the child in and playing with him at a table.
    2. Leave him alone in the room and hope it gets better.
    3. Take the child back to his room so he can watch television.
    4. Tell the child to find a game and ask someone to play with him.

23. A 10-year-old child broke her left leg, and the whole end of the bone protrudes through the skin. The nurse understands this fracture to be:
    1. Compound
    2. Greenstick
    3. Incomplete
    4. Simple

24. A school-age child is in traction. When the nurse enters the room, the child is twisted in bed. She says she's trying to reach her radio. The nurse should:
    1. Arrange games, toys, snacks, and call signal within reach.
    2. Take the radio out of the room.
    3. Tell her parents that they need to stay with her all the time.
    4. Tell the child to call whenever she needs anything.

25. A new cast is applied to a school-age child's leg in preparation for discharge. Nursing care of the newly applied cast would include:
    1. Lower the extremity until the cast dries.
    2. Keep the cast moist and clean.
    3. Provide ROM exercises to fractured joint.
    4. Tell the child not to put anything inside the cast.

26. A 14-year-old adolescent has a new diagnosis of diabetes. The nurse would expect this to be:
    1. Glucose intolerance
    2. Insulin-dependent diabetes
    3. Maturity-onset diabetes
    4. Plain diabetes

27. An adolescent with a new diagnosis of diabetes is learning to administer her own medication by injection. The adolescent has drawn up the correct dose, but she cannot give herself a shot. The nurse should:
   1. Give the shot and let her get more practice with an orange.
   2. Assist her by guiding her hand, then insert the needle for her.
   3. Tell her that she does not need the shot as long as she follows her diet.
   4. Tell her that this is a problem that the physician should be made aware of.

28. The nurse understands that planning care for an adolescent with diabetes would include:
   1. Balancing diet, exercise, and insulin
   2. Increasing exercise and activity to lower blood glucose
   3. Limiting dietary intake to lower the blood glucose
   4. Limiting exercise and activity to decrease insulin needs

29. Signs and symptoms of ketoacidosis that the nurse would teach a diabetic with a new diagnosis of diabetes would include:
   1. Glucose in urine
   2. Headache
   3. Low blood sugar
   4. Thirst

30. A toddler had an URI last week. Today, the toddler is crying and pulling at his left ear. The nurse would expect a diagnosis of:
   1. Otitis media
   2. Diphtheria
   3. Pertussis
   4. Tonsillitis

31. With a diagnosis of otitis media, the nurse would not anticipate which of the following in nursing care for the child?
   1. Antibiotic administration
   2. Analgesic administration
   3. Oxygen therapy
   4. Surgical intervention

32. The nurse would identify which outcome when evaluating care of the child with otitis media?
   1. Comfort and ear canal status
   2. Completion of antibiotics
   3. Family's ability to give injections
   4. Prevention of secondary infection

33. A teenage girl is admitted to the adolescent unit with a diagnosis of cystic fibrosis. The nurse determines that the adolescent has a typical sign of this disease when which of the following is noted?
   1. Cool, dry skin
   2. Frequent urination
   3. Large, bulky, foul-smelling stools
   4. Poor appetite

34. The nurse knows that the primary cause of the serious pulmonary problems that children with cystic fibrosis can develop is:
   1. Bronchial constriction
   2. Inadequate surfactant
   3. Pulmonic stenosis
   4. Thick, tenacious mucus

35. If pancreatic enzymes are prescribed for a child with cystic fibrosis, the nurse should administer these by which route?
   1. Intramuscularly
   2. Intavenously
   3. Orally
   4. Intradermally

36. The nurse promotes exercise in an adolescent with cystic fibrosis because it is therapeutically important to help promote a sense of well-being and to:
   1. Aid digestion and absorption of nutrients
   2. Enhance heart muscle and vascular tone
   3. Promote mobilization of lung secretions
   4. Stimulate exocrine gland secretions

37. A child with cystic fibrosis may be treated with a mist tent at home. The nurse would want the family to identify the reason for the mist is to help:
   1. Dilate alveoli
   2. Minimize secretions
   3. Prevent dehydration
   4. Relieve dyspnea

38. Postural drainage is prescribed for home care. The family and child need to learn about the therapy and all positions for treatments. The nurse would teach the family and child which position to help move secretions from the right lower lobes?
   1. Lying on back with head lowered
   2. Lying on left side with head lowered
   3. Lying on left side with head raised
   4. Sitting with left knee bent

39. As a nurse, you know that a child with cystic fibrosis must learn to avoid:
   1. Dog and cat hair
   2. Bacterial infections
   3. Sodium chloride
   4. Ultraviolet light

40. A 6-year-old child is admitted to the pediatric unit with a diagnosis of rheumatic fever (RF). The nurse associates the probable cause of the child's recent sore throat with:
   1. Pneumococci
   2. Staphylococci
   3. Streptococci
   4. Influenza B

41. An initial nursing intervention for a child with RF would include:
   1. Administering corticosteroids
   2. Assisting child into squatting position

3. Encouraging visits by school friends
4. Protecting from sunlight

42. The mother of a child with a diagnosis of RF is concerned that the physician ordered aspirin for her 6-year-old child. The nurse would explain to the mother that aspirin is important to reduce:

1. Carditis
2. Itching
3. Headaches
4. Joint tenderness

43. Evaluation of care for a child with RF would include assessing family knowledge of:

1. Coughing and deep breathing
2. Fluid and diet restrictions
3. Long-term penicillin administration
4. Oxygen therapy

44. A 2-year-old child had a tonsillectomy yesterday. The nurse would be least concerned about:

1. Halitosis
2. Increased pulse
3. Nausea
4. Restlessness

45. The second day after a tonsillectomy, a child is receiving a full-liquid diet. Which of the following should be discouraged?

1. Chocolate milk
2. Ice cream
3. Orange juice
4. Popsicles

46. A child is admitted with bronchial asthma. The respiratory signs that the nurse would expect to see include:

1. Sleep apnea
2. Inspiratory stridor
3. Productive cough
4. Prolonged expirations

47. In the management of an episode of acute asthma, the nurse would not expect to include:

1. Antibiotics
2. Antiemetics
3. Corticosteroids
4. Bronchodilators

48. An infant was given a diagnosis of a lumbar myelomeningocele at birth. The nurse knows that this is a:

1. Defect in closure of spinal vertebral column with varying degrees of tissue protrusion through the opening
2. Failure of complete closure of the vertebral column with no outpouching
3. Hernial protrusion of saclike cyst of meninges containing spinal fluid
4. Hernial protrusion of saclike cyst of meninges containing spinal fluid and a portion of the spinal cord with nerves

49. For an infant with myelomeningocele, nursing care before surgery to close the defect would include:

1. Meticulous skin care, especially in the area of sac
2. Supine positioning whenever possible
3. Securing a diaper firmly over buttocks to avoid contamination
4. Taping a dry dressing over the sac

50. The nurse knows that which of the following is frequently associated with myelomeningoceles?

1. Hydrocephalus
2. Intussusception
3. Mental retardation
4. Pneumonia

51. A mother brings her 2-year-old child to the clinic. The child is drooling, agitated, and appears to be in respiratory distress. The pediatrician suspects epiglottitis. Which action by the nurse is best?

1. Allow the mother to hold the child.
2. Insist that the mother leave the examination room.
3. Give the child cool fruit juice to drink.
4. Obtain a throat culture.

52. The nurse explains to the mother that the usual cause of epiglottitis is:

1. β-Hemolytic streptococcus
2. *Haemophilus influenzae*
3. Respiratory syncytial virus
4. *Staphylococcus aureus*

53. A toddler is being admitted to the pediatric unit with epiglottitis. Which intervention would be the most important for the nurse?

1. Have tracheostomy equipment available.
2. Notify the respiratory therapist of the admission.
3. Have the antibiotics prepared when the child arrives on the unit.
4. Make the child NPO.

54. An infant is being admitted for a cleft lip repair tomorrow morning. The nurse collecting data from the mother will expect to obtain information about:

1. Drooling
2. Noisy respirations
3. Sucking problems
4. Swallowing difficulty

55. During the first 24 hours postoperatively after a cleft lip repair, the nurse would:

1. Apply elbow restraints to the infant.
2. Position the infant prone.
3. Keep the infant upright in an infant seat.
4. Use a mist tent to facilitate the infant's breathing.

56. An 18-year-old adolescent is being admitted to the pediatric unit with a low platelet count. The nurse planning care would:

1. Assess temperature with rectal thermometers.
2. Encourage brushing teeth after each meal and at bedtime.

3. Reduce aspirin intake to once daily.
4. Teach the adolescent the importance of using creams to remove hair on legs.

57. When planning care for a child with neutropenia, the nurse would:

1. Include raw vegetables and fruit in meal plans.
2. Maintain bed rest.
3. Report any temperature elevation to the physician.
4. Restrict visitors.

58. A toddler with a diagnosis of sickle cell disease is being discharged home with his parents. Which nursing intervention should take priority?

1. Assessing the parents' knowledge of pain management
2. Consulting home health care for follow-up
3. Identifying a support group for the family
4. Teaching measures to prevent sickle cell crisis

59. The nurse planning care for a preschooler postoperatively would identify which behavior as being characteristic of pain response in this age group?

1. Demanding explanations
2. Stoic behavior
3. Clinging to parents
4. Stalling behaviors

60. The nurse planning care for a postoperative child receiving meperidine (Demerol) would:

1. Not administer meperidine longer than 48 hours.
2. Give meperidine on the second postoperative day.
3. Prefer meperidine to morphine because it has fewer side effects.
4. Use naloxone (Narcan) to reverse any side effects of meperidine.

61. The nurse planning care for a school-age child immobilized with traction would:

1. Avoid isometric exercises.
2. Force fluids.
3. Limit peer visitation.
4. Offer detailed description of procedures.

62. A child is 12 hours postoperative after repair of a compound fracture of the arm. The nurse would identify which data as requiring immediate attention?

1. Bruising of the fingers
2. Capillary refill of 2 seconds
3. Pallor at the nailbeds
4. Edema of the extremity

63. The nurse would be concerned that a child could develop compartment syndrome if pain is:

1. Radiating distally
2. Responsive to repeated oral medication
3. Unresponsive to oral medication and responsive to narcotics
4. Unresponsive to narcotics

64. The nurse is teaching parents cast care. The nurse would identify which of the following as a sign of infection?

1. Increased pain in the extremity
2. Temperature of 100°F (37.7°C) orally
3. Hot areas felt on the cast
4. Blood-tinged drainage on the cast

65. An adolescent is less than 24 hours postoperative from reduction of a compound fracture. The nurse would be most concerned with:

1. Blood pressure (BP) 100/60 mm Hg
2. Petechiae noted on the chest
3. Moderate amount of pain relief from narcotic
4. Urine output of 600 mL

66. Which action by the nurse is the most important in maintaining Buck's traction on a 4-year-old child?

1. Assessing the weights to ensure that they are hanging freely
2. Conducting neurovascular checks every 4 hours
3. Monitoring the effectiveness of a muscle relaxant
4. Readjusting the fit of the bandage daily to promote countertraction

67. Evaluation of care for a child with a diagnosis of juvenile rheumatoid arthritis would include objectives related to:

1. Preserving joint function
2. Preventing side effects of corticosteroid therapy
3. Minimizing growth to prevent deformities
4. Promoting home schooling

68. Evaluation of care for a child with lupus would include assessing the family's knowledge of:

1. High-protein and high-fat diet
2. Restricting sun exposure
3. Reducing exercise
4. Yearly eye examinations

69. The nurse knows that ritualistic behavior provides security for which age group?

1. Infant
2. Toddler
3. Preschool
4. Adolescent

70. The nurse is aware that which of the following age groups fears body mutilation?

1. Toddler
2. Preschool
3. School-age
4. Adolescent

71. As the nurse planning care for a school-age child, which activity would be the most appropriate for this age?

1. Reading stories to the child
2. Giving the child hospital supplies to collect
3. Playing a card game
4. Listening to a tape from peers

72. A child with a history of allergic rhinitis is scheduled for skin testing today. What measure by the nurse would promote the accuracy of the results?

1. Making sure that the child has no nasal congestion
2. Making sure that the child has not taken antihistamines in the last several days
3. Testing for food allergens
4. Using the posterior legs for testing

73. The nurse would recognize which early sign of anaphylactic shock in a client who received an allergy shot?

    1. Abdominal cramping
    2. Bradycardia
    3. Elevated BP
    4. Sense of doom

74. Which measure would the nurse teach the mother to limit dust mite exposure for her child?

    1. Disinfecting the bath area daily
    2. Limiting the child's exposure to animals
    3. No smoking in the home
    4. Restricting the child from playing on the carpet

75. A child with lupus has been placed on corticosteroids for an indefinite period. Which diet would the nurse teach the family to follow?

    1. Bland
    2. High-protein, high-fiber
    3. Low-sodium
    4. Reduced fat

76. The nurse knows that which symptom is associated with disease activity in a child with lupus?

    1. Abdominal cramping
    2. Chest congestion
    3. Excessive fatigue
    4. Sore throat

77. The nurse would teach a mother to avoid giving which food to a child who is allergic to wheat?

    1. Instant drink mixes
    2. Chocolate-covered peanuts
    3. Salad dressings
    4. Wieners

78. A child has been given a diagnosis of allergy to eggs. The nurse would teach the child to avoid which food?

    1. Cola
    2. Gravy
    3. Instant breakfast drinks
    4. Mayonnaise

79. The nurse would teach the mother to introduce cereal into the infant's diet at what age?

    1. 2 months
    2. 4 months
    3. 9 months
    4. 12 months

80. A mother brought her 6-month-old infant to the well-baby clinic. The mother is interested in starting her infant on cereal. Which cereal would the nurse instruct the mother to introduce first in the infant's diet?

1. Barley
2. Oat
3. Rice
4. Wheat

81. A mother began her 14-month-old child on cow's milk 4 weeks ago. Which symptom would the nurse identify as a possible allergy to cow's milk?

    1. Chronic runny nose
    2. Excessive urination
    3. Irritability
    4. Refusal to drink milk

82. A child admitted with a respiratory infection has been placed on continuous pulse oximetry. The nurse would identify which following situation as best for obtaining an accurate pulse oximetry reading?

    1. Normal hemoglobin level
    2. Room with a cool temperature
    3. Very active child
    4. A child with a capillary refill of 3 seconds or more

83. An infant is admitted to the pediatric unit with a respiratory infection. Which of the following could indicate to the nurse that the infant might be developing respiratory distress?

    1. Heart rate = 100 bpm
    2. Grunting on expiration
    3. Capillary refill of 2 seconds
    4. Urine output of 80 mL for last 4 hours

84. A 4-year-old child is receiving a blood transfusion. Which sign would indicate to the nurse that the child might be having a reaction to the blood?

    1. BP = 90/50 mm Hg
    2. Heart rate = 90 bpm
    3. Oral temperature = 100°F (37.7°C)
    4. Respiratory rate = 26/min

85. The order for a 4-year-old child reads "Gentamicin 1 drop OS qid." Which action by the nurse is appropriate to administer the medicine?

    1. Pull the left lower eyelid down, instill drop, and repeat on other eye.
    2. Pull the right pinna back and upward to instill drop.
    3. Pull the left lower eyelid down to form a reservoir, then instill drop.
    4. Pull the right pinna back and down to instill the drop, then repeat with the left.

86. Which action by the nurse is appropriate when instilling eardrops into an infant's ear?

    1. Pull the pinna back and down to instill drops.
    2. Hold the child still for 10 minutes after the drops are instilled.
    3. Increase the head of the bed to facilitate absorption of the drops.
    4. Tape a piece of cotton in the child's ears once the drops have been instilled.

87. The physician orders a saline enema for a 4-year-old child. The nurse knows that the appropriate amount of fluid to administer would be:
    1. 100 mL
    2. 300 mL
    3. 500 mL
    4. 700 mL

88. The nurse is making midmorning rounds on a child to whom she administered insulin at 7:30 AM. What symptom would alert the nurse that the child might be hypoglycemic?
    1. Confused state
    2. Irritability and crying
    3. Flushed face
    4. Fruity breath

89. A nurse is teaching the child and parents when to administer a combination of regular and NPH insulin injections. The nurse would teach the appropriate time as:
    1. Just before meals
    2. Thirty minutes before meals
    3. Just after meals
    4. In the morning and the evening

90. The nurse knows that repeated vaginal yeast infection in an adolescent girl is a classic sign of:
    1. Diabetes mellitus
    2. Poor hygiene
    3. Sexual activity
    4. Urinary tract dysfunction

91. The nurse knows that full-term infants are at a high risk for developing iron-deficiency anemia at what age?
    1. 6 weeks
    2. 4 months
    3. 6 months
    4. 9 months

92. An 11-month-old infant has been given a diagnosis of iron-deficiency anemia. The nurse would use which of the following criteria to evaluate the outcome of teaching a mother about iron supplements?
    1. The mother acknowledges that the iron should be given with fruit juice.
    2. The mother acknowledges that the iron should be given alone.
    3. The mother acknowledges that the iron should be given with meals.
    4. The mother acknowledges that the iron should be given with milk.

93. The nurse could use which of the following to determine if a mother is administering iron supplements to her infant?
    1. The absence of jaundice in the infant
    2. The observance of a tarry stool in the infant's diaper
    3. The mother saying that she is not having difficulty administering the iron
    4. The mother notifying the nurse that the infant no longer has diarrhea

94. The nurse would instruct the mother of a 6-year-old who is receiving iron to administer the iron:
    1. At bedtime
    2. Early in the morning
    3. By straw
    4. With protein

95. A mother complains that her daughter, who has juvenile rheumatoid arthritis, has stiffness in the morning. The nurse would advise the mother to:
    1. Give her warm baths each morning.
    2. Administer a pain medication before the child gets up.
    3. Do passive ROM with the child before she gets out of bed.
    4. Have the child wake up 1 hour early to allow the stiffness to go away.

96. The nurse would identify which criterion to evaluate the outcome of discharge teaching with a mother of a child with a diagnosis of rheumatic fever?
    1. Compliance with monthly penicillin shots
    2. Compliance with monthly throat cultures
    3. Compliance with yearly echocardiograms
    4. Compliance with a regular exercise program

97. The mother of a child with a diagnosis of Kawasaki disease asks the nurse, "Why does my child need aspirin when he no longer has a fever"? The nurse would explain that aspirin:
    1. Is given to reduce inflammation
    2. Is given for its antipyretic effects
    3. Prevents valve damage
    4. Decreases the chances of thrombus formation

98. The nurse would identify which child as being at high risk for developing iron-deficiency anemia?
    1. A 4-month-old child who is breast-feeding
    2. A 2-year-old child who drinks 48 oz of milk a day
    3. An 8-year-old child who refuses to drink milk
    4. A 15-year-old adolescent who refuses to eat chicken

99. The nurse would instruct the mother of a child on long-term steroid therapy to:
    1. Add vitamins to diet
    2. Limit social contacts
    3. Reduce sodium and fat in the diet
    4. Restrict physical activity

100. The nurse would identify a complication of meningitis as being:
    1. Hearing loss
    2. Spinal damage
    3. Urinary incontinence
    4. Memory loss during the acute illness

101. A newborn is receiving phototherapy because of elevated bilirubin levels. Nursing care would include **(select all that apply)**:
    1. Applying patches to shield the newborn's eyes
    2. Avoiding oily applications to the skin
    3. Maintaining infant in prone position

4. Monitoring hydration status
5. Providing supplemental oxygen via nasal cannula
6. Using a knitted cap for the newborn's head

102. The nurse has completed the assessment of a 2 year old. Which of the following reflexes are considered normal? (**Select all that apply.**)

    1. Babinski
    2. Blink
    3. Moro
    4. Ortolani
    5. Tonic neck
    6. Yawn

103. The nurse is discussing routine immunizations with the parents of a 3-day-old girl. After her first immunization in the nursery the next immunizations are given at 2, 4, and 6 months of age. Which immunizations are recommended for 2, 4, and 6 months of age? (**Select all that apply.**)

    1. DTaP
    2. HiB
    3. Influenza
    4. MMR
    5. Polio
    6. Varicella

104. The nurse would withhold an immunization for DTaP if the child's history included (**select all that apply**):

    1. Anaphylactic reaction to previous injection
    2. Breast milk as only dietary intake
    3. Mild upper respiratory infection
    4. Nonprogressive neurological disorder
    5. Severe croup (laryngotracheobronchitis)
    6. Temperature of 101°F by mouth

105. Interdisciplinary members a nurse would expect to be a part of the team involved with an infant who has a cleft lip and his or her family are (**select all that apply**):

    1. Dietitian
    2. Occupational therapist
    3. Pediatric urologist
    4. Pharmacist
    5. Registered nurse
    6. Schoolteacher

106. A 6-year-old is receiving Lanoxin (digoxin). The nurse would withhold the drug if the (**select all that apply**):

    1. Child is scheduled for an radiograph
    2. Child is sleeping
    3. Child is teething
    4. Child is vomiting repeatedly
    5. Pulse is below 70 bpm
    6. Respiratory rate >40/minute

107. The nurse is preparing to suction a child with a tracheostomy. Put the following steps in order:

    1. Clear suction tubing with water.
    2. Cover thumb hole to apply suction.
    3. Gather equipment.
    4. Insert suction catheter.

5. Wash hands.
6. Withdraw catheter.

108. Expected outcomes for a child diagnosed with a seizure disorder would be the following (**select all that apply**):

    1. Child cooperates with care
    2. Child remains seizure free
    3. Child shows no signs of physical injury
    4. Family follows instructions
    5. Family treats the child as special
    6. Family keeps padded tongue blade available

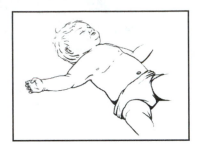

109. The nurse finds a 1 year old unresponsive. Put an X in the area in the figure above where the nurse would assess the pulse:

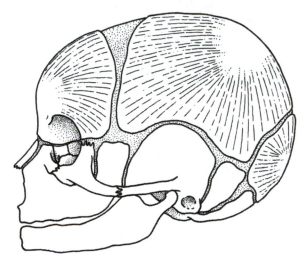

110. A 9-month-old girl is at the clinic for a routine visit. The nurse is preparing to assess the anterior fontanel. Put an X in the area in the figure above where the nurse would locate the fontanel.

111. The first immunization a normal newborn should receive is one to prevent (**select all that apply**):

    1. Chickenpox
    2. Diphtheria
    3. Hepatitis B
    4. Influenza
    5. Polio
    6. Tetanus

112. An adolescent is on the pediatric unit following a ventriculoperitioneal (VP) shunt revision. The nurse is completing the I&O (intake and output) record for the shift.

Intake: Output:

IV - D$_5$RL   720 mL   600 mLc urine
Apple juice   240 mL
Ginger ale   120 mL
Water   8 oz
Beef broth   1 cup

The nurse should document the client's intake as _____ mL.

113. Working as a member of a team on a pediatric unit the nurse may delegate which of the following tasks to a certified nursing assistant (CNA)? **(Select all that apply.)**

1. Bathing a toddler
2. Changing an IV bag
3. Comforting a crying infant
4. Feeding an infant
5. Giving an enema
6. Obtaining vital signs

114. Nursing care for an infant after placement of a ventriculoperitioneal (VP) shunt for hydrocephalus includes **(select all that apply)**:

1. Irrigate shunt tubing
2. Maintain constant pressure on shunt valve
3. Measure head circumference
4. Monitor body temperature
5. Monitor intake and output
6. Place in Trendelenburg position

115. Masturbation in prepubescent children is considered **(select all that apply)**:

1. An illness
2. Developmentally harmful
3. Normal
4. Precocious
5. Socially inappropriate
6. Suggestive of homosexual tendencies

116. The nurse encourages the hospitalized child to engage in therapeutic play. The purposes for this are to allow the child to **(select all that apply)**:

1. Educate other pediatric clients
2. Express feelings about being hospitalized
3. Get to know other children
4. Have fun
5. Learn about procedures and treatments
6. Maintain a sense of control

117. During a visit to the pediatrician's office the mother of a 16-month-old girl tells the nurse she is tired of changing diapers and wants to start toilet training. The nurse then talks with the mother about the signs that a child is ready to learn toilet training. These include **(select all that apply)**:

1. Able to sit on toilet for 5–10 minutes without fussing
2. Able to recite first five letters of the alphabet (a–e)
3. Fine motor skills of holding a spoon
4. Gross motor skills of sitting, walking, and squatting
5. Mother's plans to start working
6. Verbal or nonverbal communication skills to indicate needs

118. The nurse is caring for a 16-year-old boy admitted for chemotherapy. The nurse recognizes that adolescents are most interested in which psychosocial issues? **(Select all that apply.)**

1. Fear of mutilation
2. Fear of separation
3. Loss of independence
4. Privacy
5. Self-identity
6. Separation from peers

119. A 9-year-old girl who has a known seizure disorder is admitted to the hospital for adjustment of medication dosage. A nurse witnesses the onset of a grand mal seizure and implements the seizure plan. This would include which steps? **(Select all that apply.)**

1. Document history of the seizure.
2. Loosen the child's clothing.
3. Move the child to a safe location.
4. Move hard or sharp objects away from child.
5. Place a padded tongue blade between the child's teeth.
6. Put a blanket under the child's head.

120. A child is admitted with a diagnosis of R/O Sepsis; Fever of Unknown Origin. Her temperature is 102°F. Motrin (ibuprofen) 75 mg q 4–6 hr is ordered for temp >101°F. Motrin is supplied in a suspension 100 mg/5 mL. How many milliliters would you give?

_____ mL

121. The hydration status of an infant can be estimated by observing which of the following parameters? **(Select all that apply.)**

1. Appetite
2. Reflexes
3. Skin turgor
4. Stools
5. Urine
6. Weight

122. Which of the following are signs and symptoms of overhydration? **(Select all that apply.)**

1. Bulging fontanels
2. Cold, mottled skin
3. Decreased urine output
4. Difficulty breathing
5. Edema of eyes and scrotum
6. Increased pulse

123. An adolescent is admitted for a severe infection. The physician ordered gentamicin 81 mg to be given every 12 hours. The IVBP (bag) with the medication prepared by pharmacy has 50 mL of fluid. The medication needs to infuse per pump in 30 minutes. How many mililiters per hour would you administer?

_____ mL

124. A 16-year-old student and his friends are drinking beer and swimming in a river near their home. He climbs a tree and dives head first into the river. After a few seconds his friends realize something is wrong. They pull him onto the river bank. He is conscious and breathing, but unable to move. What should they do first? (**Select all that apply.**)

1. Check his pulse.
2. Get the AED (Automatic External Defibrillator).
3. Immobilize him and call for help.
4. Remove his wet clothing.
5. Turn him onto his stomach to allow water to drain from is lungs.
6. Use a four-man carry to take him to safety.

125. A 1-day-old newborn of average gestational age is hospitalized in the well-baby nursery. Which of the following vital sign parameters is most important to report to the physician?

1. Apical pulse 118 to 148 beats/minute
2. Respirations 48–52 breaths/minute
3. Axillary temperature 97.9°F–98.1°F.
4. Blood pressure 65/41 mm Hg (upper extremity) and 56/36 mm Hg (lower extremity)

126. Which of the following explanations by the nurse is most accurate regarding the reason not to defrost frozen breast milk in the microwave?

1. High-temperature microwaving significantly destroys the anti-infective factors.
2. The baby can be burned by the hot breast milk.
3. The glass container may explode from the heat.
4. The warm milk may cause indigestion in the newborn.

127. Because of the client's history of being born prematurely, which of the following nursing measures is important in administration of childhood immunizations to the hospitalized infant of 2 months?

1. Administer only half-doses until age 1 year.
2. Immunization schedule should be adjusted based on the number of weeks the client was premature.
3. Give oral polio vaccine (OPV) only while still in the nursery.
4. Initiate at the appropriate, actual chronological age.

128. Because of the possibility of mild local side effects from the DPT injection, the nurse should administer the medication using which technique?

1. Subcutaneously in the deltoid area
2. Deep intramuscular in the vastus lateralis or ventrogluteal
3. Using an air lock and a new sterile needle
4. After application of a topical anesthetic (EMLA)

129. The nurse would expect to find which of the following cardinal symptoms in an infant with colic?

1. A duration of crying longer than 3 hours/day with drawing up of the legs
2. A history of projectile vomiting and diarrhea
3. Formula intolerance and weight loss
4. Only late night, loud crying and fussiness

130. Which of the following explanations by the nurse would be the most accurate regarding sudden infant death syndrome (SIDS)?

1. A higher percentage of girls are affected.
2. The peak time of year when it occurs is fall (November).
3. The time of death is typically during sleep in a supine position.
4. The peak age of affected infants is 2–4 months, with 95% occurring within the first 6 months.

131. Which of the following notations is more accurate for the nurse to chart on a child who is lying quietly in bed watching television yet who states his pain is a 4 on a scale of 1– 5?

1. Client rates pain a 4 on a scale of 1–5.
2. Client rates pain incorrectly on the scale for pain.
3. Client resting quietly without pain.
4. Client is faking pain.

132. Assessment of pain is subjective to the degree that it is what the client says it is; however, pain rating scales may be used in clients beginning at which age?

1. 1 year old
2. 2 years old
3. 3 years old
4. 4 years old

133. Which of the following nursing interventions would best monitor fluid levels in an immediately postoperative child who had undergone cardiac surgery?

1. Strictly measuring the intake of oral fluids and urine output every shift
2. Strictly measuring the intake of oral and IV fluids and urine output hourly via Foley catheter
3. Asking the parents to count all diapers used and bottles given
4. Restricting all fluids and placing the child on the bedpan hourly

134. Which of the following statements by the mother indicates the need for further teaching about the administration of digoxin to her infant?

1. "If my child vomits, I should not give a second dose."
2. "I can place the medication in a small amount of milk."
3. "I should administer the medication slowly to the side and back of the mouth."
4. "If I forget a dose and only 3 hours has passed since the scheduled time, I should give the medication."

135. To promote optimal respirations and maximum chest expansion, the nurse places the infant with cardiovascular disease in which position?

1. Supine
2. Side-lying
3. Prone with the head down
4. With head of the bed up 45 degrees

136. Because of the possibility of pulmonary emboli in an adolescent with multiple long-bone fractures, the nurse would have which of the following supplies readily accessible for initial treatment?

1. Oxygen
2. Heparin

3. Corticosteroids
4. IV fluids

137. When assessing a child, which of the following information is more reliable in determining if a child has a fracture?

1. The child will not be able to move a broken extremity.
2. The child who refuses to walk should be strongly suspected of having a fracture.
3. Radiological examination with a comparison film of the unaffected extremity is diagnostic.
4. If bruising and swelling are present, it is soft tissue trauma only.

138. Which of the following is the first early response for the child with an impending airway obstruction?

1. Decreasing pulse and respirations
2. Substernal, suprasternal, and intercostal retractions
3. Decreasing responsiveness
4. Nasal congestion and drainage

139. Which of the following diagnostic tests is commonly used to measure the asthmatic client's greatest flow velocity during an acute asthmatic attack?

1. Peak expiratory flow rate (PEFR)
2. Arterial blood gases (ABGs)
3. Peripheral oxygen saturation (SaO_2)
4. Auscultation of anterior and posterior lung fields

140. Which of the following observations would indicate that the client in the immediate postoperative period after tonsillectomy and adenoidectomy (T&A) was worsening?

1. Frequent swallowing
2. Complaints of moderate pain
3. Pulse of 100 to 110 bpm
4. Dark brown blood in the emesis

141. Which of the following commonly used nursing actions best determines the amount of urine and stool excreted by a hospitalized infant in diapers?

1. An external collection bag to measure exact milliliters
2. Counting the number of soiled diapers per day
3. Weighing the diapers and subtracting a dry diaper weight (1 g = 1 mL lost)
4. An internal Foley catheter measured hourly

142. The nurse would expect to find which of the following in a client experiencing a first-degree burn?

1. Blisters
2. Pain
3. Waxy white or brown skin
4. Dull and dry wounds

143. Which of the following statements would indicate the need for further teaching in the emergency treatment of minor burns?

1. "I should not apply butter."
2. "I should not rupture the blisters."
3. "I should immediately apply a loose gauze dressing."
4. "I should run cool water over the area."

144. To increase the infant's resistance to infection, the nurse should provide which of the following information about feeding to the mother?

1. Promote breast-feeding for the first year of life through objective information.
2. Remain entirely neutral—offer no information to the mother on breast- or bottle- feeding.
3. Provide written information packets only and ask for the mother's decision.
4. Take the infant a bottle, and if the mother wants to use it, she can.

145. Which of the following parent statements indicates a proper understanding of when the child with chickenpox may return to school?

1. When vesicles have dried
2. When crusts have fallen off
3. When new lesions have stopped appearing
4. When 7 days have passed since the first vesicle appeared

146. What is the purpose of applying lotions such as calamine (Caladryl) sparingly over open lesions?

1. Excessive absorption may lead to toxicity.
2. It prevents the oatmeal baths from being soothing.
3. It keeps the area moist and prevents crusting.
4. It prolongs the period of outbreak.

147. Which of the following tests is the most common in diagnosing pinworms in the child?

1. A rectal swab and culture
2. The tape test
3. A skin scraping
4. A stool specimen

148. Congenital heart defects that typically produce cyanosis are (**select all that apply**):

1. Aortic stenosis
2. Atrial septal defect
3. Coarctation of aorta
4. Patent ductus arteriosus
5. Tetralogy of Fallot
6. Transposition of the great vessels

149. The nurse would expect to find the greatest cyanosis in a child with which cardiovascular condition?

1. A defect of decreased pulmonary flow like tricuspid atresia
2. An obstructive defect like coarctation of the aorta
3. A defect of increased pulmonary blood flow like atrioventricular canal defect
4. A mixed defect like transposition of the great vessels (TGV) with a large patent ductus arteriosus (PDA).

150. Which of the following information would be most important to remember in assessing a child with poisoning?

1. Determine any allergies to medications.
2. Determine what was taken and any treatments initiated by parents.
3. Give ipecac before activated charcoal.
4. Place sweetener in the activated charcoal to improve palatability.

ANSWERS

1. **(3)** Integrated processes: nursing process — data collection; client need: physiological integrity; physiological adaptation; content area: pediatrics.
   RATIONALE
   (1) This infant does not weigh at least 2500 g. **(2)** The data do not give information on an ill child. **(3)** This infant is <2500 g, which describes a low-birth-weight infant. **(4)** A very-low-birth-weight infant is one that is <1500 g.

2. **(1)** Integrated processes: nursing process — planning; client need: physiological integrity; basic care and comfort; content area: pediatrics.
   RATIONALE
   (1) It is very important to conserve warmth and energy in an infant with low birth weight. **(2)** Too much bathing can result in loss of body heat. **(3)** Daily shampooing is not necessary to prevent cradle cap and can cause heat loss. **(4)** Neonates should be placed in an environment with minimal stimulation.

3. **(3)** Integrated processes: nursing process — data collection; client need: physiological integrity; physiological adaptation; content area: pediatrics.
   RATIONALE
   (1) The nurse must learn to identify behaviors that indicate discomfort in neonates. **(2)** Neonates do respond to painful stimuli. **(3)** Crying and flexing are means of responding to pain in neonates. **(4)** Change in VSs can indicate pain but can also indicate other problems.

1. **(3)** Integrated processes: nursing process — planning; client need: physiological integrity; physiological adaptation; content area: pediatrics.
   RATIONALE
   (1) Acne does not occur in neonates. **(2)** Chickenpox has an incubation of approximately 2 weeks, and the neonate would be protected by maternal antibodies. **(3)** Jaundice is a common occurrence in newborns and low-birth-weight infants. **(4)** Scoliosis is not common in neonates.

5. **(2)** Integrated processes: nursing process — implementation; client need: physiological integrity; basic care and comfort; content area: pediatrics.
   RATIONALE
   (1) Bathing can stimulate circulation, but this is not desired in the neonate. **(2)** Bathing two or three times weekly can remove bacteria. **(3)** Oils are not needed because the neonate has natural protection. **(4)** Cleansing of soiled areas would minimize irritation; frequency is limited because of increased temperature loss during bathing.

6. **(1)** Integrated processes: nursing process — evaluation; client need: physiological integrity; physiological adaptation; content area: pediatrics.
   RATIONALE
   (1) This would indicate that treatment was successful and the problem is resolving. **(2)** Surgery is not a treatment for respiratory distress syndrome. **(3)** Respiratory distress syndrome is not genetic. **(4)** This type of respiratory illness is not contagious.

7. **(2)** Integrated processes: nursing process — planning; client need: physiological integrity; basic care and comfort; content area: pediatrics.
   RATIONALE
   (1) Corticosteroids may be used for their anti-inflammatory effect, but they are not among the first measures taken with croup. **(2)** Cool humidification is usually the first measure taken. Cool temperature constricts the edematous blood vessels. Oxygen is supplemented when necessary. **(3)** Prophylactic intubation is no longer a trend. Intubation equipment should be on standby if respiratory failure occurs. **(4)** Whirlpool therapy is not indicated with croup.

8. **(3)** Integrated processes: nursing process — data collection; client need: health promotion and maintenance; content area: pediatrics.
   RATIONALE
   (1) Adolescents are concerned the most with privacy. **(2)** School-age children focus on external causes of illnesses. **(3)** Preschool children focus on illness as punishment for wrongdoing. **(4)** Infants have greater anxiety toward separation.

9. **(4)** Integrated processes: nursing process — data collection; client need: psychosocial integrity; content area: pediatrics.
   RATIONALE
   (1) Attachment is not a phase of separation anxiety. **(2)** The initial phase is protest, demonstrated by crying. Acceptance is only superficial if this phase is demonstrated. **(3)** Acceptance is not a phase of separation anxiety. **(4)** Protest is demonstrated through crying. Despair is observed in depression of the child. Detachment, which seldom occurs, is demonstrated by an appearance of adjustment.

10. **(1, 2, 3, 6)** Integrated processes: nursing process — implementation; communication and documentation; client need: pyschosocial integrity; content area: pediatrics.
    RATIONALE
    (1) Mimicking health-care procedures can promote toddler cooperation and adaption. **(2)** Parents should be discouraged from leaving when the child falls asleep to minimize associating sleep with parental abandonment. **(3)** Sibling visitation reduces anxiety and isolation. **(4)** Parental involvement should be maximized and families should be encouraged to bring familiar toys and home supplies like music tapes. **(5)** Explanations should be simple and in lay terms. Use of dolls is beneficial. **(6)** Side rails should be used at all times.

11. **(2)** Integrated processes: nursing process — implementation; communication and documentation; client need: physiological integrity; basic care and comfort; content area: pediatrics.
    RATIONALE
    (1) A favorite toy is appropriate, but the tent separates him from his mother. The tent might frighten the child. The child in respiratory distress needs the comfort of his mother. **(2)** This choice would provide his mother's comfort while giving him the benefit of humidification and a quiet activity. **(3)** Sedation is contraindicated because it could mask some signs of respiratory distress. **(4)** Threatening the child with separation from his mother is inappropriate.

12. **(2)** Integrated processes: nursing process — evaluation; client need: health promotion and maintenance; content area: pediatrics.

RATIONALE

(1) Promotion of family involvement is good. Not all families are involved at this level of care. The goal should be family adaptation, not to relieve nurses of responsibility. **(2)** Before discharge, the family should demonstrate the ability to provide care for their child. **(3)** The family should be involved in care. The child is too young to be ultimately responsible for his or her own care. **(4)** Rejection of family indicates an adjustment problem.

13. **(1)** Integrated processes: nursing process — data collection; client need: health promotion and maintenance; content area: pediatrics.

RATIONALE

(1) Chickenpox is characterized by itching and vesicular skin eruptions over the body; first occurring on the torso. Incubation is 13–17 days. **(2)** Diphtheria is characterized by respiratory involvement and a membrane on the pharynx. **(3)** Measles is characterized by a macular rash that begins on the face and spreads to the trunk. **(4)** Mumps is characterized by swelling of the parotid glands.

14. **(3)** Integrated processes: nursing process — implementation; client need: physiological integrity; basic care and comfort; content area: pediatrics.

RATIONALE

(1) Aspirin is contraindicated because of the increased chance of developing Reye's syndrome. **(2)** Using soothing lotions is encouraged to decrease scratching, which can increase chances of secondary infection. **(3)** Keeping the fingernails short decreases the chance of breaking the skin by scratching. **(4)** Child should be isolated for approximately 6 days after the eruptions until crusty patches begin to form. This is a highly contagious disease.

15. **(4)** Integrated processes: nursing process — data collection; client need: psychosocial integrity; content area: pediatrics.

RATIONALE

(1) Endocrine dysfunction is related to growth failure. **(2)** GI dysfunction indicates an organic FTT. **(3)** Neurological dysfunction is associated with organic FTT. **(4)** These are signs and symptoms of nonorganic FTT associated with neglect.

16. **(3)** Integrated processes: nursing process — planning; caring; client need: psychosocial integrity; content area: pediatrics.

RATIONALE

(1) Limiting the number of caregivers promotes consistency and helps to establish trust. **(2)** Parental decisions should be incorporated to promote parental self-esteem. **(3)** Developing the trust of both the child and the family establishes an appropriate environment in which to promote parenting skills. **(4)** Stimulation should be provided in an appropriate manner.

17. **(2)** Integrated processes: nursing process — evaluation; client need: psychosocial integrity; content area: pediatrics.

RATIONALE

(1) The family demonstrates an ability to care for the child without depending on nursing staff. **(2)** To develop appropriately, the child should be in a family that is able to provide a nurturing environment. **(3)** The infant should be gaining weight. **(4)** Although the nurse wants to see progress toward developmental milestones, it may take longer than this hospital admission. If the family is nurturing and providing for the child appropriately, the milestones will be achieved.

18. **(4)** Integrated processes: nursing process — implementation; client need: physiological integrity; pharmacological therapies; content area: pediatrics.

RATIONALE

(1) Absorbing the remaining substance would not be recommended, and this is not the action of ipecac. **(2)** Dilution of the poisonous substance would not be recommended. **(3)** Ipecac is not administered to prevent aspiration. **(4)** Ipecac is administered to induce vomiting and remove stomach contents.

19. **(3)** Integrated processes: nursing process — planning; client need: physiological integrity; basic care and comfort; content area: pediatrics.

RATIONALE

(1) A burn involving the dermis would be a first-degree, superficial burn that is expected to heal without scarring. **(2)** The epidermis is the middle layer, and this layer alone could not be burned. A burn which involes the dermis is a second-degree burn. **(3)** Partial- and full-thickness burns involve all layers of the skin. **(4)** A fourth-degree full-thickness burn involves all layers of skin, subcutaneous tissue, and muscle.

20. **(1)** Integrated processes: nursing process — implementation; client need: physiological integrity; reduction of risk potential; content area: pediatrics.

RATIONALE

(1) The nurse should promote mobility of the area as long as it would not interfere with grafts or healing. **(2)** The nurse should help the child to avoid scratching wound so that injury and delayed healing will not occur. **(3)** The nurse should encourage the child to take fluids and eat nutritious, high-protein meals and not to limit fluids. **(4)** The nurse should keep the wound clean and take care not to damage the crusts and eschar when cleaning.

21. **(1)** Integrated processes: nursing process — implementation; communication and documentation; client need: physiological integrity; physiological adaptation; content area: pediatrics.

RATIONALE

(1) Children respond to pain differently. One way is sleep or withdrawal. The best response is to assess for increased pulse and respirations, facial grimacing, and restlessness. **(2)** The child should be assessed before administration of the medication. **(3)** This response is acceptable, but the child should be assessed first. **(4)** This response required nursing judgment without input from a physician.

22. **(1)** Integrated processes: nursing process — implementation; caring; client need: psychosocial integrity; content area: pediatrics.

RATIONALE

(1) The bandages could be scary and the child may need some help adjusting. The best response is to stay with him until he feels comfortable in asking other children to play. **(2)** This intervention does not promote interaction among the children. **(3)** This response will not help to break the ice and initiate interaction. **(4)** This child may need help in interacting initially because of his different appearance.

23. **(1)** Integrated processes: nursing process — data collection; client need: physiological integrity; physiological adaptation; content area: pediatrics.

RATIONALE

(1) A compound fracture occurs when the bone protrudes through the skin. **(2)** A greenstick fracture is an incomplete one in which the bone bends. **(3)** In an incomplete fracture, the bone fragments remain attached. (4) A simple fracture does not cause a break in the skin.

24. (1) Integrated processes: nursing process — implementation; client need: physiological integrity; reduction of risk potential; content area: pediatrics.

    RATIONALE
    (1) The child's activity needs should be met without jeopardizing her traction. (2) The child needs activities appropriate to age. It would be better to assist her to identify how far she can move without assistance by marking the bed with tape to alert her to a limitation. (3) The parents may not be able to be present all the time, and it is not necessary that the do so. (4) Things should be arranged to promote some independence in the child. If needed, she can call.

25. (4) Integrated processes: nursing process — implementation; teaching/learning; client need: physiological integrity; reduction of risk potential; content area: pediatrics.

    RATIONALE
    (1) Lowering the extremity could cause edema and should be discouraged. (2) The cast should stay dry and clean. (3) The child should be mobile when the cast is dry, but ROM exercises to the extremity would be dangerous. (4) The child should be instructed not to put anything inside the cast. Objects inside the cast could cause pressure points and sores.

26. (2) Integrated processes: nursing process — data collection; client need: physiological integrity; physiological adaptation; content area: pediatrics

    RATIONALE
    (1) Glucose intolerance is not recognized as a form of diabetes. (2) This type of diabetes usually occurs in childhood. (3) This type of diabetes occurs in adult life. (4) Plain diabetes not recognized as a form of diabetes.

27. (1) Integrated processes: nursing process — implementation; client need: psychosocial integrity; content area: pediatrics.

    RATIONALE
    (1) Give the shot and allow the child to get more practice. It is better to wait until she is comfortable. This would be a time for the nurse to allow the child to express her feelings. (2) This could be done when the child is ready to try on her own. (3) A balanced diet would help to control the disease, but she will still require medication. (4) This is not a physician's problem. The nurse should allow the child more time.

28. (1) Integrated processes: nursing process — planning; client need: health promotion and maintenance; content area: pediatrics.

    RATIONALE
    (1) Balancing diet, exercise, and insulin is the focus of therapeutic diabetic management that promotes optimal functioning. (2) Exercise is important in lowering blood glucose, but it must be considered in relation to the overall picture of diet and insulin therapy. (3) An adequate amount of nutrition is required to promote growth. (4) Exercise, not limiting exercise, decreases insulin needs.

29. (1) Integrated processes: nursing process — planning; client need: physiological integrity; physiological adaptation; content area: pediatrics.

    RATIONALE
    (1) Ketoacidosis results if glucose control is not maintained and blood glucose levels rise. Signs and symptoms include ketonuria, glucosuria, dehydration, vomiting, electrolyte imbalance, metabolic acidosis, abdominal pain, fruity acetone breath, and drowsiness progressing to coma. (2) Headache is a symp-

tom of low blood glucose. (3) Ketoacidosis is the result of high blood glucose levels. (4) Thirst does occur in hyperglycemia, but glucose in urine is more specific for ketoacidosis.

30. (1) Integrated processes: nursing process — data collection; client need: physiological integrity; physiological adaptation; content area: pediatrics.

    RATIONALE
    (1) It is common for an ear infection to follow a respiratory infection in a toddler. Signs and symptoms include crying, restlessness, rolling head from side to side, and pulling on the affected ear. (2) Diphtheria is a respiratory illness that can affect this age group. (3) Pertussis is accompanied by a "whooping" cough. (4) Tonsillitis is accompanied by difficulty swallowing.

31. (3) Integrated processes: nursing process — planning; client need: physiological integrity; physiological adaptation; content area: pediatrics.

    RATIONALE
    (1) Antibiotics are part of the management of otitis media. (2) Analgesics may be required. (3) Oxygen therapy is usually not a part of management. (4) Myringotomy may be required in some children, most commonly after multiple ear infections.

32. (1) Integrated processes: nursing process — evaluation; client need: physiological integrity; basic care and comfort; content area: pediatrics.

    RATIONALE
    (1) Comfort and absence of drainage would take priority for measuring evaluation of care. (2) Completion of antibiotics is an outcome, but it does not indicate status of ear or comfort. (3) Family may be required to give medications orally, but usually not injections for ear infections. (4) Prevention of secondary infections is also a means of evaluating care, but comfort and absence of infection are more specific.

33. (3) Integrated processes: nursing process — data collection; client need: physiological integrity; physiological adaptation; content area: pediatrics.

    RATIONALE
    (1) Cool, dry skin is not a sign of cystic fibrosis. A salty taste to the skin is a sign of cystic fibrosis. (2) Frequent urination is not a sign of cystic fibrosis. (3) Large, bulky, foul-smelling stools are a sign of cystic fibrosis. These are attributed to decrease in or absence of pancreatic enzymes, resulting in faulty absorption of nutrients. In addition, salty taste of sweat, weight loss in the presence of a good appetite, distended abdomen, and marked tissue wasting are signs of cystic fibrosis. (4) Poor appetite is not a symptom.

34. (4) Integrated processes: nursing process — data collection; client need: physiological integrity; physiological adaptation; content area: pediatrics.

    RATIONALE
    (1) Bronchial constriction is not a problem associated with cystic fibrosis. (2) Inadequate surfactant is associated with premature infants. (3) Pulmonic stenosis is associated with cardiovascular problems that involve a narrowing of heart vessels. (4) Thick, tenacious mucus is a classic sign of cystic fibrosis that leads to pulmonary obstruction.

35. (3) Integrated processes: nursing process — implementation; client need: physiological integrity; pharmacological therapies; content area: pediatrics.

    RATIONALE
    (1) Intramuscular administration is an inappropriate route. (2) IV administration is an inappropriate route. (3) Pancreatic enzymes are available in capsule form. An adolescent would

swallow the capsule. For a child who has difficulty swallowing a capsule, the capsule could be opened and the enzyme sprinkled on the child's food. (4) Intradermal administration is inappropriate.

36. **(3)** Integrated processes: nursing process — planning; teaching/learning; client need: health promotion and maintenance; content area: pediatrics.

    RATIONALE

    (1) Enzymes are given to aid in the digestion and absorption of nutrients. (2) Heart muscle and vascular tone are not the focus for medical concerns. (3) Exercise promotes mobilization of pulmonary secretions and enhances pulmonary treatments. (4) Cystic fibrosis produces secretions; therefore stimulation of secretions is not a goal.

37. **(4)** Integrated processes: nursing process — planning; teaching/learning; client need: physiological integrity; basic care and comfort; content area: pediatrics.

    RATIONALE

    (1) Mist does not dilate alveoli. (2) Mist does not reduce secretions. (3) Mist does not prevent dehydration. (4) Mist helps to liquefy the thick secretions, making it easier for the child to bring the secretions up.

38. **(2)** Integrated processes: nursing process — planning; teaching/learning; client need:physiological integrity; reduction of risk potential; content area: pediatrics.

    RATIONALE

    (1) This position is not the best for draining the right lower lobe. (2) This position is the best for draining the right lower lobe. Postural drainage uses gravity to help move secretions. This position would help secretions move into the larger bronchi toward the mouth. (3) This position would not facilitate drainage of the lower lobes into the bronchi. (4) This position would not affect the drainage from the lungs.

39. **(2)** Integrated processes: nursing process — planning; client need: physiological integrity; reduction of risk potential; content area: pediatrics.

    RATIONALE

    (1) If the child is allergic to dog and cat hair, then these animals should be avoided. (2) Therapeutic management of cystic fibrosis includes prevention and treatment of pulmonary infections. Persons with any kind of infection, bacterial, viral, or fungal, should be avoided. (3) Sodium may become depleted because the sweat glands fail to reabsorb sodium; salt should not be avoided and may need to be supplemented. (4) Sunlight is not a problem with cystic fibrosis.

40. **(3)** Integrated processes: nursing process — data collection; client need: physiological integrity; physiological adaptation; content area: pediatrics.

    RATIONALE

    (1) Pneumococci do not cause RF. (2) Staphylococci do not cause RF. (3) RF is caused by a group A β-hemolytic streptococcus. (4) Influenza B is not the cause of RF.

41. **(1)** Integrated processes: nursing process — implementation; client need: physiological integrity; pharmacological therapies; content area: pediatrics.

    RATIONALE

    (1) Corticosteroids may be administered for pancarditis and valvular involvement. (2) Squatting positions are useful in treating certain types of heart defects in children. (3) Rest is important for these children. Visits by friends during the acute phase are discouraged. (4) Sunlight does not affect this disease process.

42. **(4)** Integrated processes: nursing process — planning; teaching/learning; client need: physiological integrity; pharmacological therapies; content area: pediatrics.

    RATIONALE

    (1) Aspirin is not the treatment for carditis in RF. (2) The rash associated with RF is nonitching. (3) Headaches are not a major complaint of RF. (4) Polyarthritis; migratory, swollen, hot, red, painful joints; and fever are symptoms of this disease. Aspirin is prescribed as an anti-inflammatory agent to suppress joint inflammation.

43. **(3)** Integrated processes: nursing process — evaluation; teaching/learning; client need: physiological integrity; pharmacological therapies; content area: pediatrics.

    RATIONALE

    (1) Coughing and deep breathing are not home-care interventions for rheumatic fever. (2) There are no diet and fluid restrictions for home care. (3) Penicillin therapy is prophylactic to prevent recurrences of RF. (4) Oxygen therapy is not a home intervention with RF.

44. **(1)** Integrated processes: nursing process — data collection; client need: physiological integrity; basic care and comfort; content area: pediatrics.

    RATIONALE

    (1) Halitosis is common for 10–14 days after surgery and can be relieved with oral fluids and mouthwash. This would be the nurse's least concern. (2) Increased pulse could be associated with pain or blood loss and requires close observation. (3) Nausea can be associated with blood loss and would be of concern. (4) Restlessness can be a sign of pain or blood loss, and the child should be observed closely.

45. **(3)** Integrated processes: nursing process — implementation; client need: physiological integrity; basic care and comfort; content area: pediatrics.

    RATIONALE

    (1) Chocolate milk is appropriate in a full-liquid diet. (2) Ice cream is appropriate in a full-liquid diet. (3) Acidic fluids and foods such as orange juice should be avoided because they can cause irritation to the throat during healing. (4) Popsicles are an appropriate clear liquid. Red or brown popsicles should be avoided because they might mask signs of bleeding.

46. **(4)** Integrated processes: nursing process — data collection; client need: physiological integrity; physiological adaptation; content area: pediatrics.

    RATIONALE

    (1) Sleep apnea is not a sign of asthma. (2) Inspiratory stridor is not a sign of asthma. (3) Productive cough is not a sign of asthma. (4) A prolonged expiratory phase of respiration with shortness of breath, nasal flaring, audible wheezing, and a hacking, nonproductive cough are signs of asthma.

47. **(2)** Integrated processes: nursing process — planning; client need: physiological integrity; pharmacological therapies; content area: pediatrics.

    RATIONALE

    (1) Antibiotics may be administered if infection is thought to be the cause of the attack or if secondary infection is a concern. (2) Nausea and vomiting are not associated with asthma. (3) Hypersensitivities and inflammation are a concern with asthma. (4) Bronchospasms are of concern with asthma.

48. **(4)** Integrated processes: nursing process — data collection; client need: physiological integrity; physiological adaptation; content area: pediatrics.

RATIONALE

(1) This defect is spina bifida. (2) This defect is spina bifida occulta. (3) This anomaly is meningocele. (4) This anomaly is myelomeningocele.

49. (1) Integrated processes: nursing process — implementation; client need: safe, effective, care environment; safety and infection control; content area: pediatrics.

RATIONALE

(1) Meticulous skin care, especially in sac and genital areas, is critical. (2) Supine positioning should be avoided because pressure could be placed on the sac. (3) The diaper should not be secured around the infant, only placed under him or her. (4) A sterile moist dressing should be placed over the sac.

50. (1) Integrated processes: nursing process — planning; client need: physiological integrity; physiological adaptation; content area: pediatrics.

RATIONALE

(1) A large number of children with myelomeningocele develop hydrocephalus and require shunting. (2) Intussusception is not associated with neural tube defects. (3) The majority of children with myelomeningocele have normal IQs. (4) Pneumonia can be a potential problem, but is not the appropriate choice.

51. (1) Integrated processes: nursing process — implementation; Caring; client need: psychosocial integrity; content area: pediatrics.

RATIONALE

(1) It is best that the mother hold the child so that the child will not become more upset. Her presence will be a comfort. (2) Having the mother leave the examination room could cause the child to become further upset and could further compromise respiratory status. (3) Cool fruit juice is appropriate once the immediate distress is over and the inflammation is going down. (4) A throat culture could cause complete obstruction in a child with epiglottitis who is in distress. Examination of the throat should take place only if someone is available to intubate the child.

52. (2) Integrated processes: nursing process — data collection; Teaching/learning; client need: physiological integrity; physiological adaptation; content area: pediatrics.

RATIONALE

(1) This organism is not the cause of epiglottitis, but it is the cause of scarlet fever. (2) This organism is the usual cause of epiglottitis. (3) This virus is frequently associated with laryngitis. (4) This organism is the usual cause of bacterial tracheitis.

53. (1) Integrated processes: nursing process — implementation; client need: physiological integrity; reduction of risk potential; content area: pediatrics.

RATIONALE

(1) This is the most important intervention. Epiglottitis can cause complete airway obstruction. Emergency equipment would be needed immediately. (2) This intervention is appropriate, but the tracheostomy equipment is the most important for a new admission. (3) Antibiotics are usually given to the child, but the nurse should wait for the physician's order. (4) Initially the child will be NPO, but the tracheostomy equipment is the most important intervention.

54. (3) Integrated processes: nursing process — data collection; client need: physiological integrity; physiological adaptation; content area: pediatrics.

RATIONALE

(1) The infant should be able to handle saliva without drooling. (2) The infant will more than likely be a mouth breather, but noisy respirations are not expected. (3) The infant will have difficulty sucking because of the inability to create a vacuum with the lips. (4) The cleft lip should not affect the infant's ability to swallow.

55. (1) Integrated processes: nursing process — implementation; client need: safe, effective, care environment; safety and infection control; content area: pediatrics.

RATIONALE

(1) Restraints should be applied to keep the infant from putting fingers in the mouth and causing trauma to the incision. (2) The infant should not be placed on the abdomen because the incision site could be traumatized in this position. (3) It would be acceptable to position in an infant seat, but the major concern is to avoid trauma to the incision. (4) A mist tent is unnecessary.

56. (4) Integrated processes: nursing process — implementation; teaching/learning; client need: physiological integrity; basic care and comfort; content area: pediatrics.

RATIONALE

(1) Rectal thermometers should be avoided. (2) Brushing could cause gums to bleed. (3) Aspirin should not be given because aspirin affects platelet function and increases risk of bleeding. (4) Using creams is an appropriate means to remove hair, because shaving with a razor could cause bleeding if the skin was cut.

57. (3) Integrated processes: nursing process — planning; client need: physiological integrity; reduction of risk potential; content area: pediatrics.

RATIONALE

(1) Raw vegetables and fruit should be avoided because bacteria can be introduced to the child. (2) Strict bed rest is unnecessary. (3) Temperature elevations should be reported to the physician. (4) Visitors should be limited to those without infections, but not restricted.

58. (4) Integrated processes: nursing process — implementation; teaching/learning; client need: health promotion and maintenance; content area: pediatrics.

RATIONALE

(1) It would be important for parents to understand pain management, but preventing sickle cell crisis is the priority. (2) Home health care would not be necessary. (3) Support groups can be beneficial to the family, but would not be the priority intervention. (4) Teaching measures to prevent sickle cell crisis is most important to maintain physiological integrity of the child.

59. (3) Integrated processes: nursing process — planning; client need: health promotion and maintenance; content area: pediatrics.

RATIONALE

(1) The child may be loud and crying, but demanding explanations would be characteristic of an older child. (2) The preschooler would be physical, requiring restraint, not stoic. (3) Clinging to parents is a typical behavior of the preschooler. (4) Stalling behaviors are typical of school-age children.

60. (1) Integrated processes: nursing process — planning; client need: physiological integrity; pharmacological therapies; content area: pediatrics.

RATIONALE

(1) Meperidine should not be administered for longer than 48 hours because of build-up of a toxic metabolite. (2) An oral dose of meperidine would be four times the dose of morphine and might not get the same analgesic effects. (3) Morphine can

be administered for a longer time than meperidine with fewer side effects. (**4**) Naloxone should not be used with meperidine because it can alter the seizure threshold.

61. (**2**) Integrated processes: nursing process — planning; client need: physiological integrity; reduction of risk potential; content area: pediatrics.

RATIONALE

(**1**) Isometric exercises should be encouraged. (**2**) Forcing fluids is important to prevent constipation and to promote removal of calcium from the body. (**3**) Peer visitation is important at this age, and engaging in table games is a good activity for this age group. (**4**) An explanation of procedures and their effects on the body is important, but a detailed description is not necessary.

62. (**3**) Integrated processes: nursing process — data collection; client need: physiological integrity; reduction of risk potential; content area: pediatrics.

RATIONALE

(**1**) Bruising can be expected with compound fracture. The fingers should be observed for further discoloration that would indicate decreased circulation. (**2**) Capillary refill of 2 seconds is normal. (**3**) Pallor suggests a decrease in circulation to the extremity. The surgeon should be notified. (**4**) Edema is expected but should be watched for an increase that might impair circulation.

63. (**4**) Integrated processes: nursing process — data collection; client need: physiological integrity; physiological adaptation; content area: pediatrics.

RATIONALE

(**1**) Pain is expected and pressure on nerves can cause pain to radiate. (**2**) Pain responding to oral medication is acceptable. (**3**) Pain responding to a narcotic is acceptable. (**4**) Pain unresponsive to a narcotic indicates deteriorating neuromuscular status. This requires immediate attention.

64. (**3**) Integrated processes: nursing process — implementation; teaching/learning; client need: safe, effective care environment; safety and infection control; content area: pediatrics.

RATIONALE

(**1**) Increased pain can suggest infection, but other symptoms should be present with pain. (**2**) This temperature should be watched. A low-grade fever can be expected with inflammation. (**3**) Infected areas are hot to touch, and the heat can radiate through the cast. (**4**) Bloody drainage on the cast does not mean infection, but drainage can lead to infection.

65. (**2**) Integrated processes: nursing process — data collection; client need: physiological integrity; reduction of risk potential; content area: pediatrics.

RATIONALE

(**1**) This is an acceptable BP for an adolescent. (**2**) Petechiae on the chest is a classic symptom of pulmonary fat embolism. This would require immediate attention. (**3**) Pain management is important; additional medication may be required. (**4**) This is an acceptable urinary output.

66. (**1**) Integrated processes: nursing process — implementation; client need: physiological integrity; reduction of risk potential; content area: pediatrics.

RATIONALE

(**1**) Weights should be hanging freely to get the desired effect. (**2**) Neurovascular checks have no effect on the traction. (**3**) Relaxed muscles will not affect this traction. (**4**) Countertraction is achieved by the body weight, not tightness of the bandage.

67. (**1**) Integrated processes: nursing process — evaluation; client need: health promotion and maintenance; content area: pediatrics.

RATIONALE

(**1**) The disease directly affects joint capsules; therefore, the goal would be directed toward preserving joint functioning. (**2**) Side effects cannot be prevented but can be minimized. (**3**) Normal growth is important. Minimizing growth will not prevent deformities. (**4**) The child should attend school with peers if at all possible.

68. (**2**) Integrated processes: nursing process — evaluation; teaching/learning; client need: health promotion and maintenance; content area: pediatrics.

RATIONALE

(**1**) Diet should be low in fat to reduce chances of weight gain. (**2**) Sun exposure should be restricted—especially between 10 AM and 2 PM—by use of sunscreen, hats, and clothing that covers the extremities. (**3**) Exercise should be encouraged, but should not be strenuous. (**4**) Yearly eye examinations are essential if the child is taking hydroxychloroquine sulfate (Plaquenil). Hydroxychloroquine sulfate has been associated with retinal damage.

69. (**2**) Integrated processes: nursing process — data collection; client need: health promotion and maintenance; content area: pediatrics.

RATIONALE

(**1**) Infants are in the stage of trust versus mistrust, and a consistent primary caregiver is important. (**2**) Toddlers are developing a sense of autonomy, and ritualistic behavior provides a sense of comfort. (**3**) Preschoolers are developing a sense of initiative and exploration. (**4**) Adolescents are interested in peer support and identification.

70. (**2**) Integrated processes: nursing process — data collection; client need: health promotion and maintenance; content area: pediatrics.

RATIONALE

(**1**) Toddlers fear separation. (**2**) Preschoolers fear body mutilation. (**3**) School-age children fear the physical nature of the illness. (**4**) Adolescents are concerned with loss of independence.

71. (**3**) Integrated processes: nursing process — planning; client need: health promotion and maintenance; content area: pediatrics.

RATIONALE

(**1**) School-age children would prefer to be more active. (**2**) Preschool children are interested in collecting. (**3**) School-age children are at an age for competitive games. This would be an appropriate activity. (**4**) Peer relationships are very important to the adolescent.

72. (**2**) Integrated processes: nursing process — data collection; client need: physiological integrity; reduction of risk potential; content area: pediatrics.

RATIONALE

(**1**) This would not affect the testing. (**2**) Antihistamines could alter the results of testing. It is best to wait 48–96 hours after the last dose of antihistamine. (**3**) Only testing for food allergens would limit results for sensitivities to environmental allergens and pollens. (**4**) Forearms and upper back are the best sites for testing.

73. (**4**) Integrated processes: nursing process — data collection; client need: physiological integrity; physiological adaptation; content area: pediatrics.

RATIONALE

(1) Abdominal cramping is a late sign of anaphylaxis. (2) Tachycardia is a sign of anaphylaxis. (3) Hypotension is seen in anaphylaxis. (4) A sense of doom voiced by the client is an early sign of anaphylaxis.

74. **(4)** Integrated processes: nursing process — implementation; teaching/learning; client need: health promotion and maintenance; content area: pediatrics.

RATIONALE

(1) Disinfecting the bath area reduces exposure to molds. (2) Restricting pets does not affect allergies to dust mites. (3) Cigarette smoking is an irritant, not an allergen. (4) Dust mites are attracted to carpets. Avoiding playing on carpets reduces exposure.

75. **(3)** Integrated processes: nursing process — implementation; teaching/learning; client need: physiological integrity; basic care and comfort; content area: pediatrics.

RATIONALE

(1) There are no data to support the need for a bland diet. (2) A high-protein, high-fiber diet is not necessary. (3) A low-sodium diet would be recommended because of fluid gain with corticosteroids. (4) A reduced-fat diet is good, but there is no indication that the child is consuming too much fat.

76. **(3)** Integrated processes: nursing process — data collection; client need: physiological integrity; physiological adaptation; content area: pediatrics.

RATIONALE

(1) Abdominal cramping is usually not associated with disease activity in lupus. (2) Chest congestion does not indicate disease activity with lupus. (3) Excessive fatigue is a sign of disease activity with lupus. (4) Sore throat does not indicate disease activity with lupus.

77. **(4)** Integrated processes: nursing process — implementation; teaching/learning; client need: health promotion and maintenance; content area: pediatrics.

RATIONALE

(1) Instant drink mixes should not contain wheat products. (2) Chocolate-covered peanuts would not affect an allergy to wheat. (3) Wheat is usually not contained in salad dressings. (4) Wieners do contain wheat. Teach the mother how to read food labels.

78. **(4)** Integrated processes: nursing process — implementation; teaching/learning; client need: health promotion and maintenance; content area: pediatrics.

RATIONALE

(1) Cola should be avoided with allergy to chocolate. (2) Gravy should be avoided with wheat allergy. (3) Instant breakfast drinks should be avoided with milk allergy. (4) Mayonnaise is made with eggs and should be eliminated from the child's diet.

79. **(2)** Integrated processes: nursing process — implementation; teaching/learning; client need: health promotion and maintenance; content area: pediatrics.

RATIONALE

(1) Two months is too soon. (2) Four to 6 months is an appropriate time to introduce cereal. (3) By 9 months of age, fruit, vegetables, and junior foods can be introduced. (4) By 12 months of age, cow's milk can be introduced.

80. **(3)** Integrated processes: nursing process — implementation; teaching/learning; client need: health promotion and maintenance; content area: pediatrics.

RATIONALE

(1) Barley is not the first choice. (2) Oat is not the first choice. (3) Rice is the first choice because it is easier to digest and has the least potential of allergy than other cereals. Cereals should be introduced one at a time in case allergies develop. This would make it easier to identify the allergen. (4) Wheat should be introduced after rice cereal.

81. **(1)** Integrated processes: nursing process — data collection; client need: physiological integrity; physiological adaptation; content area: pediatrics.

RATIONALE

(1) Chronic runny nose is an allergic response to cow's milk. (2) Excessive urination is not indicative of an allergy. (3) Irritability can be the result of symptoms of an allergy. (4) Refusal to drink milk does not imply an allergy.

82. **(1)** Integrated processes: nursing process — data collection; client need: physiological integrity; reduction of risk potential; content area: pediatrics.

RATIONALE

(1) Normal hemoglobin levels give a more accurate pulse oximetry reading. (2) Cool temperature can cause vascular constriction, and the reading would not be as accurate. (3) Excessive motion can interfere with the reading. (4) Poor perfusion can interfere with an accurate reading.

83. **(2)** Integrated processes: nursing process — data collection; client need: physiological integrity; physiological adaptation; content area: pediatrics.

RATIONALE

(1) This is an appropriate heart rate for an infant. (2) Expiratory grunting can indicate respiratory distress. (3) This is a desirable capillary refill time. (4) This is a satisfactory urinary output.

84. **(3)** Integrated processes: nursing process — data collection; client need: physiological integrity; pharmacological therapies; content area: pediatrics.

RATIONALE

(1) This is a normal BP. (2) This is a normal heart rate. (3) This temperature is elevated, which indicates an allergic response to blood. (4) This is an acceptable respiratory rate.

85. **(3)** Integrated processes: nursing process — implementation; client need: physiological integrity; pharmacological therapies; content area: pediatrics.

RATIONALE

(1) The abbreviation OS means left eye, not both eyes. (2) The order is to instill drops in the eye, not the ear. (3) The abbreviation OS means left eye, and pulling lower lid down and forming a reservoir are proper actions. (4) The order is to instill drops in the eye, not the ear.

86. **(1)** Integrated processes: nursing process — implementation; client need: physiological integrity; pharmacological therapies; content area: pediatrics.

RATIONALE

(1) This is the proper way to administer eardrops when the child is less than 3 years old. For individuals older than 3 years, the proper earlobe position is pulled up and back. (2) The child should be held still for a few minutes, but 10 minutes is not necessary. (3) It is not necessary to raise the head of the bed. (4) This is acceptable, but not required.

87. **(2)** Integrated processes: nursing process — implementation; client need: physiological integrity; basic care and comfort; content area: pediatrics.

RATIONALE

(1) This is too small an amount. Infants are given approximately 200 mL. (2) This is the appropriate amount for a 4-year-old child. (3) This amount would be in the range for a school-age child. (4) This amount is in the range for a school-age child.

88. **(2)** Integrated processes: nursing process — evaluation; client need: physiological integrity; physiological adaptation; content area: pediatrics.

RATIONALE

(1) Confusion is a symptom of hyperglycemia. (2) An irritable, weepy, and nervous child is consistent with hypoglycemia. (3) Flushed face is a symptom of hyperglycemia. (4) Fruity breath is a sign of hyperglycemia.

89. **(2)** Integrated processes: nursing process — implementation; teaching/learning; client need: physiological integrity; pharmacological therapies; content area: pediatrics.

RATIONALE

(1) The insulin should be administered 30 minutes before meals. (2) Administering the insulin 30 minutes before meals coordinates the peak of the insulin with the ingestion of food. (3) This would be too late; insulin is given before meals. (4) Insulin is usually administered to children in the morning and the evening, but this answer does not give information on the time for each of the doses in relation to meals.

90. **(1)** Integrated processes: nursing process — data collection; client need: physiological integrity; physiological adaptation; content area: pediatrics.

RATIONALE

(1) Vaginal yeast infections and urinary tract infections are early signs of diabetes in adolescent girls. (2) This is not the cause of yeast infections in girls with diabetes. (3) Sexual activity can result in vaginal infections, but a hyperglycemic state contributes to yeast infections in girls with diabetes. (4) Urinary tract dysfunction does not cause vaginal yeast infections.

91. **(4)** Integrated processes: nursing process — planning; client need: physiological integrity; physiological adaptation; content area: pediatrics.

RATIONALE

(1) Iron stores are adequate for the first 5–6 months of age in the term infant. (2) Iron stores from the mother are still adequate when an infant is 4 months old. (3) At 6 months, maternal iron stores are depleting, but iron levels are maintained for an additional 120 days through the life of these RBCs. (4) The infant receives iron from the mother in utero that can be stored for up to 6 months. The majority of the iron is stored in the hemoglobin of RBCs, and an additional supply is stored in the liver, spleen, and bone marrow. The life of a normal RBC is 120 days. If the infant is not receiving iron supplements or an adequate amount of iron in the diet, iron-deficiency anemia will show up at 9 months, after the life of the RBCs stored from the mother.

92. **(1)** Integrated processes: nursing process — evaluation; teaching/learning; client need: physiological integrity; pharmacological therapies; content area: pediatrics.

RATIONALE

(1) Fruit juice contains vitamin C, which enhances the absorption of iron. (2) Iron should be given with juice or a multivitamin to increase its absorption. (3) Iron should be administered between meals because the bulk of a meal can decrease the absorption of the iron in the upper GI tract. (4) Milk decreases the absorption of iron.

93. **(2)** Integrated processes: nursing process — evaluation; client need: physiological integrity; physiological adaptation; content area: pediatrics.

RATIONALE

(1) Jaundice does not indicate iron deficiency. (2) Iron supplements can cause green, tarry stools. (3) It is good for a mother to identify the fact that she is compliant, but evidence of the tarry stool is objective data. (4) Iron deficiency does not produce diarrhea. Iron supplements can result in constipation.

94. **(3)** Integrated processes: nursing process — implementation; teaching/learning; client need: physiological integrity; pharmacological therapies; content area: pediatrics.

RATIONALE

(1) Iron should be administered in divided doses throughout the day to maximize absorption. (2) Dividing the dose throughout the day maximizes absorption. (3) Iron should be given through a straw or by a dropper or syringe to prevent staining the teeth. (4) Iron absorption is enhanced if given with vitamin C, not protein.

95. **(1)** Integrated processes: nursing process — implementation; teaching/learning; client need: physiological integrity; basic care and comfort; content area: pediatrics.

RATIONALE

(1) Soaking in warm water decreases stiffness in the joints. (2) Pain medication does not reduce stiffness. (3) Doing passive ROM reduces stiffness but does not soothe the joint as the warm water does. (4) Waking up early does not reduce stiffness.

96. **(1)** Integrated processes: nursing process — evaluation; teaching/learning; client need: health promotion and maintenance; content area: pediatrics.

RATIONALE

(1) Penicillin shots are usually administered for an indefinite period after the occurrence of RF to prevent reinfection with streptococcus. (2) Monthly throat cultures are not necessary. (3) Yearly echocardiograms can evaluate the status of the heart but do nothing to prevent reinfection. (4) A regular exercise program is good for the child, but the aim of therapy is to prevent reinfection with streptococcus.

97. **(4)** Integrated processes: nursing process — implementation; teaching/learning; client need: physiological integrity; pharmacological therapies; content area: pediatrics.

RATIONALE

(1) Aspirin controls inflammation, but the reason for aspirin at this time is to decrease thrombus formation. (2) Because fever is gone, the aspirin is not needed as an antipyretic. (3) Aspirin cannot prevent valve damage, but it can help to control inflammation that contributes to valve damage. (4) Aspirin is continued in an antiplatelet dose once fever has subsided to decrease thrombus formation.

98. **(2)** Integrated processes: nursing process — data collection; client need: health promotion and maintenance; content area: pediatrics.

RATIONALE

(1) This child is not at high risk because of maternal iron stores. (2) A 2-year-old child's diet should be limited to 24 oz of milk per day. Intake of large quantities of milk decreases intake of a balanced diet. (3) Refusing to drink milk does not cause iron-deficiency anemia. (4) Refusing to eat chicken does not cause iron-deficiency anemia.

99. **(3)** Integrated processes: nursing process — implementation; teaching/learning; client need: physiological integrity; pharmacological therapies; content area: pediatrics.

RATIONALE

(1) This would not be necessary because of steroid therapy. (2) The child needs to be around peers for support and normal development. (3) Steroids cause water retention and increase appetite. Weight gain is common. (4) The child still needs to be active, and exercise is encouraged.

100. **(1)** Integrated processes: nursing process — data collection; client need: physiological integrity; physiological adaptation; content area: pediatrics.
   RATIONALE
   (1) Hearing loss can occur from damage to nerves. (2) Spinal damage is not likely. (3) Urinary incontinence is not a complication. (4) Memory loss is not a complication.

101. **(1, 2, 4)** Integrated processes: nursing process — implementation; client need: physiological integrity; reduction of risk potential; content area: pediatrics
   RATIONALE
   (1) Patches must be applied to prevent corneal irritation. (2) Oily substances applied to the skin can promote burns. (3) The infant's position should be changed frequently to increase exposure to the phototherapy. (4) The nurse must monitor for signs of dehydration. (5) Supplemental oxygen is not indicated with hyperbilirubinemia. (6) A knitted cap would decrease the surface area and reduce the effectiveness of the phototherapy. The lights produce heat; therefore concerns about heat loss are not warranted.

102. **(2, 6)** Integrated processes: nursing process — planning; client need: health promotion and maintenance; content area: pediatrics.
   RATIONALE
   Reflexes serve as primitive responses that protect human bodies from danger and help with adjustment to surroundings. (1) The Babinski reflex disappears after age 1 year. (2) An eye blink occurs with the sudden appearance of a bright light or object directed toward the eye and persists throughout life. (3) The Moro or startle reflex disappears by 3–4 months of age. (4) A positive Ortolani's reflex refers to an audible click on abduction which is associated with a dislocated or subluxated hip. (5) The tonic neck reflex disappears by 3–4 months of age. (6) A yawn is a spontaneous response to decreased oxygen levels which persists throughout life.

103. **(1, 2, 5)** Integrated processes: nursing process — planning; teaching/learning; client need: health promotion and maintenance; content area: pediatrics.
   RATIONALE
   (1) DTaP is given at 2, 4, 6, and 15 months of age. (2) HiB is given at 2, 4, and 6 months of age. (3) The influenza vaccine is given once yearly to at-risk populations. (4) MMR is given at 12 months of age. (5) Polio is given at 2, 4, and 6 months of age. (6) Varicella is given at 12 months of age.

104. **(1, 5)** Integrated processes: nursing process — planning; client need: physiological integrity; reduction of risk potential; content area: pediatrics.
   RATIONALE
   (1) Anaphylactic reaction to previous injection is an absolute contraindication for that immunization. (2) Breast milk is the preferred infant formula and is not a contraindication. (3) A mild illness is not a contraindication. (4) A nonprogressive neurological disorder is not a contraindication. (5) A moderate or severe illness is a contraindication to immunization because it may be difficult to differentiate responses to the vaccine and worsening of an illness. (6) A

fever of 101°F is considered a mild illness and is not a contraindication.

105. **(1, 2, 5)** Integrated processes: nursing process — planning; communication and documentation; client need: safe, effective care environment; coordinated care; content area: pediatrics.
   RATIONALE
   (1) Nutrition is an important part of planning when an infant has a cleft lip. (2) An occupational therapist can help with oral motor skills and feeding techniques. (3) A pediatric urologist is a physician who specializes in diseases of the urinary system; a pediatric surgeon, plastic surgeon, or eye, ear, nose, and throat specialist would be involved. (4) There is no pharmacologic therapy for a cleft lip. (5) A registered nurse, often a clinical specialist or advanced practitioner, would be involved with the team. (6) A schoolteacher is usually not involved with an infant but should be involved with the school-age child.

106. **(4, 5)** Integrated processes: nursing process — implementation; client need: physiological integrity; pharmacological therapies; content area: pediatrics.
   RATIONALE
   (1) The drug should be given before the child goes to radiology. (2) Digoxin should be given at regular intervals 1 hour before or 2 hours after eating even if the child is sleeping. (3) Teething is not a reason to withhold digoxin; however, the teeth should be brushed after administration of the medication to prevent tooth decay from sweet liquid. (4) Vomiting is one of the most common signs of toxicity. A single episode of vomiting is not a reason to withhold the drug but repeated episodes are a reason to withhold the dose and consult with the physician. (5) Digoxin should not be given if a child's pulse is below 70 bpm. (6) Respiratory distress is often associated with congestive heart failure and must be reported but is not a reason to withhold the drug.

107. **(3, 5, 4, 2, 6, 1)** Integrated processes: nursing process — implementation; client need: safe, effective care environment; safety and infection control; content area: pediatrics.
   RATIONALE
   (1) When the procedure is complete, the suction tubing is rinsed with water to minimize collection of debris inside the tubing. (2) The thumb hole should not be covered until the catheter is in place to minimize trauma to the trachea and must be covered to apply suction in order to remove secretions. (3) All equipment should be gathered before starting a procedure. (4) Insert the suction catheter into the tracheostomy. (5) Hand washing is the first step in any procedure done after gathering equipment to minimize spread of disease. (6) After the thumb hole is covered, the catheter is withdrawn.

108. **(1, 2, 3, 4)** Integrated processes: nursing process — evaluation; teaching/learning; client need: psychosocial integrity; content area: pediatrics.
   RATIONALE
   (1) A child's cooperation and participation with the treatment plan is important to optimize control of seizures. (2) Control of seizures is the primary goal. (3) Absence of signs of physical injury would provide evidence that there is lack of injury during a seizure should it occur; e.g. there is appropriate management of the seizure. (4) A seizure disorder may require multiple visits to health-care providers, medications, a special diet, and/or environmental modifications. (5) For optimal

growth and development, the child should not be viewed as handicapped and should exhibit no evidence of overprotection or abuse. (6) The use of tongue blades is no longer recommended during a seizure.

109. Integrated processes: nursing process — implementation; client need: physiological integrity; physiological adaptation; content area: pediatrics.

RATIONALE
The brachial pulse of a 1 year old is the proper location to assess cardiac status when an individual is unresponsive (CPR).

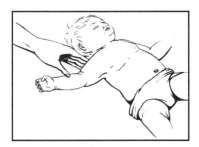

110. Integrated processes: nursing process — data collection; client need: health promotion and maintenance; content area: pediatrics.

RATIONALE
The anterior fontanel is located at the junction of the frontal and parietal bones. It can be palpated midline above the forehead until about 14 months of age.

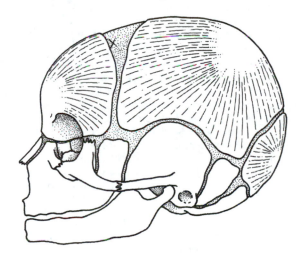

111. (3) Integrated processes: nursing process — planning; client need: health promotion and maintenance; content area: pediatrics.

RATIONALE
(1) The first chickenpox (varicella) vaccine is given at 12 months of age. (2) Diphtheria is included in the DTaP vaccine started at 2 months of age. (3) Hepatitis B vaccinations should start shortly after birth and before a newborn leaves the hospital. (4) Influenza protection is recommended annually for high-risk populations. (5) The inactivated polio vaccine is started at 2 months of age. (6) Tetanus is included in the DTaP vaccine started at 2 months of age.

112. (**1560 mL**) Integrated processes: nursing process — implementation; communication and documentation; client need: physiological integrity; basic care and comfort; content area: pediatrics.

RATIONALE
The intake is the total of the IV (720 mL) and oral fluids (apple juice 240 mL; ginger ale 120 mL; water 240 mL (1 oz = 30 mL), beef broth 240 mL (1 cup = 8 oz) = 1560 mL.

113. (**1, 3, 4, 6**) Integrated processes: nursing process — planning; communication and documentation; client need: safe, effective care environment; coordinated care; content area: pediatrics.

RATIONALE
(1) A CNA is trained to bathe a toddler. (2) Only a nurse may change an IV bag. This is not appropriate for a CNA under any circumstance. (3) Comforting a crying infant is appropriate to delegate to a CNA. (4) A CNA is trained to feed an infant. (5) Giving an enema is medication administration and may not be delegated to a CNA. (6) A CNA is trained to obtain vital signs.

114. (**3, 4, 5**) Integrated processes: nursing process — implementation; client need: physiological integrity; reduction of risk potential; content area: pediatrics.

RATIONALE
(1) Irrigating the shunt tubing is a medical/surgical procedure performed by a physician. (2) The child must be positioned carefully to prevent any pressure on the shunt site and valve. (3) Rapid changes in head circumference may be indicative of problems, and the head circumference must be assessed regularly using the same landmarks for comparison. A marking pen may be used to designate the landmarks. (4) Infection is the most common complication with shunt placement. (5) After surgery, infants are often NPO with IV fluids ordered and they must be monitored carefully for dehydration and fluid overload. (6) The Trendelenburg position with the head lower than the body would increase pressure on the shunt site and valve.

115. (**3**) Integrated processes: nursing process — data collection; client need: health promotion and maintenance; content area: pediatrics.

RATIONALE
(1) Masturbation is not an illness. (2) Self-stimulation can occur at any age, and it is not developmentally harmful. (3) This behavior is considered a normal part of sexual curiosity and is most common for 4 year olds and adolescents. (4) Precocious puberty refers to the development of secondary sex characteristics before 8 years of age; e.g., breast development or sperm production. (5) Masturbation in public is not appropriate and teaching children safe, appropriate behavior may be necessary. (6) Excessive masturbation may reflect boredom, anxiety, or unresolved conflicts which need to be addressed. Sexual orientation develops primarily during adolescence.

116. (**2, 5, 6**) Integrated processes: nursing process — implementation; communication and documentation; client need: psychosocial integrity; content area: pediatrics.

RATIONALE
(1) Therapeutic play is an individual intervention and is not directed at sharing information about a diagnosis with other children. (2) Therapeutic play promotes the expression of feelings about illness and hospitalization. (3) Getting to know other children with an illness may promote adaptation but is not a purpose of therapeutic play. (4) Play is the work of a child, but having fun is not a purpose here. (5) Play can provide a child with an opportunity to learn about procedures and equipment (6) Therapeutic play can assist the child in maintaining a sense of control.

117. **(1, 4, 6)** Integrated processes: nursing process — implementation; teaching/learning; client need: health promotion and maintenance; content area: pediatrics.

RATIONALE

(1) The ability is sit without fussing is a sign of psychological readiness for toilet training. **(2)** This cognitive skill is not related to readiness. **(3)** Fine motor skills are not signs of readiness for toilet training. **(4)** These gross motor skills are signs of physical readiness.**(5)** These plans may be a reason to defer the training because the family needs to be willing to invest the time required and the training should be done when other stresses are minimized. **(6)** This is a sign of mental readiness.

118. **(3, 4, 5)** Integrated processes: nursing process — planning; client need: health promotion and maintenance; content area: pediatrics.

RATIONALE

(1) Fear of mutilation is a concern of preschoolers. **(2)** Fear of separation from a favorite toy or family is a concern of infants and toddlers. **(3)** Loss of independence is a concern of adolescents. **(4)** Privacy is a major concern for the adolescent. **(5)** The adolescent often expresses anxiety regarding loss of independence, control, and identity with illness and hospitalization. **(6)** Separation from peers and the ability to maintain a position in a group is a concern of the school-age child.

119. **(1, 2, 4)** Integrated processes: nursing process — implementation; communication and documentation; client need: physiological integrity; reduction of risk potential; content area: pediatrics.

RATIONALE

(1) Documenting the history of a seizure is an important nursing responsibility which can assist in developing strategies to control the disorder. **(2)** Restrictive clothing should be loosened to minimize the risk of injury. **(3)** The child should not be restrained or forced to move. **(4)** If the child is standing or sitting, he or she should be eased down to prevent falling. **(5)** Nothing should be placed in the child's mouth. **(6)** The child should not be moved.

120. **(3.75 mL)** Integrated processes: nursing process — implementation; client need: physiological integrity; pharmacological therapies; content area: pediatrics.

RATIONALE

To calculate the dosage set up the problem:

$$\frac{x}{75} = \frac{5 \text{ mL}}{100 \text{ mg}} = 100x: 375; x = 3.75$$

121. **(3, 4, 5, 6)** Integrated processes: nursing process — data collection; client need: physiological integrity; physiological adaptation; content area: pediatrics.

RATIONALE

(1) Appetite is not related to hydration. **(2)** Reflexes are not affected by hydration status. **(3)** Skin turgor is an excellent indicator of hydration status. **(4)** The consistency of stools is directly related to hydration. **(5)** The amount of urine output is directly related to hydration status. **(6)** Weight is one of the most sensitive indicators of hydration status.

122. **(1, 4, 5, 6)** Integrated processes: nursing process — data collection; client need: physiologic integrity; physiological adaptation; content area: pediatrics.

RATIONALE

Causes of fluid overload or water intoxication include incorrectly mixed infant formula, excessive water ingestion, rapid IV fluid administration, or administration of an inappropriate hypotonic IV solution. **(1)** Bulging fontanels are associated with fluid excess. **(2)** Cold, mottled skin is associated with fluid volume deficit. **(3)** A large urine output is a sign of water intoxication. **(4)** Dyspnea is associated with fluid volume excess. **(5)** Swelling is a manifestation of overhydration, particularly in the face, perineum, and torso. **(6)** Decreased pulse rate is a sign of overhydration; a rapid pulse rate is a sign of dehydration.

123. **(100 ml)** Integrated processes: nursing process — implementation; client need: physiological integrity; pharmacological therapies; content area: pediatrics.

RATIONALE

To calculate the dosage set up the problem:

$$\frac{50 \text{ mL}}{30 \text{ min}} = \frac{x}{60 \text{ min}}; \frac{3000}{30 \text{ x}}; x = 100$$

124. **(3)** Integrated processes: nursing process — implementation; client need: safe, effective care environment; coordinated care; content area: pediatrics.

RATIONALE

(1) If the student is conscious and breathing, checking the pulse would not be the first step. **(2)** The AED is used when there is a cardiac arrest. **(3)** With a potential head or neck injury, the most important thing to do is not increase any damage. Immobilization is essential until help arrives. **(4)** Wet clothing could only be removed if the student's extremities were moved. **(5)** The student should not be turned. **(6)** The student should not be moved.

125. **(4)** Integrated processes: nursing process — data collection; communication and documentation; client need: physiological integrity; physiological adaptation; content: pediatrics.

RATIONALE

(1) A normal heart rate for a newborn is 120–140 bpm. Crying may increase it and sleeping may decrease it. **(2)** The normal respiratory rate for a newborn is 30–60 breaths/min. Crying may increase it and sleeping may decrease it. **(3)** Axillary temperature is 97.9–98.0° F in the newborn and may be altered by environmental factors. **(4)** Coarctation of the aorta may be present if the systolic blood pressure in the upper extremity is 6–9 mm Hg less than the lower extremity. This discrepancy, as well as weaker femoral pulses, needs to be reported.

126. **(1)** Integrated processes: nursing process — implementation; teaching/learning; client need: physiological integrity; basic care and comfort; content: pediatrics.

RATIONALE

(1) High temperatures from microwaves destroy the anti-infective properties. **(2)** The risk of burns to the newborn is true for breast milk or formula heated in a microwave; however, the most accurate reason is that high tempperatures destroy the anti-infective properties. **(3)** There is risk of exploding glass containers for any food or milk product if microwaved at too high a temperature; however, the most accurate reason is that high temperatures destroy the anti-infective properties. **(4)** Breast milk is warm by nature and does not increase indigestion.

127. **(4)** Integrated processes: nursing process — implementation; client need: health promotion and maintenance; content: pediatrics.

RATIONALE

(1) Full-strength doses are recommended for premature as well as full-term infants. **(2)** Dosages should be given based on the actual, not corrected, chronological age. These must be initiated in the hospital. (3) The OPV is the one vaccine not given in the hospital due to the risk of transmission to other infants in the nursery. (4) The actual chronological age is used to administer vaccines to preterm infants.

128. (2) Integrated processes: nursing process — implementation; client need: physiological integrity; pharmacological therapies; content: pediatrics.

RATIONALE

(1) Subcutaneous injection is not recommended for DPT. (2) Deep intramuscular injection with an appropriate-length needle into the ventrogluteal or vastus lateralis is the recommended method. The deltoid is used only after 18 months of age. (3) An air lock is theoretically helpful but not proven to be beneficial. The needle change after drawing up the medicine does not decrease local reactions. (4) The application of a local anesthetic may decrease pain, but not local reactions.

129. (1) Integrated processes: nursing process — data collection; client need: physiological integrity; physiological adaptation; content: pediatrics.

RATIONALE

(1) The typical colicky infant does cry more than usual and does have abdominal cramping. (2) Although abdominal pain and gastric distention may be present, projectile vomiting and diarrhea are not typical. (3) Typically, the formula is tolerated well and the infant thrives with adequate weight gain. (4) Some studies indicate late evening fussiness in infants. For some infants, the time is altered.

130. (4) Integrated processes: nursing process — implementation; teaching/learning; client need: health promotion and maintenance; content: pediatrics.

RATIONALE

(1) Males are affected at higher percentages. (2) The peak time of year is winter (January). (3) The time of death is usually during sleep, but most often in a prone, not supine, position. (4) The peak age is 2–4 months with 95% occurring in the first 6 months.

131. (1) Integrated processes: nursing process — data collection; communication and documentation; client need: safe, effective care environment; coordinated care; content: pediatrics.

RATIONALE

(1) This statement accurately documents what the client states. (2) The fact that your opinion of the client's pain and the client's opinion of the pain differ should not be considered. If the physical appearance differs from the stated value, chart the stated value. (3) The client may be lying in bed, but he states that he is in pain, which is what should be documented. (4) The statement that the client is faking pain is a judgment and should not be documented.

132. (3) Integrated processes: nursing process — data collection; client need: physiological integrity; basic care and comfort; content: pediatrics.

RATIONALE

(1) During infancy, the client presents generalized responses to pain by crying loudly and assuming a look of pain, but she cannot "objectify" it. (2) A young child can anticipate painful procedures and try to resist, but cannot objectively describe it. (3) By age 3 years, the Faces pain scale can be used to point to the face best depicting the child's own pain. (4) By age 4 years, the child can associate meaning with numbers and can use tools like the poker-chip tool or numerical-value tool.

133. (2) Integrated processes: nursing process — planning; client need: physiological integrity; reduction of risk potential; content: pediatrics.

RATIONALE

(1) Because the child is often NPO for the first 24 hours, this option does not include measuring the IV fluids. (2) Strictly measuring the intake of all oral and IV fluids, including medication diluents and flushes for lines in addition to hourly Foley catheter measurements, gives the best input and output pictures. (3) Parents should not be requested to keep accurate counts in the immediate postoperative period. (4) Fluids are restricted, but offering the bedpan hourly would be inaccurate, inappropriate, unnecessary, and tiring for the immediate postoperative period.

134. (2) Integrated processes: nursing process — evaluation; teaching/learning; client need: physiological integrity; pharmacological therapies; content: pediatrics.

RATIONALE

(1) If vomiting occurs, the dose should not be repeated. (2) Because of binding, the medication should not be given with milk products. It should be given 1 hour before meals or 2 hours after meals. (3) Oral medication is properly administered to the side and back. (4) If a dose is forgotten and less than 4 hours has passed, the dose can be given.

135. (4) Integrated processes: nursing process — implementation; client need: physiological integrity; basic care and comfort; content: pediatrics.

RATIONALE

(1) Supine is a position recommended by the American Association of Pediatrics (AAP) for well infants. (2) Side lying is a position recommended by the AAP for well infants. (3) Prone is recommended for infants, with a tendency to spit up or with respiratory problems, but not with the head down. (4) The head of the bed up 45 degrees or an infant seat is recommended along with loose clothing for optimal chest expansion.

136. (1) Integrated processes: nursing process — planning; client need: physiological integrity; physiological adaptation; content: pediatrics.

RATIONALE

(1) Oxygen via mask or cannula needs to be administered immediately to treat the severe dyspnea. (2) Heparin may be given as part of the management plan. (3) Corticosteriods may be given as part of the management plan. (4) An IV will be established to treat shock and administer medication.

137. (3) Integrated processes: nursing process — data collection; client need: physiological integrity; reduction of risk potential; content: pediatrics.

RATIONALE

(1) A child may be able to use the affected extremity. (2) A child who does not want to walk may have a fracture, so it should not be ruled out. However, it is not diagnostic. (3) A radiograph with comparison films is still the best way to compare extremities for fractures. (4) Bruising and swelling may be present over fractures.

138. (2) Integrated processes: nursing process — data collection; client need: physiological integrity; physiological adaptation; content: pediatrics.

RATIONALE

(1) Pulse and respirations typically increase with early airway obstructions. (2) Retractions are a common finding in early airway obstructions. (3) Restlessness usually increases early.

(4) Nasal flaring is evident but not necessarily congestion and drainage.

139. **(1)** Integrated processes: nursing process — data collection; client need: physiological integrity; reduction of risk potential; content: pediatrics.

RATIONALE

(1) PEFR measures peak flow velocity and is compared to the client's personal best. **(2)** ABGs measure artery blood gases of PaO_2, $PaCO_2$, pH, and base excess. **(3)** SaO_2 measures peripheral oxygen saturation and is presented in a percentage. **(4)** Ausculation will help determine wheezing and any decrease in breath sounds.

140. **(1)** Integrated processes: nursing process — data collection; client need: physiological integrity; reduction of risk potential; content: pediatrics.

RATIONALE

(1) An early sign of bleeding and potential hemorrhage in a T&A client is frequent swallowing. **(2)** Moderate pain is common, especially in the first 24 hours. **(3)** A pulse of greater than 120 bpm may indicate hemorrhage. **(4)** Dark brown blood is expected in emesis secretions and in the nose and teeth. Bright red blood is indicative of hemorrhage.

141. **(3)** Integrated processes: nursing process — implementation; client need: physiological integrity; basic care and comfort; content: pediatrics.

RATIONALE

(1) An infant often has an external urine collection bag to retrieve urine specimens. **(2)** The number of wet diapers gives a broad estimate as to whether output is adequate. **(3)** A diaper can be weighed to determine better the milliliters of fluid lost (1 g = 1 mL or 1 cc). Because evaporation is possible, frequent checks are needed, especially if the client is under a radiant warmer or if the diaper leaks. **(4)** Catheters are not routinely inserted without adequate rationale.

142. **(2)** Integrated processes: nursing process — data collection; client need: physiological integrity; physiological adaptation; content: pediatrics.

RATIONALE

(1) Blisters occur in second-degree burns. **(2)** Pain is the predominant symptom in first-degree burns. **(3)** Waxy white skin may be present in second- or third-degree burns. Brown skin is present in third-degree burns. **(4)** Burns of full-thickness, fourth-degree burns, appear dull and dry with bones or ligaments noted.

143. **(3)** Integrated processes: nursing process — evaluation; teaching/learning; client need: physiological integrity; physiological adaptation; content: pediatrics.

RATIONALE

(1) Butter and oils should not be applied. **(2)** Blisters should be left intact. **(3)** Loose gauze is not necessarily applied. **(4)** Cool water should be run over the burn.

144. **(1)** Integrated processes: nursing process — implementation; teaching/learning; client need: health promotion and maintenance; content: pediatrics.

RATIONALE

(1) Benefits to mother and infant should be provided, and the parents of the infant should be allowed to make an informed decision. **(2)** Providing no information will not lead the parents to make an informed decision. **(3)** Written packets would not allow for questions and answers. **(4)** The mother should have some input into the type of formula used if she opts to bottle feed. The nurse should not assume bottle feeding.

145. **(1)** Integrated processes: nursing process — evaluation; teaching/learning; client need: physiological integrity; physiological adaptation; content: pediatrics.

RATIONALE

(1) When the vesicles have dried, the child can be released from home isolation. **(2)** Crusts may still be present when the child returns to school. Support and conferences with the teacher may be needed for the child's psychological security. **(3)** New lesions may appear for a few days. **(4)** It does take an average of 1 week for lesions to dry.

146. **(1)** Integrated processes: nursing process — implementation; client need: physiological integrity; basic care and comfort; content: pediatrics.

RATIONALE

(1) If oral diphenydramine (Benadryl) is given simultaneously, toxicity can result from the increased topical absorption. **(2)** Cool baths with oatmeal or soap are still comforting according to some. **(3)** Calamine does not prevent crusting. **(4)** According to the literature, calamine can be very comforting and does not prolong the outbreak.

147. **(2)** Integrated processes: nursing process — implementation; client need: physiological integrity; reduction of risk potential; content: pediatrics.

RATIONALE

(1) Rectal swabs are used to determine the causative organisms of diarrhea. **(2)** The tape test, which involves placing transparent tape, sticky side out, around a tongue depressor, which is then secured to the anus of the sleeping child. Specimens are collected in the early morning before stooling or awakening. **(3)** A skin scraping is used for many rashes and infestations like scabies. **(4)** A stool specimen is often used for diarrhea complaints.

148. **(5, 6)** Integrated processes: nursing process — planning; client need: physiological integrity; physiologic adaptation; content area: pediatrics.

RATIONALE

(1) Aortic stenosis is the narrowing of the aortic valve which does not cause cyanosis. **(2)** Atrial septal defect is an acyanotic defect; it is an abnormal opening between the right and left atria. **(3)** Coarctation of aorta is a narrowing of the aorta, an acyanotic defect which causes decreased circulation to the body. **(4)** Patent ductus arteriosus is failure of the fetal ductus arteriosus to close, an acyanotic defect which causes decreased circulation to the lungs. **(5)** Tetralogy of Fallot is a major cyanotic defect which includes a ventricular septal defect, pulmonic stenosis, overriding aorta, and right ventricular hypertrophy. **(6)** Transposition of the great vessels is a major cyanotic defect in which there is no blood flow between the systemic and pulmonary circulatory systems. Systemic blood enters the right ventricle and returns to the body via the aorta. Pulmonary blood enters the left ventricle and returns to the lungs in pulmonary vessels.

149. **(1)** Integrated processes: nursing process — data collection; client need: physiological integrity; physiologic adaptation; content area: pediatrics.

RATIONALE

(1) A newborn with tricuspid atresia is usually cyanotic. **(2)** Infants with obstructive defects often have the signs and symptoms of congestive heart failure (CHF). Mild cases may be asystematic. **(3)** With conditions like atrioventricular canal defect, cyanosis may be mild, but worsened with crying. A characteristic murmur is present and CHF may be severe. **(4)** Infants with TGV who have minimal mixing of the blood become severely cyanotic; however, if a large PDA is present, the signs and symptoms of CHF are more characteristic than those of cyanosis.

150. **(2)** Integrated processes: nursing process — data collection; client need: physiological integrity; reduction of risk potential; content: pediatric.

RATIONALE

(1) Allergies are important to know; however, first what was taken and when it was taken needs to be determined to plan treatment. **(2)** Because there is no universal antidote for "poison," what was taken, amount, when, and anything that caregivers may have done to improve or worsen the situation all need to be determined. **(3)** Ipecac is given before activated charcoal if both are to be given. However, ipecac is contraindicated if the client takes calcium channel blockers, benzodiazepines, and other drugs. **(4)** Activated charcoal is black, tasteless, and odorless medicine that may hold sweetener, but it is lower priority.

CHAPTER 5

Medical-Surgical Nursing: Content Review and Test

Jennifer Couvillion, RN, PhD
Deborah Garbee, RN, APRN, MN, BC
Judith Gentry, RN, APRN, MSN, OCN
Karen Silady, RN, MN

Respiratory System

Basic Information

All body cells depend on adequate oxygen level and carbon dioxide removal. The respiratory system is regulated by the central nervous system (CNS) and depends on the cardiovascular system for its blood supply. Diseases of the respiratory system can be either primary (direct) or secondary (caused by diseases in other body systems). The licensed practical nurse (LPN) needs to make a respiratory assessment of all clients and include this information in the nursing care plan even when secondary to disease in other body systems. In this chapter, "Diagnostic tests and methods" replaces "Planning" step.

I. Basic data collection
  A. Subjective observations (client description)
    1. Cough
    2. Difficulty in breathing
    3. Pain
    4. Weakness, tiredness
    5. Sputum
  B. Client history
    1. Respiratory illness or difficulty
    2. Injuries
    3. Use of extra pillows when sleeping
    4. Smoking
    5. Occupation
    6. Use of medications
  C. Objective observations (LPN description)
    1. Respirations
      a. Rate
      b. Depth
      c. Breath sounds
      d. Difficulty in breathing
    2. Symptoms of lack of oxygen
      a. Yawning

      b. Restlessness
      c. Drowsiness
      d. Anxiety
      e. Confusion
      f. Disorientation
    3. Skin
      a. Color
        1) Pale or ruddy (reddened)
        2) Cyanotic (bluish): color of lips, nails, inside of mouth
      b. Temperature
      c. Excessive sweating
    4. Cough
      a. Frequency: continuous, sporadic (on and off)
      b. Type: productive, moist, hacking, dry, nonproductive
    5. Sputum
      a. Presence or absence
      b. Type: thick, frothy, watery
      c. Color: white, yellow, rusty, blood-tinged, purulent
      d. Amount: scant, moderate, abundant
      e. Odor
    6. Vital signs
      a. Pulse: rate, quality, type
      b. Blood pressure (BP)
      c. Temperature: tympanic membrane
  D. Recording and reporting of all observations

Major Respiratory Diagnoses

Epistaxis (Nosebleed)

I. Description
  A. Bleeding from the nose
  B. Causes
    1. Direct trauma to nose: blow to nose, insertion of foreign object

2. Nasal polyps
3. Acute or chronic infections: sinusitis or rhinitis
4. Systemic diseases such as hypertension
5. Local irritation: inhalation of chemicals (nasal spray use or illicit drug use)
6. Varicosities within nasal cavity
7. Chronic use of aspirin/nonsteroidal anti-inflammatory drugs (NSAIDs)
8. High altitudes, dry climates
9. Hodgkin's disease
10. Scurvy
11. Vitamin K deficiency
12. Rheumatic fever
13. Blood dyscrasias: hemophilia, purpura, leukemia, some anemias

II. Data collection
  A. Subjective symptoms
    1. Bleeding
    2. Pain
    3. Lightheadedness, dizziness
    4. Difficulty in breathing through the nose
  B. Objective symptoms
    1. Observation of bleeding from nose
    2. Trauma around nose
    3. Decrease in blood pressure (BP)
    4. Rapid, bounding pulse
    5. Dyspnea
    6. Pallor
    7. Other indications of progressive shock

III. Diagnostic tests and methods
  A. Client history
  B. Physical examination
    1. Examination of nasal cavity
    2. Bruises or bleeding elsewhere
  C. Laboratory tests
    1. Repeated hemoglobin (Hgb) and hematocrit (Hct) tests
    2. Platelet count
    3. Prothrombin time (PT)

IV. Implementation
  A. Check nasal packing.
  B. Keep airway open (have client breathe through mouth).
  C. Control bleeding.
    1. Pinch soft part of nose firmly for 10–15 minutes.
    2. Tilt head slightly forward.
    3. Apply ice collar or cold wet compresses to nose.
  D. Encourage expectoration of blood (swallowing blood causes vomiting).
  E. Monitor skin color.
  F. Monitor vital signs.
    1. Report and record vital signs.
    2. Report any changes in vital signs immediately.
  G. Provide mouth care.
  H. Administer medications as ordered.
  I. Instruct client not to drink hot fluids.
  J. Provide reassurance to client and family.
  K. Explain home care
    1. Instruct client not to pick nose or insert foreign objects in nose.
    2. Emphasize need for follow-up examinations and periodic blood studies for nosebleeds.

3. Suggest use of humidifiers if client lives in dry climate or at high elevation, or both, or in home heated with circulating hot air.

V. Evaluation
  A. Client maintains effective airway and breathing pattern.
  B. Bleeding is absent.
  C. Client reports increased comfort.
  D. Vital signs remain stable.
  E. Laboratory blood values remain within normal range.
  F. Pain is decreased or absent.
  G. Client demonstrates an understanding of disease process, treatment, and home care.

Laryngitis

I. Description
  A. Acute or chronic inflammation and swelling of mucous membrane lining of the larynx and vocal cords (enlarged upper end of the trachea).
  B. Acute form possibly occurring as an isolated infection or as part of a generalized bacterial or viral upper respiratory tract infection.
  C. Possibly leading to decreased secretion and shrinking of the mucous membrane.
  D. Difficulty in breathing if crusts accumulate in laryngeal area and vocal cords, narrowing the breathing area.
  E. Possibly becoming chronic because of recurrent irritation after the acute form.
  F. Causes
    1. Excessive use of voice; talking or singing
    2. Exposure to cold and wet
    3. Spread of infection from nose and throat
    4. Local irritation caused by smoking
    5. Inhalation of irritating chemicals, dust, fumes
    6. Aspiration of caustic chemicals
    7. Preexisting nose and throat pathology
    8. Association with other diseases such as whooping cough, measles
    9. Alcohol abuse

II. Data collection
  A. Subjective symptoms
    1. Pain on swallowing or speaking
    2. Complaints of hoarseness
    3. Complaints of dry cough
    4. Tickling sensation in throat
    5. Fever
    6. Malaise
    7. Complaints of difficulty in breathing (because of crust formation)
  B. Objective symptoms
    1. Loss of voice
    2. Hoarseness
    3. Dry cough
    4. Increase in temperature
    5. Edema of larynx
    6. Difficulty in breathing (because of crust formation and narrowing of breathing space)

III. Diagnostic tests and methods
  A. Client history
  B. Physical examination

C. Indirect laryngoscopy (use of mirror visualization to examine the larynx)
 1. Determines presence of red, inflamed, and occasionally hemorrhagic vocal cords and exudate (fluid, pus, or serous material)
 2. Checks for swelling
IV. Implementation
 A. Mark intercom to inform other hospital personnel that the client cannot answer.
 B. Explain to client why he or she should not talk.
 C. Provide a "magic slate" or pad and pencil for communication.
 D. Minimize need to talk by anticipating the client's needs.
 E. Provide vaporizer or humidifier.
 F. Administer medications as ordered.
 G. Discourage smoking.
 H. Explain disease process, treatment, and home care
 1. Use of humidifier during winter
 2. Avoidance of air conditioning during summer (because air conditioning dehumidifies room)
 3. Use of medicated throat lozenges
 4. No smoking
V. Evaluation
 A. Client reports increased comfort.
 B. Laryngitis is absent.
 C. Client demonstrates an understanding of disease process, treatment, and home care.

Carcinoma of the Larynx

I. Description
 A. Most common form (95%) is squamous cell carcinoma.
 B. Rare forms include adenocarcinoma, sarcoma, and others.
 C. Intrinsic tumors are found on the true vocal cord and do not tend to spread because nearby tissues lack lymph nodes.
 D. Extrinsic tumors are found on the larynx outside of the true vocal cord and tend to spread early.
 E. Cancer of the larynx is nine times more common in men than in women and usually occurs between the ages of 50 and 65 years.
 F. Causes
 1. Major predisposing factors
 a. Smoking (especially heavy)
 b. Alcoholism
 c. Chronic inhalation of noxious fumes
 d. Familial tendency
 e. Genetic (mutation tumor supressor gene on chromosome 17)
 f. History of frequent laryngitis and vocal straining
 G. Classification by location
 1. Supraglottis (posterior surface of epiglottis, false vocal cords)
 2. Glottis (true vocal cords)
 3. Subglottis (downward from vocal cords [rare])
II. Data collection
 A. Subjective symptoms
 1. Hoarseness lasting >2weeks
 2. Cough

3. Pain or burning in throat after drinking citrus juice or hot liquid
4. Difficulty in breathing
5. Pain radiating to ear
6. Anxiety
 B. Objective symptoms
 1. Hoarseness
 2. Lump in throat
 3. Dysphagia (difficulty in swallowing)
 4. Cough
 5. Enlarged lymph nodes in neck
III. Diagnostic tests and methods
 A. Client history
 B. Visual examination (indirect laryngoscopy)
 C. Direct laryngoscopy and biopsy
 D. Computed tomographic (CT) scan or magnetic resonance imaging (MRI)
 E. Chest radiograph to detect metastases
IV. Implementation
 A. Provide emotional support.
 B. Provide general preoperative and postoperative care for
 1. Laryngectomy (removal of larynx, partial or complete)
 2. Radical neck dissection (excision that includes lymph nodes, entire larynx, epiglottis, and possible excision of muscle tissue, thyroid, internal jugular vein, mandible, and submaxillary gland)
 a. Permanent tracheostomy
 3. Radiation therapy
 C. Preoperative care
 1. Before partial or total removal of larynx
 a. Instruct client to maintain good mouth care.
 b. Instruct bearded male client to shave off beard (helps in giving postoperative care).
 c. Encourage client to talk about concerns and problems in communicating after surgery.
 d. Encourage client to choose method of communication
 1) Pencil and paper
 2) Magic slate
 3) Sign language
 4) Alphabet board
 e. Explain postoperative procedures
 1) Suctioning
 2) Nasogastric (NG) feeding or gastrostomy feeding
 3) Care of largyngectomy tube
 4) Breathing through neck
 5) Speech alteration
 D. Immediate postoperative care
 1. Maintain open airway (care of tracheostomy, if present).
 2. Place client in Fowler's position.
 3. Check dressing every hour.
 4. Prevent movement of client's head.
 5. Connect wound drain to suction as ordered.
 6. Maintain intravenous (IV) fluids as ordered.
 7. After partial laryngectomy
 a. Provide tube feedings (starting 2 days postoperatively as ordered).
 b. Encourage oral fluids after tube feedings are discontinued.

c. Keep tracheostomy tube in place until edema subsides
   1) Encourage client not to use voice until physician orders otherwise.
   2) Caution client to whisper until healing is complete.

8. After total laryngectomy
   a. On return from recovery room, position client on side, elevate head 30–45 degrees.
   b. Monitor vital signs.
   c. Record fluid intake (tube feedings and IV fluids) and fluid output (Foley catheter, drains) (I&O).
   d. Provide frequent mouth care.
   e. Support back of neck to prevent tension on sutures and possible wound rupture.
   f. Suction gently as ordered; do not use deep suctioning (may damage suture line)
      1) Suction through both tube and nose (client can no longer blow air through nose).
      2) Suction mouth gently.
   g. Give pain medication as ordered.
   h. If tube feeding is ordered, check tube placement, residuals, and elevate client's head to prevent aspiration
      1) Have suction available after removal of feeding tube (client may have difficulty swallowing).
   i. Watch for crusting and secretions around stoma (tracheostomy opening).
   j. Provide room humidification (helps prevent crust formation).
   k. Remove crusting (use prescribed ointments, moist gauze).
   l. Check for and report complications
      1) Redness, swelling, secretions on suture line
      2) Bleeding (may be a ruptured carotid artery: apply pressure to site; *call for help*)
      3) Tracheostomy stenosis (narrowing of opening causing shortness of breath)
      4) Presence of fistula (abnormal opening around tube)

E. Provide reassurance to client that speech rehabilitation can help him or her speak again.
F. Support client through grieving process.
G. Watch for depression.

V. Evaluation
   A. Client reports decreased anxiety.
   B. There are no avoidable complications from surgery.
   C. Client learns alternative forms of communication.
   D. Client uses effective coping strategies regarding altered body image.
   E. Pain is controlled.
   F. Client maintains adequate nutritional intake.

Pneumonia

I. Description
   A. Acute inflammation of lung tissue, with secretions filling the alveolar sacs (air cells of the lungs), allowing bacterial or viral growth
   B. Inflammation spreading to neighboring sacs, resulting in consolidation accompanied by thick exudate in the lung spaces
   C. Sputum having a characteristic rusty color; breathing becoming difficult
   D. Causes
      1. Inhalation of respiratory secretions (droplets) containing bacteria, viruses; inhalation of irritating chemicals, fungi or parasites
      2. Classifications
         a. Community-acquired pneumonia (CAP)
         b. Hospital-acquired pneumonia (HAP)
      3. Types of bacteria
         a. *Streptococcus pneumoniae*
         b. *Staphylococcus aureus*
         c. *Haemophilus influenzae*
         d. *Mycoplasma pneumoniae*
         e. *Pseudomonas aeruginosa*
      4. Viral infections
      5. Irritating chemicals
         a. Aspiration of chemicals in stomach contents
         b. Inhalation of chemicals (e.g., chlorine)

II. Data collection
   A. Subjective symptoms
      1. Productive cough
      2. Difficulty in breathing
      3. Chills
      4. Pain on inspiration (breathing in)
      5. Weakness
   B. Objective symptoms
      1. Painful, dry cough, changing to a productive cough with green, yellow, or rusty sputum depending on organism
      2. Marked elevation in temperature
      3. Elevated white blood cell (WBC) count
      4. Positive diagnosis by chest radiograph
      5. Positive sputum culture analysis
      6. Presence of crackles
      7. Hypoxemia (decreased amount of oxygen in blood)
      8. Confusion in the elderly

III. Diagnostic tests and methods
   A. Client history
   B. Physical examination with auscultation of chest (listening to chest with a stethoscope)
   C. Chest radiograph and examination
   D. Complete blood count (CBC) and white blood count (WBC)
   E. Sputum culture and sensitivity test
   F. Sputum Gram stain
   G. Arterial blood gases (ABGs) and pulse oximetry

IV. Implementation
   A. Keep personal items and call signal within client's easy reach.
   B. Provide mouth care.
   C. Help client conserve energy; schedule rest periods.
   D. Encourage eating small meals and increasing fluid intake.
   E. Place client in semi-Fowler's to high-Fowler's positions.
   F. Give oxygen with humidity as prescribed.
   G. Check vital signs every 4 hours using tympanic thermometer.
   H. Check breathing effort.

I. Check sputum color and thickness.
J. Collect sputum specimens.
K. Encourage good handwashing technique.
L. Isolate as indicated; provide for proper disposal of oral and nasal secretions.
M. Suction as necessary.
N. Have client turn, cough, and breathe deeply every 2 hours, or as prescribed.
O. Maintain IV fluids and medication schedule as ordered.
P. Administer prescribed antibiotics, antipyretics, analgesics, expectorants, and bronchodilators as ordered.
Q. Document all observations and treatments.
R. Explain disease process, treatment, and home care.
V. Evaluation
A. Client reports increased comfort and decreased anxiety.
B. There are no complications from infection.
C. Client maintains adequate nutritional and fluid intake.
D. Client understands how to take medications as ordered.
E. Client demonstrates an understanding of disease process, treatment, and home care.

Empyema, Suppurative Pleurisy, Pleural Effusion

I. Description of empyema
A. A collection of pus and necrotic (dead) tissue within the pleural space, which normally contains a small amount of extracellular fluid (ECF) that lubricates the surfaces of the pleura.
B. Causes
1. Pneumonia
2. Lung abscess
3. Chest trauma or surgery
4. Liver disease with ascites
5. Peritoneal dialysis
6. Fungal infections
II. Description of suppurative pleurisy
A. Purulent inflammation of the pleura, causing pain and a pleural friction rub.
B. Causes
1. Pneumonia
2. Lung abscess
3. Infection
4. Pulmonary infarction
5. Chest trauma or surgery
6. Pulmonary tuberculosis
7. Neoplasm
III. Description of pleural effusion
A. Accumulation of fluid within the pleural space
B. Causes
1. Pulmonary tuberculosis
2. Lung cancer
3. Other infections of lung: pneumonia, lung abscess
4. Congestive heart failure
5. Liver disease with ascites
6. Chronic renal disease
7. Chest trauma
IV. Data collection
A. Subjective symptoms

1. Chest pain
a. Empyema
1) Unilateral (one sided)
b. Suppurative pleurisy
1) Sharp pain on inspiration: referred to shoulder, abdomen, or affected side
2. Malaise
3. Difficulty in breathing
4. Cough
B. Objective symptoms
1. Elevated temperature
2. Cough
3. Decreased breath sounds
4. Chest expansion not symmetrical (one side does not expand to same degree as other side of chest)
5. Increase in WBC count
6. Presence of pleural friction rub (coarse, creaky sound heard during inspiration and early expiration directly over area of inflammation present in pleurisy)
7. Findings from chest radiograph
V. Diagnostic tests and methods
A. Client history
B. Chest radiograph
C. Physical examination (including listening to lung sounds)
D. Laboratory study of pleural fluid specimen obtained via thoracentesis
VI. Implementation
A. Monitor respirations, breath sounds, and vital signs.
B. Administer antibiotic, anti-inflammatory, and analgesic medications as ordered.
C. Place client in semi-Fowler's or high-Fowler's position to assist in breathing.
D. Provide adequate rest.
E. Demonstrate how to splint chest for coughing.
F. Encourage coughing and deep-breathing exercises.
G. Encourage good handwashing technique.
H. Encourage fluid intake.
I. Prepare client and assist with thoracentesis or chest tube insertion, or both, as ordered for pleural effusion and empyema.
J. Explain disease process, treatment, and home care to client and family.
VII. Evaluation
A. Client reports increased comfort.
B. Client maintains effective breathing pattern.
C. Chest tube systems work correctly.
D. There are no complications from infection.
E. Client and family demonstrate an understanding of the disease process, treatment, and home care.

Asthma

I. Description
A. Sudden narrowing of the trachea (windpipe) and bronchi, obstructing airflow.
B. Airway inflammation and hyperresponsiveness
C. Spasms of the muscle of the bronchi, edema, and swelling of mucous membrane producing thick secretions
D. Air that enters is trapped

E. Characteristic wheeze when client tries to exhale (breathe out) through narrowed bronchi

F. Difficulty in breathing

G. Inability to expectorate in sufficient amounts through coughing

H. Attacks lasting 30–60 minutes with normal breathing between attacks

I. Possibility of status asthmaticus, which is difficult to control

J. Causes
1. Inhalation of irritating chemicals such as those found in cigarette smoke, polluted air
2. Recurrent respiratory infections, sinusitis
3. Allergic reaction
4. Physical or emotional stress
5. Exercise and cold, dry air
6. Seasonal occurrence
7. Gastroesophageal reflux disease (GERD)

II. Data collection
A. Subjective symptoms
1. Shortness of breath
2. Wheezing
3. Thick, tenacious sputum (after an acute attack)
4. Chest tightness
5. Anxiety (feeling of suffocation)
B. Objective symptoms
1. Dyspnea
2. Wheezing on expiration or inspiration, prolonged expiration
3. Thick, tenacious sputum
4. Flaring nostrils
5. Use of accessory muscles of respiration
6. Tachypnea
7. Tachycardia
8. Diaphoresis (perspiration)
9. Flushing
10. Cough

III. Diagnostic tests and methods
A. Client history
B. Physical examination
C. Chest radiograph
D. Sputum analysis if indicated
E. ABGs
F. Electrocardiogram (ECG) if arrhythmias
G. Skin tests for allergies
H. Pulmonary function tests (PFT)
I. Serum IgE and eosinophil count

IV. Implementation
A. Decrease anxiety; provide time to listen, and do not leave client alone during attack.
B. Keep environment free from dust and allergens.
C. Place client in semi- to high-Fowler's position with arms supported by overbed table.
D. Prevent infection; discourage visits by persons with upper respiratory infections.
E. Discourage smoking.
F. Monitor vital signs; assess respirations and skin color frequently. Monitor oxygen saturation.
G. Administer prescribed medications as ordered, especially bronchodilators
H. Give oxygen as ordered.
I. Note sputum characteristics.

J. Encourage adequate fluid intake.
K. Monitor fluid I&O.
L. Encourage adequate nutritional intake (small, frequent, high-protein, high-calorie meals).
M. Explain disease process, treatment, prevention, and home care
1. Importance of taking medications on time
2. Breathing exercises
3. Diet and fluids
4. Client and family assist in planning care
5. Importance of signs and symptoms indicating immediate follow-up

V. Evaluation
A. Client reports increased comfort and decreased anxiety.
B. There are no complications from exacerbation.
C. Client maintains effective breathing pattern, PFT, and peak expiratory flow rate (PEFR).
D. Client maintains open airway and adequate gas exchange.
E. Client verbalizes feelings regarding disease.
F. Client discusses intention to stop smoking.
G. Client discusses intention to check home and work environment for triggers.
H. Client maintains fluid balance.
I. Client maintains undisturbed sleep pattern.
J. Client maintains adequate nutritional intake.

Chronic Obstructive Pulmonary Disease

I. Description
A. Chronic obstructive pulmonary disease (COPD) includes a group of lung conditions that are frequently progressive and obstruct pulmonary airflow.
B. COPD affects expiratory (breathing out) airflow.
C. COPD comprises two major conditions: emphysema and chronic bronchitis.

EMPHYSEMA

I. Description
A. Emphysema is a chronic, progressive condition in which the air sacs (alveolar sacs) distend, rupture, and destroy the capillaries.
B. The alveoli lose elasticity, resulting in trapping of inspired air.
C. Inspiration (breathing in of air) becomes difficult; expiration (breathing out) is prolonged.
D. Lung tissue becomes fibrotic (formation of scar tissue).
E. Exchange of oxygen and carbon dioxide decreases (destruction of alveolar walls decreases surface area for gas exchange).
F. Causes
1. Cigarette smoking
2. Family tendency, alpha-antitrypsin (AAT) deficiency
3. Recurrent inflammation or infection: pneumonia, air pollution
4. Aging
5. Family tendency

II. Data collection
A. Subjective symptoms

1. Chronic cough
2. Difficulty in breathing
3. Anorexia (loss of appetite)
4. Weight loss
5. Malaise
 B. Objective symptoms
    1. Minimal cough
    2. Barrel chest
    3. Use of accessory muscles of respiration
    4. Prolonged expiratory period: grunting, pursed-lips breathing, abnormal rapidity of breathing
    5. Peripheral cyanosis of extremities
    6. Clubbing of fingers
    7. Dyspnea on exertion
    8. Orthopnea
    9. Difficulty in talking: short, jerky sentences
    10. Drowsiness, confusion, possible unconsciousness caused by lack of oxygen to brain
    11. Hypoxia
    12. Thin and underweight from hypermetabolic state
III. Diagnostic tests and methods
 A. Client history
 B. Physical examination
 C. Chest radiograph
 D. Pulmonary function tests
 E. ABGs
 F. Sputum analysis if indicated
 G. ECG if cardiac symptoms
IV. Implementation
 A. Encourage coughing and deep-breathing exercises to increase respiratory function such as pursed-lip breathing and huff coughing.
 B. Prevent and control infections.
 C. Discourage smoking.
 D. Avoid air pollution.
 E. Administer antibiotics on time as ordered.
 F. Discourage visits from persons with upper respiratory infections.
 G. Give OXYGEN in low concentrations (1–2 L)
    1. Higher levels of OXYGEN are dangerous when CARBON DIOXIDE level is high.
    2. Respiratory center of brain becomes used to low blood OXYGEN level.
    3. Increases in OXYGEN level causes respiratory rate to decrease (may lead to unconsciousness and death).
 H. Encourage adequate fluid intake.
 I. Provide humidity.
 J. Use nebulizers and bronchodilator drug therapy.
 K. Administer expectorants as ordered.
 L. Provide adequate rest.
 M. Organize care
    1. Limit exertion.
    2. Assist with turning and getting in and out of bed.
    3. Explain disease process, diagnostic procedures, treatment, and home care.
 V. Evaluation
 A. Client reports increased comfort and decreased anxiety.
 B. Client remains free of injury or infection.
 C. Client maintains effective airway clearance and gas exchange.

 D. Client maintains adequate tissue perfusion.
 E. Client maintains adequate nutritional intake.
 F. Client maintains undisturbed sleep pattern.
 G. Client verbalizes feelings regarding disorder and intentions to stop smoking.
 H. Client uses effective coping strategies.
 I. Client demonstrates an understanding of disease process, diagnostic procedures, treatment, and home care.

CHRONIC BRONCHITIS

I. Description
 A. Chronic, progressive condition accompanied by excessive secretions from overactive mucus glands in lung
 B. Edema and infection within bronchi obstructing airflow and gas exchange
 C. Chronic inflammatory changes, disappearance of cilia, and narrow airways, emphysema
 D. Causes
    1. Inhalation of irritating chemicals such as those in cigarette smoke
    2. Recurrent respiratory infections
    3. Air pollution
II. Data collection
 A. Subjective symptoms
    1. Cough
    2. Thick, gray, white, yellow, or blood-tinged sputum
    3. Dyspnea on exertion
    4. Weight gain or normal weight
    5. Swelling of legs if cor pulmonale present
    6. Tachypnea (abnormally rapid breathing)
    7. Wheezing
    8. Anxiety
    9. Bluish red color of skin
 B. Objective symptoms
    1. Productive cough with tenacious gray, white, or blood-tinged sputum
    2. Tachypnea
    3. Use of accessory respiratory muscles
    4. Dyspnea on exertion
    5. Wheezing
    6. Neck vein distention and edema of cor pulmonale present
    7. Hypoxia and hypercapnia (increased carbon dioxide)
III. Diagnostic tests and methods
 A. Client history
    1. Cough for 3 months of the year for 2 consecutive years
 B. Physical examination
 C. Chest radiograph
 D. Pulmonary function tests
 E. ABGs
IV. Implementation
 A. Provide safe, effective care environment.
 B. Loosen, liquefy, and remove secretions.
 C. Perform postural drainage, clapping, chest physiotherapy as ordered.
 D. Force fluids as ordered.
 E. Provide adequate rest.
 F. Provide high-protein diet.

G. Discourage visits from persons with upper respiratory infections.
H. Administer bronchodilators, antibiotics, corticosteroids as ordered.
I. Administer diuretics for edema as ordered.
J. Give oxygen as ordered for relief of hypoxia (1-2 L/min)
K. Discourage smoking.
L. Include client and family in planning care.
M. Explain disease process, treatment, prevention, and home care to client and family.

V. Evaluation
A. Client reports increased comfort and decreased anxiety.
B. Client maintains open airway for increased gas exchange.
C. Client has no complications from infection.
D. Client's sleeping pattern improves.
E. Client maintains adequate nutritional and fluid intake.
F. Client verbalizes intention to stop smoking.
G. Client and family demonstrate an understanding of disease process, treatment, prevention, and home care.

Pneumothorax and Hemothorax

I. Description
A. Pneumothorax is an accumulation of air in the pleural space causing collapse of the lung.
   1. The amount of air trapped in the pleural space determines the degree of lung collapse.
   2. The collapse may be partial or complete.
   3. In tension pneumothorax, air in the pleural space causes higher pressure, which causes a mediastinal shift leading to compression of the opposite lung and vascular structures.
   4. In an open pneumothorax, air flows between pleural space and outside of body; also called a sucking chest wound.
   5. In a closed pneumothorax, there is no external wound.
   6. Prompt treatment is required for tension or large pneumothorax:
      a. Without prompt treatment, fatal pulmonary and circulatory impairment will result.
B. Hemothorax is an accumulation of blood in pleural space.
   1. Blood from intercostal, pleural, mediastinal, and sometimes blood vessels in the lung enters the pleural cavity.
   2. Amount of lung collapse and mediastinal shift depends on amount of bleeding and underlying cause.
   3. Pneumothorax often accompanies hemothorax and is called a hemopneumothorax.
C. Causes
   1. Spontaneous (air in pleural space from rupture of blebs next to pleural surface, rupture of emphysematous bulla [large vesicle], exercise, coughing, tubercular lesions, or cancerous lesions that erode into pleural space)
   2. Trauma (stab wound, fractured ribs, subclavian catheter insertion, gunshot wound, mechanical ventilation)
   3. Postoperative procedure where chest cavity is entered (thoracotomy)
   4. Diagnostic and treatment procedures
      a. Thoracentesis
      b. Insertion of central venous line line
      c. Thoracoscopy

II. Data collection
A. Subjective symptoms
   1. Spontaneous: sudden sharp pleuritic pain increased by breathing and coughing
   2. Anxiety
   3. Dizziness
B. Objective symptoms
   1. Shortness of breath.
   2. Dizziness.
   3. Decreased oxygen saturation.
   4. Cyanosis.
   5. Neck vein distention, tracheal deviation, distant heart sounds (tension pneumothorax).
   6. Asymmetrical (uneven) chest movements.
   7. Crackling under skin (subcutaneous emphysema).
   8. Hypotension.
   9. Tachycardia, tachypnea.
   10. Decreased vocal fremitus.
   11. Decreased or absent breath sounds over collapsed lung.
   12. ABG findings: pH <7.35, PO_2 <80 mm Hg, PCO_2 >45 mm Hg.
   13. Respiratory distress.
   14. Chest pain and cough with or without hemoptysis (blood in sputum).
   15. Spontaneous pneumothorax with only a small amount of air in pleural space may cause no symptoms or few symptoms.

III. Diagnostic tests and methods
A. Client history
B. Physical examination
C. Chest radiograph

IV. Implementation
A. For spontaneous pneumothorax with no signs of increased pleural pressure, lung collapse of <30%, and no signs of dyspnea or other indications of compromise or complications
   1. Maintain bed rest.
   2. Monitor vital signs hourly for indications of shock and/or change in respiratory status.
   3. Give oxygen as prescribed.
B. For lung collapse >30%
   1. Prepare client for placement of chest tube.
   2. Prepare client for possible surgical repair.
C. Watch for pallor, gasping respirations, and sudden chest pain.
D. Check for increased respiratory distress or mediastinal shift.
E. Listen for breath sounds over both lungs.
F. Encourage client to control coughing and gasping during thoracentesis.
G. Encourage coughing and deep-breathing exercises

once chest tubes are in place to facilitate lung expansion.

H. For clients undergoing chest tube drainage:
1. Watch for air leak (increased bubbling), which indicates that lung has not reexpanded.
2. Check tube insertion site for crackling beneath the skin, which is a sign of subcutaneous emphysema.
I. Check, record, and report amount and color of drainage.
J. Assist in changing dressings around chest tube insertion site if ordered.
1. Do not reposition chest tube.
2. If chest tube becomes disconnected, attach new (sterile) water seal system.
3. If chest tube falls out, treat as an open pneumothorax and cover with a vented dressing (4 × 4 taped with only three sides) to prevent a tension pneumothorax.
4. Provide reassurance to client and family.
5. Explain disease process, treatment, and home care.
K. Keep tubing straight, DO NOT elevate drainage system to chest level.

V. Evaluation
A. Client reports increased comfort and decreased anxiety.
B. Vital signs stabilize.
C. Lungs reexpand.
D. Pain is absent.
E. Respiratory problems are absent.
F. Client maintains effective breathing pattern.
G. Client maintains effective gas exchange (ABGs are normal).
H. Client demonstrates an understanding of disease process, treatment, and home care.

Pulmonary Tuberculosis

I. Description
A. Pulmonary tuberculosis (TB) is an acute or chronic infection caused by *Mycobacterium tuberculosis*, which leads to an immune response and formation of a granuloma also called a tubercle.
B. An infected person harbors the bacillus for life. It is dormant but viable. It becomes reactivated when the immune system is weakened or the patient becomes immunosuppressed.
C. The granulomas become fibrosed and the area becomes calcified and can be identified by radiography.
D. The incidence of tuberculosis is currently increasing, and multi-drug–resistant strains are harder to treat. Individuals with acquired immunodeficiency syndrome (AIDS), those infected with human immunodeficiency virus (HIV), the homeless, and others living in crowded, poorly ventilated conditions have a higher than average incidence of this disease.
E. Transmission of the organism is by airborne droplets.
F. Cause
1. Inhalation of airborne droplets containing the tubercle bacillus from an infected person
G. Factors contributing to activation of infection
1. Uncontrolled diabetes mellitus

2. Hodgkin's disease
3. Leukemia
4. Treatment with corticosteroids
5. Treatment with immunosuppressive drugs

II. Data collection
A. Subjective symptoms
1. Early phase may be asymptomatic
2. Fatigue
3. Weakness
4. Weight loss
5. Anorexia
6. Night sweats
7. Low-grade fever
8. Cough with micropurulent sputum
9. Occasional hemoptysis (coughing up of blood from the lungs) with advanced cases
10. HIV patient with TB may have atypical symptoms attributed to *Pneumocystis carinii* pneumonia (PCP) or other opportunistic diseases
11. Chest pain
12. Anxiety; fear of public rejection
B. Objective symptoms
1. Productive cough with micropurulent sputum
2. Elevated temperature
3. Positive chest radiograph
4. Sputum positive for acid-fast bacilli (AFB)
C. Presence of hemoptysis
D. Positive tuberculin skin test

III. Diagnostic tests and methods
A. History of tuberculin exposure
B. Physical examination
C. Chest radiograph
D. Tuberculin skin test
E. Sputum smears and cultures for AFB
F. Auscultation of chest
G. Chest percussion
H. Nucleic acid amplification (NAA)
I. Antigen skin testing with *Candida* and mumps for immunosuppressed patients

IV. Implementation
A. If in-hospital care required, use respiratory isolation in well-ventilated room until sputum cultures are negative.
B. Assist with comfort measures.
C. Assess respirations, breath sounds, and vital signs.
D. Instruct client to cough, sneeze, or laugh into tissue.
E. Instruct client to dispose of tissues in receptacle provided for this purpose.
F. Instruct client to wear mask when outside room.
G. Instruct visitors to wear masks and staff to wear high-efficiency particulate air (HEPA) masks.
H. Provide adequate rest.
I. Encourage client to eat well-balanced meals.
J. Encourage client to eat small, frequent meals.
K. Record weight weekly.
L. Observe, report, and record hemoptysis.
M. Administer antituberculosis drugs as ordered for 6–9 months.
N. Explain need for taking medications (combination of at least four drugs) as ordered to prevent resistant strains.

O. Watch for drug side effects and monitor compliance with drug regimen.

P. Explain disease process, treatment, prevention, and home care to client and family:
   1. Report side effects of medications immediately.
   2. Emphasize importance of regular follow-up examinations.
   3. Report signs and symptoms of recurrent tuberculosis.
   4. Emphasize need for long-term treatment (6–9 months).
   5. Advise persons exposed to infected clients to receive tuberculin skin tests, and, if ordered, chest radiographs and prophylactic antituberculosis medications.

V. Evaluation
   A. Client reports increase in comfort.
   B. Hemoptysis is absent.
   C. Client maintains adequate nutritional intake.
   D. Cough and sputum are absent.
   E. Client maintains effective airway clearance.
   F. Client and family demonstrate an understanding of disease process; mode of transmission; treatment, including medications and need for long-term treatment; and home care.

Adult Respiratory Distress Syndrome

I. Description
   A. Adult respiratory distress syndrome (ARDS) is respiratory failure that occurs as a result of massive trauma to the lungs.
   B. ARDS results from increased permeability of alveolar capillary membrane.
   C. Fluid accumulates in the tissues of the lung, alveolar spaces, and small airways.
   D. Decreased lung compliance occurs, which prohibits adequate oxygenation of pulmonary capillary blood.
   E. Condition characterized by hypoxia (low oxygen levels), dyspnea, pulmonary edema, destruction of alveoli, inflammation, and pulmonary infiltrates, resulting in decreased oxygen and carbon dioxide exchange.
   F. Severe ARDS can cause irreversible and fatal hypoxia; however, clients who recover usually have little or no permanent damage.
   G. Three phases of ARDS
      1. Exudative — increased capillary permeability, decreased surfactant, and compliance.
      2. Proliferative — fibrosis develops.
      3. Fibrotic — scarring and fibrosis continues and results in pulmonary hypertension.
   H. Contributing factors
      1. Aspiration of gastric contents
      2. Infection
      3. Sepsis
      4. Shock
      5. Drug overdose
      6. Blood transfusion reaction
      7. Smoke or chemical inhalation
      8. Pancreatitis, uremia
      9. Near-drowning
      10. Disseminated intravascular coagulation (DIC)
      11. Oxygen toxicity
      12. Trauma: lung contusion, head injury, long bone fracture with fat emboli

II. Data collection
   A. Subjective symptoms
      1. Rapid breathing
      2. Dyspnea
      3. Confusion, anxiety
      4. Restlessness, apprehension
      5. Mental sluggishness
      6. Increased heart rate
      7. Decreased urinary output
   B. Objective symptoms
      1. Dyspnea
      2. Cough
      3. Tachypnea
      4. Cyanosis
      5. Elevated temperature
      6. Rapid, shallow breathing
      7. Intercostal and suprasternal retractions
      8. Presence of crackles and rhonchi
      9. Restlessness, confusion, and apprehension caused by hypoxia
      10. Motor dysfunction caused by hypoxia
      11. Decreased urinary output
      12. Hypoxia and hypercapnia with vital organ hypoxia despite oxygen therapy
      13. Evidence of more severe ARDS

III. Diagnostic tests and methods
   A. No specific tests for ARDS
   B. ABGs
   C. Pulmonary artery catheterization
   D. Chest radiographs
   E. Laboratory tests
      1. Sputum culture and sensitivity
      2. Blood cultures to detect infections
      3. Toxicology screen for drug ingestion
      4. Serum amylase determination if pancreatitis suspected

IV. Implementation
   A. Maintain bed rest in high-Fowler's position. Some patients improve with prone (face down) position or lateral rotation therapy (bed frame slowly turns side-to-side).
   B. Administer humidified oxygen via a tight-fitting mask (allows for use of continuous positive airway pressure [CPAP]) as ordered. Maintain PaO_2 60 mm Hg or higher.
   C. Assist with intubation and mechanical ventilation support if needed:
      1. Administer sedatives, narcotics, and neuromuscular blocking agents as ordered to minimize restlessness and oxygen consumption and to facilitate mechanical ventilation.
   D. Monitor ventilator, ABGs, and vital signs hourly.
   E. Administer prescribed IV fluids, bronchodilators, and vasodilators to facilitate ventilation.
   F. Maintain open airway; suction as necessary.
   G. Check extremities for color, temperature, and capillary refill hourly.
   H. Restrict fluids as ordered.
   I. Administer diuretics to reduce edema as ordered.

J. Monitor I&O hourly.

K. Administer a short course of high-dose steroids as ordered in clients in whom fat emboli or chemical injuries are the cause of ARDS.

L. Assist with administration of IV fluids, vasopressors, and/or inotropic drugs as ordered to maintain BP and cardiac output if hypotension occurs.

M. Administer antimicrobial drugs as ordered for infections.

N. Monitor respiratory status at least every hour:
1. Watch for retractions on inspiration.
2. Note rate, rhythm, and depth of respirations.
3. Watch for use of accessory muscles of respiration.
4. Using stethoscope, listen for abnormal breath sounds.
5. Check characteristics of sputum (clear, frothy sputum is indicative of pulmonary edema).

O. Monitor for signs of confusion caused by hypoxia.

P. Prepare client and assist with insertion of Swan-Ganz catheter.

Q. Monitor placement and dressing of Swan-Ganz catheter.

R. Provide emotional support to client and family.

S. Communicate frequently with client using appropriate communication aids if intubated.

T. Explain condition, treatment, prevention, and home care to client and family.

V. Evaluation
A. Client reports decreased anxiety.
B. Client maintains effective gas exchange (oxygen and carbon dioxide).
C. Client maintains effective breathing pattern.
D. Client maintains adequate nutritional intake.
E. Edema is absent.
F. Client maintains PaO_2 60 mm Hg or greater during acute phase.
G. Client maintains normal ABGs as condition improves.
H. Client verbalizes feelings regarding condition.
I. Client communicates needs.
J. Client and family demonstrate an understanding of condition, treatment, prevention, and home care.

Respiratory Failure

I. Description
A. In clients with normal lung tissue, acute respiratory failure usually means PCO_2 >45 mm Hg and PO_2 <60 mm Hg as a result of inadequate ventilation.
B. Predisposing factors
1. COPD
2. Pulmonary edema
3. Chest trauma
4. Infections: pneumonia, bronchitis
5. Asthma
6. Cystic fibrosis
7. ARDS
8. Cancer
9. Pulmonary embolism
10. Congestive heart failure
11. Anatomic shunt (ventricular septal defect)
12. Spinal cord injury and neuromuscular diseases
13. Head injury
14. Shock
15. Morbid obesity
16. Drug overdose leading to CNS depression

II. Data collection
A. Subjective symptoms
1. Severe morning headache
2. Confusion
3. History of contributing factors
4. Difficulty in breathing
5. Increased heart rate
6. Restlessness
B. Objective symptoms
1. ABGs: PaO_2 <60 mm Hg, $PaCO_2$ >45 mm Hg, and pH <7.35
2. Dyspnea
3. Cyanosis, decreased oxygen saturation
4. Hypertension and tachycardia or hypotension and bradycardia
5. Tachypnea
6. Arrhythmias and decreased cardiac output
7. Restlessness, combative behavior
8. Confusion
9. Sodium retention and edema
10. Decreased level of consciousness
11. Alterations in respirations and breath sounds (accessory muscle use and inspiration:expiration ratio of 1:3 or 1:4)

III. Diagnostic tests and methods
A. ABGs
B. Chest radiographs
C. ECG
D. PFT
E. Complete blood count (CBC)
F. Serum electrolytes
G. Urinalysis

IV. Implementation
A. Maintain bed rest with high-Fowler's position.
B. Monitor vital signs and breath sounds.
C. Monitor ABGs.
D. Give oxygen as prescribed.
E. Monitor for signs of hypoxia.
F. Suction only when secretions are present (preoxygenize before suctioning).
G. Administer prescribed bronchodilators and corticosteroids.
H. Prepare client and assist with intubation and mechanical ventilation if necessary:
1. Administer sedatives, narcotics, and neuromuscular blocking agents as ordered to minimize restlessness and oxygen consumption and to facilitate ventilation.
2. Give sedatives to promote relaxation while client is being mechanically ventilated.
3. Have resuscitation bag with mask available (clients are temporarily pharmacologically paralyzed).
4. Make sure ventilator alarms are *on*.
5. Make sure endotracheal tube is secured with a commercial tube holder.
6. Assess client for retained secretions (while temporarily paralyzed, cough reflex is lost).
7. Keep eyes lubricated to avoid corneal abrasions (temporary loss of corneal reflex).

I. Continuously monitor ECG monitor, vital signs, and pulmonary artery catheter for changes in cardiovascular status.

J. Monitor CNS (level of consciousness, movement, and sensation).

K. Monitor renal status (urine output, blood urea nitrogen [BUN], and serum creatinine levels).

L. Check nutritional status; assist with administration of supplementation or total parenteral nutrition (TPN) as ordered:

1. Provide amount of protein and calories based on client's metabolic state.

2. Poor gastrointestinal (GI) perfusion and motility interfere with absorption of nutrients.

3. Avoid gastric distention because it may lead to respiratory insufficiency as a result of upward pressure against diaphragm.

4. Check fluid balance and electrolytes (sodium, potassium, carbon dioxide, chloride, calcium, phosphate, and magnesium blood levels).

M. Give emotional support to client and family.

N. Explain disease process, contributing factors, treatment, and home care to client and family.

V. Evaluation

A. Client reports increased comfort and decreased anxiety.

B. Client maintains effective airway clearance.

C. Client maintains adequate exchange of oxygen and carbon dioxide.

D. Client maintains effective breathing patterns.

E. Client maintains improved ABGs and pH.

F. Client maintains adequate nutritional intake.

G. Client maintains adequate cardiac output.

H. Client maintains adequate CNS function.

I. Client maintains adequate renal function.

J. Client and family demonstrate an understanding of disease process, contributing factors, treatment, and home care.

Carcinoma of the Lung

I. Description

A. A primary or secondary (metastatic from a primary site) malignant tumor in the lung or bronchi.

B. Bronchogenic carcinoma, usually developing within wall or epithelium of the bronchial tree, is most common primary tumor

1. Usually without symptoms until late stages when metastasis has spread to brain, liver, bones, lymph nodes, and adrenal glands.

2. Treatment in late stages usually symptomatic.

3. Prognosis poor unless detected and treated early.

C. Types

1. Non–small-cell lung cancer
   a. Squamous-cell (epidermoid) carcinoma
   b. Adenocarcinoma
   c. Large-cell carcinoma

2. Small cell lung cancer
   a. Small-cell (oat-cell) carcinoma

D. Risk factors

1. Cigarette smoking

2. Exposure to asbestos

3. Exposure to other carcinogens: uranium, arsenic, nickel, iron oxides, chromium, radon, and coal dust

4. Heredity

5. Primary prevention beginning with cessation or avoidance of cigarette smoking and avoidance of particular industrial and air pollutants

6. Pulmonary diseases such as TB, fibrosis, COPD

II. Data collection

A. Subjective symptoms

1. Asymptomatic in early stages

2. Depend on location of lesion

B. Objective symptoms

1. Pneumonitis secondary to obstructed bronchi

2. Cough

3. Wheezing

4. Dyspnea

5. Hemoptysis late in disease

6. Chest pain

7. Fever

8. Weakness

9. Weight loss

10. Anorexia

C. Later symptoms of metastasis

1. Pleural friction rub

2. Pleural effusion

3. Clubbing of fingers

4. Hoarseness

5. Paralysis of diaphragm

6. Dysphagia

7. Superior vena cava obstruction

8. Cardiac tamponade

III. Diagnostic tests and methods

A. Chest radiograph

B. Examination of sputum for cells

C. Bronchoscopy and biopsy

D. Positron emission tomography (PET) scan

E. MRI

F. Thoracentesis

G. CT Scan

H. Pulmonary angiography and fine-needle aspiration (FNA)

I. Tests to detect metastasis

1. Bone scan

2. Bone marrow biopsy

3. CT scan of brain

4. Liver function tests

5. Mediastinoscopy

6. Staging (using tumor, node, metastases [TNM] system to determine extent of disease and aids in planning treatment)

IV. Implementation

A. Prevent avoidable complications.

B. Encourage adequate nutritional intake.

C. Reduce anxiety.

D. Assist client and family in coping with fear.

E. Monitor vital signs, breath sounds, and skin color.

F. Monitor cough and sputum.

G. Monitor for development of paraneoplastic syndrome.

H. Explain postoperative procedures:

1. Foley catheter insertion

2. Endotracheal tube

3. IV therapy
4. Dressing changes
5. Coughing, deep breathing, turning
6. Range-of-motion (ROM) exercises
7. Chest tube

I. After chest surgery (thoracotomy)
  1. Maintain open airway for adequate gas exchange.
  2. Monitor chest tubes and drainage system.
  3. Prevent postoperative and pulmonary complications.
  4. Check vital signs every 15 minutes for first hour, every 30 minutes for next 4 hours, then every 4 hours.
  5. Observe and report abnormal respirations and other changes immediately.
  6. Suction as necessary; encourage deep breathing and coughing.
  7. Check secretions (initial sputum will be thick and contain dark blood, changing to thin and clearer).
  8. Monitor and record closed chest drainage: watch for air leaks, report immediately.
  9. Position client in semi-Fowler's position.
  10. Monitor I&O; maintain adequate hydration.
  11. Check for potential infection, shock, hemorrhage, dyspnea, mediastinal shift, atelectasis, and/or pulmonary embolus.
  12. Use antiembolism stockings and encourage ROM exercises to prevent pulmonary embolus.
  13. Teach incentive spirometry; use every hour while awake.

J. For clients receiving chemotherapy and radiation:
  1. Encourage client to eat soft, nonirritating foods high in protein.
  2. Explain and watch for possible side effects of chemotherapy and radiation.
  3. Administer antiemetics and antidiarrheals as ordered.
  4. Provide good skin care to decrease skin breakdown.
  5. Use reverse isolation technique if bone marrow suppression occurs (leukopenia or neutrophil)

K. Before discharge:
  1. Assist with instruction of client receiving radiation therapy as outclient to avoid sunburn and tight-fitting clothes.
  2. Teach exercises for prevention of shoulder stiffness.
  3. Discourage smoking.
  4. Explain disease process, diagnostic procedures, treatment, and home care.

V. Evaluation
A. Client reports increased comfort and decreased anxiety.
B. Client maintains effective airway for gas exchange.
C. Client uses effective coping mechanisms.
D. Client verbalizes feelings regarding disease.
E. Client exhibits acceptable ABGs.
F. There are no complications.
G. Client maintains adequate nutritional intake.
H. Client demonstrates an understanding of disease process, diagnostic procedures, treatment, and home care.

Chest Injuries

I. Description
A. Trauma to rib cage, diaphragm, mediastinum, or pleura possibly caused by blunt or penetrating injuries
  1. Blunt chest injuries
    a. Damage to internal structures without chest wall penetration
    b. Commonly caused by motor vehicle crashes
    c. Types
      1) Myocardial contusion: bruising of heart muscle
      2) Pulmonary contusion: bruising of lung tissue or pleura
      3) Rib and sternal fractures: displacement of ribs and sternum resulting from fractures caused by a powerful impact
      4) Flail chest: asymmetrical (uneven) chest movement during respiration owing to multiple rib fractures
        a) Possibility that fractures may cause fatal complications, such as hemorrhagic shock, diaphragmatic rupture, pneumothorax, and hemothorax.
  2. Penetrating chest injuries
    a. Pierce chest wall causing injury and damage to chest cavity contents.
    b. Depending on size of injury, may cause varying degrees of damage to soft tissue, bones, nerves, and blood vessels.
    c. Commonly caused by stab wounds or gunshot wounds.

II. Data collection
A. Blunt chest injuries
  1. Rib fracture location
    a. Pain at site of injury, increasing with deep breathing and movement
    b. Shallow, splinted respirations that may lead to hypoventilation
    c. Evidence of fracture noted on radiograph
  2. Sternal fractures
    a. Paradoxical chest movements
    b. Damage to liver, spleen
  3. Flail chest
    a. Paradoxical chest movements
    b. Damage to liver, spleen
  4. Pulmonary contusion
  5. Myocardial contusion
B. Penetrating chest injuries
  1. Pneumothorax
    a. Dyspnea
    b. Tachycardia
    c. Absent breath sounds on affected side
    d. Sucking sound with open wound
    e. Cyanosis
    f. Hypotension
    g. Mediastinal shift with tension pneumothorax
    h. Varying levels of consciousness
    i. Weak, thready pulse
    j. Tachycardia
    k. Possible hemothorax (blood in pleural space)

III. Diagnostic tests and methods
   A. Client history
   B. Chest radiograph
   C. Auscultation of chest
   D. ECG
   E. Aspartate transaminase (AST), Alanine transaminase (ALT), lactate dehydrogenase (LDH), and creatine phosphokinase (CPK)
   F. Contrast studies and liver and spleen scans to detect injuries
   G. ABGs
   H. CBC
   I. Palpation and auscultation of abdomen to evaluate damage to nearby organs and structures
IV. Implementation
   A. Assess airway, breathing, and circulation (ABCs).
   B. Place an sterile dressing taped on three sides over sucking wound.
   C. Check level of consciousness.
   D. Evaluate color and temperature of skin.
   E. Look for distended jugular veins.
   F. Have blood typed and cross-matched.
   G. Check breath sounds and vital signs.
   H. Assist in establishing an open airway and support ventilation as needed.
   I. Monitor for signs of tension pneumothorax.
   J. Stabilize injury:
      1. Assist with insertion of chest tubes for pneumothorax.
      2. Support flail chest or fractured ribs with taping.
   K. Monitor pulses frequently.
   L. Control blood loss (remember to look under client to estimate amount of loss).
   M. Monitor for shock.
   N. Give oxygen as ordered.
   O. Place client in Fowler's position unless shock position is required.
   P. Monitor telemetry for suspected cardiac damage.
   Q. Administer analgesics, antibiotics, and supportive medications as ordered.
   R. Provide emotional support.
   S. Prepare client for surgical intervention if required.
   T. Follow specific postoperative procedures.
   U. Explain condition, treatment, and home care.
V. Evaluation
   A. Client maintains adequate oxygenation and chest expansion.
   B. Client reports pain relief.
   C. Client maintains stable vital signs.
   D. Client resumes prior lung capacity.
   E. Client maintains adequate nutritional intake.
   F. Client demonstrates an understanding of condition, treatment, and home care.

Cardiovascular System

Basic Information

The heart, arteries, veins, and lymphatic system form the cardiovascular system, which serves as the body's transport system. It brings life-supporting oxygen and nutrients to cells, removes metabolic waste products, and transports hormones from one part of the body to another. It is divided into two branches: pulmonary circulation and systemic circulation. Circulation requires normal function of the heart, which pushes blood through the system by continuous rhythmic contractions.

Diseases related to the cardiovascular system constitute the leading cause of death in the United States. Conditions affecting this system occur across the age continuum. Three major strategies to reduce death and disability resulting from disorders of the cardiovascular system include early detection, appropriate treatment to control the progress of the disease, and a reduction of risk factors that predispose individuals to the disease.

I. Basic data collection
   A. Subjective symptoms
      1. Chest pain during periods of physical and emotional stress
      2. Dyspnea on exertion
      3. Dizziness, fainting
      4. Hemoptysis
      5. Fatigue
      6. Family history of heart disease and hypertension
   B. Objective symptoms
      1. Irregular pulse
      2. Abnormal respirations
      3. Skin temperature, color (pallor, cyanosis)
      4. Distended neck veins
      5. Abnormal heart sounds
      6. Clubbing of fingers and toes
      7. Presence of edema
      8. Abnormal peripheral pulses
      9. Bruits or thrills over carotid arteries
      10. Pulsations in jugular vein
      11. Pericardial friction rub

Major Cardiovascular Diagnoses

Angina Pectoris

I. Description
   A. Episodes of acute chest pain as a result of an inadequate oxygen supply to the myocardium owing to a decrease in blood flow from the coronary arteries.
   B. Condition occurs with either gradual or sudden onset; pain usually lasts <15 minutes and not >30 minutes (average 3 minutes).
   C. Chest pain located behind or under sternum, often radiating to back, neck, left arm, jaws, even upper abdomen or fingers.
   D. Mild to moderate pressure, deep sensation; varied pattern of attacks, "tightness," "squeezing," "crushing" sensations.
   E. Predisposing factors
      1. Exercise
      2. Cigarette smoking
      3. Eating a heavy meal
      4. Environmental temperature extremes: cold, hot, or humid weather
      5. Alcohol use
      6. Drugs

F. Causes
   1. Atherosclerotic plaque within coronary arteries major cause
   2. Thrombus formation within vessel
   3. Vasospasm
   4. Hypotension
   5. Low blood volume
   6. Cardiac arrhythmia
   7. Sustained hypertension
   8. Aortic stenosis
   9. Cardiomyopathy
   10. Mitral valve disease

II. Data collection
   A. Subjective symptoms
      1. Substernal chest pain lasting an average of 3–5 minutes
      2. Report of exertion before episode
      3. Radiation of pain to neck, jaw, left arm
      4. Anxiety
      5. Sensation of heaviness, tightness, suffocation
      6. Indigestion
      7. Desire to void
      8. Belching
      9. Pain alleviated by nitroglycerin or rest
      10. Verbalizing feelings of fear, impending doom, or apprehension
   B. Objective symptoms
      1. Presence of nausea or vomiting
      2. Dyspnea
      3. Potential increase in heart rate
      4. Potential increase in BP
      5. Skin condition: warm and dry or cool and clammy

III. Diagnostic tests and methods
   A. Client history
   B. Physical examination
   C. ECG
   D. Electrocardiogram
   E. Coronary angiography
   F. Treadmill exercise test
   G. Serum lipid and enzyme values
   H. Noninvasive cardiac output monitoring

IV. Implementation
   A. Monitor vital signs, especially during attack.
   B. Monitor ECG; record and report any changes.
   C. Provide environment conducive to rest (remove stressors such as noise, bright lights, interruptions).
   D. Give oxygen as ordered.
   E. Decrease activity level.
   F. Monitor weight.
   G. Provide diet (fat- and cholesterol-restricted) as prescribed.
   H. Monitor angina attacks:
      1. Instruct client to notify staff at the onset of an anginal attack.
      2. Record and report onset, duration, location, symptoms, quality, and intensity.
      3. Administer vasodilating medication as prescribed; observe, record, and report results and any side effects.
   I. Provide emotional support to client and family.
   J. Explain disease process, predisposing factors, treatment including medication, prevention by avoidance

of risk factors, home care including diet and lifestyle modifications to client and family.

V. Evaluation
   A. Client reports increased comfort.
   B. Vital signs remain stable.
   C. ECG remains within normal limits.
   D. Client uses effective coping strategies.
   E. Client and family demonstrate an understanding of disease process, treatment, prevention, and home care.

Hypertension (High Blood Pressure)

I. Description
   A. Intermittent or sustained elevation in diastolic or systolic blood pressure: systolic pressure >140 mm Hg and diastolic pressure >90 mm Hg
   B. Arterioles primarily affected, resulting in an increase in peripheral resistance with rise in blood pressure, which may be caused by responses of the sympathetic nervous system and stimulation of the renin angiotensin mechanism
   C. Damage occurring to organ supplied by these blood vessels over time
   D. Two major types: essential (primary or idiopathic) hypertension, the most common, and secondary hypertension, resulting from renal disease or other identifiable cause
      1. Essential hypertension
         a. Cause unknown
      2. Secondary hypertension
         a. Predisposing factors
            1) Smoking
            2) Obesity
            3) Diet
            4) Stress
            5) Family history
            6) Sex: primarily among men >35 years old and women >45 years old
            7) Race: primarily among blacks: twice the incidence of whites
            8) Birth control pills, estrogen use
         b. Associations with other diseases
            1) Renal disease
            2) Pheochromocytoma
            3) Atherosclerosis
            4) Cushing's syndrome
            5) Thyroid, parathyroid, or pituitary dysfunction
            6) Primary aldosteronism
            7) Peripheral vascular disease
            8) Diabetes
   E. Malignant hypertension: a severe form of hypertension common to both types
   F. A major cause of cardiac disease, renal failure, decreased supply of blood to coronary arteries, and cerebrovascular accident (CVA)
   G. Prognosis is good if condition detected early and treatment begins before the development of complications
   H. Hypertensive crisis (profoundly elevated BP) may be fatal

II. Data collection
   A. Subjective symptoms
      1. Asymptomatic or vague symptoms; may have condition and not know it
      2. Chest pain
      3. Fatigue
      4. Blurred vision
      5. Morning headache
      6. Irritability
      7. Dizziness
      8. Ringing in ears
      9. Tachycardia and palpitations
      10. Nausea or vomiting
      11. Shortness of breath
      12. Anxiety
   B. Objective symptoms
      1. BP readings >140/90 mm Hg
      2. Epistaxis
      3. Evidence of other associated diseases
      4. Hematuria
      5. Proteinuria
      6. Restlessness
III. Diagnostic tests and methods
   A. Client history
   B. Physical examination
   C. Series of resting BP readings
   D. Tests and examinations to check for other organ involvement
      1. Chest radiograph
      2. ECG
      3. Routine urinalysis and testing of BUN and serum creatinine levels
      4. Serum potassium levels
      5. IV pyelogram
      6. Serum electrolytes
      7. Blood glucose levels
IV. Implementation
   A. Assess, report, and record signs and symptoms and any reaction to treatments.
   B. Schedule rest periods.
   C. Provide quiet, calm environment.
   D. Give emotional support to decrease anxiety.
   E. Administer prescribed medications (antihypertensives, sedatives, diuretics).
   F. Observe, record, and report side effects of medications.
   G. Monitor weight daily to assess results of diuretic therapy.
   H. Monitor I&O to evaluate results of diuretic therapy.
   I. Monitor vital signs, including BP at same time every day.
   J. Provide diet as ordered.
   K. Discourage smoking.
   L. Explain to client:
      1. Risk factors
      2. Disease process
      3. Monitoring BP
      4. Medications
      5. Weight
      6. Diet restrictions
      7. Exercise
      8. Stress management

V. Evaluation
   A. Client reports decreased anxiety.
   B. BP readings decrease to normal limits.
   C. Client understands risk factors.
   D. Client explains reasons for dietary restriction.
   E. Client explains reasons for complying with treatment and medications.
   F. Number of existing risk factors decreases.
   G. Client states plan for taking BP measurements.
   H. Client explains methods to control stress.

Myocardial Infarction (Heart Attack)

I. Description
   A. Myocardial infarction (MI) is necrosis (death) of an area of the myocardium as a result of obstruction to blood flow through the coronary artery or one of its branches.
   B. The myocardium tissue dies as a result of oxygen deprivation, which causes cell ischemia.
   C. The location and size of the necrosed area affects the heart's ability to regain or maintain its function.
   D. The leading cause of death in cardiovascular disease; death usually results from cardiac damage or complications of MI.
   E. Mortality is high when treatment is delayed.
   F. Approximately one-half of sudden deaths caused by MI occur within 1 hour after onset of symptoms and before hospitalization.
   G. Prognosis improves if vigorous treatment is started immediately, unless location and size of infarct are profound.
   H. Complications
      1. Cardiogenic shock
      2. Arrhythmias
      3. Congestive heart failure
      4. Ventricular aneurysm
      5. Ventricular rupture
      6. Pericarditis
      7. Pulmonary embolism
      8. Postmyocardial infarction
   I. Risk factors
      1. Smoking
      2. Family history
      3. Hypertension
      4. Elevated serum triglycerides and cholesterol levels
      5. Obesity or excessive intake of saturated fats
      6. Sedentary lifestyle
      7. Aging
      8. Stress
      9. Sex: men more susceptible, although incidence in women is increasing
      10. Diabetes mellitus
   J. Causes
      1. Atherosclerosis: approximately 90% of cases
      2. Constriction or spasm of the coronary artery
      3. Coronary artery embolus
      4. Coronary artery thrombus
II. Data collection
   A. Subjective symptoms
      1. Chest pain
         a. Tightness, heaviness, squeezing, or crushing

sensation in substernal area, which may radiate to other areas such as neck, jaw, left arm, or shoulder

    b. Pain not relieved by rest or drugs and possibly lasting 30 minutes or more

    c. In elderly and those with diabetes, pain possibly absent, mild, potentially confused with indigestion

  2. Precipitating factors

    a. Exertion

    b. Stress

    c. Exercise

  3. Predisposing factors

    a. Respiratory tract infection

    b. Pulmonary emboli

    c. Hypoxemia

    d. Blood loss

  4. Anxiety, fear, apprehension, feeling of doom, denial, depression

B. Objective symptoms

  1. Dyspnea

  2. Nausea and vomiting

  3. Profuse diaphoresis and pallor

  4. Presence of rales

  5. Tachycardia, decreased BP

  6. Rise in temperature after 24–48 hours

  7. Elevation of cardiac enzymes

    a. CPK peaks 1–8 hours after onset.

    b. CPK-MB elevated 2–4 hours after onset.

    c. AST peaks 24–36 hours after onset.

    d. LDH peaks 48–72 hours after onset.

    e. LDH_1 and LDH_2 may show a flipped pattern, in which case LDH_1 is greater than LDH_2; present in 48 hours in most infarctions.

III. Diagnostic tests and methods

  A. Client history

  B. Physical examination

  C. ECG Monitoring

  D. Cardiac enzyme studies: AST, LDH, CPK-MB

  E. Serial chest radiographs

  F. Erythrocyte sedimentation rate (ESR) and WBC count

  G. Scans

IV. Implementation

  A. Provide quiet, calm environment; explain tests, procedures, equipment.

  B. Keep client on bed rest for first 24–48 hours; then allow progressive activity as prescribed:

    1. Turn client every 2 hours, with assistance.

    2. Use antiembolism stockings to prevent venostasis and thrombophlebitis.

    3. Client may be allowed out of bed to use commode (less strain placed on cardiovascular system).

    4. Avoid activities that may cause stress on the cardiovascular system:

      a. Administer stool softeners as prescribed.

      b. Instruct client not to strain during bowel movement.

      c. Monitor pulse during periods of activity.

  C. Administer sedatives as prescribed to decrease anxiety and apprehension.

  D. Administer vasopressor drugs as prescribed.

  E. Perform internal monitoring of BP and pulmonary artery pressure (hemodynamic monitoring).

  F. Keep IV line open as ordered to provide means for IV drug administration.

  G. Relieve chest pain with prescribed medications.

  H. Monitor heart rhythm to detect arrhythmias.

  I. Administer and monitor oxygen to relieve respiratory distress.

  J. Administer anticoagulant medications.

  K. Record vital signs every hour during acute episode.

  L. Monitor pulmonary artery catheter readings for cardiac function.

  M. Assist with progressive activity when condition stabilizes.

  N. Continue assessment and documentation of symptoms and reactions to treatments.

  O. Monitor for signs of complications:

    1. Pulmonary edema: left ventricle failure resulting in decrease in blood pumped out by the diseased heart to the body per minute

    2. Congestive heart failure

    3. Cardiogenic shock caused by a decrease in cardiac output

  P. Assist with cardiopulmonary resuscitation in event of cardiac arrest.

  Q. Explain disease process, risk factors, treatment including medication compliance, and home care including lifestyle modifications, activity, diet, and stress management to client and family:

    1. Advise client and family to report to the physician any chest pain immediately.

    2. Educate client on the importance of smoking cessation.

V. Evaluation

  A. Client reports increased comfort.

  B. Client reports decrease or absence of chest pain.

  C. Hemodynamic status remains stable.

  D. Client shows progress with activity, with decreased fatigue.

  E. Client and family demonstrate an understanding of disease process, treatment including medication compliance, and home care including lifestyle modifications, activity, diet, and stress management.

Congestive Heart Failure

I. Description

  A. Congestive heart failure (CHF) is a condition in which the pumping mechanism of the heart is impaired, resulting in an insufficient blood supply to meet the metabolic needs of the body.

  B. A buildup pressure occurs in the vascular beds of the affected side of the heart.

  C. Congestion of systemic venous circulation results in peripheral edema or enlarged liver.

  D. Congestion of pulmonary circulation may result in pulmonary edema.

  E. CHF usually occurs in the left ventricle (left heart failure) but can occur in the right ventricle (right heart failure) primary or secondary to left heart failure or to COPD.

  F. Sometimes left and right heart failure occur at the same time.

  G. CHF is generally considered a chronic disorder with retention of salt and water by the kidneys.

H. CHF may be acute as a direct result of MI.

I. Prognosis depends on underlying cause and response to treatment.

J. Causes
1. MI
2. Cardiomyopathy
3. Myocarditis
4. Ventricular aneurysm
5. Aortic or mitral regurgitation or stenosis
6. Cardiac tamponade
7. Arrhythmias
8. Ventricular or atrial septal defects
9. Condition may become progressively worse from:
   a. Respiratory tract infections
   b. Pulmonary embolism
   c. Added emotional stress
   d. Increased salt or water intake
   e. Failure to comply with prescribed therapy

II. Data collection
A. Subjective symptoms
1. Anxiety or restlessness
2. Fatigue
3. Dyspnea
4. Confusion

B. Objective symptoms
1. Left-sided heart failure
   a. Dyspnea
   b. Orthopnea
   c. Nonproductive cough: worsens at night
   d. Later, productive cough with frothy, blood-tinged sputum
2. Right-sided heart failure
   a. Weight gain caused by fluid accumulation in tissues
   b. Pitting, dependent edema (ankle and leg edema or sacral edema, or both)
   c. Ascites from portal hypertension, resulting in accumulation of fluid in abdominal cavity, which may interfere with respirations owing to pressure against diaphragm
   d. Decreased urine output
   e. Distended neck veins
   f. Nausea, vomiting, and anorexia

III. Diagnostic tests and methods
A. Client history
B. Physical examination
C. Chest radiograph
D. ECG
E. Pulmonary artery monitoring
F. ABGs
G. Renal function tests
H. Liver function tests

IV. Implementation
A. Give and monitor oxygen as ordered.
B. Place client in high-Fowler's position and elevate extremities.
C. Record vital signs every 15 minutes to 2 hours during acute phase.
D. Restrict fluids as ordered.
E. Provide adequate nutritional intake:
   1. Restrict salt intake.
F. Record I&O every hour during acute phase.

G. Provide quiet, calm environment.

H. Provide adequate rest (conserves energy, prevents fatigue).

I. Monitor and record daily weights (report any changes).

J. Monitor mental status.

K. Monitor IV intake as prescribed.

L. Monitor BUN, creatinine, serum potassium, sodium, chloride, and magnesium levels.

M. Assess amount of activity that results in the least discomfort to client.

N. Monitor for pitting dependent edema (ankle, leg, and sacral edema).

O. Assist with use of rotating tourniquets as ordered:
1. Check radial and pedal pulses often to ensure tourniquets are not too tight.
2. Remove one tourniquet at a time to prevent sudden upsurge in circulating volume.

P. Assist with ROM exercises to prevent deep vein thrombosis caused by vascular congestion.

Q. Apply antiembolism stockings; watch for calf pain and tenderness.

R. Assist with activities of daily living (ADLs) until client is able to show gradual progress.

S. Administer medications such as digitalis, diuretics, and vasodilators as prescribed:
1. Check apical-radial pulse when giving digitalis.
2. Monitor, record, and report response to medications, including any side effects.

T. Monitor digitalis toxicity test.

U. Assist client to turn, cough, and breathe deeply.

V. Explain disease process, treatment, home care, and follow-up care to client and family:
1. Advise to avoid foods high in sodium, such as canned prepared foods and dairy products, to reduce fluid overload.
2. Reinforce information regarding loss of potassium through use of diuretics and replacement with prescribed potassium supplement and eating high-potassium foods.
3. Emphasize need for regular checkups.
4. Emphasize importance of taking digitalis exactly as prescribed.
5. Instruct client to watch for signs of toxicity (anorexia, nausea, vomiting, yellow vision, cardiac arrhythmias).
6. Emphasize importance of notifying physician immediately for following: irregular pulse or pulse <60 beats per minute (bpm), persistent dry cough, palpitations, increased fatigue, paroxysmal nocturnal dyspnea, swollen ankles, decreased urinary output, or weight gain of 3–5 lb in a week.

V. Evaluation
A. Client reports decreased anxiety.
B. Client displays decreased confusion.
C. Respiratory difficulties are decreased.
D. Client tolerates progressive increases in activity level.
E. Edema is decreased.
F. Client and family demonstrate an understanding of disease process, treatment including medication compliance, home care including need for daily weight monitoring and lifestyle modifications, and follow-up care.

Shock

I. Description
  A. Insufficient cardiac output or tissue perfusion
  B. Three types
    1. Cardiogenic shock
      a. Occurs if cardiac function is less than 15%
      b. May lead to cardiac arrest
    2. Hypovolemic shock
      a. Occurs because of reduction in intravascular blood volume resulting in insufficient perfusion of the tissues (loss of fluid within vascular space)
      b. May lead to irreversible cerebral and renal damage, cardiac arrest, and death
      c. Requires immediate recognition of signs and symptoms and prompt aggressive treatment to improve prognosis
    3. Vasogenic (or neurogenic) shock
      a. Occurs from acute vasodilation of vascular beds with pooling of blood within peripheral blood vessels.
      b. Results in inadequate perfusion of tissues.
  C. Complications
    1. ARDS
    2. Renal failure
    3. DIC
    4. Cerebral infarction
    5. Liver dysfunction
    6. GI ulcerations
II. Data collection
  A. Subjective symptoms
    1. Confusion, lethargy, restlessness
  B. Objective symptoms
    1. BP: initially normal; then drops
    2. Rapid, weak pulse
    3. Cold, clammy skin
    4. Low urine output
    5. Diaphoresis, pallor
    6. Increased respiratory rate, dyspnea, cough
    7. Decreased level of consciousness
    8. Abnormal clotting with DIC
    9. Decreased or absent bowel sounds (paralytic ileus)
III. Diagnostic tests and methods
  A. Client history
  B. Physical examination
  C. Cardiogenic shock
    1. ECG
    2. Serum enzyme levels
    3. Radiograph to identify internal bleeding sites
  D. Hypovolemic shock
    1. Laboratory tests
    2. Gastroscopy
    3. Aspiration of gastric contents
    4. Coagulation studies
IV. Implementation
  A. Monitor BP and heart rate immediately.
  B. Keep IV line open as ordered for IV drug instillation.
  C. Keep airway open.
  D. Give oxygen as ordered to promote adequate oxygenation of tissues.
  E. Monitor vital signs:

    1. Cardiac arrhythmias or cardiac ischemia may be produced.
    2. Report hypotension immediately.
  F. Monitor ABGs.
  G. Monitor CBC and serum electrolyte levels.
  H. Monitor urinary output.
  I. Administer prescribed vasoactive drugs.
  J. Monitor urinary output (use Foley catheter); notify registered nurse (RN) if output drops to 30 mL/hr.
  K. Administer diuretic as prescribed.
  L. Turn client every 2 hours to prevent skin breakdown.
  M. Monitor for signs of infection.
  N. Provide safe environment for client who is confused and restless.
  O. Provide environment for client to rest; assist in comfort measures.
  P. Provide mouth care.
V. Evaluation
  A. Vital signs remain within normal range.
  B. Client maintains urine output of >30 mL/hr.
  C. Anxiety, confusion, and restlessness are reduced.
  D. Serum electrolyte levels remain within normal range.
  E. BUN and creatinine levels remain within normal range.
  F. Client maintains good skin hygiene.

Acquired Inflammatory Diseases of the Heart

These diseases occur because of an acute or chronic inflammation of the heart, lining of the heart, and heart valves, caused by bacteria, viruses, trauma, or other factors (four types: pericarditis, myocarditis, endocarditis, and rheumatic heart disease).

Pericarditis

I. Description
  A. Inflammation of the pericardium, the fibroserous sac that envelops and protects the heart; can be acute or chronic
  B. Causes
    1. Bacterial, fungal, or viral infections
    2. Neoplasms: primary or secondary from lungs, breasts, and other organs
    3. High-dose radiation to chest
    4. Hypersensitivity or autoimmune disease such as rheumatic fever, systemic lupus erythematosus, and rheumatoid arthritis
    5. Postcardiac injury
    6. Medications
    7. Idiopathic factors (unknown cause)
    8. Aortic aneurysm with pericardial leakage
    9. Myxedema
II. Data collection
  A. Subjective symptoms
    1. Sharp pain over sternum radiating to neck, shoulders, back, and arms
    2. Pain increases with deep inspiration, decreases when sitting up or leaning forward (pulls heart away from diaphragmatic pleurae of lungs)
    3. Difficulty in breathing

4. Tachycardia
5. Feeling of fullness in chest
B. Objective symptoms
   1. Signs of pericardial effusion
   2. Dyspnea
   3. Orthopnea
   4. Tachycardia
   5. Substernal chest pain
   6. Pallor; cold, clammy skin
   7. Hypotension
   8. Jugular venous distention
   9. Hypotension
   10. Signs of constrictive pericarditis
   11. Increase in systemic venous pressure
   12. Pericardial friction rub
   13. Symptoms similar to right-sided heart failure: fluid retention, hepatomegaly, ascites

III. Diagnostic tests and methods
A. Client history
B. Physical examination
C. WBC count
D. ESR
E. Serum cardiac enzymes
F. Cardiocentesis
G. ECG
H. BUN level
I. Pericardial fluid culture
J. Echocardiography to assess valvular disease

IV. Implementation
A. Assess pain in relation to respiration and body position.
B. Place client in upright position to relieve dyspnea and pain.
C. Provide adequate bed rest.
D. Administer salicylates, antibiotics, and other prescribed medications.
E. Give oxygen as prescribed.
F. Assist with procedures as necessary.
G. Monitor for signs of infection.
H. Explain diagnostic procedures.
I. Monitor BP and venous pressure (decreased BP and increased venous pressure indicate pericardial effusion).
J. Follow postoperative care procedures.
K. Explain disease process, surgical procedure, treatment, home care, and follow-up care.

V. Evaluation
A. Pericardial friction rub is absent.
B. Pericardial effusion and signs of infection are absent.
C. Client reports increased comfort.
D. Pain is absent.
E. Vital signs remain within normal range.
F. Laboratory studies remain within normal range.
G. Client demonstrates an understanding of disease process, surgical procedure, treatment, home care and follow-up care.

Myocarditis

I. Description
A. Inflammation of the cardiac muscle; may be acute or chronic and may occur at any age.

B. Resultant impairment of contractility; often does not produce specific symptoms or ECG abnormalities.
C. Recovery can be spontaneous without residual effects.
D. Complications including congestive heart failure, myocardial ischemia, necrosis, and, rarely, cardiomyopathy.
E. Causes
   1. Viral infections: influenza, measles, German measles, echoviruses
   2. Bacterial infections: diphtheria, tuberculosis, typhoid fever, tetanus, staphylococci, pneumococci, and gonococci
   3. Hypersensitive immune reactions: acute rheumatic fever
   4. Radiation therapy: large doses to chest for treatment of lung or breast cancer
   5. Chemical poisons: chronic alcoholism
   6. Parasitic infections

II. Data collection
A. Subjective symptoms
   1. Fatigue
   2. Difficulty in breathing
   3. Feeling of soreness in chest
B. Objective symptoms
   1. Dyspnea
   2. In severe cases, neck vein distention, tachycardia, fever, arrhythmia

III. Diagnostic tests and methods
A. Client history
B. Physical examination
C. Serum cardiac enzymes
D. WBC count and ESR
E. ECG
F. Throat culture
G. Stool culture

IV. Implementation
A. Assess cardiovascular status frequently.
B. Listen for rales.
C. Take vital signs.
D. Weigh daily.
E. Record I&O.
F. Monitor cardiac rhythm and conduction.
G. Observe for signs of digitalis toxicity.
H. Check serum electrolyte levels.
I. Emphasize importance of bed rest.
J. Assist with activities; schedule rest periods.
K. Provide bedside commode.
L. Instruct client to resume normal activities slowly.
M. Explain disease process, treatment, and home care to client and family.

V. Evaluation
A. Client reports increased comfort.
B. Cardiovascular status remains within normal range.
C. Signs of infection are absent.
D. Client and family demonstrate an understanding of disease process, treatment, and home care.

Endocarditis

I. Description
A. An inflammation of the endocardium, heart valves, or cardiac prosthesis caused by infectious organisms

B. Usually fatal if untreated, but with treatment approximately 70% of affected individuals have a full recovery.

C. Prognosis is worse when severe vascular damage occurs, resulting in insufficiency of blood flow and congestive heart failure, or when a prosthetic valve is involved

D. Causes
  1. In acute form, bacteremia after septic thrombophlebitis, open-heart surgery involving prosthetic valve, or skin, bone, and pulmonary infections
  2. Group A nonhemolytic *Streptococcus* (rheumatic endocarditis), *Pneumococcus,* and *Staphylococcus* organisms most common
  3. Condition caused by organisms such as staphylococci and *Streptococcus viridans* producing vegetative growths on the heart valves, endocardial lining of the heart chambers, or endothelium of blood vessels that may break off and embolize to the CNS, spleen, kidneys, and lungs

E. Occurrence in IV drug users as a result of infections with *Staphylococcus aureus, Pseudomonas* organisms, or *Candida* organisms

II. Data collection
  A. Subjective symptoms
    1. Anorexia, weight loss
    2. Malaise, weakness
    3. Chest pain
    4. Chills
    5. Night sweats
  B. Objective symptoms
    1. Low-grade fever (99–102°F [37.2–38.8°C]): subacute endocarditis.
    2. High-grade fever (103–104°F [39.4–40°C]): acute infective endocarditis.
    3. Positive blood cultures.
    4. Heart murmurs.
    5. Clubbing of fingers.
    6. Petechiae: in 49% of cases.
    7. Complications caused by emboli reaching other organs, including spleen, kidney, lungs, peripheral vascular beds. Common symptoms include hematuria, pleuritic chest pain, and upper left quadrant pain.

III. Diagnostic tests and methods
  A. Blood culture studies
  B. WBC count
  C. Histiocyte studies
  D. ESR
  E. Rheumatoid factor
  F. Echocardiography to identify valvular damage
  G. ECG
  H. Cardiac output

IV. Implementation
  A. Obtain client history of allergies.
  B. Administer antibiotics to maintain consistent antibiotic blood levels.
  C. Monitor for signs of heart failure.
  D. Provide mouth care; avoid invasive procedures.
  E. Watch for signs of embolization.
  F. Monitor renal status (BUN, creatinine levels, and urinary output to check for signs of renal emboli or drug toxicity).
  G. Provide reassurance.
  H. Explain disease process, treatment, precautions, and home care to client and family:
    1. Watch for symptoms of relapse.
    2. Instruct need for prophylactic antibiotics before, during, and after dental work, childbirth, genitourinary and GI procedures.
    3. Instruct client to notify physician immediately if symptoms reappear.

V. Evaluation
  A. Fever and signs of infection are absent.
  B. Client remains free of complications.
  C. Client maintains adequate cardiac output.
  D. Client and family demonstrate an understanding of disease process, treatment, precautions, and home care.

Rheumatic Heart Disease

I. Description
  A. Inflammatory process that may affect the myocardium, pericardium, and/or endocardium
  B. Severe pancarditis (involvement of myocardium, pericardium, and endocardium), which occasionally produces fatal congestive heart failure during acute phase
  C. Usually resulting in distortion, scarring, and stenosis of valves; may lead to adhesions of adjacent tissue
  D. Frequent cause of mitral stenosis

II. Data collection
  A. Subjective symptoms
    1. Prior history of rheumatic fever
    2. General malaise, fatigue
    3. Pain: may or may not be present
  B. Objective symptoms
    1. Temperature increase
    2. Murmurs over affected valves
    3. Dyspnea
    4. Polyarthritis: red, swollen, painful large joints
    5. Sydenham's chorea: abrupt, purposeless involuntary movements

III. Diagnostic tests and methods
  A. Client history
  B. Physical examination
  C. WBC count and ESR
  D. C-reactive protein
  E. Cardiac enzymes
  F. ECG
  G. Chest radiograph
  H. Echocardiography
  I. Cardiac catheterization
  J. Cardiac output

IV. Implementation
  A. Monitor vital signs.
  B. Provide quiet, calm environment.
  C. Provide adequate rest.
  D. Administer prescribed medication (penicillin, digitalis, diuretics).
  E. Provide prescribed nutrition.
  F. Monitor I&O.

G. Explain disease process, treatment, and home care to client and family.
V. Evaluation
   A. Client reports increased comfort.
   B. Client remains free of complications.
   C. Cardiovascular status remains within normal range.
   D. Client and family demonstrate an understanding of disease process, treatment, and home care.

Valvular Heart Disease

I. Description
   A. Valvular heart disease results in either stenosis or insufficiency of heart valves.
   B. In valvular stenosis, the valve cusps become fibrotic and thicken, hindering blood flow.
   C. In valvular insufficiency, valve cusps become inflamed and scarred, and no longer close completely.
   D. Alteration of blood flow through the heart results in a decrease in cardiac output, systemic and pulmonary congestion, and dilation of heart chambers.
   E. Any of these conditions can lead to heart failure.
   F. Types
      1. Mitral stenosis: mitral valve becoming calcified and stiff; leading to left atrial hypertrophy with an increase in left atrial and pulmonary pressures; resultant right-sided heart failure
         a. Causes
            1) Rheumatic fever
         b. Complications: atrial fibrillation, thrombus formation, and congestive heart failure
      2. Mitral regurgitation: insufficient valves allowing blood to backflow from ventricle to atria during systole, with resultant atrial and left ventricular hypertrophy
         a. Causes
            1) Rheumatic fever
            2) MI
            3) Ventricular aneurysm
            4) Papillary muscle rupture
            5) Endocarditis
         b. Complications: atrial fibrillation, elevated left-sided heart pressures, CHF, systemic embolization
      3. Aortic stenosis: aortic valve becoming stiffened and fibrotic, impeding blood flow during left ventricular emptying; resultant left ventricular hypertrophy, increased oxygen demands, and pulmonary congestion
         a. Causes
            1) Rheumatic fever
            2) Congenital valve defects
            3) Atherosclerosis
         b. Complications: right-sided heart failure, pulmonary edema, atrial fibrillation
      4. Aortic regurgitation: aortic valve becoming insufficient owing to deformed or contracted valve cusps; inability of valves to close completely, resulting in backflow of blood into left ventricle; resultant left ventricular hypertrophy
         a. Causes

            1) Rheumatic fever
            2) Congenital defects
            3) Endocarditis
         b. Complications: left-sided heart failure, arrhythmias
      5. Tricuspid stenosis: chordae tendinae becoming fused and shortened, resulting in a narrowing of the valvular opening; blood flow obstruction to the right atrium, causing right-sided heart failure and decreased cardiac output
         a. Causes
            1) Rheumatic fever
            2) Right atrial myxomata
      6. Tricuspid regurgitation: valve becoming insufficient as a result of papillary muscle dysfunction or dilation of the valvular ring; blood flow returning to the right atrium, with resultant venous overload and decreased cardiac output
         a. Causes
            1) Rheumatic fever
            2) Congenital defect
            3) Dilation of right ventricle
            4) Endocarditis
II. Data collection
   A. Subjective symptoms
      1. Fatigue, weakness
      2. General malaise
      3. Dyspnea on exertion
      4. Dizziness
      5. Chest pain, discomfort
      6. Weight gain
      7. Prior history of rheumatic fever
   B. Objective symptoms
      1. Orthopnea
      2. Dyspnea, rales
      3. Pink-tinged sputum (mitral stenosis)
      4. Heart murmurs
      5. Palpitations
      6. Cyanosis, capillary refill
      7. Edema
      8. Arrhythmias
      9. Restlessness
      10. Left- or right-sided elevated pressures
III. Diagnostic tests and methods
   A. Client history
   B. Physical examination
   C. ECG
   D. Chest radiograph to determine size of heart
   E. Cardiac catheterization: identification of pressure changes
   F. Echocardiogram for information regarding structure and function of valves
IV. Implementation
   A. Assess, report, and record signs and symptoms and any reaction to treatment.
   B. Elevate head of bed.
   C. Give oxygen as prescribed.
   D. Provide emotional support to client and family.
   E. Administer prescribed medication (antibiotics, digitalis, diuretics, and anticoagulants); assess results and any side effects.
   F. Check digitalis toxicity reports.

G. Provide quiet, calm environment to conserve client's energy.
H. Monitor and record vital signs.
I. Monitor I&O.
J. Check for edema and capillary refill.
K. Weigh daily.
L. Provide sodium-restricted diet as prescribed.
M. Provide cardiac rehabilitation.
N. Explain disease process, treatment including medication and need for compliance, precautions, and home care including diet and activity to client and family.

V. Evaluation
A. Client maintains adequate cardiac output.
B. Client maintains effective breathing pattern.
C. Client reports increased comfort.
D. Anxiety and edema are reduced.
E. Client demonstrates an understanding of disease process, treatment including medication and need for compliance, precautions, and home care.

Acute Pulmonary Edema

I. Description
A. In cardiogenic pulmonary edema, fluid accumulation in alveoli, bronchioles, and bronchi is a result of elevations in pulmonary venous and capillary pressures. Gas exchange is compromised.
B. Pulmonary edema is a common complication of cardiac disorders; it can occur as a chronic condition or develop quickly with rapidly fatal consequences.
C. Causes
1. CHF
2. Valvular heart disease
3. Fluid overload
4. Inhalation of irritating chemicals
5. Nephrosis, extensive burns, liver disease, and nutritional deficiency owing to decreased serum colloid osmotic pressure
6. Hodgkin's disease: impaired lung lymphatic drainage

II. Data collection
A. Subjective symptoms
1. Difficulty in breathing
2. Anxiety, apprehension
3. Weakness
4. Cough
B. Objective symptoms
1. Dyspnea
2. Restlessness, confusion
3. Productive cough with frothy pink sputum
4. Weak, rapid pulse
5. Wheezing
6. Cyanosis
7. Increased central venous pressure (CVP) readings
8. Tachycardia
9. Orthopnea
10. Arrhythmias
11. Cold, clammy skin
12. Decreased blood pressure

III. Diagnostic tests and methods
A. Client history
B. Physical examination

C. ABGs
D. Chest radiograph
E. Pulmonary artery catheterization

IV. Implementation
A. Provide complete bed rest.
B. Place client in high-Fowler's position.
C. Monitor vital signs.
D. Monitor breath sounds.
E. Check for peripheral edema.
F. Give oxygen as ordered.
G. Administer prescribed medications such as morphine, diuretics, digitalis, and vasodilators.
H. Observe effects of medications, including side effects.
I. Assess client's condition frequently.
J. Monitor ABG values.
K. Check cardiac monitor frequently; report any changes.
L. Assist with rotating tourniquets if prescribed; record sequence and timing.
M. Provide reassurance to client and family; explain procedures.
N. Explain disease process, treatments, prevention, and home care.

V. Evaluation
A. Venous return decreases.
B. Client maintains effective gas exchange.
C. Client maintains effective cardiovascular function.
D. Client reports increased comfort and decreased anxiety and apprehension.
E. Client demonstrates an understanding of disease process, treatment, prevention, and home care.

Cardiopulmonary Arrest

I. Description
A. Sudden cessation of the heart's pumping function, stopping ventilation and circulation; rapidly fatal if untreated; delay in treatment of 3–5 minutes possibly producing irreversible brain damage
B. Condition accounting for >350,000 deaths in the United States each year, with most occurrences outside of the hospital
C. Prompt, aggressive treatment and early hospitalization necessary to prevent death
D. Causes
1. Severe MI with necrosis
2. Ventricular fibrillation resulting from MI, heart failure, anesthetics, electrolyte disturbances (hyperkalemia and hypokalemia, acidosis), acute hemorrhage, electrical shock, ventricular irritation (from cardiac pacing wires, cardiac catheterization)

II. Data collection
A. Objective symptoms
1. Unconsciousness
2. Absence of pulse and respiration
3. Absence of heart sounds
4. Pupillary dilation
5. Cyanosis

III. Diagnostic tests and methods
A. Client history
B. Physical examination
C. ECG and enzyme studies, after emergency treatment

IV. Implementation
  A. Perform basic life support measures (cardiopulmonary resuscitation [CPR]):
    1. ABCs.
    2. Establish airway; assist with ventilation measures.
    3. Assist with circulation measures:
      a. Continue ventilation and circulation measures.
    4. Interrupt ventilatory and circulatory measures (CPR) when:
      a. Client begins to breathe spontaneously
      b. Another person giving CPR replaces you
      c. Client is transferred (resume CPR during transport to hospital)
    5. Stop CPR when client is pronounced dead by physician or resuscitation is effective.
  B. During recovery from cardiac arrest
    1. Keep IV lines open as ordered to allow administration of IV drugs.
    2. For clients with ventricular arrhythmias, keep IV lidocaine at bedside for bolus administration.
    3. Monitor ABGs frequently.
    4. Watch for arrhythmias, hypoxia, acidosis, and hypokalemia.
    5. Assess renal status: monitor urine output and specific gravity hourly.
    6. Monitor electrolyte, BUN, and creatinine levels daily.
    7. Administer osmotic diuretics, if prescribed.
    8. Assess cardiac status (level of consciousness, skin color, temperature, peripheral pulses; also monitor pulmonary artery catheter readings and cardiac output).
    9. Assess neurological status (signs of cerebral edema, elevated temperature, wide pulse pressures, decreased responsiveness, or presence of seizures, changes in level of consciousness, pupil changes).
    10. Observe for complications of CPR (rib or sternal fractures, cardiac tamponade, pneumothorax).
    11. Give emotional support to family.
V. Evaluation
  A. Spontaneous ventilation and circulation return.
  B. Client remains free of injury or complications.
  C. Client and family are instructed in performing CPR.

Peripheral Vascular System

Basic Information

Peripheral vascular disease refers to vascular disorders other than those specifically affecting the heart. Blood flow is decreased because of narrowed or obstructed blood vessels. The underlying factor is the arteriosclerotic process. The decreased blood flow causes changes in the tissues.
II. Basic data collection
  A. Subjective symptoms
    1. Aching calves
    2. Numbness in legs
    3. Leg cramps
    4. Loss of sensation in legs
    5. Pain in legs during exercise (intermittent claudication)

    6. History of diabetes mellitus, thrombophlebitis, hypertension, alcoholism
  B. Objective symptoms
    1. Skin of lower extremities
      a. Cold or blue feet
      b. Redness of leg in dependent position
      c. Sparse hair distribution
      d. Edema
      e. Stasis ulcers
      f. Varicose veins
      g. Diminished or absent pulses
      h. Delay in capillary filling
      i. Bruits heard in major arteries
      j. Differences in circumference of legs

Major Peripheral Vascular Diagnoses

Raynaud's Disease (Thromboangiitis)

I. Description
  A. Disease characterized by episodic vasospasm in small peripheral arteries and arterioles, resulting in interruptions of blood flow to distal parts of affected extremities
  B. Occurring bilaterally, usually affecting hands; feet less often affected
  C. Most prevalent in women, especially between puberty and age 40 years
  D. Precipitating factors
    1. Cold, stress, smoking
    2. Associated with collagen diseases in women
  E. Contributing factors
    1. Pressure to fingertips: typists, pianists, users of hand-held vibrating equipment
II. Data collection
  A. Subjective symptoms
    1. Numbness, coldness of hands or feet
    2. Pain in hands or feet
  B. Objective symptoms
    1. Hands or feet feel cold to touch
    2. Color changes: pallor, cyanosis
    3. Numbness and tingling
    4. Dryness and atrophy of nails
    5. Ulcerations or gangrene, especially on fingertips
III. Diagnostic tests and methods
  A. Client history
  B. Physical examination
  C. Arteriography
  D. ECG
  E. Doppler ultrasonography
  F. Chest radiograph
IV. Implementation
  A. Record location and characteristics of pain.
  B. Administer prescribed vasodilators and analgesics; record results and any side effects.
  C. Observe affected areas every shift for color, sensation, diminished pulse.
  D. Keep extremities warm and protected.
  E. Provide safe environment to prevent injury.
  F. Instruct client to avoid exposure of hands and feet to cold and to use gloves and warm socks.
  G. Instruct client to avoid constrictive clothing and to maintain adequate caloric intake.

H. Encourage rest after exercise.
I. Discourage smoking.
J. Provide emotional support.
K. Explain disease process, avoidance of cold, protection from trauma, cessation of smoking, and prevention of spasms to client and family.

V. Evaluation
A. Client verbalizes relief of pain.
B. Client maintains effective tissue perfusion and good skin hygiene.
C. Client and family demonstrate an understanding of disease process, treatment including medication, and prevention.

Thrombophlebitis

I. Description
A. Thrombophlebitis: characterized by inflammation and thrombus formation; may occur in deep or superficial veins
   1. Superficial thrombophlebitis begins with localized inflammation alone (phlebitis); thrombus formation is frequently provoked by the inflammatory process.
   2. Platelets, red blood cells (RBCs), and fibrin form a clot within the vein, which potentially can break loose and lead to emboli.
   3. Deep vein thrombophlebitis frequently leads to pulmonary embolism.
   4. Causes of deep vein thrombophlebitis:
      a. Damage to vessel lining
      b. Venous pooling and stasis
      c. Increased clotting ability of blood
   5. Predisposing factors:
      a. Prolonged bed rest
      b. Trauma
      c. Surgery
      d. Prolonged periods of standing
      e. Increased abdominal pressure: pregnancy, obesity
      f. Use of oral contraceptives
   6. Causes of superficial thrombophlebitis:
      a. Trauma
      b. Infection
      c. IV drug abuse
      d. Chemical irritation: extensive use of IV route for medications and diagnostic tests

II. Data collection
A. Subjective symptoms
   1. Pain in affected extremity
   2. History of causes and contributing factors
B. Objective symptoms
   1. Warmth and redness of extremity
   2. Elevation of body temperature
   3. Swelling
   4. Positive Homans' sign (pain on dorsiflexion of foot)
   5. Area sensitive to touch
   6. Decreased pulse in affected extremity

III. Diagnostic tests and methods
A. Client history
B. Physical examination
C. Homans' sign
D. Doppler ultrasonography
E. Venography
F. Phlebography
G. Laboratory studies: CBC, ESR, coagulation studies
H. Lung scan to rule out pulmonary embolism

IV. Implementation
A. Assess, report, and record signs and symptoms and any reaction to treatment.
B. Provide bed rest.
C. Use moist heat as prescribed to reduce swelling and to provide comfort.
D. Elevate affected limb to decrease swelling and to prevent blood stasis.
E. Administer analgesics as ordered; monitor for side effects.
F. Monitor thigh and calf measurements daily.
G. Monitor vital signs every 4 hours.
H. Avoid massaging affected leg.
I. Use antiembolism stocking on unaffected leg.
J. Administer anticoagulants, vasodilators, and anti-inflammatory medications as prescribed; monitor results.
K. Assist with ROM exercises to unaffected extremity.
L. Monitor for bleeding tendencies:
   1. Check gums.
   2. Check skin for bruises and petechiae.
   3. Watch for nosebleeds.
   4. Monitor Hgb and Hct levels.
M. Monitor for signs and symptoms of complications such as embolism.
N. Explain to client and family:
   1. Avoidance of long periods of sitting or standing
   2. Routine exercise plan
   3. Avoidance of tight, constrictive clothing
   4. Use of elastic or support hose for extended periods of sitting or standing

V. Evaluation
A. Client reports increased comfort and decreased anxiety.
B. Swelling is decreased or absent.
C. Redness along affected superficial vein disappears.
D. Pain is relieved.
E. Client maintains effective tissue perfusion.
F. Client and family demonstrate an understanding of disease process, treatment, prevention, and home care.

Varicose Veins

I. Description
A. Dilated, tortuous leg veins owing to backflow of blood caused by incompetent venous valve closure, resultant venous congestion, and further vein enlargement
B. Usually affects subcutaneous leg veins (saphenous veins and branches)
C. Causes
   1. Basic cause unknown
   2. Contributing factors

a. Congenital weakness of venous valves or venous wall

b. Diseases of venous system, such as thrombophlebitis

c. Conditions that produce venostasis: pregnancy, prolonged standing

d. Familial tendency

II. Data collection

A. Subjective symptoms

1. Aching

2. Cramping and pain

3. Feeling of heaviness

B. Objective symptoms

1. Palpable nodules

2. Ankle edema

3. Dilated veins

4. Pigmentation of calves and ankles

III. Diagnostic tests and methods

A. Client history

B. Physical examination

C. Venography

D. Trendelenburg's test

IV. Implementation

A. Provide adequate rest with client's legs elevated.

B. Apply support stockings.

C. Discourage prolonged standing, sitting, and crossing legs.

D. Encourage weight management.

E. Instruct client to avoid constrictive clothing.

F. Prepare client for surgical procedure (surgical vein stripping, ligation, vein sclerosing).

G. After surgical procedure

1. Administer analgesics as prescribed to alleviate pain.

2. Elevate affected leg.

3. Check circulation in toes frequently (color and temperature).

4. Observe elastic bandages for bleeding.

5. Rewrap bandage once per shift if ordered (wrap from toe to thigh with leg elevated).

6. Watch for signs of complications:

a. Sensory loss in leg (indicative of saphenous nerve damage)

b. Calf pain (indicative of thrombophlebitis)

c. Fever (indicative of infection)

V. Evaluation

A. Pain is relieved.

B. Client reports increased comfort.

C. Client maintains adequate tissue perfusion.

D. Client remains free of complications.

E. Client demonstrates an understanding of the condition, prevention, and home care.

Aneurysms

I. Description

A. The enlargement or ballooning of an artery.

B. Some aneurysms progress to serious and eventually fatal complications, such as rupture.

C. Types

1. Dissecting aneurysm: a hemorrhagic separation of the inner layer of the arterial wall

2. Saccular aneurysm: an outpouching of one side of the arterial wall with a narrow neck

3. Fusiform aneurysm: a spindle-shaped enlargement including the entire circumference of the artery

D. Causes

1. Arteriosclerosis primary cause: plaque formation causing degenerative changes, with resultant loss of vessel elasticity, weakness, and dilation

2. Infections

3. Congenital disorders

4. Trauma

5. Syphilis

6. Hypertension

II. Data collection

A. Thoracic aneurysm involves the transverse or descending portion of the aorta and is most common in men 50–70 years old. Dissecting aneurysms are most common in the black race.

1. Subjective symptoms

a. Possibly asymptomatic

b. Dyspnea

c. Severe chest pain

d. Dysphagia (difficulty in swallowing)

e. Hoarseness or cough

f. Dizziness

2. Objective symptoms

a. Diaphoresis

b. Increased pulse rate

c. Cyanosis

d. Neck vein distention

e. Leg weakness or transient paralysis

f. Diastolic murmur caused by aortic regurgitation

g. Abrupt loss of femoral and radial pulses or wide variations in pulses of arms and legs

h. Symptoms of shock but systolic BP often normal or significantly increased

i. Varying symptoms according to size and location of defect, the effects of compression, and erosion of surrounding structures

B. Abdominal aneurysm usually occurs between the renal arteries and iliac branches; is approximately four times more common in white men 50–80 years old than in the general population.

1. Subjective symptoms

a. Tenderness or pain in abdomen or back

b. Chest pain in dissecting aneurysms

2. Objective symptoms

a. Pulsating mass in periumbilical area of abdomen

b. Systolic bruit over aorta

c. Elevated BP

d. Pulse changes in lower extremities

e. Possibly mimicking renal calculi, lumbar disk disease, or duodenal compression, if large

III. Diagnostic tests and methods

A. Client history

B. Physical examination

C. Angiograph to determine location of aneurysm

D. Radiograph

E. Ultrasonography
F. Routine ECG
G. Laboratory studies: Hgb, Hct

IV. Implementation
A. Monitor vital signs and peripheral pulses every 15 minutes until stable.
B. Monitor for signs of decreased tissue perfusion: low BP, bleeding, rapid weak pulse.
C. Assess pain, respirations, and carotid, radial, and femoral pulses.
D. Administer prescribed medications to decrease pain.
E. Administer prescribed antibiotics.
F. Listen to lung and bowel sounds at least every 4 hours.
G. Monitor for arrhythmias.
H. Apply antiembolism stockings; do not massage lower extremities.
I. Compare extremities for warmth and color.
J. Administer IV fluids as ordered.
K. Monitor oxygen therapy.
L. Assist with monitoring of CVP.
M. Monitor I&O for fluid balance.
N. Provide emotional support to client and family.
O. Provide information in regard to postoperative care, activity, and incisional management.
P. Encourage coughing and deep-breathing exercises.
Q. Maintain bed rest.
R. Encourage prescribed leg exercises to prevent venous stasis.

V. Evaluation
A. Client reports increased comfort and decreased anxiety.
B. Vital signs remain stable.
C. Fluid balance remains stable.
D. Pain is relieved.
E. Client remains free of complications.
F. Client demonstrates an understanding of disease process, surgical treatment, and home care.

Hematological System

Basic Information

- Blood is a major body fluid tissue that continuously circulates through the heart and blood vessels, carrying vital elements to all parts of the body.
- Erythrocytes (RBCs) carry oxygen to the tissues and remove carbon dioxide from them.
- Leukocytes (WBCs) assist in inflammatory and immune responses.
- Plasma carries antibodies and nutrients to tissues and wastes from tissues.
- Coagulation factors found in plasma along with thrombocytes (platelets) control blood clotting.
- The average individual has 5–6 L of circulating blood, which constitute 5%–7% of body weight.
- The pH of blood ranges from 7.35–7.45 and is either dark red (venous blood) or bright red (arterial blood), depending on the level of Hgb and the degree of oxygen saturation.
- Malfunction of the hematological system has far-reaching effects on the body.

I. Basic data collection
A. Subjective symptoms
1. Weakness, fatigue
2. Nausea
3. Dyspnea
4. Irritability
5. Bleeding from nose and mouth
6. Headache
7. Numbness, burning of feet
8. Vertigo
B. Objective symptoms
1. Tachycardia and tachypnea
2. Pallor and jaundice
3. Pruritus
4. Impaired thought processes
5. Mouth ulcerations
6. Smooth tongue
7. Hypotension

Major Hematological Diagnoses

Anemia Caused by Decreased Red Blood Cell Production

I. Description
A. Deficiency of RBCs (anemia) because of conditions affecting production of RBCs
B. Types
1. Pernicious anemia
a. Condition caused by lack of intrinsic factor in GI system, which is required for the absorption of vitamin B_{12}.
b. Deficiency of mucosal surface of GI tract, which secretes intrinsic factor.
c. Those who have had gastrectomies and small bowel resections are at risk.
2. Folic acid deficiency
a. Folic acid necessary for synthesis of DNA; DNA required for production and maturation of RBCs
b. Condition caused by poor nutrition (lack of citrus fruits, liver, grains, leafy green vegetables), drugs, alcohol abuse, hemodialysis, and malabsorption disorders, which interfere with absorption of folic acid
3. Iron-deficiency anemia
a. Condition caused by insufficient intake of dietary iron, necessary for production of Hgb and RBCs
b. Condition possibly caused by malabsorption, hemolysis of RBCs, and blood loss
4. Aplastic anemia
a. Decrease in all blood types: RBC, WBC, and platelets. Also called pancytopenia
b. Condition caused by congenital problems or acquired from radiation, chemicals, infection, or medications.

II. Data collection
A. Subjective symptoms
1. Pallor
2. Fatigue
3. Dyspnea

4. Anginal pain
5. Blurred vision
6. Vertigo
7. Irritability
8. Depression
9. Nausea
10. Anorexia
11. Weight loss
12. Bone pain
13. Numbness, tingling of feet
   B. Objective symptoms
      1. CHF
      2. Positive bone marrow findings
      3. Impaired thought processes
      4. Confusion
      5. Vomiting
      6. Splenomegaly
      7. Hepatomegaly
III. Diagnostic tests and methods
   A. Client history
   B. Physical examination
   C. RBC count and morphology
   D. CBC
   E. Reticulocyte count
   F. Serum iron and ferritin
   G. Total iron binding capacity
IV. Implementation
   A. Assess, report, and record signs and symptoms and any reaction to treatments.
   B. Monitor vital signs, I&O, skin color and oxygen saturation.
   C. Provide planned activity; schedule rest periods.
   D. Administer prescribed supplemental oxygen.
   E. Administer prescribed medications such as iron supplements, vitamin B_{12}, and oral folic acid.
   F. Assist with comfort and hygiene needs.
   G. Monitor blood transfusions; check for reactions.
   H. Provide mouth care.
   I. Provide prescribed diet and fluid intake.
   J. Support client; allay anxiety.
   K. Provide emotional support.
   L. Explain condition, diagnostic procedures, treatment, prevention, home care including planned activities, and follow-up care to client and family.
V. Evaluation
   A. Client reports increased comfort and decreased anxiety.
   B. Client maintains adequate cardiac output and tissue perfusion.
   C. Laboratory values remain within normal range.
   D. Client and family demonstrate an understanding of disease process, diagnostic procedures, treatments, prevention, home care, and follow-up care.

Anemia Caused by Red Blood Cell Destruction

I. Description
   A. Condition caused by RBCs being destroyed faster than they are being produced
   B. Causes
      1. Infections
      2. Drugs, chemicals

3. Snake venom
4. Antigen-antibody reactions
5. Disorders of the spleen
6. Organic compounds
7. Congenital disorders
II. Data collection
   A. Subjective symptoms
      1. Weakness, fatigue
      2. Pallor
      3. Weight loss
      4. Painful episodes; history of stress (sickle cell anemia)
   B. Objective symptoms
      1. Positive Coombs' test result: acquired anemia caused by drugs or autoimmune disorder
      2. Elevated serum bilirubin level
      3. Elevated reticulocyte count
      4. Enlarged spleen
      5. Low-grade fever
      6. Renal insufficiency
      7. Jaundice
III. Diagnostic tests and methods
   A. Client history
   B. Physical examination
   C. Laboratory studies: serum bilirubin, CBC, Coombs' test
   D. Renal studies to check renal status
   E. Routine chest radiograph
   F. Routine ECG
   G. Bone marrow biopsy
   H. Presence of abdominal sickle cells in blood or other abnormal cells (macrophytic, microcytic, hypochromic)
IV. Implementation
   A. Assess, report, and record signs and symptoms and any reaction to treatment.
   B. Schedule rest periods to avoid fatigue.
   C. Protect client from exposure to infection sources.
   D. Monitor for bleeding and bruising.
   E. Assist in administration of blood transfusions; check reaction to transfusion.
   F. Administer prescribed medications; check for side effects.
   G. Give oxygen as prescribed.
   H. Monitor fluid I&O.
   I. Monitor laboratory studies.
   J. Provide for genetic counseling.
   K. Caution client to avoid postural hypotension; advise him or her to get up slowly.
   L. Explain disease process, treatment, prevention, home care, and follow-up care to client and family.
V. Evaluation
   A. Client reports increased comfort and decreased anxiety.
   B. Client maintains adequate gas exchange.
   C. Client maintains adequate cardiac output and tissue perfusion.
   D. Client verbalizes feelings regarding disease.
   E. Client and family demonstrate an understanding of disease process, treatment, prevention, home care, and follow-up care.

Leukemia

I. Description
   A. Disorder of the hematological system characterized by an overproduction of immature WBCs
   B. Fewer normal WBCs produced as disease progresses
   C. Increase in abnormal WBCs, infiltrating and damaging bone marrow, lymph nodes, spleen, and other organs
   D. RBC production disrupted, leading to anemia, immature cells, thrombocytopenia, and decline in immunity
   E. Cause unknown; considered to be a neoplastic process.
   F. Predisposing factors
      1. Viral origin
      2. Exposure to radiation
      3. Exposure to chemicals
      4. Familial tendency
      5. Congenital disorders such as Down's syndrome, Fanconi's anemia, and congenital agammaglobulinemia
      6. All forms fatal if untreated
   G. Classification as acute or chronic, and according to cell type
      1. Acute lymphocytic leukemia (ALL)
         a. Lymphoblasts mostly present in bone marrow.
         b. Incidence peaks at 2–4 years of age.
         c. Remission induced in 40%–65% of adults as a result of treatment.
         d. Average survival 1–2 years.
      2. Acute myelogenous leukemia (AML)
         a. Myeloblasts are present mostly in bone marrow.
         b. Incidence peaks at 12–20 and >55 years of age.
         c. Average survival is 1 year after diagnosis even with aggressive therapy.
      3. Chronic myelogenous leukemia (CML)
         a. Granulocytes mostly present in bone marrow.
         b. Incidence peaks at 30–50 years of age.
      4. Chronic lymphocytic leukemia (CLL)
         a. Lymphocytes mostly present in bone marrow.
         b. Incidence peaks at 50–70 years of age.

II. Data collection
   A. Subjective symptoms: ALL and AML
      1. Sudden onset of high fever
      2. Abnormal bleeding such as nosebleeds, easy bruising, prolonged menses
      3. Fatigue
      4. Chills
      5. Recurrent infections
      6. Dyspnea
      7. Abdominal or bone pain
      8. Confusion, lethargy, headache when leukemic cells cross blood-brain barrier
   B. Subjective symptoms: CLL and CML
      1. Fatigue
      2. Weakness
      3. Anorexia
      4. Weight loss
      5. Lymph node enlargement
      6. Recurrent infections
      7. Bone tenderness
   C. Objective symptoms: ALL and AML
      1. Anemia
      2. Elevated temperature
      3. Abnormal bleeding
      4. Lymphadenopathy
      5. Ecchymoses
      6. Tachycardia
      7. Palpitations
      8. Systolic ejection murmur
      9. Positive bone marrow biopsy
      10. Normal, elevated, or decreased WBC count
   D. Objective symptoms: CLL and CML
      1. Skin lesions
      2. Elevated WBC count
      3. Anorexia
      4. Enlarged spleen and liver
      5. Petechiae
      6. Positive bone marrow biopsy
      7. Anemia
      8. Dyspnea
      9. Tachycardia
      10. Palpitations
      11. Recurrent opportunistic fungal, viral, and bacterial infections

III. Diagnostic tests and methods
   A. Client history
   B. Physical examination
   C. Laboratory studies: CBC, Hgb, Hct, platelet count
   D. Differential leukocyte count for determination of cell type
   E. Bone marrow biopsy
   F. Routine chest radiograph
   G. Routine ECG
   H. Lumbar puncture for detection of meningeal involvement

IV. Implementation
   A. Assess, report, and record signs and symptoms and any reaction to treatment.
   B. Provide comfort measures.
   C. Monitor laboratory data.
   D. Check for signs of bleeding or infection.
   E. Monitor vital signs.
   F. Assist in administration of prescribed medications such as chemotherapeutic drugs, antiemetics, analgesics, IV fluids, and blood or blood-product transfusions.
   G. Monitor for side effects of medications and transfusions.
   H. Minimize side effects of chemotherapy.
   I. Monitor fluid I&O.
   J. Prevent exposure to infection.
   K. Assist client with activities; schedule rest periods.
   L. Provide emotional support.
   M. Allay anxiety and fears.
   N. Monitor supplemental oxygen, if ordered.
   O. Provide and encourage prescribed diet.
   P. Provide oral hygiene.
   Q. Provide skin care; use protective devices.
   R. Provide environment that allows client to verbalize feelings.

S. Request discharge planning regarding available community resources and support groups.
T. Explain disease process, treatment including medication, home care including diet, activity, avoidance of injury and infection, and checking for abnormal bleeding, and follow-up care.

V. Evaluation
A. Client reports increased comfort and decreased anxiety.
B. Client maintains adequate tissue perfusion and gas exchange.
C. Client remains free of injury or infection.
D. Client demonstrates an understanding of disease process, treatment including medication and side effects, home care, and follow-up care.

Multiple Myeloma

I. Description
A. A disseminated neoplasm of immature plasma cells that infiltrate bone to produce tumors throughout the skeleton (vertebrae, skull, pelvis, flat bones, ribs).
B. During the late stages, infiltrates body organs (lungs, liver, spleen, adrenals, lymph nodes, GI tract, kidneys, skin).
C. Men 50–70 years old mostly affected.
D. Prognosis poor because diagnosis often made after widespread skeletal destruction.
E. Vertebral collapse without treatment.
F. In approximately 50% of clients, death within 3 months of diagnosis; in 90%, death within 2 years.
G. Life prolonged for 3–5 years with early treatment.
H. Death usually after complications such as infection, fractures, hypercalcemia, hyperuricemia, or renal failure.
I. Cause unknown.

II. Data collection
A. Subjective symptoms
1. Bone pain
2. Fatigue
3. Achiness
4. Joint swelling
5. Tenderness
6. Fever
7. Weight loss
8. Decreased body height
B. Objective symptoms
1. Anemia
2. Deformities of thorax
3. Renal complications: pyelonephritis resulting from tubular damage
4. Elevated serum calcium and uric acid levels
5. Severe recurrent infections, such as pneumonia, as a result of damaged nerves associated with respiratory function
6. Pathological fractures
7. Symptoms of vertebral compression
8. Decreased platelet count
9. Elevated ESR
10. Hypercalciuria possibly present
11. Presence of Bence Jones protein in urine
12. Positive bone marrow aspiration for myeloma cells
13. Elevated globulin

III. Diagnostic tests and methods
A. Client history
B. Physical examination
C. CBC: determines presence of anemia
D. ESR
E. Urine studies
F. Bone marrow biopsy
G. Serum electrophoresis for abnormal globulin
H. Radiographs of skeleton
I. IV pyelography (IVP)

IV. Implementation
A. Assess, report, and record signs and symptoms and any reaction to treatment.
B. Monitor vital signs, I&O, and laboratory studies.
C. Check for bleeding, infection, or presence of fractures.
D. Encourage fluid intake.
E. Monitor I&O (immediately report daily output of <1500 mL).
F. Encourage client to ambulate (decreases potential for bone demineralization and pneumonia).
G. Assist client in walking with use of walker or other supportive devices to prevent falls.
H. Protect client from others with infections.
I. Administer prescribed medications such as melphalan and prednisone, cyclophosphamide, antibiotics, and analgesics.
J. Assist with good hygienic measures to prevent infection.
K. Provide emotional support to client and family.
L. Prevent complications; watch for presence of fever or malaise.
M. If client is to receive complete bed rest, turn him or her every 2 hours.
N. Give passive ROM and deep-breathing exercises.
O. Ensure that blood is drawn as ordered for platelet count and WBC count before administration of melphalan (derivative of nitrogen mustard, which depresses bone marrow).
P. Prepare client and family for laminectomy if spinal cord compression occurs.
Q. Prepare client and family for dialysis if renal complications occur.
R. Provide comfort measures.
S. Provide information regarding appropriate community resources for additional support.
T. Explain disease, treatment including medication, prevention, and home care.

V. Evaluation
A. Client remains free of avoidable infections or injuries.
B. Client reports increased comfort and decreased anxiety.
C. Client maintains adequate I&O.
D. Client has access to community resources for support.
E. Client maintains adequate urine output.
F. Client demonstrates an understanding of disease process, treatment including medication, prevention, home care, and follow-up care.

Hodgkin's Disease

I. Description
   A. Neoplastic disease with painless progressive enlargement of lymph nodes, spleen, and other lymphoid tissue.
   B. Disease results from proliferation of Reed-Sternberg giant cells, lymphocytes, eosinophils, and histocytes.
   C. Disease potentially curable because of recent advances in therapeutic measures.
   D. Prognosis dependent on stage of the disease.
   E. Four stages defined by the Ann Arbor clinical staging classification of Hodgkin's disease.
   F. Five-year survival rate in approximately 54% of clients with treatment.
   G. Disease occurs most often in young adults, with a higher incidence in men than in women.
   H. Disease occurs in all races but is slightly more common in whites.
   I. Incidence peaks in two age groups (15–38 and >50 years of age).

II. Data collection
   A. Subjective symptoms
      1. Fatigue
      2. Loss of appetite
      3. Weakness
      4. History of recent upper respiratory infection
      5. Persistent fever
      6. Night sweats
      7. Weight loss
      8. Malaise
      9. Pruritus
   B. Objective symptoms
      1. Enlarged lymph nodes, spleen, and liver
      2. Positive biopsy of lymph nodes: cervical nodes most often affected
      3. Anemia
      4. Positive CT scan of liver and spleen
      5. Elevated temperature
      6. Thrombocytopenia
      7. Elevated serum alkaline phosphatase level: indicating liver or bone involvement
      8. Evaluation of stage by results of lymphangiography and laparotomy
      9. Positive bone marrow biopsy (if affected)

III. Diagnostic tests and methods
   A. Client history
   B. Physical examination
   C. Lymph node biopsy
   D. Bone marrow, liver, and spleen biopsies
   E. CT scan of lung, bone, liver, spleen
   F. Lymphangiography for detection of involved lymph nodes or organ involvement
   G. Hematological tests: CBC, blood chemistries to check serum alkaline phosphatase levels
   H. Staging laparotomy for clients <55 years old or with no obvious stage III or IV disease or other medical contraindications
   I. Measures to rule out other disorders that also cause enlarged lymph nodes

IV. Implementation
   A. Assess, report, and record signs and symptoms and any reaction to treatment.
   B. Assist with comfort measures for night sweats, itching, and fever.
   C. Prepare and explain to client and family treatments such as radiation, chemotherapy, and surgical procedures, if needed.
   D. Monitor vital signs and I&O.
   E. Protect client from contact with others who have infections.
   F. Provide safe environment.
   G. Provide emotional support to client and family.
   H. Monitor for signs of infection and changes in skin integrity.
   I. Minimize radiation side effects by good nutrition.
   J. Monitor for radiation and chemotherapeutic side effects (anorexia, nausea, vomiting, diarrhea, hair loss).
   K. Administer good oral hygiene using a soft toothbrush, cotton swab, or anesthetic mouthwash (if prescribed) to control pain and bleeding from stomatitis.
   L. Provide appropriate counseling and reassurance.
   M. Provide information regarding local chapter of American Cancer Society to assist in financial matters and supportive counseling, if needed.
   N. Explain disease, diagnostic procedures, treatment including medication, home care, and follow-up care to client and family.

V. Evaluation
   A. Client remains free of injury or infection.
   B. Client reports increased comfort and decreased anxiety.
   C. Client maintains good hygienic measures and skin integrity.
   D. Client uses effective coping strategies.
   E. Client and family demonstrate an understanding of disease process, treatment, home care, and follow-up care.

Thrombocytopenia

I. Description
   A. Most common cause of hemorrhagic disorders.
   B. Condition characterized by a decreased number of circulating platelets.
   C. Poses a serious threat to hemostasis.
   D. Prognosis good if thrombocytopenia is drug induced, by withdrawing drug.
   E. Prognosis in other cases dependent on response to treatment of underlying cause.
   F. Abnormally low platelet count (normal range 150,000–400,000/mm^3)
   G. Causes
      1. Congenital or acquired
      2. Condition usually results from:
         a. Decreased production of platelets in marrow (leukemia, aplastic anemia, or toxicity of certain drugs)
         b. Increased destruction of platelets outside the marrow (cirrhosis of liver, DIC, severe infections)
         c. Reduction in platelet survival time
         d. Collection of blood (sequestration) in spleen
         e. Acquired thrombocytopenia possibly caused by certain drugs, such as quinine, quinidine,

chlorothiazide, sulfisoxazole, phenylbutazone, rifampin, heparin, and cyclophosphamide)
II. Data collection
    A. Subjective symptoms
        1. History of current medication intake
        2. Bleeding from oral cavity and nose
        3. Easy bruising
        4. Malaise
        5. Fatigue
        6. General weakness
    B. Objective symptoms
        1. Petechiae
        2. Ecchymoses
        3. Epistaxis or gingival bleeding
        4. Low platelet count
        5. Blood-filled bullae in oral cavity
        6. Presence of megakaryocytes (platelet precursors) in bone marrow aspirations
        7. Hematuria
        8. Tachycardia, dyspnea, loss of consciousness, and death from hemorrhage
III. Diagnostic tests and methods
    A. Client history
    B. Physical examination
    C. Laboratory (coagulation) tests, platelet count, Hgb, Hct
    D. Bone marrow biopsy
IV. Implementation
    A. Assess, report, and record signs and symptoms and any reaction to treatment.
    B. Monitor for signs of bleeding.
    C. Protect from injury or trauma.
    D. Avoid invasive procedures such as venipuncture, intramuscular injections, urinary catheterization, and taking rectal temperature readings, if possible.
    E. If venipuncture is used, exert pressure on puncture site for at least 20 minutes, or until bleeding stops.
    F. Assist in administration of prescribed platelet transfusions.
    G. Monitor vital signs.
    H. Monitor platelet count, blood count, and bleeding times.
    I. Test stool for presence of blood; use a dipstick to test urine and emesis for blood.
    J. Instruct client to avoid aspirin and other drugs that decrease clotting.
    K. Instruct client to avoid straining at stool or when coughing (increases intracranial pressure [ICP] with potential for causing cerebral hemorrhage); provide stool softener, if necessary.
    L. Enforce bed rest if bleeding occurs.
    M. Provide safe environment.
    N. Provide emotional support.
    O. Explain disease process, diagnostic procedures, treatment including medication, prevention, home care, and follow-up care to client and family.
V. Evaluation
    A. Client reports increased comfort and decreased anxiety.
    B. Client remains free of injury.
    C. Client maintains adequate tissue perfusion.
    D. Client maintains good skin integrity.
    E. There is no bleeding.

F. Client and family demonstrate an understanding of disease process, diagnostic procedures, treatment including medication, prevention, home care, and follow-up care.

Acquired Immunodeficiency Syndrome

I. Description
    A. Human immunodeficiency virus (HIV): disorder that disrupts T lymphocytes, eventually destroying them and causing an immune deficiency
    B. Disease resulting in inability of body to defend itself against infection
    C. Progressive and fatal, with death occurring as result of opportunistic complications
    D. Causes
        1. HIV is spread by sexual contact, sharing of infected needles, and transfusions using blood or blood product containing HIV.
        2. The virus may also be transmitted by contaminated blood or body fluids in contact with broken skin surfaces.
        3. Infected mothers can pass the virus to their unborn infant.
II. Data collection
    A. Subjective symptoms
        1. Recurrent fever and night sweats
        2. Weight loss
        3. Anorexia
        4. Chronic diarrhea
        5. Fatigue, weakness
    B. Objective symptoms
        1. Swollen lymph glands
        2. White spots or lesions in oral cavity
        3. Dry cough
        4. Shortness of breath
        5. Presence of opportunistic infections such as Kaposi's sarcoma (purplish skin lesions) and *Pneumocystis carinii* pneumonia
III. Diagnostic tests and methods
    A. Client history
    B. Physical examination
    C. HIV or human T-cell lymphotropic virus type III (HTLV III) in serum
    D. Presence of opportunistic infections
    E. Lumbar puncture
    F. CT scan
    G. Bronchial biopsy
IV. Implementation
    A. Assess, report, and record signs and symptoms and any reaction to treatment.
    B. Protect client from opportunistic infections.
    C. Administer zidovudine (AZT) and other prescribed medications; check for side effects.
    D. Provide nutritional support.
    E. Monitor vital signs.
    F. Use blood and body fluid precautions:
        1. Protective clothing (e.g., gloves, masks, gowns)
        2. Good handwashing technique
        3. Careful labeling of specimens
        4. Appropriate disposal of contaminated articles
    G. Encourage physical independence.
    H. Monitor oxygen therapy.

I. Administer analgesics for pain.
J. Schedule rest periods.
K. Provide emotional support to client and family.
L. Provide information for support network.
M. Explain disease, mode of spread, protective measures, home care, and community resources.

V. Evaluation
A. Client reports increased comfort.
B. Client remains free of injury.
C. Client maintains adequate tissue perfusion.
D. Client demonstrates an understanding of disease process, mode of spread, protective measures, home care, and follow-up care.

Gastrointestinal System

Basic Information

- Breaks down food — carbohydrates, fats, and proteins — into molecules small enough to pass through cell membranes.
- Provides cells with necessary energy to function properly; prepares food for cellular absorption by altering its physical and chemical composition.
- Influenced by other systems: the endocrine, central nervous, and autonomic nervous systems, which serve as regulators.
- Malfunction of the GI tract has far-reaching metabolic effects on the body.

I. Basic data collection
A. Subjective symptoms
1. Nausea and vomiting
2. Difficulty in swallowing
3. Difficulty in chewing
4. Weight changes
5. Indigestion
6. Appetite change
7. Gas
8. Changes in bowel habits
9. Intolerance to certain foods
10. Personal and family history of GI-related problems
B. Objective symptoms
1. Stomatitis
2. Hematemesis
3. Abdominal distention
4. Jaundice
5. Constipation or diarrhea
6. Edema
7. Hemorrhoids
8. Stool changes: clay-colored, black, frothy
9. Dark urine

Major Gastrointestinal Diagnoses

Esophageal Varices

I. Description
A. Dilatation of blood vessels (varicose veins) at lower end of esophagus
B. Causes
1. Elevated pressure in portal vein (vessel bringing blood into liver) because of:

a. Cirrhosis of the liver
b. Mechanical obstruction of portal vein by blood clot or tumor or obstruction of the hepatic veins
C. Possibility that varices may rupture, causing hemorrhage and shock
D. Death from hemorrhage approximately 67%

II. Data collection
A. Subjective symptoms
1. Anxiety
2. History of cirrhosis, portal hypertension
3. Weakness, vertigo
B. Objective symptoms
1. Blood in emesis
2. Melena (black, tarry stools caused by bleeding)
3. Low Hgb and Hct values
4. Elevated AST, ALT, amylase, bilirubin levels; low albumin level
5. Hypotension
6. Tachycardia
7. Decreased level of consciousness
8. Signs of shock

III. Diagnostic tests and methods
A. Client history
B. Physical examination
C. Endoscopy to identify bleeding site
D. Laboratory studies: Hct, Hgb, liver function tests
E. Angiography

IV. Implementation
A. Monitor for hemorrhage and hypotension.
B. Monitor emesis and stool for presence of blood.
C. Monitor laboratory test results, and report abnormal findings.
D. Give oxygen, if prescribed.
E. Monitor vital signs at least every 4 hours (every half-hour if bleeding occurs).
F. Monitor I&O and CVP for volume determination.
G. Evaluate level of consciousness.
H. Provide emotional support and reassurance to client and family.
I. Provide mouth care.
J. Administer prescribed medications and monitor for side effects.
K. Administer and monitor IV infusion and blood transfusions as prescribed.
L. Keep client quiet and comfortable.

NOTE: Tolerance to sedatives and tranquilizers may be decreased because of liver disease.

M. Control bleeding by:
1. Giving ice water lavages
2. Assisting with insertion of Sengstaken-Blakemore tube if ordered (keep scissors taped to head of bed in case of emergency)
3. Administering vitamin K as prescribed
4. Monitoring vasopressin (Pitressin) effects (used to constrict splanchnic vessels)
N. Monitor client with Sengstaken-Blakemore tube for:
1. Bleeding in gastric drainage
2. Signs of asphyxiation
3. Tube displacement
4. Proper inflation of balloons
5. Correct traction to keep tube in correct placement

O. Assist with injection of sclerosing agent to control bleeding as ordered.
P. Monitor for signs of hepatic encephalopathy.
Q. Prepare client for surgery, if required to control bleeding.
R. Provide postoperative care; explain care to client and family.
S. Assist with preparation of client for discharge and self-care.
T. Explain disease process, prevention, and home care.

V. Evaluation
A. Client reports increased comfort and decreased anxiety.
B. Hematemesis is decreased or absent.
C. Melena is decreased or absent.
D. Vital signs remain stable.
E. Client maintains adequate fluid I&O.
F. Client maintains adequate nutritional intake.
G. Laboratory values remain within normal range.
H. Client demonstrates an understanding of disease process, prevention, and home care.

Hiatal Hernia

I. Description
A. Protrusion of part of stomach through weakened area of diaphragm into thoracic cavity
B. Gastric reflux (regurgitation) when the lower esophageal sphincter (muscle) pressure is less than the pressure in the stomach
C. Possibility of gastric reflux entering esophagus, resulting in inflammation and ulceration
D. Causes
1. Congenital weakness of diaphragm
2. Trauma
E. Related factors
1. Increased abdominal pressure
2. Relaxed esophageal sphincter
3. Pregnancy
4. Obesity
5. Smoking and alcohol and caffeine ingestion

II. Data collection
A. Subjective symptoms
1. Heartburn
2. Regurgitation
3. Dysphagia (difficulty in swallowing)
4. Feeling of fullness
5. History of trauma, obesity, pregnancy
6. Anxiety
B. Objective symptoms
1. Dyspnea (difficulty in breathing)
2. Discovered via diagnostic methods

III. Diagnostic tests and methods
A. Client history
B. Physical examination
C. Chest radiograph
D. Upper GI series (barium swallow)
E. Esophagoscopy

IV. Implementation
A. Provide small, frequent meals (bland diet: high protein, low fat).

B. Keep head of bed elevated when client is eating and up to 3 hours after meal.
C. Administer medications such as bethanechol (Urecholine), cimetidine (Tagamet), and antacids as prescribed.
D. Instruct client not to perform activities that increase abdominal pressure, such as lifting heavy objects, bending over, and wearing tight clothing around waist.
E. Instruct obese clients regarding weight management.
F. Keep head of bed slightly elevated during sleep periods.
G. Instruct client to avoid alcohol and caffeine.
H. Prepare client and family for surgical intervention, if conservative measures fail.
I. Provide postoperative care:
1. Assist with administration of and monitor IV therapy and blood transfusions.
2. Assist in insertion of NG tube and monitor effects.
3. Administer analgesics and antiemetics as prescribed.
4. Monitor medications for side effects.
5. Monitor fluid I&O.
6. Monitor vital signs.
7. Report incidence of gastric reflux immediately.
J. Explain condition and medication compliance to client and family.

V. Evaluation
A. Client reports increased comfort and decreased anxiety.
B. Client maintains adequate nutritional intake.
C. Symptoms disappear.
D. Client and family demonstrate an understanding of condition and medication compliance.

Peptic Ulcer

I. Description
A. Ulcerations in the gastric mucosal membrane.
B. Ulcerations can develop in lower esophagus, stomach, pylorus, duodenum, or jejunum:
1. Duodenal ulcer: approximately 80% occur in this area (proximal part of small intestine)
a. Ulcer occurs most often in men 20–50 years old.
b. Ulcer often becomes chronic, with remissions and exacerbations.
c. Complications requiring surgical intervention possible.
2. Gastric ulcer (stomach)
a. Ulcer occurs most often in middle-aged and elderly men.
b. Especially common among poor and undernourished.
c. Tendency of benign gastric ulcers to recur.
C. Both types of ulcers possibly asymptomatic.
D. Complications
1. Penetration to pancreas, causing severe back pain
2. Perforation of area involved
3. Hemorrhage
4. Pyloric obstruction
E. Possible causes:

1. Decreased mucus resistance
2. Inadequate mucosal blood flow
3. Defective mucus
4. Acid hypersecretion, possibly from overactive vagus nerve, likely to contribute to duodenal ulcer formation
5. Bacteria in stomach lining (*Helicobacter pylori*)

F. Related factors
   1. Chronic use of aspirin and alcohol
   2. Cigarette smoking
   3. Heredity
   4. Emotional stress
   5. Chronic use of drugs such as ibuprofen and corticosteroids

II. Data collection
   A. Subjective symptoms
      1. Gastric ulcer
         a. Heartburn
         b. Indigestion
         c. Feeling of fullness and distention after a large meal
      2. Duodenal ulcer
         a. Heartburn
         b. Pain (gnawing, burning) in middle-upper abdomen relieved by food ingestion
         c. Sensation of water bubbling in back of throat
         d. "Attacks" approximately 2 hours after meals or when stomach is empty
         e. Ingestion of citric juices, coffee, aspirin, or alcohol causing pain
   B. Objective symptoms
      1. Gastric ulcer
         a. Loss of appetite
         b. Possible repeated episodes of GI bleeding
         c. Weight loss
         d. Anemia
         e. Melena
         f. Vomiting: coffee-grounds appearance with bleeding
      2. Duodenal ulcer
         a. Weight gain from eating to relieve discomfort
         b. Vomiting and other digestive symptoms rare
         c. Possibility of complications: watch for GI bleeding, melena

III. Diagnostic tests and methods
   A. Client history
   B. Physical examination
   C. Upper GI series
   D. Gastric analysis
   E. Gastroscopy
   F. Laboratory studies: Hct, Hgb, electrolytes, CBC
   G. Biopsy of tissue to rule out malignancy/*H. pylori*

IV. Implementation
   A. Assess, report, and record signs and symptoms and any reactions to treatment.
   B. Provide quiet environment, and assist with comfort measures.
   C. Administer prescribed medications such as analgesics, sedatives, antacids, anticholinergics, histamine receptor antagonists (ranitidine [Zantac], cimetidine) to neutralize or inhibit gastric secretions, sedatives, and bismuth preparations.

D. Monitor and report medication side effects such as dizziness, rash, mild diarrhea, muscle pain, leukopenia, gynecomastia, dry mouth, blurred vision, headache, constipation, and urinary retention.
E. Monitor vital signs.
F. Monitor laboratory test results (Hct, Hgb, CBC, electrolytes).
G. Watch for signs of bleeding:
   1. Changes in vital signs
   2. Vomiting (coffee-ground appearance)
   3. Anemia
   4. Black and tarry or bloody stools
H. Provide prescribed diet: avoid irritating foods such as coffee and spices.
I. Discourage cigarette smoking.
J. Assist with preparation of client and family for surgical intervention, if required for recurrent ulcers, perforation, or hemorrhage.
K. Provide preoperative care:
   1. Assist in administration of blood replacement.
   2. Assist with insertion of nasogastric tube for gastric decompression.
   3. Provide reassurance to client and family.
L. Explain surgical intervention:
   1. Closure if perforation has occurred
   2. Total or partial resection of stomach or duodenum to remove ulcerated area(s)
   3. Pyloroplasty and vagotomy if gastric outlet is obstructed
M. Provide postoperative care
   1. Monitor vital signs (report abnormalities immediately).
   2. Administer narcotics and analgesics as prescribed for pain.
   3. Monitor fluid I&O.
   4. Assess for signs of dehydration, sodium deficiency, and metabolic alkalosis (may occur secondary to gastric suction).
   5. Assist in administration of blood transfusions and IV infusions, and monitor for side effects.
   6. Monitor patency of nasogastric tube; check, record, and report characteristics of drainage.
   7. Monitor and report signs of bleeding.
   8. Encourage coughing and deep breathing.
   9. Monitor elimination. Check bowel sounds. Keep client nothing by mouth (NPO) until peristalsis resumes and NG tube is removed or clamped.
   10. Watch for complications
       a. Hemorrhage, shock
       b. Iron folate, or vitamin B_{12} deficiency anemia (from continued blood loss or malabsorption)
       c. Dumping syndrome (weakness, nausea, diarrhea, gas pains, distention, and palpitations within 30 minutes after a meal)
   11. Begin nursing interventions if complications such as hemorrhage occur
       a. Monitor vital signs every half-hour, and report abnormalities immediately.
       b. Monitor fluid I&O.
       c. Provide complete bed rest, and keep client NPO as ordered.
       d. Provide quiet environment; allay anxiety.

e. Monitor NG drainage, presence of vomitus, bloody stools; report changes immediately.

f. Assist in administration of blood, IV fluids, and medications as prescribed.

N. Instruct client in prevention of dumping syndrome
1. Eating four to six small, high-protein, low-carbohydrate meals during the day
2. Sitting up or standing after meals
   a. Drink fluids between rather than with meals.
   b. Avoid eating large amounts of carbohydrates.

O. Instruct client that magnesium-containing antacids may cause diarrhea and that aluminum-containing antacids may cause constipation.

P. Instruct client to avoid drugs containing aspirin, as they irritate gastric mucosa.

Q. Advise client to avoid excessive use of coffee and alcohol and to avoid stressful situations.

R. Advise client to stop smoking, as it stimulates gastric secretions.

S. Explain condition, treatment including need for compliance, and home care.

V. Evaluation
A. Client reports increased comfort and decreased anxiety.
B. Client maintains adequate nutritional intake.
C. Symptoms disappear.
D. Laboratory values remain within normal range.
E. Client and family demonstrate an understanding of condition, treatment including need for compliance, and home care including lifestyle modification.

Crohn's Disease (Regional Enteritis)

I. Description
A. Inflammation of any part of the GI tract (usually the terminal ileum)
1. Lacteal blockage in intestinal wall, leading to edema.
2. Disease eventually leads to inflammation, ulceration, stenosis, abscess, and fistula formation.
B. Inflammation extending through all layers of the intestinal wall
C. "Cobblestone" ulcerations in intestinal lining, forming scar tissue
D. Bowel becoming thick and narrow
E. Possibly also involving regional lymph nodes and the mesentery
F. Possibility that ulcerations may perforate, resulting in fistulas leading to colon, bladder, vagina, and perianal area, as well as perirectal abscesses and perforations
G. Normal absorption of nutrients decreased owing to scar tissue formation
H. Possibility that strictures may develop, with potential for intestinal obstruction
I. Most prevalent in adults 20–40 years old
J. Two to three times more common in those of Jewish ancestry and least common in blacks
K. In up to 5% of affected clients, pattern of one or more affected relatives (inheritance pattern is not clear)
L. Possible causes (exact cause unknown)
1. Allergies and other immune disorders
2. Lymphatic obstruction

3. Infection
4. Environmental or genetic factors
5. Emotional stress
6. Heredity (genetic cause)

II. Data collection
A. Subjective symptoms
1. Abdominal pain and cramping
2. Tenderness
3. Gas pains
4. Nausea
5. Loss of appetite
6. Malaise, weakness, fatigue
7. Anxiety
8. Inability to cope with everyday stress
B. Objective symptoms
1. Elevated temperature
2. Diarrhea (four to six stools a day) containing pus, mucus, or blood
3. Marked weight loss
4. Anemia
5. Laboratory test results
   a. Elevated WBC count and ESR
   b. Hypokalemia
   c. Hypocalcemia
   d. Hypomagnesemia
   e. Depressed Hgb
6. Signs of dehydration (poor skin turgor, dry mucous membranes)
7. Results of stool specimen studies
8. Lower right quadrant tenderness

III. Diagnostic tests and methods
A. Client history
B. Physical examination
C. Stool specimen examination for occult blood
D. Laboratory studies: CBC, ESR, electrolytes, Hgb, Hct
E. Barium enema showing string sign (segments of stricture separated by normal bowel)
F. Endoscopy
G. Sigmoidoscopy or colonoscopy: patchy areas of inflammation possible (helps rule out ulcerative colitis)
H. Biopsy: for definitive diagnosis
I. Colonoscopy

IV. Implementation
A. Assess, report, and record signs and symptoms and any reaction to treatment.
B. Provide emotional support and adequate rest.
C. Record I&O (include amount of stool).
D. Weigh daily.
E. Watch for dehydration (decrease in urinary output, poor skin turgor).
F. Monitor fluid and electrolyte balance.
G. Monitor vital signs every 4 hours.
H. Watch for signs of intestinal bleeding (bloody stools):
1. Check stools daily for occult blood.
I. Provide prescribed diet
1. Restricted fiber diet with no fruit or vegetables for intestinal stenosis
2. Low-fat diet to decrease fatty stools as ordered
3. Elimination of dairy products for lactose deficiency
J. Administer prescribed medications, and monitor for side effects

1. Sulfasalazine for anti-inflammatory effects
2. Steroids to reduce inflammation (watch for GI bleeding, as steroids mask signs of infection)
3. Antibiotics to reduce risk of infection from peritoneal irritation, abscess, or fistulas
4. Sedatives
5. Analgesics
6. Anticholinergics
7. Bulk hydrophilic drugs to treat diarrhea

K. Check Hgb and Hct daily
   1. Administer iron supplements and blood transfusions as prescribed.
L. Provide mouth care.
M. Provide good skin care after each bowel movement.
N. Keep clean, covered bedpan within client's reach.
O. Ventilate room to eliminate odors.
P. Monitor client for fever or pain on urination (may indicate a bladder fistula).
Q. Monitor client for abdominal pain, fever, and hard, distended abdomen (may indicate intestinal obstruction).
R. Provide information regarding surgical intervention and postoperative course, if required (colectomy with ileostomy often required in clients with extensive disease of large intestine and rectum).
   1. Before ileostomy, request that an enterostomal therapist visit client.
S. Care during postoperative period
   1. Monitor IV infusion and NG tube for proper functioning.
   2. Monitor fluid I&O.
   3. Monitor vital signs.
   4. Watch for wound infection.
   5. Provide meticulous stoma care.
   6. Teach stoma care to client and family.
   7. Provide reassurance and emotional support (ileostomy changes client's body image).
T. Encourage reduction in stress (may need to refer client for counseling).
U. Explain disease process, diagnostic procedures, treatment including medication, home care including diet and bed rest, stoma care, sexuality, and follow-up care.

V. Evaluation
   A. Client reports increased comfort and decreased anxiety.
   B. Client maintains adequate nutritional and fluid intake.
   C. Client tolerates progressive activity.
   D. Client verbalizes concerns and problems.
   E. Client uses effective coping strategies.
   F. Client demonstrates an understanding of disease process, treatment, prevention, home care, and follow-up care.

Ulcerative Colitis

I. Description
   A. Inflammatory, often chronic, disorder of the large bowel, with rectal and sigmoid colon mucosae and submucosae becoming edematous and developing small bleeding lesions that result in ulcerations

   B. Inflammation often extending upward into entire colon; rarely affecting small intestine except for the terminal ileum
   C. Condition producing congestion, edema (resulting in mucosal friability)
   D. Ulcerations developing into abscesses
   E. Eventual loss of elasticity of colon, with a reduction in nutrient absorptive capability
   F. Severity ranging from a mild, localized condition to a severe disease that may result in a perforated colon, progressing to potentially fatal peritonitis and toxemia
   G. At risk for development of colorectal cancer
   H. Condition occurring primarily in young adults, especially women
   I. More prevalent in Jews and upper socioeconomic groups
   J. Overall, incidence rates increasing
   K. Causes unknown
   L. Possible predisposing factors
      1. Family history of disease
      2. Bacterial infection
      3. Allergic reaction to food, milk, or substances that release inflammatory histamine in the bowel
      4. Overproduction of enzymes that break down mucous membrane
      5. Autoimmune reactions such as arthritis and hemolytic anemia
      6. Environmental factors
      7. Emotional stress

II. Data collection
   A. Subjective symptoms
      1. Abdominal cramping pain
      2. Nausea
      3. Loss of appetite
      4. Irritability
      5. Anxiety
      6. Weakness
   B. Objective symptoms
      1. Bloody diarrhea containing pus and mucus
      2. Spastic rectum and anus
      3. Weight loss
      4. Vomiting

III. Diagnostic tests and methods
   A. Client history
   B. Physical examination
   C. Stool examination
   D. Sigmoidoscopy: shows increased mucosal friability; thick inflammatory exudate
   E. Colonoscopy with biopsy to determine extent of disease and evaluate strictures and pseudopolyps
   F. Barium enema to assess extent of disease and detect complications
   G. Laboratory studies: electrolytes, CBC, Hgb, Hct, ESR

IV. Implementation
   A. Assess, report, and record signs and symptoms and any reaction to treatment.
   B. Provide emotional support and adequate rest.
   C. Provide good skin care to prevent anal excoriation.
   D. Monitor the number, amount, time, and characteristics of stools.
   E. Provide client with air mattress or sheepskin to prevent skin breakdown.

F. Monitor bowel sounds every 4 hours in all four quadrants.

G. Administer prescribed medications, and monitor for side effects:

1. Corticosteroids (prolonged therapy causing "moonface," hirsutism, edema, gastric irritation)

H. Monitor vital signs.

I. Monitor I&O.

J. Watch for signs of dehydration (dry skin and mucous membranes, sunken eyes, fever).

K. Monitor Hgb, Hct, and electrolyte levels.

L. Assist with blood transfusions and IV therapy as prescribed.

M. Provide mouth care for those kept NPO.

N. Weigh daily.

O. Provide prescribed diet.

P. Assist with ADLs.

Q. Monitor for signs of complications such as perforated colon or peritonitis:

1. Fever
2. Severe abdominal pain
3. Rigid and tender abdomen
4. Cool, clammy skin
5. Abdominal distention and decreased or absent bowel sounds
6. Preparation of client for surgery if complications occur:
   a. Arrange for visit by an enterostomal therapist.

R. Provide postoperative care:

1. Give meticulous care and teach correct stoma care to client and family.
2. Monitor NG tube for patency.
3. After NG tube removal, provide a clear-liquid diet; advance to low-residue diet.

S. Prepare client for discharge; encourage regular physical examinations.

T. Explain disease process, treatment including compliance, prevention, and home care to client and family.

V. Evaluation

A. Client reports increased comfort and decreased anxiety.

B. Client maintains adequate nutritional and fluid intake.

C. Client continues progressive activity.

D. Client verbalizes concerns.

E. Client explains or demonstrates self-care.

F. Client and family demonstrate an understanding of disease process, treatment including compliance, prevention, home care, and follow-up care.

Diverticulosis and Diverticulitis

I. Description

A. Bulging pouches (diverticula) found in the GI wall.

B. Mucosal lining pushed through surrounding muscle by diverticula.

C. Most common site is sigmoid colon, although it may develop from proximal end of pharynx to anus.

D. Diverticular disease of ileum (Meckel's diverticulum) most common congenital anomaly of GI tract.

E. Two clinical forms of diverticular disease:

1. Diverticulosis

   a. Diverticula present but do not cause symptoms
   b. Possibly asymptomatic; usual occurrence before age 35 years

2. Diverticulitis

   a. Diverticula are inflamed and may cause severe obstruction, infection, or hemorrhage.
      1) Retained, undigested food mixing with bacteria in diverticular sac, resulting in a hard mass.
      2) Blood supply cut off to thin walls of the diverticular sac, becoming susceptible to bacteria found in the colon.
      3) Inflammation results.
   b. Condition usually occurs between 50 and 70 years of age and may result in spasms, obstruction, perforation, or bleeding.
   c. Inflamed colon segment possibly results in a fistula leading to the bladder or other organs.

II. Data collection

A. Subjective symptoms

1. Diverticulosis
   a. Usually asymptomatic
   b. In elderly persons, rare possibility of hemorrhage from diverticula in rectum (usually mild) as complication

2. Diverticulitis
   a. Recurrent pain in lower left quadrant relieved by bowel movement or passage of gas
   b. Mild nausea
   c. Vomiting when obstruction is present

B. Objective symptoms

1. Alternating constipation and diarrhea
2. Irregular bowel movements
3. Low-grade fever
4. Increased WBC count
5. Occult bleeding
6. If rupture occurs, abdominal rigidity, severe lower left quadrant pain, signs of sepsis and shock (high fever, chills, hypotension)
7. Rupture near blood vessel: mild to severe hemorrhage based on size of affected blood vessel
8. Constipation, ribbon-like stools, intermittent diarrhea, abdominal distention (signs of incomplete bowel obstruction) usually a result of chronic condition
9. Abdominal rigidity, decreased or absent bowel sounds, nausea, vomiting, abdominal pain (signs of increasing bowel obstruction)

III. Diagnostic tests and methods

A. Client history

B. Physical examination

C. Laboratory studies: CBC, ESR, Hgb, Hct, RBC count

D. Stool for occult blood

E. Radiographic series: to reveal possible spasms of the colon

F. Upper GI series: for diverticulosis of esophagus and upper bowel

G. Barium enema: for diverticulosis of lower bowel

1. In acute diverticulitis, enema may rupture bowel.

H. Sigmoidoscopy

I. Colonoscopy

IV. Implementation
   A. Continuously assess, report, and record signs and symptoms and any reaction to treatment.
   B. Provide emotional support.
   C. For diverticulosis with pain, constipation, mild GI distress, or difficulty with bowel movements:
      1. Provide prescribed diet (liquid or soft) during acute phase (helps to relieve symptoms, decrease irritation, and decrease progression to diverticulitis).
      2. Administer stool softeners and medications as prescribed.
      3. Monitor stools: check frequency, color, and consistency.
      4. Monitor vital signs (changes may indicate progression of condition).
      5. Encourage fluid intake.
      6. Provide high-roughage diet and bulk-forming agents once pain subsides.
   D. For mild diverticulosis without complications:
      1. Provide quiet environment and bed rest.
      2. Provide a liquid diet.
      3. Administer prescribed medications such as stool softeners, broad-spectrum antibiotics, analgesics for pain, smooth muscle relaxants, antispasmodics.
      4. Observe stools and record and report abnormalities.
      5. Monitor vital signs for changes.
      6. Monitor fluid I&O.
   E. For hemorrhage:
      1. Assist with administration of blood transfusions and IV therapy as prescribed.
      2. Monitor fluid and electrolyte balance.
   F. For surgical treatment for diverticulitis that does not respond to conservative therapy:
      1. Prepare client for colon resection.
      2. Prepare client for temporary colostomy in cases of perforation, peritonitis, obstruction, or fistula formation (to drain abscesses and rest colon before anastomosis).
      3. For postoperative care:
         a. Provide meticulous wound care.
         b. Watch for signs of infection.
         c. Check drain sites frequently (observe for pus, foul odor, or fecal drainage).
         d. Change dressings as necessary.
         e. Monitor fluid I&O.
         f. Observe for postoperative bleeding (decreased Hgb and Hct).
         g. Monitor other laboratory values (electrolytes; WBC, RBC counts).
         h. Instruct client to cough and breathe deeply (to prevent atelectasis).
         i. Monitor IV therapy.
         j. Monitor patency and placement of NG tube.
   G. Education
      1. Assist with teaching of colostomy care, if needed; arrange for visit by enterostomal therapist.
      2. Instruct client to avoid any activity that increases abdominal pressure, such as bending, wearing tight clothing around waist, and straining during bowel movement.

      3. Explain disease process, treatment, prevention, home care, including diet and stress management, and follow-up care.
V. Evaluation
   A. Client reports increased comfort and decreased anxiety.
   B. Client maintains adequate nutritional and fluid intake.
   C. Signs and symptoms disappear.
   D. Client demonstrates an ability to perform colostomy care if needed.
   E. Client demonstrates an understanding of disease process, treatment, prevention, home care, and follow-up care.

Intestinal Obstruction

I. Description
   A. Partial or complete blockage of the lumen in the small or large intestine
   B. Decreased or absent peristaltic movement of intestinal contents because of mechanical or neurological disorders
   C. Mechanical disorders including such conditions as scar tissue, strangulated hernias, and tumors
   D. Neurological disorders including paralytic ileus, which interferes with innervation, preventing normal peristaltic activity
   E. Pressure increasing as peristaltic activity attempts to move intestinal contents within intestine, resulting in:
      1. Dilation, atonicity of smooth muscle
      2. Prevention of flatus because of edema and decreased blood supply for elevated pressures
      3. Collection of gas occurring in distended intestine
   F. Complete obstruction if untreated; possibly causing death within hours from ischemia, necrosis, shock, and vascular collapse
   G. Intestinal obstruction more likely to occur after abdominal surgery or in persons with congenital defects of the bowel
   H. Causes
      1. Adhesions and strangulated hernias usual causes of small bowel obstruction
      2. Carcinomas and tumors usual causes of large bowel obstruction
      3. Obstruction caused by mechanical disorders
         a. Presence of foreign bodies such as fruit pits, gallstones, worms
         b. Compression of intestinal wall caused by
            1) Stenosis
            2) Intussusception (telescoping of bowel)
            3) Volvulus (twisting) of sigmoid or cecum
            4) Tumors
            5) Atresia
      4. Obstruction caused by physiological disturbances
         a. Electrolyte imbalances
         b. Toxicity (uremia, generalized infections)
         c. Paralytic ileus
         d. Spinal cord lesions
         e. Thrombosis or embolism of mesenteric blood vessels

I. Three forms of intestinal obstruction:
   1. Simple: intestinal contents blocked from passing; no other complications
   2. Strangulated: blockage of intestinal lumen, with lack of blood supply to part or all of obstructed section
   3. Close-looped: occlusion of both ends of the bowel section, isolated from rest of intestine
II. Data collection
   A. Subjective symptoms: small bowel obstruction
      1. Nausea
      2. Colicky pain
      3. Drowsiness
      4. Thirst
      5. Aching
      6. Dry mucous membranes
      7. Intestinal spasms
      8. Persistent epigastric pain
      9. Malaise, fatigue
   B. Subjective symptoms: large bowel obstruction
      1. Constipation
      2. Colicky abdominal pain with spasms
      3. Continuous hypogastric pain
      4. Nausea
   C. Objective symptoms: small bowel obstruction
      1. Vomiting
      2. Constipation
      3. Abdominal distention
      4. Presence of bowel sounds, borborygmi (rumbling in bowels)
   D. Objective symptoms: large bowel obstruction
      1. Constipation
      2. Leakage of liquid stool around obstruction: common in partial obstruction
      3. Intestinal spasms
      4. Fecal vomiting: usually absent at first
      5. Severe abdominal distention
III. Diagnostic tests and methods
   A. Client history
   B. Physical examination
   C. Radiography: flat plate of abdomen showing presence and location of intestinal gas or fluid
   D. Upper GI series
   E. Barium enema
   F. Laboratory studies: electrolytes, WBC count, amylase levels
IV. Implementation
   A. Continuously assess, report, and record signs and symptoms and any reaction to treatment.
   B. Provide emotional support.
   C. Keep client NPO.
   D. Monitor vital signs at least every 4 hours and report changes immediately.
   E. Assist with gastric or intestinal decompression to decrease nausea and vomiting.
   F. Monitor decompression tube; check and report amount and characteristics of drainage.
   G. Monitor patency of decompression tube; irrigate with normal saline, if ordered.
   H. Listen for presence or absence of bowel sounds; report presence of flatus or mucus through the rectum.
   I. Place client in Fowler's position to facilitate breathing and to decrease respiratory distress from abdominal distention.
   J. Monitor for signs of metabolic alkalosis (changes in consciousness; slow, shallow respirations; hypertonic muscles; tetany).
   K. Monitor for signs of metabolic acidosis (shortness of breath, disorientation; and later, deep, rapid breathing, malaise, and weakness).
   L. Monitor urinary output (assessment of circulating blood volume, renal function, possible urinary retention resulting from bladder compression by distended intestine).
   M. Assist with administration of and monitor IV therapy and electrolyte supplements.
   N. Provide mouth and nose care.
V. Monitor for signs of dehydration.
   A. Administer medications as prescribed.
   B. Prepare client and family for surgery and postoperative course, if required.
   C. Provide postoperative care:
      1. Encourage coughing, turning, and deep-breathing exercises to promote ventilation.
      2. Monitor bowel sounds (return of peristalsis) and elimination.
      3. Monitor fluid and electrolyte balance.
      4. Administer pain medication as prescribed.
      5. Assist with hygiene needs.
      6. Provide quiet, restful environment.
      7. Monitor nutritional status.
      8. Encourage early ambulation.
      9. Teach client and family colostomy care if required.
   D. Explain disease process, diagnostic procedures, treatment, home care, and follow-up care to client and family.
VI. Evaluation
   A. Client reports increased comfort and decreased anxiety.
   B. Client maintains adequate hydration and electrolyte balance.
   C. Client maintains adequate nutritional intake.
   D. Abdominal distention is decreased or absent.
   E. Adequate bowel sounds are present.
   F. Signs and symptoms disappear.
   G. Client maintains normal bowel movement pattern.
   H. Client demonstrates an understanding of disease process, diagnostic procedures, treatment, home care, and follow-up.

Hernias

I. Description
   A. Protrusion of an organ or structure through an abnormal opening of the containing wall of its cavity
   B. Categories of hernias
      1. Reducible: relatively easily returned back to its normal position
      2. Irreducible: unable to be returned to its normal position
      3. Incarcerated: unable to be reduced because of formation of adhesions in hernial sac, causing an obstruction of intestinal flow

4. Strangulated: part of herniated intestine becomes twisted or edematous, cutting off blood supply and interfering with peristalsis (may lead to intestinal obstruction and necrosis)

C. Types
1. Umbilical hernia
   a. Caused by abnormal muscular structures around umbilical cord
   b. Common in infants, often closing spontaneously
   c. Severe congenital hernia in which abdominal viscera protrude—requires immediate repair
   d. Possibly occurring in women who are obese or who have had several pregnancies
2. Inguinal hernia
   a. Large or small intestine, omentum, or bladder protruding into inguinal canal
   b. Caused by increased abdominal pressure
   c. May be direct or indirect
   d. More common in men
3. Femoral hernia
   a. Occurs where femoral artery passes into femoral canal
   b. Caused by increase in abdominal pressure from pregnancy or obesity
   c. Is more common in women
   d. Usually appears as a swelling or bulge at the pulse point of the femoral artery
   e. Usually is soft, reducible, nontender mass; may become incarcerated or strangulated
4. Incisional hernia
   a. Protrusion of intestine or other structure through a previous incision
   b. Caused by increased abdominal pressure and weakened abdominal wall

D. Causes
1. Congenital weakness in containing wall
2. Weakness in containing wall because of previous incisional infections or the aging process
3. Increased intra-abdominal pressure: heavy lifting, pregnancy, obesity, or straining
4. Improper closure of opening in peritoneal sac in male clients

II. Data collection
A. Subjective symptoms
1. Presence of abdominal or inguinal mass after straining, coughing, or exertion
2. Possible pain
3. Swelling relieved by lying down
4. Sharp, steady pain in groin (inguinal hernia)
5. Severe pain and nausea (strangulated hernia)
6. Signs of intestinal obstruction (strangulated hernia)
7. Anorexia
B. Objective symptoms
1. Palpable mass in umbilical, inguinal, or femoral area
2. Signs of intestinal obstruction
   a. Vomiting
   b. Irreducible mass
   c. Diminished or absent bowel sounds
   d. Shock

e. Increased temperature
f. Bloody stools
3. Undescended testicle or hydrocele in infants

III. Diagnostic tests and methods
A. Client history
B. Physical examination

IV. Implementation
A. Continuously assess, record, and report signs and symptoms and any reaction to treatment.
B. Monitor vital signs.
C. Restrict client's activities.
D. Monitor I&O.
E. Instruct client in use of truss, if prescribed, to keep hernia in place.
F. Observe for signs of strangulation:
1. Onset of pain
2. Nausea and vomiting
3. Abdominal distention
4. Signs of shock
5. Presence of blood in stools
G. Prepare client for surgical intervention if required
1. Report symptoms of sneezing or upper respiratory tract infections before surgery (may cause tension and pressure on surgical repair site).
H. Types of surgical intervention
1. Herniorrhaphy
   a. Surgical replacement of protruding part into its containing cavity
2. Hernioplasty
   a. Surgical reinforcement of the containing wall to prevent recurrence
I. Postoperative care
1. Monitor vital signs.
2. Apply ice packs as ordered to control pain and swelling.
3. Monitor urinary output after inguinal hernia repair.
4. Monitor I&O.
5. Encourage deep-breathing exercises. *Do not let client cough.*
6. Administer pain medications as prescribed.
7. Monitor incision site for signs of infection.
8. Assist with ambulation.
9. Explain condition, treatment, and home care to client and family:
   a. Take care of incision.
   b. Check for signs of infection.
   c. Restrict driving for at least 2 weeks.
   d. Restrict activities such as heavy lifting, pulling, or pushing for 6 weeks.
   e. Assure client that sexual activity is not affected.

V. Evaluation
A. Client reports increased comfort and decreased anxiety.
B. Client maintains adequate nutritional and fluid intake.
C. Signs and symptoms disappear.
D. Client remains free of postoperative complications.
E. Client and family demonstrate an understanding of condition, treatment, and home care including activity restrictions.

Hemorrhoids

I. Description
  A. Presence of varicosities or dilated hemorrhoidal veins in the rectal and anal area that interfere with venous return
  B. Possibly occurring internally, externally, or both
  C. Incidence highest between ages of 20 and 50 years and involves both sexes
  D. Types
    1. First-degree hemorrhoids: may itch because of poor anal hygiene
    2. Second-degree hemorrhoids: may prolapse (usually painless) and return to anal canal after a bowel movement
    3. Third-degree hemorrhoids: cause constant discomfort and prolapse because of increased intra-abdominal pressure; must be manually returned to anal canal
  E. Sudden rectal pain caused by thrombosis of external hemorrhoids
  F. Severe or recurrent rectal bleeding, possibly leading to secondary anemia with signs of pallor, fatigue, and weakness
  G. Probable cause: increased intravenous pressure in hemorrhoidal vessels
  H. Predisposing factors
    1. Occupation: extended periods of sitting or standing
    2. Pregnancy
    3. Heredity
    4. Straining caused by constipation, diarrhea, coughing, sneezing, or vomiting
    5. Heart failure
    6. Hepatic disease such as cirrhosis, amebic abscesses, or hepatitis
    7. Alcoholism
    8. Anorectal infections
    9. Loss of muscle tone (aging patterns)
    10. Rectal surgery
    11. Episiotomy
    12. Anal intercourse
II. Data collection
  A. Subjective symptoms
    1. Rectal pain or itching or both
    2. History of prior episodes
    3. Painless intermittent rectal bleeding on defecation
III. Diagnostic tests and methods
  A. Client history
  B. Physical examination
  C. Digital examination
  D. Proctoscopy
IV. Implementation
  A. Assess, report, and record signs and symptoms and any reaction to treatment.
  B. Provide privacy and time for bowel elimination.
  C. Administer topical medications as prescribed to shrink mucous membranes (local anesthetic agents such as lotions, creams, or suppositories), astringents, or cold compresses.
  D. Administer stool softeners to keep stool soft and to avoid straining.
  E. Assist with sitz bath to relieve pain.
  F. Assist with comfort measures and supportive care.
  G. Provide high-fiber diet to keep stools soft.
  H. Assist with injection of sclerosing agent to produce scar tissue as ordered.
  I. Assist with manual reduction of hemorrhoids as ordered.
  J. Provide postoperative care:
    1. Check for signs of prolonged rectal bleeding.
    2. Administer analgesics as prescribed for pain.
    3. Assist with sitz baths as prescribed.
    4. Promote elimination (check stool).
    5. Monitor vital signs.
    6. Resume oral feedings as ordered (administer bulk medications after evening meal).
    7. Instruct client not to use stool softeners soon after hemorrhoidectomy (firm stool helps to dilate blood vessels and prevent anal strictures from forming scar tissue).
    8. Provide meticulous wound care.
  K. Before discharge, assist with instruction of client and family about importance of high-fiber foods, regular bowel habits, and good anal hygiene.
  L. Instruct client to use medicated astringent pads and white toilet paper (chemicals in colored toilet tissue may irritate skin).
  M. Explain disease process, treatment, prevention of constipation, and home care including increased fluid intake and high-fiber diet.
V. Evaluation
  A. Client reports increased comfort and decreased anxiety.
  B. Client has no pain, bleeding, or constipation.
  C. Client maintains adequate hydration and nutritional status.
  D. Client and family demonstrate an understanding of disease process, treatment including medication, and home care including diet and hygiene.

Appendicitis

I. Description
  A. Inflammation of the appendix
  B. Possibly resulting in edema, abscess, necrosis, and rupture causing peritonitis, the most common emergent complication of appendicitis
  C. Occurring at any age and affecting both sexes
  D. Most prevalent in men between puberty and age 30 years
  E. Decreased incidence and death rate because of use of antibiotics
  F. Fatal if untreated
  G. Causes
    1. Obstruction to lumen of appendix because of kinking, fecal mass, barium ingestion, viral infections, or foreign bodies
    2. Decreased resistance to organisms within body (intestinal flora)
II. Data collection
  A. Subjective symptoms
    1. Abdominal pain in lower right abdomen (McBurney's point)

2. Anorexia
3. Nausea
4. Increased tenderness in area

   NOTE: Sudden cessation of abdominal pain indicates rupture of appendix.

B. Objective symptoms
   1. Vomiting
   2. Abdominal rigidity
   3. Retractive respirations
   4. Severe abdominal spasms
   5. Rebound tenderness

      NOTE: Rebound tenderness on left side indicates rupture or infarction of appendix.

   6. Constipation
   7. Slight fever
   8. Decreased bowel sounds
   9. Tachycardia
   10. Elevated WBC count: 12,000–15,000 mm³
III. Diagnostic tests and methods
   A. Client history
   B. Physical examination
   C. WBC count
   D. Routine urinalysis
   E. Evaluation to rule out illnesses with similar symptoms: gastritis, colitis, diverticulitis, pancreatitis, renal colic, bladder infection, ovarian cyst, and uterine disease
IV. Implementation
   A. Assess, report, and record signs and symptoms and any reaction to treatment.
   B. Maintain bed rest.
   C. Place client in Fowler's position to decrease pain.
   D. Use ice packs to abdomen as prescribed.
   E. Keep client NPO.
   F. Assist with the administration of and monitor IV fluids to prevent dehydration.
   G. Monitor electrolytes.
   H. Administer sedatives and antibiotics as prescribed (remember that narcotics can mask symptoms).
   I. Monitor vital signs.
   J. Do not apply heat to abdomen, as it may cause appendix to rupture.
   K. Do not administer cathartics or enemas, as these may cause rupture.
   L. Prepare client and family for surgical intervention.
   M. Provide postoperative care:
      1. Monitor vital signs.
      2. Monitor I&O.
      3. Administer analgesics and antibiotics as prescribed.
      4. Monitor, report, and record bowel sounds (sign of return of peristalsis, indicating readiness to resume oral fluid intake).
      5. Encourage deep breathing, coughing, and changing position.
      6. Monitor dressing and operative site for drainage and for signs of infection.
      7. Encourage ambulation as soon as possible.
      8. Encourage progressive nutrition.
      9. Observe for complications:

         a. Continuing pain may be caused by abscess formation.
         b. Complaint of "something gave away" may be indicative of wound dehiscence.
         c. Symptoms suggestive of peritonitis may occur.
V. Evaluation
   A. Client reports increased comfort.
   B. Client remains free of infection or avoidable complications.
   C. Client demonstrates an understanding of disease process, nature of surgery, and postoperative care.

Peritonitis

I. Description
   A. Acute or chronic inflammation of the peritoneum (membrane lining the abdominal cavity and covering the visceral organs)
   B. Inflammation that may extend throughout peritoneum or be localized
      1. Possibly affecting organs of abdominal cavity (adhesions, abscesses, and obstruction)
   C. Decreasing intestinal motility, resulting in intestinal distention with gas
   D. Approximately 10% mortality, most often caused by bowel obstruction
   E. Mortality rate much higher before advent of antibiotics
   F. Causes
      1. Bacterial invasion of peritoneum, usually from inflammation and perforation of GI tract:
         a. Appendicitis, diverticulitis, peptic ulcer, ulcerative colitis, volvulus, strangulated obstruction, abdominal neoplasm, or stab wound
         b. Common organisms including streptococci, staphylococci, *Escherichia coli,* pneumococci, and gonococci
      2. Chemical inflammation: rupture of ovarian tube or bladder, perforation of gastric ulcer, or release of pancreatic enzymes.
      3. In both bacterial and chemical inflammation, the body's normal immune response results in redness, edema, accumulation of fluids containing protein and electrolytes, adhesions, and abscess.
II. Data collection
   A. Subjective symptoms
      1. Sudden, severe, and diffuse abdominal pain
      2. Nausea
      3. Weakness
      4. Oliguria
      5. Thirst
      6. Shoulder pain: inflammation of diaphragmatic peritoneum
   B. Objective symptoms
      1. Excessive sweating
      2. Vomiting
      3. Cold skin caused by excess loss of fluid, electrolytes, and protein into abdominal cavity
      4. Decreased or absent bowel sounds caused by effect of bacterial toxins on intestinal muscles
      5. Hypotension
      6. Signs of dehydration: dry swollen tongue, pinched skin

7. Abdominal rigidity
8. Rebound tenderness
9. Increased temperature: 103°F (39.4°C) or higher
10. Hiccups (inflammation of diaphragmatic peritoneum)
11. Abdominal distention with upward displacement of diaphragm
12. Decreased respiratory capacity: tendency to breathe shallowly
13. Symptoms of shock
14. Elevated WBC count: >20,000/mm³

III. Diagnostic tests and methods
   A. Client history
   B. Physical examination
   C. Laboratory studies: WBC count, electrolytes, blood cultures
   D. Abdominal radiographs
   E. Chest radiographs: may show elevated diaphragm
   F. Paracentesis: reveals bacteria, exudate, blood, pus, or urine
   G. Laporatomy: may be required to identify underlying cause

IV. Implementation
   A. Assess, report, and record signs and symptoms and any reaction to treatment.
   B. Maintain bed rest.
   C. Place client in semi-Fowler's position.
   D. Assist with intestinal decompression: explain NG tube insertion.
   E. Assist with administration of and monitor IV infusion and electrolytes.
   F. Administer antibiotics as prescribed.
   G. Keep client NPO.
   H. Monitor fluid I&O.
   I. Monitor amount and characteristic of NG drainage or vomitus.
   J. Provide mouth care.
   K. If surgery is required, assist with explanation of surgical procedure to client and family.
   L. Administer preoperative analgesics as prescribed.
   M. Provide postoperative care
      1. Administer postoperative analgesics, antibiotics, and sedatives as prescribed; monitor for side effects.
      2. Monitor IV infusion and electrolytes.
      3. Accurately record and report fluid I&O, including NG and incisional drainage.
      4. Provide emotional support and allay anxiety.
      5. Observe client for disorientation; keep side rails up.
      6. Encourage and assist with ambulation as ordered.
      7. Watch for signs of dehiscence and abscess.
      8. Assess bowel sounds frequently for peristaltic motility (abdomen soft, distended) to determine peristaltic status.
      9. After return of peristalsis, normal temperature, and pulse rate, increase oral fluids as prescribed.
   N. Explain disease process, treatment, postoperative care, and home care to client and family.

V. Evaluation
   A. Client reports increased comfort and decreased anxiety.

B. Client remains free of infection.
C. Client remains free of complications from surgery.
D. Client and family demonstrate an understanding of disease process, treatment, and home care.

Colorectal Cancer and Polyps

I. Description
   A. Cancer of the colon and rectum that may be in the form of a well-defined tumor or cancerous polyp
   B. Incidence equally distributed between men and women
   C. Tending to progress slowly and remaining localized for a long time
   D. Potentially curable in 80%–90% of clients if diagnosed early
   E. Early treatment allowing for resection before nodes become involved
   F. Causes
      1. Unknown
   G. Potential predisposing factors
      1. Relationship to diet high in animal fats and low in fiber
      2. Other diseases of GI tract
      3. Age >40 years
      4. History of ulcerative colitis
      5. History of familial polyps

II. Data collection
   A. Subjective symptoms
      1. Initially vague
      2. Abdominal aching
      3. Abdominal pressure or cramps
      4. Weakness
      5. Fatigue
      6. Dizziness
      7. Loss of appetite
      8. Nausea
      9. Change in bowel habits and shape of stool
      10. Signs of obstruction in left colon
         a. Intermittent abdominal fullness or cramping
         b. Rectal pressure
         c. Dull and constant ache in rectal or sacral region
         d. Relief of pain after passage of gas or stool
   B. Objective symptoms
      1. Black tarry stools
      2. Presence of anemia
      3. Exertional dyspnea
      4. Diarrhea, obstipation
      5. Vomiting
      6. Signs of intestinal obstruction
      7. Possible palpable tumor on right side
      8. Rectal bleeding
      9. Ribbon- or pencil-shaped stool
      10. Dark-red blood and mucus in feces
      11. Cachexia

III. Diagnostic tests and methods
   A. Client history
   B. Physical examination
   C. Digital examination for presence of abnormalities
   D. Hemoccult test (guaiac) to detect blood in stools
   E. Proctoscopy or sigmoidoscopy

F. Colonoscopy to permit visual inspection and access for biopsy of tissue

G. IVP to evaluate kidney function

H. Barium radiograph to detect lesions

I. Tumor biopsy to verify disease

IV. Implementation

A. Assess, report, and record signs and symptoms and any reaction to treatment.

B. Monitor vital signs at least every 4 hours.

C. Monitor I&O.

D. Provide emotional support.

E. Administer medications as prescribed, and monitor for side effects.

F. Prepare client and family for surgical intervention.

G. Provide postoperative care

1. Explain to family the importance of positive reaction to client's adjustment.

2. Monitor IV therapy and electrolytes.

3. Monitor I&O.

4. Monitor dressings and wound drainage.

5. Administer medications to relieve pain as prescribed.

6. Provide emotional support.

7. Monitor perineal area if drain or packing was inserted.

8. Assist with sitz baths, if ordered.

9. Arrange for visit by enterostomal therapist if client has had a colostomy

a. Encourage client to examine stoma and to participate in its care as soon as possible.

b. Teach good hygiene and skin care.

c. Encourage client to shower or bathe as soon as incision heals.

d. Arrange for visit by dietitian regarding diet.

e. Instruct client regarding physical activities.

f. Request that a visit be made by home health nurse to check on client's physical condition and ability to care for self.

g. Encourage sexual counseling, if needed.

10. Encourage yearly screening and follow-up testing.

11. Explain disease process, treatment including medications, and home care to client and family.

V. Evaluation

A. Client reports increased comfort and decreased anxiety.

B. Client demonstrates ability to irrigate and care for stoma, if present.

C. Client verbalizes concerns.

D. Client and family demonstrate an understanding of disease process, treatment, home care including diet, and follow-up care.

Cholelithiasis, Choledocholithiasis, Cholangitis, and Cholecystitis

I. Description

A. Cholelithiasis

1. Presence of stones or calculi (gallstones) in the gallbladder

2. Prognosis usually good with treatment unless infection occurs

3. With infection, prognosis according to severity and response to antibiotics

4. Causes

a. Inflammation of biliary tract resulting in increased absorption of bile salts, which in turn decrease the solubility of cholesterol

b. Metabolic alterations resulting from periods of sluggishness in gallbladder as a result of pregnancy, diabetes mellitus, oral contraception, celiac disease, cirrhosis of the liver, or pancreatitis

B. Choledocholithiasis

1. Gallstones in hepatic and bile duct

2. Obstruction of bile flow into duodenum

3. Condition leading to elevated bilirubin level, jaundice, and interference with fat and fat-soluble vitamin absorption

4. Prognosis usually good unless infection occurs

C. Cholangitis

1. Infection of the bile duct

2. Frequent association with choledocholithiasis

3. Possible occurrence after percutaneous cholangiography

4. Inflammatory process possibly causing fibrosis and stenosis of common bile duct

5. Poor prognosis

6. Predisposing factors

a. Bacterial alteration of bile salts

b. Metabolic alterations of bile salts

D. Cholecystitis

1. Acute or chronic inflammation of gallbladder

2. Usual association with impacted gallstone in the cystic duct

3. Painful distention of gallbladder

4. Acute form common in middle-aged, overweight adults

5. Chronic form common among older persons

6. Prognosis good with treatment

II. Data collection

A. Subjective symptoms

1. Acute abdominal pain in right upper quadrant after high-fat meals

2. Pain radiating to back, between shoulders, or front of chest

3. Fat intolerance

4. Indigestion

5. Flatulence

6. Nausea

7. Chills

8. Weakness

9. Fatigue

10. Pruritus

B. Objective symptoms

1. Belching

2. Profuse sweating

3. Vomiting

4. Jaundice

5. Abdominal distention

6. Absence of bowel sounds in severe cholangitis

7. Elevated WBC count

8. Elevated bilirubin level

9. Clay-colored stool

10. Dark urine
11. Increase in temperature, heart rate, respiration, and BP
12. Calculi observed on cholecystogram
13. Prolonged PT resulting from interference with vitamin K absorption
14. Easy bruising

III. Diagnostic tests and methods
   A. Client history
   B. Physical examination
   C. Laboratory studies: WBC count, total bilirubin, urine bilirubin, icteric index, alkaline phosphatase, prothrombin time (PT)
      1. Serum amylase levels to differentiate between gallbladder disease and pancreatitis
      2. Serial enzyme tests and ECG to rule out heart disease
   D. Oral cholecystography
   E. IV cholangiography

IV. Implementation
   A. Assess, report, and record signs and symptoms and any reaction to treatment.
   B. Administer analgesics for pain as prescribed.
   C. Administer antibiotics and antispasmodics as prescribed.
   D. Monitor for medication side effects.
   E. Keep client NPO.
   F. Provide mouth care.
   G. Assist with administration of and monitor IV therapy.
   H. Monitor I&O.
   I. Monitor laboratory studies.
   J. Monitor vital signs and any incidence of bleeding (e.g., urine, gums).
   K. Explain and assist with diagnostic procedures.
   L. Provide postoperative care:
      1. Monitor dressing.
      2. Monitor T-tube drainage (if T-tube present).
      3. Monitor NG tube for drainage.
      4. Assist with administration of and monitor IV therapy.
      5. Administer medications as prescribed.
      6. Assist in ambulation if ordered.
      7. Provide prescribed diet if ordered.
      8. Encourage deep breathing, coughing, and turning.
   M. Explain disease process, treatment including medication, prevention, and home care including dietary restrictions
      1. Diet: low-fat, maintain calories
      2. Activity
      3. Caring for T-tube, if present
      4. Observing for signs of infection
      5. Follow-up care

V. Evaluation
   A. Client reports increased comfort and decreased anxiety.
   B. Client remains free of infection or complications.
   C. Client maintains adequate nutritional intake.
   D. Client resumes activity gradually.
   E. Client and family demonstrate an understanding of disease process, treatment including surgical intervention, prevention, and home care.

Hepatitis A, B, C, D, and E

I. Description
   A. Viral inflammation of the liver caused by hepatotoxins, viral agents, or drugs
   B. Marked liver destruction, necrosis, and autolysis
   C. More than 70,000 cases reported annually
   D. Complications
      1. Chronic persistent hepatitis (may be benign)
      2. Chronic aggressive hepatitis
         a. Fatal in approximately 25% of cases (from hepatic failure)
      3. Fulminating hepatitis
         a. Life-threatening complication
         b. Development in about 1% of clients, causing hepatic failure with encephalopathy
         c. Progression to coma and death in approximately 2 weeks
   E. Preventive measures
      1. Enteric isolation
      2. Good handwashing technique
      3. Vaccination and immune globulin therapy
      4. Avoiding contact with blood or body fluids
   F. Five forms
      1. Hepatitis A
         a. Highly infectious (short-incubation hepatitis)
         b. Cause: hepatitis A virus (HAV)
         c. Usually transmitted by contact with feces or contaminated water or food
         d. Occasionally transmitted parenterally
         e. Outbreaks often following ingestion of contaminated seafood
         f. Incubation period 15–50 days
         g. Tending to be benign and self-limiting
         h. High-risk individuals: children, travelers to developing countries, health-care personnel
      2. Hepatitis B
         a. Serum (long-incubation hepatitis)
         b. Cause: hepatitis B virus (HBV)
         c. Rare occurrence in epidemics
         d. Higher mortality than hepatitis A
         e. Generally parenteral transmission: blood transfusion, direct contact
         f. Possible spread through contact with human secretions and feces
         g. Incidence rising among homosexuals: oral and sexual contact
         h. Incubation period 5–10 weeks
         i. High-risk individuals: parenteral drug users, health-care workers in contact with contaminated blood or body fluids
      3. Non-A, non-B hepatitis (hepatitis C)
         a. Mildest course of all types of hepatitis
         b. Cause: virus other than HAV or HBV
         c. Transmission by blood contact: usually from commercial blood donations
         d. Incubation period 14–150 days
         e. No specific diagnostic tests
         f. High-risk individuals: those receiving blood transfusions or those who come in contact with contaminated blood, persons with tattoos, body piercing, and use of cocaine (snorting)

4. Hepatitis D
   a. Cause: incomplete virus
   b. Complication of hepatitis B
5. Hepatitis E
   a. Cause: RNA virus
   b. Incubation period 2–9 weeks

II. Data collection
   A. Subjective symptoms: preicteric phase (lasts 1 week)
      1. Chills
      2. Anorexia
      3. Nausea
      4. Malaise, weakness
      5. Fatigue
      6. Headache
      7. Photophobia
      8. Pharyngitis
      9. Cough
      10. Respiratory difficulty, especially in hepatitis A
      11. Arthralgia, especially in hepatitis B
      12. Alterations in sense of taste and smell
      13. Loss of desire to smoke or to drink alcohol
   B. Subjective symptoms: icteric phase (lasts 2–6 weeks)
      1. Mild weight loss
      2. Continued anorexia
      3. Discomfort and pain in right upper abdominal quadrant
      4. Increased nausea
      5. Increased malaise and weakness
      6. Increased respiratory difficulty
      7. Pruritus
      8. Irritability
   C. Subjective symptoms: posticteric phase (lasts 2–6 weeks, with full recovery in 6 months)
      1. Decline in nausea, anorexia, and dyspnea
      2. Increased comfort
      3. Decreased weakness
   D. Objective symptoms: preicteric phase
      1. Dyspnea
      2. Vomiting
      3. Cough, coryza
      4. Elevated temperature
      5. Liver and lymph node enlargement
   E. Objective symptoms: icteric phase
      1. Dark urine
      2. Clay-colored stools
      3. Yellow sclera
      4. Liver that remains tender and enlarged
      5. Pain in right upper quadrant
      6. Splenomegaly
      7. Cervical adenopathy
      8. Bile obstruction
      9. Onset of jaundice
      10. Elevated serum bilirubin levels
      11. Elevated bilirubin and urobilinogen in urine
      12. Prolonged PT and partial thromboplastin time (PTT)
      13. Elevated aspartate aminotransferase (AST), alanine aminotransferase (ALT), alkaline phosphate levels
      14. Decreased serum albumin level
   F. Objective symptoms: posticteric phase
      1. Decreased jaundice

2. Decreased dyspnea and anorexia
3. Resolution of abnormal laboratory test results
   G. Posticteric phase
      1. Lasts 2–6 weeks
      2. Relapse may occur
      3. Remains fatigued, liver decreases

III. Diagnostic tests and methods
   A. Client history
   B. Physical examination
   C. Presence of hepatitis B surface antigens (HBsAg) and hepatitis B antibodies (anti-HBs) to confirm hepatitis B
   D. Presence of anti-HAV antibody to confirm hepatitis A
   E. Absence of anti-HAV, HBsAg, and anti-HBs to confirm non-A, non-B hepatitis
   F. PT
   G. AST and ALT levels, serum alkaline phosphatase level
   H. Serum albumin, globulin, and bilirubin levels
   I. Urine bilirubin level
   J. Liver biopsy
   K. Computed tomographic (CT) scan of liver

IV. Implementation
   A. Assess, report, and record signs and symptoms and any reaction to treatment.
   B. Provide restful environment.
   C. Assist with comfort measures.
   D. Provide emotional support.
   E. Monitor I&O.
   F. Monitor body weight.
   G. Provide and encourage adequate caloric intake (orally or IV).
   H. Limit visitors and impose Universal Precautions.
   I. Encourage fluid intake.
   J. Observe feces for color, consistency, frequency, and amount.
   K. Watch for signs of dehydration, pneumonia, vascular problems, decubitus ulcers, and hepatic coma.
   L. Administer prescribed medications such as antiemetics, antibiotics, vitamin K, antihistamines, corticosteroids, and fluid and electrolyte replacement.
   M. For clients with fulminant hepatitis:
      1. Maintain electrolyte balance.
      2. Maintain patent airway.
      3. Control bleeding.
      4. Administer prescribed medications to correct hypoglycemia.
   N. Schedule rest periods.
   O. Monitor laboratory results.
   P. Monitor for signs of bleeding.
   Q. Check skin integrity.
   R. Explain disease process, diagnostic procedures, treatments, prevention, Universal Precautions, home care, and follow-up care to client and family.

V. Evaluation
   A. Client reports increased comfort and decreased anxiety.
   B. Client remains free of infection.
   C. Client maintains adequate nutritional and fluid intake.
   D. Client demonstrates an understanding of disease process, diagnostic procedures, treatment, prevention, enteric isolation procedure, and home care.

Cirrhosis of the Liver

I. Description
  A. Chronic hepatic disease with diffuse destruction and fibrotic regeneration of liver cells
  B. Liver structure and vasculature altered, resulting in impaired blood and lymph flow, leading to hepatic insufficiency
  C. Prevalent among malnourished chronic alcoholics >50 years of age
  D. Fifty percent more common in men than in women
  E. High mortality rate
  F. Six types of cirrhosis
    1. Portal, nutritional, or alcoholic cirrhosis (Laënnec's type)
      a. Most common: occurs in 30%–50% of clients; 90% of clients have history of alcoholism
      b. Liver damage primarily from malnutrition, especially lack of protein
    2. Biliary cirrhosis
      a. Affects 15%–20% of clients
      b. Results from bile duct diseases that disrupt bile flow
    3. Postnecrotic (posthepatic) cirrhosis
      a. Affects 10%–30% of clients
      b. Results from various types of hepatitis
    4. Idiopathic cirrhosis
      a. Affects about 10% of clients
      b. Has no known cause
II. Data collection
  A. Subjective symptoms
    1. GI system: anorexia, indigestion, nausea, constipation, flatus, dull abdominal ache
    2. Respiratory difficulties
    3. CNS: lethargy, mental changes
    4. Hematological: easy bruising
    5. Endocrine: menstrual irregularities
    6. Skin: itching
    7. Miscellaneous: fatigue, pain in upper right abdomen
  B. Objective symptoms
    1. GI system: vomiting, constipation, and diarrhea or constipation
    2. Respiratory system: decreased thoracic expansion as a result of abdominal ascites
    3. Decreased gas exchange: hypoxia
    4. CNS: slurred speech, asterixis, peripheral neuritis, hallucinations, unconsciousness, and coma
    5. Hematological: nosebleeds, bruising, bleeding gums, anemia, increased bleeding time
    6. Endocrine: testicular atrophy, menstrual irregularities, loss of hair on chest and axillary region
    7. Skin: pruritus, poor tissue turgor, extreme dryness, spider angiomas, palmar erythema, jaundice
    8. Hepatic: jaundice, ascites, edema of legs, enlarged liver, hepatorenal syndrome, hypoglycemia
    9. Miscellaneous: enlarged superficial abdominal veins, muscle atrophy, palpable liver or spleen, elevated temperature, bleeding from esophageal varices resulting from portal hypertension, hypernatremia, hypoalbuminemia
    10. Elevated AST, ALT, LDH, bilirubin, ammonia levels

III. Diagnostic tests and methods
  A. Client history
  B. Physical examination
  C. Laboratory studies: WBC count, Hgb, Hct, albumin, bilirubin, alkaline phosphatase, serum ammonia, serum electrolytes, globulin, thymol turbidity, AST, ALT, LDH, PT, and PTT
  D. Bromsulfphthalein (BSP) excretion test
  E. Glucose tolerance test
  F. Urine bilirubin level
  G. Fecal urobilinogen level
  H. Liver biopsy
  I. Cholecystography
  J. Cholangiography
IV. Implementation
  A. Assess, report, and record signs and symptoms and any reaction to treatment.
  B. Monitor skin, gums, stools, and emesis for bleeding tendencies.
  C. Apply pressure to injection sites to prevent bleeding.
  D. Advise client not to take aspirin, blow nose, strain during bowel movement, or sneeze.
  E. Monitor weight daily.
  F. Measure abdominal girth daily.
  G. Monitor sacrum, legs, and ankles for presence of dependent edema.
  H. Monitor vital signs.
  I. Monitor electrolytes and other laboratory results.
  J. Monitor I&O accurately.
  K. Assist with comfort measures.
  L. Provide emotional support.
  M. Provide counseling on alcoholic consumption.
  N. Provide mouth care.
  O. Place in high-Fowler's position to assist in breathing when ascites is present.
  P. Prepare client for paracentesis, if necessary.
  Q. Administer prescribed medication such as diuretics; vitamins A, C, and K; folic acid; electrolyte supplements; IV fluids; antiemetics; antihistamines; and albumin.
  R. Use lubricating lotion in place of soap when giving skin care to prevent skin breakdown in clients who have edema and pruritus.
  S. Monitor skin integrity; avoid intramuscular injections.
  T. Provide diet high in protein, high in carbohydrates, and containing vitamins. (High-protein diet is contraindicated in presence of portal system encephalopathy [PSE] because the liver is not able to metabolize amino acids or ammonia; proteins are broken down to amino acids.)
  U. Explain disease process, diagnostic procedures, treatment including medications, prevention, home care, and follow-up care to client and family.
V. Evaluation
  A. Client reports increased comfort and decreased anxiety.
  B. Client maintains adequate fluid and electrolyte balance.
  C. Client maintains effective breathing pattern.
  D. Ascites and edema are reduced.
  E. Client remains free of injury or infection.

F. Client maintains good skin integrity.

G. Client maintains adequate nutritional intake.

H. Client and family demonstrate an understanding of disease process, diagnostic procedures, treatment, prevention, home care, and follow-up care.

Pancreatitis

I. Description

  A. Inflammation of the pancreas

  B. Acute and chronic forms

    1. Acute form: sudden occurrence, with one attack or recurrent attacks; followed by resolution

    2. Chronic form: continuous inflammation and destruction of pancreas, with proliferations of scar tissue in place of normal pancreatic tissue

  C. Common association with edema, necrosis, or hemorrhage

  D. Common association with alcoholism, trauma, or peptic ulcer in men

  E. Common association with biliary tract disease in women

  F. Prognosis poor when cause is alcoholism

  G. Prognosis good when cause is biliary tract disease

  H. Mortality up to 60% when condition associated with necrosis and hemorrhage

  I. Causes

    1. Most common causes are biliary tract disease and alcoholism.

    2. Other causes include pancreatic carcinoma, trauma, certain drugs, complication of peptic ulcer, mumps, or hypothermia.

  J. Increased permeability of the vascular bed, leading to further edema

  K. Damaged islets of Langerhans, possibly leading to complications including diabetes mellitus.

  L. Fulminant pancreatitis, causing massive hemorrhage and destruction of pancreatic tissue, ending in diabetic acidosis, shock, coma, and/or death

II. Data collection

  A. Subjective symptoms

    1. Abdominal discomfort or pain centered close to umbilicus and unrelieved by vomiting

    2. Severe attack: severe abdominal pain

    3. Relief of pain by drawing knees up

    4. Malaise

    5. Restlessness

    6. Nausea

    7. History of alcohol intake, previous trauma, surgery, gallbladder disease

    8. Chills

    9. Weight loss

  B. Objective symptoms

    1. Severe attack: persistent vomiting, abdominal rigidity, diminished bowel sounds, rales at bases of lungs, left pleural effusion

    2. Dehydration

    3. Elevated temperature

    4. Tachycardia

    5. Cold, sweaty extremities

    6. Elevated enzyme levels

    7. Elevated WBC count, bilirubin, blood glucose, serum amylase, serum lipase, Hct

    8. Decreased serum calcium level

    9. ECG changes: prolonged QT segment, normal T wave

    10. Abdominal radiograph: dilation of small or large intestine

    11. GI series: pressure on duodenum or stomach because of edema of pancreas head

    12. Paracentesis: exceedingly high amylase levels

    13. Positive stool test results for meat fibers, fat in chronic pancreatitis

    14. Chronic form showing calcification on CT scan or ultrasound

III. Diagnostic tests and methods

  A. Client history

  B. Physical examination

  C. Laboratory tests: serum amylase, serum lipase, serum calcium, WBC count, serum glucose, Hct

  D. Routine ECG

  E. Abdominal radiographs

  F. GI series

  G. Chest radiographs

  H. Paracentesis

IV. Implementation

  A. Position client to relieve pain.

  B. Keep client NPO to allow pancreas to rest.

  C. Explain and assist in insertion of NG tube to allow pancreas to rest.

  D. Monitor I&O.

  E. Monitor vital signs continuously.

  F. Provide meticulous supportive care.

  G. Monitor pulmonary artery pressure closely if present.

  H. Monitor CVP line closely if present.

  I. Monitor fluid I&O.

  J. Monitor electrolyte, BUN, and creatinine levels.

  K. Assist in administration of IV fluids or blood as ordered.

  L. Assist in administration of plasma to maintain BP if ordered.

  M. Assess for rales and decreased breath sounds.

  N. Maintain constant NG suctioning to decompress bowel if required.

  O. Provide good oral and nose hygiene.

  P. Provide emotional support.

  Q. Start client on clear liquids, progressing to bland low-fat diet in small feedings daily once oral intake is ordered.

  R. Monitor for signs and symptoms of complications such as hyperglycemia or hypoglycemia and respiratory difficulties.

  S. Explain condition, diagnostic procedures, treatment including medication, health maintenance procedures such as avoidance of alcohol and adequate nutrition, home care, and follow-up care to client and family.

V. Evaluation

  A. Client reports increased comfort and decreased anxiety.

  B. Client maintains adequate nutritional intake.

  C. Client maintains fluid and electrolyte balance.

  D. Client and family demonstrate an understanding of

disease process, treatment including medications, health maintenance procedures, home care, and follow-up care.

Integumentary System (Skin)

Basic Information

The skin acts as the body's barrier and protector against the environment. The functions of the skin include temperature regulation, sensation, and excretion of small amounts of water and sodium chloride. It protects the body tissues and organs from external insults such as injury. Proper nutrition, hydration, exercise, rest, and electrolyte balance are required to maintain a healthy integumentary system.

I. Basic data collection
  A. Subjective symptoms
    1. History: onset of problem, changes, presence of pain, burning, itching sensations
    2. Allergic reactions
    3. Changes in lifestyle: e.g., diet, medications, environment, detergents
    4. Change in body image
    5. Changes in activities because of disease or condition
  B. Objective symptoms
    1. Skin
      a. Color: deviations from normal such as pallor, jaundice, cyanosis
      b. Temperature: differences in feeling of warmth, coolness
      c. Turgor: elasticity (hydration)
      d. Pressure sores: location, size, odor, color, edema, open wound
      e. Cleanliness of skin
    2. Hair
      a. Texture: coarse, fine
      b. Lice
      c. Absence of body hair
    3. Scalp
      a. Scars
      b. Parasites
    4. Nails
      a. Shape
      b. Cleanliness
      c. Brittleness

Major Integumentary Diagnoses

Burns

I. Description
  A. Injury to the skin from dry or moist heat, chemicals, electrical currents, or radiation that destroys the skin's normal protective function
  B. Physiological changes
    1. Depend on the severity of the burn; exposure to heat source
      a. Loss of protective barrier against infection
      b. Decreased sensory perception
      c. Loss of body fluids and electrolytes
      d. Loss of body temperature regulation
      e. Damage to sweat and sebaceous glands
  C. Two stages of physiological changes
    1. Hypovolemic stage
      a. Intravascular fluid shifting into interstitial space around burn, resulting in increased permeability of capillaries and cells; resultant vasodilation
      b. Leakage of protein and sodium into area, with edema and blister formation
      c. Occurring at onset of injury
      d. Possibly leading to dehydration of healthy tissue, oliguria, hypoproteinemia, hypovolemic shock, hyperkalemia, hyponatremia, respiratory distress, and metabolic acidosis, depending on burn severity
    2. Diuretic stage
      a. Beginning after initial injury
      b. Intravascular volume and capillary integrity restored
      c. Resulting in increased blood volume, increased renal function, and diuresis
      d. Possibly causing hypokalemia, fluid overload, sodium deficit, metabolic acidosis, anemia, and malnutrition
  D. Classification of burns
    1. Superficial partial thickness burn (first degree)
      a. Involve epidermis
      b. Presence of erythema (redness), edema, and pain
    2. Deep partial-thickness burn (second degree)
      a. Involve epidermis and part of dermis
      b. Presence of blisters and mottled, white, or red skin
      c. Mild or moderate edema and pain
      d. Heals with undamaged epithelial cells
    3. Full-thickness burn (third degree)
      a. Involve both epidermis and dermis
      b. Presence of white, leathery tissue (eschar) and thrombosed blood vessels
      c. Possibly extending through subcutaneous tissue to muscle and bone (fourth degree)
      d. Presence of charred, white, dark, black, or red skin
      e. Absence of pain because of total nerve damage
      f. Requiring skin grafting to repair injury because of extent of damage
  E. Use of "Rule of Nines" chart, taking into account client's age
    1. Measured by percentage of body surface area (BSA) covered by burn
    2. Allows estimate of size of burn
    3. Correlation of size and depth of burn allows estimation of severity
  F. Classification of severity of burn
    1. Minor
      a. Third-degree burn on <2% of BSA
      b. Second-degree burn on <15% of adult BSA (10% in children)
    2. Moderate
      a. Third-degree burn on 2%–10% of BSA

b. Second-degree burn on 15%–25% of adult BSA (>10% in children)
3. Major
  a. Third-degree burn on >10% of BSA
  b. Second-degree burn on >25% of adult BSA (>20% in children)
  c. Burns of eyes, ears, face, hands, feet, or genitalia
  d. Electrical burns
  e. Burns in presence of fractures or with respiratory damage
  f. All burns in poor-risk clients
    1) Children <4 years old; adults >60 years old
    2) Clients with history of complicating medical problems (e.g., disorders that impair peripheral circulation, such as diabetes and coronary artery disease)

II. Data collection
  A. Subjective symptoms
    1. Pain (depending on degree of burn)
    2. Anxiety
    3. Confusion
  B. Objective symptoms
    1. Skin appearance: indicative of type of burn
    2. Infection
    3. Loss of body tissue (protein)
    4. Hypoproteinemia (protein shifts into tissue space around injury)
    5. Electrolyte imbalance
    6. Decreased serum sodium levels
    7. Dehydration
    8. Edema
    9. Oliguria
    10. Hypovolemic shock caused by fluid loss or shift
    11. Hematuria caused by hemolysis of RBCs and decreased blood flow
    12. Signs of neurogenic shock
    13. Respiratory distress caused by hypovolemic shock, inhalation injury, or airway obstruction

III. Diagnostic tests and methods
  A. Client history
  B. Physical examination

IV. Implementation
  A. Anticipate and prevent respiratory distress
    1. Maintain airway (may be intubated if head or neck or both are involved, or for inhalation injury).
    2. Monitor breathing every hour; then every 4 hours when stable.
    3. Keep tracheostomy equipment available.
  B. Keep client NPO for first 24 hours as ordered.
  C. Monitor vital signs and CNS status frequently.
  D. Insert catheter and urinary drainage as ordered.
  E. Assist in insertion of CVP lines and other IV lines.
  F. Assist in administration of rapid fluid replacement as prescribed.
  G. Monitor I&O hourly.
  H. Monitor for presence of hematuria.
  I. Monitor serum and urine electrolytes and Hct.
  J. Monitor weight daily.

    NOTE: Weight gain of 15%–20% is expected in first 72 hours related to fluid shifts.

K. Administer analgesics for pain as prescribed.
L. Avoid heavy sedation to prevent respiratory complications.
M. Administer prophylactic tetanus as prescribed.
N. Monitor burn site for appearance, fluid loss, infection, and damage extent.
O. Monitor pulses in all extremities if possible.
P. Monitor oxygen.
Q. Dress burned area and change dressings:
  1. Administer analgesic for pain before dressing changes.
  2. Clean and debride burn area with antiseptic agents and prescribed dressing.
  3. Apply appropriate wet dressings as prescribed.
R. Anticipate infection: maintain asepsis; reverse isolation; administer antibiotics; monitor vital signs frequently.
S. Anticipate shock: assess level of consciousness and mental state; monitor vital signs.
T. Prevent complications of immobilization: provide proper alignment to prevent deformities; prevent skin surfaces from touching by use of turning frames, cradles.
U. Assess for GI distress or bleeding.
V. Administer topical agents such as mefenide acetate (Sulfamylon cream), silver sulfadiazine (Silvadene cream), or silver nitrate to prevent infection and assist in the healing process as ordered.
W. Monitor for presence of paralytic ileus and impaction.
X. Assist with preparation of client for skin grafts if required.
Y. Provide adequate nutritional intake (after acute phase) (diet high in protein, vitamins, carbohydrates, fat, and calories).
Z. Provide frequent mouth and skin care.
AA. Encourage coughing and deep-breathing exercises.
BB. Assist in use of coping measures.
CC. Allow client to discuss feelings regarding condition.
DD. Explain home care and follow-up care:
  1. Caring for burn
  2. Skin care
  3. Medications
  4. Protective measures against irritants and infection
  5. Signs of complications
  6. Need for follow-up care
EE. Provide for counseling.

V. Evaluation
  A. Client remains free of infection or injury.
  B. Client reports increased comfort and decreased anxiety.
  C. Client maintains effective airway and breathing patterns.
  D. Client maintains fluid and electrolyte balance.
  E. Client maintains adequate cardiac output.
  F. Client maintains adequate I&O.
  G. Client maintains adequate nutritional intake.
  H. Client resumes social interaction.
  I. Client adapts to change in family process.
  J. Client demonstrates an understanding of condition, treatment including medication, home care, and follow-up care.

Neoplasms of the Skin

I. Description
- A. Malignant lesions of the skin
- B. May or may not metastasize to other tissues
- C. May cause destruction of cells
- D. May result in infection
- E. Types of neoplasms
  1. Basal cell epithelioma
     - a. Slow-growing destructive skin tumor
     - b. Usually occurs in individuals >40 years old
     - c. Is more prevalent in blond, fair-skinned men
     - d. Appears as an opaque light pink or tan nodule
     - e. Seen mostly on hairy skin areas
     - f. Usually does not metastasize but may become invasive
     - g. Causes
       1) Prolonged sun exposure
       2) Radiation
       3) Burns
       4) Vaccinations
  2. Squamous cell carcinoma
     - a. Invasive tumor of the epidermal surface with metastatic potential
     - b. Usually located on arms or face
     - c. May develop from preexisting skin lesions such as keratosis or leukoplakia
     - d. Occurs most often in white men >60 years old
     - e. Risk increased in occupations necessitating outdoor employment in sunny, warm climate
  3. Malignant melanoma
     - a. Most serious type of skin neoplasm
     - b. Relatively rare: accounts for only 1%–2% of all malignancies
     - c. Slightly more common in women than in men; rare in children
     - d. Peak incidence occurs between ages 50 and 70 years
     - e. Occurrence mostly on skin areas exposed to sunlight
     - f. Color of lesion varies (blue, black, or yellow) with irregular shapes and pigmentation
     - g. Spreads through the lymphatic and vascular systems
     - h. Metastasizes to regional lymph nodes, liver, lungs, and CNS (course unpredictable)
     - i. Prognosis according to tumor thickness
     - j. Superficial lesions generally curable; deeper lesions tending to metastasize
     - k. Prognosis better for involvement on an extremity (drained by one lymphatic network) than for involvement of head, neck, or trunk (drained by several lymphatic networks)

II. Data collection
- A. Subjective symptoms
  1. History of prior skin tumors or lesions
  2. Soreness around site
  3. Itching
- B. Objective symptoms
  1. Presence of skin lesions
  2. Change in appearance, size, or shape of existing mole or nodule
  3. Drainage or bleeding from lesion
  4. Positive biopsy of lesion

III. Diagnostic tests and methods
- A. Client history
- B. Physical examination
- C. Skin biopsy with histological examination
- D. Baseline laboratory studies: CBC with differential, ESR, platelet count, urinalysis, liver function studies
- E. Chest radiographs
- F. CT scan of body

IV. Implementation
- A. Assess, report, and record signs and symptoms and any reaction to treatment.
- B. Monitor skin lesions for appearance, size, shape, color, and drainage.
- C. Administer prescribed topical agents such as chemotherapeutic drugs and antibiotics.
- D. Provide skin care to lesion:
  1. Avoid use of metal-containing powders or creams.
  2. Use aseptic technique in cleaning area.
  3. Monitor for local reaction to topical medications.
- E. Explain condition, treatment such as irradiation, chemotherapy, and other medication, prevention, home care, and follow-up care.

V. Evaluation
- A. Client reports increased comfort and decreased anxiety.
- B. Client maintains good skin integrity.
- C. Client demonstrates an understanding of condition, diagnostic procedures, and treatment, prevention, home care, and follow-up care.

Renal and Urological Systems

Basic Information

The renal system maintains homeostasis through the production and elimination of urine. The kidneys regulate the volume, acid-base balance, and electrolyte balance of body fluids. This system is responsible also for detoxification of the blood, elimination of wastes, aiding in erythropoiesis, and regulating BP. Body wastes are eliminated by the kidneys via urine formation, tubular reabsorption, and tubular excretion. Disorders of these systems affect the body's normal function.

I. Basic data collection
- A. Subjective symptoms
  1. Problems with elimination
  2. Changes in voiding habits
  3. Discharge from the urethra
  4. Pain in the suprapubic area or back
  5. Burning sensation on voiding
- B. Objective symptoms
  1. Bladder distention (rigid, tender abdomen)
  2. Urine color, odor, cloudiness, presence of mucus, sediment, blood, casts, bacteria
  3. Genital irritation
  4. Amount of urinary output
  5. Electrolyte studies
  6. Edema of extremities, scrotum
  7. Vital signs

8. History of:
   a. Previously normal urinary habits
   b. Health problems with urinary system and other body systems
   c. Presence and location of edema
   d. Medications
   e. Food or medication allergies
   f. Spasms or pain (or both) in bladder region
   g. Presence of discharge

Major Renal and Urological Diagnoses

Renal Calculi (Kidney Stones)

I. Description
   A. Most commonly develop in renal pelvis or calyces of the kidney but possible anywhere in the urinary tract
   B. Result from precipitation of substances such as calcium oxalate, calcium phosphate, urate, or cystine, which are normally dissolved in the urine
   C. Vary in size and may be solitary or multiple
   D. May stay in renal pelvis or descend into ureter
   E. Result in possible damage to renal and urinary tract tissue
   F. Possibly produce large calculi, causing pressure necrosis
   G. May cause obstruction along urinary tract, resulting in hydronephrosis
   H. Tend to recur
   I. Are more common in white men 30–50 years old; rare in blacks
   J. Are more prevalent in southeastern United States (the "stone belt"), possibly because of:
      1. Regional dietary habits
      2. Dehydration as a result of hot climate
   K. Unknown cause
   L. Predisposing factors
      1. Dehydration: decrease in urine production, allowing concentration of calculus-forming substances
      2. Prolonged immobilization: causing urinary stasis with accumulation of calculus-forming substances
      3. Infection: pH changes resulting in a medium favorable for calculus formation
      4. Obstruction: allowing calculus-forming substances to collect; promoting infection and further obstruction
      5. Metabolic factors: excessive intake of calcium or vitamin D; hyperparathyroidism; renal tubular acidosis; elevated uric acid; defective metabolism of oxalate

II. Data collection
   A. Subjective symptoms
      1. Severe pain in flank area, suprapubic area, pelvis, or external genitalia (renal colic)
      2. Urgency, frequency of urination
      3. Nausea
      4. Chills
   B. Objective symptoms
      1. Increased temperature
      2. Pallor
      3. Hematuria
      4. Abdominal distention

   5. Pyuria
   6. Anuria (from bilateral obstruction)
   7. Evidence of urinary tract infection (UTI) via diagnostic procedures
   8. Evidence of presence of calculi via diagnostic procedures

III. Diagnostic tests and methods
   A. Urinalysis
   B. Urine culture
   C. 24-hour urine examination
   D. Kidney-ureter-bladder (KUB) radiograph
   E. Calculi analysis
   F. IVP (less frequently)
   G. Renal CT
   H. Kidney ultrasonography
   I. Cystoscopy
   J. Serial blood calcium and phosphorus levels to detect hyperparathyroidism and increased calcium level compared with normal serum protein

IV. Implementation
   A. Assess, report, and record signs and symptoms and any reaction to treatment.
   B. Maintain a 24- to 48-hour record of urine pH (test with nitrazine pH paper) as ordered.
   C. Strain all urine through gauze.
   D. Save all solid material in urine for analysis.
   E. Provide and encourage intake of fluids for a urinary output of 3–4 L/day.
   F. Offer fruit juices—especially cranberry juice—to acidify alkaline urine.
   G. Assist with administration of supplemental IV fluids as prescribed.
   H. Record I&O accurately.
   I. Weigh client and record weight daily.
   J. Have dietitian instruct client regarding importance of proper diet.
   K. Instruct client regarding need for compliance with drug therapy.
   L. Prepare client for:
      1. Cystoscopy or passage of ureteral catheter surgery for crushing or dislodging calculi
      2. Extracorporeal shockwave lithotripsy: with client sitting in large warm bath, ultrasound waves delivered to area of calculus to disintegrate it
   M. Prepare client for surgery to remove ureteral or kidney stone
      1. Nephrolithotomy: incision through kidney and removal of calculus
      2. Pyelolithotomy: removal of calculi from renal pelvis
      3. Ureterolithotomy: removal of calculus in the ureter
   N. Provide general preoperative and postoperative nursing care.
   O. Provide analgesics as ordered.
   P. Maintain patency of catheters: irrigate renal or ureteral catheters with strict sterile technique per order only. No more than 5-mL aliquots.
   Q. Maintain gravity urinary drainage from catheter: do not clamp ureteral or nephrostomy catheters.
   R. Record output from ureteral and nephrostomy catheters separately; report and record urine output from each.

S. Monitor for bleeding, vital signs, and signs of urinary obstruction.

T. Keep client NPO if nausea, vomiting, or abdominal distention occurs.

U. Assist with comfort measures.

V. Protect against infection.

W. Encourage activity.

X. Explain disease process, treatment, prevention, home care, and follow-up care.

V. Evaluation

A. Client reports increased comfort and decreased anxiety.

B. Client remains free of infection.

C. Client maintains adequate urinary elimination pattern.

D. Client demonstrates an understanding of condition, diagnostic procedures, treatment, prevention, home care, and follow-up care.

Acute Renal Failure

I. Description

A. Sudden interruption of kidney function resulting from obstruction, reduced circulation, or disease of renal tissue

B. Results in retention of toxins, fluids, and end products of metabolism

C. Usually reversible with medical treatment

D. May progress to end-stage disease, uremic syndrome, and death without treatment

E. Causes

1. Prerenal failure associated with decreased blood flow to kidneys
   a. Hypovolemia
   b. Shock
   c. Blood loss
   d. Embolism
   e. Pooling of fluid because of ascites or burns
   f. Cardiovascular disorders: CHF, arrhythmias
   g. Sepsis

2. Intrarenal renal failure owing to damage to kidneys
   a. Acute tubular necrosis
   b. Acute poststreptococcal glomerulonephritis
   c. Sickle cell disease
   d. Bilateral renal vein thrombosis
   e. Nephrotoxins
   f. Ischemia
   g. Renal myeloma
   h. Acute pyelonephritis

3. Postrenal failure caused by bilateral obstruction of urinary outflow
   a. Renal calculi
   b. Blood clots
   c. Benign prostatic hypertrophy
   d. Urethral edema from catheterization

II. Data collection

A. Subjective symptoms
1. Nausea
2. Loss of appetite
3. Headache
4. Lethargy
5. Tingling in extremities

B. Objective symptoms
1. Oliguric phase
   a. Vomiting
   b. Disorientation
   c. Edema
   d. Hyperkalemia
   e. Hyponatremia
   f. Elevated BUN and creatinine levels
   g. Acidosis
   h. Arrhythmias
   i. CHF, pulmonary edema
   j. Hypertension caused by hypervolemia
   k. Anorexia
   l. Sudden drop in urine output
   m. Convulsions, coma
   n. Pruritus
   o. Altered clotting mechanisms
   p. Diarrhea or constipation
   q. Stomatitis
   r. Hematemesis
   s. Uremic breath

2. Diuretic phase
   a. Increased urine output: 4–5 L/day
   b. Gradual decline in BUN and creatinine levels
   c. Hyponatremia
   d. Hypokalemia
   e. Tachycardia
   f. Improved level of consciousness

III. Diagnostic tests and methods

A. Client history

B. Physical examination

C. Laboratory blood studies: BUN, serum creatinine, sodium, potassium, pH, bicarbonate, Hgb, and Hct

D. Urine studies

E. Ultrasound of kidneys

F. Plain films of abdomen (KUB radiographs)

G. Abdominal/renal CT

H. IVP

I. Renal scan

J. Retrograde pyelography

K. Nephrotomography

IV. Implementation

A. Assess, report, and record signs and symptoms and any reaction to treatment.

B. Monitor fluid I&O:
1. Oral fluids
2. All body fluids, such as wound drainage, NG output, diarrhea

C. Monitor laboratory test results.

D. Assist in administering parenteral blood products as ordered.

E. Monitor vital signs.

F. Check for signs of pleuritic chest pain, tachycardia, and pericardial friction rub indicative of pericarditis.

G. Monitor electrolyte study results
1. Observe for symptoms of hyperkalemia, such as malaise, anorexia, paresthesia, or muscle weakness and changes in ECG readings (and report immediately).

2. Watch for signs of hyperglycemia or hypoglycemia in clients receiving hypertonic glucose and insulin infusions.

H. Maintain nutritional status; provide high-calorie, low-protein, low-sodium, and low-potassium diet with vitamin supplements as ordered
    1. Provide small, frequent meals to clients with anorexia.
    2. Limit fluid intake.

I. Provide good mouth care (dry mucous membranes)
    1. Administer antibiotics for stomatitis as prescribed.

J. Check stools for blood.

K. Prevent complications from immobilization
    1. Encourage frequent coughing and deep-breathing exercises.
    2. Assist the client to ambulate when ordered.

L. Use safety measures, such as side rails, for clients who are confused or dizzy.

M. Prepare client for peritoneal dialysis if ordered
    1. Elevate head of bed to reduce pressure on diaphragm and aid respiration.
    2. Monitor for signs of infection (elevated temperature, cloudy drainage).
    3. Monitor blood glucose periodically; administer insulin as ordered.
    4. Monitor for complications, such as peritonitis, hypokalemia, pneumonia, and shock.

N. Prepare client for hemodialysis, if ordered
    1. Check site of arteriovenous shunt every 4 hours for thrill and bruit.
    2. Use opposite arm for drawing blood or taking BP readings.
    3. Monitor temporary central line site.
    4. Monitor vital signs, clotting time, vascular access site, arterial and venous pressures, and blood flow during dialysis procedure.
    5. Monitor for complications such as embolism, hepatitis, septicemia, electrolyte loss, and disequilibrium syndrome.

O. After hemodialysis
    1. Monitor vital signs.
    2. Monitor vascular access site.
    3. Observe for signs of fluid and electrolyte imbalance.

P. Provide reassurance and emotional support to client and family.

Q. Explain condition, diagnostic procedures, treatment, prevention, home care, and follow-up care to client and family.

V. Evaluation
A. Client reports increased comfort and decreased anxiety.
B. Client remains free of infection.
C. Client maintains adequate renal perfusion.
D. Client maintains adequate urinary elimination pattern.
E. Client maintains good skin integrity.
F. Client maintains adequate nutritional and fluid balance.
G. Client demonstrates an understanding of disease process, diagnostic procedures, treatment, prevention, home care, and follow-up care.

Chronic Kidney Disease

I. Description
A. Resulting from a gradually progressive loss of renal function
B. Occasionally caused by rapidly progressive disease of sudden onset
C. Symptoms apparent once 75% of glomerular filtration is lost
D. Progressive destruction of the nephrons, resulting in cellular hypertrophy, retention of fluid and waste products with resultant loss of renal function
E. Accumulation of uremic toxins, producing physiological changes in major organ systems if not treated
F. Maintenance dialysis and transplantation to support life temporarily
G. Causes
    1. Recurrent infections, pyelonephritis
    2. Congenital anomalies such as polycystic kidneys
    3. Vascular disorders such as renal nephrosclerosis
    4. Toxic agents such as antibiotics overdose
    5. Endocrine disorders such as diabetic neuropathy
    6. Urinary obstruction such as calculi and strictures
    7. Chronic glomerular disease such as glomerulonephritis
    8. Acute renal failure that does not respond to treatment

II. Data collection
A. Subjective symptoms
    1. Anorexia
    2. Nausea
    3. Lethargy
    4. Headache
    5. Pruritus
    6. Anxiety
B. Objective symptoms
    1. Renal
        a. Hyponatremia
        b. Initially resulting in hypotension, dry mouth, loss of skin turgor
        c. Progression to confusion, salt overload, accumulation of potassium with muscle irritability and muscle weakness
        d. Fluid overload and metabolic acidosis
        e. Proteinuria
        f. Glycosuria
        g. Erythrocytes (RBCs), leukocytes (WBCs), and casts
    2. Cardiovascular
        a. Hypertension
        b. Arrhythmias
        c. Pericardial effusion
        d. CHF
        e. Peripheral edema
    3. Neurological
        a. Restless leg syndrome with burning, pain, and itching
        b. Paresthesia
        c. Motor nerve dysfunction
        d. Muscle cramping
        e. Shortened memory span
        f. Apathy

g. Drowsiness
h. Confusion
i. Convulsions
j. Coma
k. Electroencephalographic (EEG) changes
4. GI
   a. Stomatitis, gum ulceration, and bleeding
   b. Parotitis
   c. Esophagitis, gastritis, duodenal ulcers
   d. Ulcerative lesions on small and large bowel
   e. Pancreatitis
   f. Ammonia smell to breath (uremic fetor)
   g. Vomiting
   h. Constipation
5. Respiratory
   a. Pulmonary changes with increased susceptibility to infection
   b. Pulmonary edema
   c. Pleural friction rub and effusion
   d. Pleural pain
   e. Uremic pneumonitis
   f. Dyspnea caused by CHF
   g. Kussmaul's respirations caused by acidosis
6. Endocrine
   a. Stunted growth patterns in children
   b. Amenorrhea and cessation of menses
   c. Male impotence
   d. Increased aldosterone secretion
   e. Impaired blood glucose levels because of impairment of carbohydrate metabolism
   f. Thyroid and parathyroid abnormalities
7. Hemopoietic
   a. Anemia
   b. Decrease in RBC survival time
   c. Blood loss from dialysis and GI bleeding
   d. Platelet deficits
   e. Bleeding and clotting disorders: purpura, hemorrhage from body orifices, ecchymoses
8. Skeletal
   a. Muscle and bone pain
   b. Bone demineralization
   c. Pathological fractures
   d. Calcifications in blood vessels, myocardium, joints, gums, eyes, and brain
9. Cutaneous
   a. Pallid, yellowish-bronze, scaly skin
   b. Pruritus
   c. Purpura
   d. Uremic frost
   e. Thin, brittle fingernails
   f. Dry, brittle hair: may change color and fall out

III. Diagnostic tests and methods
   A. Client history
   B. Physical examination
   C. Creatinine clearance test
   D. BUN, serum creatinine, potassium levels
   E. Arterial pH and bicarbonate
   F. Hgb and Hct
   G. Urine specific gravity
   H. Urinalysis
   I. KUB radiographs
   J. Renal CT
   K. Renal scan
   L. Renal arteriography
   M. Nephrotomography
   N. Kidney biopsy

IV. Implementation
   A. Assess, report, and record signs and symptoms and any reaction to treatment.
   B. Provide emotional support.
   C. Provide meticulous skin care.
   D. Provide good perineal care.
   E. Pad side rails to prevent ecchymoses.
   F. Turn client often; use egg-crate mattress.
   G. Provide mouth care.
   H. Offer small nutritious meals high in calories.
   I. Instruct client and family to avoid high-potassium and high-sodium foods.
   J. Monitor for signs of hyperkalemia (leg and abdominal cramps, diarrhea, muscle irritability, weak pulse rate and ECG changes, muscle weakness and paralysis at higher levels).
   K. Monitor for bone and joint complications, such as pathological fractures.
   L. Monitor hydration status:
      1. Check jugular vein distention.
      2. Auscultate lungs for rales.
      3. Measure I&O, including all drainage.
      4. Record daily weight.
      5. Assess for thirst.
      6. Monitor for signs of hypertension.
      7. Check for peripheral edema.
      8. Encourage deep breathing and coughing to prevent pulmonary congestion.
   M. Monitor for signs of pulmonary edema (dyspnea, restlessness, rales).
   N. Administer diuretics and other prescribed medications.
   O. Maintain strict aseptic technique.
   P. Watch for signs of infection (increased temperature, leukocytosis, malaise).
   Q. Monitor for convulsions and coma:
      1. Assist with administration of IV sodium bicarbonate for acidosis.
      2. Administer sedatives or anticonvulsants as ordered.
      3. Keep suction at bedside.
      4. Assess neurological status frequently.
      5. Check for Trousseau's and Chvostek's signs (indicate low serum calcium).
   R. Monitor for signs of bleeding (ecchymoses, petechiae):
      1. Check IV sites for prolonged bleeding.
      2. Monitor Hgb and Hct values.
      3. Monitor stool, urine, and emesis for blood.
   S. Prepare client for hemodialysis if required
      1. Instruct client regarding care of arteriovenous shunt if present.
      2. Check vascular access site every 4 hours for thrill and bruit.
      3. Check upper extremity (temperature, pulse rate, capillary refill, and sensation to determine blood supply; nervous function).
      4. Notify charge nurse if clotting is suspected.

5. Avoid using arm with vascular access for drawing blood or taking BP.
6. Monitor Hgb and Hct values.
7. Monitor temporary central line per policy.

T. After dialysis
1. Monitor for disequilibrium syndrome caused by sudden correction of blood chemistry abnormalities (headache, seizures).
2. Check dialysis site for excessive bleeding.
3. Apply pressure dressing as ordered.
4. Monitor BP readings.

U. Prepare client for kidney transplantation if indicated
1. Selection criteria
2. Immediate postoperative period
3. Reverse isolation and protection against infection
4. Fluid balance maintenance
5. Use of immunosuppressive drugs and their side effects

V. Refer client and family to appropriate counseling for assistance in coping with condition.

W. Explain disease process, treatment, health maintenance procedures, home care, and follow-up care:
1. Preventive measures
2. Dietary restrictions
3. Skin care
4. Treatment (dialysis, transplant, medication)

V. Evaluation
A. Client reports increased comfort and decreased anxiety.
B. Client remains free of infections.
C. Client maintains adequate nutritional intake.
D. Client maintains adequate fluid and electrolyte balance.
E. Client maintains adequate urinary elimination pattern.
F. Client maintains good skin hygiene.
G. Client demonstrates an understanding of disease process, treatment, health maintenance procedures, home care, and follow-up care.

Lower Urinary Tract Infection (Cystitis and Urethritis)

I. Description
A. Two forms of lower UTI: cystitis and urethritis
B. Usually responding well to treatment
C. Possibly recurring because of presence of resistant bacteria
D. More common in women than in men
E. Prevalent in children—especially girls
F. Frequent association with anatomical or physiological abnormalities in children and men
G. Causes
1. Gram-negative bacterial infection caused by organisms such as *Proteus, Enterobacter, Pseudomonas,* and *Escherichia coli* ascending from the urethra
2. Contamination of lower urinary tract during catheterization or instrumentation
3. Breakdown in bladder's defense mechanisms, allowing bacteria to invade bladder mucosa
4. Bacterial flare-up caused by resistance of organisms to antimicrobial therapy
5. If recurrent, majority caused by reinfection by same or new pathogen

6. Small number of recurrent cases caused by perseverant infection from conditions such as kidney stones or chronic prostatitis
7. High incidence in women possibly caused by shortness of urethra
8. Bacterial invasion from vagina, perineum, rectum, or sexual partner

II. Data collection
A. Subjective symptoms
1. Urgency
2. Frequency of urination
3. Cramps or bladder spasms
4. Dysuria
5. Itching
6. Nocturia
7. Burning on urination
8. Low back pain
9. Malaise
10. Nausea
11. Abdominal or flank pain
12. Chills
B. Objective symptoms
1. Hematuria
2. Increased temperature
3. Vomiting
4. Tenderness over bladder region
5. Purulent urine

III. Diagnostic tests and methods
A. Client history
B. Physical examination
C. Routine urine examination
D. Urine culture and sensitivity to identify pathogen and correct antimicrobial agent to use
E. Culture of discharge from urethra (especially in men)
F. IVP, or cystoscopy, to detect congenital abnormalities that may be a cause for recurrent UTIs

IV. Implementation
A. Assess, report, and record signs and symptoms and any reaction to treatment.
B. Force fluids unless contraindicated.
C. Provide diet that acidifies urine as ordered.
D. Monitor temperature and administer antipyretics as prescribed.
E. Administer antimicrobial agent as prescribed.
F. Monitor results of urine examination and culture.
G. Provide perineal care.
H. Provide sitz baths.
I. Prepare client for dilatation if stricture is present.

V. Evaluation
A. Client reports increased comfort and decreased anxiety.
B. Client remains free of infection.
C. Client maintains adequate elimination pattern.
D. Client demonstrates an understanding of condition, diagnostic procedures, and treatment including medication.

Cancer of the Bladder

I. Description
A. Malignant lesions of the bladder
B. Possibly developing on surface of bladder wall (papil-

lomas, benign or malignant) or growing within bladder (usually more virulent)

C. Invasion of underlying muscles
D. More prevalent in individuals >50 years old; more common in men than women
E. Incidence increased in densely populated industrial areas with high number of chemical plants
F. High-risk individuals: rubber workers, weavers, aniline dye workers, hairdressers, petroleum workers, spray painters, and leather finishers
G. Accounting for about 2%–4% of all cancers
H. Predisposing factors
    1. Specific environmental carcinogens such as benzidine, tobacco, and nitrates (latent period between exposure and development of symptoms about 18 years)

II. Data collection
A. Subjective symptoms
    1. Urinary urgency
    2. Dysuria
B. Objective symptoms
    1. Signs of cystitis
    2. Gross, painless, intermittent hematuria
    3. Suprapubic pain after voiding (when invasive lesions occur)
    4. Signs of renal failure
    5. Positive bladder biopsy
    6. Positive cystoscopic examination
    7. Urinary frequency, nocturia, and dribbling

III. Diagnostic tests and methods
A. Client history
B. Physical examination
C. Cystoscopy
D. Bladder tissue biopsy
E. IVP
F. Urinalysis
G. Excretory urography
H. Pelvic arteriography
I. Abdominal CT

IV. Implementation
A. Assess, report, and record signs and symptoms and any reaction to treatment.
B. Provide emotional support.
C. Monitor urine output for evidence of bleeding.
D. Obtain urine specimen for culture and sensitivity.
E. Prepare client and family for surgical procedure:
    1. Transurethral fulguration or excision: removal of small tumors with little tissue-layer infiltration
    2. Cystectomy: various types of complete removal of bladder with permanent alteration of urinary elimination
        a. Ureterostomy: excision of ureters from bladder and connection of ureters to abdominal wall to form stomas for urinary drainage
        b. Colonic conduit: excision of ureters from bladder to a resected portion of the colon, which is passed through abdominal wall to construct a stoma for urinary drainage
        c. Ileal conduit: similar to colonic conduit except a portion of the ileum is used instead of the colon
        d. Ureterosigmoidostomy: anastomosis of ureters to sigmoid colon for urinary drainage through the rectum
        e. Nephrostomy: insertion of catheter into kidney for drainage
        f. Continent urinary diversion: internal pouch created from bowel to prevent peristaltic action. Must be catheterized.
F. Provide postoperative care if required
    1. Monitor urinary drainage and patency of conduits.
    2. Monitor for abdominal distention due to hemorrhage.
    3. Monitor for signs of hemorrhage.
    4. Assist in promotion of adequate respiratory ventilation.
    5. Provide frequent meticulous skin care around stomas.
    6. Encourage fluid intake when ordered.
    7. Protect client from infection.
G. Prepare client for radiation treatment and/or chemotherapy.
H. Assist with and explain care of stoma and skin care.
I. Explain drainage equipment and application.
J. Provide visit with ostomy therapist.
K. Provide information regarding local ostomy organization.
L. Explain disease process, diagnostic procedures, treatment, and home care to client and family.

V. Evaluation
A. Client reports increased comfort and decreased anxiety.
B. Client remains free of infection.
C. Client maintains adequate urinary elimination pattern.
D. Client uses effective coping strategies.
E. Client and family demonstrate an understanding of condition, diagnostic procedures, treatment, home care, and follow-up care.

Male Genitourinary System

Benign Prostatic Hypertrophy

I. Description
A. Slow enlargement of prostate gland (hypertrophy) with extension into bladder
B. Obstruction of urinary outflow through the urethra
C. Urinary stream decreases, with dysuria
D. Stasis of urine in bladder
E. Gradual dilation of ureters and kidneys because of the obstruction
F. Possible hydronephrosis, calculi formation, or cystitis
G. Acute urinary retention if obstruction is complete
H. Frequent occurrence in men >50 years old
I. Cause unknown
J. Theoretical causes
    1. Link between benign prostatic hypertrophy (BPH) and hormonal activity: androgenic hormone decreases with age, causing an imbalance between androgen and estrogen levels and high levels of dihydrotestosterone
    2. Neoplasms
    3. Arteriosclerosis

4. Inflammation
5. Metabolic or nutritional disturbances

II. Data collection
  A. Subjective symptoms
    1. Urgency, frequency, burning, and hesitancy on urination
    2. Decreased force on urination
    3. Nocturia
  B. Objective symptoms
    1. Voiding small amounts
    2. Hematuria possible
    3. Urinary retention
    4. Infection
    5. Enlarged prostate gland on palpation and proctoscopic examination
    6. Renal insufficiency secondary to obstruction

III. Diagnostic tests and methods
  A. Client history
  B. Physical examination
  C. IVP
  D. BUN and creatinine levels
  E. Urinalysis and urine culture
  F. Cystourethroscopy immediately before surgery

IV. Implementation
  A. Assess, report, and record signs and symptoms and any reaction to treatment.
  B. Monitor urinary elimination pattern, intake, output, and characteristics of urine.
  C. Prepare client for surgical intervention (transurethral prostatectomy [TURP] or suprapubic, retropubic, or perineal prostatectomy), brachytherapy (prostatic cancer), radiation therapy (prostatic cancer).
  D. Assist with explanation of postoperative course, including bladder spasms, hemorrhage, pain, and catheter.
  E. Provide postoperative care
    1. Explain reason for sensation of bladder fullness from retention balloon on catheter.
    2. Instruct client to avoid attempting to urinate around catheter.
    3. Monitor three-way irrigation catheter patency; keep bladder free of clots.
    4. Keep catheter system sterile.
    5. Monitor urine output and characteristics (red to light pink for first 24 hours).
    6. Monitor and maintain accurate I&O; record all drainage tubes separately.
    7. Change dressing around suprapubic catheter frequently.
    8. Administer analgesics or antispasmodics as prescribed.
    9. Avoid use of rectal thermometer.
    10. Administer analgesics for pain as prescribed.
    11. After catheter removal, monitor urinary output, retention, and continence.
    12. Encourage oral fluid intake.
  F. Explain disease process, diagnostic procedures, treatment, prevention, home care, and follow-up care.

V. Evaluation
  A. Client reports increased comfort and decreased anxiety.
  B. Client remains free of infection.

C. Client maintains adequate urinary elimination pattern.
D. Client demonstrates an understanding of diagnostic process, diagnostic procedures, treatment, prevention, home care, and follow-up care.

Cancer of the Prostate

I. Description
  A. Malignant tumor of the prostate gland
  B. After skin cancer, prostatic cancer most common neoplasm found in men >50 years old
  C. Seldom produces symptoms until well advanced
  D. Seldom results from BPH
  E. Accounts for 17% of all cancers
  F. Five-year survival rate 70% when treated in its localized form
  G. Five-year survival rate <35% if treatment occurs after metastases
  H. Fatal when widespread bone metastasis occurs
  I. Cause unknown

II. Data collection
  A. Subjective symptoms
    1. Early tumor: no symptoms
    2. Back pain
    3. Symptoms from metastases
  B. Objective symptoms
    1. Difficulty in starting urinary stream
    2. Dribbling
    3. Urinary retention
    4. Unexplained cystitis
    5. Hematuria (rare)

III. Diagnostic tests and methods
  A. Client history
  B. Physical (digital) rectal xamination (DRE)
  C. Biopsy examination
  D. Ultrasound
  E. Serum acid phosphatase levels
  F. PSA (prostate-specific antigen)
    1. Elevated in prostatic cancer
    2. Used as baseline to determine effectiveness and treatment
  G. Serum alkaline phosphatase levels
    1. Elevated levels point to bone metastasis
  H. Bone scan

IV. Implementation
  A. Assess, report, and record signs and symptoms and any reaction to treatment.
  B. Provide emotional support to client and family.
  C. Explain expected effects of surgery, such as possible incontinence, impotence, and treatment of radiation side effects.
  D. Encourage client to express his fears.
  E. Explain postoperative procedures such as dressing changes and placement of tubes.
  F. Teach perineal exercises to decrease incontinence.
  G. After prostatectomy:
    1. Monitor dressing, incision, and drainage system for excessive bleeding.
    2. Monitor for signs of bleeding (cold, clammy skin; pallor; restlessness; decreasing BP readings; and rising pulse rate).

3. Administer antispasmodics as ordered (control of postoperative bladder spasms).
4. Monitor for signs of infection (chills, increased temperature, inflamed incisional site).
5. Maintain adequate fluid intake (minimum of 2000 mL daily).
6. Provide good skin care (incontinence is a frequent problem).

H. After suprapubic prostatectomy:
1. Encourage family's psychological support.
2. Keep skin around drain clean and dry.
3. Encourage perineal exercises 24–48 hours after surgery.
4. Provide meticulous catheter care (check tubing for kinks, mucous plugs, clots).
5. Explain reason for avoiding pulling on tubes or catheter.

I. After perineal prostatectomy:
1. Avoid taking temperature rectally or inserting rectal tubes.
2. Provide frequent sitz baths to relieve pain and inflammation.
3. Use pads to absorb urinary drainage.

J. After transurethral resection:
1. Monitor for abdominal distention (caused by urethral stricture or blockage of catheter by blood clot).
2. Irrigate catheter as ordered.
3. Monitor for signs of urethral stricture (straining to urinate, dysuria).

K. Monitor for radiation effects, such as nausea and vomiting, dry skin, and alopecia.
L. Watch for side effects of diethylstilbestrol (DES) (estrogen therapy), such as gynecomastia, fluid retention, nausea, and vomiting.
M. Monitor for presence of thrombophlebitis in clients receiving DES.
N. Explain condition, diagnostic procedures, treatment, home care, and follow-up care.

V. Evaluation
A. Client reports increased comfort and decreased anxiety.
B. Client maintains adequate urinary elimination pattern.
C. Client remains free of infection.
D. Client demonstrates an understanding of condition, diagnostic tests, treatment, home care, and follow-up care.

Female Reproductive System

Basic Information

Nursing care of the gynecological client is a reflection of the interest in improving the quality of health for women. Multiple gynecological abnormalities may occur at the same time. For example, a client with vaginitis may also have dysmenorrhea, dysuria, and infertility. There may also be complications associated with the urological disorders because of the proximity of the reproductive system to the urinary system. Disorders of the reproductive system may interfere with sexuality, conception, and self-image.

I. Basic data collection
A. Subjective symptoms
1. Lower abdominal pain and cramping
2. Backache
3. Urinary frequency and urgency
4. Stress incontinence
5. Tenderness and burning of breasts
6. Tenderness and burning of nipples
7. Itching and burning of external genitalia
8. Burning, itching, tenderness, and pain during intercourse
9. Pain, headache, irritability, depression, and insomnia related to menstrual cycle

B. Objective symptoms
1. General appearance
2. Vital signs
3. Weight
4. Breasts
   a. Shape
   b. Skin dimpling
   c. Presence of nodules
      1) Size
      2) Consistency
      3) Fixed or mobile
   d. Nipples
      1) Asymmetry
      2) Discharge
      3) Retraction
      4) Ulceration
5. External genitalia
   a. Irritation
   b. Redness
   c. Excoriation
6. External vaginal orifice
   a. Irritation
   b. Redness
   c. Nodules
   d. Excoriation
7. Vaginal discharge
   a. Color
   b. Consistency
   c. Odor

Major Female Reproductive System Diagnoses

Endometriosis

I. Description
A. Presence of endometrial tissue outside the lining of the uterine cavity
B. Endometrial cells bleeding into nearby spaces to cause inflammation, adhesions, tumor, or cystic formation as a result of stimulation by ovarian hormones
C. Condition usually confined to the pelvic area, most commonly around the ovaries, the cul-de-sac, uterosacral ligaments, and the uterovesical peritoneum, but can appear anywhere in the body
D. Usually occurring between the ages of 30 and 40 years, especially in women who postpone pregnancy; uncommon before age 20 years
E. Severe endometriosis with abrupt onset or with slow development over a period of years

F. Usually becoming progressively severe during the menstrual years
G. Treatment variable depending on stage of the disease
1. Conservative treatment in stages 1 and 2 possible in young women who wish to have children
2. Surgical intervention conducted in stages 3 and 4 when ovarian masses are present, in order to rule out malignancy
3. Possible conservative surgical intervention conducted to resect cysts and remove adhesions
4. For women not wishing to bear children, or when the condition is in stages 3–5, total abdominal hysterectomy with bilateral salpingo-oophorectomy performed as treatment of choice
H. Usually subsides after menopause
I. Direct cause unknown
J. Predisposing factors
1. Familial susceptibility or recent surgery necessitating opening of the uterus, such as cesarean section
II. Data collection
A. Subjective symptoms
1. Abdominal fullness
2. Dysmenorrhea: constant pain in lower abdomen, vagina, posterior pelvis, and back
a. Begins approximately 5 days before menses; lasts 2–3 days
3. Different from primary dysmenorrhea, which is more cramplike and located in the midline of the abdomen
4. Affecting ovaries or cul-de-sac: dyspareunia
5. Affecting ovaries and fallopian tubes: profuse menses
6. Affecting cervix, vagina, and perineum: bleeding from endometrial implants. Ovarian implants also called chocolate cysts.
7. Affecting rectovaginal septum and colon: nausea
8. Affecting small bowel: nausea, worsening before menses; abdominal cramps
9. Irregular menses
10. Menorrhagia
B. Objective symptoms
1. Infertility
2. Nodular, tender uterosacral ligaments; enlarged uterus per pelvic examination
3. Positive findings on laparoscopy
III. Diagnostic tests and methods
A. Client history
B. Physical examination
C. Pelvic examination
D. Palpitation
E. Laparoscopy
F. Cul-de-sac aspiration
G. Barium enema to rule out bowel disorders
IV. Implementation
A. Assess, report, and record signs and symptoms and any reaction to treatment.
B. Allow client to verbalize feelings.
C. Administer prescribed medication that suppresses ovulation, such as danazol, oral contraceptives, or leuprolide acetate (Lupron).
D. Advise adolescents to use sanitary napkins in place of tampons to assist in prevention of retrograde

(backward) menstrual flow in girls who have a narrow vagina or small introitus (external vaginal orifice).
E. Reassure client that condition is not normally life threatening.
F. Prepare client and family for surgical intervention such as laparoscopy, laser lysis of endometrial implants and adhesions, hsterectomy, salpingectomy, or oophorectomy if needed.
G. Provide appropriate postoperative care
1. Monitor for vaginal bleeding.
2. Monitor for signs of hemorrhage.
H. Monitor urinary output for dysuria.
I. Recommend an annual pelvic examination and Papanicolaou (Pap) smear to all female clients for early diagnosis and more effective treatment.
J. Explain condition, diagnostic procedures, treatment, home care, and follow-up care to client and family
1. Medications
2. Hygiene
3. Activity
4. Estrogen therapy, if premenopausal
V. Evaluation
A. Client reports increased comfort and decreased anxiety.
B. Client remains free of injury or infection.
C. Client uses effective coping strategies.
D. Client demonstrates an understanding of condition, diagnostic procedures, treatment, home care, and follow-up care.

Carcinoma of the Cervix

I. Description
A. Malignant lesion of the cervix; classified as either precancerous changes or dysplasia
B. Precancerous changes ranging from minimal cervical dysplasia to carcinoma in situ
C. Cervical dysplasia: cervical intraepithelial neoplasia (CIN) divided into three stages
1. CIN I: mild to moderate dysplasia
2. CIN II: moderate to severe dysplasia
3. CIN III: severe to malignant
D. Precancerous changes curable 75%–90% of the time with early detection and proper treatment
E. Precancerous changes if untreated possibly progressing to invasive cervical cancer
F. In invasive carcinoma, spread of cancer cells directly to adjacent pelvic structures or to distant sites via lymphatic system
G. Invasive carcinoma responsible for approximately 8000 deaths per year in the United States
H. About 95% of all cases squamous cell carcinomas; only 5% adenocarcinomas
I. Invasive carcinoma generally occurring between ages 30 and 50 years; rarely before age 20 years
J. Mortality declining with early detection and Pap smear examinations
K. Asymptomatic in early stages; treatment dependent on stage of disease, health status, age, and presence of complications
L. Related risk factors
1. Sexual intercourse at early age; before 17 years old

2. Lower socioeconomic status
3. Infection with human papillomavirus (HPV)
4. Multiple sexual partners
5. Smoking

II. Data collection
   A. Subjective symptoms
      1. Mild bleeding after intercourse or between menstrual cycles
      2. Pain is a late symptom
      3. Anorexia
      4. Weight loss
   B. Objective symptoms
      1. Watery discharge
      2. Foul vaginal discharge with disease progression
      3. Leakage of urine and feces from a fistula
      4. Evidence of malignancy via Pap smear
      5. Evidence of dysplasia via Pap smear indicating need for follow-up studies

III. Diagnostic tests and methods
   A. Client history
   B. Physical examination
   C. Pap smear
   D. Colposcopy and biopsy
   E. Schiller's iodine test

IV. Implementation
   A. Assess, report, and record signs and symptoms and any reaction to treatment.
   B. Allow client to verbalize feelings in regard to condition.
   C. Assist with preparation of client for appropriate treatment, such as conization, laser treatments, hysterectomy, radiation, and/or chemotherapy.
   D. Provide appropriate postoperative care for simple or radical hysterectomy
      1. Monitor I&O; patency of Foley catheter.
      2. Monitor for postoperative complications, such as thrombophlebitis and abdominal distention, vaginal hemorrhage, or vaginal discharge other than serosanguineous.
      3. Monitor for urinary retention if Foley catheter is not used.
      4. Monitor for grief response related to image as female.
      5. Monitor for surgical menopause if ovaries are removed.
      6. Change perineal pads every 3–4 hours and as needed.
      7. Monitor for return of bowel sounds.
   E. For clients who receive an internal radium implant
      1. Provide radiation precautions.
      2. Instruct client to maintain a side-lying or supine position to prevent displacement of implant.
      3. Provide perineal hygiene.
      4. Monitor for radiation sickness (nausea, vomiting, malaise, fever, diarrhea).
      5. Administer prescribed medications, including antiemetics.
      6. Provide a high-protein, low-residue diet to avoid straining during defecation as ordered.
      7. Encourage high fluid intake (2000–3000 mL daily).
      8. Explain to client, family, and visitors that time spent with client will be limited in order to avoid overexposure to radiation.
      9. Provide emotional support for feelings of alienation.
      10. Monitor patency of Foley catheter and I&O.
      11. Monitor vaginal packing used to protect bladder and rectum from radiation.
      12. Monitor for complications such as cystitis, hemorrhage, and vaginal fistula.
   F. Explain condition, diagnostic procedures, treatment, home care, and follow-up care
      1. Avoidance of heavy lifting for approximately 2 months
      2. Avoidance of sexual intercourse for 4–6 weeks after surgery
      3. Checking for vaginal discharge or bleeding, which may appear after radiation therapy
      4. Engaging in activities that do not cause straining
      5. Keeping appointment for follow-up care

V. Evaluation
   A. Client reports increased comfort and decreased anxiety.
   B. Client remains free of complications.
   C. Client remains free of injury or infection.
   D. Client maintains good skin integrity.
   E. Client develops a positive self-image.
   F. Client demonstrates an understanding of condition, diagnostic procedures, treatment, home care, and follow-up care.

Ovarian Cancer

I. Description
   A. Primary ovarian cancer: fourth most common cause of cancer deaths among women in United States after those of cancer of the breast, colon, and lung
   B. Metastatic ovarian cancer more common than cancers at other sites in women who have had previously treated breast cancer.
   C. Rapid spread by local extension, surface seeding, and occasionally via the lymph system and the bloodstream
   D. Prognosis generally poor because ovarian tumors tend to spread rapidly
   E. Five-year survival is about 25%
   F. Incidence higher in women
      1. Between ages 55 and 65 years
      2. With family history of ovarian cancer
      3. Have BRCA gene mutation
      4. Eat high-fat diet
   G. Exact causes unknown

II. Data collection
   A. Symptoms variable according to size of tumor
   B. In early stages
      1. Vague abdominal discomfort and pelvic heaviness
      2. Dyspepsia
      3. Other mild GI disturbances
   C. In later stages
      1. Urinary frequency
      2. Bowel dysfunction
      3. Pelvic discomfort
      4. Abdominal distention, increased abdominal girth

5. Weight loss
6. Palpable mass
    D. Advanced stage
        1. Ascites
        2. Symptoms relating to metastatic sites, such as symptoms of pleural effusion
        3. Rarely causes postmenopausal bleeding or pain
III. Diagnostic tests and methods
    A. Client history
    B. Physical examination, bimanual pelvic exam
    C. CA 125
    D. Abdominal and vaginal ultrasound
    E. Diagnostic tests for metastasis
        1. CBC, blood chemistry, and ECG
        2. Culdoscopy
        3. Chest radiograph
        4. Lymphangiography to determine lymph node involvement
        5. Mammography to rule out primary breast cancer
        6. Liver function tests or liver scan for clients with ascites
        7. Ascites fluid aspiration for identification of cells by histology
        8. Biopsy examination
        9. Barium enema for clients with GI symptoms to determine presence of obstruction and size of tumor
        10. Exploratory laparotomy for accurate diagnosis: includes tumor resection and lymph node evaluation
        11. Histological studies
IV. Implementation
    A. Assess, report, and record signs and symptoms and any reaction to treatment.
    B. Prepare client for surgical intervention.
    C. Provide emotional support.
    D. Allow client to verbalize feelings regarding condition.
    E. Provide appropriate postoperative nursing care (total abdominal hysterectomy, salpingoophorectomy)
        1. Monitor vital signs frequently.
        2. Monitor IV fluid therapy.
        3. Monitor I&O.
        4. Maintain patent Foley catheter.
        5. Check dressings for excessive bleeding or drainage.
        6. Observe for signs of infection.
        7. Provide abdominal support, and check for signs of abdominal distention.
        8. Administer prescribed analgesics for pain.
        9. Administer prescribed chemotherapeutic drugs; monitor for side effects.
        10. Reposition client at least every 2 hours.
        11. Encourage coughing and deep-breathing exercises.
        12. Encourage and assist with ambulation as necessary.
    F. If stage III or IV, monitor for complications of pelvic exenteration (radical hysterectomy, vaginectomy, removal of bowel and bladder, colostomy, and urostomy)
    G. Monitor and treat side effects of radiation and chemotherapy, if applicable

1. Provide emotional support for client and family.
2. Request supportive care from chaplain, social worker, and other health-care team members as appropriate.
3. Assist client in dealing with changes of body image.
4. Assist client in developing coping strategies.
    H. Explain condition, diagnostic procedures, treatment including medication, home care management, and follow-up care.
V. Evaluation
    A. Client reports increased comfort and decreased anxiety.
    B. Client remains free of complications.
    C. Client remains free of injury or infection.
    D. Client maintains good skin integrity.
    E. Client develops a positive self-image.
    F. Client demonstrates an understanding of condition, diagnostic procedures, treatment, home care, and follow-up care.

Breast Mass

I. Description
    A. Nodule or mass in the breast, which may or may not be malignant
    B. Nonmalignant breast lesion
        1. Fibroadenomas
            a. Round, encapsulated, movable, firm, and nontender on palpation
        2. Dysplasia
            a. Thick, nodular lumps within the breast
            b. Association with pain during menses
            c. Nodule is soft, movable, and tender on palpation
            d. Possibly multiple nodules
            e. Occurring most often in women between 30 years of age and menopause
    C. Malignant breast tumors
        1. Most common form of cancer in women
        2. Incidence increases with age
        3. Affecting white women more than African American women, but African American women have lower survival rates
        4. High-risk factors
            a. Nulliparity: women who have not been pregnant
            b. BRCA 1 or BRCA 2 gene mutation
            c. Family history, first-degree maternal relative
            d. Early menarche and late menopause
            e. History of breast cancer, colon cancer, or endometrial cancer
            f. First pregnancy after age 30 years
            g. Obesity
            h. Exposure to radiation
        5. Possibly firm, nonmovable, tender, and nontender on palpation
        6. Most frequently located in upper, outer portion of the breast.
        7. Metastasis occurring early, transported by lymph system, spreading to lung, bone, and/or brain

II. Data collection
   A. Subjective symptoms
      1. Small mass felt during breast self-examination
   B. Objective symptoms
      1. Palpable mass in breast tissue
      2. Presence of tumor on mammography
      3. Nipple retraction or elevation
      4. Skin dimpling, peau d'orange
      5. Nipple discharge
      6. Abnormal findings on ultrasound
      7. Positive malignant breast biopsy through fine-needle aspiration or surgical removal of tumor and microscopic examination for malignant cells

III. Diagnostic tests and methods
   A. Client history
   B. Physical examination
   C. Mammography: radiograph of breast tissue
   D. Ultrasound
   E. Stereotactic core biopsy
   F. Fine needle aspiration
   G. Prognostic factors
      1. Axillary lymph node status
      2. Tumor size and histology
      3. Estrogen and progesterone receptors
      4. DNA content (ploidy)
      5. Cell proliferative indexes
      6. HER-2/neu genetic marker

IV. Implementation
   A. Assess, report, and record signs and symptoms and any reaction to treatment.
   B. Allow client to verbalize feelings regarding condition.
   C. Provide emotional support.
   D. Provide frequent contact and encourage illness adjustment.
   E. Provide for visit by individuals from Reach to Recovery with approval of physician.
   F. Prepare client for biopsy procedure.
   G. Prepare client for surgical intervention, if required
      1. Provide preoperative teaching.
      2. Explain type of surgical intervention
         a. Lumpectomy: excision and removal of mass
         b. Simple mastectomy: removal of breast tissue, leaving anterior skin, underlying chest muscle, and axillary lymph nodes intact
         c. Modified radical mastectomy: total removal of breast tissue and nipple with partial excision of skin, surrounding tissue, and lymph nodes
         d. Radical mastectomy: total removal of breast tissue and nipple with partial removal of overlying skin, chest muscles, axillary lymph tissue, and surrounding adipose tissue
         e. Oophorectomy, adrenalectomy, or hypophysectomy: to remove source of estrogen and hormones that stimulate the breast
   H. Provide postoperative care
      1. Administer prescribed analgesics.
      2. Monitor dressing and drainage and/or Hemovac drainage system; check client's back for pooling of blood.
      3. Empty Hemovac and measure every 8 hours.
      4. Elevate affected arm above level of right atrium of heart to prevent edema.
      5. Monitor circulatory status of affected arm.
      6. Measure upper arm and forearm of affected arm twice daily to detect presence of edema.
      7. Avoid drawing blood, administering parenteral fluids, or taking BP in affected arm.
      8. Encourage exercises of affected arm when ordered; avoid abduction:
         a. Squeezing ball
         b. Brushing hair
         c. Feeding self
         d. "Climbing" wall with fingertips
         e. Rope pull
         f. Elbow spread
         g. Arm swing
      9. Encourage adequate nutritional intake when appropriate.
      10. Administer prescribed hormone therapy, such as tamoxifen, an antiestrogen to alter cancer that is estrogen-receptor positive.
      11. Request representative from Reach to Recovery to revisit client with approval of physician.
      12. Provide information on breast prosthesis if requested.
      13. Provide emotional support; assist with adjustments to body image.
      14. Assist in development of coping strategies.
   I. Provide appropriate nursing care for clients receiving radiation therapy
      1. Apply prescribed lotion to skin.
      2. Monitor for skin problems such as radiation burns.
   J. Administer adjuvant chemotherapeutic agents, if prescribed (vincristine, doxorubicin [Adriamycin], methotrexate, 5-fluorouracil, prednisone).
   K. For clients receiving radiation and chemotherapeutic therapy:
      1. Explain and assist with potential side effects: nausea and vomiting
         a. Anorexia
         b. Stomatitis
         c. Malaise
         d. Hair loss
         e. Itching
         f. Reduced energy
         g. Heartburn
         h. Cough
         i. Bone marrow depression
         j. Anemia
   L. Prepare client for breast reconstruction if indicated.
   M. Explain condition, diagnostic procedures, treatment, prevention, home care, and follow-up care to client and family
      1. Correct technique for breast self-examination
      2. Arm exercises and activity level
      3. Resumption of sexual activity
      4. Medication
      5. Information on community resources such as Reach to Recovery

V. Evaluation
   A. Client reports increased comfort and decreased anxiety and fear.
   B. Client remains free of injury or infection.
   C. Client maintains adequate level of mobility.

D. Client develops a positive self-image.
E. Client and family demonstrate an understanding of condition, diagnostic procedures, treatment, home care, and follow-up care.

Endocrine System

Basic Information

Together with the nervous system, the endocrine system regulates and integrates the metabolic activities of the body. The hypothalamus controls endocrine organs by hormonal and neural pathways. Hormones are chemical transmitters that are released from certain types of cells in the bloodstream and then carried to its organ-receptor cells. These latter cells respond to the specific hormone.

The pathways of the nervous system connect the hypothalamus to the posterior pituitary gland. Neural stimulation causes the posterior pituitary gland to secrete two hormones: antidiuretic hormone (ADH) and oxytocin.

The hypothalamic hormones stimulate the anterior pituitary to emit the following tropic hormones: adrenocorticotropic hormone (ACTH), thyroid-stimulating hormone (TSH), follicle-stimulating hormone (FSH), and luteinizing hormone (LH). The hypothalamic hormones are also responsible for the release or inhibition of the human growth hormone (hGH), melanocyte-stimulating hormone (MSH), and prolactin. The atropic hormones in turn stimulate the adrenal cortex, thyroid, and gonads.

The endocrine system is regulated by a negative simple or complex feedback system. In a simple feedback system, the level of one substance regulates the secretion of a hormone. For example, high serum calcium inhibits the secretion of the parathyroid hormone (PTH), while low serum calcium levels stimulate the secretion of PTH. An example of the complex feedback system is that of the stimulation of the release of ACTH as a result of the secretion of the hypothalamic corticotropin-releasing hormone (CRH). ACTH then stimulates the adrenal gland to secrete cortisol. Once serum cortisol rises, it inhibits the secretion of ACTH by decreasing CRH.

Careful evaluation of each level of the endocrine system is necessary in clients whose clinical condition suggests endocrine dysfunction owing to the involvement of the complex hormonal sequence. A disturbance in one of the secreting endocrine glands can affect the regulation of another gland. The client with an endocrine dysfunction may experience multiple problems.

I. Basic data collection
  A. Subjective symptoms
    1. Pain: skeletal, back, abdominal, muscle spasms, headache
    2. Weakness
    3. Lethargy
    4. Numbness
    5. Mood swings
    6. Tingling
    7. Intolerance to cold or heat
    8. Polyuria, dysuria, nocturia
    9. Impotence, infertility, decreased libido
    10. Menstrual disturbances
    11. Anorexia or polyphagia
    12. Frequent infections
    13. Nausea
  B. Objective symptoms
    1. General appearance
    2. Skin color
      a. Flushed
      b. Pale
      c. Bronze pigmentation
      d. Yellow pigmentation
    3. Skin temperature
      a. Excess perspiration or lack of perspiration
      b. Dry
      c. Moist
    4. Poor wound healing
    5. Nails
      a. Thin
      b. Thick
      c. Brittle
      d. Dry
    6. Hair
      a. Brittle
      b. Thin
      c. Dry
    7. CNS
      a. Alterations in consciousness
        1) Lethargy
        2) Decreased cognition
        3) Seizures
        4) Confusion
        5) Stupor
        6) Coma
      b. Personality changes
      c. Abnormal reflexes: Chvostek's or Trousseau's sign
      d. Slowed, sluggish speech
    8. Eyes
      a. Protruding eyeball (exophthalmos)
      b. Drooping eyelids (ptosis)
      c. Edema around eyes (periorbital)
    9. Respiratory system
      a. Kussmaul's respirations
      b. Acetone breath
      c. Tachypnea
    10. Cardiovascular system
      a. Tachycardia
      b. Bradycardia
      c. Hypertension
      d. Hypotension
    11. GI system
      a. Anorexia
      b. Polyphagia
      c. Polydipsia
      d. Diarrhea
      e. Constipation
    12. Renal system
      a. Oliguria
      b. Anuria
      c. Polyuria
    13. Musculoskeletal system
      a. Weight loss or gain
      b. Stature (excessive or delayed growth)
      c. Bone density
    14. Vital signs

Major Endocrine Diagnoses

Hyperthyroidism (Graves' Disease; Thyrotoxicosis)

I. Description
   A. Metabolic imbalance caused by thyroid hormone overproduction
   B. Most common form, Graves' disease, in which thyroxine production is increased, with enlargement of the thyroid gland, resulting in multiple system changes
   C. Thyroid storm: an acute exacerbation of this condition, possibly leading to life-threatening cardiac, renal, or hepatic failure if not treated immediately
   D. Incidence highest in individuals between the ages of 30 and 40 years
   E. Incidence high in individuals with a family history of thyroid disorders
   F. Possible for most clients to lead normal life with treatment
   G. Causes and predisposing factors
      1. Presence of genetic and immunological factors
      2. Abnormal iodine metabolism
      3. Other endocrine disorders such as thyroiditis, hyperparathyroidism, and diabetes mellitus
      4. Excessive dietary iodine intake
      5. Stressful conditions: surgery, infection, toxemia of pregnancy, and diabetic ketoacidosis, especially in clients with untreated or inadequately treated hyperthyroidism, possibly precipitating thyroid storm

II. Data collection
   A. Subjective symptoms
      1. Fatigue
      2. Weakness
      3. Vision problems
      4. Intolerance to heat
      5. Increased appetite
      6. Diarrhea
      7. Palpitations
      8. Nervousness
      9. Menstrual abnormalities
      10. Difficulty in concentrating
      11. Clumsiness
      12. Nausea
      13. Loss of appetite
      14. Irritability
   B. Objective symptoms
      1. Enlarged thyroid gland (goiter)
      2. Weight loss
      3. Profuse diaphoresis
      4. Diarrhea
      5. Tremors
      6. Exophthalmos
      7. Shaky handwriting
      8. Smooth, warm, flushed skin
      9. Fine, soft hair
      10. Premature graying with increased hair loss
      11. Friable nails
      12. Thickened skin
      13. Tachycardia
      14. Bounding pulse
      15. Cardiomegaly
      16. Dyspnea on exertion and at rest
      17. Increased defecation
      18. Liver enlargement
      19. Muscle atrophy
      20. Oligomenorrhea or amenorrhea
      21. Gynecomastia in men caused by increased estrogen levels
      22. Increased serum thyroxine (T_4) and triiodothyronine (T_3) concentrations
      23. Thyroid storm: extreme irritability, hypertension, tachycardia, vomiting, temperature up to 106°F (41.1°C), delirium, and coma

III. Diagnostic tests and methods
   A. Client history
   B. Physical examination
   C. Radioactive iodine uptake (RAIU)
   D. Thyroid scan
   E. Thyroid suppression test for evaluation of pituitary control of thyroid gland
   F. Thyroid-releasing hormone (TRH) stimulation test for evaluation of TSH levels
   G. Basal metabolism rate (BMR)
   H. Serum protein-bound iodine (PBI)
   I. Serum cholesterol and total lipids
   J. Ultrasonography to evaluate subclinical ophthalmopathy

IV. Implementation
   A. Assess, report, and record signs and symptoms and any reaction to treatment.
   B. Monitor vital signs and neurological status.
   C. Monitor weight daily.
   D. Monitor serum electrolytes.
   E. Monitor for signs of hyperglycemia and glycosuria.
   F. Monitor cardiac function.
   G. Monitor fluid I&O.
   H. Monitor pregnant women for signs of spontaneous abortion (spotting, occasional mild cramps).
   I. Mix prescribed iodine medication with milk to prevent GI distress.
   J. Administer prescribed iodine medication through a straw to prevent tooth discoloration.
   K. Administer other prescribed medications, such as digitalis, propranolol (Inderal), sedatives, and sleep aids.
   L. Assist with comfort measures.
   M. Assist with activities as needed.
   N. Encourage adequate intake of high-calorie, high-carbohydrate, high-protein, and high-vitamin diet.
   O. Explain and understand mood swings.
   P. Monitor for signs of thyroid storm:
      1. Tachycardia
      2. Elevated temperature
      3. Tremors and restlessness
      4. Vomiting
      5. Hypertension
      6. Delirium
      7. Coma
   Q. Treat thyroid storm as prescribed:
      1. Administer medications as prescribed:
         a. Saturated solution of potassium iodide (SSKI) or ^{131}I to inhibit thyroid hormone (instruct client to expectorate or cough freely after ^{131}I therapy; saliva remains radioactive for 24 hours)

b. Glucocorticoids to inhibit release of thyroid hormone

c. β-Adrenergic blockers for increased adrenergic stimulation

d. Medications for CHF

2. For clients taking methimazole (Tapazole):

a. Monitor CBC periodically to detect leukopenia, thrombocytopenia, and agranulocytosis.

b. Instruct client to take medication with meals to decrease GI distress.

c. Instruct client to avoid over-the-counter cough preparations because they may contain iodine.

d. Instruct client to report signs of blood dyscrasia, such as enlarged cervical lymph nodes, fever, mouth sores, sore throat, skin rash, or skin eruptions.

3. Monitor BP and cardiac rate and rhythm.

4. Monitor temperature.

5. Administer hypothermic measures for high fever (sponging, hypothermia blankets, and acetaminophen; avoid aspirin as it raises thyroxine levels).

6. Maintain IV line.

R. For clients with exophthalmos:

1. Advise use of sunglasses, shields, or eye patches to protect eyes.

2. Moisten conjunctivas with isotonic eyedrops.

3. Advise client with severe lid retraction to avoid sudden movement (may cause lid to slip behind eyeball).

4. Monitor for corneal damage.

S. Prepare client and family for surgical intervention, if required.

T. Provide postoperative care:

1. Monitor for signs of respiratory distress frequently.

2. Keep tracheostomy tray at bedside.

3. Monitor for signs of hemorrhage into neck, such as tight dressing with absence of blood.

4. Change dressing and perform wound care as ordered (check back of dressing for drainage).

5. Place client in semi-Fowler's position (support head and neck to ease tension on the incision).

6. Monitor for signs of thyroid storm.

7. Monitor for signs of hypocalcemia (tetany, numbness) caused by accidental removal of parathyroid gland during surgery.

8. Emphasize importance of follow-up care after discharge (hypothyroidism may develop 2–4 weeks postoperatively).

9. Emphasize importance of repeated measurement of serum thyroxine levels.

U. Explain condition, diagnostic procedures, treatment including medication, home care, diet, and follow-up care to client and family.

V. Evaluation

A. Client reports increased comfort and decreased anxiety.

B. Client remains free of injury or infection.

C. Client maintains adequate nutritional intake.

D. Client maintains adequate rest and undisturbed sleep pattern.

E. Client participates in self-care activities.

F. Client uses effective coping strategies.

G. Client and family demonstrate an understanding of condition, diagnostic procedures, treatment including medication, home care, and follow-up care.

Hypothyroidism

I. Description

A. Condition characterized by low serum thyroid hormone level resulting from hypothalamic, pituitary, or thyroid insufficiency

B. Leads to a decline in the metabolic rate and affects almost all systems

C. Clinical effects ranging from mild fatigue and loss of appetite to life-threatening myxedema coma

D. Most prevalent in women

E. Incidence rising in individuals between the ages of 40 and 50 years

F. Infection, use of sedatives, and exposure to cold may precipitate myxedema coma

G. Causes

1. Dysfunction of thyroid gland caused by:

a. Thyroidectomy

b. Irradiation therapy (especially ^{131}I)

c. Inflammation

d. Chronic autoimmune thyroiditis

e. Inflammatory conditions such as sarcoidosis and amyloidosis

2. Failure of pituitary gland to produce TSH

3. Failure of hypothalamus to produce TRH

4. Inborn errors of thyroid hormone synthesis

5. Iodine deficiency: usually dietary, resulting in inability to synthesize the hormone

6. Use of antithyroid medications such as propylthiouracil

II. Data collection

A. Subjective symptoms

1. Fatigue

2. Forgetfulness

3. Sensitivity to cold

4. Loss of appetite

5. Decreased libido, menstruation changes

6. Muscle stiffness and pain

7. Chest pain

8. Headache

9. Drowsiness or apathy

10. Numbness or tingling

11. Decreased mental status

B. Objective symptoms

1. Weight gain

2. Decreased bowel sounds

3. Constipation

4. Dry, flaky, cool, coarse, inelastic skin

5. Puffy face, hands, and feet

6. Sparse body hair

7. Immature body development

8. Decreased BMR

9. Bradycardia

10. Hoarseness

11. Periorbital edema

12. Dry, sparse, brittle hair

13. Upper eyelid droop

14. Thick, brittle nails
15. Abdominal distention
16. Infertility
17. Ataxia
18. Intention tremor
19. Nystagmus
20. Reflexes: delayed reaction time
21. Decreased urine output
22. Low body temperature
23. Decreased T_4, T_3; increased TSH
24. Pleural effusion on chest radiograph
25. Elevated serum cholesterol, carotene, alkaline phosphatase, and triglyceride levels
26. Signs of myxedema coma
    a. Progressive stupor
    b. Hypoventilation
    c. Hypoglycemia
    d. Hypotension
    e. Hyponatremia
    f. Hypothermia

III. Diagnostic tests and methods
   A. Client history
   B. Physical examination
   C. RAIU
   D. TSH levels, T_4, T_3
   E. Serum cholesterol, carotene, alkaline phosphatase, triglyceride levels, and basic chemistry panel
   F. CBC with differential
   G. For myxedema coma
      1. Serum sodium levels (decreased)
      2. ABGs (decreased pH and elevated PCO_2)

IV. Implementation
   A. Assess, report, and record signs and symptoms and any reaction to treatment.
   B. Monitor vital signs, respirations, GI functions, and neurological status.
   C. Orient to environment as needed.
   D. Provide safe, warm environment.
   E. Provide a high-bulk, low-calorie diet.
   F. Encourage activity to promote weight loss and to combat constipation.
   G. Administer prescribed thyroxine replacement, analgesics for pain, laxatives or stool softeners for constipation, and IV fluids.
   H. Monitor for signs of hyperthyroidism caused by thyroxine replacement:
      1. Restlessness
      2. Nervousness
      3. Sweating
      4. Excessive weight loss
   I. Instruct client to report signs of cardiovascular diseases such as chest pain and tachycardia.
   J. Instruct client to report signs of infection immediately.
   K. Encourage fluid intake.
   L. Provide meticulous skin care; monitor for skin breakdown.
   M. Monitor for signs of myxedema coma:
      1. Decreased urinary output (sign of decreased cardiac output)
      2. Decreased temperature (hypothermia)
         a. Provide extra blankets and clothing.
         b. Provide a warm room.

c. Avoid rapid rewarming as it may cause vasodilation and vascular collapse.
3. Monitor daily I&O and weight.
4. Turn client every 2 hours.
5. Provide meticulous skin care.
6. Avoid sedation or reduce dosage (hypothermia delays metabolism of many drugs).
7. Maintain patent IV line:
   a. Monitor serum electrolytes while client is receiving IV therapy.
   b. Monitor vital signs—especially if client is receiving levothyroxine (too-rapid correction of hypothyroidism may cause adverse cardiac effect).
8. Report chest pain or tachycardia immediately.
9. Monitor elderly clients for hypertension and CHF.
10. Monitor ABGs for signs of hypoxia and respiratory acidosis.
11. Monitor for need of ventilatory assistance.
12. Monitor urine and sputum for sources of infection.
13. Check possible sources of infection (blood, urine, sputum), as coma may have been triggered by infection.

   N. Explain condition, diagnostic procedures, treatment, home care, and follow-up care to client and family:
      1. Monitor vital signs, elimination, activity, skin care, reaction to medications.
      2. Emphasize compliance to prescribed treatment.
      3. Emphasize need for follow-up visits to physician.

V. Evaluation
   A. Client reports increased comfort and decreased anxiety.
   B. Client remains free of injury or infection.
   C. Client maintains good skin integrity.
   D. Client maintains adequate level of mobility.
   E. Client maintains adequate cardiac output.
   F. Client maintains adequate elimination pattern.
   G. Client demonstrates improvement in thought process.
   H. Client develops positive self-image.
   I. Client complies with thyroid medication routine.
   J. Client and family demonstrate an understanding of condition, diagnostic procedures, treatment including medication, home care, and follow-up.

Hyperparathyroidism

I. Description
   A. Condition characterized by overactivity of one or more of the four parathyroid glands, which results in an abnormal increase in the secretion of PTH
   B. Increased levels of PTH, which promotes resorption of bone and results in hypercalcemia (elevated serum calcium levels) and hypophosphatemia (diminished levels of phosphorus)
   C. Resultant increase in renal and GI absorption of calcium
   D. Classification as either primary or secondary hyperparathyroidism
   E. Primary type: increased PTH secretion caused by the enlargement of one or more of the parathyroid glands, which results in increased serum calcium levels

F. Secondary type: increased PTH secretion caused by a hypocalcemia-producing abnormality excluding the parathyroid gland, which causes resistance to the metabolic action of PTH

II. Data collection
   A. Subjective symptoms
      1. Fatigue
      2. Weakness
      3. Anorexia
      4. Nausea
      5. Chronic low back pain
      6. Bone tenderness
      7. Constipation
      8. Abdominal pain
      9. Pruritus
     10. Marked muscle weakness
   B. Objective symptoms
      1. Elevated PTH levels
      2. Marked muscle atrophy
      3. Elevated serum calcium, chloride, and alkaline phosphatase levels
      4. Diminished serum phosphorus levels
      5. Elevated urine calcium levels
      6. Bone fractures or cysts on radiographs because of osteoporosis
      7. Polyuria
      8. Polydipsia
      9. Arrhythmias
     10. Hypertension
     11. Renal calculi
     12. Polynephritis
     13. Hematemesis
     14. Vomiting
     15. Signs of pancreatitis, peptic ulcer
     16. Stupor, coma
     17. Necrosis of skin
     18. Cataracts
     19. Calcium microthrombi in lungs and pancreas
     20. Negative Trousseau's or Chvostek's signs
     21. Subcutaneous calcification
     22. Memory loss
     23. Symptoms of secondary hyperparathyroidism
        a. Decreased serum calcium levels
        b. Variable serum phosphorus levels
        c. Skeletal deformities
        d. Symptoms of underlying disease

III. Diagnostic tests and methods
   A. Client history
   B. Physical examination
   C. Serum PTH
   D. Total serum calcium
   E. Serum phosphorus
   F. Quantitative urinary calcium
   G. Uric acid and creatinine levels
   H. Tests for underlying disease for secondary hyperparathyroidism

IV. Implementation
   A. Assess, report, and record signs and symptoms and any reaction to treatment.
   B. Monitor vital signs, respiratory, and cardiovascular status frequently.
   C. Monitor skeletal, renal, and neurological status frequently.
   D. Administer prescribed diuretics and medications to inhibit bone resorption.
   E. Provide safe environment; assist with comfort measures.
   F. Administer prescribed analgesics for pain.
   G. Record I&O.
   H. Encourage fluid intake of 3000 mL daily; include cranberry juice to acidify urine.
   I. To help prevent spontaneous fractures:
      1. Assist with ambulation.
      2. Keep bed at lowest position with side rails up.
      3. Lift immobilized client carefully to decrease stress on bones.
      4. Check radiographic reports to determine which bones are the weakest.
   J. Explain rationale for moderate-calcium, low-phosphorus diet.
   K. Strain urine to monitor for presence of stones; check for signs of hematuria.
   L. Prepare client and family for surgical intervention (parathyroidectomy), if indicted.
   M. Explain condition, diagnostic procedures, and treatment.

V. Evaluation
   A. Client reports increased comfort and decreased anxiety.
   B. Client remains free of injury or infection.
   C. Client maintains adequate cardiac output.
   D. Client maintains adequate nutritional intake.
   E. Client maintains adequate elimination patterns.
   F. Client demonstrates an understanding of condition, diagnostic procedures, and treatment.

Hypoparathyroidism

I. Description
   A. Condition characterized by a deficiency of PTH
   B. Resultant decrease in bone resorption because low serum calcium levels (hypocalcemia) and increase in levels of phosphorus (hyperphosphatemia)
   C. Hypocalcemia producing neuromuscular symptoms ranging from paresthesia to severe tetany
   D. Clinical effects generally corrected with PTH replacement therapy
   E. Some complications, such as cataracts, possibly irreversible
   F. Either idiopathic or acquired

II. Data collection
   A. Subjective symptoms
      1. Numbness and tingling
      2. Dyspnea
      3. Depression or irritability
      4. Confusion
      5. Headache
      6. Visual problems, photophobia
      7. Muscle cramps and spasms
      8. Muscle pain
      9. Difficulty in walking
     10. Abdominal pain

B. Objective symptoms
   1. Positive Trousseau's and Chvostek's signs (tetany)
   2. Convulsions
   3. Laryngeal stridor
   4. Arrhythmias
   5. CHF
   6. Calcification of skull on radiography
   7. Dry, scaly skin
   8. Decreased calcium levels
   9. Elevated serum phosphorus levels
   10. Decreased urine calcium levels
   11. Increased bone density on radiograph
   12. Increased QT interval and ST segment on ECG as a result of hypocalcemia
   13. Cataracts

III. Diagnostic tests and methods
   A. Laboratory serum values: calcium, phosphorus
   B. Qualitative urinary calcium (Sulkowitch's) test
   C. Radiographs of skeletal system
   D. ECG
   E. Trousseau's and Chvostek's tests

IV. Implementation
   A. Assess, report, and record signs and symptoms and any reaction to treatment.
   B. Monitor vital signs; maintain patent airway.
   C. Monitor serum calcium and phosphorus levels and urinary calcium levels.
   D. Maintain patent IV line; keep IV calcium available.
   E. Maintain seizure precautions.
   F. Keep tracheotomy tray and endotracheal tube at bedside (in case of laryngospasm).
   G. Assist in administration of prescribed IV diazepam; monitor vital signs frequently to ascertain BP and heart rate.
   H. Monitor for cardiac rhythm, if indicated.
   I. Monitor for signs of tetany; check Trousseau's or Chvostek's sign.
   J. Assist in administration of calcium gluconate or calcium chloride, and vitamin D as prescribed.
   K. Monitor I&O.
   L. Monitor for signs of heart block and signs of decreasing cardiac output.
   M. Provide adequate nutrition with high-calcium, low-phosphate diet.
   N. Apply prescribed cream to soften scaly skin.
   O. Explain condition, diagnostic procedures, treatment including medication compliance, home care, and follow-up care to client and family.

V. Evaluation
   A. Client reports increased comfort and decreased anxiety.
   B. Client remains free of injury or infection.
   C. Client maintains effective breathing pattern.
   D. Client maintains adequate cardiac output.
   E. Client maintains adequate nutritional and fluid intake.
   F. Client shows improvement in thought process.
   G. Client demonstrates an understanding of condition, diagnostic procedures, treatment including medication compliance, home care, and follow-up care.

Addison's Disease (Adrenal Hypofunction)

I. Description
   A. Condition characterized by hyposecretion of cortisol by the adrenal cortex
   B. Classification as primary or secondary
   C. Occurring at any age and in both sexes
   D. Incidence of secondary type increasing with use of steroid therapy
   E. Prognosis good with early diagnosis and appropriate treatment
   F. Adrenal crisis (addisonian crisis) a result of extreme deficiency of mineralocorticoids and glucocorticoids because of acute stress in individuals with chronic Addison's disease
   G. Adrenal crisis: requires immediate emergency treatment
   H. Causes
      1. Fungal infections such as histoplasmosis
      2. Bilateral adrenalectomy
      3. Hemorrhage into adrenal gland
      4. Tuberculosis
      5. Adrenal carcinoma
      6. Idiopathic atrophy
      7. Impaired circulation
      8. Autoimmune response (circulating antibodies react against adrenal tissue)

II. Data collection
   A. Subjective symptoms
      1. Weakness
      2. Fatigue
      3. Nausea
      4. Anorexia
      5. Inability to concentrate
      6. Muscle pain
      7. Menstrual changes, impotence
      8. Decreased tolerance for minimal stress
      9. Craving for salty food
   B. Objective symptoms
      1. Lethargy
      2. Bronze skin
      3. Weight loss
      4. Vomiting
      5. Chronic diarrhea
      6. Areas of absent skin pigmentation
      7. Decreased plasma ACTH
      8. Low serum sodium levels
      9. High serum potassium and BUN levels
      10. Elevated Hct, lymphocyte, and eosinophil counts
      11. Evidence of small heart and adrenal calcification on radiograph
      12. Hypoglycemia (fasting blood glucose)
      13. Poor skin turgor, sunken eyeballs, dry mucous membrane as a result of dehydration
      14. Hypotension
      15. Weak, irregular pulse
      16. Decreased concentration of corticosteroids in plasma or urine
      17. Decreased 17-hydroxysteroid, 17-ketosteroid and 17-hydroxycorticosteroid (17-OHCS) in 24-hour urine test
      18. Sparse body hair in women

III. Diagnostic tests and methods
  A. Client history
  B. Physical examination
  C. Plasma and urine corticosteroid levels
  D. Serum sodium, potassium, and BUN levels
  E. Fasting blood glucose test
  F. ACTH stimulation test
  G. Radiography
Implementation
  H. Assess, report, and record signs and symptoms and any reaction to treatment.
  I. Monitor for electrolyte imbalance and hypoglycemia.
  J. For clients with diabetes, check blood glucose level periodically (steroid replacement therapy may require an adjustment of insulin dosage).
  K. Provide diet that maintains sodium and potassium balance.
  L. Administer prescribed glucocorticoid and mineralocorticoid replacement.
  M. Administer antacids to prevent ulcers.
  N. Provide safe, calm environment, limit visitors, avoid potential stressors.
  O. Provide emotional support.
  P. Monitor client receiving steroids for cushingoid symptoms, such as edema of face and around eyes.
  Q. Observe client for signs of petechiae.
  R. Monitor for facial growth and other masculinization signs in female clients who are on testosterone injections for muscle weakness and decreased libido.
  S. Explain need for lifelong therapy and need to watch for symptoms of overdosage and underdosage.
  T. Advise client to avoid infections, injury, or heat, which may precipitate an adrenal crisis.
  U. Monitor for signs of addisonian crisis:
    1. Acute hypotension, tachycardia
    2. Profound weakness
    3. Nausea, vomiting, diarrhea, vague abdominal pain
    4. Dehydration
    5. Vascular collapse, shock
    6. Renal failure
    7. Coma
    8. Hyponatremia, hyperkalemia, hypoglycemia
  V. Provide care for addisonian crisis
    1. Assist in administration of prescribed IV hydrocortisone immediately.
    2. Administer prescribed intramuscular (IM) hydrocortisone after initial IV therapy or assist in administration of prescribed hydrocortisone diluted with IV saline or dextrose until condition stabilizes.
    3. Monitor vital signs every 15 minutes.
    4. Monitor urine output hourly.
    5. Monitor weight.
    6. Monitor serum sodium levels.
    7. Monitor fluid intake.
  W. Instruct client to carry a medical identification card.
  X. Instruct client and family on how to inject hydrocortisone.
  Y. Advise client and family to keep hydrocortisone in a prepared syringe for use in case of stress.
  Z. Provide comfort measures, such as backrubs and relaxation techniques.
  AA. Assist with gradual return to activities.
  BB. Explain condition, diagnostic procedures, treatment, home care, and follow-up care to client and family.
IV. Evaluation
  A. Client reports increased comfort and decreased anxiety.
  B. Client remains free of injury or infection.
  C. Client maintains adequate fluid balance.
  D. Client maintains adequate nutritional intake.
  E. Client uses effective coping strategies.
  F. Client and family demonstrate an understanding of condition, diagnostic procedures, treatment including medication compliance, home care, and follow-up care.

Cushing's Syndrome and Disease

I. Description
  A. Characterized by a cluster of abnormalities caused by excessive levels of adrenocortical hormones (especially cortisol), androgens, and aldosterone
  B. Affecting women more than men
  C. Affecting:
    1. Protein, carbohydrate, and fat metabolism
    2. Inflammatory and immune response
    3. Mineral and water metabolism
    4. Blood components
    5. Emotional status
  D. Prognosis depends on underlying cause: poor in individuals who have not received treatment and in those with metastatic adrenal malignancy or untreatable ectopic ACTH-producing malignancy
  E. Causes
    1. Overproduction of ACTH with resultant hyperplasia of adrenal cortex (Cushing's syndrome)
    2. Overproduction of ACTH from pituitary hypersecretion
    3. ACTH-producing tumor (ectopic ACTH secretion) in another organ external to the adrenal gland such as pancreatic or bronchogenic carcinoma
    4. Administration of synthetic glucocorticoids or ACTH
    5. Cortisol-secreting adrenal tumor: usually benign
II. Data collection
  A. Subjective symptoms
    1. Fatigue
    2. Muscle weakness
    3. Irritability
    4. Insomnia
    5. Poor wound healing
    6. Changes in menstrual cycle and libido
    7. Bone pain
    8. Emotional disturbances
  B. Objective symptoms
    1. Evidence of steroid diabetes: decreased glucose tolerance, glucosuria, and fasting hyperglycemia
    2. Moon face (from fat deposits)
    3. Buffalo hump: fat pads over upper back
    4. Fat pads over clavicle
    5. Truncal obesity with slender arms and legs
    6. Little or no scar formation
    7. Acne and hirsutism in women

8. Muscle atrophy caused by increased catabolism
9. Pathological fractures caused by decreased bone mineral
10. Skeletal growth retardation in children
11. Striae (stretch marks on skin)
12. Evidence of peptic ulcer, resulting from increased gastric secretions and production of pepsin
13. Hypertension caused by sodium and water retention
14. Left ventricular hypertrophy
15. Capillary weakness caused by protein loss: leads to petechiae and ecchymosis
16. Infections caused by suppressed antibody formation and decreased lymphocyte production
17. Sodium (and secondary fluid) retention
18. Increase in potassium excretion
19. Ureteral calculi caused by increased bone demineralization
20. Elevated urine calcium levels
21. Enlargement of breasts in men and clitoral hypertrophy, virilism, and amenorrhea in women

III. Diagnostic tests and methods
A. Client history
B. Physical examination
C. Plasma and urinary steroid levels
D. Low-dose dexamethasone suppression test for Cushing's syndrome
E. High-dose dexamethasone suppression test for Cushing's disease
F. Ultrasound, CT scan, and angiography to localize adrenal tumors
G. CT scan of head to identify presence of pituitary tumors

IV. Implementation
A. Assess, report, and record signs and symptoms and any reaction to treatment.
B. Monitor vital signs and neurological status every 4 hours.
C. Monitor serum electrolyte, blood glucose, and cortisol levels.
D. Monitor urinary glucose levels.
E. Monitor daily weight and check for edema.
F. Monitor I&O carefully.
G. Provide diet high in protein and potassium and low in calories, sodium, and carbohydrates.
H. Monitor for signs of infection
   1. Check temperature every 4 hours.
   2. Check skin, oral cavity, and lungs for signs of infection.
   3. Encourage coughing and deep-breathing exercises.
   4. Turn client frequently.
   5. Provide proper hygienic measures.
   6. Avoid individuals with upper respiratory infections.
I. Assist in reducing stressors
   1. Maintain continuity of nursing care.
   2. Avoid excessive noise or temperature changes.
   3. Limit visitors.
   4. Provide privacy.
   5. Allow adequate rest periods.
J. Monitor and record instances of emotional lability.

K. Provide a restful environment; allow client to verbalize feelings.
L. Administer prescribed medications, such as potassium replacements and inhibitors of cortisol production or release; monitor for side effects.
M. Prepare client and family for surgical intervention, if indicated
   1. Bilateral adrenalectomy
   2. Total hypophysectomy
   3. Transsphenoidal adenectomy
N. Provide postoperative care
   1. Monitor wound drainage or fever immediately.
   2. Use strict aseptic technique in changing dressings when ordered.
   3. Administer analgesics and replacement steroids as ordered.
   4. Monitor urinary output.
   5. Monitor vital signs; check for shock symptoms (decreased BP, increased pulse rate, pallor, cold clammy skin)
      a. Administer prescribed vasopressors and increase IV flow rate as ordered.
      b. Monitor for decreased mental alertness and for signs of physical weakness.
      c. Assess neurological and behavioral status.
      d. Monitor for signs of nausea, vomiting, and diarrhea.
   6. Monitor laboratory reports for signs of hypoglycemia caused by removal of cortisol source (cortisol maintains normal blood glucose levels).
   7. Monitor for signs of adrenal hypofunction indicative of inadequate steroid replacement
      a. Orthostatic hypotension
      b. Apathy, weakness, fatigue
   8. Monitor for signs of abdominal distention and recurrence of bowel sounds.
   9. For clients undergoing pituitary surgery, monitor and report signs of increased ICP (agitation, changes in level of consciousness, confusion, nausea, vomiting).
O. Advise client to take steroid replacements with antacids or meals to decrease gastric irritation.
P. Advise client to carry a medical identification card.
Q. Advise client to monitor for and immediately report signs of inadequate steroid dosage (weakness, vertigo, fatigue).
R. Instruct the client and family that discontinuation of the steroid replacement medications may produce a fatal adrenal crisis.
S. Encourage a positive self-image.
T. Explain condition, diagnostic procedures, treatment including medication, home care including activities and prevention of complications, and follow-up care to client and family.

V. Evaluation
A. Client reports increased comfort and decreased anxiety.
B. Client remains free of injury or infection.
C. Client maintains adequate activity.
D. Client maintains adequate fluid balance.
E. Client uses effective coping strategies.

F. Client develops a positive self-image.

G. Client maintains adequate nutritional intake.

H. Client maintains compliance with medication replacement therapy.

I. Client and family demonstrate an understanding of condition, diagnostic procedures, treatment including medications, prevention, home care, and follow-up.

Diabetes Mellitus

I. Description

A. Condition characterized by insulin deficiency or resistance, with disturbances in carbohydrate, protein, and fat metabolism followed by chronic neuropathies and microvascular change

B. Insulin responsible for transporting glucose into body cells for use as energy and for storing glycogen

C. Insulin causing stimulation of protein synthesis and free fatty acid storage

D. Deficiency in insulin that jeopardizes access of body cells to essential nutrients

E. Incidence approximately equal in men and women, rising with age

F. Predisposing client to renal failure, as well as to peripheral vascular, cerebrovascular, and coronary artery disease.

G. A leading cause of blindness

H. Three forms
1. Type I (insulin-dependent diabetes mellitus)
   a. Usually occurring before age 30 years (although may occur at any age)
   b. Individual usually thin, requiring endogenous insulin and dietary management
2. Type II (non–insulin-dependent diabetes mellitus)
   a. Most prevalent among obese. Children rapidly becoming larger section of this population.
   b. Responds to dietary treatment alone or in combination with hypoglycemic agents or insulin
   c. Three major abnormalities: insulin resistance, impaired glucose tolerance, inappropriate production of glucose by the liver.
3. Type 3 (secondary diabetes)
   a. Secondary to another medical condition such as pregnancy, tumors, or removal of the pancreas.

I. Effects of insufficient endogenous insulin includes
1. Elevated serum blood glucose level as a result of impaired intake by liver; high blood levels of glucose pulling fluid from body tissues, causing osmotic diuresis
2. Lipolysis resulting from changes in fat metabolism causing ketone formation, possibly leading to ketonuria

J. Glucose content in epidermis (skin) and urine, stimulating bacterial growth

K. Causes
1. Heredity
2. Environmental
3. Autoimmune factors
4. Precipitating factors
   a. Obesity: causes resistance to endogenous insulin
   b. Physiological or emotional stress: causes prolonged increased levels of cortisol, epinephrine, glucagon, and growth hormone, which in turn raise blood glucose levels, thereby increasing demands on the pancreas
   c. Pregnancy and use of oral contraceptives: increase levels of estrogen and placental hormones, which are antagonists of insulin
   d. Use of other insulin antagonists such as thiazide diuretics and renal corticosteroids

II. Data collection

A. Subjective symptoms
1. Fatigue
2. Polyphagia
3. Polydipsia
4. Nocturia, polyuria
5. Visual disturbances as a result of edema and sugar deposits, which cause changes in lens
6. Anxiety
7. Abdominal pain
8. Prolonged wound healing
9. Recurrent infections

B. Objective symptoms
1. Lethargy
2. Weight loss (type I); obesity (type II)
3. Elevated fasting serum glucose level
4. Glycosuria
5. Dehydration
6. Dry mucous membranes
7. Poor skin turgor
8. Long-term effects
   a. Retinopathy
   b. Nephropathy
   c. MI
   d. Stroke
   e. Peripheral neuropathy
   f. Nocturnal diarrhea
   g. Skin infections
   h. UTIs
   i. Vaginitis
   j. Anal pruritus

III. Diagnostic tests and methods

A. Client history

B. Physical examination

C. Fasting blood glucose test

D. Urinalysis

E. Urine tests for glucose and acetone

F. Glucose tolerance test

G. Hemoglobin A1C; also known as glycosolated hemoglobin

H. Twenty-four-hour urine quantitative glucose specimen

I. C-peptide

IV. Implementation

A. Assess, report, and record signs and symptoms and any reaction to treatment.

B. Emphasize importance of compliance with prescribed program.

C. Provide safe and hazard-free environment.

D. Provide comfort measures.

E. Monitor I&O.

F. Monitor serum glucose, urine glucose levels, and electrolytes.

G. Monitor vital signs every 4 hours or as needed as condition warrants.

H. Monitor for signs of hypoglycemia (abnormally low blood glucose levels caused by an excess of insulin or oral hypoglycemic medication in relation to activity or dietary intake or the result of insufficient glucose to supply CNS needs)
1. Pallor
2. Weakness, numbness
3. Confusion or irritability
4. Fatigue
5. Vertigo
6. Blurred vision
7. Tachycardia
8. Diaphoresis
9. Hunger
10. Seizures
11. Coma

I. Instruct client and family on carbohydrate foods to treat hypoglycemia
1. Fruit juice
2. Hard candy
3. Honey
4. Cola

J. If unconscious, assist in administration of IV dextrose or IM glucagon.

K. Continue to monitor vital signs and neurological status frequently.

L. Monitor blood glucose level frequently.

M. Provide safe, hazard-free environment.

N. Continue to monitor I&O and nutritional status.

O. Facilitate use of effective coping strategies.

P. Explain self-care and prevention.

Q. Teach correct self-glucose testing.

R. Monitor for signs of hyperglycemia (ketoacidosis: acute or gradual insulin deficiency precipitated by emotional stress, infection, trauma, or other stressors; occurs in clients with insulin-dependent diabetes; leads to protein catabolism, release of potassium and urea nitrogen, and ketone formation from fat breakdown).
1. Increased thirst
2. Nausea, vomiting
3. Abdominal pain
4. Drowsiness
5. Headache
6. Acetone breath: fruity breath odor from respiratory compensation for elevated serum acetone level
7. Elevated serum glucose level
8. Elevated serum acetone level and osmolarity
9. Decreased arterial pH and bicarbonate level
10. Dehydration
11. Weak, rapid pulse
12. Kussmaul's respirations
13. Osmotic diuresis
14. Electrolyte imbalance

S. Monitor for signs of hyperglycemic nonketonic coma
1. Polyuria

2. Thirst
3. Neurological abnormalities
4. Stupor

T. Both diabetic ketoacidosis and hyperosmolar coma are hyperglycemic crises
1. Assist in administration of prescribed IV fluids.
2. Assist in administration of prescribed insulin and electrolyte replacement.
3. Assist in administration of potassium replacement, if required.
4. Monitor for signs of hypoglycemia as a result of insulin administration.
5. Monitor vital signs every 4 hours.
6. Monitor I&O hourly.
7. Monitor serum glucose levels, electrolytes, and ABGs.
8. Monitor for correction of dehydration.
9. Provide a safe, calm environment.
10. Monitor for diabetic effects on the cardiovascular system
    a. Symptoms of cerebrovascular disease
    b. Symptoms of coronary artery and peripheral vascular disease

U. Monitor for and treat all injuries, cuts, and blisters (especially on lower extremities) as prescribed.

V. Monitor for signs of UTI and renal failure.

W. Assess client for diabetic neuropathy
1. Numbness
2. Pain in arms and legs
3. Footdrop
4. Neurogenic bladder
5. Instruct client to avoid trauma; client may injure himself or herself unknowingly because of decreased sensation in arms and legs.

X. Assist with instruction of client and family about insulin and explain that it is administered to control serum glucose metabolism and thereby control diabetes:
1. Types of insulin
   a. Rapid acting (lispro); onset 15 minutes; peak 60–90 minutes; solution clear.
   b. Rapid-acting (regular): onset within 1 hour, peak action in 1–4 hours; solution appears clear.
   c. Intermediate-acting (neutral protamine Hagedorn [NPH], Lente): onset begins in 2–4 hours, with peak action in 6-8 hours; solution appears cloudy.
   d. Long-acting (protamine zinc, Ultralente): onset begins in 4–8 hours, peak action in 16–18 hours; solution appears cloudy. Rarely used.
   e. Long-acting (glargine); onset 1–2 hours, no pronounced peak, duration 24 hours; clear; cannot be mixed nor given IV.
2. Strength or concentration
3. Source: pork, beef, Humulin insulin
4. Purity
5. Regimen prescribed
6. Rotation sites and subcutaneous injection
7. Mixing of different types

Y. Explain condition, diagnostic procedures, complications, treatment including medication, prevention, and home care including self-care and activity.

V. Evaluation
   A. Client reports increased comfort and decreased anxiety.
   B. Client remains free of injury or infection.
   C. Client maintains adequate serum glucose level.
   D. Client maintains adequate fluid and nutritional intake.
   E. Client maintains adequate fluid balance and tissue perfusion.
   F. Client maintains good skin integrity.
   G. Client develops a positive self-image.
   H. Client reports reduction in feeling of powerlessness.
   I. Client verbalizes plan for compliance.
   J. Client uses effective coping strategies.
   K. Client demonstrates an understanding of condition, diagnostic procedures, complications, and treatment including medication, prevention, and home care including self-care and activity.

Musculoskeletal System

Basic Information

The musculoskeletal system is a complex system of bones, muscles, ligaments, tendons, and other connective tissue. This system gives the body shape and form. It also makes movement possible, protects vital organs, provides the site for hemopoiesis, and stores calcium and other minerals.

Muscle tissue has contractility that makes movement of bones and joints possible. Muscles also move food through the intestines, pump blood through the blood vessels of the body, and make breathing possible. The activity of muscles aids in temperature regulation by producing heat. Muscles also assist in maintaining body position such as standing and sitting. Muscles are classified as skeletal (attached to bones), visceral (provide function of internal organs), and cardiac (forming the wall of the heart). Muscles are also classified as voluntary and involuntary. Involuntary muscles are controlled by the autonomic nervous system, which includes the cardiac and visceral muscles. Voluntary muscles are controlled by deliberate intention and influenced by the somatic nervous system. These latter muscles are classified as skeletal muscles. Muscle mass accounts for about 40% of the weight of humans.

The human skeleton has 206 bones composed of organic salts, such as calcium and phosphate, which are imbedded in fibers of collagen. Bones are classified as long, short, flat, or irregular. Musculoskeletal disorders can be either acute or chronic. Acute problems are usually caused by simple injuries; chronic conditions often result in loss of mobility and changes in self-image.

I. Basic data collection
   A. Subjective symptoms
      1. Weakness
      2. Pain
      3. Complaints of joint stiffness
      4. Weight loss
      5. Anorexia
      6. Limited movement
   B. Objective symptoms
      1. General appearance
      2. Abnormal gait
      3. Impaired neurovascular status
      4. Differences between affected and unaffected sides
      5. Absence of extremity
      6. Decreased handgrip
      7. Abnormal spinal curvature
      8. Joint enlargement
      9. Presence of edema, redness, warmth over affected area
      10. Decreased ROM
      11. Changes in vital signs
      12. Nonalignment of extremities
      13. Inability to move a body part

Major Musculoskeletal Diagnoses

Systemic Lupus Erythematosus

I. Description
   A. A chronic inflammatory disorder of connective tissues
   B. Usually affecting multiple organ systems as well as the skin
   C. Possibly fatal
   D. Condition characterized by recurring remissions and exacerbations
   E. Affecting women eight times as often as men; incidence increases during childbearing years
   F. Exacerbations more common during the spring and summer
   G. Prognosis improved with early detection and treatment
   H. Prognosis poor for clients who develop complications: severe infections, renal and neurological problems
   I. Causes unknown
   J. Theoretical causes
      1. Autoimmune: antibodies entering tissue suppress normal immunity response of body
      2. Certain predisposing factors causing susceptibility
         a. Physical or mental stress
         b. Streptococcal or viral infections
         c. Immunization
         d. Exposure to sunlight or ultraviolet light
         e. Pregnancy
         f. Genetic predisposition
      3. Triggered or aggravated by certain drugs
         a. Anticoagulants
         b. Hydralazine
         c. Procainamide
         d. Sulfa drugs
         e. Penicillin
         f. Oral contraceptives
II. Data collection
   A. Subjective symptoms
      1. Photosensitivity
      2. Fatigue
      3. Weakness
      4. Weight loss
      5. Joint pain and stiffness of hands, feet, or large joints
      6. Tenderness of affected joints
      7. Anorexia

8. Abdominal pain
9. Nausea
10. Irregular menstrual periods
11. Headaches, irritability
B. Objective symptoms
   1. Nondeforming arthritis
   2. Facial erythema (butterfly rash)
   3. Oral or nasopharyngeal ulcerations
   4. Pleuritis, pericarditis, neuritis, glomerulonephritis, peritonitis
   5. Convulsions
   6. Hemolytic anemia, thrombocytopenia, leukopenia
   7. Positive antinuclear antibody (ANA) or systemic lupus erythematosus (SLE) cell test result
   8. Proteinuria
   9. UTIs
   10. Increased cellular casts in urine
   11. Alopecia
   12. Chronic false-positive serological test result for syphilis
   13. Increased temperature
   14. Vomiting
   15. Lymph node enlargement
   16. Diarrhea or constipation or both
   17. Dyspnea
III. Diagnostic tests and methods
   A. Client history
   B. Physical examination
   C. CBC with differential
   D. Platelet count
   E. ESR
   F. Serum electrophoresis
   G. ANA and SLE cell tests
   H. Urine studies
   I. Chest radiograph
   J. ECG
   K. Kidney biopsy
IV. Implementation
   A. Assess, report, and record signs and symptoms and any reaction to treatment.
   B. Provide emotional support to client and family.
   C. Monitor for dyspnea, chest pain, and edema of extremities.
   D. Note size, type, and location of skin lesions.
   E. Monitor urine for signs of hematuria.
   F. Monitor scalp for hair loss (alopecia).
   G. Monitor skin and oral mucous membrane for bleeding, ulceration, petechiae, and bruising.
   H. Provide a well-balanced diet.
   I. Provide a low-sodium, low-protein diet if renal disorder is present.
   J. Administer prescribed medications such as
      1. Ointments or creams for rash
      2. Corticosteroids for inflammatory response and renal or neurological complications
      3. Analgesics for arthritic pain
      4. Cytotoxic drugs, if prescribed
   K. Prepare client and family for dialysis or kidney transplant if renal failure occurs.
   L. Advise use of protective clothing, screening agent, and sunglasses when out in sun.
   M. Apply heat packs for relief of joint pain and stiffness.
   N. Encourage full ROM exercises to prevent contractures.
   O. Arrange for physical therapy and occupational counseling.
   P. Provide frequent skin and mouth care.
   Q. Monitor vital signs, I&O, laboratory reports, and weight.
   R. Monitor GI secretions and stools for presence of blood.
   S. Monitor for signs of renal involvement (hypertension, weight gain).
   T. Assess for signs of neurological involvement (personality changes, ptosis, double vision, seizures).
   U. Explain use of cosmetics to women (hypoallergenic cosmetics).
   V. Refer client to Lupus Foundation of America and Arthritis Foundation.
   W. Explain diagnostic condition, diagnostic procedures, treatment, home care, and follow-up care.
V. Evaluation
   A. Client reports increased comfort and decreased anxiety.
   B. Client remains free of injury or infection.
   C. Client maintains good skin integrity.
   D. Client uses effective coping strategies.
   E. Client remains free of organ-specific complications.
   F. Client demonstrates an understanding of condition, diagnostic procedures, treatment, home care, and follow-up care.

Rheumatoid Arthritis

I. Description
   A. Chronic, systemic, inflammatory disease that primarily involves peripheral joints and surrounding muscles, tendons, ligaments, and blood vessels
   B. Eventual depletion of joint cartilage results in joint dislocation
   C. Condition characterized by spontaneous remissions and unpredictable exacerbations
   D. Usually requiring lifelong treatment and occasionally surgery
   E. Possible for majority of clients to carry on with normal activity
   F. Occurring worldwide; affecting women three times more than men
   G. Occurring at any age but most prevalent in women aged 20 to 60 years, with peak onset between ages 35 and 45 years
   H. Inflammatory process within joints occurring in four stages if left untreated
      1. First stage: synovitis developing from congestion and edema of synovial membrane and joint capsule
      2. Second stage: formation of thickened layers of granulation tissue, in which thickened layers cover and invade cartilage, destroying joint capsule and bone
      3. Third stage: formation of fibrous ankylosis; fibrous invasion of thickened layers of granulation tissue with scar formation, which occludes the joint space; visible deformities caused by bone atrophy

and malalignment, resulting in muscle atrophy and imbalance
  4. Fourth stage: calcification of fibrous tissue, with bony ankylosis causing total immobility
I. Cause unknown
J. Theoretical causes
  1. Susceptibility caused by genetic defects impairing autoimmune system
  2. Bacterial or viral infection
  3. Environmental factors
  4. Endocrine, nutritional, and metabolic factors
  5. Occupational and psychosocial influences

II. Data collection
  A. Subjective symptoms
     1. Morning stiffness of joints
     2. Sore, stiff, swollen red joint(s)
     3. Weakness
     4. Fatigue
     5. Malaise
     6. Numbness, tingling in feet, hands
     7. Loss of sensation in fingers and toes
     8. Inability to perform usual activities
     9. Pain with ROM
     10. Loss of appetite
  B. Objective symptoms
     1. Limited ROM of joint
     2. Weakened grip
     3. Low-grade fever
     4. Anemia
     5. Weight loss
     6. Subcutaneous nodes
     7. Enlarged lymph nodes
     8. Muscle atrophy
     9. Appearance of joints bilaterally
     10. Elevated ESR
     11. Positive rheumatoid factor (RF) or latex fixation test
     12. Radiograph evidence of joint deterioration
     13. Spindle-shaped fingers
     14. Flexion deformities of affected joints
     15. Skin lesions and leg ulcers as a result of vasculitis
     16. Peripheral neuropathy
     17. Complications such as infection, osteoporosis, and temporomandibular disease (which impairs chewing and causes earaches)

III. Diagnostic tests and methods
  A. Client history
  B. Physical examination
  C. Radiography of joints
  D. Rheumatoid factor (RF) test
  E. ANA and SLE cell tests
  F. Synovial fluid analysis
  G. CBC with differential
  H. Serum protein electrophoresis
  I. C-reactive protein

IV. Implementation
  A. Assess, report, and record signs and symptoms and any reaction to treatment.
  B. Provide emotional support.
  C. Encourage adequate nutritional intake; assist with meals as needed.
  D. Schedule undisturbed rest periods.

E. Administer heat applications such as paraffin dip, hot packs, and warm tub baths or showers for relief of pain and muscle relaxation as ordered.
F. Administer analgesics, anti-inflammatory, and disease modifying antirheumatic medications as ordered.
G. Allow verbalization of feelings and support positive body image.
H. Provide ROM exercises within limits of pain tolerance.
I. Provide meticulous skin care; use lotion or cleaning oil in place of soap for dry skin.
J. Apply splints correctly, if ordered; observe for pressure sores.
K. Encourage mobility
  1. Encourage client to perform ADLs with assistance as necessary.
  2. Assist with active ROM exercise.
  3. Instruct client to protect joints and conserve energy.
  4. Encourage client to ambulate with assistance as necessary.
  5. Coordinate care with physical therapy department.
L. Explain disease process and chronic pain, as well as medical or surgical treatment (synovectomy, arthrotomy, arthroplasty, or arthrodesis).

V. Evaluation
  A. Client reports increased comfort and decreased anxiety.
  B. Client participates in ADLs.
  C. Client develops a positive self-image.
  D. Client maintains adequate nutritional intake.
  E. Client remains free of injury or infection.
  F. Client demonstrates an understanding of disease process, diagnostic procedures, treatment, home care, and follow-up care.

Osteoarthritis

I. Description
  A. Most common form of arthritis, a progressive disorder causing deterioration of the joint cartilage and formation of reactive new bone at margins of joints
  B. Most often affecting weight-bearing joints such as the hips and knees
  C. Incidence rising among older people
  D. Earliest symptoms generally beginning in middle age, becoming progressively severe with advancing age
  E. Affecting both sexes
  F. Prognosis that depends on site and severity of involvement; may range from minor limitations involving the fingers to severe disability involving knees and hips
  G. Varying rate of progression
  H. Causes
     1. Primary osteoarthritis: resulting from genetic predisposition, a normal part of aging
     2. Secondary osteoarthritis: an acquired form resulting from joint damage caused by trauma, stress, excessive "wear and tear," infection, underlying joint disease, and/or metabolic disorders

II. Data collection
  A. Subjective symptoms
     1. Pain after exercise or weight bearing
     2. Morning stiffness

3. Aching during changes in weather
4. "Grating" of joint during movement
B. Objective symptoms
1. Limited ROM
2. Crepitant joint
3. Prominent bony enlargement
4. Heberden's nodes on distal joints of phalanges and Bouchard's nodes on proximal joints of phalanges: initially painless; then red, swollen, and tender
III. Diagnostic tests and methods
A. Client history
B. Physical examination
C. Radiography of affected joints
IV. Implementation
A. Assess, report, and record signs and symptoms and any reaction to treatment.
B. Encourage client to verbalize feelings about condition.
C. Provide adequate rest, especially after activity.
D. Assist with physical therapy.
E. Care for affected joint.
1. Hand: apply hot soaks and paraffin dips to relieve pain as ordered.
2. Spine (lumbar and sacral): provide firm mattress or bedboard to decrease morning pain.
3. Spine (cervical): provide cervical collar for constrictions; monitor for signs of redness.
4. Hip
a. Apply moist heat pads to relieve pain.
b. Administer antispasmodic medications as ordered.
c. Assist with ROM and strengthening exercises.
d. Check assistive devices such as crutches, braces, and walker for proper fit.
e. Advise use of elevated toilet seat and cushions when sitting.
5. Knee
a. Assist with prescribed ROM exercises.
b. Encourage exercises to maintain muscle tone.
F. Explain condition, diagnostic procedures, treatment, home care, and follow-up care.
1. Avoid overexertion.
2. Take medications as prescribed.
3. Obtain adequate rest.
4. Wear well-fitting supportive shoes.
5. Use guardrails in bathroom
a. Minimize weight-bearing activities.
V. Evaluation
A. Client reports increased comfort and decreased anxiety.
B. Client remains free of injury or infection.
C. Client participates in self-care activities.
D. Client develops a positive self-image.
E. Client demonstrates an understanding of condition, diagnostic procedures, treatment, home care, and follow-up care.

Gout

I. Description
A. A metabolic disease resulting in an acute inflammation of synovial tissue characterized by deposits of urate crystals

B. Increased concentration of uric acid resulting in urate deposits (tophi) in joints and tissues, causing local necrosis or fibrosis
C. Primary gout occurring in men, with onset at approximately age 50 years, and in postmenopausal women
D. Secondary gout occurring in elderly clients
E. Following an intermittent course, with most clients free of symptoms for years between attacks
F. Possibly leading to chronic disability
G. In rare instances, possibly leading to severe hypertension and progressive renal disease
H. Affecting any joint, but found mostly in joints of feet and legs
I. Development in four stages: asymptomatic, acute, intercritical, and chronic
J. Prognosis good with treatment
K. Causes
1. Primary gout
a. Exact cause unknown
b. Condition linked to a genetic defect in purine metabolism, resulting in an overproduction of uric acid (hyperuricemia), retention of uric acid, or both
2. Secondary gout
a. Follows course of other diseases such as polycythemia vera or multiple myeloma
b. Caused by breakdown of nucleic acid
c. May also follow drug therapy, such as hydrochlorothiazide, which interferes with urate excretion
II. Data collection
A. Subjective symptoms
1. Onset of pain in joint of the great toe, feet, ankles, or knees
2. Pruritus
3. Headache
4. Malaise
5. Severe back pain
B. Objective symptoms
1. Elevated serum uric acid level
2. Normal or elevated 24-hour urinary uric acid level
3. Positive for monosodium urate crystals in synovial fluid
4. Inflamed joints
5. Elevated WBC count and ESR
C. Asymptomatic stage: serum urate levels increase with no apparent symptoms
1. Acute stage
a. Hypertension, kidney stones: attack sudden, peaking quickly
b. Affected joints: hot, inflamed, dusky-red, cyanotic
c. Joint of great toe usually affected first, followed by the instep, ankle, heel, knee, or wrist joints
2. Intercritical stage: symptom-free between gout attacks
3. Chronic stage
a. Persistent painful polyarthritis
b. Large, subcutaneous tophaceous deposits in cartilage, synovial membranes, tendons, and soft tissues (urate deposits above earlobe, fingers, hands, knees, feet, and ulnar sides of forearms)

c. Ulcerations over tophi, with presence of chalky white exudate or pus
d. Joint degeneration or deformity, and disability
e. Kidney involvement, resulting in symptoms of chronic renal dysfunction
f. Urolithiasis (urinary calculi)

III. Diagnostic tests and methods
   A. Client history
   B. Physical examination
   C. Serum uric acid levels
   D. Urinary uric acid levels
   E. WBC count
   F. ESR
   G. Analysis of aspirated synovial fluid or of tophaceous material
   H. Radiographs of joints
   I. RF test to rule out rheumatoid arthritis

IV. Implementation
   A. Assess, report, and record signs and symptoms and reaction to treatment.
   B. Provide bed rest during acute attacks.
   C. Provide adequate fluid to prevent calculi formation; monitor I&O.
   D. Monitor appearance of joints (ROM ability).
   E. Administer analgesics such as aspirin or acetaminophen as prescribed to relieve pain of mild attacks.
   F. Provide bed rest; use bed cradle to keep bedcovers off affected joints.
   G. Position affected joint in mild flexion position during acute attack; assist with mobility.
   H. Administer prescribed medications such as colchicine, anti-inflammatory drugs such as phenylbutazone (Butazolidin), probenicid (Benemid), indomethacin (Indocin), or sulfinpyrazone (Anturane) to facilitate uric acid secretion; allopurinol (Zyloprim) to decrease formation of uric acid; monitor for side effects.
   I. Administer corticosteroids for resistant inflammation as prescribed.
   J. Assist with joint aspiration and injection of intra-articular corticosteroid injection, if needed.
   K. Apply hot or cold packs to inflamed joints as ordered; monitor serum uric acid levels on a regular basis.
   L. Encourage weight loss in obese clients (obesity places additional stress on painful joints).
   M. Prepare client for excision and drainage of infected or ulcerated tophi.
   N. Monitor for acute gout attacks 24–96 hours after surgery.
   O. Explain disease process, diagnostic procedures, treatment, prevention, and home care
      1. Checking serum uric acid levels periodically
      2. Avoiding use of high-purine foods such as anchovies, kidneys, sweetbreads, lentils, and alcoholic beverages
      3. Dieting to gradually decrease weight in obese clients
      4. Complying with prescribed medication regimen
      5. Reporting side effects of medications immediately

V. Evaluation
   A. Client reports increased comfort and decreased anxiety.
   B. Client remains free of injury or infection.

C. Client maintains adequate nutritional and fluid intake.
D. Client maintains adequate level of mobility.
E. Client demonstrates an understanding of disease process, diagnostic procedures, treatment including medication, prevention, and home care.

Osteoporosis

I. Description
   A. Metabolic bone disorder with an acceleration of bone resorption rate and a slowing down in the rate of bone formation, resulting in loss of bone mass
   B. Calcium and phosphate salts lost from affected bones
   C. Affected bones becoming brittle, vulnerable to fractures
   D. Either primary or secondary to an underlying disease
   E. Primary osteoporosis (senile or postmenopausal): most common in postmenopausal women
   F. Usually affected sites: vertebrae, pelvis, and femur
   G. Causes of primary osteoporosis
      1. Unknown
   H. Predisposing factors involving primary osteoporosis
      1. Prolonged negative calcium balance because of inadequate dietary intake of calcium
      2. Decline in gonadal adrenal function
      3. Faulty protein metabolism resulting from estrogen deficiency and sedentary lifestyle
   I. Causes of secondary osteoporosis
      1. Prolonged therapy with steroids or heparin
      2. Total immobilization or disuse of bone, as with hemiplegia
      3. Alcoholism: malnutrition
      4. Lactose intolerance
      5. Hyperthyroidism
      6. Scurvy
      7. Osteogenesis imperfecta

II. Data collection
   A. Subjective symptoms
      1. Backache
      2. Pain radiating around trunk
   B. Objective symptoms
      1. Vertebral compression
      2. Kyphosis
      3. Loss of height
      4. Pathological fractures: neck, femur, hip, Colles' fracture
      5. Changes in skull, ribs, and long bones owing to severe or advanced osteoporosis, as in hyperthyroidism or Cushing's syndrome

III. Diagnostic tests and methods
   A. Client history
   B. Physical examination
   C. Skeletal radiographs
   D. Serum calcium, phosphorus, and alkaline phosphatase levels within normal limits
   E. Elevated parathyroid hormone level
   F. Bone biopsy
   G. Dexa Scan

IV. Implementation
   A. Assess, report, and record signs and symptoms and any reaction to treatment.

B. Encourage exercise and other weight bearing physical activity to prevent disuse atrophy.
C. Administer estrogen replacement as ordered to improve calcium balance.
D. Administer biphosphates to inhibit bone resorption.
E. Provide diet high in protein and calcium.
F. Administer vitamin D supplements and calcium as ordered to support normal bone metabolism.
G. Encourage fluid intake of 2000–3000 mL daily to avoid formation of renal calculi (unless contraindicated).
H. Provide support of spine with brace or corset as ordered.
I. Monitor daily for redness, warmth, and new sites of pain.
J. Perform passive ROM exercises as appropriate.
K. Coordinate care with physical therapist.
L. Provide safety precautions such as side rails, moving client gently and carefully.
M. Administer analgesics as prescribed for pain.
N. Encourage use of walker or cane to stabilize balance when client is ambulating.
O. Encourage early mobilization after surgical procedure or trauma.
P. Monitor for signs of malabsorption.
Q. Encourage avoidance or decrease of alcohol consumption.
R. Instruct client and family in importance of following prescribed daily activity.
S. Advise client and family on importance of sleeping on a firm mattress and avoiding excessive bed rest.
T. For women receiving estrogen, emphasize need for routine gynecological checkups, including Pap smears. Instruct client to report any abnormal bleeding and presence of breast lumps.
U. Instruct client regarding good body mechanics, such as stooping before lifting and avoiding twisting motions and prolonged bending.
V. Explain disease process, diagnostic procedures, treatment, prevention, home care, and follow-up care.

V. Evaluation
A. Client reports increased comfort and decreased anxiety.
B. Client remains free of injury or infection.
C. Client maintains adequate level of mobility.
D. Client maintains adequate nutritional and fluid intake.
E. Client participates in self-care activities.
F. Client demonstrates an understanding of disease process, diagnostic procedures, treatment, prevention, home care, and follow-up care.

Herniated Nucleus Pulposus (Slipped or Ruptured Disk)

I. Description
A. Protrusion of the nucleus pulposus (soft, mucoid central portion of an intervertebral disk), resulting in compression of nerve roots of spinal cord or spinal cord itself
B. Nucleus pulposus forced through the disk's weakened or torn outer ring

C. Compressed nerve roots or spinal cord, resulting in back pain and other signs of nerve root irritation
D. Usually occurring in adults (mostly men) under age 45 years
E. Occurring anywhere along the spine; however, sites usually affected between L4 and L5, L5 and sacrum, C5 and C6, and C6 and C7
F. After trauma in lumbosacral area: pain possibly beginning suddenly, subsiding briefly, recurring at shorter intervals with progressive intensity; sciatic pain following; Valsalva's maneuver, sneezing, coughing, or bending magnifying pain, accompanied by muscle spasms
G. Possibly causing sensory and motor loss in area innervated by compressed spinal nerve root followed by weakness and atrophy of affected muscles
H. Causes
   1. Severe trauma or strain
   2. Intervertebral joint degeneration
   3. Congenitally small lumbar spinal canal

II. Data collection
A. Subjective symptoms
   1. Cervical disk
      a. Stiff neck
      b. Shoulder pain descending down arm into hand
      c. Numbness of arm and hand
   2. Lumbosacral disk
      a. Severe low back pain radiating down buttocks, legs, and feet—usually unilaterally
      b. Can have bowel or urinary incontinence
B. Objective symptoms
   1. Cervical disk: sensory disturbances of neck, arm, and hand
   2. Lumbosacral disk
      a. LeSegue's signs: pain in back and legs, loss of ankle or knee-jerk reflex with client lying flat, thighs and knees flexed 90 degrees while raising heel with knee straight
      b. Straight-leg raising test: pain in posterior leg (sciatic pain) with client lying supine, examiner placing one hand on client's ilium and other hand under ankle, while slowly raising client's leg
      c. Difficulty in ambulating
      d. Numbness of leg and foot

III. Diagnostic tests and methods
A. Client history
B. Physical examination
C. Neurological examination
D. Radiography of spine
E. CT scan or MRI of spine
F. Peripheral vascular status check: posterior tibial and dorsalis pedis pulses, and skin temperature of extremities to rule out ischemic vascular disease
G. Myelography
H. Electromyography

IV. Implementation
A. Assess, report, and record signs and symptoms and any reaction to treatment.
B. Encourage verbalization of fears and other feelings related to immobility.
C. Assess allergies to iodides (such as seafood) before

myelography (may indicate sensitivity to radiopaque dye used in diagnostic test).

D. After myelography
   1. Have client remain supine in bed, with knees raised.
   2. Provide increased fluid intake to prevent renal stasis; monitor I&O.
   3. Monitor for allergic reaction to dye.
E. Encourage deep breathing, coughing, and use of blow bottles to prevent pulmonary complications.
F. Provide meticulous skin care.
G. Assess bowel function and use fracture bedpan when client is receiving complete bed rest.
H. Monitor for abnormal neurological signs.
I. Apply antiembolism stockings as ordered.
J. Provide diet high in fiber with adequate fluid intake to prevent constipation and straining.
K. Encourage client to move legs.
L. Provide high-topped sneakers to prevent footdrop.
M. Coordinate prescribed exercises with physical therapist to ensure consistent regimen.
N. Prepare client for surgical intervention, if required (laminectomy or spinal fusion).
O. Provide postoperative care
   1. Enforce bed rest.
   2. Monitor for leakage of cerebrospinal fluid (CSF) on surgical dressing; reinforce dressing until checked by physician.
   3. Log-roll client to change position to prevent motion of spinal column.
   4. Check tubing of Hemovac blood-draining system for kinks and patent vacuum.
   5. Empty Hemovac at end of each shift; record amount and color of drainage.
   6. Monitor neurovascular status of involved extremities; color, temperature, sensation, and mobility. Monitor for incontinence.
   7. Monitor bowel sounds and abdomen for distention.
   8. Administer prescribed analgesics.
   9. Assist client during first ambulation attempt.
   10. Instruct client with spinal fusion on how to wear a brace.
   11. Assist with straight-leg raising and toe-pointing exercises as ordered.
P. Prepare client for chemonucleolysis, if required
   1. Check for allergic reaction to radiopaque dyes or meat tenderizers, which are similar to chemical used (chymopapain) for procedure.
Q. After chemonucleolysis procedure
   1. Enforce bed rest.
   2. Administer analgesics for pain as prescribed.
   3. Apply heat to area, if ordered.
   4. Assist with special exercises as prescribed.
R. Instruct client and family regarding proper body mechanics.
S. Advise client to use a firm mattress and to sleep on side rather than abdomen.
T. Encourage weight loss if client is obese to prevent lordosis.
U. Explain condition, diagnostic procedures, treatment, prevention, and home care.

V. Evaluation
   A. Client reports increased comfort and decreased anxiety.
   B. Client remains free of injury or infection.
   C. Client maintains adequate elimination patterns.
   D. Client maintains adequate level of mobility.
   E. Client verbalizes feelings and devlops a positive self-image.
   F. Client understands reason for weight reduction if obese.
   G. Client demonstrates an understanding of condition, diagnostic procedures, treatment, prevention, home care including activity, and follow-up care.

Fractures

I. Description
   A. Usually resulting from trauma and often causing substantial muscle, nerve, and other soft-tissue damage
   B. Prognosis varies with
      1. Extent of disability or deformity
      2. Amount of tissue and vascular damage
      3. Adequacy of reduction and immobilization
      4. Client's health status, age, and nutritional status
   C. Possibility of bones of adults in poor health, along with impaired circulation, not to heal properly
   D. Severe open fractures, especially those involving the femoral shaft, possibly causing considerable bleeding and life-threatening hypovolemic shock
   E. Types of fractures
      1. Incomplete: break extending only partially through bone
      2. Complete: bone breaking into two or more pieces.
      3. Closed (simple): overlying skin remaining unbroken
      4. Open (compound): wound present over fractured area; fractured bone breaking through skin
      5. Nondisplaced: fractured bone remaining in proper alignment
      6. Transverse: break running transversally (straight across) the bone shaft
      7. Spiral: break encircling bone like a coil
      8. Oblique: bone broken at a diagonal angle
      9. Comminuted: bone shattered or compressed into bone fragments
      10. Impacted: bone ends driven into each other
      11. Compression: bone (vertebrae) collapsing under excessive pressure
      12. Linear: break running length of bone
      13. Greenstick: bone splintering fibers on one side of bone, leaving other side intact
      14. Avulsion: overexertion resulting in tearing of a muscle or ligament from a bone, pulling a small bone fragment with it
      15. Depression: bone fragments driven inward by trauma (usually referring to fracture of the skull)
   F. Complications of fractures of the extremities
      1. Permanent deformity and dysfunction caused by failure of bones to heal (nonunion) or bones healing improperly (malunion)

2. Hypovolemic shock as a result of blood vessel damage
3. Muscle contractures
4. Aseptic necrosis of bone segments because of decreased circulation
5. Renal calculi forming decalcification because of prolonged immobilization
6. Fat embolism
7. Compartment syndrome

G. Causes
1. Most fractures occur from major trauma.
2. Pathological fractures occur because of underlying conditions of osteoporosis, bone tumors, or metabolic disease.
3. Prolonged standing, walking, or running may cause stress fractures of foot and ankle (usually seen in postal workers, nurses, soldiers, and joggers).

II. Data collection
A. Subjective symptoms
1. Pain: usually intense and acute; worsening with pressure or movement
2. Loss of movement of affected extremity
3. Loss of sensory perception distal to fracture site
4. Point tenderness
5. Numbness and tingling

B. Objective symptoms
1. Pallor
2. Limited motion or paralysis of affected limb distal to fracture site
3. Deformity of affected limb
4. Edema; discoloration
5. Crepitus on movement of limb
6. Warmth over site
7. Possible arterial compromise or nerve damage
   a. Mottled cyanosis
   b. Cool skin at end of extremity
   c. Loss of pulses distal to injury
   d. Signs of shock
8. Evidence of fracture on radiography

III. Diagnostic tests and methods
A. Client history
B. Physical examination
C. Radiography of suspected fracture sites and associated joints

IV. Implementation
A. Assess, report, and record signs and symptoms and any reaction to treatment.
B. Splint or immobilize injured area.
C. Monitor vital signs; observe for shock symptoms (rapid pulse, decreased BP, cool clammy skin, and pallor).
D. Assist in administration of IV fluids as ordered.
E. Administer analgesics and/or muscle relaxants as prescribed.
F. Apply ice compress to injured area as ordered.
G. Discuss use of relaxation techniques.
H. Prepare client for surgical intervention and provide postoperative care as indicated.
I. Assist with passive and active ROM of unaffected limbs; maintain mobility.
J. Assist with appropriate exercise to affected limb as ordered.

K. Encourage client to participate in self-care activities.
L. Provide a well-balanced nutritional diet: high in protein and vitamins, high in bulk. Encourage adequate fluid intake to prevent bowel and urinary problems.
M. Monitor for signs of compartment syndrome (pain out of proportion, swelling with tight shiny skin, numbness or tingling, cool or mottled extremity, loss of pulse as a late sign).
N. Monitor for signs of fat embolism (apprehension, sweating, fever, tachycardia, pallor, dyspnea, petechial rash on chest and shoulders, pulmonary effusion, tissue hypoxia, cyanosis, convulsions, coma).
O. Turn client, if not contraindicated, every 2 hours, maintaining proper alignment.
P. Encourage use of isometric exercises to prevent muscle atrophy.
Q. Types of traction
1. Buck's traction: used to ease muscle spasm and immobilize limb by maintaining a straight pull on limb using weights
2. Russell's traction: used to alleviate muscle spasm and immobilize limb by maintaining a pull at knee and foot with use of knee sling
3. Skeletal traction: direct application of traction to bone with use of wires or pins (Steinmann pin, Kirschner wire) that are pulled by traction weights
4. Crutchfield tongs: tongs inserted into shallow holes in the skull and joined to skeletal traction for fractures of the cervical vertebrae

R. Care for long-term immobilization with traction
1. Reposition client often to increase comfort and to prevent formation of decubitus ulcers.
2. Assist with ROM exercises to prevent muscle atrophy.
3. Encourage deep breathing and coughing to prevent pulmonary complications.
4. Encourage adequate fluid intake to prevent urinary stasis and constipation.
5. Monitor for signs of renal colic (flank pain, nausea, and vomiting).
6. Maintain proper body alignment.
7. Check ropes and weights for proper placement (ropes in middle of pulley and weights should hang freely).
8. Provide meticulous skin care.
9. Avoid bumping into or manipulating traction device.
10. Inspect site of pins and affected limb frequently.
11. Monitor site of cervical tongs: provide meticulous skin care using aseptic technique.
12. Use footboard to prevent footdrop; use high-topped sneaker on unaffected leg.
13. Monitor circulation; check for signs of thrombophlebitis.

S. Cast care
1. Support cast with pillows while still wet.
2. Observe for skin irritation near cast edges.
3. Check for foul odors or discharge.
4. Instruct client to report signs of decreased circulation to the part (skin coldness, tingling, numbness, discoloration of toes or fingers).
5. Instruct client to keep cast dry.

6. Instruct client to avoid inserting foreign objects under the cast.
T. Encourage movement as soon as possible.
U. Assist with ambulation.
V. Demonstrate the correct method of walking with crutches (placing weight on hands and not on axillary region) to prevent damage to nerves.
W. After cast removal, refer to physical therapist for assistance in restoring limb mobility.
X. Explain condition, diagnostic procedures, treatment, prevention, home care including activity, and follow-up care.

V. Evaluation
   A. Client reports increased comfort and decreased anxiety.
   B. Client remains free of injury or infection.
   C. Client maintains safe environment.
   D. Client maintains adequate level of mobility.
   E. Client maintains good skin integrity.
   F. Client maintains adequate elimination pattern.
   G. Client maintains adequate tissue perfusion.
   H. Client maintains adequate nutritional intake.
   I. Client demonstrates an understanding of condition, diagnostic procedures, treatment, prevention, home care, and follow-up care.

Amputation

I. Description
   A. Two types of amputation: surgical and traumatic
   B. Surgical amputation: surgical removal of part or all of an extremity.
      1. Majority resulting from vascular disorders causing an inadequate oxygen supply to the tissue
      2. Other reasons for amputation: septic wounds, gas gangrene, malignant tumors, severe trauma, burns
   C. Traumatic amputation: the accidental loss of a body part, such as an arm, leg, finger, or toe
      1. In complete amputation, the part is completely severed.
      2. In partial amputation, some soft tissue remains.
      3. Prognosis has improved because of
         a. Improved emergency and critical care management
         b. New surgical techniques
         c. New prosthetic designs
         d. Early rehabilitation
         e. Innovative limb reimplantation techniques used but their usefulness limited by incomplete nerve regeneration
      4. Causes: accidents involving farm, factory, motor vehicles, use of power tools, or war

II. Data collection
   A. Subjective symptoms (surgical amputation)
      1. Peripheral vascular diseases: pain, tingling
      2. Septic wounds and gas gangrene: pain
   B. Objective symptoms (surgical amputation)
      1. Peripheral vascular diseases
         a. Pallor
         b. Edema
         c. Diminished pulses
         d. Cyanosis
         e. Ulcer formation
         f. Hyperpigmentation
      2. Septic wounds, gas gangrene
         a. Foul odor
         b. Blackened wound
         c. Edema
         d. Fever
         e. Necrosis
   C. Subjective symptoms (traumatic amputation)
      1. Pain
   D. Objective symptoms (traumatic amputation)
      1. Profuse bleeding
      2. Hypovolemic shock
         a. Hypotension
         b. Narrowing pulse pressure
         c. Tachycardia
         d. Rapid, shallow respirations
         e. Oliguria
         f. Cold, clammy skin
         g. Metabolic acidosis
         h. Missing tissue or limb

III. Diagnostic tests and methods
   A. Both surgical and traumatic amputations
      1. Client history
      2. Physical examination
   B. Surgical amputations
      1. Arteriography
      2. Oscillometry
      3. Radiography
      4. Skin temperature studies

IV. Implementation
   A. Surgical amputation
      1. Assess, report, and record signs and symptoms and any reaction to treatment.
      2. Prepare client and family for surgical intervention.
      3. Encourage verbalization of feelings.
      4. Provide emotional support.
      5. Explain phantom pain (pain in amputated limb).
      6. Explain postoperative plan
         a. Program of exercises
            1) Exercises for strengthening upper extremities
            2) Transferring from bed to chair and vice versa
            3) Ambulating with walker or crutches
      7. Provide postoperative care
         a. Provide routine postoperative care.
         b. Provide reassurance to help client cope with altered body image.
         c. Apply Ace bandages in a figure-eight pattern only.
         d. Monitor for signs of bleeding; have a tourniquet at bedside for emergency use.
         e. Elevate stump 8–12 hours on a pillow.
         f. Remove pillow after 12 hours to prevent hip contracture.
         g. Place client in prone position every 4 hours to prevent hip contracture.
         h. Place trochanter roll along outer side of stump to prevent outward rotation.
         i. Instruct client to massage the stump to improve vascularity.
         j. Instruct client regarding conditioning of the stump to prepare for application of a prosthesis

1) Push stump against a pillow.
2) Progress by pushing stump against a harder surface.
  k. Instruct client to avoid letting stump hang over edge of bed or chair to prevent stump contracture.
    1) Use transcutaneous electrical nerve stimulator (TENS) for relief of phantom pain if ordered.
  8. Explain condition, diagnostic procedures, treatment, prevention, home care, and follow-up care.
B. Traumatic amputation
  1. Emergency treatment
    a. Monitor vital signs.
    b. Cleanse wound.
    c. Administer prescribed tetanus prophylaxis, antibiotics, and analgesics.
    d. After complete amputation
      1) Preserve extremity wrapped in gauze moistened with sterile saline, within a sterile plastic bag, then place bag on ice.
      2) Notify reimplantation surgeon.
    e. After partial amputation
      1) Position limb in normal alignment.
      2) Drape with sterile towels moistened with sterile normal saline solution.
  2. Preoperative care: assist with thorough wound irrigation and debridement.
  3. Postoperative care
    a. Change dressing using sterile technique.
    b. Provide reassurance to help client cope with altered body image.
    c. Provide rehabilitation as in postoperative care of surgical amputation.
V. Evaluation
  A. Client reports increased comfort and decreased anxiety.
  B. Client remains free of injury or infection.
  C. Client maintains adequate level of mobility.
  D. Client maintains good skin integrity.
  E. Client verbalizes feelings, develops positive self-image and self-concept.
  F. Client uses effective coping strategies to cope with altered body image.
  G. Client participates in self-care activities.
  H. Client demonstrates an understanding of condition, treatment, home care, and follow-up care.

The Eyes

Basic Information

Visual acuity depends on general good health, CNS regulation of movement and conduction, and condition of eye structures. Vision disorders frequently indicate systemic disease. Disorders that affect the eye usually lead to impairment or loss of vision. Routine eye examination can provide information regarding disease in other body systems. The incidence of visual impairment and blindness increases with age; however, individuals of all ages can be affected. Vision has recently been the focus of innovative medical and surgical treatment.

Routine and early eye examinations, along with early treatment, are essential.

I. Basic data collection
  A. Subjective symptoms
    1. Double vision
    2. Blurred or clouded vision
    3. Decreased or absent vision
    4. Sensitivity to light
    5. Spots, halos around lights
    6. Flashes of light
    7. Problems seeing in dark
    8. Itching, pain, tearing, burning, headache
  B. Objective symptoms
    1. Tearing, discharge: clear or purulent
    2. Color of sclera: white, yellow, or pink
    3. Glasses or contact lenses
    4. Accuracy and range of vision
    5. Crusts, blinking, rubbing
    6. Edema of eyelids
    7. Squinting or drooping of lid
    8. Symmetry
    9. History of
      a. Trauma to eyes
      b. Contact lenses
      c. Eye medications
      d. Changes in vision
      e. Systemic medications in use

Major Diagnoses Related to the Eyes

Cataract

I. Description
  A. Clouding or opacity of the lens, which prevents light rays from reaching the retina
  B. Can occur in one or both eyes, with each progressing independently resulting in a gradual decrease in vision
  C. Most prevalent as part of the aging process in persons over age 65 years
  D. Surgical improvement of vision in 95% of affected individuals
  E. Causes
    1. Aging process (senile cataract)
    2. Injury to eye (traumatic cataract)
    3. Resulting from another eye disease (secondary cataract)
    4. Inherited trait (congenital cataract) such as maternal rubella
    5. In metabolic disease, such as diabetes mellitus, they develop at a younger age
    6. Infections and inflammation
    7. Radiation or ultraviolet (UV) light exposure
    8. Systemic or topical corticosteroids
II. Data collection
  A. Subjective symptoms
    1. Progressive decreased vision
    2. Altered color perception
    3. Blinding glare from headlights at night
    4. Loss of vision with mature cataract; thick, white, hard central opacity

    B. Objective symptoms
      1. Opaque or cloudy-white pupil
      2. Decreased visual acuity
 III. Diagnostic tests and methods
    A. Client history
    B. Physical examination
    C. Examination with ophthalmoscope
    D. Slit-lamp examination
    E. Glare test
    F. A-scan ultrasound
    G. Keratometry
 IV. Implementation
    A. Assess, report, and record signs and symptoms and any reaction to treatment.
    B. Provide a safe environment; keep necessary items in specific areas within reach.
    C. Administer prescribed preoperative eye medication (mydriatic) to dilate pupil for surgery.
    D. Administer prescribed preoperative cycloplegic agent to paralyze accommodation muscles
    E. Administer prescribed antianxiety medications
    F. Provide postoperative care to prevent increased intraocular pressure
      1. Position client supine or on unoperative side with head of bed elevated.
      2. Administer prescribed antibiotic eye drops to prevent infection.
      3. Instruct client to avoid any actions that may increase intraocular pressure, such as straining, bending, or performing rapid head movements, or lift anything heavy.
      4. Administer stool softener if ordered to prevent straining during bowel movement.
      5. Monitor dressing if present.
      6. Administer prescribed steroid eyedrops to reduce inflammation.
    G. Assist with self-care activities and ambulation.
    H. Instruct client and family in correct instillation of eyedrops.
    I. Monitor for complications such as increased intraocular pressure, or sudden sharp pain in eye.
    J. Explain condition, diagnostic procedures, and treatment, home care, and follow-up care
      1. Avoiding heavy lifting for several weeks
      2. Activity
      3. Use of eye shield at night
      4. Medications
      5. Use of sunglasses to protect from UV light.
  V. Evaluation
    A. Client reports increased comfort and decreased anxiety.
    B. Client remains free of injury or infection.
    C. Client maintains adequate sensory perception.
    D. Client demonstrates an understanding of condition, diagnostic procedures, treatment, home care, and follow-up care.

Retinal Detachment

  I. Description
    A. Sensory layer of the retina pulling away from pigmented layer

    B. Vitreous humor leaks into space between the separated layers
    C. Usually unilateral; most commonly affects men
    D. New surgical techniques used to reattach retinal layers in about 90% of clients
    E. Causes
      1. Degenerative changes of aging, resulting in a spontaneous retinal break caused by: (a) shrinkage and pulling away of the vitreous that pulls on retina (retinal tear); or (b) atropic, spontaneous breaks (retinal hole)
      2. Traction detachment
      3. Secondary or exudative detachment
    F. Predisposing factors
      1. Myopia
      2. Aphakia
      3. Surgical disturbance of vitreous
      4. Trauma
      5. Result of systemic diseases, such as diabetic retinopathy
      6. Retinal lattice degeneration
 II. Data collection
    A. Subjective symptoms
      1. Floating spots from blood or retina cells as a result of tears
      2. Recurrent flashes of light (photopsia)
      3. Gradual, painless loss of peripheral or central vision
      4. Ring in visual field
    B. Objective symptoms
      1. Loss of vision
      2. Retina separation on ophthalmoscopic exam
 III. Diagnostic tests and methods
    A. Client history
    B. Physical examination
    C. Ophthalmoscopy after full pupil dilation
    D. Visual acuity
    E. Slit lamp
    F. Ultrasound
 IV. Implementation
    A. Assess, report, and record signs and symptoms and any reaction to treatment.
    B. Position head to relieve stress on tear.
    C. Restrict activity based on procedure anticipated.
    D. Provide emotional support.
    E. Provide a calm, safe, restful environment, with side rails up and call signal within easy reach if patient is hospitalized.
    F. Instruct client to avoid activities that cause sudden movement of head, such as sneezing, coughing, or vomiting.
    G. Administer cough medications or antiemetics as ordered.
    H. Assist client with ADLs if indicated.
    I. Administer prescribed eye medications, such as mydriatics, antibiotics, or steroids.
    J. Administer prescribed analgesics.
    K. Prepare client and family for surgical intervention
      1. Administer antibiotics and mydriatic eyedrops as prescribed.
      2. Obtain appropriate consent forms.
    L. Provide postoperative care

1. Position client as ordered (usually by elevating head of bed about 30 degrees).
2. Instruct client to avoid bending over, straining, or rubbing eyes.
3. Assist with ambulation when ordered.
4. If restricted to bed rest after pneumatic retinopexy, encourage leg exercises to prevent thrombophlebitis and head position as ordered to keep intravitreal bubble in position against retina.
5. Monitor for possible complications, such as signs of bleeding or retinal detachment in opposite eye.
6. Instruct client and family in instillation of eyedrops and ointments.
7. Advise client to use dark glasses in bright light.
   M. Explain condition, diagnostic procedures, treatment, home care, and follow-up care.
V. Evaluation
   A. Client reports increased comfort and decreased anxiety.
   B. Client maintains adequate sensory perception.
   C. Client demonstrates an understanding of condition, diagnostic procedures, treatment, home care, and follow-up care.

Glaucoma

I. Description
   A. Abnormal increase in intraocular pressure, which may result in severe and permanent vision defects
   B. Increased intraocular pressure caused by disturbance in circulation of aqueous humor resulting from imbalance between production and drainage.
   C. Possibly secondary to injuries and infections
   D. Most preventable cause of blindness
   E. Affecting approximately 2 million people in the United States
   F. Affecting 1 in 10 African Americans
   G. Normal intraocular pressure ranges from 10 to 21 mm Hg
   H. Requires early diagnosis to prevent damage to the optic nerve and blindness
   I. Prognosis usually good with early diagnosis and treatment
   J. Several forms
      1. Primary open-angle glaucoma (most common)
         a. Caused by overproduction of aqueous humor or obstruction to its outflow in the trabecular meshwork
         b. Frequently familial in origin, affecting 90% of all individuals with glaucoma
         c. Usually bilateral, with insidious onset
         d. Symptoms usually appearing late in the disease
      2. Primary angle-closure glaucoma (narrow-angle): obstruction to outflow of aqueous humor
         a. Resulting from
            1) Anatomically narrow angle between anterior iris and posterior corneal surface
            2) Shallow anterior chamber
            3) Bulging iris that presses on the trabeculae meshwork closing the angle
            4) Thickened iris causing closure of the angle on pupil dilation

b. Rapid onset; produces blindness in 3–5 days if not treated promptly
c. Symptoms possibly misinterpreted as GI distress
      3. Secondary glaucoma
         a. Resulting from
            1) Inflammatory process damaging trabecular meshwork
            2) Trauma
            3) Intraocular neoplasms
         b. Gradual onset
         c. Progressing to absolute glaucoma with pain and blindness
         d. Enucleation necessary to relieve extreme pain
II. Data collection
   A. Subjective symptoms (primary open-angle glaucoma)
      1. Asymptomatic early in disease
      2. Mild aching in eyes
      3. Loss of peripheral vision
      4. Tunnel vision
   B. Subjective symptoms (acute angle-closure glaucoma)
      1. Unilateral pain, sudden, excruciating pain in eye
      2. Occular redness
      3. Blurred vision
      4. Decreased visual acuity
      5. Seeing halos around lights
      6. Nausea and vomiting
   C. Subjective symptoms (chronic angle-closure glaucoma)
      1. Usually producing no symptoms
      2. Blurred vision
      3. Seeing colored halos around lights
      4. Occular redness
      5. Eye or brow pain
   D. Objective symptoms
      1. Elevated intraocular pressure with tonometry
      2. Inflammation
      3. Decreased peripheral vision on visual fields test
      4. Optic-disk cupping on ophthalmoscopic examination
      5. Vomiting
      6. Narrow or flat anterior chamber angle
III. Diagnostic tests and methods
   A. Client history
   B. Physical examination
   C. Tonometry
   D. Gonioscopy: to differentiate between primary open-angle glaucoma and acute or chronic angle-closure glaucoma
   E. Ophthalmoscopy
   F. Slit-lamp examination
   G. Visual acuity
   H. Perimetry or visual field tests: to evaluate extent of primary angle or angle-closure deterioration
   I. Fundus photography
IV. Implementation
   A. Assess, report, and record signs and symptoms and any reaction to treatment.
   B. Explain and administer prescribed eyedrops to decrease aqueous humor production or facilitate drainage (miotic agent pilocarpine; beta-blocker timolol maleate).

C. Explain the need for lifetime compliance in the use of eye medications to prevent disk changes, loss of vision, and need for surgery.
D. Prepare client and family for surgical intervention, if required.
E. Provide postoperative care
1. Administer cycloplegic eyedrops to affected eye
a. Decrease inflammation and relax ciliary muscle.
b. Prevent adhesions.
2. Administer prescribed analgesics for eye pain.
3. Administer prescribed eye medications to constrict pupil.
4. Administer prescribed steroids to rest the pupil.
5. Protect eye with eye patch or eye shield.
6. Assist with positioning on unoperative side.
7. Provide safe environment, with side rails up and call signal within easy reach.
F. Educate client and family in the importance of glaucoma screening for early detection and prevention.
G. Explain condition, diagnostic procedures, treatment, home care, and follow-up care
1. Explain lifetime medication regimen.
2. Explain type of medication, including any side effects.
3. Instruct client to report to physician any eye pain, changes in vision, or seeing halos around lights immediately.
V. Evaluation
A. Client reports increased comfort and decreased anxiety.
B. Client remains free of injury, infection, and further loss of peripheral vision.
C. Client maintains adequate sensory perception.
D. Client demonstrates an understanding of condition, diagnostic procedures, treatment, home care, and follow-up care.
E. Intraocular pressure within normal limits.

Conjunctivitis

I. Description
A. Infection or inflammation of the conjunctiva because of infection, allergy, or chemical reactions
B. Usually benign and self-limiting
C. Possibly chronic, indicative of degenerative changes or damage from repeated attacks
D. Most common eye disorder in the Western Hemisphere
E. Very contagious (especially in young children)
F. Usually beginning in one eye and spreading to other eye via contaminated towels, washcloths, or client's own hands
G. Causes
1. Bacterial infections
2. Chlamydial infections
3. Viral infections
4. Allergic reactions to pollen, grass, air pollutants (e.g., cigarette smoke), topical medication, unknown seasonal allergens, occupational irritants, and rickettsial and parasitic diseases
II. Data collection
A. Subjective symptoms
1. Itching

2. Burning
3. Sensation of foreign body in eye
4. Pain
B. Objective symptoms
1. Photophobia
2. Tearing
3. Sticky, mucopurulent discharge
4. Profuse, purulent discharge if caused by *Neisseria gonorrhoeae*
5. Enlarged preauricular lymph node if caused by viral infection
III. Diagnostic tests and methods
A. Client history
B. Physical examination
C. Conjunctival scrapings
D. Culture and sensitivity tests for bacterial infections
IV. Implementation
A. Assess, report, and record signs and symptoms and any reaction to treatment.
B. Apply warm compresses to affected eye.
C. Cleanse affected eyelid, using warm compresses and removing crusts, before administering eye medications.
D. Administer prescribed ointment or drops.
E. Instruct client in correct instillation of eyedrops and ointments.
F. Advise client to wear safety glasses when working near chemical irritants.
G. Educate client and family regarding spread of infection
1. Teach proper handwashing technique.
2. Avoid sharing washcloths, towels, and pillows.
3. Isolate personal items (washcloths, towels, pillows).
4. Instruct client to avoid rubbing affected eye.
5. Instruct client not to irrigate eye.
6. Use clean washcloths and towels frequently to avoid infecting other eye.
H. Explain condition, diagnostic procedures, treatment, and home care including medication.
V. Evaluation
A. Client reports increased comfort and decreased anxiety.
B. Client remains free of injury or infection.
C. Client demonstrates an understanding of condition, treatment, infection control, and home care.

The Ears

Basic Information

Hearing is initiated by sound waves reaching the tympanic membrane, causing a vibration of the ossicles in the middle ear. The stapes transmit the vibrations to the perilymphatic fluid in the inner ear by vibrating against the oval window. These vibrations then pass across the cochlea's fluid receptor cells, stimulating movement of the hair cells of the organ of Corti and initiating auditory nerve impulses to the brain.

The inner ear structure also maintains the equilibrium and balance of the body. The fluid in the semicircular canals is set into motion by body movement and stimulates nerve cells lining the canal. These cells transmit impulses to the brain via the vestibular branch of the acoustic nerve.

The sense of hearing contributes to well-being and safety. Initially, hearing problems are usually not as obvious as other disorders. Many individuals refuse to wear hearing aids because they associate hearing loss with dependency or disfigurement. Hearing should be assessed for each client.

Conductive hearing loss is a result of injury, obstruction, or disease that interferes with sound wave conduction to the inner ear (e.g., foreign body or wax in the ear canal). Sensory hearing loss is a result of a malfunction of the inner ear, the auditory nerve, or the auditory center in the brain.

I. Data collection
  A. Subjective symptoms
    1. Difficulty in hearing
    2. Vertigo
    3. Pain
    4. Blurred vision
    5. Headache
    6. Itching, pressure (or "full" feeling)
    7. Ringing, popping, buzzing
  B. Objective symptoms
    1. Drainage
    2. Hearing loss
    3. Nonresponse to loud noises
    4. Vomiting
    5. Tenderness
    6. Dried secretions
    7. Deformities of ear
    8. Presence of hearing aid
    9. Notation of history of
      a. Ear infections
      b. Ear surgery
      c. Head injury
      d. Medications

Major Diagnoses Related to the Ears

Ménière's Disease

I. Description
  A. Chronic disease of the inner ear characterized by sudden attacks of vertigo, tinnitus (ringing in the ears), and hearing loss, which results in alterations in body equilibrium and balance
  B. Attacks lasting a few minutes to several weeks
  C. Usually affecting men more often than women, between the ages of 30 and 60 years
  D. Possibly leading to residual tinnitus and hearing loss if attacks continue over time
  E. Symptoms possibly not apparent between attacks (except for tinnitus, which worsens during an attack)
  F. Attacks several times per year or remissions possible, which can last several years
  G. Attacks eventually becoming less frequent with increasing hearing loss
  H. Attacks possibly ceasing entirely with total hearing loss
  I. Surgical destruction of the affected labyrinth possibly required to relieve symptoms permanently if disorder persists for >2 years of treatment or produces constant vertigo (resulting in permanent, irreversible hearing loss)

  J. Unknown causes but have accumulation of endolymph in membranous labyrinth.
  K. Precipitating factors
    1. Autonomic nervous system dysfunction resulting in a temporary constriction of blood vessels that supply inner ear
    2. Premenstrual edema
    3. Viral infection
II. Data collection
  A. Subjective symptoms
    1. Vertigo
    2. Nausea
    3. Tinnitus, hearing loss
    4. Headache
    5. History of ear infection
    6. Fullness or blocked feeling in ear
    7. Loss of balance
  B. Objective symptoms
    1. Nystagmus
    2. Vomiting
    3. Diaphoresis
    4. Sensorineural hearing loss demonstrated with audiometry and vestibular testing
III. Diagnostic tests and methods
  A. Client history
  B. Physical examination
  C. Neurological assessment
  D. Caloric testing (vestibular test)
  E. Glycerol test
  F. Audiometric studies
  G. Electronystagmography
IV. Implementation
  A. Assess, report, and record signs and symptoms and any reaction to treatment.
  B. Provide bed rest during attacks in dark, quiet room.
  C. Advise client to avoid reading and exposure to bright lights to minimize vertigo (avoid fluorescent or flickering lights and televison).
  D. Provide a safe environment; keep side rails up.
  E. Assist with ADLs and ambulation to prevent falls.
  F. Instruct client to move slowly to prevent vertigo.
  G. Instruct client to avoid sudden position changes.
  H. Administer prescribed medications, such as diuretics, antihistamines, vasodilators, antibiotics, antiemetics, steroids, anticholingergics, diazepam (Valium), and meclizine hydrochloride (Antivert).
  I. Provide a low-sodium diet.
  J. Provide care same as that for client with limited hearing (see under Basic Information).
  K. Prepare client and family for surgical intervention, if necessary.
  L. Provide postoperative care
    1. Give general postoperative care.
    2. Record fluid I&O.
    3. Advise client to expect vertigo and nausea for 1–2 days.
    4. Administer prophylactic antibiotics and antiemetics as ordered.
    5. Instruct client to move slowly.
    6. Assist with ambulation while equilibrium is impaired.
  M. Assist with coping and comfort measures.

N. Explain condition, diagnostic procedures, treatment, and home care including activities.
V. Evaluation
  A. Client reports increased comfort and decreased anxiety.
  B. Client remains free of injury or infection.
  C. Client maintains adequate auditory sensory perception.
  D. Client use effective coping strategies.
  E. Client demonstrates an understanding of condition, diagnostic procedures, treatment, and home care.
  F. No hearing loss

Otosclerosis

I. Description
  A. Disorder of the middle ear characterized by fixation of the stapes in the oval window caused by spongy bone formation.
  B. Prevents normal movement of the stapes, resulting in disruption of the conduction of vibrations from the tympanic membrane to the cochlea, which causes progressive hearing loss of the affected ear, possibly progressing to the unaffected ear
  C. Affects approximately 10% of whites between the ages of 15 and 30 years
  D. Prevalence 50% higher in women, accelerated during pregnancy.
  E. Prognosis good with surgery (stapedectomy)
II. Data collection
  A. Subjective symptoms
    1. Hearing loss
    2. Ability to hear conversation better in a noisy environment than a quiet one (paracusis of Willis)
  B. Objective symptoms
    1. Positive findings on audiometric testing
    2. Conductive loss, as demonstrated by Weber and Rinne tests
    3. Reddish blush to tympanic membrane (Schwartz's sign)
Diagnostic tests and methods
  C. Client history
  D. Physical examination
  E. Rinne's test
  F. Weber's test
  G. Audiometric testing
  H. Tympanometry
  I. Otoscopic exam
III. Implementation
  A. Assess, report, and record signs and symptoms and any reaction to treatment.
  B. Monitor for degree of hearing loss.
  C. Provide a safe environment, and assist with ADLs as necessary.
  D. Prepare client and family for stapedectomy (removal of stapes) and insertion of titanium prosthesis for the purpose of restoring hearing in the middle ear.
  E. Provide postoperative care
    1. Keep client with head of bed elevated and head turned so that affected ear is turned upward.
    2. Instruct client to avoid sneezing, coughing, blowing nose (if sneezing unavoidable, instruct client to keep mouth open to equalize ear pressure).
    3. Administer prescribed antibiotics, analgesics, and antiemetics.
    4. Instruct client to move slowly to decrease vertigo episodes.
    5. Monitor for presence of nausea, vomiting, vertigo, headache, or abnormal ear sensations.
    6. Assist with activities as necessary.
    7. Reassure client that hearing will improve when packing is removed and edema resolves.
  F. Provide discharge instructions
    1. Instruct client to avoid loud noises and sudden pressure changes (flying or diving) until healing is complete (usually 6 months).
    2. Instruct client to avoid blowing nose for at least 1 week to prevent air from entering the eustachian tube and dislodging prosthesis.
    3. Advise client to protect ears against cold.
    4. Advise client to avoid contact with individuals who have upper respiratory infections.
    5. Instruct client to avoid any activities that produce vertigo, such as bending, heavy lifting, straining.
    6. Teach client and family to change the external ear dressing and care for the surgical incision.
    7. Advise the client and family of the necessity to complete the prescribed antibiotic regimen.
  G. Explain condition, diagnostic procedures, treatment, home care, and follow-up care.
IV. Evaluation
  A. Client reports increased comfort.
  B. Client remains free of injury or infection.
  C. Client maintains adequate auditory perception.
  D. Client demonstrates an understanding of condition, diagnostic procedures, treatment, home care, and follow-up care.

Neurological System

Basic Information

The neurological system consists of the communication network responsible for coordinating and organizing the functions of all body systems. There are three main divisions: the CNS, which is the control center of the body (brain and spinal cord); the peripheral nervous system, which includes nerves communicating with distant body parts, relaying and receiving messages from them; and the autonomic nervous system, regulating involuntary functions of the internal organs.

The pathology involving the CNS arises from injuries, vascular insufficiency, tumors, infections, and disorders from other diseases. Neurological medical problems are caused by interference with normal functioning of the affected cells.

I. Basic data collection
  A. Subjective symptoms
    1. History of head injury, vertigo, weakness, headache, loss of consciousness, paralysis, seizures, double vision
    2. Pain, numbness, difficulty concentrating, memory loss, drowsiness, difficulty with elimination

B. Objective symptoms
1. Orientation to person, time, and place
2. Mental status (alert, drowsiness, lethargy)
3. Level of consciousness (arousal status to verbal and physical stimuli)
   a. Use of Glasgow coma scale to describe level of consciousness
      1) Eye opening
      2) Verbal response
      3) Motor response
4. Emotional response
5. Speech: presence of aphasia, appropriate speech patterns
6. Behavior: appropriate for situation
7. Ability to follow simple instructions
8. Vital signs (temperature, pulse, respirations, and BP)
9. Motor function: gait, balance, coordination, strength, posture, and function
10. Eyes
    a. Movement of lids and pupils
    b. Size, configuration, and reaction of pupils to light
    c. Comparison from baseline assessment
11. Ears: drainage
12. Facial symmetry
13. Sensation for pain, smell, and light touch
14. Bladder and bowel control
15. Cranial nerve assessment (CN I to CN XII)
16. Reflexes

Major Neurological Diagnoses

Cerebrovascular Accident (Stroke)

I. Description
A. Sudden impairment of the circulation in one or more of the blood vessels supplying the brain; blood vessels occluded, stenosed, ruptured, or thrombus
B. Oxygen supply to the affected brain tissue interrupted or diminished, often causing severe damage or necrosis of the involved tissue
C. Sudden or gradual onset
D. Symptoms related to location and size of brain area affected
E. Approximately 50% of survivors permanently disabled
F. High proportion experiencing recurrence within weeks to years
G. Chances for complete recovery depending on the circulation returning to normal soon after the initial episode
H. Third most common cause of death in the United States and most common cause of neurological disability
I. Predisposing factors
1. History of transient ischemic attacks (TIAs)
2. Hypertension
3. Arrhythmias, atrial fibrillation
4. Atherosclerosis and carotid artery stenosis
5. Rheumatic heart disease

6. Myocardial enlargement
7. Diabetes mellitus
8. High serum triglyceride levels, hyperlipidemia, hypercoagulability
9. Lack of exercise, obesity
10. Cigarette smoking
11. Family history
12. Alcohol use
13. Oral contraceptive use
14. Sickle cell disease
J. Causes
1. Thrombosis
   a. Obstruction of blood vessel by blood clot formed within vessel
   b. Most common cause of CVA in middle-aged and elderly individuals
   c. Tendency to develop while individual is awake or shortly after awakening
   d. Individuals at risk including clients with a history of atherosclerosis, diabetes, and hypertension
   e. Risk increasing with smoking or obesity or both
2. Embolus
   a. Occlusion of blood vessel in brain by a fragmented clot, tumor, fat, air, or bacteria
   b. Can occur at any age and is the second most common cause of CVA
   c. Individuals at risk include clients with a history of rheumatic heart disease, atrial fibrillation, other arrhythmias, or endocarditis, myocardial infarction, clients who have just undergone open-heart surgery, or valvular prosthesis.
   d. Usually developing rapidly (10–20 seconds) and without warning
   e. Most often affecting middle cerebral artery
   f. If embolus septic, infection may extend beyond blood vessel wall, with development of abscess or encephalitis
      1) Infection within blood vessel wall may develop into an aneurysm, with potential cerebral hemorrhage.
3. Hemorrhage
   a. Sudden rupture of a cerebral blood vessel
   b. Occurring at any age and is the third most common cause of CVA
   c. Individuals at risk including clients with chronic hypertension, aneurysms, vascular malformations, trauma, or tumors
   d. Blood supply to the affected brain tissue decreasing with accumulation of blood deep within brain substance, with subsequent compression of nerve tissue and further damage
K. Classification of CVA (least severe to complete stroke)
1. TIA
   a. "Little stroke" caused by temporary interruption of blood flow
   b. Occurring most often in carotid and vertebrobasilar arteries
2. Progressive stroke
   a. Thrombus in evolution begins with slight neurological deficit.

b. Condition exacerbates within 1–2 days.

c. Lasts 15 minutes to 24 hours.

3. Complete stroke: maximum neurological deficits occur immediately at onset

I. Data collection

A. Depending on artery affected, area of brain involved, severity of damage, and extent of collateral circulation, which develops to compensate the brain for diminished blood supply

B. Left hemisphere involvement resulting in symptoms on right side of body; right hemisphere in symptoms on left side of body

C. CVA causing cranial nerve damage, which produces neural dysfunction on same side of the body

D. Subjective symptoms

1. Changes in motor function—sensation and strength

2. Headache

3. Dizziness

4. Difficulty in speaking

5. Visual disturbances

E. Objective symptoms

1. Middle cerebral artery

a. Aphasia, hemiparesis, visual field cuts

b. Hemiparesis more severe in face and arm than in leg

2. Anterior cerebral artery

a. Numbness, confusion, weakness (especially lower limb)

b. Incontinence

c. Personality changes

d. Loss of coordination

e. Impaired motor and sensory functions

3. Posterior cerebral artery

a. Visual field cuts

b. Dysphagia

c. Cortical blindness

d. Sensory impairment

e. Ataxia

f. Alert to comatose

g. Dysarthria

h. Hoarseness

4. Carotid artery

a. Weakness, paralysis

b. Sensory changes

c. Altered level of consciousness

d. Headache

e. Aphasia

f. Ptosis

g. Visual disturbances on affected side

5. Vertebrobasilar artery

a. Numbness around lips

b. Weakness on affected side

c. Double vision

d. Slurred speech

e. Dysphagia

f. Poor coordination

g. Vertigo

h. Amnesia

i. Ataxia

III. Diagnostic tests and methods

A. Client history

B. Physical examination

C. Neurological assessment

D. CT scan

E. MRI

F. Lumbar puncture, CSF analysis

G. Electroencephalogram (EEG)

H. Cerebral angiography, carotid Doppler ultrasonography

I. ECG, chest radiograph, echocardiogram

J. Baseline laboratory studies

1. Coagulation studies (platelets, PT, activated partial thrombboplastin time [APTT])

2. Urinalysis

3. Serum osmolality

4. CBC

5. Triglycerides, lipid profile

6. Serum electrolytes

7. Creatinine and BUN levels, liver function test (LFT)

8. Cardiac enzymes

9. ABG

IV. Implementation

A. Assess, report, and record signs and symptoms and any reaction to treatment, such as complications from angiogram or surgery.

B. Provide bed rest; provide complete care.

C. Maintain patent airway and oxygen therapy.

D. Check for ballooning of cheek with respiration (side affected by stroke).

E. Keep unconscious client in a lateral (sidelying) position to allow secretions to drain by gravity or use suction as necessary (prevents aspiration of saliva).

F. Monitor vital signs and neurological status.

G. Monitor BP, voluntary and involuntary movements, changes in pupils, level of consciousness, speech, skin color, sensory function, and neck rigidity or flaccidity.

H. Monitor for signs of pulmonary emboli, such as chest pain, shortness of breath, increased temperature, and tachycardia; and check ABGs for signs of increased PCO_2 or decreased PO_2.

I. Monitor for signs of increased ICP.

J. Keep precautionary respiratory equipment at bedside.

K. Provide a safe environment and elevate side rails.

L. Administer prescribed medications such as antihypertensives, diuretics, and anticoagulants; monitor for side effects.

M. Maintain fluid and electrolyte balance

1. Encourage fluid intake orally as ordered.

2. Assist in IV administration as ordered.

N. Monitor ability to swallow (check gag reflex).

O. Place bedside stand in client's visual field so that client can see what is on stand.

P. Provide meticulous mouth care; clean and care for dentures.

Q. Provide meticulous eye care; patch affected eye if client cannot close lid.

R. Maintain adequate nutritional intake (make sure gag reflex has returned)

1. Place food in client's visual field so that client can see what is on tray.

2. Assist in insertion of NG feeding tube if unable to intake food by mouth.

S. Position client, align extremities correctly; use draw sheet to turn client every 2 hours.

T. Use padded footboard to prevent footdrop and contracture.

U. Assist client with ROM exercises for both affected and unaffected sides.

V. Instruct client in how to use unaffected side to exercise affected side, collaborate with physical therapy.

W. Provide egg-crate, pulsating, or flotation mattress to prevent skin breakdown (decubitus).

X. Facilitate communication with client
  1. Allow client sufficient time to communicate.
  2. Anticipate needs; speak slowly and clearly.
  3. If client is aphasic, set up other means of communication such as drawing, writing, use of pictures, gestures.
  4. Assure client that intellect has not been impaired; include family members in communicating methods.
  5. Encourage speech therapy.

Y. Involve family members in client's care when possible.

Z. Monitor elimination pattern
  1. Offer bedpan frequently for urinary or fecal incontinence.
  2. Assist client as necessary; provide privacy by not exposing client.
  3. Be alert for signs of straining at stool (which increases ICP).
  4. Check with dietitian to modify diet and to administer stool softener and/or prescribed laxatives.
  5. Encourage adequate fluid intake.
  6. Provide roughage in diet.

AA. Begin rehabilitation of client on admission
  1. Amount of teaching varies depending on neurological deficit present.
  2. If necessary, teach client to bathe, comb hair, and dress; collaborate with occupational therapy.
  3. Encourage client to begin speech therapy as soon as possible (if needed).
  4. Involve family in all aspects of rehabilitation.
  5. Coordinate care with physical therapist; use walking frames, handbars on toilet, and ramps.

BB. Instruct client and family regarding signs of CVA.

CC. Instruct client and family to watch for possible GI bleeding if aspirin is prescribed to decrease the risk of embolus stroke.

DD. Explain disease process, treatment, home care, and follow-up to client and family.

EE. Explain prevention of CVAs
  1. Stress
    a. Need to control diseases such as hypertension or diabetes mellitus
    b. Emphasis on importance of eating a low-salt, low-cholesterol diet
    c. Need to control weight
    d. Need to increase activity
    e. Avoidance of smoking and prolonged bed rest

V. Evaluation
  A. Client reports increased comfort and decreased anxiety.

B. Client remains free of injury or infection.

C. Effective communication is established.

D. Client maintains effective airway clearance and breathing pattern.

E. Client maintains effective elimination (urinary and bowel) patterns.

F. Client maintains good skin integrity.

G. Client maintains adequate cerebral tissue perfusion.

H. Client and family demonstrate an understanding of disease process, diagnostic procedures, treatment, home care, and follow-up care.

Increased Intracranial Pressure

I. Description
  A. Fluid accumulation or lesion taking up space in the cranial cavity, producing an increase in blood, cerebrospinal fluid (CSF), and/or brain tissue
  B. Resulting in gradual compression of the brain, with potential cessation of life-sustaining functions
  C. Progressing slowly or occurring suddenly
  D. Causes
    1. Head injury
    2. Cranial surgery
    3. Cerebral infections
    4. Tumor/mass/lesion
    5. Cerebral ischemia/infarction
    6. Encephalopathy (metabolic or toxic)

II. Data collection
  A. Subjective symptoms
    1. Related to primary disorder
    2. Headache, anxiety
    3. Blurred or double vision
    4. Lethargy
    5. Weakness
  B. Objective symptoms
    1. Vomiting: projectile, recurrent, unrelated to nausea
    2. Headache
    3. Changes in level of consciousness
    4. Change in pupil response to light
    5. Change in vital signs—Cushing's triad (widening pulse pressure, bradycardia, irregular respiratory pattern)
    6. Decreased motor function
    7. Posturing—decorticate and decerebrate

III. Diagnostic tests and methods
  A. Client history
  B. Physical examination
  C. Neurological assessment
  D. ICP monitoring
  E. MRI and CT scan
  F. Skull radiographs
  G. Chest radiograph
  H. Spinal radiograph
  I. Electroencephalogram (EEG)
  J. Cerebral blood flow
  K. CBC, ABGs, coagulation, electrolytes
  L. Positron emission tomography (PET)

IV. Implementation
  A. Assess, report, and record signs and symptoms and any reaction to treatment.
  B. Elevate head to semi-Fowler's position—30 degrees

C. Maintain patent airway; provide oxygen therapy.

D. Prevent aspiration; position client on side.

E. Monitor vital signs every 15 minutes.

F. Monitor neurological responses frequently.

G. Monitor laboratory values.

H. Monitor I&O.

I. Turn client every 2 hours.

J. Provide hygienic care frequently, including mouth care, skin care, and hair care.

K. Provide passive ROM exercises.

L. Use footboard or high-topped sneakers for prevention of footdrop and contractures.

M. Use splints to prevent wrist deformities.

N. Monitor pupillary response (usually unequal and may not react to light).

O. Provide safe environment (elevate side rails).

P. Report any change in level of consciousness immediately.

Q. Assist in administration of prescribed medications or devices.

R. Provide usual care and observation for unconscious client or one with seizures.

S. Keep suctioning and coughing at a minimum.

T. Explain condition, diagnostic procedures, treatment, home care, and follow-up care to client and family.

V. Evaluation

A. Client reports increased comfort and decreased anxiety.

B. Client remains free of injury or infection.

C. Client maintains adequate cerebral tissue perfusion.

D. Client maintains adequate airway clearance, breathing patterns, and gas exchange.

E. Client maintains adequate cardiac output.

F. Client maintains adequate fluid and electrolyte balance.

G. Client maintains adequate nutritional intake.

H. Client maintains adequate elimination pattern.

I. There are no deformities or contractures.

J. Client and family demonstrate an understanding of condition, treatment, home care, and follow-up care.

Intracranial Tumors

I. Description

A. Malignant or benign lesion within the brain that may displace or destroy adjacent structures or increase ICP

B. Either lesion originating within brain tissue (primary lesion) or one originating elsewhere in the body and metastasizing to the brain (secondary lesion)

C. ICP possible because of displacement of space by tumor, cerebral edema, and vasodilation resulting from impairment of the cerebral blood flow

D. More common in men than in women

E. Occurring at any age; in adults, incidence usually highest between the ages of 40 and 60 years

F. Classification according to tissue origin

1. Gliomas: arise in cerebral connective tissue; unencapsulated
   a. Characterized by rapid growth with infiltration of the brain tissue
   b. Are not well defined for surgical removal
   c. Occur most often in cerebral hemispheres, especially frontal and temporal lobes
   d. Prognosis: mean survival rate 6 months; maximum 1–2 years

2. Meningiomas: originate within meningeal layers
   a. Constituting 15% of primary brain tumors
   b. Peak incidence among 50 year olds; rare in children, more common in women than in men
   c. Occurring most often in sphenoidal ridge, anterior part of the base of the skull, and spinal canal
   d. Tumors benign, well circumscribed, and highly vascular
   e. Compression of adjacent underlying brain tissue by invading overlying skull
   f. Prognosis: median survival rate 1–2 years or less; if treated, neurological deficits potentially completely reversible

3. Neuromas: originate on cranial nerves
   a. Benign but often classified as malignant because of growth pattern: slow-growing, present for years before symptoms appear
   b. Accounting for approximately 10% of all intracranial tumors
   c. Incidence higher in women
   d. Onset of symptoms approximately 30–60 years of age
   e. Affecting craniospinal nerve sheath: usually eighth cranial nerve; also affecting fifth and seventh cranial nerves, although to a lesser extent
   f. Prognosis: if adequately treated, potential for permanent cure

4. Pituitary tumors: originate most often in anterior pituitary gland
   a. Accounting for 10% of intracranial tumors
   b. Occurring in adults of both sexes ages 30–50 years
   c. Three types: chromophobe adenoma, basophilic adenoma, and eosinophilic adenoma
   d. Amenable to surgical treatment
   e. Prognosis: fair to good, depending on extent of tumor spread beyond sella turcica

5. Metastatic tumors: originate elsewhere in body, often from lung
   a. Prognosis: poor

G. Gliomas and meningiomas most common type among adults

H. Brain tumors one of the most common causes of death from cancer in children

1. Incidence usually highest in <1 year olds and then in children 2–12 years of age

2. Astrocytoma (type of glioma), medulloblastomas (rare type of glioma), and brainstem gliomas most common types

I. Cause unknown

II. Data collection

A. Subjective symptoms

1. Alterations in judgment or personality

2. Visual disturbances
3. Headache
4. Numbness, tingling sensations
5. Difficulty and loss of hearing
6. Family or personal history
B. Objective symptoms
   1. Vomiting
   2. Orientation to person, place, and time
   3. Movement and strength of extremities
   4. Reaction of pupils to light
   5. Changes in vital signs
   6. Changes in level of consciousness
   7. Presence of papilledema
   8. Presence of seizures
   9. Abnormal cranial nerve reflexes
   10. Signs of increased ICP
   11. Presence of protein and decreased glucose and occasional tumor cells in spinal fluid
   12. Signs associated with tumor location
       a. Frontal lobe: personality changes, hemiparesis, visual problems, seizures, memory deficit
       b. Temporal lobe: seizures and dysphagia
       c. Parietal lobe: inability to write, spatial disorder, unilateral neglect, inability to differentiate between left and right, speech disturbance
       d. Occipital lobe: blindness, convulsions

III. Diagnostic tests and methods
A. Client history
B. Physical examination
C. Neurological assessment
D. CT scan
E. Skull radiograph
F. Brain scan
G. EEG
H. Biopsy of lesion
I. Cerebral angiography
J. Lumbar puncture
K. MRI
L. PET scan

IV. Implementation
A. Assess, report, and record signs and symptoms and any reaction to treatment.
B. Monitor and record baseline information regarding neurological status.
C. Check continuously for changes in neurological status
   1. Watch for and immediately report sudden unilateral dilation of pupil with loss of light reflex (indicates transtentorial herniation).
D. Monitor for signs of increased ICP
   1. Rising systolic pressure
   2. Widening pulse pressure
   3. Decrease in pulse rate
   4. Changes in level of consciousness
   5. Abnormal respiratory patterns
   6. Elevation of temperature
E. Assist with mobility and exercise.
F. Monitor respiratory changes (anoxia, abnormal respiratory rate and depth), which may indicate rising ICP or herniation of cerebellar tissue from expanding mass.

G. Monitor temperature (increased temperature often follows hypothalamic anoxia and might also indicate meningitis).
   1. Use hypothermia blankets, if prescribed, to decrease temperature and decrease metabolic demands of brain tissue.
H. Discuss effects of treatment with client and family.
I. Document seizure activity.
J. Maintain patent airway.
K. Provide safe and hazard-free environment (elevate side rails).
L. Administer anticonvulsants, diuretics, and steroids as prescribed.
M. Assist with administration and monitoring of IV therapy.
N. Monitor fluid I&O and electrolyte balance; restrict fluids as ordered (rapid diuresis may lead to heart failure).
O. Prepare client and family for surgical intervention.
P. Monitor for side effects of radiation therapy, if ordered (check for wound breakdown, infection, signs of rising ICP).
Q. Monitor for side effects of prescribed medication adjuncts to radiotherapy and surgery
   1. Cause delayed bone marrow depression (watch for signs of infection or bleeding)
R. Assist with instruction of client and family in early signs of recurrence; encourage compliance with therapy.
S. Begin rehabilitation early; encourage independence in ADLs.
T. Provide aids for self-care, if necessary.
U. Arrange for consultation with speech therapist if client is aphasic.
V. Explain diagnosis, treatment, potential disabilities, lifestyle alterations, home care, and follow-up care to client and family.

V. Evaluation
A. Client reports increased comfort and decreased anxiety.
B. Client remains free of injury or infection.
C. Client maintains adequate cerebral tissue perfusion.
D. Client maintains adequate airway clearance and breathing pattern.
E. Client participates in rehabilitation therapy (exercise, ambulation, ADLs).
F. Client demonstrates an understanding of disease process, diagnostic tests, treatment including medication, prevention, and home care.

Parkinson's Disease

I. Description
A. Condition characterized by progressive muscle rigidity, akinesia, and involuntary tremor
B. Caused by damage to neurons in the substantia nigra, which is located within the basal ganglia
C. Unknown cause
D. Predisposing factors
   1. Deficiency in dopamine, which interferes with inhibition of excitatory impulses

2. May be related to certain viruses, drugs, arteriosclerosis
   E. Progression of deterioration for an average of 10 years
   F. Death usually caused by aspiration pneumonia or other infection
   G. More common in men than in women
II. Data collection
   A. Subjective symptoms
      1. Drooling
      2. Fatigue
      3. Intolerance to heat
      4. Muscular pain
      5. Problems with coordination
      6. Changes in emotion and judgment
   B. Objective symptoms
      1. Muscle rigidity: resistance to passive muscle stretching ("lead pipe" or jerky)
      2. Akinesia (loss of movement) causing shuffling gait, loss of posture control, altered reflexes, masklike facial expression, high-pitched monotone voice, and dysphagia
      3. Difficulty performing ADLs
      4. Tremors of fingers (unilateral "pill-roll" tremor) increasing with stress
III. Diagnostic tests and methods
   A. Client history
   B. Physical examination
   C. Neurological assessment
   D. Urinalysis (dopamine levels)
IV. Implementation
   A. Assess, report, and record signs and symptoms and any reaction to treatment.
   B. Encourage client to maintain independence in ADLs as much as possible.
   C. Assist client while eating; have him or her use utensils with large handles for easy grip.
   D. Encourage client to continue with previous work, social, and diversionary activities as much as possible.
   E. Maintain effective airway clearance.
   F. Provide safe, hazard-free environment.
   G. Administer levodopa (dopamine replacement) as prescribed; monitor for side effects.
   H. Administer alternate drug therapy such as anticholinergics and antihistamines as prescribed.
   I. Assist in establishment of a regular bowel routine (encourage fluid intake, high-bulk foods).
   J. Provide emotional support to client and family.
   K. Prepare client and family for stereotactic neurosurgical procedure (electrical coagulation, freezing, radioactivity, or ultrasound to destroy the ventrolateral nucleus of thalamus to prevent involuntary movement) if necessary.
   L. After surgery, monitor for signs of hemorrhage and increased ICP.
   M. Coordinate care with physical therapist (used to assist in maintenance of normal muscle tone and function).
   N. Instruct family members how to prevent contracture formation (use of firm mattress without a pillow; lying in prone position to facilitate proper posture during rest).
   O. Maintain good skin integrity, and instruct client and family in prevention of skin breakdown.
   P. Instruct family to establish long- and short-term goals; awareness of need for intellectual stimulation and diversion for client.
   Q. Explain disease process, treatment, home care, and follow-up care.
V. Evaluation
   A. Client reports increased comfort and decreased anxiety.
   B. Muscular tremors and rigidity are reduced.
   C. Client maintains good skin integrity.
   D. Client maintains effective airway clearance.
   E. Client maintains adequate nutritional and fluid intake.
   F. Client performs some ADLs and participates in physical therapy.
   G. Client demonstrates an understanding of disease process, treatment, home care, and follow-up care.

Paraplegia

I. Description
   A. Spinal cord trauma or disease resulting in motor or sensory loss in the lower extremities with or without involvement of abdominal and back muscles
   B. Possibly complete or incomplete paralysis, which may be flaccid or spastic, permanent or temporary, and symmetrical or asymmetrical
   C. Complete severing of spinal cord resulting in permanent paralysis of body parts below site of injury
   D. Approximately 50% of spinal cord injuries resulting in paraplegia
   E. More prevalent in men than in women; incidence highest between ages 16 and 35 years
   F. Causes
      1. Trauma: automobile, diving, motorcycle, gunshot wounds, falls, other sporting accidents
      2. Nontraumatic lesions such as spina bifida, spinal tumors, scoliosis, and chordoma
II. Data collection
   A. Subjective symptoms
      1. Loss of sensation
      2. Loss of voluntary movement
   B. Objective symptoms
      1. Immediate phase
         a. Areflexia as a result of spinal shock
         b. Complete loss of sensation
         c. Complete loss of voluntary (motor) function
         d. Flaccid paralysis below site of injury
         e. Hypotonia
      2. Later phase
         a. Spasticity of muscles below site of injury
         b. Hyperreflexia: hyperactive responses
      3. Level of injury
         a. Lower thoracic level
            1) Loss of movement of bowel, bladder, and lower extremities, depending on level of injury
            2) Paralysis of legs
         b. Lumbar and sacral level

1) Loss of movement and sensation of lower extremities
2) S2–4 center of micturation: injury or lesion above this level permitting bladder to empty involuntarily; lesions below this level resulting in bladder contraction without emptying (autonomous neurogenic bladder)

4. Injury above S2 (in men): allowing erection to occur without ejaculation because of sympathetic nerve damage
5. Injury between S2 and S4: prevention of erection or ejaculation because of damaged sympathetic and parasympathetic nerves
6. Associated injuries such as fractures, hemorrhage, shock

III. Diagnostic tests and methods
  A. Client history
  B. Physical examination
  C. Neurological assessment
  D. Lumbar puncture
  E. Laboratory studies: CBC, PT, electrolytes, urinalysis
  F. After stabilization: hip, knee, chest radiographs, IVP to provide baseline information for detection of pathological changes
  G. Weekly urine culture and sensitivity tests

IV. Implementation
  A. Emergency care
    1. Assess for
      a. Pain, tenderness
      b. Numbness, tingling
      c. Weakness
      d. Alterations of sensation and motor function below level of injury
    2. Monitor for signs of shock.
    3. Provide supportive treatment to control systemic shock and hemorrhage.
    4. Immobilize client (movement may further damage spinal cord).
    5. Stabilize head and spine by strapping client on board.
    6. Place client on stretcher in emergency department without removing him or her from board.
    7. Insert Foley catheter to ensure uninterrupted urine drainage.
  B. Phase after emergency intervention
    1. Assess, report, and record signs and symptoms and any reaction to treatment.
    2. Provide meticulous catheter care; use intermittent catheterization to re-establish bladder capacity and to prevent infection once spinal shock period is over.
    3. Maintain proper body alignment and position to prevent contractures in immobilized client.
    4. Provide meticulous skin care, inspect pressure areas daily, and have client shift position at least every 15 minutes while sitting in wheelchair.
    5. Administer prescribed medications, such as corticosteroids, to reduce spinal cord edema, and analgesics for pain.
    6. Monitor fluid I&O; restrict fluids to 2000-2500 mL/day if client is on an intermittent catheterization program. Increase fluids for clients with indwelling Foley catheters to 4000 mL/day.
    7. Assist with active and passive ROM exercises; coordinate care with physical therapist.
    8. Monitor for symptoms of orthostatic hypotension as client progresses from bed rest to wheelchair; use antiembolism hose to assist in compensation for a sitting position after being restricted to a lying position for a long time.
    9. Provide a high-bulk diet to prevent constipation; give protein supplements to build up body tissues.
    10. Establish a bowel elimination routine
      a. Provide stool softeners, suppositories, and laxatives as ordered.
      b. Administer stool softeners and suppositories on a regular timed schedule.
      c. Use digital stimulation, if necessary.
      d. Teach muscle strengthening.
      e. Monitor for abdominal distention, flatus, and fullness in rectum, which indicates need to defecate.
      f. Teach client to use intra-abdominal compression by leaning forward and use of Valsalva's maneuver except if cardiac problems are present.
    11. Monitor for UTIs.
    12. For autonomic or spastic bladder reflex, instruct client regarding possible stimuli to initiate urination; use external catheters for men. Teach client to report signs of UTI.
    13. For atonic or areflexic bladder, instruct client to observe for distention. Use intermittent catheterization. Teach use of Credé's maneuver or abdominal straining to initiate urination.
    14. Provide postoperative wound care if a laminectomy is performed.
    15. Encourage family involvement in rehabilitation.
    16. Monitor for psychological problems (altered body image, loss of self-esteem, denial, anger).
    17. Provide emotional support to client and family.
    18. Provide counseling on sexual dysfunction or alterations.
    19. Provide client and family with information regarding community resources.
    20. Explain condition, treatment including medication, home care, and follow-up care.

V. Evaluation
  A. Client reports increased comfort and decreased anxiety.
  B. Client remains free of injury or infection.
  C. Client maintains good skin integrity.
  D. Client maintains adequate (bowel and bladder) elimination patterns.
  E. Client copes effectively with alterations in sensory and motor function.
  F. Client verbalizes feelings regarding self-image, self-concept, and sexual concerns.
  G. Client participates in self-care activities.
  H. Client demonstrates an understanding of condition, diagnostic procedures, treatment including medications, home care, and follow-up care.

Quadriplegia

I. Description
   A. A permanent injury that affects all body systems
   B. Condition characterized by paralysis of the arms, legs, and body below the level of injury to the spinal cord
   C. Affecting 150,000 individuals in the United States
   D. Incidence highest in men ages 20–40 years
   E. Causes flaccidity of the arms and legs and loss of movement and sensation below the level of injury
   F. Injury above the fifth cervical vertebra also causes blockage of the sympathetic nervous system, which allows the parasympathetic system to dominate; complications that may result from this phenomenon include
      1. Hypotension with BP <90/60 mm Hg caused by vasodilation allowing blood to pool in veins of extremities, resulting in slowing of the venous blood return to the heart
      2. Bradycardia (decreased heartbeat) as a result of stimulation of the heart by the vagus nerve and the absence of the inhibiting effects of the sympathetic system
      3. Decrease in body temperature because of inability of blood vessels to constrict effectively; allows blood vessel to contact with body surface; results in heat loss
      4. Respiratory complications: caused by damage to upper cervical cord
      5. Decreased peristalsis
      6. Autonomic dysreflexia (injuries above the fourth thoracic vertebra): connections between the brain and spinal cord are severed; produces an exaggerated autonomic response to specific stimuli such as distended bladder or bowel, presence of infection, decubitus ulcers, and/or surgical manipulation; key symptom is severe hypertension
   G. Causes
      1. Spinal cord injury; especially involving the fifth to seventh cervical vertebrae
      2. Vertebral pressure from tumors, degenerative spinal cord lesions
II. Data collection
   A. Subjective symptoms
      1. Loss of sensation
      2. Difficulty in breathing
      3. Pain
      4. Nature of injury
      5. Orientation
   B. Objective symptoms
      1. Symptoms of spinal shock
      2. Complete loss of sensation below level of injury
      3. Complete loss of movement below level of injury
      4. Unconsciousness
      5. Flaccid paralysis
      6. Hypotonia
      7. Respiratory difficulty
      8. Level of injury
         a. Cervical lesion with paralysis of trunk and all extremities

         b. Possible shoulder movement if at C5 or below
         c. Decreased perspiration
         d. Decrease in touch sensation
         e. Respiratory failure at level of C4 or above
III. Diagnostic tests and methods
   A. Client history
   B. Detailed history of trauma
   C. Physical examination
   D. Neurological assessment
   E. Spinal radiographs
   F. Myelography to identify fractures, dislocations, subluxation, and blockage in spinal cord
   G. Radiographs of head, chest, and abdomen to rule out underlying injuries
   H. Laboratory studies to assess respiratory, hepatic, and pancreatic function
IV. Implementation
   A. Assess, report, and record signs and symptoms and any reaction to treatment.
   B. Monitor respirations, chest movement, and vital signs frequently (injury at C4 or above requires permanent ventilatory support).
   C. Monitor PCO_2 and pH for signs of respiratory insufficiency.
   D. Assist with administration of IV therapy (do not overhydrate if vasodilation and venous pooling are present below level of injury).
   E. Assist with insertion of NG tube, if needed.
   F. Observe for signs of GI complications, such as paralytic ileus, bleeding, and pancreatic dysfunction
      1. Listen for bowel sounds every 8 hours.
      2. Record amount and type of NG drainage; check for coffee-ground secretions.
   G. Assist with intubation and ventilatory support as ordered.
   H. Connect client to cardiac monitor if bradycardia occurs.
   I. Place client in slight Trendelenburg position if signs of hypotension occur (constantly assess respiratory function).
   J. Use abdominal binder and antiembolism stockings when placing client in upright position (aid venous return and prevent orthostatic hypotension).
   K. Warm client with blankets if hypothermia occurs (temperature <90°F [32.2°C]). Do not use hot-water bottles or mechanical heat devices, as these may result in burning caused by sensory deficit.
   L. Maintain proper body alignment and immobilization of spine.
   M. Monitor neurological status, level of consciousness, sensations, movement, and pupil response frequently.
   N. Monitor for severe hypertension, which may lead to heart failure, intracranial bleeding, and retinal hemorrhage (sign of autonomic dysreflexia in client with injury above C4):
      1. In presence of hypertension
         a. Elevate head of bed to decrease BP.
         b. Check for bladder distention; obstructed catheter.

c. Check for fecal impaction; do not manipulate rectum, as it worsens symptoms.
   1) Before removal of impaction, apply topical anesthetic ointment, which decreases risk of further increasing the BP.
   2) Administer a smooth muscle relaxant or antihypertensive, if prescribed.
   3) Administer a β-adrenergic blocking agent for persistent hypertension as prescribed.
O. Maintain skeletal traction, tongs, or CircOlectric bed or Stryker frame.
P. Prepare client for surgical intervention such as spinal decompression; provide postoperative care.
Q. Administer medications as prescribed.
R. Provide frequent skin care to prevent formation of decubitus ulcers and infection.
S. Turn client every 2 hours.
T. Maintain firm mattress support.
U. Assist with passive ROM exercises; coordinate care with physical therapist.
V. Assist with urinary elimination.
W. Explain condition, diagnostic procedures, treatment, home care, follow-up care, and community resources.

V. Evaluation
   A. Client reports increased comfort and decreased anxiety.
   B. Client remains free of injury or infection.
   C. Client maintains effective breathing pattern and gas exchange.
   D. Client maintains adequate level of mobility in wheelchair.
   E. Client maintains good skin integrity.
   F. Client participates in self-care activities.
   G. Client copes effectively with alterations in sensory perception and motor function.
   H. Client maintains adequate elimination pattern.
   I. Client demonstrates an understanding of condition, treatment, home care, follow-up care, and community resources.

Pain: The Fifth Vital Sign

I. Description
   A. Pain is
      1. "An unpleasant sensory and emotional experience associated with actual or potential tissue damage" (International Association for the Study of Pain [IASP])
      2. Whatever the person says it is.
   B. The most common sources of non–cancer-related pain include, e.g., back, head joints, extremity, chest, and abdomen. Untreated pain results in decreased ability to concentrate, work, exercise, socialize, and sleep.
   C. Acute pain
      1. Occurs in a limited time, usually under 3–6 months.
      2. Objective symptoms
         a. Quality: sharp, stabbing
         b. Edema, erythemia at site
         c. Increased heart rate, increased blood pressure, and increased respirations

      3. Subjective symptoms
         a. Complaints of being anxious and fearful
         b. Moans, grimaces
   D. Chronic pain
      1. Occurs longer than 3–6 months
      2. Objective symptoms
         a. Quality: burning, throbbing
         b. No change in vital signs
      3. Subjective symptoms
         a. Depressed, angry, fearful, anxious
         b. Few verbal complaints
         c. Sleep disturbance
         d. Social isolation
         e. Inability to concentrate
         f. Hopeless/helpless
         g. Impaired job performance

II. Data collection
   A. An effective pain treatment strategy requires a thorough pain assessment.
   B. Assessment (PQRST)
      1. P = Palliative/provocative factors
      2. Q = Quality of pain
         a. What kind of pain—e.g., sore, aching, deep, cramping, burning, shooting
      3. R = Region/radiation
         a. Where is the pain? Does it radiate?
      4. S = Severity of pain
         a. Rate your pain on a scale from 0 to 10, with 0 representing "no pain" and 10 being the "worst imaginable pain."
      5. S = Severity of pain
         a. Would you describe your pain as none, mild, moderate, severe, or excruciating?
      6. T = Temporal (time) aspects to pain sensation
         a. Is your pain better or worse at any time during the day or night?
         b. When does it start and when does it stop?
         c. Is it intermittent or constant or does it occur only when you are moving?
   C. Initial assessment should also include
      1. A detailed history including
         a. Medicine use
         b. Treatment history
         c. Previous surgeries and injuries
         d. Impact on quality of life (QOL) and activities of daily living (ADL)
      2. Physical examination, emphasizing the system involved in pain complaint
      3. Psychosocial assessment, including family history of depression and/or chronic pain
      4. Appropriate diagnostic workup to determine cause of pain and to rule out treatable causes.

III. Pain management
   A. Goals of chronic pain management
      1. Patient education
      2. Improve function
      3. Minimize suffering with minimal side effects
      4. Maintain or improve quality of life and activities of daily living
   B. Principle of pharmacotherapy for the treatment of chronic pain

1. A = Ask about regularly
2. B = Believe the patient and family about the intensity of the pain and what relieves it.
3. C = Choose pain therapies that are appropriate for the patient and the setting.
4. D = Deliver the medications in a timely (not prn), logical fashion, with the aim of preventing rather than "chasing pain."
5. E = Empower patients through the use of active self-management interventions to enable them to control increased pain throughout the day.

C. Pharmacology therapy
1. Nonopioid analgesics
2. Acetaminophen
3. Nonsteroidal anti-inflammatory drugs (NSAIDs)
4. Opioid analgesics
5. Adjuvant agents
   a. Anticonvulsants
   b. Benzodiazepines
   c. Antidepressants
6. Neural blockade
   a. Local anesthetic, opioid, steroid, other
   b. Neuroablation (chemical, thermal)

D. Nonpharmacological therapy
1. Education
2. Comfort therapy
   a. Heat/cold application
   b. Exercise
   c. Relaxation/imagery
   d. Pastoral counseling
   e. Music, art, or drama therapy
3. Psychosocial therapy/counseling
4. Physical and occupational therapy
   a. Aquatherapy
   b. Tone and strengthening
   c. Desensitization
5. Neurostimulation
   a. Transcutaneous electrical nerve stimulation (TENS)
   b. Acupuncture

E. WHO Analgesic Ladder
1. Step I (nonmalignant pain)
   a. Provide appropriate and concurrent treatment for cause of pain; use adjuvant drugs as needed.
   b. Nonopioids for mild pain (e.g., aspirin, acetaminophen, NSAIDs)
   c. Examples of adjuvant drugs: tricyclic antidepressants, antiseizure drugs, anxiolytics, antihistamines, benzodiazepines, caffeine, dextroamphetamine, corticosteroids
2. Step II (malignant pain)
   a. Pain persists or increases.
   b. Add step 2 opioid; continue step 1 drugs and adjuvant drugs as needed.
   c. Opioids for mild to moderate pain (e.g., codeine, oxycodone).
3. Step III
   a. Pain persists or increases.
   b. Replace step 2 opioid with step 3 opioid.
   c. Continue step 1 drugs and adjuvant drugs as needed.
   d. Opioids for moderate or severe pain (e.g., morphine, hydromorphone, methadone).

F. Nursing diagnoses
1. Activity intolerance
2. Acute pain
3. Anxiety
4. Chronic pain
5. Constipation
6. Disturbed sleep pattern
7. Disturbed thought processes
8. Fatigue
9. Fear
10. Hopelessness
11. Ineffective coping
12. Ineffective role performance
13. Interrupted family processes
14. Powerlessness
15. Risk for self-mutilation
16. Social isolation

G. Patient and family teaching
1. Maintain a diary of level of pain and effectiveness of medications/non-medications.
2. Take pain medications around the clock to maintain a blood level.
3. Tolerance will develop with opioids after a time: dosages may need to be adjusted.
4. Teach about potential side effects of opioid medications: nausea and vomiting, constipation, sedation, itching, urinary sweating.
5. Aggressively treat constipation: schedule a bowel program.
6. Need to report pain when pain is not relieved.
7. Definition of tolerance: the need for an increased opioid dose to maintain the same degree of analgesia. Tolerance is not addiction.
8. Definition of physical dependence: expected physiologic response to ongoing exposure to opioids manifested by a withdrawal syndrome that occurs when blood levels of the drug are abruptly decreased. When opioids are no longer needed to provide pain relief, a tapering schedule should be used with careful monitoring.
9. Definition of addiction: complex psychosocial condition characterized by a drive to obtain and take substances for other than the prescribed therapeutic use for pain

H. Barriers to effective pain management
1. Fear of addiction
2. Fear of side effects
3. Desire to be a "good" patient (not to be a "bother" to health care team)
4. Concern that pain signifies disease progression

Cultural Considerations

Good nursing care is always culturally sensitive. Table 5–1 presents biological variations and special health considerations for a variety of cultural and ethnic groups found in North America.

Table 5-1. Diseases and Health Conditions of Various Cultural/Ethnic Groups

Cultural Group	Biological Variations	Diseases and Health Conditions
African American Heritage	• Skin color varies from light to very dark • Tendency toward the overgrowth of connective tissue associated with the protection against infection and repair after injury • Have a higher bone density • Pseudofolliculitis ("razor bumps") is more common in males • Melasma ("mask of pregnancy") is more common in darker-skinned females during pregnancy • Birthmarks are more common • Genetically more prone to retain sodium	• High intake of sodium, overweight, sedentary lifestyle, smoking, alcohol, and high stress levels are associated with increased blood pressure • Causes of death include accidents, cancer, infant mortality, and cardiovascular diseases, homicide, cirrhosis, malnutrition, chemical dependency, and diabetes • At greater risk for many diseases, especially those associated with low income, stressful life conditions, lack of access to primary health care, and negating health behaviors • Examples are violence, poor dietary habits, lack of exercise, and lack of importance placed on seeking primary health-care early • Leading causes of death in women are cancer, stroke, chronic obstructive pulmonary disease, pneumonia, unintentional injuries, diabetes, suicide, HIV/AIDS, alcohol, illicit drug use, and depression • Leading cause of death among young men is homicide • Minorities suffer the most from environmental pollution • Many suffer from genetic conditions such as sickle cell disease and glucose-6-phosphate dehydrogenase deficiency, which interferes with glucose metabolism • AIDS contributes to lower life expectancy
Amish Heritage	• Skin variations range from light to olive tones • Hair and eye colors vary • No specific health-care precautions	• Hereditary diseases found include dwarfism, cartilage hair hypoplasia, pyruvate kinase anemia, and hemophilia B • Other health conditions include neurological diseases and manic-depressive disorders
Appalachian Heritage	• Skin color varies. • Mixture of white ancestry and Cherokee or Apalachee Indian • Influence of Native Americans can be seen in skin color • Those with Scotch-Irish background have lighter skin color	• Industrial pollution increases the risk for respiratory diseases • Other health conditions include hypochromic anemia, otitis media, cardiovascular diseases, female obesity, non–insulin-dependent diabetes mellitus, and parasitic infections • Children are at greater risk for sudden infant death syndrome, congenital malformations, and infections • Cancer, suicide, and accidents are greater in some parts of Appalachia
Arab Heritage	• May have dark or olive skin • May also have blonde or auburn hair, blue eyes, and fair complexions	• Major public health concerns are trauma related to motor vehicle accidents, maternal-child health, and control of communicable diseases • Infectious diseases include tuberculosis, malaria, trachoma, typhus, hepatitis, typhoid fever, dysentery, and parasitic infections • Schistosomiasis has been called Egypt's number one health problem • Glucose-6-phosphate dehydrogenase (G-6-PD) deficiency, sickle cell anemia, and the thalassemias are common • Hypertension, diabetes, and coronary artery disease have emerged
Chinese Heritage	• Skin color similar to Westerners with pink undertones • Some have a yellow tone, while others are very dark • Mongolian spots, dark bluish spots over the lower back and buttocks, are present in 80% of the infants	• Three major causes of death are heart disease, other circulatory diseases, and cancers • Thalassemia is found • Increased incidence of lactose intolerance, resulting in diarrhea, indigestion, and bloating when milk and milk products are consumed

(Continued on following page)

Table 5–1. Diseases and Health Conditions of Various Cultural/Ethnic Groups (Continued)

Cultural Group	Biological Variations	Diseases and Health Conditions
	• Differences in bone structure • Hip measurements are significantly smaller • Bone density is less • Elderly have a high hard palate • Many males do not have much facial or chest hair • Rh-negative blood type is rare • Twins are not common	• Increased incidence of hepatitis B and tuberculosis • Higher rates of suicide over the age of 45 years in women
Cuban Heritage	• Have no Indian ancestry • 80% are white, 5% are black • Skin, hair, and eye colors vary from light to dark • African Cuban extraction are dark-skinned and may have physical features similar to African Americans	• Health problems include overweight, hypertension, high rate of nonalcoholic cirrhosis, chronic bronchitis among smokers, and total tooth loss is significantly higher • Gingival inflammation and periodontitis is higher
Filipino Heritage	• Aboriginal tribes are Negroid and petite in stature • Typical native-born or immigrant Filipinos may be of Malay stock (brown complexion) with a multiracial genetic background • Physical features may include jet black to brunette or light brown hair, dark to light brown pupils with eyes set in almond-shaped eyelids, deep brown to very light tan skin tones, and mildly flared nostrils and slightly low to flat nose bridges • Height ranges from under 5 feet to the height of average Americans • Commonly gain weight when they come to the United States. • Have a smaller thoracic cavity • 40% have blood type B and a low incidence of Rh-negative factor	• Infant mortality is associated with respiratory conditions, congenital anomalies, diarrhea, birth injury, septicemia, measles, meningitis, and nutritional deficiencies • Leading causes of maternal mortality include complications of pregnancy, delivery, and puerperium such as hemorrhage and hypertension • Ten leading causes of morbidity in adults are diarrhea, bronchitis/bronchiolitis, pneumonia, influenza, hypertension, respiratory tuberculosis, malaria, heart disease, chickenpox, and typhoid fever • Ten leading causes of mortality are heart disease, vascular system disease, pneumonia, accidents, malignancy, TB, COPD, other respiratory diseases, diabetes mellitus, and renal disease
French Canadian Heritage	• Canadians of French descent are white	• Primary causes of death are cardiac diseases, lung cancer in men, breast cancer in women, premature birth rates, and trauma for those under age 30 years • Suicide rates are higher • Have a higher number of hereditary and genetic diseases
Iranian Heritage	• White Indo-Europeans with skin tones and facial features resembling those of other Mediterranean and southern European groups • Coloring ranges from blue or green eyes, light brown hair, and fair skin to nearly black eyes, black hair, and brown skin	• Heat and humidity provide fertile ground for the spread of cholera and malaria • Other diseases include viral and bacterial meningitis, hookworm, and gastrointestinal dysenteries • Hypertension is widespread • Ischemic heart disease is rising • Diseases and birth defects associated with marriages between cousins include epilepsy, blindness, several forms of anemia, and hemophilia • Large number suffer from acute psychological illnesses
Irish Heritage	• Most have either dark hair and fair skin or red hair, red cheeks, and fair skin • Irish are taller and broader in stature than average European Americans	• Increased risk of respiratory illnesses due to mining • Heart disease and cancer are the leading causes of premature mortality • Osteoporosis is a significant health problem affecting older women • Major cause of infant mortality is congenital abnormalities
Italian Heritage	• Those from northern background have lighter skin, lighter hair, and blue eyes • Those from south of Rome have dark, often curly hair, dark eyes, and olive-colored skin	• Genetic diseases, such as Mediterranean fever, G-6-PD, and thalassemias • High incidence of hypertension and coronary artery disease • Increased incidence of ventricular septal defects in children • Increased risk of multiple sclerosis

(Continued on following page)

Cultural Group	Biological Variations	Diseases and Health Conditions
Japanese Heritage	• "Yellow" skin that varies markedly • Hair is straight and naturally black with differences in shade • Average stature of adults is smaller than that of Americans • Northern Japan has fair-skinned people • Japanese island peoples are darker-skinned and have a stockier build	• Leading causes of death include cancers, heart disease, stroke, pneumonia, accidents, motor vehicle accidents, suicide, renal disease, liver disease, diabetes, hypertension, and tuberculosis • Asthma related to straw mats that cover floors in Japan is one of the few endemic diseases
Jewish Heritage	• Ashkenazi Jews' skin color ranges from fair skin and blonde hair to darker skin and brunette hair • Sephardic Jews have darker skin tones and hair coloring • Jewish groups from Ethiopia are black	• Genetic diseases such as Tay-Sachs disease and Gaucher's disease • Other conditions include inflammatory bowel disease, colorectal cancer, and breast cancer in women
Korean Heritage	• Physical characteristics include dark hair and dark eyes, with variations in skin color and degree of hair darkness • Skin color ranges from fair to light brown	• Schistosomiasis and other parasitic diseases are common • Immigrants to United States need to be evaluated for asbestos-related health problems • High prevalence of stomach and liver cancer, tuberculosis, hepatitis, and hypertension • High incidence of stomach cancer • High incidence of lactose intolerance • High incidence of gum disease and oral problems
Mexican Heritage	• Some with predominant Spanish background have light-colored skin, blond hair, and blue eyes • People with indigenous Indian backgrounds may have black hair, dark eyes, and cinnamon-colored skin	• Common health problems include malnutrition, malaria, cancer, alcoholism, drug abuse, obesity, hypertension, diabetes, heart disease, adolescent pregnancy, dental disease, and HIV and AIDS • Migrant worker populations, infectious, communicable, and parasitic diseases continue to be major health risks • Cardiovascular disease is the leading cause of death and disability • High incidence of diabetes mellitus
Navajo Indians	• Skin color varies from light brown to very dark brown depending on the tribe • Newborns and infants have Mongolian spots on the sacral area • Navajo are taller and thinner than other American Indian tribes	• Water on tribe predisposes Indians to waterborne bacterial infections such as *Shigella* infection • *Salmonella* infection is common because of the lack of refrigeration • Hypothermia is a problem • Common diseases related to living in close contact with others include upper respiratory illnesses and acute otitis media • Higher incidence of alcoholism, tuberculosis, diabetes mellitus, type II, unintentional injuries, suicide, pneumonia and influenza, homicide, gastrointestinal disease, infant mortality, and heart disease • Other health problems include the plague, tick fever, and Muerto Canyon Hanta virus infection. • Cardiovascular diseases are on the increase among the Navajo • High incidence of severe combined immunodeficiency syndrome (SCIDS), an immunodeficiency syndrome unrelated to AIDS • Navajo neuropathy is unique to this population—an autosomal recessive gene originating from a single common ancestry may explain this • Albinism occurs in the Navajo and Pueblo tribes • Genetically prone blindness that develops in individuals during their late teens and early 20s.

(Continued on following page)

	Table 5–1. **Diseases and Health Conditions of Various Cultural/Ethnic Groups** (Continued)	
Cultural Group	Biological Variations	Diseases and Health Conditions
Polish Heritage	• Most are of medium height with a medium-to-large bone structure • Many may be dark and Mongol looking or fair and delicate with blue eyes and blond hair	• Common health problems are obesity, smoking, and low leisure-time physical activity • Miners and workers in heavy industry are at risk for development of pulmonary disease • Other health problems include dental and cardiac diseases, alcoholism, respiratory conditions, thyroid disorders, and cancer, particularly, leukemia
Puerto Rican Heritage	• This heritage is a mixture of Native Indian, African, and Spanish ancestry • Some may have dark skin, thick kinky hair, and a wide flat nose • Others are white skinned with straight auburn hair and hazel or black eyes • Diseases are posulated to be the result of indigenous Indian and African heritage	• Health conditions are the same for the United States: heart disease, malignant neoplasm, diabetes mellitus, unintentional injuries, and AIDS are the leading causes of death • Aging populations have increasing chronic conditions such as hypertension, diabetes, asthma, and cardiovascular disease • In United States, decreased mortality rates for lung, breast, and ovarian cancers are seen in Puerto Ricans • In United States, an increased incidence of stomach, prostatic, esophageal, pancreatic, and cervical cancers • High incidence of chronic conditions such as mental illness among younger adults and cardiopulmonary and osteomuscular diseases among the elderly • Acute conditions include a disproportionate number of acute respiratory illnesses, injuries, infectious and parasitic diseases, and diseases of the digestive system • Women have a high incidence of being overweight • Dengue, a mosquito-transmitted disease, is found in those migrating to the United States • Highest incidence of HIV
Vietnamese Heritage	• Are members of the Mongolian or Asian race • Skin color ranges from pale ivory to dark brown • Mongolian spots, bluish discolorations on the lower back of a newborn child, are normal hyperpigmented areas in many Asians • Usually small in physical stature and light in build • Typical physical features include inner eye folds that make the eyes look almond shaped, sparse body hair, and coarse head hair • Also have dry earwax, which is gray and brittle • Generally have larger teeth; may have a torus, bony protuberance, on the midline of the palate or on the inner side of mandible near the second premolar	• Women have the highest incidence of cervical cancer • Have higher rates of depression, generalized anxiety disorders, and post-traumatic stress • Chronic personal and emotional problems often stem from post-traumatic stress experiences • High incidence of TB • Other endemic diseases include hepatitis B, leprosy, high levels of parasitism, and malaria • Two clinical illnesses that may mimic tuberculosis, melioidosis and paragonimiasis, have also been reported • Moderate to severe dental problems may occur, especially in children

Data from Purnell, LD, and Paulanka, BJ: Transcultural Health Care: A Culturally Competent Approach, ed 2. Phialdelphia, FA Davis, 2003.

QUESTIONS

Jennifer Couvillion, RN, PhD, Deborah Garbee, RN, APRN, MN, BC,
Judith Gentry, RN, APRN, MSN, OCN, and Golden Tradewell, RN, PhD

1. A 49-year-old woman was admitted to a physical rehabilitation unit 2 weeks before surgery for a below-the-knee amputation on her right leg. She asks, "Why do I have to keep wrapping my stump?" The nurse's best response is:

   1. "You will have to shrink and shape the residual limb to fit the prosthesis."
   2. "You want to increase the size of the residual limb to fit the prosthesis."
   3. "You need to because it is what your physical therapist wants."
   4. "You need to speak to your doctor."

2. To prevent flexion contraction of the hip after a below-the-knee amputation, the nurse should encourage the client to be:

   1. In supine position with a pillow between the legs
   2. In a semi-Fowler's position most of the day
   3. In supine position with a pillow under the knees
   4. In prone position

3. After a below-the-knee amputation, a client states, "Please tell me I am not crazy because it still feels like my right foot is still there." The nurse's best response is:

   1. "Since your leg is not there, you should not feel anything."
   2. "You are experiencing phantom limb sensation, which is normal."
   3. "It might be best for you to see a psychiatrist to help you deal with your loss."
   4. "Next you will be telling me you can see your toes."

4. In caring for a residual limb after a below-the-knee amputation, the nurse knows that which of the following statements by the client indicates a need for further teaching? "I should

   1. Inspect the stump for redness and abrasions."
   2. Apply lotion or alcohol to the stump."
   3. Use a stump sock or Ace bandage."
   4. Clean the stump with mild soap."

5. A 65-year-old man with hypertension has suffered a stroke and has right hemiplegia. When assessing the client, the nurse expects to find:

   1. Weakness on one side of the body
   2. Paralysis of the lower extremities
   3. Total body paralysis
   4. Paralysis of one side of the body

6. A client has dysphagia. The nurse would include in the plan of care which of the following?

   1. Promote exercises to decrease facial rigidity.
   2. Allow extra time for speaking.
   3. Institute special feeding precautions.
   4. Increase light in the environment.

7. When assessing a client after a stroke, the nurse notes that there is an impairment of the ability to read, write, speak, listen, and comprehend. The nurse identifies this as:

   1. Ataxia
   2. Aphasia
   3. Dysphagia
   4. Agnosia

8. A client's entire posterior chest and buttocks have full-thickness burns. Using the Rule of Nines, the nurse would calculate the BSA burned as:

   1. 9
   2. 18
   3. 27
   4. 36

9. Which of the following is the most characteristic symptom of the disequilibrium syndrome associated with hemodialysis?

   1. Seizures
   2. Hypertension
   3. Chest pain
   4. Shortness of breath

10. A wife whose husband has suffered an MI states, "My husband's favorite foods are fried chicken and french-fried potatoes. Would it be okay for me to bring him some?" The nurse's best response is:

    1. "That's a good idea; he has a hearty appetite."
    2. "If you bring him only a small amount, it will be okay."
    3. "First let's speak to the dietitian about his diet."
    4. "No, you can't bring food into the hospital."

11. The nurse is preparing a 42-year-old man for hospital discharge after an MI. Which of the following statements indicates the need for further teaching?

    1. "I will take my medications as prescribed."
    2. "I will follow a low-cholesterol, low-fat diet."
    3. "I can exercise as much as I want."
    4. "I can have a small glass of wine with the evening meal."

12. A wife whose husband has suffered a stroke notices that he cries and laughs inappropriately. She asks, "Why does he do that?" The nurse's best response is:

1. "He is experiencing emotional lability, which is common after a stroke."
2. "Ignore him; he likes to play games."
3. "Don't you also cry when something is funny and laugh when it is not?"
4. "I don't know; maybe he needs a psychiatrist."

13. A 17-year-old girl was injured in a car accident. She now has paraplegia secondary to a T11 spinal cord injury. The nurse identifies the four divisions of the spinal column as:

    1. Coccygeal, cranial, thoracic, lumbar
    2. Cervical, thoracic, lumbar, sacral
    3. Cervical, trochanter, ischial, sacral
    4. Thoracic, coccygeal, femur, ulnar

14. The nurse assesses for which of the following symptoms in a T11 spinal cord injury?

    1. Loss of movement in both the upper and lower extremities
    2. Loss of bladder control
    3. Loss of movement in the upper extremities
    4. Loss of respiratory control

15. Humulin NPH insulin is administered at 7 AM. At what time would the nurse anticipate the peak action to take place?

    1. 9 AM
    2. 12 noon
    3. 5 PM
    4. 11 PM

16. While the client is in the prone position, which site is most likely to develop a pressure area?

    1. Occiput
    2. Buttocks
    3. Heels
    4. Toes

17. When performing endotracheal suctioning, suctioning should be limited to how many seconds?

    1. 5
    2. 10
    3. 20
    4. 30

18. A 56-year-old man is walking down the hall and complains of chest pain. Before administering nitroglycerin sublingually, what action should be performed first?

    1. Call for a stat 12 lead ECG.
    2. Lower the head of the bed.
    3. Start oxygen with a nasal cannula.
    4. Tell client to stop and rest.

19. Which position facilitates the greatest expansion of the lungs for the client restricted to bed rest?

    1. High-Fowler's
    2. Low-Fowler's
    3. Sims'
    4. Trendelenburg

20. For adults, the diastolic BP is recorded when:

    1. The first sound is heard during cuff deflation
    2. The muffled sound is heard during cuff deflation
    3. The muffled sound is heard during cuff inflation
    4. The last sound is heard during cuff deflation

21. When teaching a female client the proper technique for cleaning the perineum before intermittent self-catheterization, the nurse would teach her to separate the labia and:

    1. Wipe from back to front
    2. Wipe in a circular motion
    3. Wipe from side to side
    4. Wipe from front to back

22. When administering which medication does the nurse frequently obtain peak-and-trough levels?

    1. Digoxin
    2. Heparin
    3. Aminophylline
    4. Vancomycin

23. What is the minimum time established for a health-care worker to properly wash the hands?

    1. 10 seconds
    2. 30 seconds
    3. 45 seconds
    4. 60 seconds

24. Which of the following is a common symptom of constipation?

    1. Increase in appetite
    2. Suprapubic distention
    3. Vomiting
    4. Firm abdomen

25. What directions should the nurse give a client who has just been given a suppository for complaints of constipation?

    1. Get up and go to the toilet immediately.
    2. Wait 5–10 minutes before going to the toilet.
    3. Wait 20–30 minutes before going to the toilet.
    4. Remain in the prone position before getting up and going to the toilet.

26. The physician has ordered povidone-iodine (Betadine) for wound care. When pouring povidone-iodine onto the 4 × 4 bandages, the nurse should:

    1. Hold the bottle with the label facing the sterile field.
    2. Pour while holding the bottle high over the sterile field.
    3. Pour 1–2 mL into another container before pouring onto the sterile bandages.
    4. Pour some into a cap and then over the sterile bandages.

27. The major cause of nosocomial infection in the hospital setting is:

    1. Excessive use of disposable equipment
    2. Proximity of beds in a semiprivate room

3. Infrequent handwashing
4. Excessive use of oral antibiotics

28. A surgical incision has become infected and now requires wound care every 8 hours. When packing the incision with saline-soaked 4 × 4 bandages, the nurse accidentally drops the dressing on the client's chest. The nurse should:

1. Use the bandage if the client has just bathed.
2. Resoak the bandage in sterile saline and place it in the incision.
3. Discard that bandage and prepare a fresh one.
4. Use the bandage on top of other sterile bandages.

29. The nurse knows the best place to assess for pallor in a very dark-skinned person is:

1. Sclera
2. Nailbed
3. Mucous membranes
4. Lips

30. While charting, the nurse makes an error while writing in the nurse's notes. The nurse should:

1. Write with erasable ink to correct the entry easily.
2. Draw lines through the entry until the entry is no longer readable.
3. Draw one straight line through the erroneous entry, initial it, and write "error."
4. Draw one straight line through the erroneous entry and initial it.

31. Your client has left-leg weakness and needs to use a cane. You observe proper ambulation with the cane when the client:

1. Keeps one point of support on the floor at all times
2. Keeps two points of support on the floor at all times
3. Leans slightly to the left with the cane in the left hand
4. Uses the proper-length cane—the top of the cane should be at waist level

32. To measure BP accurately, the nurse should:

1. Position the client's arm above the level of the heart.
2. Position the cuff at least 2 inches above the site of the radial artery pulsation.
3. Position the client's arm extended, with the palm down.
4. Center the arrow marker on the cuff over the brachial artery pulsation.

33. The most accurate technique used to assess the apical pulse is:

1. Inspection
2. Palpation
3. Auscultation
4. Percussion

34. The nurse is giving discharge instructions to a client who will be receiving oxygen at home, including placing a "No Smoking" sign at all entrances to the home. The rationale for using the sign is:

1. Oxygen can cause a fire to ignite.
2. Oxygen can cause an explosion.
3. The sign alerts visitors to enter the home at their own risk.
4. Smoking causes lung cancer.

35. The nurse plans to give a complete bed bath to a 70-year-old woman. When cleansing the face area, the nurse should use:

1. Warm water only
2. Tissues instead of a washcloth
3. Liquid soap on all areas except the eyes and lips
4. The client's preference of facial soap and warm water

36. While receiving a soapsuds enema, the client complains of abdominal cramps. The nurse should:

1. Temporarily stop the flow of the enema.
2. Tell the client to breathe slowly through the mouth.
3. Raise the height of the enema container.
4. Clamp the tubing and withdraw the rectal tube.

37. The nurse auscultates a BP of 180/99 mm Hg in the right arm and decides to double-check the reading. Before reinflating the cuff, the nurse should wait:

1. 10 seconds
2. 30 seconds
3. 1 minute
4. 2 minutes

38. The nurse obtains a report from the laboratory stating her client's serum potassium is 4.3 mEq/L. Which action should she perform next?

1. Notify the doctor immediately, because the value is dangerously low.
2. Note the value in her notes, and notify the doctor when he makes rounds.
3. This is a panic value. The level is dangerously high, and the doctor must be notified immediately.
4. Offer the client potassium-rich foods such as orange juice and bananas.

39. Postoperatively, a client has not voided in more than 8 hours. The nurse feels the lower abdomen and finds it to be distended. The method of physical examination used by the nurse is termed:

1. Auscultation
2. Percussion
3. Palpation
4. Inspection

40. A sterile specimen would be obtained from an indwelling Foley catheter by:

1. Taking urine from the urinometer
2. Taking urine from the drainage bag
3. Disconnecting the catheter from the drainage tubing
4. Withdrawing urine from the latex port

41. The nurse knows that an enteric-coated oral medication:

1. Dissolves rapidly when placed under the tongue
2. Needs to be shaken before being administered

3. Does not dissolve until it reaches the small intestine
4. Needs to be chewed and taken with a full glass of water

42. A client is ordered to receive an IM injection by the Z-track method. The rationale for the use of this method is that it:

1. Prevents the drug from irritating the skin
2. Allows faster absorption of the drug
3. Eliminates discomfort caused by the needle
4. Allows slower absorption of the drug

43. Medications are absorbed most rapidly through which of the following routes?

1. Topical
2. IV
3. IM
4. Oral

44. After abdominal surgery, your client has a Salem sump tube that is draining excessive amounts of fluid. Which acid-base disturbance is most likely to occur?

1. Metabolic acidosis
2. Metabolic alkalosis
3. Respiratory acidosis
4. Respiratory alkalosis

45. Your client is being discharged and has been instructed how to lift objects to avoid lower back strain. Which of the following statements made by the client is correct? "I must

1. Narrow my base of support."
2. Move away from the object to be lifted."
3. Position my center of gravity high above the object to be lifted."
4. Maintain alignment of the head, neck, and back while lifting."

46. The nurse knows that evaluation is:

1. The final phase of the nursing process
2. Not related to client goals of care
3. The first phase of the nursing process
4. A continuous and ongoing process

47. To administer oral care to an unconscious client, the nurse should:

1. Use a toothbrush and floss after every meal.
2. Squirt 30 mL of mouthwash into the mouth and then suction the oral cavity.
3. Scrape secretions from inside the mouth with a tongue blade.
4. Use a padded tongue blade to keep the mouth open.

48. According to the American Heart Association (AHA), which of the following is the most prevalent form of cardiovascular disease?

1. Stroke
2. Coronary artery disease (CAD)
3. Hypertension
4. Rheumatic heart disease

49. A 65-year-old man is admitted to the hospital with the diagnosis of congestive heart failure (CHF). Which of the following is an expected symptom of CHF?

1. Shortness of breath
2. Decrease in tissue turgor
3. Flat neck veins
4. Left upper quadrant abdominal tenderness

50. Which of the following would be an appropriate nursing intervention for a client in CHF?

1. Assess daily weight.
2. Encourage fluids.
3. Position the head of the bed <30 degrees upright.
4. Teach the importance of a diet enriched with sodium.

51. Which of the following is the usual adult daily dose of digoxin?

1. 0.025 mg
2. 0.25 mg
3. 2.5 mg
4. 25 mg

52. Which symptom represents a toxic side effect of digoxin?

1. Ringing in the ears
2. Fluid retention
3. Anorexia, nausea, vomiting
4. Hair loss

53. Which of the following is a symptom of thrombophlebitis of the leg?

1. Negative Homans' sign
2. Weak or absent pedal pulses
3. Cool temperature and mottled appearance of the foot
4. Calf pain with dorsiflexion of the foot

54. Which intervention would be indicated for a client with thrombophlebitis of the leg?

1. Encourage fluids by mouth.
2. Gently massage the affected leg.
3. Keep the leg positioned below the level of the heart.
4. Start antibiotic therapy.

55. The rationale for starting a heparin infusion for a client with thrombophlebitis is:

1. Heparin dissolves blood clots.
2. Heparin dilates the vessels to increase blood flow in the leg.
3. Heparin prevents additional clots from forming.
4. Heparin constricts the vessels to increase blood flow in the leg.

56. A heparin drip consists of 25,000 units of heparin in 250 mL D_5W. The infusion is being delivered via an infusion pump at a rate of 10 mL/hr. How many units per hour are infusing?

1. 10
2. 100
3. 1000
4. 2500

57. Your client will be discharged from the hospital on warfarin (Coumadin). Which of the following statements do you want to include in teaching about this drug?

1. Decrease your dietary intake of green leafy vegetables.
2. When you have a headache, aspirin may be taken to relieve the discomfort.
3. You will need to have periodic PTT drawn.
4. Shave with a straight-edge razor.

58. Which of the following is the best site for assessing skin turgor in an 80-year-old client?

1. Dorsal hand
2. Forearm
3. Sternum
4. Ankles

59. When would you advise someone with unknown heart disease who is experiencing chest pain to seek emergency care?

1. If the chest pain persists more than 2 minutes
2. If three nitroglycerin tablets taken 3–5 minutes apart do not relieve the pain
3. If more than six nitroglycerin tablets are taken in a 24-hour period
4. When the chest pain goes away

60. A 55-year-old female client has been diagnosed with CAD. Which therapeutic intervention would offer a cure for this disease?

1. Coronary artery bypass graft (CABG) surgery
2. Placement of a coronary artery stent
3. Balloon angioplasty of the coronary artery blockage
4. No cure currently available

61. Which of the following would be a major modifiable risk factor for the development of CAD?

1. Obesity
2. Family history of CAD
3. Cigarette smoking
4. Diabetes

62. Which of the following is the best site to assess for edema in a client confined to bed?

1. Ankles
2. Pretibial
3. Hands
4. Sacrum

63. The nurse is teaching a client nutritional aspects of a low-cholesterol diet. Which statement made by the client indicates understanding of the diet?

1. "Broiled chicken, with the skin removed, contains no cholesterol."
2. "Eat fish rather than red meat because it contains no cholesterol."
3. "It is permissible to use polyunsaturated oils to fry food."
4. "Egg whites do not contain cholesterol."

64. The discomfort of angina pectoris most commonly radiates to what area of the body?

1. Left arm
2. Both arms
3. Neck bilaterally
4. Jaw unilaterally

65. The nurse is caring for a client 2 days after percutaneous coronary angioplasty (PTCA). During the morning assessment, a pulse deficit is detected. A pulse deficit is best described as:

1. The absence of a particular pulse
2. The difference between the systolic and diastolic BP
3. The difference between the apical and radial heart rates
4. The radial pulse minus the apical pulse rate

66. Which nursing intervention is appropriate when caring for a client immediately after cardiac catheterization?

1. Allow to ambulate to bathroom with assistance only.
2. Monitor pedal pulses frequently.
3. Maintain the head of bed in a high-Fowler's position.
4. Restrict fluids.

67. Which pulse is located behind the medial malleolus?

1. Radial
2. Popliteal
3. Dorsalis pedis
4. Posterior tibial

68. A 38-year-old man has hypertension. He is interested in starting an exercise program. What form of exercise would be best for him?

1. Bicycling
2. Water skiing
3. Weight lifting
4. Calisthenics

69. Which condiment would the nurse recommend to a client who is on a low-sodium diet?

1. Catsup
2. Lemon juice
3. Garlic salt
4. Soy sauce

70. A 39-year-old man was admitted to the hospital 4 days ago with an acute MI. He is expected to be discharged tomorrow. Suddenly, he calls you to his room and complains of chest pain. Which action should you perform first?

1. Assess the vital signs.
2. Administer nitroglycerin sublingually stat.
3. Raise the head of the bed to a 30- to 45-degree angle.
4. Call the physician stat.

71. A 56-year-old woman was placed on strict I&O. Her diagnosis is renal insufficiency. The I&O for the last 24 hours was 3000 mL in and 1000 mL out. Based on this information, the nurse anticipates her weight to:

1. Increase by 2 kg
2. Increase by approximately 2 lb

3. Decrease by approximately 2 lb
4. Remain the same

72. A client with chronic CHF is being discharged on furosemide (Lasix). The dietitian advises a diet high in potassium. Which food choice listed below has the most potassium content?

1. Peanuts
2. Peaches
3. Broccoli
4. Milk

73. A 60-year-old man has an ileostomy. He is admitted to the hospital with nausea, vomiting, diarrhea, and severe dehydration. What IV fluids would this nurse expect the physician to order?

1. 0.9 normal saline (NS) with added potassium
2. 0.9 NS
3. 0.45 (1/2 NS) with added potassium
4. 3% NS with added potassium

74. Which of the following would be included in the routine care of an ileostomy?

1. Bowel training, thus eliminating need to wear appliance
2. Irrigating the stoma daily to promote continence
3. Providing a skin barrier around the stoma
4. Administering a stool softener daily

75. A 75-year-old man has a diagnosis of oat cell cancer of the lung. After several courses of chemotherapy, the tumor has not responded. There are no other treatment options available, and he is dying. Which of the following is the most appropriate action for the nurse to take while caring for this dying client?

1. Limit visitors to no more than two at a time.
2. Request frequent reassignments to prevent becoming too attached to client and family.
3. Advise the client and family to settle unfinished business.
4. Request reassignments when client displays angry behavior.

76. A client with a diagnosis of terminal cancer states, "If I can just beat this thing, I'll go back to church every Sunday." Which stage of the dying process does this statement represent?

1. Denial
2. Anger
3. Depression
4. Bargaining

77. For which of the following infusions must the nurse use an electronic controlling device delivery system?

1. Dopamine
2. Packed RBCs
3. Vancomycin
4. One liter D$_5$W with 40 mEq KCl

78. A breathing pattern in which respirations gradually wax and wane in a regular pattern (increase and decrease in rate and depth) with periods of apnea is known as:

1. Kussmaul's
2. Biot's
3. Cheyne-Stokes
4. Eupnea

79. While a nurse is bathing a terminally ill client, he stops breathing. He has told the nurse many times that he does not want to live on machines. The physician has not written a "do not resuscitate" order. The nurse's best response is to:

1. Continue bathing him for 5 minutes and then call a full code.
2. Start CPR immediately and then call a full code.
3. Start artificial respiration, but if asystole occurs, stop trying to revive him.
4. Stop the bath, and consult with the charge nurse for further instructions.

80. While providing postmortem care, the nurse will:

1. Place an incontinence pad under the buttocks.
2. Place the body in a flat position.
3. Remove the dentures.
4. Remove the hospital armband.

81. The most characteristic assessment finding for the client in pulmonary edema is:

1. Nondistended neck veins
2. Anxiety
3. Generalized edema
4. Pink, frothy sputum

82. Vancomycin 500 mg in 250 mL of IV solution is to be administered over 90 minutes IV piggyback. Calculate the rate in drops per minute using a drop factor of 20 gtt/mL.

1. 20 gtt/min
2. 56 gtt/min
3. 83 gtt/min
4. 90 gtt/min

83. A 76-year-old female client informs you that she has been having vaginal bleeding for the last several days. Which of the following is the most appropriate response?

1. Reassure her that vaginal bleeding is normal for her age.
2. Explain that the bleeding will stop in a few days.
3. Encourage her to notify her doctor.
4. Encourage her to notify her daughter.

84. A 60-year-old man is scheduled for suprapubic resection of the prostate in the morning. He discusses with you that he is worried about his sexual functioning after surgery. Your most appropriate response would be:

1. Assume he is joking and chuckle at his statement.
2. "Don't worry, the surgery will not affect your sexual functioning."
3. "I understand your concern, but most men do not experience a problem after surgery."
4. "I understand your concern. Most men do experience sexual functioning problems after this type of surgery."

85. Which of the following interventions would be appropriate when caring for a client with hypercalcemia?
    1. Encourage fluids.
    2. Promote bed rest.
    3. Administer calcium supplement tablets.
    4. Administer antibiotics.

86. Which of the following would be an appropriate food choice for a neutropenic client?
    1. Bananas
    2. Carrot sticks
    3. Garden salad
    4. Canned pears

87. Which of the following does the nurse recognize as being the only diagnostic parameter for cancer?
    1. Elevated carcinoembryonic antigen (CEA) level
    2. Positive tissue biopsy
    3. Sore that does not heal
    4. Nagging cough or hoarseness

88. A 40-year-old man has developed stomatitis after chemotherapy treatment. He should be encouraged to:
    1. Eat hot, spicy foods.
    2. Brush his teeth after each meal and at bedtime.
    3. Rinse his mouth with commercial mouthwash after each meal.
    4. Drink plenty of orange juice.

89. When irrigating a descending colostomy with 1000 mL of warm tap water, the nurse would expect:
    1. Complete return of the solution plus soft or formed feces
    2. Complete return of the solution mixed with liquid stool
    3. Evacuation of soft and formed feces only
    4. Evacuation of tap water only

90. Which acid-base disturbance would be most characteristic of a narcotic overdose?
    1. Metabolic acidosis
    2. Respiratory acidosis
    3. Metabolic alkalosis
    4. Respiratory alkalosis

91. The nurse recognizes which of the following as early signs of hypoxemia?
    1. Restlessness, yawning, tachycardia
    2. Dyspnea, restlessness, hypotension
    3. Yawning, confusion, bradycardia
    4. Bradycardia, hypotension, dyspnea

92. In compliance with standard (universal) blood and body fluid precautions, the nurse would wear which of the following when giving an IM injection?
    1. Mask, gown, gloves, goggles
    2. Gloves and gown only
    3. Gloves
    4. Gloves and goggles

93. Before beginning intermittent feeding via NG tube, the nurse will first:

    1. Auscultate for bowel sounds and instill 100 cc of air.
    2. Auscultate for bowel sounds and instill 10 mL of tap water.
    3. Confirm tube placement with an abdominal radiograph.
    4. Aspirate and reinstill the stomach contents.

94. What side effects would you expect a client to experience receiving external beam irradiation for esophageal cancer?
    1. Nausea, dysphagia, bone marrow suppression
    2. Diarrhea, dysphagia, bone marrow suppression
    3. Alopecia, nausea, dysphagia
    4. Dysphagia, alopecia, constipation

95. A female client is receiving external beam irradiation for squamous cell cancer of the lung. After 2 weeks of treatment, her skin in the treatment field is red and warm to touch. Your best response would be to apply which of the following?
    1. Solarcaine, and notify the doctor
    2. A&D ointment, and notify the doctor
    3. Desitin, and notify the doctor
    4. Nothing, but notify the doctor

96. A 49-year-old Jehovah's Witness was recently given a diagnosis of multiple myeloma. The Hgb level is 6.3, and the doctor writes an order to infuse 4 units of RBCs. The client refuses the transfusion on religious grounds. The nurse's most appropriate response would be to:
    1. Do nothing.
    2. Notify the doctor of the client's refusal.
    3. Convince the client to take the transfusion.
    4. Administer the transfusion as ordered.

97. A 50-year-old female client is thrombocytopenic (decreased platelets) secondary to chemotherapy. She complains of nausea and vomiting. All of the following medications are ordered on an as-needed basis. Which medication would be the most appropriate for the client to receive?
    1. Promethazine (Phenergan) 25 mg PO
    2. Thiethylperazine maleate (Torcan) 10 mg IM
    3. Promethazine 25 mg suppository
    4. Prochlorperazine maleate (Compazine) 10 mg IV push

98. Your client is receiving continuous enteral nutrition via an NG tube. Which of the following interventions is the most important to prevent aspiration?
    1. Adding blue food coloring to the formula
    2. Keeping the head of the bed elevated
    3. Administering at rates less than 50 mL/hr
    4. Hanging no more formula than the client will receive in a 4-hour period

99. While assisting a client with right-sided hemiparesis to ambulate, the nurse should stand on the client's:
    1. Left side and hold the left hand
    2. Right side and hold the right hand
    3. Left side and hold one arm around the client's waist
    4. Right side and hold one arm around the client's waist

100. After an eye operation, the client may experience partial loss of sight. The nurse should assist at mealtime by:
    1. Feeding the client everything on the tray
    2. Encouraging the family to feed the client
    3. Orienting the client to the location of all foods on the tray
    4. Encouraging the client to use a spoon only

101. A 33-year-old client has pneumonia. When the nurse assesses this client, the following data will receive highest priority:
    1. Size of pupil, presence of sneezing, location of pain
    2. Presence of hiccups, amount of sweating, BP
    3. Capillary refill, amount of sputum, trembling
    4. Restlessness, chest wall movement, color of nails

102. A 42-year-old client has pneumonia and is receiving oxygen by nasal cannula. The quickest way to obtain an accurate reading of his temperature is to take it by:
    1. Mouth
    2. Axilla
    3. Rectum
    4. Feeling the forehead

103. The nurse is teaching a first-aid class for parents. The topic is treatment for a nosebleed. One of the parents indicates a need for further teaching with the following statement:
    1. "Pinch the soft part of the nose firmly."
    2. "Administer some warm milk or cocoa."
    3. "Apply ice to the back of the neck or to the nose."
    4. "Consult a physician as needed."

104. A 56-year-old client is scheduled for a partial laryngectomy. The nurse recognizes that he needs more preparation for surgery when the following statement is heard:
    1. "I will be able to talk by covering the tracheostomy tube."
    2. "I will be fed through a tube for a few days after surgery."
    3. "My bed should be in Fowler's position."
    4. "I should hold my head still after surgery."

105. A 26-year-old client is experiencing an attack of asthma. The following outcome will receive the highest priority in the care of this client:
    1. The client's anxiety level will be reduced.
    2. The client should maintain an open airway with adequate gas exchange.
    3. The client should talk about how he feels about his disease.
    4. The client should maintain adequate fluid balance.

106. A 46-year-old client is on a ventilator and is receiving positive end-expiratory pressure. He starts sweating profusely, the pulse increases to 122 bpm, the trachea is deviated to the right, and breath sounds on the left are diminished. The nurse would prepare for a possible:

    1. Cor pulmonale
    2. Cardiac tamponade
    3. Pneumothorax
    4. Pleural effusion

107. The following laboratory test result indicates that a client is infectious for pulmonary tuberculosis:
    1. A positive Mantoux
    2. A negative Gram stain
    3. Lesion seen on radiograph
    4. Positive sputum for acid-fast bacillus

108. The nurse is teaching a 56-year-old client about hypertension. This nurse recognizes a need for more instruction when the client makes the following statement:
    1. "I need to learn to manage stress better."
    2. "As long as my pressure gets no higher than 140/90, I'm OK."
    3. "High blood pressure can lead to heart attack and/or stroke."
    4. "I can stop taking my blood pressure medicine when I feel all right."

109. A friend calls and states that he has taken three nitroglycerin tablets for his chest pain, but the pain is still there. The nurse advises him to:
    1. Call his doctor
    2. Drive to the nearest emergency room
    3. Lie down and rest to see if the pain goes away
    4. Call 911

110. A 47-year-old client is in acute CHF after an MI. The goal of highest priority for this client at this time is to:
    1. Decrease the workload of the heart.
    2. Breathe easily.
    3. Decrease edema.
    4. Know his medications.

111. This is the second postoperative day for a 54-year-old client who had a CABG. At 8 AM her BP is normal; the pulse rate is 123 bpm (normally 82 bpm) and weak. The client is cold, clammy, and confused. Her respiratory rate is 44/min; bowel sounds are absent, and the urinary output is 22 mL/hr. The nurse prepares for the treatment of:
    1. CHF
    2. MI
    3. Shock
    4. Cardiac tamponade

112. The nurse is about to administer a dose of digoxin to a client. The client states that she has not eaten her breakfast and complains of being nauseated and having visual changes. After checking her apical and radial pulses and the serum digoxin level, the nurse would:
    1. Call the physician
    2. Check tissue perfusion
    3. Review the latest electrolyte report
    4. Administer an ordered antiemetic

113. A 33-year-old client is admitted to a nursing unit complaining of pain and swelling in her left leg. She has a positive Homans' sign and is diagnosed with deep vein thrombosis (DVT). An appropriate nursing intervention would be:

1. Apply antiembolism stockings to both legs.
2. Administer aspirin for pain.
3. Massage both legs to promote comfort.
4. Provide bed rest.

114. A 46-year-old client recently had a radical mastectomy. She will not look at the surgical site and refuses to see her visitors. An appropriate action for the nurse to suggest is:

1. See a minister.
2. Talk about her feelings.
3. Join a support group.
4. Face reality.

115. A 48-year-old client with leukemia is receiving chemotherapy. Depression of bone marrow is a possible side effect. The nurse would assess for any signs of infection and/or anemia. The nurse would also observe for:

1. Decrease in cardiac output
2. Drop in urinary output
3. Broken bones
4. Bleeding

116. A client with AIDS indicates that more teaching about the condition is needed when the nurse hears the following statement:

1. "This disease is spread by sexual contact."
2. "I'm afraid to touch anyone; I might give them my disease."
3. "The virus may also be spread through body fluids."
4. "Infected mothers can pass the virus to their unborn infants."

117. A nurse explains to a family that the Sengstaken-Blakemore tube is used for the treatment of:

1. Esophageal varices
2. Cirrhosis of the liver
3. Renal stones
4. Hiatal hernia

118. The nurse recognizes that a client needs more teaching about prevention of peptic ulcer disease (PUD) after he states:

1. "I shouldn't use aspirin-like drugs too often."
2. "I will miss my morning coffee so much."
3. "I have to stop smoking."
4. "I need to manage stress better."

119. A 36-year-old client recently returned from the operating room after having a partial gastrectomy for peptic ulcer disease. He has an NG tube that has been connected to low, intermittent suction for 2 days. A nurse would observe for:

1. High serum potassium level
2. Respiratory alkalosis

3. Metabolic alkalosis
4. Metabolic acidosis

120. A 46-year-old client has his first meal after a Billroth II surgical procedure. About 30 minutes after the meal, he becomes nauseated, feels very weak, and complains of severe gas pains and distention. The nurse prepares for treatment of:

1. Shock after perforation of the GI tract
2. Paralytic ileus
3. GI obstruction
4. Dumping syndrome

121. A 34-year-old client is hospitalized for Crohn's disease; the nurse should assess this client frequently for:

1. Vital signs, bleeding, and diarrhea
2. Skin turgor, urinary output, and electrolyte report results
3. Breath sounds, pupil size, and change in mental status
4. Peripheral perfusion, skin color, and muscle twitching

122. A 39-year-old client has an ileal conduit after recent surgery for cancer of the bladder. The nurse assesses the amount and characteristics of the drainage, the fluid and electrolyte balance of the client, and the condition of the stoma and surrounding skin and for:

1. Adventitious lung sounds
2. Pulse deficits
3. Renal stones
4. Bowel sounds

123. A 27-year-old client has chest tubes connected to a Pleur-evac after a stab wound to the left chest. When the client goes to radiology via wheelchair, the nurse would manage the Pleur-evac in the following way:

1. Disconnect the Pleur-evac from the drainage tubing.
2. Clamp the drainage tubing before disconnecting the Pleur-evac.
3. Replace wall suction with a portable suction machine.
4. Attach the Pleur-evac to the side of the wheelchair.

124. While assessing a client who has a possible bowel obstruction, the nurse hears very loud, rumbling bowel sounds (a stethoscope is not needed). The nurse would chart these sounds as:

1. Excess flatus
2. Acini
3. Hypoactive
4. Borborygmi

125. A 33-year-old client recently had an inguinal hernia repair. The nurse modifies postoperative care from that given most general surgery clients as follows:

1. Antiembolism stockings are not used for this client.
2. Hemorrhage is not as likely in this client.
3. This client should not cough.
4. Infection is less likely in this client.

126. A 27-year-old client returns to the hospital room after a barium enema. An important part of his nursing care at this point in time is to:

1. Obtain an order for a cleansing enema.
2. Observe for signs of renal damage.
3. Maintain bed rest until a physician orders otherwise.
4. Observe for an allergic reaction to the barium.

127. A 16-year-old client complains of abdominal pain. The nurse:

1. Recommends a laxative
2. Checks for rebound tenderness
3. Applies a heating pad
4. Calls the physician

128. A 44-year-old client is diagnosed with peritonitis after a small bowel obstruction. The nurse would:

1. Encourage ambulation
2. Place the client in a supine position
3. Check the mouth for ulcerations
4. Keep the client NPO

129. A client admitted for a diagnostic workup passes a stool that is of normal size in some areas but string-like in others. The nurse would:

1. Document the finding on the chart.
2. Ignore the appearance of the stool.
3. Obtain an order for a laxative.
4. Check for fecal impaction.

130. A nurse is teaching a client about choledocholithiasis. The nurse explains that the term means:

1. Infection of the bile duct
2. Stones in the hepatic and bile duct
3. Inflammation of the gallbladder
4. Stones in the gallbladder

131. When the nurse is giving emotional support to a comatose client, this nurse would:

1. Disturb the client as little as possible
2. Explain all nursing actions to the family
3. Encourage the client to express feelings
4. Explain all nursing actions to the client

132. A nurse is doing preoperative teaching for a client who will have a cholecystectomy. The nurse teaches that special care must be taken to prevent the following postoperative complication:

1. Hypostatic pneumonia
2. Thrombosis
3. Hemorrhage
4. Paralytic ileus

133. A nurse is teaching a client with newly diagnosed hepatitis A. The client asks, "How did I catch this disease?" The best response by the nurse is which of the following?

1. Blood or contaminated needles
2. Body fluids
3. Sexual intercourse
4. Feces or contaminated food or water

134. A client has been given a diagnosis of hepatitis A. The nurse would use which of the following precautions for preventing transmission of the disease to self and others?

1. Reverse isolation
2. A mask and gown
3. Universal Precautions
4. Isolation precautions for trash

135. A 44-year-old client has cirrhosis of the liver with severe ascites. The nurse plans for the following intervention:

1. Apply prolonged pressure to injection sites.
2. Administer aspirin for headache as needed.
3. Measure abdominal girth weekly.
4. Provide a low-protein, high-carbohydrate diet.

136. A client has been given a diagnosis of acute pancreatitis. The nurse will assess this client for:

1. Hyperkalemia
2. Metabolic acidosis
3. Hypocalcemia
4. Hyperglycemia

137. A nurse assesses the surgical wound of a client who recently had an appendectomy. The wound is red and swollen with pus oozing from the lower edge. The nurse would:

1. Clean the wound with an antibiotic solution.
2. Report the findings to a physician.
3. Clean the wound with hydrogen peroxide.
4. Irrigate the wound with NS.

138. A 34-year-old client has third-degree burns on 10% of the BSA. A dressing change is scheduled for 10 AM. The nurse would:

1. Force fluids by mouth.
2. Use clean technique for changing the dressing.
3. Administer the analgesic as needed at about 9 AM.
4. Monitor I&O each shift.

139. A 23-year-old client received multiple superficial injuries in a motorcycle accident. The nurse in the emergency room will:

1. Ask when the client had the last tetanus shot.
2. Administer a tetanus injection as prescribed.
3. Treat the injuries and send the client home.
4. Administer morphine as prescribed for pain.

140. A 47-year-old man enters the emergency room complaining of severe pain in the left flank, which radiates to the suprapubic area. He is nauseated and gives a history of renal stones. The nurse would:

1. Save all of the client's urine
2. Keep the client NPO
3. Record I&O
4. Strain all urine through gauze

141. A 41-year-old client has a ureteral catheter because of a stone in the left lower ureter. The nurse would:

1. Clamp the catheter and change the drainage tubing as needed

2. Record output from the ureteral catheter separately
3. Irrigate the ureteral catheter every 4 hours
4. Maintain bed rest until the catheter is removed

142. A client with chronic renal failure in the early stage of uremia is instructed on diet. The nurse recognizes a need for more instruction when the following statement is heard:

1. "I will need meat three times a day and all the milk I can drink."
2. "I need a lot of calories to provide energy for healing."
3. "I need to avoid foods high in potassium, like bananas and raisins."
4. "I can't add salt to my food or eat foods high in salt."

143. A 33-year-old client is undergoing peritoneal dialysis for acute renal failure. To prevent one of the most common complications of peritoneal dialysis, the nurse

1. Makes certain that the drain time is adequate
2. Checks the dwelling time to see that it is precise
3. Uses strict aseptic technique
4. Adds calcium gluconate to the solution

144. A 44-year-old client with chronic renal failure has an arteriovenous shunt in the right arm for access to hemodialysis. The nurse would:

1. Check BP in the left arm
2. Start an IV in the right arm
3. Irrigate the shunt every 4 hours
4. Draw blood from the shunt

145. A 46-year-old client is scheduled to go for hemodialysis at 9:30 AM. The physician has ordered cimetidine, digoxin, and docusate for 9 AM. The nurse would:

1. Give all medications as ordered.
2. Hold all medications until dialysis has been completed.
3. Check to see which medications are removed by dialysis.
4. Check with the physician.

146. A nurse is writing a care plan for a 45-year-old client with chronic renal failure. An important goal would be to:

1. Detect fluid or electrolyte imbalances
2. Protect the perianal area from excoriation
3. Detect respiratory changes caused by alkalosis
4. Observe for signs and symptoms of hypokalemia

147. A 56-year-old client just returned from the operating room after having a TURP for cancer. The nurse will give highest priority to assessing for:

1. Urinary output
2. Bowel sounds
3. Abnormal lung sounds
4. Clot formation in an extremity

148. A 62-year-old client is receiving radiation treatments for lung cancer. The field for radiation therapy is clearly outlined with purple ink. The nurse would treat this field as follows:

1. Bathe it the same as any other part of the body.
2. Apply moisturizing lotion to prevent dryness.
3. Wipe it with clear water and pat dry as needed only.
4. Treat as a stage I decubitus ulcer.

149. A 49-year-old client just returned from the operating room after having a total abdominal hysterectomy. The nurse will:

1. Encourage the client to void.
2. Apply antiembolism stockings PRN.
3. Change perineal pads every 8 hours.
4. Change the abdominal dressing to check for bleeding.

150. A 44-year-old male client recently had a lumbosacral laminectomy to repair a herniated nucleus pulposus. The nurse would:

1. Get the client out of bed the first day of surgery.
2. Apply a brace before getting the client out of bed.
3. Teach the client not to raise his legs or point his toes.
4. Log-roll the client when changing his position in bed.

151. A client has a diagnosis of epiglottitis. It would be most important for the nurse to keep which of the following at the bedside?

1. Oxygen
2. An oral airway
3. Suction equipment
4. Tracheostomy set

152. After a liver biopsy, the nurse should place the client in which of the following positions?

1. Right side
2. Left side
3. High-Fowler's
4. Trendelenburg

153. A 50-year-old man complains of chills, low back pain, and nausea 10 minutes after a blood transfusion has begun. An hour later, his temperature increases to 102°F (38.8°C), he is hypotensive, and he voids urine red in color. Which type of blood transfusion reaction is occurring?

1. Febrile
2. Allergic
3. Septic
4. Hemolytic

154. An 18-year-old client is experiencing a sickle cell crisis. Which of the following interventions is indicated for this client?

1. ROM exercises every 2 hours
2. Fluid restriction of <1 L/day
3. Administration of antidiarrheal medications
4. Pain assessments every 4 hours

155. An 80-year-old client who had a left cerebrovascular accident (CVA) is experiencing continuous oozing of small amounts of liquid stool and has not had a bowel movement in 4 days. He eats only 20% of meals served to him. The oozing of stool is most likely a result of:

1. Decreased intake
2. Spinal cord trauma
3. Fecal impaction
4. Dehydration

156. A client has been diagnosed with epilepsy. Which of the following is an appropriate action for the nurse to take when a client is having a seizure?

    1. Administer oxygen via nasal cannula.
    2. Apply vest and wrist restraints to prevent injury.
    3. Pry the jaw open to maintain an airway.
    4. Place the client on the side with the head flexed forward.

157. A client who has received continuous enteral tube feedings for a week has pulled her NG tube out. Within an hour, she develops tachycardia, diaphoresis, and tremors of her hands. The nurse correctly identifies her symptoms as:

    1. Hypoglycemia
    2. Hyperglycemia
    3. Hypokalemia
    4. Hyperkalemia

158. A client in a nursing home is at high risk to develop pressure ulcers because of immobility, incontinence, and low serum albumin. Which of the following would the nurse assess for as a first sign of a pressure ulcer?

    1. Breakdown of the skin
    2. Erythema of the skin
    3. Clear-colored drainage
    4. Exposure of underlying muscle

159. A client has been placed on oral anticoagulants after an MI. Which of the following instructions should the nurse give to the client?

    1. The client will need to have a PTT monitored periodically.
    2. The client should carry identification indicating that he or she is taking an anticoagulant.
    3. The client should take aspirin instead of acetaminophen for headaches and minor pain.
    4. One or two alcoholic beverages per week will not interfere with the effectiveness of the anticoagulant.

160. A client is scheduled to receive morphine sulfate. Which of the following is an appropriate nursing action?

    1. Monitor the pulse rate and withhold administration if <60 bpm.
    2. Monitor the respiratory rate and withhold administration if <12/min.
    3. Monitor the temperature and administer if >101°F (38.3°C).
    4. Monitor the BP and administer if <90/60 mm Hg.

161. A 74-year-old woman is admitted with symptoms of vaginal bleeding. The nurse identifies this bleeding as most likely a result of:

    1. An irregular menstrual cycle
    2. An increase in estrogen production

3. A sexually transmitted disease
4. Uterine cancer

162. The nurse is assessing a client who has recently been found to be hyperthyroid. The nurse would expect to find which of the following symptoms?

    1. Progressively gains weight
    2. Cannot tolerate cold temperatures
    3. Has a rapid pulse on rest and exertion
    4. Often develops myxedema

163. The nurse is teaching a class on wound healing. Which of the following is an accurate statement concerning wound healing?

    1. Accumulation of blood in a wound becomes a growth medium for infection.
    2. A tight dressing increases the blood supply carrying nutrients to the area.
    3. Clients taking steroids have a heightened inflammatory response.
    4. Activity promotes wound healing.

164. The nurse is assessing the client for hypovolemic shock. Which of the following symptoms would the nurse expect to find?

    1. A slow, thready pulse
    2. Deep, slow respirations
    3. Cold, moist skin
    4. Urinary output of 100 mL/hr or more

165. A client with a DVT suddenly cries out with sharp, stabbing pains in the chest and becomes dyspneic, anxious, and cyanotic. The nurse correctly identifies this as which of the following?

    1. MI
    2. Anaphylaxis
    3. Pulmonary embolism
    4. Bronchopneumonia

166. A client has been given a diagnosis of esophageal stricture. It is important for the nurse to teach him to:

    1. Eat hot, spicy foods to relax the stricture.
    2. Lie supine after eating.
    3. Eat just before bedtime.
    4. Eat small amounts frequently.

167. When planning for care of the client with a percutaneous endoscopic gastrostomy (PEG) tube, it would be important for the nurse to include which of the following:

    1. Nasal assessment for skin irritation from the tube
    2. Securing the tube to the client's cheek
    3. Assessing for tube displacement after coughing or suctioning
    4. Assessing bowel elimination patterns

168. A client has a bowel movement that consists of dark, tarry stools. The nurse would expect that the client is experiencing bleeding from:

    1. Hemorrhoids
    2. Stomach

3. Rectum
4. Sigmoid colon

169. A client is admitted with a diagnosis of peptic ulcer disease (PUD). Which of the following symptoms would alert the nurse that the ulcer has perforated?

1. The client complains of chronic continuous pain persisting for a week.
2. Bowel movements are painful and the stool is white.
3. Pain is noted in the right shoulder.
4. Gastric pain is noted after eating.

170. A client has light-colored stools and dark urine. The nurse correctly identifies these symptoms as being associated with:

1. Hepatitis B
2. PUD
3. Renal failure
4. Small bowel obstruction

171. Four units of regular insulin are given subcutaneously to a client at 4 PM for an elevated glucose level. The client is at greatest risk for rebound hypoglycemia at:

1. 4:01 PM
2. 8 PM
3. Midnight
4. 6 AM the following morning

172. Which of the following statements made by a client indicates a need for additional diabetic teaching?

1. "If I ever get shaky, hungry, and sweaty, I should drink some juice or eat some sugar."
2. "I could go blind from the diabetes."
3. "My blood sugar level will remain the same throughout the day now that I am on insulin."
4. "I draw up the regular insulin first, then the intermediate-acting NPH insulin when I put them both in one syringe."

173. After a thyroidectomy, a client develops spasms of the hands and feet accompanied by muscle twitching. The nurse identifies these symptoms as signs of:

1. Hypocalcemia
2. Hypercalcemia
3. Hypokalemia
4. Hyperkalemia

174. A client has received steroid therapy for 1 year. Which of the following is caused by long-term steroid therapy?

1. Weight loss
2. Masking of signs of infection
3. Addison's disease
4. Improvement in facial acne

175. The nurse is developing a plan of care for a client who has a diagnosis of acute pancreatitis. The rationale for maintaining the client on bed rest is to:

1. Reduce pancreatic and gastric secretions
2. Minimize the effects of hypoglycemia

3. Reduce the risk of DVT
4. Decrease the likelihood of orthostatic hypotension

176. The physician has ordered a urinalysis for a client. The nurse gives which of the following instructions?

1. Women should cleanse the perineum from back to front.
2. Hands should be washed before collecting the specimen.
3. The container should be pressed gently against the genitalia.
4. The first portion of the voiding should not be collected.

177. The nurse is doing discharge planning with a quadriplegic client. Which of the following instructions should be given to the client with an indwelling urinary catheter connected to gravity drainage?

1. Drainage bag should be placed above the level of the heart when the client is in bed.
2. Drainage bag should rest on the floor while the client is sitting in a chair.
3. Drainage bag should be emptied when completely full.
4. Tubing of the drainage bag should be inspected for kinks or twists frequently.

178. Which of the following statements made by a client indicates that a complication of peritoneal dialysis is occurring?

1. "The dressing around the peritoneal catheter is completely dry."
2. "A little bit of blood comes out of the peritoneal catheter on the days I menstruate."
3. "The drainage from my catheter is cloudy and white in color."
4. "I haven't gained any weight over the past week."

179. A client with a history of recurrent UTIs is being evaluated in the clinic. Which of the following actions indicates that the client is adhering to instructions?

1. Limits fluids to 32 oz/day
2. Voids every 2–3 hours while awake
3. Discontinues antibiotics when symptom-free
4. Takes daily tub baths

180. A client is placed on hemodialysis. The nurse would best assess the client's progress by:

1. Monitoring the client's weight
2. Performing a calorie count
3. Measuring the client's exercise tolerance
4. Inspecting the client's skin for bruising

181. A client is evaluated in the clinic 2 years after having a kidney transplant. The nurse expects this client to be most concerned about:

1. Fear of kidney rejection
2. Developing an infection
3. Uncertainty about the future
4. Effects of immunosuppressive therapy

182. Which of the following is an applicable nursing diagnosis for a client admitted with renal stones?

1. Impaired gas exchange
2. Fluid volume deficit
3. Risk for infection
4. Disturbance in self-concept

183. A 34-year-old recently married man is admitted for an ileal conduit urinary diversion. The nurse should:

1. Teach the client how to perform intermittent urinary catheterization.
2. Explore the client's self-concept and self-esteem before surgery.
3. Explain the rationale for peritoneal dialysis.
4. Inform the client that urine and stool will be redirected to a stoma on the abdominal wall.

184. A male client has a diagnosis of herpes genitalis infection. The nurse should instruct him to:

1. Avoid condom use to reduce irritation.
2. Take all prescribed antibiotic doses.
3. Avoid touching the blister-like lesions.
4. Apply antifungal cream sparingly.

185. An 80-year-old man states that he experiences dribbling of clear yellow urine, hesitancy in starting urination, and a sensation of incomplete emptying of the bladder. The nurse identifies which of the following as the most likely cause of the symptoms?

1. The aging process
2. An enlarged prostate gland
3. A UTI
4. Chronic constipation

186. A client with AIDS is unable to cough because of weakness and fatigue. The client is at risk for:

1. Impaired gas exchange
2. Pain
3. Altered thought processes
4. Ineffective airway clearance

187. The nurse is changing the dressing covering an infected abscess that has been drained. The gauze is saturated with a foul-smelling yellow exudate. The nurse removes the dressing:

1. With bare hands
2. After donning nonsterile gloves
3. After donning sterile gloves
4. After double-gloving

188. A client states that his eyes and skin itch 10 minutes after a penicillin derivative is administered. Hives are noted on the client's arms, trunk, and legs. The nurse can anticipate that which of the following may occur?

1. Hypertensive crisis
2. Laryngeal edema
3. Paralytic ileus
4. Liver failure

189. During the physical assessment of a woman with an exacerbation of systemic lupus erythematosus (SLE), the nurse is likely to note which of the following?

1. Bulging eyes
2. Butterfly-shaped rash across the bridge of the nose
3. Jaundice
4. Kaposi's lesions

190. A nurse is conducting a physical assessment on a client. Which of the following characteristics of a mole on the skin warrants further evaluation by a physician?

1. Brown color
2. Irregular shape
3. Located on the neck
4. Skin around area sunburned

191. A child sustains a burn injury when a boiling pot of water is knocked off a stove. The skin on the child's chest appears sunburned and is dry. The nurse describes the burn injury as a:

1. Smoke inhalation injury
2. Superficial (first-degree) injury
3. Partial-thickness (second-degree) injury
4. Full-thickness (third-degree) injury

192. The nurse identifies which of the following as care of the client during the rehabilitation phase of burn care?

1. Monitoring urine output hourly
2. Maintaining NG suction
3. Applying topical antibacterials
4. Applying pressure garments

193. A medication is ordered to be administered "1 gtt to OD." The nurse administers 1 drop to:

1. The right eye
2. The left eye
3. Both eyes
4. Each ear

194. To reduce intraocular pressure in the client who has undergone retinal surgery, the nurse would:

1. Apply a hot compress to the eye.
2. Provide bright lighting and teaching tools in large print.
3. Instruct the client to press gently on the eye if discomfort occurs.
4. Elevate the head of the bed 30 degrees or higher.

195. A client has undergone ear surgery. The nurse should instruct the client to:

1. Blow nose frequently.
2. Shampoo on the day after surgery.
3. Report altered taste and mouth dryness.
4. Keep the ear packing moist.

196. A client has sustained a head injury from a motor vehicle accident. The nurse would assess for which of the following early signs of increasing ICP?

1. Reaction only to loud auditory or painful stimuli
2. Absence of reflexes and flaccidity of extremities
3. Fixed and dilated pupils
4. Lethargy and changing levels of consciousness

197. A client is unconscious after a severe head injury. The nurse's most important action is to:
    1. Provide meticulous skin care
    2. Maintain an airway and adequate ventilation
    3. Turn the client every 2 hours to reduce infection risk
    4. Elevate the head of the bed to prevent aspiration of secretions

198. After a CVA, a client experiences memory loss, inability to concentrate, altered judgment, and impaired decision making. The nurse identifies these as which type of deficit?
    1. Sensory
    2. Verbal
    3. Cognitive
    4. Emotional

199. The nurse is planning a bowel program for a client with multiple sclerosis. This would include:
    1. Fluid restriction
    2. A high fiber diet
    3. Daily irrigation of the colostomy
    4. Intermittent self-catheterization

200. After a total hip replacement, the nurse should assess the neurovascular status of the leg by:
    1. Monitoring vital signs
    2. Noting the amount of wound drainage
    3. Assessing capillary refill of the toes
    4. Performing ROM exercises

201. Chronic pain is defined as an unpleasant sensory and emotional experience associated with:
    1. Actual tissue damage.
    2. Actual or potential tissue damage.
    3. Only observable pain behaviors.
    4. Physiological signs and symptoms that the pain exists.

202. A client taking opioids for cancer pain begins to require more medication to provide the same amount of analgesia. This is known as:
    1. Physical dependence.
    2. Drug tolerance.
    3. Addiction.
    4. Equianalgesia.

203. Physical dependence or drug dependence is which type of phenomenon?
    1. Psychologic
    2. Physiologic
    3. Addiction
    4. Obsessive-compulsive

204. Cancer pain is best managed with the use of:
    1. A patient-controlled analgesia pump.
    2. Short-acting opioids administered around the clock.
    3. Frequent administration of breakthrough medications.
    4. Long-acting opioids administered around the clock.

205. In keeping with the World Health Organization's statement: "Every client has a right to adequate pain control," a nurse educator instructs staff to:
    1. Rely only on observable signs of pain.
    2. Always consider clients as potential malingerers.
    3. Assume that they will become addicted.
    4. Believe that clients may have pain without observable signs.

206. To evaluate adequately the effectiveness of therapies for pain control, the nurse should:
    1. Be casual and informal.
    2. Not bother if the client is quiet.
    3. Use a pain assessment tool.
    4. Rely on the client's feedback.

207. A client is admitted to the ICU with a diagnosis of an acute myocardial infarction and the following hemodynamic evaluation: arterial B/P = 100/80; heart rate = 135, CO = 3.5 L/min, and CI 2 L/min. Reviewing this data, your goal for hemodynamic stability is:
    1. Increase heart rate and cardiac output.
    2. Decrease heart rate to increase oxygen supply to the coronary arteries.
    3. Increase blood pressure to increase cardiac index.
    4. Decrease cardiac output.

208. Which of the following hemodynamic variables gives the best indication of left ventricular afterload and right ventricular afterload?
    1. Central venous pressure, systemic vascular resistance
    2. Pulmonary capillary wedge pressure, systemic vascular resistance
    3. Systemic vascular resistance, pulmonary vascular resistance
    4. Mean arterial blood pressure; pulmonary capillary wedge pressure

209. A client has an intra-aortic balloon pump in the 1:2 mode. He wants to get out of bed to use the commode. What is the *best* explanation as to why this is not recommended?
    1. The position of the balloon catheter will be altered in the upright position blocking left subclavian artery perfusion.
    2. The balloon will not function if the patient's position changes.
    3. An increase in heart rate decreases myocardial oxygen consumption.
    4. The balloon insertion site may become infected.

210. The client's heart rate is 60 beats per minute per internal pacemaker, cardiac output is 6 L per minute, pulmonary capillary wedge pressure is 12 mm Hg, and systemic vascular resistance is 900 dynes. If the cardiologist increases the intrinsic rate of the pacemaker to 75 beats per minute, which of the following is the nurse likely to see in the client's hemodynamic monitoring:
    1. Systemic vascular resistance will increase.
    2. Pulmonary capillary wedge pressure will increase.
    3. Cardiac output will increase.
    4. Heart rate will decrease.

211. A 56-year-old man is admitted to your unit from the cardiac catherization laboratory where an angioplasty of the right coronoary artery was performed. He currently has a balloon pump in place, set at an inflation ratio of 1:2. His cardiac output is 5:1, with a blood pressure of 142/82. He calls you to his room complaining of bleeding from the catherization site. Your initial action would be to:

1. Rush the client to the operating room.
2. Apply direct pressure to the site.
3. Call the physician stat.
4. Place the client on his left side.

212. A 75-year-old client presents with confusion, fever, chills, cough, and pleuritic chest pain. Community acquired pneumonia is diagnosed. Which of the physician's orders should the nurse perform first?

1. Ascultation of lung sounds.
2. Collection of sputum specimen for culture and sensitivity.
3. Administer levofloxacin (Levaquin) 500 mgm IVPB.
4. Draw blood for CBC.

213. A 26-year-old male presents to the ER with exercise-induced asthma. Assessment findings that confirm his diagnosis are: (**Select all that apply.**)

1. Wheezing
2. Chest tightness
3. Cough
4. "Silent chest"
5. Peak expiratory flow rate (PEFR) 80%
6. Calm behavior
7. Diminished breath sounds

214. A patient with COPD develops the complication of cor pulmonale. Indicate with an X on this figure where you would auscultate to make this determination.

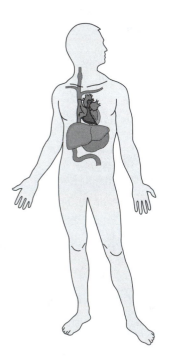

215. When teaching a client with COPD interventions to decrease air trapping, which statement made by the client indicates a need for further instruction?

1. "I will use my oxygen at 2 liters per minute."
2. "Pursed-lip breathing is only for times when I am short of breath."
3. "Chest physiotherapy every day will make it easier to breath."
4. "Diaphragmatic breathing gives me more control over my breathing."

216. What complication of oxygen therapy can occur with high levels of oxygen and result in the development of ARDS?

1. Carbon dioxide narcosis
2. Absorption atelectasis
3. Infection
4. O_2 toxicity

217. Select the chamber in a Pleur-evac that provides a water seal and also shows tidaling.

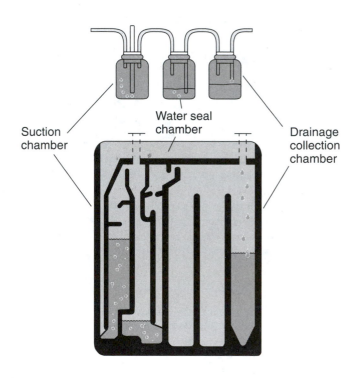

Suction chamber   Water seal chamber   Drainage collection chamber

218. Select all possible treatments for tuberculosis.

1. INH
2. 3TC
3. Rifampin
4. Ethambutol
5. Streptomycin
6. Pyrazinamide
7. Lamivudine

219. Identify a positive response to tuberculosis (TB) testing.

1. 15 mm

2. 10 mm
3. 5 mm
4. Negative candidiasis and negative TB

220. A client with a tracheostomy has rhonchi in both lungs and a cough. You determine the client needs suctioning. What is the proper technique for suctioning?

1. Insert the suction catheter 10 inches.
2. Remove oxygen mask while sterile set-up is prepared.
3. Limit suctioning to no more than 10 seconds.
4. Use new catheter for each suctioning until airway is clear.

221. Which lab value alerts the nurse that the client has iron deficiency anemia?

1. WBC 11,500
2. MCV 84
3. RBC 5
4. Hgb 6

222. Choose the proper route and site for administration of parenteral iron preparation.

1. Subcutaneous, arm
2. Intramuscular, gluteus
3. Intramuscular, arm
4. Intramuscular, Z track, gluteus

223. Select all treatment options for iron deficiency anemia.

1. Ferrous sulfate
2. Ascorbic acid
3. Docusate
4. Folic acid
5. Thiamine
6. Eggs, milk, cheese
7. Legumes
8. Whole blood transfusions

224. The 19-year-old female client complained of leukorrhea and intermenstrual bleeding. After obtaining a negative pregnancy test, you take a health history. Identify all risk factors, that if present, may increase the risk of cervical cancer.

1. Human papillomavirus
2. Sexually active since age 14 years
3. Multiple sexual partners
4. Nonsmoker

225. The client has ovarian cancer and underwent a total abdominal hysterectomy with bilateral salpingo-oophorectomy. Postoperative assessment includes: (**Select all that apply.**)

1. Monitoring Foley catheter output
2. Administering a vaginal douche and enema
3. Assessing for bowel sounds
4. Encouraging leg exercises or use of compression devices
5. Removal of sutures in 4 days

226. Approximately 50% of all breast cancers develop in one quadrant of the breast. Place an X on the quadrant.

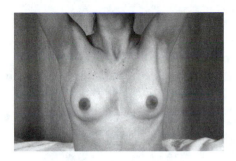

227. You are teaching the client in preparation for discharge after a cataract extraction. Choose all appropriate teaching topics:

1. Wear sunglasses outdoors.
2. How to instill eye medications.
3. When to take opioids.
4. Avoidance of bending, coughing, and lifting over 5 lb.
5. Importance of follow-up in 1 week.
6. Signs and symptoms of infection.
7. Signs and symptoms of increased intraocular pressure.

228. A client presents to the clinic with a chief complaint of sudden excruciating pain in his left eye. He also has nausea and vomiting and blurred vision. Based on these data, what is the client experiencing?

1. Angle closure glaucoma
2. Cataract
3. Meniere's isease
4. Retinal detachment

229. A client has Meniere's disease and asks you for interventions to reduce the symptoms during an attack. Choose all the interventions that apply:

1. High protein diet
2. Restrict caffeine, nicotine, and alcohol
3. Diuretics
4. Antihistamines
5. Antiemetic
6. Meclizine hydrochloride (Antivert)
7. Quiet dark room
8. Watching television

230. The client had a thrombotic stroke and is having trouble with dysphagia during her recovery. Identify interventions to assist your client to overcome this problem.

1. Assess communication deficits and plan strategies to increase verbal skills.
2. Sit client upright for meals (90-degree angle).
3. Assist client when ambulating.
4. Reinforce bladder training.

231. A client is admitted to your unit with a diagnosis of brain tumor. He is awake and alert on admit, but later in the shift, he became hard to arouse. What other assessment finding makes you suspect increased intracranial pressure?

1. Glasgow Coma Scale of 15
2. Hyperresponsive reflexes
3. Dilated pupil
4. BP 120/80

232. The client had a craniotomy for removal of a glioma 48 hours ago. Identify all priority nursing assessments;

1. Level of consciousness
2. Pupil response
3. Vital signs
4. Condition of the surgical dressing
5. Turning and positioning
6. Encouraging adequate nutrition
7. Assessing pain

233. A client is in traction for a fractured femur. Which of the following statements indicates understanding of the nurse's instruction?

1. "The weights must hang freely at all times."
2. "I'm free to move about in bed as I wish."
3. "I'll be in a lot of pain and will need narcotics frequently."
4. "I won't have the time or energy to work on my paintings."

234. During the evening following a partial gastrectomy, a client's oral temperature is 100°F. Other data include a blood pressure of 134/68, a pulse of 88, and a respiratory rate of 18. The nurse should:

1. Notify the physician immediately.
2. Take the temperature every hour until it is normal.
3. Perform a respiratory assessment.
4. Remove the dressing and check the operative site.

235. A client with insulin-dependent diabetes mellitus (IDDM) is being discharged. The nurse knows that the client has understood essential teaching when the following statement is heard:

1. "I need to cut my nails straight across."
2. "I can't make any substitutions in my diet."
3. "My insulin should be given into my arms."
4. "I should eat less before exercising."

236. A 45-year-old client has recently been told that she has acute myelocytic leukemia. She seems quite happy and laughs and jokes about everything. The nurse should:

1. Remind her of the seriousness of her diagnosis.
2. Encourage her to continue with her laughter and joking.
3. Wait and allow her to explore her feelings.
4. Reprimand her for not taking her treatment seriously.

237. Radioactive iodine is being used to treat a client with cancer of the thyroid gland. The nurse knows that the client has understood teaching about the treatment when the following statement is heard:

1. "Only my thryoid gland will be radioactive."
2. "I need not be concerned with radioactivity."
3. "My whole body will be radioactive."
4. "My body fluids will be radioactive for a short time."

238. A client's total parenteral nutrition is 6 hours behind schedule. The nurse would:

1. Run the fluid at a rate to make up for the lost time.
2. Report the situation to the physician.
3. Run the IV at the prescribed site.
4. Check the blood glucose level.

239. A 44-year-old client is in acute congestive heart failure. The nurse and client establish a goal of highest priority as:

1. Rest mentally as well as physically.
2. Learn stress management.
3. Train for a less demanding job.
4. Prevent complications of immobility.

240. A 33-year-old client is having a routine physical examination. The nurse evaluates which of the following data on a urinalysis report as normal?

1. Positive for ketones
2. Trace of protein
3. Positive for glucose
4. Cloudy

241. A client with chronic renal failure has an arteriovenous shunt in the left arm. The nurse makes which of the following assessments of the left arm each shift?

1. Blood pressure and pulse
2. Detection of a thrill and bruit
3. Venous and arterial distention
4. Skin turgor and skin integrity

242. A 17-year-old client's mother has recently been diagnosed with pulmonary tuberculosis. The nurse would expect the physician to order which of the following tests *initially?*

1. The Mantoux
2. A radiograph
3. A sputum culture
4. Gram stain of the sputum

243. A 49-year-old client with cancer of the lung just had a thoracentesis. The nurse would position the client:

1. On the affected side
2. Sitting
3. On the unaffected side
4. In Fowler's position

244. A 55-year-old client has a chest tube connected to a Pleur-evac system to remove blood from the pleural cavity. While returning the client, the nurse remembers to:

1. Keep the Pleur-evac below the level of the wound.
2. Remove the suction from the Pleur-evac.
3. Clamp the tubing connected to the Pleur-evac.
4. Drain the sterile water from the Pleur-evac.

245. A client has recently been told about a diagnosis of cancer. The nurse plans which of the following as a priority action?

1. A schedule of regualar exercise
2. Activities for diversional therapy
3. Time for the client to share feelings
4. Social activities with a variety of people

246. A 42-year-old client returned from the operating room 2 hours ago after having a lumbar diskectomy. The nurse would:

1. Allow the client to remain in the same position.
2. Encourage the client to turn himself.
3. Obtain a trapeze to help the client turn himself.
4. Turn the client every 2 hours by log-rolling him.

247. A 53-year-old client is scheduled for an arteriogram to evaluate a femoral-distal bypass in the right leg. In order to protect the kidneys from the effects of the iodine-based contrast medium to be used, the nurse should:

1. Check for allergies to the contrast medium.
2. See that the client gets a low protein diet prior to the test.
3. Administer enemas until clear the evening before the test.
4. See that the client is as well-hydrated as possible.

248. A client on antineoplastic therapy has a platelet count of 20,000/mm³. An appropriate intervention for the nurse to use would be:

1. Administering vitamin K intramuscularly
2. Massaging injection sites to aid absorption
3. Encouraging the use of firm toothbrushes and vigorous flossing
4. Avoiding rectal temperatures and other rectal procedures

249. A client who is receiving radiation to the abdomen for a malignant tumor is having diarrhea. Which of the following statements would indicate to the nurse that the client has understood teaching about management of diarrhea?

1. "I should eat foods rich in potassium."
2. "I need a quart of milk a day or its equivalent."
3. "I should drink liquid and eat a healthy diet."
4. "I can have what I want of my favorite beverages."

250. A client has frequent nausea and vomiting following radiation therapy to the abdomen. An appropriate intervention for the nurse to use is:

1. Administer antiemetics with meals.
2. Monitor fluid intake and output.
3. Serve the diet while food is hot.
4. Provide music and conversation during meals.

ANSWERS

1. **(1)** Integrated processes: nursing process — implementation; client need: physiological integrity; basic care and comfort; content area: medical-surgical

RATIONALE

(1) Shrinking the residual limb and shaping it into a conical form help to ensure the comfort and fit of the prosthetic device; wrapping helps to shrink the size. **(2)** The residual limb needs to be decreased, not increased in size. **(3)** Telling a client that it is what the therapist wants is not a sufficient answer. **(4)** It is inappropriate to tell her to call her doctor when the nurse can answer the question.

2. **(4)** Integrated processes: nursing process — implementation; client need: physiological integrity; reduction of risk potential; content area: medical-surgical

RATIONALE

(1) Lying supine with a pillow between the legs does not prevent flexion contraction of the hip. **(2)** A semi-Fowler's position promotes development of flexion contraction. **(3)** Although the limb should be elevated the first 24 hours to reduce swelling and edema around the incision site, placing a pillow under the knees not only promotes venous stasis but also contributes to flexion contraction. **(4)** Lying prone stretches the flexor muscles and prevents flexion contraction of the hip.

3. **(2)** Integrated processes: nursing process — implementation; client need: physiological integrity; physiological adaptation; content area: medical-surgical

RATIONALE

(1) Although the leg has been severed, the nerve tracts sending messages to the brain are still functioning. **(2)** This response explains phantom limb sensation, which is pain in the amputated limb. It is a real sensation caused by nerve tracts that register pain still sending their messages to the brain. **(3)** Most people are able to get over the loss of a body part without severe emotional problems necessitating the help of a psychiatrist. **(4)** This response demonstrates the nurse's unfamiliarity with the phantom limb phenomenon.

4. **(2)** Integrated processes: nursing process — planning; client need: health promotion and maintenance; prevention and early detection of disease; content area: medical-surgical

RATIONALE

(1) Redness can be a sign of infection, and abrasions are susceptible to the development of infection. **(2)** Alcohol dries and cracks the skin, and lotion softens the skin too much; therefore, both create a risk for safe prosthesis use. No ointments, antiseptics, or lotions should be used unless ordered by the physician. **(3)** The stump sock helps to prevent skin breakdown; Ace bandages are used the first 24–48 hours to prevent swelling and edema. **(4)** The stump should be cleaned with a mild soap and a soft cloth.

5. **(4)** Integrated processes: nursing process — data collection; client need: physiological integrity; physiological adaptation; content area: medical-surgical

RATIONALE

(1) This response is the definition of hemiparesis, not hemiplegia. **(2)** Paraplegia is the paralysis of the lower extremities. **(3)**

Quadriplegia is total body paralysis. **(4)** Hemiplegia is the paralysis of one side of the body.

6. **(3)** Integrated processes: nursing process — planning; client need: safe, effective care environment; safety and infection control; content area: medical-surgical.

RATIONALE

(1) Exercises to decrease facial rigidity would not help the dysphagia problem. **(2)** Dysarthria, not dysphagia, is the lack of coordination in speech. **(3)** Dysphagia is the inability to swallow or difficulty in swallowing; therefore, instituting special feeding precautions would need to be included in the plan of care. **(4)** Increasing the light in the environment would have absolutely no influence on the dysphagia problem.

7. **(2)** Integrated processes: nursing process — data collection; client need: physiological integrity; physiological adaptation; content area: medical-surgical

RATIONALE

(1) Ataxia is unsteady gait. **(2)** Aphasia is the inability to express oneself through speech and language. **(3)** Dysphagia is difficulty swallowing. **(4)** Agnosia is difficulty smelling.

8. **(2)** Integrated processes: nursing process — data collection; client need: physiological integrity; reduction of risk potential; content area: medical-surgical.

RATIONALE

(1) This response represents a miscalculation of the percent burned. **(2)** The Rule of Nines is a quick method to calculate the percentage of BSA burned. The entire posterior chest and buttocks represent 18%. The total body is divided into nine sections of multiples of nine. The head and neck equals 9%, each arm 9%, each leg 18%, anterior chest 18%, posterior chest including buttocks 18%, perineum 1%. **(3)** This represents a miscalculation of the percent burned. **(4)** This represents a miscalculation of the percent burned.

9. **(1)** Integrated processes: nursing process — data collection; client need: physiological integrity; reduction of risk potential; content area: medical-surgical.

RATIONALE

(1) The disequilibrium syndrome is caused by rapid fluid shifts occurring as the result of hemodialysis, especially during one of the first treatments. When solutes such as urea and sodium are removed from the blood faster than from the CSF, seizures are most likely to occur. Other associated symptoms are nausea and vomiting, headache, restlessness, and confusion. **(2)** Hypertension is not commonly associated with the syndrome. **(3)** Chest pain is not associated with the syndrome; but it can occur with cardiac clients if the speed of blood flow is high. **(4)** Shortness of breath is not associated with the syndrome. If present, it usually represents a symptom of fluid overload.

10. **(3)** Integrated processes: nursing process — planning; client need: health promotion and maintenance; prevention and early detection of disease; content area: medical-surgical.

RATIONALE

(1) A hearty appetite is no reason to eat high-fat foods. **(2)** The diet to prevent coronary artery disease (CAD) is lifelong. Clients and spouses should be encouraged to eat foods low in fat, cholesterol, and sodium. (3) The client and his wife need diet instruction. A diet high in fat and cholesterol will further contribute to the CAD process. (4) Some hospitals allow foods to be brought in, but oftentimes a doctor's order is needed.

11. (3) Integrated processes: nursing process — evaluation, client need: health promotion and maintenance; prevention and early detection of disease; content area: medical-surgical.
RATIONALE
(1) Taking medications as prescribed is a desired response. (2) This is the recommended post-MI diet. (3) Although exercise is recommended after MI, it is usually done in a cardiac rehabilitation program where the client is monitored. Exercise is gradually increased over several weeks. (4) Consuming a small glass of wine with the evening meal complies with the current literature.

12. (1) Integrated processes: nursing process — implementation; client need: psychosocial integrity; coping and adaptation; content area: medical-surgical.
RATIONALE
(1) Emotional lability (inappropriate laughing and crying) is an emotional change that is common after a stroke and may or may not be appropriate to the situation. (2) Ignoring a client would not be a correct action; nor should the nurse assume he is playing games. (3) This is a nonsense answer. People do not typically cry when something is funny or laugh when it is not. (4) The emotional lability after a stroke does not typically warrant a psychiatric consultation.

13. (1) Integrated processes: nursing process — data collection; client need: physiological integrity; physiological adaptation; content area: medical-surgical
RATIONALE
(1) Cranial is not a division of the spinal canal. (2) The four divisions of the spinal column are cervical (neck), thoracic (upper back), lumbar (lower back), and sacrum and coccyx (tailbone). (3) Trochanter and ischial are not divisions of the spinal canal; they refer to parts of a bone. (4) Femur and ulnar are not divisions of the spinal canal; they refer to bones.

14. (3) Integrated processes: nursing process — data collection; client need: physiological integrity; physiological adaptation; content area: medical-surgical.
RATIONALE
(1) The client would have movement of the upper extremities. An injury above C5 would indicate loss of control of the arms. (2) The client with a T11 injury is paraplegic and loses all function below this level. (3) Movement in the upper extremities would remain intact. (4) Respiratory control would remain intact.

15. (3) Integrated processes: nursing process — planning; client need: physiological integrity; pharmacological therapies; content area: medical-surgical.
RATIONALE
(1) Peak action of NPH insulin would not occur within 2 hours (9 AM). (2) Peak action of NPH insulin would not occur within 5 hours (12 noon). (3) NPH is an intermediate-acting insulin. The peak action takes place 8–12 hours after administration. If NPH was given at 7 AM, the peak action would occur between 3 PM and 7 PM. (4) Peak action of NPH insulin would not take this long to occur (11 PM).

16. (4) Integrated processes: nursing process — data collection; client need: physiological integrity; reduction of risk potential; content area: medical-surgical.

RATIONALE
(1) The occiput is a posterior structure. (2) The buttocks are located on the posterior surface. (3) The heels are located on the posterior surface. (4) When the client is prone, the anterior structures of the body receive pressure. The toes are the only anterior features among the choices.

17. (3) Integrated processes: nursing process — implementation; client need: physiological integrity; reduction of risk potential; content area: medical-surgical.
RATIONALE
(1) Five seconds is too little time spent suctioning. The result would not be effective. (2) To prevent hypoxemia, time spent suctioning should be no longer than 10–15 seconds, and no more than 80–120 mm Hg suction should be used. (3) Twenty seconds exceeds the recommended time and is more likely to result in hypoxemia. (4) Thirty seconds greatly exceeds the acceptable limits of time spent suctioning.

18. (4) Integrated processes: nursing process — implementation; client need: physiological integrity; physiological adaptation; content area: medical-surgical.
RATIONALE
(1) Although a 12-lead ECG is important to obtain when a client is having chest pain, the question focuses on what should be done before administering nitroglycerin. (2) Based on the information that has been given, there is no reason to lower the head of the bed. (3) Although a client experiencing chest pain should receive supplemental oxygen, the question focuses on what should be done before administering nitroglycerin. (4) Rest reduces the need for oxygen.

19. (1) Integrated processes: nursing process — planning; client need: physiological integrity; basic care and comfort; content area: medical-surgical.
RATIONALE
(1) High-Fowler's position allows gravity to assist in dropping the diaphragm. If the client is allowed to dangle the legs at the bedside, chest expansion would be facilitated even further because posterior chest movement is not inhibited by the bed. (2) The gravitational pull on the diaphragm is not as great in the low-Fowler's position because the head of the bed is elevated to only 30 degrees. (3) Sims' position is a side-lying position and therefore restricts chest movement on the dependent side. (4) The Trendelenburg position is a head-down, feet-up position. As a result, abdominal contents tend to be pushed up on the diaphragm, thus resulting in less chest expansion.

20. (4) Integrated processes: nursing process — data collection; client need: physiological integrity; physiological adaptation; content area: medical-surgical.
RATIONALE
(1) The first sound heard when the cuff is deflating is the systolic pressure. (2) In children, the diastolic pressure is the muffled sound heard when deflating the cuff. (3) One does not listen to the sounds as the cuff inflates. (4) For adults, the diastolic pressure is recorded when the last sound is heard during cuff deflation.

21. (4) Integrated processes: nursing process — implementation; client need: safe, effective care environment; safety and infection control; content area: medical-surgical.
RATIONALE
(1) Wiping from back to front greatly increases the chance of fecal contamination and consequent development of a urinary tract–vaginal infection. (2) Circular motion increases risk of

fecal contamination when movement, especially with the swing from back to front, occurs. (3) Side to side does not indicate whether the swab is progressing from front to back or back to front. (4) Wiping from front to back decreases fecal contamination of the vagina and urinary meatus. Fecal contamination greatly increases the chance of developing an infection.

22. (4) Integrated processes: nursing process — implementation; client need: physiological integrity; pharmacological therapies; content area: medical-surgical.

RATIONALE
(1) Digoxin has a narrow therapeutic margin; therefore, periodic serum levels are drawn. (2) The therapeutic effect of heparin is monitored by drawing periodic partial thromboplastin time (PTT). (3) Serum theophylline levels are often drawn when a client is receiving aminophylline, especially the IV form. (4) For the choices given, only vancomycin requires the periodic drawing of peak-and-trough levels. When a peak-and-trough level is ordered, the trough is drawn immediately before the administration of the scheduled dose. Peak levels are usually drawn 30 minutes after the medication has completely infused.

23. (1) Integrated processes: nursing process — evaluation; client need: safe, effective care environment; safety and infection control; content area: medical-surgical.

RATIONALE
(1) Proper handwashing by health-care workers reduces the risk of nosocomial infections. Ten seconds of vigorous handwashing will remove most transient flora and is the minimum amount of time one should spend washing. (2) Although washing for 30 seconds will remove more flora, it does not represent the minimum time one should spend washing. (3) Forty-five seconds is longer than the minimum acceptable time. (4) Sixty seconds is longer than the minimum acceptable time.

24. (4) Integrated processes: nursing process — data collection; client need: physiological integrity; basic care and comfort; content area: medical-surgical.

RATIONALE
(1) Constipation tends to cause a decrease rather than an increase in appetite. (2) Suprapubic distention is a symptom associated with bladder fullness. (3) Nausea may infrequently be associated with constipation, but vomiting is a rare occurrence. (4) Symptoms of constipation include abdominal firmness, distention, hard-formed stools, fewer stools than normal, headache, and a decrease in appetite.

25. (3) Integrated processes: nursing process — implementation; client need: physiological integrity; pharmacological therapies; content area: medical-surgical.

RATIONALE
(1) Getting up and going to the toilet immediately causes premature, ineffective evacuation of the bowel. (2) Waiting 5–10 minutes results in less effective evacuation of the bowel when compared to waiting 20–30 minutes. (3) Waiting 20–30 minutes gives the suppository time to dissolve and irritate the colon, and the irritation stimulates the bowel evacuation. (4) Being in the prone position may or may not help retention of the suppository.

26. (3) Integrated processes: nursing process — implementation; client need: safe, effective care environment; safety and infection control; content area: medical-surgical.

RATIONALE
(1) The label is obliterated when the fluid is poured facing the sterile field. The bottle is held with the label in the palm of the hand. (2) To avoid splashing the fluid when poured, the bottle is held rather low over the sterile field. (3) Before pouring sterile solution onto a sterile field, 1–2 mL of the fluid is discarded to remove organisms from the lip of the bottle. (4) The cap is in contact with the lip and may harbor organisms.

27. (3) Integrated processes: nursing process — implementation; client need: safe, effective care environment; safety and infection control; content area: medical-surgical.

RATIONALE
(1) Disposable equipment does not cause nosocomial infections. (2) Semiprivate rooms do not cause nosocomial infections. (3) The most common cause of nosocomial infections is infrequent handwashing by health-care workers. (4) Oral antibiotics do not cause nosocomial infections.

28. (3) Integrated processes: nursing process — implementation; client need: safe, effective care environment; safety and infection control; content area: medical-surgical.

RATIONALE
(1) The bandage became contaminated once it touched the skin. (2) Placing the bandage in the sterile saline would contaminate the sterile saline. (3) To maintain surgical asepsis, remember: sterile touching clean becomes contaminated; sterile touching contaminated becomes contaminated. (4) Once a sterile item is contaminated, the only option is to discard it and prepare a fresh one. Using the contaminated bandage would contaminate the other sterile bandages.

29. (3) Integrated processes: nursing process — data collection; client need: physiological integrity; physiological adaptation; content area: medical-surgical.

RATIONALE
(1) Pallor can be assessed in the conjunctiva, not the sclera. (2) Assessing pallor in the nailbeds is not as reliable as assessing the mucous membranes. (3) It is more difficult to assess changes such as pallor (paleness indicating decreased amounts of oxygen-carrying Hgb) in clients with dark skin tones. Pallor is most easily perceived in the buccal mucous membranes of the mouth. (4) Assessing pallor of the lips is not as reliable as assessing the mucous membranes.

30. (4) Integrated processes: nursing process — implementation; client need: safe, effective care environment; coordinated care; content area: medical-surgical.

RATIONALE
(1) Black, permanent ink is used, not erasable ink or pencil. (2) Inking over an entry may appear to be an attempt to hide information. (3) Writing "error" is no longer advised because it can be interpreted to mean an error or mistake was made in the client's care. (4) The acceptable method of correcting an erroneous entry is to draw one straight line through the erroneous entry and initial it. A nurse can be charged with fraud for otherwise altering a client's record.

31. (2) Integrated processes: nursing process — evaluation; client need: safe, effective care environment; safety and infection control; content area: medical-surgical.

RATIONALE
(1) Keeping one point of support does not provide enough stability to prevent the client from falling. (2) Two points of support are on the floor at all times. The cane is kept on the stronger (right side). First the cane is moved forward, keeping body weight on both legs. Second, the weaker left leg is moved forward to the cane (body weight evenly divided between the stronger leg and the cane). Third, the stronger right leg is advanced past the cane (weaker leg and body weight are supported by the cane and weaker leg). (3) The client should stand upright, not leaning to the side. The cane should be in the right

hand if the left leg is weak. (4) The top of the cane should be at the level of the greater trochanter of the client's femur.

32. **(4)** Integrated processes: nursing process — data collection; client need: health promotion and maintenance; prevention and early detection of disease; content area: medical-surgical.
RATIONALE
(1) The client's arm should be positioned at the level of the heart. If the arm is above the heart level, the measurement results in a falsely low reading. If the arm is positioned below the heart level, the measurement results in a falsely high reading. (2) The cuff is traditionally positioned 1 inch above the brachial, not the radial, artery. If the BP is obtained at the radial site, the cuff is placed 1 inch above the artery. (3) The client's arm should be extended with the palm up. (4) To ensure an accurate BP measurement, proper pressure is applied to the brachial artery by inflating the bladder of the cuff directly over the artery.

33. **(3)** Integrated processes: nursing process — data collection; client need: health promotion and maintenance; prevention and early detection of disease; content area: medical-surgical.
RATIONALE
(1) Although in some individuals the pulsatile force of the heart can be seen, it is not easily visible. (2) Although the apical pulse can be palpated (felt), especially in thin people, it is not as accurate as the amplified sound heard with the stethoscope. (3) The stethoscope amplifies the sound of the heart (apical pulse) when placed over the precordium. (4) Percussion is performed by tapping to produce sounds in underlying organs and tissues. The apical pulse cannot be obtained with this method.

34. **(1)** Integrated processes: nursing process — implementation; client need: safe, effective care environment; safety and infection control; content area: medical-surgical.
RATIONALE
(1) Oxygen is a highly combustible gas. Oxygen can easily cause a fire to ignite if it contacts a spark. (2) Oxygen does not spontaneously burn or cause an explosion. (3) Oxygen use in the home does not represent a health risk to others who may visit. (4) The statement that smoking causes lung cancer is true, but it is not the correct rationale in this specific example.

35. **(4)** Integrated processes: nursing process — planning; client need: physiological integrity; basic care and comfort; content area: medical-surgical.
RATIONALE
(1) The nurse should use warm water only if it is the client's preference. (2) Using tissues may be a preference for some people. (3) The nurse should use soap if it is the client's preference. (4) Whenever possible, the client should be asked about personal preferences of skin care and hygiene products. The client's preference determines the regimen to be followed when washing the face.

36. **(1)** Integrated processes: nursing process — implementation; client need: physiological integrity; basic care and comfort; content area: medical-surgical.
RATIONALE
(1) Cramping is temporarily relieved by lowering the container and/or clamping the tubing to temporarily stop the flow of enema solution. Once cramping passes, the enema is continued until the entire amount of fluid is administered. (2) Mouth breathing may help to relax the client, but it does not relieve cramping. (3) Raising the height of the enema container would increase the rate of flow and increase the degree of cramping.

(4) It is not appropriate to clamp and withdraw the tube; cramping is very commonly experienced. The nurse simply stops the flow until the cramping subsides and then resumes the enema.

37. **(4)** Integrated processes: nursing process — implementation; client need: health promotion and maintenance; prevention and early detection of disease; content area: medical-surgical.
RATIONALE
(1) Waiting only 10 seconds increases venous congestion and may make the reading erroneous. (2) Waiting only 30 seconds tends to increase venous congestion in the arm and may make the reading erroneous. (3) The American Heart Association (AHA) recommends waiting 2 minutes, not 1 minute, before repeating the pressure. (4) The AHA recommends waiting 2 minutes before repeating a BP reading in the same arm. This decreases venous congestion.

38. **(2)** Integrated processes: nursing process — implementation; client need: physiological integrity; reduction of risk potential; content area: medical-surgical
RATIONALE
(1) The value is not low; it is within normal limits. (2) A normal serum potassium level is 3.8–5.0 mEq/L; therefore, a potassium level of 4.3 is within the normal limits. Unless ordered to notify the physician of a laboratory value, the nurse would note the potassium result in her notes and inform the physician when he makes rounds. (3) The value is not high; it is within normal limits. (4) It is not necessary to offer potassium-rich foods because the potassium value is well within the normal limits.

39. **(3)** Integrated processes: nursing process — data collection; client need: health promotion and maintenance; prevention and early detection of disease; content area: medical-surgical.
RATIONALE
(1) Auscultation uses the sense of hearing to assess clients. The stethoscope is used with this technique. (2) Percussion uses a striking motion to elicit sounds and thus assess underlying structures. (3) Palpation uses the sense of touch to perform physical assessments. The nurse when feeling the lower abdomen is using the palpation technique. (4) Inspection uses the sense of sight to assess clients.

40. **(4)** Integrated processes: nursing process — implementation; client need: health promotion and maintenance; prevention and early detection of disease; content area: medical-surgical.
RATIONALE
(1) The urinometer is considered contaminated. The urinometer rapidly grows bacteria as urine collects and therefore should not be used as a site for collecting a urine specimen for culture. (2) The drainage bag, like the urinometer, is considered contaminated. Bacteria grow rapidly as urine collects in the bag. (3) Disconnecting the catheter disrupts the closed sterile system and allows introduction of additional bacteria into the system. (4) The correct procedure for collecting a sterile urine specimen is to use a sterile needle and syringe and use the latex sampling port on the tubing.

41. **(3)** Integrated processes: nursing process — implementation; client need: physiological integrity; pharmacological therapies; content area: medical-surgical.
RATIONALE
(1) The enteric coating does not dissolve in the mouth. (2) This is a nonsense answer. Enteric coatings are placed on pills and do not apply to liquids. (3) The enteric coating on an oral medication consists of materials that do not dissolve in the mouth or the stomach. The coating dissolves in the intestine, where the medication is absorbed. (4) The enteric coating

is destroyed when it is chewed. The medication is then absorbed from the stomach and not from the intestine as designed.

42. **(1)** Integrated processes: nursing process — planning; client need: physiological integrity; pharmacological therapies; content area: medical-surgical.

    RATIONALE

    (1) By displacing the tissue laterally using the Z-track method, the needle track is sealed as the needle is removed. The medication cannot escape from the deep muscle, and irritation to sensitive tissues is avoided. **(2)** The Z-track method does not affect the speed of absorption of the medication into the body. **(3)** The Z-track method does not eliminate discomfort caused by the needle. **(4)** The Z-track method does not affect absorption rate from the muscle.

43. **(2)** Integrated processes: nursing process — implementation; client need: physiological integrity; pharmacological therapies; content area: medical-surgical.

    RATIONALE

    (1) Topical absorption is usually the slowest. **(2)** A medication administered IV begins to act immediately as it directly enters the bloodstream. **(3)** IM absorption is slower than IV, but usually faster than oral. **(4)** Oral absorption is slower than IM, but usually faster than topical.

44. **(2)** Integrated processes: nursing process — data collection; client need: physiological integrity; physiological adaptation; content area: medical-surgical.

    RATIONALE

    (1) Metabolic acidosis is caused by an excessive amount of acid or not enough base in the body. The GI tract is predominantly "base." When excessive base is lost (diarrhea), metabolic acidosis usually results. **(2)** The Salem sump tube drains stomach contents that are acidic because of the hydrochloric acid. The loss of stomach acid sets up a situation in which the body then has too much base for the amount of acid present. This situation can also occur when excessive vomiting occurs. This is a metabolic problem; thus, metabolic alkalosis occurs. **(3)** The primary cause of respiratory acidosis is a respiratory problem. When too much acid (carbon dioxide) accumulates, as with hypoventilation, respiratory acidosis occurs. **(4)** The primary cause of respiratory alkalosis is also a respiratory problem. The problem now is not enough acid (carbon dioxide). This occurs in hyperventilation states.

45. **(4)** Integrated processes: nursing process — evaluation; client need: health promotion and maintenance; prevention and early detection of disease; content area: medical-surgical.

    RATIONALE

    (1) An enlarged base of support maintains better body balance. **(2)** By moving close to the object to be lifted, one increases body balance. **(3)** The center of gravity should be low, not high. **(4)** The head, neck, and back should be maintained in proper alignment, along with a low center of gravity and a wide base of support. The muscle groups can then work in a synchronized manner, and risk of injury to the lumbar spine and muscles is reduced.

46. **(4)** Integrated processes: nursing process — evaluation; client need: safe, effective care environment; coordinated care; content area: medical-surgical.

    RATIONALE

    (1) Evaluation is not final; it is ongoing and continuous. **(2)** Evaluation is always related to client goals of care. **(3)** Data collection is considered the first phase. **(4)** Evaluation is a continuous and ongoing process that interacts with other phases of the nursing process. Evaluation indicates effectiveness of the care plan through assessment of the client's response.

47. **(4)** Integrated processes: nursing process — implementation; client need: physiological integrity; basic care and comfort; content area: medical-surgical

    RATIONALE

    (1) Unconscious clients are not able to chew food; therefore, food particles would not get trapped between teeth, necessitating the need to floss. Putting food in the mouth of an unconscious person would greatly increase the risk of aspiration. **(2)** 30 mL of fluid squirted into the mouth is a large volume and could easily cause aspiration. **(3)** Scraping secretions with a tongue blade is not recommended. Not only is it ineffective, but it could cause mucosal trauma. **(4)** A padded tongue blade keeps the mouth open and teeth separated during oral care without traumatizing the oral cavity. The teeth are cleaned with a sponge, toothbrush, or gauze-wrapped tongue blade to gently stimulate the gums and mucosa. To prevent aspiration, the sponge or gauze is moistened (not soaked).

48. **(3)** Integrated processes: nursing process — data collection; client need: physiological integrity; reduction of risk potential; content area: medical-surgical.

    RATIONALE

    (1) Stroke is not the most prevalent form of cardiovascular disease. **(2)** CAD is not the most prevalent form of cardiovascular disease. **(3)** The AHA states the most prevalent form of cardiovascular disease is hypertension, followed in descending order by CAD, rheumatic heart disease, and stroke. **(4)** Rheumatic heart disease is not the most prevalent form of cardiovascular disease.

49. **(1)** Integrated processes: nursing process — data collection; client need: physiological integrity; physiological adaptation; content area: medical-surgical.

    RATIONALE

    (1) Shortness of breath is an expected symptom with CHF. The heart is an ineffective pump and less blood is ejected with each beat. The extra volume of blood left in the heart exerts a pressure. As the pressure increases, it is exerted backward from the left ventricle to the left atrium and finally to the lungs. The alveoli start to fill with fluid as the capillary pressure increases, leading to shortness of breath. **(2)** There is a decrease in tissue turgor with hypovolemic, not hypervolemic, states. **(3)** Neck veins become distended as the pressure on the left side of the heart is exerted backward to the right heart. More blood (volume) stays in the peripheral circulation, eventually leading to systemic edema. **(4)** Right, not left, upper quadrant abdominal tenderness develops as the liver becomes engorged with extra circulation volume from the right side of the heart.

50. **(1)** Integrated processes: nursing process — implementation; client need: physiological integrity; basic care and comfort; content area: medical-surgical.

    RATIONALE

    (1) Fluid lost or gained would be reflected as a loss or gain in weight. One liter equals 1 kg (2.2 lb). A rapid rise in weight would indicate that the CHF is getting worse. **(2)** Fluids are usually limited or restricted (not encouraged) because of the hypervolemia. **(3)** To help alleviate the shortness of breath, most clients are more comfortable in an upright position (head of bed elevated >30–45 degrees). **(4)** Sodium in the diet should be limited, not enriched. Sodium fosters the retention of fluid, thus making the volume overload problem worse.

51. **(2)** Integrated processes: nursing process — implementation; client need: physiological integrity; pharmacological therapies; content area: medical-surgical.
RATIONALE
(1) This dose is well below the usual adult daily dose. **(2)** The usual dose of digoxin for adults is 0.25 mg every day. **(3)** This dose well exceeds the usual dose. **(4)** This dose well exceeds the usual dose and would probably result in death.

52. **(3)** Integrated processes: nursing process — implementation; client need: physiological integrity; pharmacological therapies; content area: medical-surgical.
RATIONALE
(1) Ringing in the ears is not a typical symptom of digoxin toxicity. **(2)** Fluid retention is not a typical sign of digoxin toxicity. **(3)** Digoxin has a very narrow therapeutic margin, and toxic effects are frequently seen. Anorexia, nausea, and vomiting are often the first signs of developing toxicity. **(4)** Hair loss is not a typical symptom of digoxin toxicity.

53. **(4)** Integrated processes: nursing process — data collection; client need: physiological integrity; physiological adaptation; content area: medical-surgical.
RATIONALE
(1) A positive, not negative, Homans' sign is a symptom of thrombophlebitis. **(2)** Thrombophlebitis involves the venous system. Because the arterial flow is not impaired, the pedal pulses would not be affected. **(3)** Cool temperature of the extremity and a mottled appearance indicate impaired arterial flow. Arterial circulation is not the problem. **(4)** Calf pain on dorsiflexion of the foot (positive Homans' sign) is a symptom of thrombophlebitis. Other common symptoms include stiffness and redness over the inflamed site.

54. **(1)** Integrated processes: nursing process — implementation; client need: physiological integrity; reduction of risk potential; content area: medical-surgical.
RATIONALE
(1) Efforts should be made to ensure that clients are adequately hydrated. Dehydration and/or fluid volume deficit increase the viscosity of the blood. The increased viscosity is a causative factor in the development of thrombophlebitis. **(2)** Massaging the affected leg is never done because this action can dislodge a thrombus and cause an embolus. The nurse should be alert for the signs and symptoms of a pulmonary embolus. **(3)** The leg should be positioned above, not below, the level of the heart to aid venous return. **(4)** Antibiotics are not usually indicated in thrombophlebitis.

55. **(3)** Integrated processes: nursing process — data collection; client need: physiological integrity; pharmacological therapies; content area: medical-surgical.
RATIONALE
(1) Heparin cannot dissolve existing clots. **(2)** Heparin has no vasoactive properties; therefore, it cannot dilate vessels. **(3)** Heparin prevents additional clots from forming. **(4)** Heparin has no vasoactive properties; therefore, it cannot constrict vessels.

56. **(3)** Integrated processes: nursing process — implementation; client need: physiological integrity; pharmacological therapies; content area: medical-surgical.
RATIONALE
(1) This answer indicates a miscalculation. **(2)** This answer indicates a miscalculation. **(3)** 25,000 : 250 : : x : 10; 250x = 25,000; x = 1000 units/10 mL. **(4)** This answer indicates a miscalculation.

57. **(1)** Integrated processes: nursing process — implementation; client need: physiological integrity; pharmacological therapies; content area: medical-surgical.
RATIONALE
(1) Green leafy vegetables and other foods high in vitamin K (asparagus, broccoli, cabbage, brussels sprouts) should be limited. Vitamin K counteracts the therapeutic effects of warfarin. **(2)** Aspirin inhibits platelet aggregation by decreasing the synthesis of substances that mediate platelet aggregation. Aspirin can thus cause bleeding and is contraindicated in connection with other anticoagulant medications. **(3)** PTT values monitor the therapeutic effects of heparin. PT monitors the effects of warfarin. **(4)** Cuts are more likely to occur when shaving with a straight-edge razor and should be discouraged.

58. **(3)** Integrated processes: nursing process — data collection; client need: physiological integrity; physiological adaptation; content area: medical-surgical.
RATIONALE
(1) The skin elasticity over the dorsal hand is lost early in the aging process and therefore is not a reliable indicator of turgor in the elderly client. **(2)** The skin elasticity of the forearm is lost during the aging process and is not a reliable indicator of turgor in the elderly client. **(3)** The elasticity of the skin decreases as one ages. The skin over the sternum retains elasticity longer than the skin on other areas of the body. **(4)** The skin is normally very taut over the ankle, making it difficult to pinch and painful for the client of any age.

59. **(1)** Integrated processes: nursing process — implementation; client need: physiological integrity; pharmacological therapies; content area: medical-surgical.
RATIONALE
(1) A person with no history of heart disease should seek emergency care if chest pain persists longer than 2 minutes. **(2)** This is the recommended procedure for people with a history of CAD who have been prescribed nitroglycerin. **(3)** A person with undiagnosed heart disease should not be taking nitroglycerin that has been prescribed for someone else. **(4)** It would be absolutely wrong to wait until the chest pain goes away before seeking care.

60. **(4)** Integrated processes: nursing process — data collection; client need: physiological integrity; reduction of risk potential; content area: medical-surgical.
RATIONALE
(1) CABG surgery is not a cure. This disease in the native vessels continues to progress. The disease can also occur in the bypass graft vessels. **(2)** Coronary artery stent is not a cure. It is a mechanical device to keep the coronary artery patent at the blockage site. **(3)** Angioplasty is not a cure. The balloon dilation at the blockage site reduces the severity of the lesion. **(4)** CAD is a lifelong process that currently has no cure. Risk factor modification will help to slow the disease process.

61. **(3)** Integrated processes: nursing process — data collection; client need: health promotion and maintenance; prevention and early detection of disease; content area: medical-surgical.
RATIONALE
(1) Obesity is a modifiable risk factor, but is not considered a major risk factor. **(2)** Family history, gender, sex, and age are the nonmodifiable risk factors. **(3)** The three major modifiable risk factors in the development of CAD are hypertension, hypercholesteremia, and cigarette smoking. **(4)** Diabetes is a contributing factor in the development of CAD. Diabetes can be controlled, but it is not considered one of the major modifiable risk factors.

62. **(4)** Integrated processes: nursing process — data collection; client need: physiological integrity; physiological adaptation; content area: medical-surgical.

RATIONALE

(1) The ankles are one of the first places for edema to accumulate when a client is predominantly in the upright position. **(2)** In the upright position, edema first accumulates in the ankles. As the condition advances, edema starts accumulating in the legs (distal to proximal). **(3)** The hands become edematous as the edema accumulates, but the edema first appears in the sacrum of the bedridden client. **(4)** The sacrum is the most dependent area of the body for the client confined to bed rest. Edema accumulates in a dependent area first.

63. **(4)** Integrated processes: nursing process — implementation; client need: health promotion and maintenance; prevention and early detection of disease; content area: medical-surgical.

RATIONALE

(1) Broiled chicken does contain cholesterol, but less than red meat. **(2)** Fish also contains cholesterol, but in much smaller amounts than red meat. **(3)** Polyunsaturated oils are recommended for use, but heating them changes their polyunsaturated states. Fried foods are not recommended. **(4)** Egg yolks contain cholesterol; egg whites do not.

64. **(1)** Integrated processes: nursing process — data collection; client need: physiological integrity; physiological adaptation; content area: medical-surgical.

RATIONALE

(1) The discomfort of angina most commonly radiates to the left arm, along with feelings of arm numbness and heaviness. Radiation to both arms, the jaw, and the neck does occur but less frequently than to the left arm. **(2)** Although radiated pain may be in both arms, it is most often in the left arm. **(3)** Although radiated pain may be in the neck, it is usually unilateral. **(4)** Although radiated pain may be in the jaw, it is most often in the left arm.

65. **(3)** Integrated processes: nursing process — data collection; client need: physiological integrity; reduction of risk potential; content area: medical-surgical.

RATIONALE

(1) Although certain beats in the peripheral pulse cannot be palpated (felt) when a pulse deficit is present, it is not the absence of a pulse. **(2)** The difference in systolic and diastolic pressures is known as the pulse pressure. **(3)** The difference in the apical and radial heart rates is known as a pulse deficit. The heartbeat can be auscultated apically but cannot be felt in the radial (peripheral) pulse. **(4)** Because it is the peripheral pulse that has a deficit, the peripheral pulse rate is subtracted from the apical rate.

66. Integrated processes: nursing process — implementation; client need: physiological integrity; reduction of risk potential; content area: medical-surgical.

RATIONALE

(1) Bed rest is maintained for 4–6 hours after this procedure because the clot that has sealed the insertion site may burst with activity. **(2)** Immediately after the procedure, vital signs are assessed every 15 minutes. Assessing distal circulation (pedal pulses), especially in the cannulated leg, is performed as frequently as assessment of vital signs. **(3)** The head of the bed is usually ordered to be no higher than 30 degrees (low-Fowler's position). **(4)** Fluids are encouraged to aid in eliminating the dye used in the procedure.

67. **(4)** Integrated processes: nursing process — data collection; client need: physiological integrity; physiological adaptation; content area: medical-surgical.

RATIONALE

(1) The radial pulse lies just medial to the radius at the wrist. **(2)** The popliteal pulse lies in the posterior fossa behind the knee. **(3)** The dorsalis pedis runs along the anterior surface of the foot. **(4)** The posterior tibial pulse is located behind the medial malleolus (ankle bone).

68. **(1)** Integrated processes: nursing process — evaluation; client need: health promotion and maintenance; prevention and early detection of disease; content area: medical-surgical.

RATIONALE

(1) Of the choices given, bicycling represents the only isotonic (dynamic) exercise, which is the form recommended for hypertensive clients. There are two types of exercise: isotonic and isometric. Isotonic exercise involves change in the muscle length, shortening of muscle fibers, and moving joints and bones. Isometric exercise involves development of tension within the muscle length, which increases BP during the process. **(2)** Water skiing represents a form of isometric exercise. **(3)** Weight lifting represents a form of isometric exercise. **(4)** Calisthenics represents a form of isometric exercise.

69. **(2)** Integrated processes: nursing process — implementation; client need: health promotion and maintenance; prevention and early detection of disease; content area: medical-surgical.

RATIONALE

(1) Catsup is high in sodium content. **(2)** Lemon juice represents the only choice that has no sodium; all of the other choices are high in sodium content. **(3)** Garlic salt is very high in sodium content. **(4)** Soy sauce is very high in sodium content.

70. **(1)** Integrated processes: nursing process — implementation; client need: physiological integrity; physiological adaptation; content area: medical-surgical.

RATIONALE

(1) Although nitroglycerin is indicated for clients with chest pain, before it is administered, the BP should be assessed. If the pressure is low, nitroglycerin is contraindicated. **(2)** Nitroglycerin has vasodilating properties and will lower the BP. Before administering nitroglycerin, the BP should be taken. If the client is hypotensive, nitroglycerin should not be given because it lowers the pressure even further. **(3)** Raising the head of the bed may ease the effort of breathing if shortness of breath and dyspnea are present, but the question does not give this information. **(4)** Before calling the physician, additional assessment data must be obtained, such as vital signs.

71. **(1)** Integrated processes: nursing process — data collection; client need: physiological integrity; physiological adaptation; content area: medical-surgical.

RATIONALE

(1) Intake greater than output would reflect an increase in weight. One liter of fluid is equal to 1 kg (2.2 lb) in weight. Intake exceeds output by 2000 mL (2 kg). The nurse would anticipate the weight to increase by 2 kg or 4.4 lb. **(2)** The weight would be increased by approximately 4.5 lb, not 2. **(3)** The weight would increase, not decrease, because more fluid was taken in. **(4)** The weight would not remain the same because there is a difference in the 24-hour I&O.

72. **(2)** Integrated processes: nursing process — implementation; client need: physiological integrity; reduction of risk potential; content area: medical-surgical.

RATIONALE

(1) Peanuts are high in magnesium content. Depending on the preparation, peanuts may also be high in sodium. **(2)** The following foods are rich in potassium: bananas, cantaloupe, apricots, peaches, dates, raisins, orange juice, tomato juice, avocados, navy beans, potatoes, squash, carrots, and cauliflower.

(3) Broccoli is high in calcium content. (4) Milk is not a potassium-rich food.

73. **(3)** Integrated processes: nursing process — planning; client need: physiological integrity; pharmacological therapies; content area: medical-surgical.

    RATIONALE

    (1) Although potassium is needed, NS is not the needed solution. NS exerts equal pressure on the cell and does not aid in rehydration. **(2)** NS is not the needed solution, as stated in rationale 1. **(3)** Because of fluid loss from vomiting and diarrhea, the client needs a hypotonic solution (0.45 NS). Hypotonic fluids allow fluid to reenter the cell. Potassium should be added because of the loss of potassium-rich fluid through vomiting and diarrhea. **(4)** Hypertonic solutions (3%) pull additional fluid out of the cell, thus making the dehydration worse.

74. **(3)** Integrated processes: nursing process — implementation; client need: physiological integrity; basic care and comfort; content area: medical-surgical.

    RATIONALE

    (1) Bowel training is not done with ileostomies because the contents are liquid and contain digestive enzymes. The client must wear an appliance to collect the fluid. **(2)** Ileostomies are not routinely irrigated; doing so always makes the client incontinent. **(3)** To maintain skin integrity, the nurse would ensure that the skin is clean and dry and then apply a skin barrier and a properly fitting appliance. **(4)** Because the contents of the ileum are liquid, stool softeners are not necessary.

75. **(3)** Integrated processes: nursing process — implementation; client need: psychosocial integrity; coping and adaptation; content area: medical-surgical.

    RATIONALE

    (1) Instituting steadfast rules limiting visitors should not be done routinely. Restricting visitors can be done at intervals if the client seems to be adversely affected. **(2)** Although caring for dying clients can be extremely difficult, consistent nursing assignments are imperative for the development of therapeutic relationships with the terminally ill. **(3)** Once the nurse, terminally ill client, and family establish a therapeutic relationship, the nurse is often the one to advise completion of unfinished business. **(4)** Anger is one of the stages in the dying process. Although difficult for some clients to identify, their outward behavior is often indicative of internal emotions. The nurse assists the client and family to understand these emotions.

76. **(4)** Integrated processes: nursing process — data collection; client need: psychosocial integrity; coping and adaptation; content area: medical-surgical.

    RATIONALE

    (1) There is no evidence of denial in the statement. **(2)** There is no evidence of anger in the statement. **(3)** There is no evidence of depression in the statement. **(4)** Kubler-Ross has identified five stages in the dying process: denial, anger, bargaining, depression, acceptance. By promising to return to church every Sunday, the client is bargaining with God to prolong life.

77. **(1)** Integrated processes: nursing process — planning; client need: physiological integrity; pharmacological therapies; content area: medical-surgical.

    RATIONALE

    (1) Dopamine is a very potent vasopressor and must always be delivered via an electronic device. **(2)** Electronic pumps should not be used to infuse RBCs; damage to the cells can occur, causing hemolysis. **(3)** Vancomycin, although a very potent antibi-

otic, does not have to be infused via an electronic pump. **(4)** Only very strong concentrations of KCl should be administered via a pump. Forty mEq in 1 L is not a strong concentration; therefore, a pump is not mandatory.

78. **(3)** Integrated processes: nursing process — data collection; client need: physiological integrity; physiological adaptation; content area: medical-surgical.

    RATIONALE

    (1) Kussmaul's respiration is a hyperventilation pattern. There is an increase in both rate and depth. **(2)** Biot's breathing is similar to Cheyne-Stokes except the pattern is irregular. **(3)** The observed breathing pattern is known as Cheyne-Stokes. **(4)** Eupnea is normal breathing: regular, quiet, effortless.

79. **(2)** Integrated processes: nursing process — implementation; client need: safe, effective care environment; coordinated care; content area: medical-surgical.

    RATIONALE

    (1) The nurse could be charged with murder or manslaughter because there is no written "no-code" order. **(2)** Although it is always preferable to obtain a no-code order before an emergency situation occurs, in its absence, unless a living will has been signed, the nurse's only legal recourse is to begin CPR and call a code. **(3)** In the absence of a written no-code order, if the client stops breathing but has a pulse, artificial respiration alone is in order. Once the client becomes pulseless or asystole occurs, both breathing and compressions must be performed. **(4)** Consulting with the charge nurse is wasting time. In the absence of a written no-code order, the nurse must begin CPR and call a code.

80. **(1)** Integrated processes: nursing process — implementation; client need: physiological integrity; basic care and comfort; content area: medical-surgical.

    RATIONALE

    (1) Incontinence pads should be placed under the deceased individual's buttocks because bowel and bladder evacuation may continue even after death has occurred because of relaxation of the bowel and bladder muscles. **(2)** The deceased client's head should remain slightly elevated to prevent pooling of blood and interstitial fluid in the head or face or both. **(3)** Dentures should not be removed. If the client dies not wearing dentures, they should be placed in the mouth during postmortem care. It is very difficult to open the mouth after rigor mortis occurs. **(4)** The identification armband should not be removed because positive identification is required before the body can be released to the morgue.

81. **(4)** Integrated processes: nursing process — data collection; client need: physiological integrity; physiological adaptation; content area: medical-surgical.

    RATIONALE

    (1) The neck veins would be distended in pulmonary edema. **(2)** Clients do display anxiety when in pulmonary edema. There are many causes of anxiety; therefore it is not the most characteristic symptom. **(3)** Clients in pulmonary edema often do have peripheral edema, but this is not always the case. **(4)** Pink, frothy sputum is the characteristic finding with pulmonary edema.

82. **(2)** Integrated processes: nursing process — implementation; client need: physiological integrity; pharmacological therapies; content area: medical-surgical.

    RATIONALE

    (1) This answer indicates a miscalculation. **(2)** x gtt/min = 250 mL/90 min × 20 gtt/mL. **(3)** This answer indicates a miscalculation. **(4)** This answer indicates a miscalculation.

83. **(3)** Integrated processes: nursing process — implementation; client need: health promotion and maintenance; prevention and early detection of disease; content area: medical-surgical.

    RATIONALE
    (1) Vaginal bleeding is not normal after menopause. **(2)** The bleeding is abnormal at her age; she needs to see her physician. **(3)** Vaginal bleeding after menopausal onset is highly abnormal and usually indicates the presence of gynecological malignancy. Although the bleeding may become intermittent, continue, or get worse, the most appropriate response would be to recommend that she consult her physician for medical follow-up. **(4)** Notifying her daughter could be done if the client wishes, but doing so does not solve the vaginal bleeding problem. Physician notification is the most appropriate answer.

84. **(3)** Integrated processes: nursing process — implementation; client need: psychosocial integrity; coping and adaptation; content area: medical-surgical.

    RATIONALE
    (1) It is inappropriate to joke and chuckle. Doing so may inhibit expression of his feelings. **(2)** It is inappropriate to tell him not to worry; there is a chance that sexual functioning will be influenced by surgery. **(3)** When the suprapubic or retropubic approach is used in the removal of the prostate gland, erectile function is preserved. However, if a perineal prostatectomy is performed, innervation of the penile shaft can possibly be affected and impotence ensue. **(4)** It is inappropriate to tell him that most men do have sexual functioning problems after surgery; this is not true.

85. **(1)** Integrated processes: nursing process — implementation; client need: physiological integrity; reduction of risk potential; content area: medical-surgical.

    RATIONALE
    (1) Hypercalcemia is a condition in which serum calcium is elevated. By providing increased amounts of fluid, calcium excretion is promoted and the amount of circulating calcium decreased. **(2)** When caring for client with hypercalcemia, ambulation, not bed rest, should be encouraged. During periods of bed rest and immobility, the bone releases calcium into the peripheral circulation. **(3)** Administering calcium supplements would only make the condition worse. **(4)** Antibiotics have no effect on hypercalcemia.

86. **(4)** Integrated processes: nursing process — implementation; client need: physiological integrity; basic care and comfort; content area: medical-surgical.

    RATIONALE
    (1) A banana is a raw fruit and not allowed on the diet. **(2)** Raw vegetables such as carrot sticks are not allowed on the diet. **(3)** Garden salads are made of raw vegetables and are not allowed on the diet. **(4)** Neutropenic clients have a decreased number of circulating WBCs, and therefore have an increased potential for developing an infection. Raw fruits and vegetables are not allowed on a neutropenic diet because they may contain microbial contamination. All fruits and vegetables must be thoroughly cooked before the client eats them. Canned fruits and vegetables are permitted. The safety of dairy products remains controversial.

87. **(2)** Integrated processes: nursing process — data collection; client need: health promotion and maintenance; prevention and early detection of disease; content area: medical-surgical.

    RATIONALE
    (1) Although some clients with malignant disease processes have an elevated CEA level, it is not diagnostic. **(2)** A positive tissue biopsy is the only reliable diagnostic measure. **(3)** A sore that does not heal is an early warning sign of cancer, but is not diagnostic. **(4)** A nagging cough or hoarseness is an early warning sign of cancer, but is not diagnostic.

88. **(2)** Integrated processes: nursing process — implementation; client need: physiological integrity; basic care and comfort; content area: medical-surgical.

    RATIONALE
    (1) Eating spicy food causes further oral discomfort for clients with stomatitis. **(2)** Stomatitis is inflammation of the mucous membranes of the mouth. Although the oral mucosa might be tender, clients with stomatitis should be encouraged to brush their teeth after each meal and before bedtime with a soft toothbrush or toothettes to prevent secondary infections. **(3)** Although commercial mouthwashes may kill the germs commonly found in the oral cavity, they are not recommended because of their alcohol content and irritating nature. **(4)** Orange juice is acidic and will cause further oral discomfort.

89. **(1)** Integrated processes: nursing process — evaluation; client need: physiological integrity; reduction of risk potential; content area: medical-surgical.

    RATIONALE
    (1) Complete return of the solution should occur with the evacuation of soft or formed feces. Soft or formed stool is found in the descending colon. **(2)** Liquid or semisoft stool is found in the ascending and transverse colon. **(3)** Lack of irrigation return could signal irrigant absorption, potentiating hypervolemia. **(4)** Evacuation of irrigant could signal only possible fecal impaction.

90. **(2)** Integrated processes: nursing process — evaluation; client need: physiological integrity; pharmacological therapies; content area: medical-surgical.

    RATIONALE
    (1) This acidosis is caused by hypoventilation (respiratory) and not by metabolic causes. **(2)** A narcotic overdose slows the rate and depth of breathing. This leads to the retention of carbon dioxide (acid). Hypoventilation problems produce respiratory acidosis. **(3)** Hypoventilation produces acidosis, not alkalosis. **(4)** Respiratory alkalosis is produced when too much carbon dioxide is blown off. The problem is retention of carbon dioxide.

91. **(1)** Integrated processes: nursing process — data collection; client need: physiological integrity; physiological adaptation; content area: medical-surgical.

    RATIONALE
    (1) Restlessness, yawning, tachycardia, and hypertension are all early signs of hypoxemia. As the oxygen deprivation continues, dyspnea, confusion, and impaired judgment occur. With the development of severe hypoxemia, tachycardia, hypotension, and bradycardia are seen. **(2)** Hypotension is a sign of severe hypoxemia. **(3)** Bradycardia is a sign of severe hypoxemia. **(4)** Bradycardia and hypotension are signs of severe hypoxemia.

92. **(3)** Integrated processes: nursing process — implementation; client need: safe, effective care environment; safety and infection control; content area: medical-surgical.

    RATIONALE
    (1) Mask, gown, and goggles are not necessary because excessive contamination is not possible in this situation. **(2)** Gowns are necessary when soiling of clothes is likely from splashes of blood and body fluids. This is not likely when giving an IM injection. **(3)** A small amount of blood may ooze from the needle puncture site after an IM injection. Therefore, the nurse should wear gloves for self-protection when massaging, holding pressure, and wiping the site. **(4)** Goggles are necessary in procedures likely to generate droplets of blood and body fluids.

93. **(4)** Integrated processes: nursing process — data collection; client need: physiological integrity; reduction of risk potential; content area: medical-surgical.

RATIONALE

(1) Although instillation of air assists in assessment of tube placement, it does not provide the nurse with a residual volume. Very high residual volumes mean the client is not absorbing and is more likely to aspirate the tube's contents. It is advisable to auscultate for bowel sounds, but no more than 20 cc of air should be used; otherwise, gastric distention is likely to occur. **(2)** One does not instill fluid first without checking placement with air and the residual volume. If the tube is not in the stomach, aspiration may occur. **(3)** Although an abdominal radiograph will confirm tube placement, it is costly and placement can be checked by other means. **(4)** It is best for the nurse to aspirate stomach contents to ascertain tube placement as well as absorption of the tube feeding. The gastric contents are reinstilled to prevent electrolyte imbalance.

94. **(1)** Integrated processes: nursing process — data collection; client need: physiological integrity; physiological adaptation; content area: medical-surgical.

RATIONALE

(1) Because radiation therapy affects fast-growing cells, the hemopoietic and GI systems would be affected. Because the treatment field incorporates the throat, esophagus, and stomach, the GI symptoms most commonly seen would include nausea and dysphagia. Bone marrow suppression would occur because the treatment field includes the sternum. **(2)** Diarrhea would not be seen because the small bowel is not included in the treatment field. **(3)** Alopecia is observed only in brain irradiation. **(4)** Radiation does not cause constipation.

95. **(4)** Integrated processes: nursing process — implementation; client need: physiological integrity; basic care and comfort; content area: medical-surgical.

RATIONALE

(1) Notify the physician; this is an over-the-counter agent. **(2)** Notify the physician; this is an over-the-counter agent. **(3)** Notify the physician; this is an over-the-counter agent. **(4)** You should never apply an over-the-counter medication to a radiation treatment field. Most of these products contain petroleum derivatives or metallic fragments, which may actually intensify the burning process. Therefore, you should notify the physician and obtain orders for a water-based emollient such as Aquaphor.

96. **(2)** Integrated processes: nursing process — implementation; client need: safe, effective care environment; coordinated care; content area: medical-surgical.

RATIONALE

(1) It would be inappropriate for the nurse to do nothing. An Hgb level of 6.3 is critical; some course of action needs to be taken. The physician needs to be notified promptly. **(2)** Jehovah's Witnesses are opposed to blood transfusions and organ donations. The physician should be informed because the client's refusal may be life threatening. **(3)** It is inappropriate for the nurse to try to convince the client to take blood and go against religious practices. **(4)** It is very inappropriate for the nurse to administer the blood without the client's consent.

97. **(4)** Integrated processes: nursing process — planning; client need: physiological integrity; pharmacological therapies; content area: medical-surgical.

RATIONALE

(1) Because the client is already vomiting, the oral route in this situation would not facilitate maximum absorption of the drug. **(2)** IM medications are not administered because of the potential for bleeding and hematoma formation. **(3)** Rectal supposi-

tories are not administered to thrombocytopenic clients because of the vascularity of the rectal mucosa and the potential for bleeding if the area were injured during the suppository insertion. **(4)** Antiemetics should be administered only IV or by mouth when the client is thrombocytopenic. The nurse would administer the IV push medication.

98. **(2)** Integrated processes: nursing process — implementation; client need: physiological integrity; pharmacological therapies; content area: medical-surgical.

RATIONALE

(1) Blue food coloring only helps to detect aspiration once it has occurred. **(2)** The head of the bed should always be elevated at least 30 degrees when continuous enteral feedings are infusing. The flat or low position facilitates gastric reflux, which increases the risk of aspiration. **(3)** Enteral feedings are often prescribed at rates greater than 50 mL/hr. As long as the gastric residuals are not high, higher infusion rates are acceptable. **(4)** This intervention helps to decrease microbial proliferation in the formula; it does not influence aspiration risk.

99. **(4)** Integrated processes: nursing process — implementation; client need: safe, effective care environment; safety and infection control; content area: medical-surgical.

RATIONALE

(1) The nurse stands on the weaker (right) side, not on the stronger (left) side. **(2)** Holding the client's hand does not give stability to the gait. **(3)** The nurse stands on the client's right (weaker) side, not on the stronger (left) side. **(4)** Hemiparesis is slight paralysis affecting one side of the body. The nurse always stands on the client's affected side and supports the client by holding one arm around the client's waist and the other arm around the client's upper arm, so that the nurse's hand supports the client's axilla. A client with right-sided weakness requires the nurse to stand on the right side.

100. **(3)** Integrated processes: nursing process — implementation; client need: physiological integrity; basic care and comfort; content area: medical-surgical.

RATIONALE

(1) There is no need for the nurse to feed the client. **(2)** There is no need for the family to feed the client. The client is capable and should be encouraged to feed himself or herself. **(3)** A client with recent visual impairment is encouraged and assisted to participate in regular ADLs. The nurse assists the client by preparing the food tray (open containers, cut meat, and so on) and orienting the client to the location of all items on the food tray. **(4)** There is no reason to encourage use of the spoon exclusively.

101. **(4)** Integrated processes: nursing process — data collection; client need: health promotion and maintenance; prevention and early detection of disease; content area: medical-surgical.

RATIONALE

(1) None of the areas is the most important respiratory assessment to make, with the possible exception of pain. **(2)** BP and sweating are important, but not the most important assessments to make. **(3)** Capillary refill is more directly related to perfusion. Trembling is irrelevant. Amount of sputum is important, but not the most important assessment. **(4)** All three of these assessments are the most essential areas to cover during a respiratory assessment; restlessness could indicate a lack of oxygen to the brain.

102. **(3)** Integrated processes: nursing process — data collection; client need: health promotion and maintenance; prevention and early detection of disease; content area: medical-surgical.

RATIONALE

(1) The oxygen would affect a temperature reading taken orally. (2) An axillary temperature is not very accurate. (3) A rectal temperature would give the most accurate reading of body temperature. (4) Feeling the forehead would not give an accurate measure of body temperature.

103. (3) Integrated processes: nursing process — implementation; client need: physiological integrity; physiological adaptation; content area: medical-surgical.

RATIONALE

(1) Pinching the soft tissue applies pressure to stop the bleeding. (2) Warm liquids should be avoided; dilatation of blood vessels could exacerbate the bleeding. (3) Cold constricts blood vessels and helps to stop the bleeding. (4) A physician should be consulted as part of follow-up care unless the cause of the bleeding is obvious.

104. (1) Integrated processes: nursing process — planning; client need: health promotion and maintenance; prevention and early detection of disease; content area: medical-surgical.

RATIONALE

(1) The client should save his voice until his physician tells him to use it. (2) The client will receive tube feedings for a few days after surgery. (3) The bed should be in a Fowler's position to promote an open airway. (4) The client should be taught that he will have to hold his head still following surgery.

105. (2) Integrated processes: nursing process — planning; client need: physiological integrity; physiological adaptation; content area: medical-surgical.

RATIONALE

(1) Reducing anxiety is a desired outcome but should not receive highest priority. (2) An open airway with adequate gas exchange takes the highest priority because it is essential to the life of the client. (3) Talking about feelings is an important outcome, but does not take highest priority. (4) Maintaining fluid balance is important, but is not the most essential outcome to maintain life.

106. (3) Integrated processes: nursing process — planning; client need: physiological integrity; physiological adaptation; content area: medical-surgical.

RATIONALE

(1) The presence of cor pulmonale would be indicated by signs and symptoms of right-sided heart failure. (2) Pulsus paradoxus or distant heart sounds would indicate cardiac tamponade. (3) The data support pneumothorax. (4) The trachea would more likely be deviated with a pneumothorax.

107. (4) Integrated processes: nursing process — data collection; client need: health promotion and maintenance; prevention and early detection of disease; content area: medical-surgical.

RATIONALE

(1) A positive Mantoux test result means only that the client has had the tubercle bacillus in the body at one time; it does not mean that the client is infectious. (2) The tubercle bacillus is gram positive. (3) The lesion could be walled off; unless the organism is in the sputum, the client will not be infectious. (4) Pulmonary tuberculosis is spread by way of airborne droplets of sputum; the organism must be in the sputum before the infection can be spread.

108. (4) Integrated processes: nursing process — evaluation; client need: health promotion and maintenance; prevention and early detection of disease; content area: medical-surgical.

RATIONALE

(1) A client with hypertension should learn how to manage stress. (2) A BP of 140/90 is the upper limit of normal. (3) Stroke and heart attack can result from untreated hypertension. (4) Antihypertensives should not be discontinued because the client feels OK.

109. (4) Integrated processes: nursing process — implementation; client need: physiological integrity; reduction of risk potential; content area: medical-surgical.

RATIONALE

(1) The client may be having an MI; calling the physician will delay treatment. (2) Driving could cause injury to himself and others. (3) Emergency care is needed. (4) A rescue squad is best equipped to give emergency treatment.

110. (1) Integrated processes: nursing process — planning; client need: physiological integrity; physiological adaptation; content area: medical-surgical.

RATIONALE

(1) Decreasing any strain on the heart is the highest priority in restoring the health of the client at this time. (2) Breathing easily is only one component of reducing the workload on the heart. (3) Decreasing edema is only one component of reducing the workload on the heart. (4) Learning about the medications is not the highest priority at this time.

111. (2) Integrated processes: nursing process — data collection; client need: physiological integrity; reduction of risk potential; content area: medical-surgical.

RATIONALE

(1) No mention is made of data indicating either left or right heart failure. (2) The data do not indicate presence of an MI. (3) The signs are classic for shock; the BP can be normal. (4) Signs of cardiac tamponade are absent.

112. (3) Integrated processes: nursing process — data collection; client need: health promotion and maintenance; prevention and early detection of disease; content area: medical-surgical.

RATIONALE

(1) It would be helpful to know the electrolyte report results when talking with the physician. (2) Signs of digoxin toxicity are present; treatment could be delayed. (3) Digoxin toxicity can occur while serum levels of the drug are normal when electrolyte imbalances occur. (4) Administering an antiemetic could mask the symptoms and delay treatment.

113. (4) Integrated processes: nursing process — implementation; client need: physiological integrity; physiological adaptation; content area: medical-surgical.

RATIONALE

(1) Antiembolism stockings should be applied only to the unaffected leg. (2) Aspirin inhibits platelet aggregation and might interfere with heparin therapy. (3) The clot could be dislodged and cause a pulmonary embolus. (4) Bed rest helps to prevent a pulmonary embolus.

114. (2) Integrated processes: nursing process — implementation; client need: psychosocial integrity; coping and adaptation; content area: medical-surgical.

RATIONALE

(1) The question does not state the client's spiritual foundation. (2) She needs most of all to talk about her feelings. (3) She may not be quite ready for a support group. (4) She needs to face the problem when she is ready to face it.

115. **(4)** Integrated processes: nursing process — data collection; client need: physiological integrity; pharmacological therapies; content area: medical-surgical.

RATIONALE

(1) No indication is given that one of the drugs might affect the heart. **(2)** Chemotherapy can be nephrotoxic, but nephrotoxicity is not part of bone marrow depression. **(3)** No data are given to indicate a need to assess for the integrity of bones. **(4)** Platelets could be depressed when bone marrow is depressed; therefore, assessment needs to be made for signs of bleeding.

116. **(2)** Integrated processes: nursing process — evaluation; client need: health promotion and maintenance; prevention and early detection of disease; content area: medical-surgical.

RATIONALE

(1) HIV can be spread by sexual contact. **(2)** The virus is not spread by casual touching, and the client needs to touch others. **(3)** The virus can be spread by way of body fluids. **(4)** A mother can pass the virus to her unborn infant.

117. **(1)** Integrated processes: nursing process — implementation; client need: physiological integrity; reduction of risk potential; content area: medical-surgical.

RATIONALE

(1) The Sengstaken-Blakemore tube is used to control bleeding in a client with esophageal varices. **(2)** A client with cirrhosis of the liver would not need a Sengstaken-Blakemore tube unless esophageal varices were present. **(3)** The Sengstaken-Blakemore tube is not used to treat renal stones. **(4)** This tube is not used to treat hiatal hernia.

118. **(2)** Integrated processes: nursing process — evaluation; client need: health promotion and maintenance; prevention and early detection of disease; content area: medical-surgical.

RATIONALE

(1) Nonsteroidal anti-inflammatory drugs (NSAIDs) have been associated with the occurrence of peptic ulcer disease in several research studies. **(2)** Coffee in moderation has not been shown to be associated with PUD. **(3)** Smoking has been associated with causing PUD. **(4)** Stress has also been associated with the development of PUD.

119. **(3)** Integrated processes: Nursing process — data collection; client need: physiological integrity; reduction of risk potential; content area: medical-surgical.

RATIONALE

(1) No data exist to suggest that hyperkalemia could be a problem. **(2)** No data exist to suggest that an acid-base disorder of respiratory origin might be a problem. **(3)** Loss of gastric acid by suction for several days could lead to metabolic alkalosis. **(4)** No data exist to suggest that acidosis might occur.

120. **(4)** Integrated processes: nursing process — planning; client need: physiological integrity; reduction of risk potential; content area: medical-surgical.

RATIONALE

(1) A rigid abdomen would be present if perforation of the GI tract occurred. **(2)** Absence of bowel sounds would be needed to support a diagnosis of paralytic ileus. **(3)** Data do not give strong support for an obstruction. **(4)** The signs and symptoms are classic for dumping syndrome.

121. **(3)** Integrated processes: nursing process — data collection; client need: physiological integrity; physiological adaptation; content area: medical-surgical.

RATIONALE

(1) Vital signs may be taken routinely, bleeding should not be a problem, and diarrhea would be monitored as it occurs. **(2)** Fluid volume deficit and electrolyte imbalances could occur; they need to be detected early. **(3)** The data do not indicate that these assessments should be made frequently. **(4)** Perfusion could be a reflection of fluid balance, and muscle twitching could indicate electrolyte imbalance, but the variables listed in rationale 2 would be more likely to detect fluid and electrolyte imbalances earlier.

122. **(4)** Integrated processes: nursing process — data collection; client need: physiological integrity; physiological adaptation; content area: medical-surgical.

RATIONALE

(1) The data do not call for more than routine assessment of lung sounds. **(2)** The data do not suggest a need to assess for a pulse deficit. **(3)** The data do not suggest a need to assess for renal stones. **(4)** Assessment for bowel sounds needs to be made frequently because a section of the GI tract was removed.

123. **(4)** Integrated processes: nursing process — implementation; client need: physiological integrity; reduction of risk potential; content area: medical-surgical.

RATIONALE

(1) The lung would collapse because the pleural cavity would be exposed to atmospheric pressure. **(2)** The tubing should not be clamped because pressure could build up in the pleural cavity or a spontaneous, closed pneumothorax could occur. **(3)** Excess suction could cause a closed pneumothorax. **(4)** The Pleur-evac should be attached to the side of the wheelchair to avoid damage to the closed chest drainage system.

124. **(4)** Integrated processes: nursing process — implementation; client need: physiological integrity; physiological adaptation; content area: medical-surgical.

RATIONALE

(1) The sounds are probably caused by peristalsis and the obstruction; excess flatus would be misleading. **(2)** Acini are small saclike structures usually found at the end of a gland. **(3)** Hypoactive would be misleading. **(4)** The loud, rumbling sounds are called borborygmi.

125. **(3)** Integrated processes: nursing process — planning; client need: physiological integrity; reduction of risk potential; content area: medical-surgical.

RATIONALE

(1) The client does need antiembolism stockings after hernia repair. **(2)** Signs of hemorrhage should be assessed the same as for other types of general surgery. **(3)** The client should not cough because the increase in pressure in the abdominal cavity could injure the repair. **(4)** Precautions against infection are just as important for the client with a hernia repair.

126. **(1)** Integrated processes: nursing process — implementation; client need: physiological integrity; reduction of risk potential; content area: medical-surgical.

RATIONALE

(1) A cleansing enema is needed to clean all of the barium out of the GI tract; it can obstruct the appendix. **(2)** Barium does not usually cause renal damage. **(3)** Activity helps to eliminate the barium. **(4)** Barium does not usually cause an allergic reaction.

127. **(2)** Integrated processes: nursing process — data collection; client need: physiological integrity; prevention and early detection of disease; content area: medical-surgical.

     RATIONALE

     (1) If the client has appendicitis, a laxative could cause the appendix to rupture. **(2)** Checking McBurney's point for rebound tenderness would be appropriate; it would provide more data about possible appendicitis. **(3)** A heating pad could cause an inflamed appendix to rupture. **(4)** More data are needed before calling a physician.

128. **(4)** Integrated processes: nursing process — implementation; client need: physiological integrity; reduction of risk potential; content area: medical-surgical.

     RATIONALE

     (1) Bed rest should be maintained. **(2)** A semi-Fowler's position is needed to facilitate respiratory movement. **(3)** The data do not support a need to check the mouth for ulcerations. **(4)** Food in the GI tract would make the obstruction worse, and the client should be prepared for surgery.

129. **(1)** Integrated processes: nursing process — data collection; client need: health promotion and maintenance; prevention and early detection of disease; content area: medical-surgical.

     RATIONALE

     (1) The stool is indicative of regional enteritis, or Crohn's disease; documentation of the stool would aid diagnosis. **(2)** The stool should not be ignored for the reason given in rationale 1. **(3)** A laxative is not indicated. **(4)** The stool is more indicative of a regional enteritis than a fecal impaction.

130. **(2)** Integrated processes: nursing process — implementation; client need: health promotion and maintenance; prevention and early detection of disease; content area: medical-surgical.

     RATIONALE

     (1) *Cholangitis* is the appropriate term for infection of the bile duct. **(2)** *Choledocholithiasis* means that stones are present in the hepatic and bile duct. **(3)** *Cholecystitis* means inflammation of the gallbladder. **(4)** *Cholelithiasis* means stones in the gallbladder.

131. **(4)** Integrated processes: nursing process — implementation; client need:psychosocial integrity; coping and adaptation; content area: medical-surgical.

     RATIONALE

     (1) All nursing actions should be explained to the client. **(2)** The client's anxiety is lessened if all actions are explained. **(3)** Encouraging someone to do something he or she is not ready to do could increase anxiety. **(4)** The client's anxiety is lessened if all actions are explained.

132. **(1)** Integrated processes: nursing process — implementation; client need: physiological integrity; reduction of risk potential; content area: medical-surgical.

     RATIONALE

     (1) The incision is located below the rib cage; therefore, the coughing and deep breathing necessary to prevent hypostatic pneumonia are especially difficult postoperatively. **(2)** The data do not indicate special precautions to prevent thrombosis. **(3)** The ordinary precautions to prevent hemorrhage are sufficient. **(4)** No special precautions are needed to prevent paralytic ileus.

133. **(4)** Integrated processes: nursing process — implementation; client need: physiological integrity; physiological adaptation; content area: medical-surgical.

RATIONALE

(1) Hepatitis A is only occasionally transmitted parenterally. **(2)** Hepatitis A is not usually transmitted through body fluids. **(3)** Hepatitis A is not usually transmitted through sexual intercourse. **(4)** Hepatitis A is usually transmitted through feces or contaminated food or water.

134. **(3)** Integrated processes: nursing process — implementation; client need: safe, effective care environment; safety and infection control; content area: medical-surgical.

     RATIONALE

     (1) Reverse isolation is used to prevent infection in the client. **(2)** A mask and gown are not required because the disease is not spread by way of the respiratory tract. **(3)** Universal Precautions provide protection except in unusual circumstances. **(4)** Trash should be isolated, but Universal Precautions are more important.

135. **(1)** Integrated processes: nursing process — implementation; client need: physiological integrity; physiological adaptation; content area: medical-surgical.

     RATIONALE

     (1) The client may have a tendency to bleed easily because clotting factors are formed in the liver. **(2)** Aspirin should not be given because it inhibits aggregation of platelets, and clotting factors may be inadequate because of a diseased liver. **(3)** The abdominal girth should be measured daily. **(4)** Unless portal system encephalopathy is present, the client needs a high-protein and high-carbohydrate diet.

136. **(4)** Integrated processes: nursing process — data collection; client need: physiological integrity; physiological adaptation; content area: medical-surgical.

     RATIONALE

     (1) The data do not indicate a need to assess for hyperkalemia. **(2)** No data suggest metabolic acidosis. **(3)** Hypocalcemia is not likely. **(4)** Hyperglycemia or hypoglycemia could occur if damage is done to the islets of Langerhans.

137. **(2)** Integrated processes: nursing process — implementation; client need: physiological integrity; reduction of risk potential; content area: medical-surgical.

     RATIONALE

     (1) Signs of infection indicate a need for medical treatment. **(2)** A physician needs to prescribe treatment. **(3)** A physician needs to prescribe treatment. **(4)** A physician needs to prescribe treatment.

138. **(3)** Integrated processes: nursing process — planning; client need: physiological integrity; pharmacological therapies; content area: medical-surgical.

     RATIONALE

     (1) Fluids are given parenterally. **(2)** Aseptic technique is needed to prevent infection. **(3)** An analgesic should be timed so that the client experiences minimal pain during the dressing change. **(4)** I&O should be monitored hourly.

139. **(3)** Integrated processes: nursing process — implementation; client need: physiological integrity; physiological adaptation; content area: medical-surgical.

     RATIONALE

     (1) Even if the client had a tetanus injection within the last 10 years, it will be more important to give a tetanus booster. **(2)** A booster is necessary after injuries to ensure inactivation of any tetanus toxin produced by entry of the tetanus bacillus. **(3)** Someone should be with the client to observe for signs of head injury. (4) Heavy sedation should be avoided in the event of a head injury.

140. **(4)** Integrated processes: nursing process — implementation; client need: physiological integrity; basic care and comfort; content area: medical-surgical.

RATIONALE

(1) Saving all urine would not be necessary. (2) Forcing fluids would be more appropriate. (3) Recording I&O would be important but not as important as straining urine. (4) The data indicate that the client may have a renal stone; it would be most important to strain the urine to obtain the stone for analysis.

141. **(2)** Integrated processes: nursing process — implementation; client need: physiological integrity; basic care and comfort; content area: medical-surgical.

RATIONALE

(1) A ureteral catheter should never be clamped. (2) The output from the ureteral catheter should be recorded separately in order to assess drainage from the left kidney. (3) The catheter is irrigated only with a physician's order and then with strict aseptic technique and with no more than 5 mL of solution. (4) Activity should be encouraged.

142. **(1)** Integrated processes: nursing process — evaluation; client need: health promotion and maintenance; prevention and early detection of disease; content area: medical-surgical.

RATIONALE

(1) A low-protein diet is needed to reduce metabolic products causing the uremia. (2) A high-calorie diet is indicated in chronic renal failure. (3) A low-potassium diet is needed. (4) A low-sodium diet is needed.

143. **(3)** Integrated processes: nursing process — implementation; client need: safe, effective care environment; safety and infection control; content area: medical-surgical.

RATIONALE

(1) Major complications of peritoneal dialysis are not related to drainage time. (2) Dwelling time needs to be accurate, not precise. (3) Infection is perhaps the most common complication of peritoneal dialysis; it can be prevented by using strict aseptic technique. (4) Calcium is not usually added to the dialysis solution unless hypocalcemia is a problem.

144. **(1)** Integrated processes: nursing process — data collection; client need: physiological integrity; basic care and comfort; content area: medical-surgical.

RATIONALE

(1) BP should be checked in the left arm to preserve the shunt. (2) An IV should not be started in the right arm. (3) The shunt should not be irrigated. (4) Blood should not be drawn through the shunt.

145. **(3)** Integrated processes: nursing process — implementation; client need: physiological integrity; pharmacological therapies; content area: medical-surgical.

RATIONALE

(1) Some medication might be removed by dialysis. (2) If these drugs are not removed by dialysis, they should be given. (3) Medications not removed by dialysis should be given. (4) It is not necessary to bother the physician.

146. **(1)** Integrated processes: nursing process — planning; client need: physiological integrity; reduction of risk potential; content area: medical-surgical.

RATIONALE

(1) Detecting fluid or electrolyte imbalances would be a high priority in the care of a client with chronic renal failure. (2) Constipation is more likely than diarrhea in chronic renal failure. (3) Acidosis is more likely in chronic renal failure. (4) Hyperkalemia is more likely in chronic renal failure.

147. **(1)** Integrated processes: nursing process — data collection; client need: physiological integrity; reduction of risk potential; content area: medical-surgical.

RATIONALE

(1) Urinary output should get highest priority because a urethral stricture or clot in the catheter could be detected early. (2) Urinary output would take a higher priority for reasons explained in rationale 1. (3) Urinary output would take a higher priority for reasons explained in rationale 1. (4) Urinary output would take a higher priority for reasons explained in rationale 1.

148. **(3)** Integrated processes: nursing process — implementation; client need: physiological integrity; physiological adaptation; content area: medical-surgical.

RATIONALE

(1) Nothing should be done to irritate the skin in the field of radiation therapy. (2) No lotions or creams are to be applied without a physician's order. (3) Most authorities allow cleaning the skin in the field of radiation therapy with water and patting dry as needed. (4) A physician's order is needed before any lotion or cream is applied.

149. **(2)** Integrated processes: nursing process — implementation; client need: physiological integrity; reduction of risk potential; content area: medical-surgical.

RATIONALE

(1) The client should have a Foley catheter in place. (2) If antiembolism stockings are not in place, they should be applied immediately; thrombus formation is one of the biggest complications of a hysterectomy. (3) Perineal pads should be changed every 3–4 hours, and bleeding should be assessed. (4) The physician usually likes to make the first dressing change; until then, nurses reinforce the dressing.

150. **(4)** Integrated processes: nursing process — implementation; client need: physiological integrity; reduction of risk potential; content area: medical-surgical.

RATIONALE

(1) The client should remain on bed rest until the physician writes an order for him to be up. (2) A brace is used only when a spinal fusion is done. (3) Raising the legs and pointing the toes may be ordered as exercises after surgery. (4) The client should be log-rolled to prevent manipulation of the spinal column and possible injury to the cord.

151. **(4)** Integrated processes: nursing process — planning; client need: physiological integrity; reduction of risk potential; content area: medical-surgical.

RATIONALE

(1) Epiglottitis, or inflammation of the flap of cartilage that covers the larynx, causes airway obstruction. Oxygen is indicated if hypoxia occurs and is effective only if a patent airway is present. (2) An oral airway assists in preventing the tongue from obstructing the airway, but it does nothing to alleviate the obstruction caused by epiglottitis. (3) Respiratory distress from the epiglottitis is caused by airway obstruction and not accumulation of secretions. (4) A tracheostomy set contains instruments that a physician can use to create an opening in the trachea below the epiglottis, thus restoring airway patency.

152. **(1)** Integrated processes: nursing process — implementation; client need: physiological integrity; reduction of risk potential; content area: medical-surgical.

RATIONALE

(1) When the client is placed on the right side, the biopsy site of the liver capsule is compressed against the chest wall, and the escape of blood or bile is impeded. **(2)** When the client is placed on the left side, the biopsy site of the liver capsule is not compressed against the chest wall, and bleeding may occur. **(3)** After a liver biopsy, the client should remain recumbent and immobile. **(4)** When feet are raised as in the Trendelenburg position, venous return is increased. The increased blood flow may cause bleeding from the biopsy site.

153. **(4)** Integrated processes: nursing process — data collection; client need: physiological integrity; pharmacological therapies; content area: medical-surgical.

RATIONALE

(1) Febrile reactions are characterized by fevers and shaking chills that occur within 30 minutes of the start of the blood transfusion. **(2)** Hives, generalized itching, and occasionally wheezing or anaphylaxis occur during allergic reactions. **(3)** Septic reactions result from transfusion of blood contaminated with bacteria and cause rapid onset of chills and high fever, vomiting, diarrhea, and hypotension. **(4)** Hemolytic reactions, which occur when the donor blood is incompatible with that of the client, cause chills, low back pain, headache, and nausea within the first 10 minutes of a transfusion. Hypotension and vascular collapse follow, and hemoglobinuria (red urine) occurs.

154. **(4)** Integrated processes: nursing process — implementation; client need: physiological integrity; basic care and comfort; content area: medical-surgical.

RATIONALE

(1) Severe joint pain occurs during a sickle cell crisis; careful movement, positioning, and support of painful areas are indicated. **(2)** Fluids should be encouraged because they promote hemodilution and reverse the clumping of sickled cells in small vessels, which causes pain. **(3)** Diarrhea is not associated with sickle cell crisis; constipation often occurs as a result of immobility and narcotic analgesic use. **(4)** Pain from sickle cell crisis, caused by clumping of sickled cells in small blood vessels, is often severe and requires narcotic analgesics. Frequent assessments of pain assist in monitoring the client's response to hydration and pain control, the mainstays of treatment for sickle cell crisis.

155. **(3)** Integrated processes: nursing process — data collection; client need: physiological integrity; basic care and comfort; content area: medical-surgical.

RATIONALE

(1) A decrease in intake causes smaller stools but does not cause seepage of liquid stool. **(2)** Spinal cord trauma is not associated with CVAs; constipation often occurs in the CVA client as a result of immobility. **(3)** Fecal impactions cause continuous oozing of liquid stool because the liquid portion of feces located high in the colon seeps around the edges of the impacted mass. **(4)** Dehydration causes hard stools and constipation.

156. **(4)** Integrated processes: nursing process — implementation; client need: physiological integrity; reduction of risk potential; content area: medical-surgical.

RATIONALE

(1) Clients having seizures are at risk for airway obstruction when the tongue occludes the airway. If they become hypoxic during a seizure, opening the airway will relieve the hypoxia; oxygen is not indicated. **(2)** Clients with seizures should not be restrained. Because muscular contractions are strong during a seizure, restraint can produce injury. **(3)** The jaw of a client having a seizure should not be pried open because broken teeth and injury to the lips and tongue may result. **(4)** When the client is placed on one side with head flexed forward, the tongue falls forward, which assists in maintaining a patent airway, and drainage of saliva and mucus is facilitated.

157. **(1)** Integrated processes: nursing process — data collection; client need: physiological integrity; physiological adaptation; content area: medical-surgical.

RATIONALE

(1) Enteral feedings contain glucose; abrupt discontinuation of glucose feedings will cause the blood glucose to drop rapidly, resulting in symptoms of hypoglycemia such as an increased heart rate, sweating, and tremors. The symptoms can progress to slurred speech, incoordination, double vision, and drowsiness. **(2)** Hyperglycemia, or high blood glucose, may occur while a client receives enteral feedings. Withdrawal of glucose causes the opposite condition, hypoglycemia. **(3)** Enteral feedings are not associated with alterations in potassium levels. Administration of parenteral fluids (IV fluids) may cause alterations in potassium levels. **(4)** Enteral feedings are not associated with alterations in potassium levels. Administration of parenteral fluids (IV fluids) may cause alterations in potassium levels.

158. **(2)** Integrated processes: nursing process — data collection; client need: physiological integrity; reduction of risk potential; content area: medical-surgical.

RATIONALE

(1) A breakdown of the skin occurs in the second stage of pressure ulcer development. **(2)** The first stage of pressure ulcer development consists of redness of the skin that blanches with pressure, complaints of discomfort, and swelling. **(3)** Drainage of pressure ulcers occurs in stages II, III, and IV. **(4)** A stage IV pressure ulcer is characterized by extension to underlying muscle and bone, infection, necrosis, and drainage.

159. **(2)** Integrated processes: nursing process — implementation; client need: health promotion and maintenance; prevention and early detection of disease; content area: medical-surgical.

RATIONALE

(1) A PTT is used to monitor response to heparin therapy. A PTT or PT is used to monitor response to oral anticoagulants. **(2)** Carrying information about oral anticoagulant therapy is helpful in an emergency situation and provides information for other health-care providers, such as dentists. **(3)** Aspirin has anticoagulation action and should not be used concurrently with other anticoagulants because it increases the risk of bleeding. **(4)** Alcohol interferes with platelet function, which increases the risk of bleeding, and therefore should be avoided.

160. **(2)** Integrated processes: nursing process — data collection; client need: physiological integrity; pharmacological therapies; content area: medical-surgical.

RATIONALE

(1) Morphine sulfate is a respiratory depressant. Digoxin is a medication that is withheld if the pulse rate is <60 bpm. **(2)** When administering morphine sulfate, a respiratory depressant, the nurse should assess the respiratory rate; if it is less than 12 bpm, the nurse should withhold the drug and call the physician. **(3)** Antipyretics, or temperature-lowering drugs, are usually administered for elevated temperatures. Morphine sulfate is a respiratory depressant. **(4)** Morphine sulfate does not increase BP; it has a hypotensive effect, and respiratory depression is its most common effect.

161. **(4)** Integrated processes: nursing process — data collection; client need: physiological integrity; physiological adaptation; content area: medical-surgical.

RATIONALE

(1) The median age of menopause is 51 years; it may occur in some women as young as 42 years or as late as 55 years. A 74-year-old woman is considered to be postmenopausal and therefore would not be menstruating. **(2)** Estrogen production decreases with advancing age and is not a cause of vaginal bleeding. **(3)** Sexually transmitted diseases cause a variety of vaginal discharges but do not cause vaginal bleeding. **(4)** Any vaginal bleeding that occurs 1 year after cessation of menses should be evaluated; the most likely cause of vaginal bleeding in a postmenopausal woman is uterine cancer.

162. **(3)** Integrated processes: nursing process — data collection; client need: physiological integrity; physiological adaptation; content area: medical-surgical.

RATIONALE

(1) Progressive loss of weight occurs with hyperthyroidism. **(2)** Hyperthyroid clients tolerate heat poorly and perspire freely; cool to cold temperatures are preferred. **(3)** The primary function of the thyroid hormones is to control cellular metabolic activity. The pulse rate, at rest and on exercise, is rapid, and clients with hyperthyroidism may experience palpitations. **(4)** Myxedema occurs with hypothyroidism.

163. **(1)** Integrated processes: nursing process — data collection; client need: physiological integrity; physiological adaptation; content area: medical-surgical.

RATIONALE

(1) Accumulation of blood creates dead spaces and dead cells that become media for infection. **(2)** Tight dressings reduce the blood supply carrying nutrients and oxygen to the wound. **(3)** Steroids may mask the presence of infection by impairing normal inflammatory response. **(4)** Activity prevents approximation of wound edges; rest favors healing.

164. **(3)** Integrated processes: nursing process — data collection; client need: physiological integrity; physiological adaptation; content area: medical-surgical.

RATIONALE

(1) Hypovolemic shock is caused by decreased fluid volume from blood or fluid loss. The pulse rate is rapid and may be irregular. **(2)** Respirations are shallow and rapid in hypovolemic shock. **(3)** In hypovolemic shock, the skin is cool, pale, and moist. The lips and nails may be cyanotic. **(4)** Urine output decreases in hypovolemic shock and may progress from 50 mL/hr to <10 mL/hr (anuria).

165. **(3)** Integrated processes: nursing process — data collection; client need: physiological integrity; physiological adaptation; content area: medical-surgical.

RATIONALE

(1) An MI may cause chest pain, but dyspnea as a primary symptom indicates a cause other than an MI. **(2)** Anaphylaxis occurs as a response to an allergic agent. **(3)** A serious complication of a DVT is pulmonary embolism. When the embolus travels to the right side of the heart and occludes the pulmonary artery, the symptoms are sudden. The client experiences chest pain and becomes breathless and cyanotic. Sudden death may occur. **(4)** Bronchopneumonia does not have a sudden onset and is characterized by an elevated temperature.

166. **(4)** Integrated processes: nursing process — implementation; client need: physiological integrity; basic care and comfort; content area: medical-surgical.

RATIONALE

(1) Hot, spicy foods should be avoided in clients with an esophageal stricture because they stimulate esophageal spasm. **(2)** The client should remain upright for 1–4 hours after each meal to prevent reflux by using gravity to decrease an elevated gastroesophageal pressure gradient. **(3)** Eating should be avoided just before bedtime to prevent reflux. **(4)** Small, frequent feedings are recommended because large quantities of food overload the stomach and promote gastric reflux.

167. **(4)** Integrated processes: nursing process — data collection; client need: physiological integrity; basic care and comfort; content area: medical-surgical.

RATIONALE

(1) A PEG tube exits from the GI tract via an abdominal incision. An NG tube, not a PEG tube, could potentially cause skin irritation of the nares. **(2)** Securing feeding tubes to the client's cheek is only applicable for nasogastrically inserted tubes. **(3)** Assessment for NG tube displacement is necessary after coughing, tracheal or NG suctioning, and airway intubation. Because a PEG tube is surgically inserted, checking for displacement after coughing, suctioning, and intubation is not indicated. **(4)** Assessment of bowel elimination patterns is indicated for the client fed via a PEG tube since feedings are often hyperosmolar and may cause diarrhea.

168. **(2)** Integrated processes: nursing process — data collection; client need: physiological integrity; physiological adaptation; content area: medical-surgical.

RATIONALE

(1) Hemorrhoids are located near or external to the anus; they usually bleed on defecation and the blood is red to bright red. **(2)** The passage of dark, tarry stools (melena) indicates bleeding from the upper GI tract. Stools appear dark and tarry because they contain digested Hgb. **(3)** The rectum and sigmoid colon are parts of the lower GI tract; dark, tarry stools are characteristic of bleeding from the upper GI tract. **(4)** The rectum and sigmoid colon are parts of the lower GI tract; dark, tarry stools are characteristic of bleeding from the upper GI tract.

169. **(3)** Integrated processes: nursing process — data collection; client need: physiological integrity; physiological adaptation; content area: medical-surgical.

RATIONALE

(1) Pain associated with a perforated peptic ulcer is sudden and severe in the upper abdominal area. **(2)** Stools are dark and tarry in PUD. **(3)** Pain, which is referred to the shoulders, especially the right shoulder, occurs when a peptic ulcer perforates because of irritation of the phrenic nerve. **(4)** Pain is relieved by eating when a peptic ulcer is located in the duodenum.

170. **(1)** Integrated processes: nursing process — data collection; client need: health promotion and maintenance; prevention and early detection of disease; content area: medical-surgical.

RATIONALE

(1) Jaundice, light-colored stools, and dark urine are associated with hepatitis B and caused by the inability of the diseased liver cells to clear bilirubin from the blood. **(2)** Dark, tarry stools are associated with PUD. **(3)** Although the urine may appear dark with renal failure, stools are not light-colored. **(4)** With small bowel obstructions, there may be no stool, and the urine would not be dark-colored.

171. **(2)** Integrated processes: nursing process — data collection; client need: physiological integrity; pharmacological therapies; content area: medical-surgical.

RATIONALE

(1) Short-acting regular insulin has an onset of action of 0.5–1.0 hour. At 4:01 PM, the insulin has not yet begun to act. (2) The peak action of regular insulin is 2–4 hours; during this time, clients are at greatest risk for developing rebound hypoglycemia. (3) Regular insulin has a duration of 6–8 hours; rebound hypoglycemia would not occur at midnight. (4) Regular insulin has a duration of 6–8 hours; rebound hypoglycemia would not occur at 6 AM the following day.

172. **(3)** Integrated processes: nursing process — evaluation; client need: health promotion and maintenance; prevention and early detection of disease; content area: medical-surgical.

RATIONALE

(1) Immediate treatment of hypoglycemia, characterized by sweating, tremor, tachycardia, nervousness, and hunger, is administration of a fast-acting sugar such as glucose tablets, fruit juice, hard candies, sugar, or honey. (2) Diabetic retinopathy is the leading cause of blindness in adults in the United States; annual eye examinations for adults with diabetes are recommended. (3) Variations in blood glucose levels are expected throughout the day, with the lowest levels before meals and the highest levels 1–2 hours after eating. The goal of diabetes treatment is to minimize wide swings in glucose levels, not to eliminate normal variations. (4) Regular (short-acting) insulin should be drawn up before the NPH insulin when combined in one syringe to keep the regular insulin vial "pure"; this practice eliminates the chance that the longer-acting NPH insulin would be introduced into the regular insulin vial.

173. **(1)** Integrated processes: nursing process — data collection; client need: physiological integrity; reduction of risk potential; content area: medical-surgical.

RATIONALE

(1) During thyroid surgery, the parathyroid glands may be injured or removed, producing a decrease in calcium production. Hyperirritability of the nerves, spasms of the hands and feet, and muscular twitching are a group of symptoms called *tetany,* and are caused by hypocalcemia. (2) Hypocalcemia causes the symptoms of tetany. (3) Although hypokalemia can cause muscular weakness, it does not cause spasms and twitching. (4) Symptoms of hyperkalemia include dysrhythmia, paresthesia, and nausea.

174. **(2)** Integrated processes: nursing process — data collection; client need: physiological integrity; pharmacological therapies; content area: medical-surgical.

RATIONALE

(1) Changes in metabolism occur as a result of long-term steroid therapy, and weight gain results. (2) Because of suppression of the immune system and inflammatory response from long-term steroid therapy, infections may occur with minimal or no symptoms. (3) Addison's disease is caused by chronic adrenocortical insufficiency; clients on longterm steroid therapy are at risk for developing Cushing's syndrome from excessive adrenocortical activity. (4) As a result of long-term steroid use, facial skin becomes oily and acne flares.

175. **(1)** Integrated processes: nursing process — planning; client need: physiological integrity; reduction of risk potential; content area: medical-surgical.

RATIONALE

(1) Bed rest decreases body metabolism and thus reduces pancreatic and gastric secretions in the client with acute pancreatitis. (2) Impairment of endocrine function of the pancreas from pancreatitis results in increased serum glucose levels. (3) Bed rest increases the risk of a DVT. (4) The rationale for bed rest for the client with pancreatitis is to reduce pancreatic and gastric secretions; clients are still at risk for orthostatic hypotension.

176. **(4)** Integrated processes: nursing process — implementation; client need: physiological integrity; reduction of risk potential; content area: medical-surgical.

RATIONALE

(1) Cleansing from the anus toward the urethra results in the introduction of rectal bacteria in the urethral area. (2) It is not necessary to wash hands before collecting the specimen. (3) The collection container should not come in contact with the genitalia; contamination may result. (4) Mid stream urine collections are the most accurate. Because the distal portion of the urethral orifice is colonized by bacteria, voiding washes away the urethral contaminants.

177. **(4)** Integrated processes: nursing process — planning; client need: physiological integrity; basic care and comfort; content area: medical-surgical.

RATIONALE

(1) A urinary drainage bag connected to an indwelling urinary catheter should never be raised above the level of the bladder; contaminated urine from the drainage bag would flow into the client's bladder. (2) The drainage bag should not lie on the floor; contamination may result. The bag should be hung from the bed frame or chair frame. (3) The drainage bag should be emptied at least every 8 hours to lessen the risk of bacterial growth. (4) A free flow of urine reduces the risk of infection. When the drainage tubing is kinked or twisted, pools of urine are allowed to collect in the loops of the tubing.

178. **(3)** Integrated processes: nursing process — evaluation; client need: physiological integrity; reduction of risk potential; content area: medical-surgical.

RATIONALE

(1) Dry peritoneal catheter dressings are desired; a wet dressing may indicate the complication of leakage. (2) A bloody effluent (drainage) may be observed occasionally, especially in young, menstruating female clients. (3) Peritonitis is the most common complication of peritoneal dialysis; indications of peritonitis include cloudy drainage and abdominal pain. (4) Rapid weight gain in clients on peritoneal dialysis occurs from fluid volume overload. A stable weight indicates that the peritoneal dialysis is effectively eliminating waste products.

179. **(3)** Integrated processes: nursing process — evaluation; client need: health promotion and maintenance; prevention and early detection of disease; content area: medical-surgical.

RATIONALE

(1) Drinking 8–10 glasses or more of fluids daily is recommended to flush out bacteria that cause UTI. (2) Voiding every 2–3 hours during the day prevents overdistention of the bladder and compromised blood supply to the bladder wall, which predispose clients to UTI. (3) Antibiotics should be taken for as long as they are prescribed; premature discontinuation (even if symptom-free) may result in repeated infection as a result of inadequate antibiotic therapy. (4) Showers are preferable to tub baths because bacteria in the bath water can enter the urethra.

180. **(1)** Integrated processes: nursing process — evaluation; client need: physiological integrity; reduction of risk potential; content area: medical-surgical.

RATIONALE

(1) Hemodialysis is indicated for clients with chronic renal failure who experience fluid volume excess and electrolyte imbalances. Removal of the excess fluid during the dialysis

process results in weight loss. Monitoring a client's weight is a simple indirect way to assess a client's fluid balance. (2) A calorie count provides information about the client's nutritional intake but is not of value for assessing response to hemodialysis. (3) Measuring exercise tolerance does not assist in assessing a client's response to hemodialysis as much as measuring the client's weight; most clients with chronic renal failure experience anemia and, as a result, are chronically fatigued. (4) Assessing for skin bruising is not a means of assessing response to hemodialysis. A skin alteration commonly associated with chronic renal failure is uremic frost, a white powdery substance that appears on the skin because of elevated urates.

181. **(4)** Integrated processes: nursing process — data collection; client need: physiological integrity; pharmacological therapies; content area: medical-surgical.

RATIONALE

(1) Kidney rejection is most likely to occur early (within 24–72 hours) or may occur within a few days or a few months. **(2)** Infection by bacterial or fungal pathogens is most likely to occur during the first few weeks following transplant. Immunosuppressive agents are gradually tapered over a period of several weeks, depending on the client's immunologic response to the transplant. **(3)** Although clients can experience uncertainty about the future at any time, the feeling of uncertainty in the kidney transplant recipient is greatest before receipt of the transplanted kidney. **(4)** Two years after a kidney transplant, a client is most likely to express concerns about the long-term effects of immunosuppressive therapy, such as developing diabetes, glaucoma, cataracts, and osteoporosis.

182. **(3)** Integrated processes: nursing process — planning; client need: physiological integrity; physiological adaptation; content area: medical-surgical.

RATIONALE

(1) Symptoms associated with renal stones include pain, nausea, hematuria, and symptoms of infection. Impairment of gas exchange is not associated with renal stones. **(2)** A renal stone obstructs flow of urine; it does not impair renal function. **(3)** Because of blockage of the urinary tract, clients are at risk for infection. **(4)** Self-concept disturbances are associated with alterations in how clients perceive themselves. Presence of an internally located renal stone would not be likely to alter a client's self-concept.

183. **(2)** Integrated processes: nursing process — implementation; client need: physiological integrity; reduction of risk potential; content area: medical-surgical.

RATIONALE

(1) In an ileal conduit, the urine is diverted by implanting the ureter into a loop of ileum that is led out through the abdominal wall. An ileostomy bag is used to collect the urine. Intermittent urinary catheterization is not indicated. **(2)** Changes in physical structure and function occur with an ileal conduit procedure; the ability to cope with these changes depends to a great degree on the client's self-concept and self-esteem. **(3)** Peritoneal dialysis is used when renal failure occurs; an ileal conduit is used when urinary diversion is needed. **(4)** Only urine is diverted via an ileal conduit; the ends of the remaining intestine are connected to provide an intact bowel.

184. **(3)** Integrated processes: nursing process — implementation; client need: physiolgical integrity; physiological adaptation; content area: medical-surgical.

RATIONALE

(1) Because herpes genitalis is a sexually transmitted disease, condoms should be used to reduce the likelihood of disease transmission to the female partner. **(2)** The herpes virus causes herpes genitalis; antibiotics are indicated for bacterial infections. **(3)** Herpes genitalis causes vesicular (blister-like) lesions in the perineum. Complications such as extragenital spread can result from touching lesions and then touching the buttocks, thighs, eyes, or other areas. **(4)** Because herpes genitalis is caused by a virus, antifungal preparations are not indicated.

185. **(2)** Integrated processes: nursing process — data collection; client need: physiological integrity; physiological adaptation; content area: medical-surgical.

RATIONALE

(1) Symptoms of dribbling, difficulty in starting urination, and sensations of incomplete emptying indicate that an obstruction is occurring between the bladder and meatus, and these symptoms are not characteristic of the normal aging process. **(2)** The prostate gland is a walnut-sized gland that is located at the base of the bladder. Enlargement causes symptoms of obstruction, such as dribbling, difficulty in starting urination, and sensations of incomplete emptying. **(3)** Enlarged prostate glands often cause stasis of urine in the bladder, which subsequently becomes infected. However, when a UTI occurs, the urine is concentrated and cloudy, and may be bloody. **(4)** Chronic constipation does not cause urinary symptoms.

186. **(4)** Integrated processes: nursing process — data collection; client need: physiological integrity; physiological adaptation; content area: medical-surgical.

RATIONALE

(1) Inability to cough results in pooling of secretions and ineffective airway clearance. Gas exchange is not impaired (the airway is impaired). **(2)** Pain may result from coughing, but inability to cough results in inability to clear the airway. **(3)** Altered thought processes may occur with hypoxia (decreased oxygen supply). However, inability to cough results in airway impairment. **(4)** Inability to cough causes secretions to pool and obstruct the airway. Coughing is a mechanism for clearing an airway; when coughing is impaired, ineffective airway clearance results.

187. **(2)** Integrated processes: nursing process — implementation; client need: safe, effective care environment; safety and infection control; content area: medical-surgical.

RATIONALE

(1) Because the exudate is a body fluid, Universal Precautions, which mandate gloving before contact with body fluids, should be instituted. **(2)** Nonsterile gloves should be used to remove dirty dressings that contain exudate, considered a body fluid. Wearing gloves reduces the risk that the nurse could acquire the infection from the client. **(3)** Sterile gloves are not indicated for removing "dirty" dressings; nonsterile gloves are sufficient, readily available, and much more cost effective. **(4)** Double gloving is not a recommended principle of Universal Precautions. Donning a single pair of nonsterile gloves is considered sufficient protection when changing soiled dressings.

188. **(2)** Integrated processes: nursing process — planning; client need: physiological integrity; pharmacological therapies; content area: medical-surgical.

RATIONALE

(1) Hypotension and shock occur with anaphylactic (immediate hypersensitivity) reactions as a result of the release of mast cell mediators. Penicillin and its derivatives have known anaphylactic potential. **(2)** Laryngeal edema, bronchospasm, cyanosis, and even cardiac arrest can occur with an anaphylactic reaction. Because less severe symptoms such as hives can progress to a life-threatening event, anticipation of this possibility enables the nurse to be prepared. **(3)** Paralytic ileus does not occur during an anaphylactic reaction. **(4)** Liver failure is typically a chronic process. Anaphylactic events occur suddenly and are usually of short duration. Liver failure is therefore unlikely.

189. **(2)** Integrated processes: nursing process — data collection; client need: physiological integrity; physiological adaptation; content area: medical-surgical.

   RATIONALE
   (1) Bulging eyes (exophthalmos) are commonly associated with Graves' disease (hyperthyroidism) and do not occur in systemic lupus erythematosus. **(2)** A butterfly-shaped erythematous rash across the nasal bridge is a classic sign of SLE. **(3)** Jaundice, or yellowing of the skin, may occur when liver function is impaired and does not occur with SLE. **(4)** Kaposi's lesions are cutaneous lesions that are brown to purple and occur in Kaposi's sarcoma, an AIDS-related malignancy.

190. **(2)** Integrated processes: nursing process — data collection; client need: health promotion and maintenance; prevention and early detection of disease; content area: medical-surgical.

   RATIONALE
   (1) Nevi (moles) are typically brown. Colors of concern include blue-black, gray, and purple. **(2)** An irregularly shaped mole warrants further evaluation, particularly if the mole was once circular and has changed. **(3)** Moles can be located all over the body. Location is of concern only when a mole is located in an area of mechanical trauma or friction, such as under a bra strap. **(4)** Sun rays, which are ultraviolet rays, cause sunburns, which increase the risk of skin cancer. However, the characteristics of the mole need to be examined, not the surrounding skin. Clients should be taught to avoid sun exposure.

191. **(2)** Integrated processes: nursing process — data collection; client need: physiological integrity; physiological adaptation; content area: medical-surgical.

   RATIONALE
   (1) Smoke inhalation injury results from the inhalation of the products of incomplete combustion. The injury is a result of chemical irritation of the pulmonary tissues at the alveolar level. Burns involving boiling water are topical and do not result in smoke inhalation. **(2)** In first-degree burns, the epidermis is destroyed or injured and a portion of the dermis may be injured. The area may be painful, appear red and dry, or it may be blistered. **(3)** In second-degree burns, the epidermis and the dermis are injured. The area is painful, appears red, and exudes fluid. **(4)** In third-degree burns, there is total destruction of epidermis and dermis; the color of the wound may be white to red to black. The burn is painless because of destruction of nerve fibers and has a leathery appearance.

192. **(4)** Integrated processes: nursing process — implementation; client need: physiological integrity; physiological adaptation; content area: medical-surgical.

   RATIONALE
   (1) Monitoring hourly urine output is performed during the immediate phase of burn care. **(2)** NG suction is maintained during the immediate phase of burn care because burn injury often produces paralytic ileus. **(3)** Topical antibiotic agents are applied during the intermediate phase of burn care to reduce the risk of bacterial colonization. **(4)** Elastic bandages or pressure garments are applied over healed areas prone to scarring to prevent hypertrophic scarring and to achieve an optimal cosmetic effect during the rehabilitation or long-term phase of burn care.

193. **(1)** Integrated processes: nursing process — implementation; client need: physiological integrity; pharmacological therapies; content area: medical-surgical.

   RATIONALE
   (1) The abbreviation *OD* refers to "oculus dexter," or "right eye." **(2)** The abbreviation *OS* refers to "oculus sinister," or "left eye." **(3)** The abbreviation *OU* refers to "oculus unitas," or "both eyes." **(4)** The abbreviation *AU* refers to "both ears."

194. **(4)** Integrated processes: nursing process — implementation; client need: physiological integrity; reduction of risk potential; content area: medical-surgical.

   RATIONALE
   (1) Cold compresses, not hot, should be applied to reduce pain and intraocular pressure. **(2)** To decrease intraocular pressure, light levels should be reduced (lights dimmed, drapes drawn), and clients should be instructed to wear dark glasses in strong light. **(3)** Pressing or rubbing the eye should be avoided to facilitate healing and reduced intraocular pressure. **(4)** Head elevation and avoiding lying on the operative side decrease eye edema and intraocular pressure.

195. **(3)** Integrated processes: nursing process — implementation; client need: physiological integrity; reduction of risk potential; content area: medical-surgical.

   RATIONALE
   (1) The client should be reminded not to blow nose or sneeze because such actions may force organisms through the auditory canal to the middle ear. **(2)** Shampoos are discouraged for about 2 weeks; moisture helps transmit organisms. **(3)** The client should be instructed to report facial paralysis, drooping of the mouth on the affected side, altered taste, drooling when drinking, and mouth dryness, which may indicate surgical trauma to the seventh cranial nerve. **(4)** Ear packing should be kept clean and dry; moist environments promote microbial growth.

196. **(4)** Integrated processes: nursing process — data collection; client need: physiological integrity; physiological adaptation; content area: medical-surgical.

   RATIONALE
   (1) Reaction only to loud noises and pain indicates serious impairment of brain circulation and is a late sign of increasing ICP. **(2)** Absence of reflexes and flaccid extremities are late signs of ICP. **(3)** Fixed and dilated pupils are very late signs of ICP; a fatal outcome is usually inevitable. **(4)** Lethargy, changing levels of consciousness, slowing of the speech, and delay in response to verbal stimuli are early indicators of increasing ICP.

197. **(2)** Integrated processes: nursing process — implementation; client need: physiological integrity; physiological adaptation; content area: medical-surgical.

   RATIONALE
   (1) An unconscious client is at risk for developing pressure ulcers and therefore requires skin care; however, the most important nursing action is to maintain an airway. **(2)** Maintaining an airway is the most important nursing action when caring for an unconscious client because the epiglottis and tongue may relax and occlude the oropharynx. If the airway becomes occluded, the brain is deprived of oxygen. **(3)** Turning a client who is unable to turn is necessary to prevent pressure ulcers and reduce infection risk, but maintaining an airway takes higher priority. **(4)** The head of the bed of an unconscious client should be elevated 30 degrees to reduce aspiration risk; however, maintaining a patent airway is the most important nursing action.

198. **(3)** Integrated processes: nursing process — data collection; client need: physiological integrity; physiological adaptation; content area: medical-surgical.
RATIONALE
(1) Sensory deficits caused by a CVA include paresthesia (numbness and tingling) and difficulty with proprioception. **(2)** Verbal deficits caused by a CVA include various types of aphasia, such as expressive, receptive, and global (both expressive and receptive). **(3)** Short- and long-term memory loss, decreased attention span, inability to concentrate, poor abstract reasoning, and altered judgment are examples of cognitive deficits caused by a CVA. **(4)** Emotional deficits after a CVA include loss of self-control, decreased tolerance to stress, depression, withdrawal, fear, hostility, and anger.

199. **(2)** Integrated processes: nursing process — planning; client need: physiological integrity; basic care and comfort; content area: medical-surgical.
RATIONALE
(1) Clients with multiple sclerosis experience altered bowel elimination because of spinal cord dysfunction. Neurogenic impairment typically causes constipation. Adequate fluid intake, not fluid restriction, is needed to prevent constipation. **(2)** A high-fiber diet increases bulk and reduces the likelihood of constipation and is a component of bowel programs designed for clients with multiple sclerosis. **(3)** Clients with multiple sclerosis have an intact bowel; they experience neurogenic impairment and do not require colostomies. **(4)** Intermittent self-catheterization is recommended as part of a bladder program for some clients with multiple sclerosis.

200. **(3)** Integrated processes: nursing process — data collection; client need: physiological integrity; reduction of risk potential; content area: medical-surgical.
RATIONALE
(1) Vital signs are monitored after a total hip replacement to assess for hemorrhage. **(2)** The wound of a client who has undergone total hip replacement is monitored for blood loss and infection. **(3)** After a total hip replacement, neurovascular status is assessed by observing the capillary refill of the toes. Rapid return of pink color indicates good capillary perfusion. **(4)** Performing ROM of the hip after a total replacement is not indicated; the hip should be kept in an abducted position and in neutral rotation to prevent dislocation.

201. **(2)** Integrated processes: nursing process — data collection; client need: physiological integrity; physiological adaptation; content area: medical-surgical.
RATIONALE
(1) Chronic pain is associated with actual or potential tissue damage. **(2)** Chronic pain is associated with actual or potential tissue damage. **(3)** Chronic pain is associated with many pain behaviors that people do not normally associate with pain. **(4)** There is no change in vital signs with chronic pain.

202. **(2)** Integrated processes: nursing process — data collection; client need: physiological integrity; pharmacological therapies; content area: medical-surgical.
RATIONALE
(1) Physical dependence is the expected physiological response to ongoing exposure to opioids manifested by a withdrawal syndrome that occurs when blood levels of the drug are abruptly decreased. **(2)** Drug tolerance is the need for an increased opioid dose to maintain the same degree of analgesia. Tolerance is not addiction. **(3)** Addiction is a complex psychosocial condition characterized by a drive to obtain and take substances for other than the prescribed therapeutic use for

pain. **(4)** Equianalgesic is having the same pain-killing effect when administered to the same individual.

203. **(2)** Integrated processes: nursing process — data collection; client need: physiological integrity; physiological adaptation; content area: medical-surgical.
RATIONALE
(1) Physical dependence is a physiological response to opioids. **(2)** Physical dependence is a physiological response to opioids. **(3)** Addiction is a complex psychosocial condition. **(4)** Obsessive-compulsive is a pyschosocial condition.

204. **(4)** Integrated processes: nursing process — planning; client need: physiological integrity; pharmacological therapies; content area: medical-surgical.
(1) Cancer pain is best managed through long-acting opioids according to the World Health Organization. **(2)** Short-acting opioids provide only short-acting responses to cancer pain. **(3)** Administration of breakthrough medications is necessary as adjuvant therapy with long-acting opioids to control cancer pain. **(4)** Cancer pain is best managed with the use of long-acting opioids administered around the clock.

205. **(4)** Integrated processes: nursing process — implementation; client need: physiological integrity; physiological adaptation; content area: medical-surgical.
RATIONALE
(1) Believe the patient and family about the intensity of the pain and what relieves it. **(2)** Believe the patient and family about the intensity of the pain and what relieves it. **(3)** Deliver medications in a timely, logical fashion, with the aim of preventing rather than "chasing pain." **(4)** According to the World Health Organization, every client has a right to adequate pain control; therefore, the nurse's responsibility is to believe that clients may have pain without observable signs.

206. **(3)** Integrated processes: nursing process — data collection; client need: physiological integrity; physiological adaptation; content area: medical-surgical.
RATIONALE
(1) The nurse needs to conduct an appropriate diagnostic workup to determine the cause of pain. **(2)** The nurse needs to ask the client regularly if she or he is in pain. **(3)** An effective pain treatment strategy requires a thorough pain assessment. **(4)** Believe the patient and family about the intensity of the pain and what relieves it.

207. **(2)** Integrated processes: nursing process — data collection; client need: physiological integrity; physiological adaptation; content area: medical-surgical.
RATIONALE
(1) Increasing heart rate will not allow blood filling to occur in the atrium and ventricle resulting in decreased cardiac output. **(2)** Decreasing heart rate will increase oxygen supply to the coronary arteries. **(3)** Increasing blood pressure will not allow for filling time in the atrium and ventricles and will increase the stress on the heart. **(4)** Decreasing heart rate will increase oxygen supply to the coronary arteries.

208. **(3)** Integrated processes: nursing process — data collection; client need: physiological integrity; physiological adaptation; content area: medical-surgical.
(1) Central venous pressure is the measure of blood flow once returned to the heart; systemic vascular resistance is the pressure used to support the veins in returning blood to the heart. **(2)** Pulmonary capillary wedge pressure is the pressure in the pulmonary artery once blood flow has been restricted with the balloon; systemic vascular resistance is the pressure used

to support the veins in returning blood to the heart. **(3)** Systemic vascular resistance is the pressure used to support the veins in returning blood to the heart; pulmonary vascular resistance is the pressure used to support the blood to the lungs. **(4)** Mean arterial blood pressure involves averaging the systolic and diastolic pressure; pulmonary capillary wedge pressure is the pressure in the pulmonary artery once blood flow has been restricted with the balloon.

209. **(1)** Integrated processes: nursing process — implementation; client need: physiological integrity; reduction of risk potential; content area: medical-surgical.

     RATIONALE
     (1) The balloon may occlude blood flow to the left subclavian. **(2)** The balloon will function if position changes. **(3)** An increase in heart rate increases myocardial oxygen consumption. **(4)** The risk of infection is directly related to the exposure to infectious bacteria or viruses.

210. **(3)** Integrated processes: nursing process — data collection; client need: physiological integrity; physiological adaptation; content area: medical-surgical.

     RATIONALE
     (1) An increase in systemic vascular resistance will increase the blood flow back to the heart. **(2)** Pulmonary capillary wedge pressure will not increase with an increase in heart rate. **(3)** Cardiac output will increase when the heart rate is increased. **(4)** Cardiac output will increase when the heart rate is increased.

211. **(2)** Integrated processes: nursing process — implementation; client need: physiological integrity; physiological adaptation; content area: medical-surgical.

     RATIONALE
     (1) It is not necessary to rush the patient to the operating room until the bleeding is assessed. **(2)** Apply direct pressure to the site to stop bleeding and avoid loss of blood flow and pressure to the vital organs. **(3)** Call a physician once the situation has been assessed. **(4)** Placing the client on the left side is not the best means to stop the bleeding at the catherization site.

212. **(2)** Integrated processes: nursing process — implementation; client need: physiological integrity; physiological adaptation; content area: medical-surgical.

     RATIONALE
     (1) Auscultation of lung sounds is a routine nursing assessment and not usually part of physician's orders. **(2)** Sputum specimens for culture and sensitivity must be collected prior to starting antibiotics as the first dose may alter the sample and culture results. **(3)** Antibiotics are started after sputum and blood cultures are obtained. **(4)** A routine CBC can be drawn any time; however, the best and most urgent order is to obtain cultures so that antibiotics can be started.

213. **(1, 2, 3, 4, 7)** Integrated processes: nursing process — data collection; client need: physiological integrity; physiological adaptation; content area: medical-surgical.

     RATIONALE
     (1) Wheezing is a classic sign of asthma. **(2)** Chest tightness occurs in response to a trigger; in this case, exercise. **(3)** Cough also occurs in response to a trigger. **(4)** A "silent chest" means that the patient is moving little air and is an ominous sign of severe obstruction. **(5)** PEFR of 80% is the lowest range of normal. Less than 80% of a client's expected peak expiratory flow rate and the presence of symptoms are indications for rescue medication use, such as an albuterol inhaler. **(6)** Most

clients are restless and show signs of anxiety. **(7)** Diminished breath sounds go along with the silent chest and may also indicate atelectasis or pneumothorax.

214. Integrated processes: nursing process — data collection; client need: physiological integrity; physiological adaptation; content area: medical-surgical.

     RATIONALE
     Cor pulmonale is right-sided hypertrophy of the heart with or without heart failure from a pulmonary disease; in this case, COPD. You should hear a gallop or click at the left sternal border.

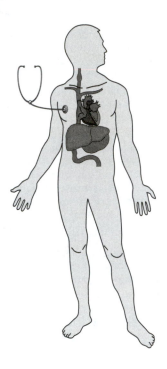

215. **(2)** Integrated processes: nursing process — evaluation; client need: physiological integrity; physiological adaptation; content area: medical-surgical.

     RATIONALE
     (1) Using oxygen increases the amount of oxygen available during respiration and does not decrease air trapping. **(2)** Pursed-lip breathing should be used 8–10 times three or four times a day to give control over breathing and decrease air trapping. **(3)** Chest physiotherapy helps clear excess bronchial secretions and does not decrease air trapping. **(4)** Pursed-lip breathing, not diaphragmatic breathing, gives control over breathing and decreases air trapping.

216. **(4)** Integrated processes: nursing process — data collection; client need: physiological integrity; reduction of risk potential; content area: medical-surgical.

     RATIONALE
     (1) CO_2 narcosis occurs when high levels of oxygen knock out the drive to breathe **(2)** High oxygen washes out the nitrogen from alveoli and they collapse. **(3)** Infection is a major complication; however, it does not lead to ARDS. **(4)** Oxygen toxicity inactivates surfactant and can lead to ARDS.

217. Integrated processes: nursing process — implementation; client need: physiological integrity; reduction of risk potential; content area: medical-surgical.

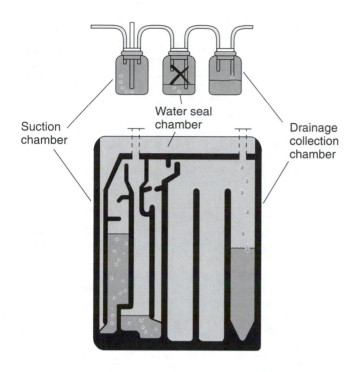

Suction chamber | Water seal chamber | Drainage collection chamber

RATIONALE

The chamber in the middle. It should be filled with sterile water up to 2 cm.

218. **(1, 3, 4, 5, 6)** Integrated processes: nursing process — data collection; client need: physiological integrity; pharmacological therapies; content area: medical-surgical.

RATIONALE

(1) INH is a pharmacological treatment for tuberculosis. **(2)** 3TC is a nucleoside reverse transcriptase inhibitor to treat HIV infection. **(3)** Rifampin is a pharmacological treatment for tuberculosis. **(4)** Ethambutol is a pharmacological treatment for tuberculosis. **(5)** Streptomycin is a pharmacological treatment for tuberculosis. **(6)** Pyrazinamide is a pharmacological treatment for tuberculosis. **(7)** Lamivudine is a nucleoside reverse transcriptase inhibitor used to treat HIV infection.

219. **(1, 2, 3, 4)** Integrated processes: nursing process — data collection; client need: health promotion and maintenance; prevention and early detection of disease; content area: medical-surgical.

RATIONALE

(1) Fifteen millimeters is a positive response in low-risk persons. **(2)** Ten millimeters is a positive response for health-care workers, patients with chronic medical problems, immigrants, and residents of long-term facilities. **(3)** One-half millimeter is a positive response in known or suspected HIV infection, transplant patients, and immunosuppressed patients. **(4)** TB must be ruled out with further testing; either two-step testing or sputum cultures and chest radiographs. These individuals do not have enough immune system to respond to the candidiasis and, therefore, the accuracy of the TB test is questionable.

220. **(3)** Integrated processes: nursing process — implementation; client need: physiological integrity; physiological adaptation; content area: medical-surgical.

RATIONALE

(1) Suction catheter should be inserted about 5–6 inches or until obstruction is felt. **(2)** Oxygen should be administered during sterile set-up. The client is preoxygenated and instructed to deep breathe prior to each suctioning. **(3)** Limit suctioning to no more than 10 seconds. **(4)** There is no need for a new suction catheter unless it has become contaminated during the procedure. The catheter is rinsed with sterile water between suctioning.

221. **(4)** Integrated processes: nursing process — data collection; client need: physiological integrity; reduction for risk potential; content area: medical-surgical.

RATIONALE

(1) An elevated white blood cell count indicates an infection. **(2)** This is a normal value. **(3)** This is a normal value. **(4)** A hemoglobin of 6 indicates a moderate to severe decrease in hemoglobin level; therefore, a decrease in oxygen-carrying capacity of the RBC.

222. **(4)** Integrated processes: nursing process — planning; client need: physiological integrity; pharmacological therapies; content area: medical-surgical.

RATIONALE

(1) Iron preparation needs to be given deep intramuscularly using the Z-track method. **(2)** Iron preparation needs to be given deep intramuscularly using the Z-track method. **(3)** Iron preparation needs to be given deep intramuscularly using the Z-track method. **(4)** Iron preparation needs to be given deep intramuscularly using the Z-track method to avoid staining the skin.

223. **(1, 2, 3, 4, 5, 6, 7)** Integrated processes: nursing process — planning; client need: physiological integrity; physiological adaptation; content area: medical-surgical.

RATIONALE

(1) Three hundred milligrams of ferrous sulfate contains 60 mg of elemental iron. **(2)** Taking iron with vtamin C (ascorbic acid) enhances absorption. **(3)** Stool softeners prevent constipation, which is common when taking iron. **(4)** Folic acid helps with RBC maturation. It is also found in green leafy vegetables, liver, meat, fish, whole grains, and legumes. **(5)** Thiamine, or vitamin B_6, aids hemoglobin synthesis. **(6)** Eggs, milk, and cheese are foods rich in amino acids. **(7)** Legumes are rich in amino acids. **(8)** Transfusions of packed red blood cells (not whole blood) may be needed if the client is symptomatic such as signs of hypoxemia, cyanosis, or low O_2 saturation.

224. **(1, 2, 3)** Integrated processes: nursing process — data collection; client need: health promotion and maintenance; prevention and early detection of disease; content area: medical-surgical.

RATIONALE

(1) The human papillomavirus increases the risk for cervical cancer. **(2)** Being sexually active before the age of 17 years old increases the risk for cervical cancer. **(3)** Multiple sexual partners increases the risk for cervical cancer. **(4)** Smokers have a 50% higher risk of cervical cancer.

225. **(1, 3, 4)** Integrated processes: nursing process — data collection; client need: physiological integrity; reduction of risk potential; content area: medical-surgical.

RATIONALE

(1) Monitoring Foley catheter output is important because the ureter may be accidently severed or ligated during surgery. The client may also experience urinary retention without a Foley catheter, and it prevents strain on the suture line. **(2)** Douche and enema are preoperative preparations. (3) Assessing bowel sounds is important because abdominal distention and paralytic ileus may develop. (4) These interventions are for prevention of deep vein thrombosis. (5) Suture removal is a physician's responsibility.

226. **(The upper outer quadrant)** Integrated processes: nursing process — data collection; client need: health promotion and maintenance; prevention and early detection of disease; content area: medical-surgical.

RATIONALE

Approximately 50% of all breast cancers develop in the upper outer quadrant of the breast.

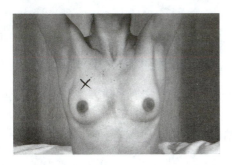

227. **(1, 2, 4, 5, 6)** Nursing process — implementation; client need: physiological integrity; reduction of risk potential; content area: medical-surgical.

RATIONALE

(1) Sunglasses protect from the ultraviolet light. (2) Proper technique for instilling eye drops is important to obtain therapeutic effects and prevent damage to the cornea. (3) Opioids are not needed following cataract surgery. Pain or discomfort is usually minimal and is relieved with nonopioid medications such as acetaminophen. If pain is severe, it is a sign of increased intraocular pressure, and the patient should notify the physician immediately. (4) These actions prevent dislocation of the implant and prevent increased intraocular pressure. (5) The client should follow-up in the physician's office 1 day after outpatient cataract surgery. (6) Reporting signs and symptoms of infection allows prompt treatment. (7) Reporting signs and symptoms of increased intraocular pressure allows prompt treatment and prevents damage to the optic nerve.

228. **(1)** Integrated processes: nursing process — data collection; client need: physiological integrity; physiological adaptation; content area: medical-surgical.

RATIONALE

(1) Angle-closure glaucoma causes excruciating pain, whereas open-angle glaucoma is painless. (2) Cataracts do not cause nausea or vomiting. Pain is rare unless the cataract enlarges to the point of occluding the canal of Schlemm, thus causing a glaucoma-like situation. (3) Meniere's disease involves the ear. (4) Retinal detachment is painless unless it is a traumatic detachment.

229. **(2, 3, 4, 5, 6, 7)** Integrated processes: nursing process — implementation; client need: physiological integrity; physiological adaptation; content area: medical-surgical.

RATIONALE

(1) The diet should be low in salt to avoid fluid retention. (2) Caffeine, nicotine, and alcohol cause vasoconstriction. (3) Diuretics remove excess fluid. (4) Antihistamines lessen the symptoms. (5) Antiemetics control nausea. (6) Antivert reduces the dizziness. (7) A quiet dark room reduces stimuli and decreases symptoms. (8) Television can exacerbate symptoms.

230. **(2)** Integrated processes: nursing process — implementation; client need: physiological integrity; basic care and comfort; content area: medical-surgical.

RATIONALE

(1) This intervention helps with aphasia, or loss of language. (2) Sitting a patient upright for meals helps prevent aspiration in patients with dysphagia, or trouble swallowing. (3) Assisting with ambulation is important with ataxia, or lack of coordinated movement. (4) Bladder training helps with bladder dysfunction such as atonic, hypotonic, or hypertonic bladders.

231. **(3)** Integrated processes: nursing process — data collection; client need: physiological integrity; reduction of risk potential; content area: medical-surgical.

RATIONALE

(1) Fifteen is a normal Glasgow Coma Scale; a score of 8 or less indicates coma. (2) With increased intracranial pressure, motor strength decreases. (3) A dilated pupil indicates compressed cranial nerve III; fixed pupil with no response indicates increased intracranial pressure. (4) This is a normal blood pressure reading. If there were a widening pulse pressure, bradycardia, and irregular respirations (Cushing's triad), it would indicate an increased intracranial pressure.

232. **(1, 2, 3, 4, 5, 6, 7)** Integrated processes: nursing process — data collection; client need: physiological integrity; reduction of risk potential; content area: medical-surgical.

RATIONALE

(1) Level of consciousness identifies changes in neurological status so that prompt reporting and interventions can occur. (2) Pupil response is an indicator of neurological status and increased intracranial pressure. (3) Vital signs give information on general condition and help identify presence of Cushing's triad. (4) Assessing the dressing determines if bleeding is occurring. (5) Turning helps prevent pulmonary and vascular complications. Positioning the client depends upon the surgical site and is usually with the head of the bed elevated, neck in body alignment, and avoidance of neck flexion. (6) Nutrition is needed for healing and malnutrition promotes cerebral edema. (7) Pain increases oxygen needs and can increase intracranial pressure.

233. **(1)** Integrated processes: nursing process — evaluation; teaching/learning; client need: physiological integrity; reduction of risk potential; content area: medical-surgical.

RATIONALE

(1) If the weights are resting on any object, the purpose of the traction is defeated. (2) The body must remain in proper alignment; some positions are contraindicated. (3) Only mild discomfort should be experienced when the muscle spasms cease. (4) Clients in traction need a lot of diversional activity.

234. **(2)** Integrated processes: nursing process — planning; client need: physiological integrity; physiological adaptation; content area: medical-surgical.

RATIONALE

(1) The physician does not need to be notified because all vital signs are normal except the temperature. A slight elevation of temperature can be caused by the inflammatory process resulting from the surgery. (2) The temperature needs to be observed frequently to rule out some cause other than the inflammatory process. (3) A thorough respiratory assessment

is not indicated at this time. The respiratory rate is normal. (4) Most physicians want to make the first dressing change themselves. Until they have an order for a dressing change, nurses should only reinforce dressings.

235. **(1)** Integrated processes: nursing process — evaluation; teaching/learning; client need: health promotion and maintenance; content area: medical-surgical.

RATIONALE

(1) Cutting nails across helps prevent ingrown toenails, which could become the site of an infection for a diabetic. **(2)** Substitutions may be made within an exchange in the diet developed by the American Diabetes Association and the American Dietetic Association. **(3)** Injection sites should be rotated according to a regular schedule. **(4)** More calories from carbohydrates are needed prior to exercise in order to keep the serum glucose within normal limits.

236. **(3)** Integrated processes: nursing process — planning; caring; client need: psychosocial integrity; content area: medical-surgical.

RATIONALE

(1) The client will face the seriousness of her diagnosis when she is ready. **(2)** Encouraging her would be offering false hope. **(3)** The client will face the seriuosness of her diagnosis when she is emotionally ready. **(4)** Denial is a stage in the grieving process; a reprimand would not be appropriate.

237. **(4)** Integrated processes: nursing process — evaluation; teaching/learning; client need: physiological integrity; reduction of risk potential; content area: medical-surgical.

RATIONALE

(1) This statement is not accurate. **(2)** Radioactivity is a concern for clients receiving treatment with radioactive isotopes. **(3)** The entire body will not become radioactive. **(4)** Body fluids will be radioactive until the isotope has been eliminated from the body.

238. **(4)** Integrated processes: nursing process — implementation; client need: physiological integrity; pharmacological therapies; content area: medical-surgical.

RATIONALE

(1) To increase rate in order to make up for lost time would result in hyperglycemia. **(2)** Notifying the physician is not necessary at this time. **(3)** Running the IV at the prescribed site does not make up for the lost time. **(4)** The level of glucose needs to be known prior to taking further action.

239. **(1)** Integrated processes: nursing process — implementation; client need: physiological integrity; physiological adaptation; content area: medical-surgical.

RATIONALE

(1) Decreasing the workload on the heart is the highest priority for someone with acute congestive heart failure; thus resting mentally as well as physically would be the best goal. **(2)** The client needs both physical and mental rest. **(3)** The data do not indicate that the client is ready to train for a new job. **(4)** Decreasing the workload on the heart takes a higher priority at this time.

240. **(2)** Integrated processes: nursing process — evaluation; client need: physiological integrity; reduction of risk potential; content area: medical-surgical.

RATIONALE

(1) Ketones would be an abnormal finding. **(2)** A trace of protein in urine is normal. **(3)** No glucose should be found in urine. **(4)** Cloudy urine indicates that infection is present.

241. **(2)** Integrated processes: nursing process — data collection; client need: physiological integrity; reduction of risk potential; content area: medical-surgical.

RATIONALE

(1) Blood pressure should never be taken in an arm where a shunt is located. **(2)** Palpation of a thrill and hearing a bruit indicate that the shunt is open. **(3)** Checking for venous and arterial distention is not indicated. **(4)** The arm with a shunt is not a good place to assess for skin turgor.

242. **(1)** Integrated processes: nursing process — data collection; client need: health promotion and maintenance; content area: medical-surgical.

RATIONALE

(1) The Mantoux test may be read in 3 days and will reveal whether the tubercule bacillus has entered the client's body. **(2)** The Mantoux test needs to be done initially. A chest radiograph does not reveal whether the tubercule bacillus has entered the client's body. **(3)** The client could have tuberculosis with a sputum negative for acid-fast bacilli. **(4)** Gram stain is only a quick method of ruling out acid-fast bacilli in the sputum.

243. **(3)** Integrated processes: nursing process — implementation; client need: physiological integrity; basic care and comfort; content area: medical-surgical.

RATIONALE

(1) It is more important to allow the punctured side to heal initially by positioning the client on the unaffected side. **(2)** The client is usually positioned in a sitting position prior to the procedure to allow fluid to pool in the base of the pleural space. **(3)** Placing the client on the unaffected side allows the puncture site to close. **(4)** Positioning the client in Fowler's position is not necessary after the procedure, but may provide comfort to the client.

244. **(1)** Integrated processes: nursing process — implementation; client need: physiological integrity; reduction of risk potential; content area: medical-surgical.

RATIONALE

(1) The Pleur-evac must be kept below the level of the wound to prevent backward flow of drainage due to gravity. **(2)** The suction should not be removed for turning. **(3)** Ths is not recommended because blood could continue to collect in the pleural cavity and collapse the lung. **(4)** The sterile water should not be drained from the Pleur-evac.

245. **(3)** Integrated processes: nursing process — implementation; caring; client need: psychosocial integrity; content area: medical-surgical.

RATIONALE

(1) Exercise is important, but not the most immediate concern. **(2)** Diversion will help, but handling feelings is the most immediate concern. **(3)** One manages feelings by talking about them; time should be planned for the client to explore and share feelings. **(4)** The client may not want to socialize with different people until after feelings are managed.

246. **(4)** Integrated processes: nursing process — implementation; client need: physiological integrity; reduction of risk potential; content area: medical-surgical.

RATIONALE

(1) Postoperative complications from immobility would result. **(2)** Turning himself could result in injury to the spine. **(3)** Ordering a trapeze could result in injury to the spine. **(4)** Log-rolling every 2 hours is safe and helps prevent postoperative complications.

247. **(1)** Integrated processes: nursing process — data collection; client need: physiological integrity; reduction of risk potential; content area: medical-surgical.
     RATIONALE
     (1) Checking for allergies to the contrast medium is the most important way to prevent allergic reactions, thus protecting the kidneys and other vital organs. **(2)** A low-protein diet is not necessary. **(3)** Enemas would make the patient less hydrated. **(4)** Checking for allergies to the contrast medium is the most important way to prevent allergic reactions. The contrast medium is potentially nephrotoxic.

248. **(4)** Integrated processes: nursing process — implementation; client need: physiological integrity; reduction of risk potential; content area: medical-surgical.
     RATIONALE
     (1) Intramuscular injections could initiate hemorrhage. **(2)** Massaging injection sites would encourage bleeding. **(3)** Firm toothbrushes and vigorous flossing could cause bleeding. **(4)** Rectal procedures could initiate hemorrhage.

249. **(1)** Integrated processes: nursing process — evaluation; teaching/learning; client need: physiological integrity; basic care and comfort; content area: medical-surgical.
     RATIONALE
     (1) Potassium will be lost in the stools and should be replaced. **(2)** Many people with diarrhea are allergic to lactose in milk or milk products. **(3)** A healthy diet is rich in fiber. People with diarrhea should have a low-residue diet, which is low in fiber. **(4)** Drinks containing caffeine could make diarrhea worse.

250. **(2)** Integrated processes: nursing process — implementation; client need: physiological integrity; reduction of risk potential; content area: medical-surgical.
     RATIONALE
     (1) Antiemetics should be administered 30 minutes before meals to give them a chance to take effect. **(2)** Fluid imbalance could easily result from nausea and vomiting; therefore, it is important to monitor fluid intake and output. **(3)** Foods cold or at room temperature are usually better tolerated. **(4)** Stimuli should be minimized in order to decrease the chances of stimulating the center for nausea and vomiting.

CHAPTER 6

Nursing Care of the Older Adult: Content Review and Test

Kathleen R. Culliton, RN, CS, MS, GNP
Golden M. Tradewell, RN, PhD

I. Facts about older people
  A. The population of older adults is the fastest growing segment of the U.S. population.
  B. More than 13% of the population is >65 years old.
  C. Older adults consume >70% of health-care services.
  D. Older adults commonly suffer from one or more chronic diseases requiring long-term treatment and life changes.
  E. Most of the older population live in the community.
  F. Only 5% of the people >65 years old live in long-term care facilities (nursing facilities).
  G. Forty percent of the residents in nursing facilities are >85 years old.
II. Beliefs about aging
  A. Society often discriminates against older people because of the value it places on youth, appearance, work performance, and functional independence.
  B. Television, greeting cards, and advertisements often portray a negative image of older people and aging.
  C. Many false beliefs about aging exist that can have an impact on the health care that an older person receives (Table 6–1).
III. Ethnicity and health-care beliefs
  A. Ethnic minority elders are more likely to
    1. Live in poverty
    2. Have a shorter life expectancy

Table 6–1. False Beliefs about Aging

All old people are sick.
All old people are alike.
All old people are senile.
Most old people are in nursing homes.
All old people are depressed.
Nurses who are not good enough to work in hospitals work in nursing homes.

    3. Experience debilitating disease processes or functional disability at a higher rate and at an earlier age.
    4. Have difficulty accessing health-care services
  B. Older adults need to be assessed within their personal cultural context
  C. American Indians/Alaskan Natives
    1. Live primarily in tribes.
    2. Many practice acute care only.
    3. Use herbs, corn, dances, and prayers to cure and balance life forces with nature.
    4. Combine Western medicine with traditional practices.
    5. Have a fear of witchcraft.
    6. Inanimate objects are believed to ward off evil.
    7. Theology and medicine are interwoven.
    8. Promote harmony with nature.
    9. Pain is something to be endured.
    10. Sick role is not usually supported.
  D. European Americans
    1. Believe humans can control nature.
    2. Have strong belief and value in technology.
    3. Practice primary acute care practices, but recent trend is moving towards prevention.
    4. Value individual responsibility for health.
    5. May use folk remedies or over-the-counter medicines before seeing a health-care practitioner.
    6. Use prayers and religious symbols for good health.
    7. Have controlled expression of pain.
    8. Need little encouragement for pain relief.
    9. Sick role not well accepted except with a major illness.
  E. African Americans/Blacks
    1. Large ethnic group—comprises 12.3% of the population.
    2. Believe diseases may be natural, caused by cold or bad air, food, or water.
    3. Believe diseases may be unnatural, caused by voodoo, witchcraft, or a hex.

4. Believe serious illness may be sent from God.
5. May resist preventive care because illness is God's will.
6. Folk and herbal medicine prevalent.
7. Use prayers for prevention and health recovery.
8. Pain is seen as a sign of illness.
9. Sick role not seen as a burden.

F. Spanish/Hispanics/Latinos
1. Large ethnic group—comprises 12.5% of the United States.
2. 90% live in cities.
3. Health beliefs strongly affected by religion.
4. Believe health and illness largely God's will.
5. May have shrines or statutes in the home to pray for good health.
6. Frequently use over-the-counter medicines and medicines brought from home country.
7. Theory of hot and cold foods used for health maintenance and treatment of disease.
8. Many are fearful and suspicious of hospitals.
9. Expressive with pain.
10. Easily enter the sick role.
11. Primarily receive acute care with little prevention.
12. Believe children and women are more susceptible to the evil eye.

G. Asians
1. The term "Asians" includes 32 different groups.
2. Good health is a gift from ancestors.
3. Imbalances in the yin and yang cause illness.
4. Believe blood is the source of life and is not replenished.
5. Amulets are worn to ward off disease.
6. Cleanliness is highly valued.

7. Prayers are used for healing.
8. Over-the-counter medicine use is common.
9. Use of herbal tea and medicine is common.
10. Commonly stoic with pain.
11. Many delay seeking help until very ill.

H. Arab Americans
1. Primarily receive acute care with little prevention.
2. Little responsibility for self-care.
3. Pray five times each day for health.
4. Combine prayers with meditation.
5. Freely use over-the-counter medication.
6. Illness is a punishment for sins.
7. Considered rude and cruel to communicate a grave diagnosis.
8. Organs may be purchased for transplantation.
9. Will display overt expression of pain.
10. Sick dependency role readily accepted.
11. Injections preferred over pills.

I. Appalachians
1. Prayer is a primary source of strength.
2. Believe good health is largely a result of God's will.
3. Biomedical care may be used as a last resort.
4. Use many folk remedies, primarily passed on by "granny" practitioners who use poultices, herbs, and teas.
5. Self-medicate first before seeking a biomedical practitioner.
6. A major health concern is the state of the blood.

IV. Loss related to aging
A. Physical changes of aging (Table 6–2)
1. All body systems are affected by the aging process.
2. It is often difficult to differentiate the normal process of physical aging from disease processes.

Table 6–2. Physical Changes: Implications of Normal Physiological Aging

Age-Related Changes by Body System	Impact on Functional Ability	Nursing Interventions to Promote Function and Decrease Disability
Vision Dry eyes ↓ Macular acuity ↑Lens size Lens yellowed ↓ Upper gaze	Increased risk of falling Increased risk of making errors in taking medications	Provide artificial tears as needed. Increase lighting. Color-code medications using reds and yellows. Use medication dosage boxes. Organize furniture, avoid clutter. Encourage eye exams and glasses.
Hearing ↓ Function of cochlear ↓ Movement of ossicles	Decreased ability to hear spoken words Increased risk of confusion	Speak clearly but do not shout. Maintain eye contact when giving instructions. Check batteries on hearing aid. Repeat instructions. Perform audiology exam.
Smell ↓ Acuity	Inability to smell smoke	Smoke detector: instruct what to do in a fire emergency.
Taste ↓ Number of taste buds	Potential weight loss	Visually stimulate appetite. Use spices to enhance food flavor.

(Continued on following page)

Age-Related Changes by Body System	Impact on Functional Ability	Nursing Interventions to Promote Function and Decrease Disability
Neurological ↓ Reaction time Mild short-term memory loss	Frustration with forgetfulness Increased errors when rushed	Reassure and allow time to remember and perform tasks. Use memory aids (calendars, pill-reminder boxes).
Respiratory Kyphosis ↓ Alveoli ↑ Inelastic tissue ↑ Dead air space	Decreased tolerance of activity	Evaluate tolerance of activity without shortness of breath. Encourage rest periods. Teach deep-breathing exercises.
Cardiovascular ↓ Vessel elasticity ↑ Peripheral resistance ↓ Stroke volume Thickening of heart valves	Increased risk of falls related to orthostatic hypertension Decreased response to exercise and stress	Assess blood pressure in lying, sitting, and standing positions. Encourage to stop between position changes and report if feeling dizzy. Encourage regular exercise and stress-reduction techniques.

Digestive
↓ Saliva
Gum atrophy
↓ Metabolism
Slowed stomach emptying
↓ Intestinal motility
Slowed absorption
	Potential decreased food intake, weight loss
	Potential adverse drug effects with ↓ metabolism
	Potential constipation
		Encourage regular dental exams.
		Make sure that dentures are in good repair.
		Food should be appropriate for dentition.
		Fluid intake is at least 1500 ml.
		Monitor drug effects.
		Prevent constipation through:
		    Fluid intake
		    Dietary fiber, bulk
		    Exercise

Urinary ↓ Renal blood flow ↓ Filtration rate ↓ Urge feeling	Potential adverse drug reactions with ↓ excretion Potential incontinence	Monitor effects of drugs. Maintain good fluid intake. Monitor urine output. Encourage regular toileting (toilet before leaving room, going to activities, and going to bed). Provide bladder training.
Muscular ↓ Muscle strength ↓ Muscle mass	Potential for decreased mobility	Provide full ROM exercises. Maintain physical exercise and activity (use least restrictive assistance).
Skeletal Bone loss Cartilage thinning Kyphosis	Potential for falls and fractures	Encourage weight bearing. Assist in ambulating with assistive devices (cane, walker). Monitor gait, balance, and transfer ability.
Skin Thinning of skin and hair Loss of subcutaneous fat ↓ Sweat Fragile blood vessels	Increased risk of bruises and skin tears Slowed wound healing	Use soap on skin minimally. Use nonscented creams and lotions. Monitor for skin breakdown and wound healing. Use a gait belt. Do not grab skin areas during transfers.

    3. Healthy lifestyle choices regarding diet, exercise, chemical exposure, stress management, and genetic exploration may change or slow the normal aging process.
  B. Social changes of aging
    1. Role changes
      a. Retirement can be a stressful life change if not thought out and planned.
      b. Widowhood can lead to loneliness and isolation.

      c. Acting as caregiver to a spouse may be a stressful burden.
      d. Moving out of one's home and into an apartment or health-care facility often means leaving social contacts, family, and valued responsibilities, which can be stressful.
      e. Loss of income or having a low income may place older adults in situations in which they have to choose among eating, buying medications, and maintaining their living situation.

C. Factors associated with loss
 1. Older adults may have problems with loneliness in response to multiple losses.
  a. Encourage socialization through community groups, senior centers, senior volunteer opportunities, shared living situations, and pets.
  b. Identify social support network of family, friends, and neighbors.
 2. Depression is common in older adults who have experienced multiple losses, such as loss of spouse, disability, social isolation, loneliness, and inability to function in previous roles.
  a. Be alert for signs of potential suicide: expressing hopelessness, giving things away, saying good-bye to friends and family, and having a plan for taking one's life.
  b. Refer client to professional counseling or crisis management.
 3. Older people often fear dependence more than they fear death.
  a. Encourage them to talk about their views and beliefs about death.
  b. Encourage future planning using living wills, estate planning, and funeral planning so client's wishes are made known.
V. Ethics and aging
 A. Social policy issues
  1. Informed consent
   a. Client or resident has the basic right to information that will allow him or her to make appropriate choices for care.
   b. When informed, the older adult has the right to refuse care.
   c. Informed consent implies that the older adult has received complete information regarding the type of procedure being done, potential complications, expected outcomes, and alternatives to the procedure.
   d. Licensed practical nurses (LPNs) often sign as witnesses to the older person's signature, implying that the person was competent (mentally able to understand and give consent), that the person was not coerced into signing, and that his or her signature was valid.
   e. Family members and others can sign consent forms if they have legal guardianship or power of attorney related to health care.
  2. Living will (advanced directives)
   a. Older people may choose to make their wishes known regarding the type and amount of treatments and care they want to receive if they are found to be terminally ill.
   b. Some states recognize a living will as a legal expression of the person's wishes.
   c. Because living wills serve only as a general guideline for care, dilemmas regarding what the older person would really want done in a specific care situation may develop.
 B. Family and family caregiver issues
  1. Caregiver burden
   a. Family caregiving can be a stressful and negative experience, as well as a rewarding and positive experience.

b. Stress is related to the amount of care required, past relationship with the frail relative, financial burden, and change in the caregiver's and family's lifestyle.
c. Support for family caregivers is provided through caregiver support groups, in-home respite care volunteers, and community-based respite and adult daycare centers.
 2. Elder abuse
  a. Elder abuse is an increasing problem, with victims most often being dependent, isolated, and frail older adults.
  b. Clues that nurses need to be aware of as indicating possible abuse include malnutrition, dehydration, bruises, fractures, pressure ulcers, burns, overmedication, cuts, scratches, and bite marks.
  c. Adult protective services should be notified of any suspected abuse situations.

Common Nursing Care Issues of Older Adults (Table 6–3)

LPNs are nursing care providers for older adults in the community, hospitals, and nursing facilities. Their primary role is assisting older adults to achieve their highest functional ability through chronic disease management, rehabilitation, and promoting function through nursing interventions. Knowledge of medical-surgical nursing practice and of the common problems associated with aging enables the nurse to fulfill this role.

Table 6–3. **Common Problems of Older Adults and Related Nursing Diagnoses**	
Problem	**Related Nursing Diagnoses**
Confusion (delirium and dementia)	Potential for injury Impaired verbal communication Impaired social interaction Social isolation Altered role performance Altered family processes Altered sexuality patterns Sleep pattern disturbance Self-care deficit Altered thought process Potential for violence Anxiety
Altered communication	Impaired verbal communication Impaired social interaction Sensory and perceptual alterations
Functional ability	Potential for injury Altered sexual patterns Impaired physical mobility Activity intolerance Diversion activity deficit Impaired home maintenance management Self-care deficit

(Continued on following page)

Problem	Related Nursing Diagnoses
	Body image disturbance Self-esteem disturbance Unilateral neglect
Bowel problems	Constipation Perceived constipation Diarrhea Bowel incontinence
Urinary dysfunction	Altered patterns of urinary elimination Urinary retention Incontinence (stress, reflex, urge, functional, or total)
Skin breakdown	Potential for infection Impaired skin integrity
Nutritional problems	Altered nutrition: more or less than body requirements Fluid volume deficit or excess Altered oral mucous membrane Feeding self-care deficit Impaired swallowing
Altered mood and behavior	Impaired social interaction Spiritual distress Ineffective individual coping Impaired adjustment Altered thought process Potential for violence Anxiety Fear
Chemical and physical restraints	Altered nutrition: less than body requirements Altered patterns of urinary elimination Diarrhea Potential fluid volume deficit Potential for injury Potential for poisoning Impaired social interaction Impaired physical mobility Sleep disturbance Self-care deficit

Confusion

I. Not a disease per se but often a symptom of an underlying problem or disease process; two types being delirium and dementia.
  A. Delirium: confusion related to a specific cause, such as medications, infection, distended bladder, fecal impaction, pain, or change in environment
    1. Related medical diagnoses
      a. Infection
      b. Fever
      c. Dehydration
      d. Circulatory, respiratory, or metabolic diseases
    2. Data collection
      a. Sudden onset, commonly at night
      b. Memory, alertness, and thinking ability changes through the day
      c. Misinterpretation of environment and care
      d. Sleepiness during the day, wakefulness at night
      e. Mood swings and agitated pacing or fidgeting
      f. Hallucinations and delusions

3. Implementation
  a. Identify cause and initiate treatment for full recovery.
  b. Often all medications are stopped, as they are a common cause of delirium.
  c. Ensure safety by close nursing supervision, possibly even one-on-one supervision.
  d. Decrease environmental stimuli such as noise, too-bright or too-dim lighting, and number of people in care area.
  e. Develop a toilet-training program.
  f. Assess for fecal impaction.
  g. Orient client to environment.
    1) Open blinds so client can look out of the window.
    2) Encourage sitting up in chair and ambulating during the day.
    3) Dress client in his or her own clothes.
    4) Place calendars and clocks in the room.
    5) Encourage family members to visit.
  h. Treat symptoms of pain.
  i. Talk in soft, reassuring tones, using simple commands and questions.
  j. Use physical and chemical restraint only if other care approaches have not worked.
B. Dementia: irreversible progressive loss of mental functioning; can be worsened by medications, pain, bowel or bladder distention, infections, physical restraints, changes in environment or environmental stimuli; most often accompanied by problem behaviors
  1. Related medical diagnoses
    a. Delirium
    b. Alzheimer's disease
    c. Multi-infarct dementia
  2. Data collection
    a. Onset usually over months or years
    b. Usually gradual steady loss of memory over time
    c. Often denial of memory problems and made-up responses to mask memory problems
    d. Identification of problems and seeking of medical care by family members rather than by client
    e. Deterioration of skills related to work, finances, and social behavior before functional ability
    f. Client generally healthy and lacking underlying disease processes
  3. Implementation
    a. Rule out any reversible cause for the change in mental functioning, such as causes of delirium.
    b. Approaches to problem behaviors are found in Table 6–4.
    c. Reassure client and orient to environment.
    d. Support family members and caregivers.
      1) Provide information about Alzheimer's disease.
      2) Refer to caregiver support groups and the Alzheimer's association.
      3) Discuss respite care and adult daycare.
      4) Discuss nursing home placement.
C. Physical and chemical restraints (see Chapter 7)
  1. Physical and chemical restraints have often been used to manage problem behaviors—especially with confused or mentally ill older adults.

Table 6–4. Approaches to Problem Behaviors

Problem Behavior	Intervention
Striking out or hitting	Prevention the best intervention
Yelling and swearing	Positive and receptive attitude
Sexual aggression	Environment 　Decrease noise level and room temperature; adjust lighting to decrease glare and maximize vision; decrease clutter and crowding, do not change room arrangements. Consistent daily routine Cues for orientation (clock, calendar) Diversional activities 　Walking, soft music, snack or drink, moving to another area or room, one-on-one talking
Constant requests or cries for help	Encouraging involvement in activities One-on-one visits with staff and volunteers Offering real choices in care Pet therapy Scheduling times for nursing interventions
Refusal to eat	Offering food and fluid choices Allowing choices of where to eat meals, time to eat, and amount of food desired Finger foods or "carry-along" foods for clients who do not sit down long enough to finish meal Small meals, with between-meal snacks Record of intake and weight daily
Refusal to perform personal hygiene	Minimizing confusion by breaking down tasks into specific instructions (task segmentation) 　*Example:* "Brush your teeth" changes to: 　1. Wet your toothbrush. 　2. Put toothpaste on your toothbrush. 　3. Put the toothbrush in your mouth. 　4. Brush up and down. 　5. Take a drink of water. 　6. Swish and spit. 　7. Rinse your toothbrush. Allowing choices such as when to bathe and type of bath desired, what to wear, whether to dress in bathroom or at bedside Leaving and requesting again later, if patient refuses Evaluating plan of care if activity is necessary at specific time or day Consistent care provider Share care 　*Example:* "You put your shirt on while I help you with your socks and shoes."
Wandering	Providing secure and safe areas to wander Closing doors to discourage going into other clients' rooms Hanging "Stop" signs or placing Velcro strips across open doorways Disguising doorways with wallpaper Placing doorknobs and latches high on the door, out of the line of vision Using door buzzers or bells that sound when door is opened Electronic beeper for client Medical alert bracelet with address and phone number and pertinent disease information Physical activities to use up energy to wander Removing clutter and other potential factors that contribute to falls Providing diversional activities: sorting tasks, laundry, music, reminiscing support groups Monitoring for toileting, hunger, pain, signs of infection

2. Recent federal and state mandates have identified the use of restraints as only a last resort when other nursing or medical interventions have failed and the client is at risk of endangering himself or herself or others.
3. Physical restraints have been related to loss of mobility, increased risk of pressure ulcers, incontinence, social isolation, falls, and deaths.
4. The use of restraints requires a physician's order.
5. All other nursing measures used to manage the problem behavior must be documented.
6. The type of restraint, when it was applied, when it was released, and the client's response to the restraint must be documented.
7. The nurse must assess skin condition and proper application of restraints.
8. Client should be toileted, given skin care, walked, and repositioned before restraint is reapplied.

9. When chemical restraints such as psychoactive drugs are used, the client must have a documented medical diagnosis that fits the drug being used.
   a. Sedatives: documented insomnia
   b. Psychotropics: psychotic behavior, hallucinations
10. Most agencies require that a consent form related to restraint use be signed by the client or guardian.
11. Alternatives to restraints
   a. Increased involvement in appropriate activities
   b. Involvement of family and volunteers
   c. Initiation of behavioral approaches (Table 6–4)
   d. Secure environment
   e. Wedge cushions and postural supports
   f. Use of reclining chairs
   g. Decreasing clutter and confusion in the environment

Communication Problems

I. Altered visual function
   A. Related medical diagnoses
      1. Diabetes
      2. Cataracts
      3. Glaucoma
      4. Macular degeneration
      5. Dry eyes
      6. Eye surgery
   B. Data collection
      1. Complaints of inability to see
      2. Unsteady ambulation; holding onto furniture, walls, and door frames when walking
      3. Isolation, refusing to leave room
      4. Wearing of mismatched or soiled clothing
      5. Making mistakes in taking medications
      6. Lack of eye contact
   C. Implementation
      1. Promote function and minimize disability.
      2. Encourage regular eye examinations and updating of glasses.
      3. Encourage use of visual aids: magnifying glass, page magnifier.
      4. Refer to agencies that support the blind.
      5. Recommend use of tape recorders, dictation machines, and tape players for letter dictating; "talking books"; and music activities.
      6. Organize room and belongings so client can find things easily and risk of falling will be minimized.
      7. Assist in clothing selection.
      8. Provide large color cues rather than written instructions to identify medications.
      9. Place medications in different-sized bottles or use medication box to assist in medication identification.
II. Communication
   A. Related medical diagnoses
      1. Alzheimer's disease
      2. Cerebrovascular accident (CVA)
      3. Parkinson's disease
      4. Deafness or hearing impairment
   B. Data collection
      1. Slurred or difficult to understand speech
      2. No verbalization or making repetitive sounds
      3. "Word salad"; use of words that do not make sense
      4. Inability to respond to commands or sounds
      5. Use of hearing aid
   C. Implementation
      1. Use hearing aid in working condition with battery.
      2. Encourage client to wear hearing aid.
      3. Use word or picture board so client can point out requests.
      4. Ask client to restate communication to ensure that message was received.
      5. Break complex tasks and commands into smaller parts.
      6. Reassure clients when they become frustrated with inability to speak or communicate.

Functional Ability and Rehabilitation Potential

I. Functional ability
   A. Related medical diagnoses
      1. Hip, wrist, and vertebral fractures
      2. Paralysis
      3. CVA
      4. Arthritis
      5. Alzheimer's disease and other dementias
   B. Data collection
      1. Inability to ambulate, transfer, bathe, toilet, eat, or perform personal care independently
      2. Unkempt appearance
      3. Isolation
      4. Skin breakdown
      5. Malnourishment and dehydration
   C. Implementation
      1. Set rehabilitative goals:
         a. To restore function to maximum self-sufficiency
         b. To replace assistance with task segmentation and verbal cuing
         c. To restore ability to support client function with fewer supports
         d. To shorten time required to provide assistance
         e. To expand the space in which self-sufficiency can be practiced
         f. To avoid or delay additional loss of independence
         g. To support the client who is certain to decline in order to lessen the likelihood of complications
      2. Select clothing that is easier to dress in (jogging suits, slip-on shoes, two-piece underwear).
      3. Help resident to use assistive devices that reduce energy expenditure and promote independence in dressing (garter ropes to pull on socks, rigid sock sleeve).
      4. Ask client to identify things that may support independence in dressing, grooming, bathing, toileting, transfers, ambulation, and eating.
      5. Encourage strengthening exercises for weakened muscle groups that client can do independently or with assistance.

6. Instruct in use of ambulation and mobility aids (walker, cane, wheelchair).
7. Encourage client to ambulate to and from activities and meals.
8. Monitor respiratory rate, pulse rate, and BP with increase in client's activity and any complaints of exhaustion.
9. Make home visits to assess appropriateness of discharge to the home environment and to instruct or recommend changes to family members (number of steps; main-floor bathroom; doorways and rooms that will accommodate walker or wheelchair).
10. Allow client and family to verbalize concerns about discharge and ability to meet functional needs.
11. Discuss slower recovery time from major illness associated with aging.

II. Falls
A. Related medical diagnoses
1. Hip fracture and vertebral fractures
2. Paralysis
3. CVA
4. Arthritis
5. Alzheimer's disease and other dementias
6. Orthostatic hypotension
7. Peripheral neuropathy
B. Data collection
1. Reduced hearing or vision or both
2. Dizziness or syncope
3. Impaired balance
4. Confusion
5. Impaired physical mobility
6. Orthostatic hypotension
7. Use of psychoactive (sedating) drugs
8. Use of diuretics, antihypertensives, anticonvulsants, cardiac antiarrhythmics, and alcohol
9. History of falls
C. Implementation
1. Assess medications for appropriate dosages and dosage times.
2. Consult with physician for medication-reduction strategy.
3. Living area is free of clutter.
4. Railings and grab bars are available in halls, stairwells, and bathrooms.
5. Bed is in low position.
6. Call signal is within easy reach at all times.
7. Personal items are within safe reach (water, television controls, radio, phone, comb, toothbrush, reading material).
8. Well-lighted rooms and night lights are available.
9. Nonskid floor surfaces are available.
10. Insruct client to move from lying to sitting to standing positions, slowly pausing at each position change.
11. Electronic bed or chair alarms are available.
12. Self-releasing seatbelts are available when client sits up in chair (if client can release them independently, they are not restraints).

13. Siderails and chest or belt restraints are available in chair and bed with a physician's order; be careful of their use, as it may lead to agitation, decreased mobility, incontinence, and skin breakdown.
14. Keep wheelchairs locked during transfers.
15. A bedside commode is present.
16. Elevated toilet seats and high-seated chairs are available.

III. Urinary incontinence; indwelling catheter
A. Related medical diagnoses
1. Fecal impaction
2. Atrophic vaginitis
3. Prostatic hypertrophy
4. Urinary tract infection (UTI)
5. Dehydration
6. Use of diuretics or psychoactive drugs
7. Alzheimer's disease or other dementias
B. Data collection
1. Inability to recognize and/or respond to the urge to void
2. Loss of urine
3. Inability to get to the toilet in time to void
4. Foul-smelling urine
5. Small amounts of concentrated urine
C. Implementation
1. Document an incontinence record to identify times or patterns of incontinence.
2. Perform urine culture to rule out UTI.
3. Perform a rectal check to assess for fecal impaction.
4. Monitor fluid intake, and encourage 1500–3000 mL of fluid per 24 hours.
5. Identify most appropriate method for toileting.
6. Toilet every 2 hours, or as appropriate for client's pattern of incontinence.
7. Monitor urine characteristics.
8. Urinary indwelling catheters are indicated only when a client is documented to be terminally ill, has stage 3 or 4 buttocks or coccygeal skin breakdown, or has no spontaneous voiding.

IV. Nutritional status
A. Factors related to nutritional problems
1. Physiological factors
a. Aging process
b. Chronic diseases
1) Diabetes mellitus
2) CVA, chronic obstructive pulmonary disease (COPD), alcoholism
3) Alzheimer's disease and other dementias
4) Nutrient deficiencies (iron, vitamin B_{12}, protein, caloric)
c. Side effects of medical treatment
d. Functional status
2. Psychosocial factors
a. Social interaction
b. Long-established food habits
c. Mental status and behavior
d. Financial need
3. Environmental factors
a. Dining room atmosphere

b. Staffing during meal times
c. Food preparation and serving
d. Alternatives to meals being served

B. Data collection
1. Loss of teeth or gum disease
2. Poorly fitting dentures
3. Refusal to eat
4. Eating <75% of meals
5. Refusal to eat in public dining area
6. Weight loss

C. Implementation
1. Provide meals with texture and appearance that are pleasing to the client yet are appropriate to the client's chewing and swallowing ability.
2. Promote a pleasant dining room environment.
3. Offer alternatives to clients who do not finish at least 75% of their meals.
4. Provide between-meal nutritional supplements.
5. Use universal cuffs and utensils with built-up handles to promote independence in feeding.
6. Allow client the opportunity to feed himself or herself before you feed him or her.
7. Encourage finger foods that may allow independence in feeding.
8. Allow client to choose foods.
9. Provide feeding tubes for clients with severely compromised nutritional status. Monitor for
   a. Aspiration and respiratory distress
   b. Placement of tube and potential dysfunction
   c. Nasal irritation
   d. Distended abdomen
   e. Gastric ulcers or hemorrhage
   f. Pain
   g. Client pulling tube out

V. Dehydration, fluid maintenance
A. Related medical diagnoses
1. Alzheimer's disease and other dementias
2. Diabetes mellitus, COPD
3. Terminal disease (cancer)
4. Urinary incontinence

B. Data collection
1. Confusion
2. Weakness
3. Poor skin turgor
4. Dry mouth, tongue, and skin
5. Concentrated urine, low urine output
6. Poor fluid intake to control incontinence

C. Implementation
1. Explain necessity of 2000–3000 ml of fluid intake a day.
2. Increase amount of fluid served with meals.
3. Give 8 oz of fluid with medications.
4. Provide water pitcher and glass at bedside.
5. Assist functionally disabled clients to drink recommended amount of fluid daily.
6. Monitor fluid intake and urinary output.

VI. Pressure ulcers
A. Related medical diagnoses and risk factors
1. Hip, wrist, and vertebral fractures
2. Paralysis, arthritis, CVA, Parkinson's disease
3. Alzheimer's disease and other dementias

4. Diabetes mellitus
5. Spasms and contracture
6. Incontinence
7. Pressure, shear, moisture, and friction
8. Terminal disease

B. Data collection
1. Areas of redness or open wounds over areas of pressure
2. Coccyx, hip, heel, and buttocks the most common areas for pressure ulcers
3. Low serum albumin level, Hgb or Hct

C. Implementation
1. Prevention is the key to treatment because pressure ulcers are very difficult to heal.
2. Turn and reposition client every 2 hours or more when in bed and even when sitting up in chair.
3. Instruct client to do small weight shifts that can change pressure over bony areas.
4. Keep skin dry and immediately remove any urine and feces from skin.
5. Do not massage reddened area of skin, as it may further traumatize or even break down the fragile capillary system under the skin.
6. Monitor and document size of wound, signs of healing, any drainage or odor, and type of treatment used.
7. Follow Agency for Health Care Policy and Research protocol.

VII. Home Health Tips
A. Schedule therapy visits and nurse visits on same day, to decrease fatiguing older adult.
B. Be aware that older persons keep their homes warm.
C. Restate your name and why you are there. Older adults forget easier.
D. Ask older client to visit in a quiet room.
E. Limit visitors or family with colds to prevent illness for the older adult.
F. Identify stressors for those older adults who live alone and report to home-care team.
G. Ask older person to take deep breaths in and out through the mouth.
H. Assess older adult's sleeping habits. Recommend ear plugs, check medications for side effects, and encourage a 15- to 30-minute nap in the early afternoon.
I. One of the first signs of infection is confusion.
J. One of the first signs of dehydration is tachycardia. Instruct on proper hydration.
K. Assess environment for safety hazards on each visit and promote safety.
L. Assess if client has dentures and how they are or are not worn.
M. Check refrigerator for outdated food to decrease food poisoning.
N. Encourage the uses of spices and herbs, such as parsley, oregano, lemon, garlic, and basil, instead of salt and sugar.
O. Encourage keeping pared apples and slices of oranges in the refrigerator for snacks.

P. Ask the older adult if he would like to be have Meals on Wheels to deliver home-cooked food.

Q. Use a warming tray when feeding an older client who takes a longer time to eat.

R. When swallowing is difficult, freezing liquids helps, so they can be eaten with a spoon or like a popsicle. Milkshakes, high-protein drinks, instant breakfast mix, or eggnog are thicker liquids that are easier to swallow.

S. Assess the degree of incontinency or amount of output by inquiring how many pads or adult briefs have been used.

T. If voiding, have older adult keep a voiding diary to assess further the degree of incontinence.

U. Suggest a bedside commode when a weakened older client is on diuretics or has a history of falling or confusion.

V. Place the bedside commode next to the bed at night to reduce the risk of falls and to ease caregiver's burden.

W. If older client reports constipation, review the diet and make suggestions regarding adequate fluid and fiber.

X. Discourage the use of mineral oil because it can make vitamins less effective.

Y. When drawing blood from the hand of an older client, use the smallest needle possible.

Z. Hold light pressure for at least 2 minutes after the needle is removed. Do not use Band-Aid on the fragile skin of the older client if the bleeding has stopped with pressure.

AA. When teaching, it is important to acknowledge the client's knowledge and life experiences. Teaching should occur with clients, not to them. Client dignity should always remain intact during home care visits and teaching sessions.

QUESTIONS

Kathleen R. Culliton, RN, CS, MS, GNP, and Golden M. Tradewell, RN, PhD

1. The nurse is assessing the client's forgetfulness to determine reversible and irreversible causes. Irreversible causes may be either Alzheimer's disease (dementia Alzheimer's type, DAT) or acquired immune deficiency syndrome (AIDS) dementia. The distinguishing characteristic betwee DAT and AIDS dementia is that in DAT:

   1. The client experiences aphasia but no definite neurological findings.
   2. The client experiences lethargy and a pronouned loss of weight.
   3. The client experiences peripheral neuropathies in all extremities.
   4. The client experiences leg weakness and tremors in all extremities.

2. The evening PN nurse for a large nursing home facility reports to the director of nursing that two clients who have recently been admitted are displaying sexual expression and signs of intimacy to each other in public areas. Both clients are recovering from a hip fracture and are receiving physical therapy. What action by the director is the most important at this time?

   1. Make arrangements for one of the clients to be moved to a different section of the nursing home.
   2. Call the family members and inform them to talk with their relatives about this recent behavior change.
   3. Perform a thorough sexual assessment on both clients including tests for sexually transmitted disease.
   4. Call a nursing conference to discuss the feelings, attitudes, and concerns of the staff members.

3. The nurse is caring for an 80-year-old client who is aphasic. The most common cause of asphasia in older adults is:

   1. Malignant brain tumors
   2. Cardiovascular accident (CVA)
   3. Head trauma
   4. Major depressive disorder

4. A 67-year-old woman reports to the nurse that she is experiencing stress incontinence. The nurse recognizes that the most common cause of stress incontinence in women is the result of:

   1. Stress brought on by menopause
   2. Pelvic floor relaxation
   3. Urinary tract infections
   4. Normal aging changes

5. The client reports feeling embarrassed by dampness due to stress incontinence. She reports that she wears a pad for protection, but always fears that others are aware of a smell. The client asks the nurse for information about treatment of stress incontinence. The nurse correctly informs the client that treatment for stress incontinence is:

   1. Behavior modification and psychological counseling
   2. Frequent change of pads and bathing twice a day
   3. Elective and depends upon the severity of the symptoms
   4. A complex surgical procedure to restore bladder support

6. The client is placed on propantheline (Pro-Banthine) 15 mg tid. Before administration of this medication, the nurse should assess:

   1. Whether the client has urinary retention
   2. Whether the client has diabetes mellitus
   3. Whether the client has a urinary tract infection
   4. Whether the client is currently on antibiotics

7. The nurse is providing instruction to the client regarding the side effects of propantheline (Pro-Banthine). Which problem should the client be instructed to report immediately to the physican?

   1. Nasal draining with enlarged lymph nodes
   2. Blurred vision with dilated pupils
   3. Dizziness when rising from a sitting position
   4. Inability to focus on near objects

8. Which statement made by the client would indicate to the nurse that the client has adequate knowledge of the cautions to be taken while on propantheline (Pro-Banthine)?

   1. "Even though I don't like green vegetables, I'll eat them."
   2. "I know I should not work in my garden on very hot days."
   3. "I know I should walk briskly for 30 minutes each day."
   4. "I know I should avoid caffeine, wine, and aged cheese."

9. A nurse is talking with a client who is being referred for a cystometrogram (CMG). The nurse instructs the client that the purpose of this procedure is to assess:

   1. The ability of the bladder to empty effectively
   2. The ability of the urethral sphincters to contract
   3. The ability of the bladder to fill and store urine
   4. The ability of the renal system to filter waste

10. A 72-year-old client is diagnosed with functional incontinence. This disorder would most likely be a result of:

    1. A cognitive deficit
    2. A peripheral field deficit
    3. A CVA
    4. A trauma to the brain

11. During a home health visit, the nurse notes a large damp spot on the clothing of a 73-year-old client. She

suspects the client may be experiencing incontinence. The client has never discussed this as a problem, but on questioning, the client indicates that these episodes have been occurring for 5 or 6 months. The nurse recognizes that the reason the client has not discussed the problem of incontinence is:

1. The client is experiencing a mild cognitive impairment.
2. The client feels discomfort and distress because of incontinence.
3. The client feels this is a normal consequence of aging.
4. The client fears placement in a long-term care facility.

12. The home health nurse is providing dietary teaching to a client with continuous ambulatory peritoneal dialysis (CAPD). The nurse instructs the client to:

1. Limit potassium-rich foods such as fruits and vegetables.
2. Limit sodium-rich foods such as kale and collard greens.
3. Limit phosphorus-rich foods such as nuts and legumes.
4. Limit protein-rich foods such as beef and chicken.

13. A nursing home client is being seen by the nurse for vague complaints of constipation. The client related numerous bouts of constipation and states, "I just don't seem to feel the urge to have a bowel movement anymore." Based on this verbal statement by the client, the nurse would investigate further to identify the possible cause of constipation as:

1. An early-stage cognitive impairment
2. A sensory neurogenic dysfunction
3. A motor neurogenic dysfunction
4. An adverse reaction of a medication

14. The client is prescribed docusate sodium (Colace) for constipation. The nurse recognizes that this type of laxative acts by:

1. Retaining and increasing water content of feces by osmotic qualities
2. Absorbing water and increasing the volume of intestinal contents
3. Increasing peristalsis in the colon by irritating nerve endings in the mucosa
4. Dispersing wetting agents and producing a soft homogeneous mixture

15. The nurse is preparing medications for a group of clients who are experiencing constipation. The physician has ordered milk of magnesia 15 mL at 8 AM. For which of the following clients would the nurse question this order?

1. A client recovering from pneumonia
2. A client recovering from arthroplasty
3. A client with end-stage renal disease
4. A client with a history of fecal impaction

16. The nurse is evaluting the bowel management program that has been implemented for 3 months. Which of the following outcomes best indicates to the nurse that the program is successful?

1. Fecal impaction decreased by 50%.
2. Bowel accidents decreased by 50%.
3. Feces occur regularly and are soft and well-formed.
4. Skin integrity is maintained and old decubitus ulcers are healed.

17. The nurse is caring for a client with neurogenic fecal incontinence. The most common cause of this dysfunction is:

1. Surgical trauma to the sphincter
2. Multiple sclerosis or spinal cord lesions
3. Psychiatric or behavioral disorders
4. Habitual use of laxatives or enemas

18. A nurse in the community has been asked for a resource for older adults to help them improve their driving skills. The most appropriate resource identified by the nurse is:

1. The local automobile insurance company
2. The local highway patrol driving program
3. The American Association of Retired Persons
4. The American Blindness Federation

19. A nurse assigned to care for a 2-day postoperative arthroplasty client notices that the client is experiencing some confusion regarding orientation to time. Although it is spring, the client states, "I've got to go home and start my holiday cooking for Christmas." The nurse recognizes that the most likely cause of this confusion is:

1. A normal aging change
2. A reaction to the medication
3. Early signs of dementia
4. Separation from familiar surroundings

20. The physician writes an order to change the operative site dressing on a 72-hour postoperative arthroplasty client. The nursing staff correctly identifies that the most important goal in carrying out this physician's orders is:

1. The need to prevent pain
2. The need to prevent infection
3. The need to be supportive
4. The need to explain the procedure to the client

21. A postoperative arthroplasty client successfully completes the physical therapy program and is scheduled for discharge. The most important area the nurse should assess before discharge is:

1. The ability to take medications as prescribed
2. The ability to manage activities of daily living
3. Support from family and friends
4. The ability to use the ambulatory aid (walker) properly

22. The arthroplasty client is discharged on a diet for weight control. The menu most reflective of the dietary needs of the older adult would be:

1. Broiled pork chop, green peas, and cantaloupe
2. Baked ham, spinach, and banana
3. Beef liver, carrots, and orange slices
4. Fried chicken, baked potato, and strawberries

23. A nurse is planning care for the client with glaucoma. priority nursing diagnosis identified by the nurse related to this client is:
    1. Alteration in nutrition related to inability to prepare food
    2. Sensory perceptual alteration related to increased peripheral vision
    3. Potential for infection related to eye drop installation
    4. Body image alteration related to thick-lensed eyeglasses

24. A 75-year-old client reports to the home health nurse that she has been having trouble sleeping. She reports going to bed at 9 PM most evenings, but always awakens at 4 AM. She asks your advice on what she can do to sleep longer in the morning. The best response by the nurse based on knowledge of the older adult would be:
    1. Have a protein-rich snack before going to bed.
    2. Obtain a comprehensive physical examination.
    3. Have a glass of milk and a sleeping pill at bedtime.
    4. Do nothing, because this is not abnormal with age.

25. The client is being assessed for an artificial prosthesis to the right leg. In assessing the rehabilitation potential for an older adult, the nurse must:
    1. Assess the ability to use unaffected extremities.
    2. Assess the ability to follow instructions.
    3. Assess the availability of support systems.
    4. Assess whether the client will return home.

26. The client is fitted with a prosthesis. He relates to the nurse that he is experiencing pain in the right leg, which was removed. The nurse recognizes this as phantom pain. The most appropriate intervention by the nurse is:
    1. Talk with the client about past experiences to get his mind off the pain.
    2. Delay ordering of the artificial limb until the pain subsides or improves.
    3. Call the doctor for pain medication and give it liberally during periods of pain.
    4. Expedite the order for an artificial limb and encourage strengthening exercises.

27. The client becomes short of breath shortly after beginning artificial limb walking. Based on the information, the nurse would modify the care plan to include:
    1. Provide crutches during the day to conserve energy.
    2. Provide a walker during the day to conserve energy.
    3. Encourage walking more frequently for shorter periods.
    4. Discontinue all activity and place on bed rest.

28. An 87-year-old client attends a community health center during the week and receives a health screening monthly. Although he can walk with a three-prong cane, he often uses a wheelchair, especially when he is in a new environment. The client relates to the nurse that he has recently been troubled with impotence. The most appropriate nursing action at this time is to:
    1. Listen and respond empathetically.
    2. Do nothing because this is normal.
    3. Do a complete health history including medications.
    4. Refer him to a physician.

29. The client is admitted to the hospital with a diagnosis of intestinal obstruction, and initial laboratory tests and radiographs are ordered. The night nurse notices that the client has been incontinent during the night. The most likely reason for the incontinence is:
    1. Frequency due to normal aging changes
    2. The inability to get to the bathroom in time
    3. Stress related to all the medical treatments
    4. Pressure from the intestinal obstruction

30. The client has surgery to relieve the intestinal obstruction. The physician ordered gentamicin (Garamycin) 75 mg every 8 hours. The nurse notes that the client has a creatinine clearance value of 70 mL/min. The most appropriate action by the nurse would be:
    1. Give the medicines as scheduled.
    2. Do nothing because the values are within the normal limits.
    3. Hold the gentamicin and inform the physician of creatinine results.
    4. Call the laboratory to see if this is an error.

31. The nurse recognizes that monitoring the creatinine clearance level is important because it is a diagnositic indicator of:
    1. Respiratory function
    2. Cardiovascular function
    3. Renal function
    4. Gastrointestinal function

32. The client is scheduled to receive carbamazepine (Tegretol) at 9 AM. In checking the laboratory reports, the nurse notes that the client has a Tegretol level of 8 μg/mL. The action by the nurse is:
    1. Administer the Tegretol as prescribed.
    2. Call the physician before giving medications.
    3. Give a reduced dose of Tegretol.
    4. Withhold the Tegretol until the level returns to 3 μg/mL.

33. A nurse is planning care for a client with left hemisphere infarction. Which plan noted by the nurse best demonstrates her knowledge of caring for cerebrovascular accident clients?
    1. Allow client to make decisions about his care.
    2. Provide a clock and calendar to maintain orientation.
    3. Encourage involvement and attendance at unit functions.
    4. Provide a structured, consistent environment.

34. A 71-year-old client is admitted to the hospital following a fall from a ladder. Admission vital signs were BP 170/98 mm Hg, pulse 92 bpm, and respirations 22/min. In performing morning care for the client, the nurse notes a brown pigmentation around both ankles. The nurse correctly identifies this to be:

1. Suggestive of earlier elder abuse
2. Suggestive of skin change in aging
3. Suggestive of lymphatic disease
4. Suggestive of venous insufficiency

35. The client becomes extremely anxious when the physician tells him he wants to perform additional tests. The most appropriate action by the nurse at this time is:
    1. Leave the room until his anxiety decreases.
    2. Encourage him to verbalize his feelings.
    3. Tell him there is nothing to worry about.
    4. Inform the client that the doctor knows best.

36. A client is diagnosed with right-sided congestive heart failure and is placed on furosemide (Lasix) and digoxin. The symptom most reflective of right-sided congestive heart failure is:
    1. Tachypnea
    2. Pink frothy sputum
    3. Korotkoff's sounds
    4. Distended jugular veins

37. Which complaint by the client would alert the nurse to digoxin toxicity?
    1. "I have to hold on to the wall to keep from falling."
    2. "My ears are ringing."
    3. "I can't see clearly and the lights have halos."
    4. "I am itching all over."

38. Laboratory values reported this morning for the client include: serum digoxin level is 2.9 mg/mL and potassium 3.2 mEq/L. The most appropriate nursing action, based upon these laboratory values, by the nurse at this time is:
    1. Give an additional dose of digoxin.
    2. Do nothing because the digoxin level is within normal limits.
    3. Give one-half the usual dose of digoxin.
    4. Call the physician and inform him or her of the laboratory values.

39. In addition to potassium supplements, the nurse would encourage the client to choose which of the following menu items to increase potassium intake?
    1. Boiled chicken, baked potato, and dried figs
    2. Beef tips, rice, and banana
    3. Roast beef, carrots, and fresh peach
    4. Fried chicken, broccoli, and fresh pear

40. The nursing diagnosis identified for the client is hypokalemia. Early symptoms indicating hypokalemia include:
    1. Muscle weakness and weak irregular pulse
    2. Diminished deep tendon reflexes
    3. Positive Trousseau's sign
    4. Positive Chvostek's sign

41. The client experiencing memory loss has lost weight. The most appropriate plan to encourage the Alzheimer's client to eat is:
    1. Eliminate distractions from the environment.
    2. Place him in the dining room for all meals.

3. Offer a variety of nourishing foods and allow him to select.
4. Serve hot foods to stimulate appetite.

42. A 67-year-old retired engineer is diagnosed with Parkinson's disease. The nurse recognizes that this disease is:
    1. Normal in persons over the age of 65 years
    2. A neurological disorder
    3. A musculoskeletal disorder
    4. A reversible condition with medical management

43. The client is placed on carbidopa/levodopa therapy. In doing dietary counseling, the nurse correctly instructs the client to avoid:
    1. Caffeine products
    2. Foods high in fats
    3. Foods high in calories
    4. Foods containing vitamin B_6

44. In addition to carbidopa/levodopa, the client with Parkinson's disease also receives digoxin 125 mg daily, haloperidol (Haldol) 20 mg HS, and temazepam (Restoril) 25 mg HS. The client begins to experience involuntary rhythmic movements of his tongue, face, and extremities. The nurse correctly identifies that these behaviors are the result of:
    1. Carbidopa/levodopa
    2. Digoxin
    3. Restoril
    4. Haloperidol

45. A nursing diagnosis related to alteration in nutrition is developed for a client with Parkinson's disease. The plan of care most appropriate to assist the client with nutrition is:
    1. Encourage liquids when chewing.
    2. Allow the client to feed himself.
    3. Place in a upright position for meals.
    4. Ask the family to bring his favorite foods from home.

46. The client with Parkinson's disease is followed by a home health nurse. The nurse finds the family willing to learn caregiving tasks, although the wife is the primary caregiver. Which action by the nurse is important in assisting the client to remain at home?
    1. Encourage him to perform activities of daily living for himself.
    2. Assist him to communicate his needs both verbally and written.
    3. Provide for physical and emotional needs of the caregiver.
    4. Keep him actively involved in day-to-day household tasks.

47. The nurse instructs the client on the need for calcium for the prevention of osteoporosis. The client states, "I drink at least three glasses of milk each day." The nurse correctly advises:
    1. That three glasses of milk does not supply enough calcium.

2. To supplement the milk with vitamin C to ensure absorption.
3. That dietary intake of calcium is not utilized by the body.
4. To increase daily oral phosphate as well as calcium.

48. A 71-year-old client complains of blurred vision and difficulty in being outside on sunny days. The nurse correctly identifies this condition to be:

1. Caused by psychotropic drug therapy.
2. An excuse to avoid exercise.
3. A symptom of cataracts.
4. Caused by diuretic therapy.

49. The client develops a stage two pressure sore. What documentation, if made by the nurse correctly, reflects the diagnosis of a stage 2 pressure sore?

1. A lesion appearing as a blister, which appears as a shallow crater.
2. A lesion appearing as a large unblanching erythema.
3. A lesion that extends into the deeper subcutaneous tissue.
4. A lesion that extends into the subcutaneous tissue with skin loss.

50. A 75-year-old client reports to a community nursing clinic for his annual flu injection. He appears tired and has a sad affect. He indicates that he is having difficulty sleeping, which results in trouble getting out of bed in the morning, and feeling tired and fatigued. He reports that he feels physically ill. What is the most important initial response of the nurse?

1. Take a complete medical history.
2. Refer him to his family physician.
3. Perform a complete physical examination.
4. Conduct a mental status examination.

51. The client is admitted to a geriatric psychiatric unit and is diagnosed as having major unipolar depressive disorder. He is prescribed with trazodone (Desyrel) 25 mg tid and lithium carbonate 300 mg HS. The nurse correctly identifies unipolar depressive disorder being characterized as:

1. Depression with no manic or hypomanic episodes
2. Depression that is followed by mania
3. A first-time experience of depression
4. A left-brain alteration leading to depression

52. The client is scheduled to receive his first dose of lithium carbonate this HS. Which action by the nurse is essential before beginning lithium therapy?

1. Check thyroid function studies (thyroid-stimulating hormone, TSH) results.
2. Check serum creatinine, blood urea nitrogen, and urinalysis results.
3. Check serum electrolytes results.
4. Check hemoglobin, hematocrit, and red blood cell count.

53. The client says to the nurse, "I feel so worthless. I'm not worth the air that I breathe." The most appropriate response by the nurse following this statement is:

1. "I understand, but I think you are a very worthy person."
2. "Don't be ridiculous, you were a very sucessful person."
3. "Have you had thoughts of harming yourself?"
4. "I don't understand; why do you feel this way?"

54. The client has received trazodone (Desyrel) for 12 days and the nurse notices little to no therapeutic results. The most appropriate action by the nurse at this time is:

1. Do nothing because therapeutic results may not be seen in this period of time.
2. Call the physician and ask him to prescribe another antidepressant medication.
3. Call the physician and ask him to discontinue the medication.
4. Observe the client at medication time to ensure he is not throwing it away.

55. A nursing diagnosis of potential altered sexuality patterns has been identified for a client taking nadolol (Corgard). The nurse is beginning to implement the plan of care. Based on the information the nurse has, which of the following nursing interventions would be most appropriate?

1. Instruct the client to notify his physician if any sexual problems occur.
2. Instruct the client on the need to use protection during sexual activity.
3. Instruct the client to rise slowly from a sitting or lying position.
4. Instruct the client to take a nitroglycerin tablet before sexual activity.

56. The spouse of a 75-year-old client asks the nurse if biofeedback would be effective in treating functional incontinence. The most appropriate response by the nurse is:

1. Biofeedback is most effective in incontinence brought about by structural causes.
2. Biofeedback is most effective in incontinence brought about by physical causes.
3. Biofeedback is most effective in incontinence brought about by major depression.
4. Biofeedback is most effective in incontinence brought about by cognitive impairment.

57. A home health nurse has been asked to see a client with end-stage renal disease for assessment of cachexia. If entered by the nurse, which documentation would correctly identify that the client is experiencing cachexia?

1. Unable to verbalize feelings or write important information
2. Unable to carry out activities of daily living without help
3. Involuntary muscular movements of the arms and legs
4. Emaciation, loss of subcutaneous fat, and lean body mass

58. A 70-year-old is attending a senior citizen center. The client engages in conversation with others but refuses to participate in recreational or social events. The client's affect is appropriate and her appearance is well groomed. The initial action by the nurse based on this information is:
    1. Assess the client for constipation.
    2. Assess the client for pain.
    3. Assess the client for depression.
    4. Assess the client for cognitive impairment.

59. The bedridden client with Alzheimer's disease is receiving decubitus ulcer care by the nurse. The nurse notes an increase in purulent wound drainage. Vital signs are temperature 99°F, pulse 78 bpm, respirations 18/min, and blood pressure 162/88 mm Hg. The most appropriate nursing action at this time is:
    1. Administer the client a prescribed antipyretic medication.
    2. Call the physician for an order for a white blood cell count.
    3. Change the decubitus ulcer care treatment regimen more often.
    4. Do nothing but continue to monitor vital signs.

60. A 79-year-old client is being admitted to the geriatrics unit of a large medical center. This is the first time the client has required hospitalization. A priority for this client at the beginning of hospitalization is:
    1. Assessment of knowledge of prescription medications.
    2. Assessment of knowledge of hospital procedures.
    3. Assessment of baseline cognitive status.
    4. Assessment of baseline functional status.

61. A nurse in a nursing clinic is approached by an older adult who says that the physician has diagnosed him with type II diabetes, but that he would be monitored for type I diabetes. The client asks, "What is the difference between type I and type II diabetes?" The nurse correctly responds:
    1. "Type I diabetes has an absence of ketosis, which signifies insulin production."
    2. "Type II diabetes has an absence of ketosis, which signifies insulin production."
    3. "Type I diabetes has an absence of ketosis, which signifies no insulin is produced."
    4. "Type II diabetes has an absence of ketosis, which signifies no insulin is produced."

62. An older adult who is diabetic calls the home health nurse and reports symptoms of a viral infection. The client indicates that she has no appetite and asks the nurse for suggestions. The most appropriate nursing action by the nurse would be to inform the client to:
    1. Drink plenty of fluids and maintain carbohydrate intake.
    2. Drink a high-protein nutritional supplement hourly.
    3. Withhold your insulin until your fever returns to normal.
    4. Report to the hospital emergency room immediately.

63. The nurse is giving dietary instruction to an older adult who is a newly diagnosed diabetic. The initial action of the nurse is to:
    1. Determine the client's usual dietary habits.
    2. Determine the client's ideal body weight.
    3. Determine the client's compliance ability.
    4. Determine the amount of insulin ordered.

64. A 70-year-old insulin-dependent diabetic client shows the nurse an area on the leg where injections have been given. This area appears as an accumulation of subcutaneous fat. The nurse identifies this as lipohypertrophy. The initial action by the nurse is to:
    1. Assess the client for signs and symptoms of infection.
    2. Assess the client for signs and symptoms of cellulitis.
    3. Assess the amount of insulin the client has been receiving.
    4. Assess the injection rotation method the client uses.

65. A newly diagnosed diabetic client is placed on tolbutamide (Orinase) 250 mg bid. The nurse reviews the medications that the client is currently taking for potential drug interactions. Which medication, if prescribed for the client and taken as prescribed, would the nurse inform the client is safe and does not need monitoring when administered with tolbutamide?
    1. Propranolol
    2. Acetaminophen
    3. Salicylate
    4. Furosemide

66. The home health nurse has recommended biofeedback for the client who is experiencing incontinence. The following information is most important in evaluating the client for biofeedback as a treatment modality:
    1. Medical factors and motivation
    2. Medical factors and family support
    3. Mental status and family support
    4. Mental status and motivation

67. The nurse completes the interview with the client who complains of dyspareunia, vaginal dryness, and diminished libido. The most appropriate action by the nurse is to:
    1. Recommend that the client place her mother in a nearby nursing home.
    2. Recommend that the client go for an appointment at a mental health center.
    3. Recommend that the client go for an immediate gynecological examination.
    4. Recommend to the client that intercourse continue at regular intervals.

68. The client is discharged home following bypass surgery. Three weeks following discharge, the client telephones the nurse to report left-sided muscle aching throughout the chest, upper back, shoulders, and neck. The most appropriate action by the nurse is:
    1. Inform the client to call the physician immediately.
    2. Inform the client to apply ice packs three times daily.
    3. Inform the client to take muscle-relaxing medications.

4. Do nothing because muscle aches are expected following surgery.

69. A client with premature ventricular contractions has been receiving procainamide hydrochloride (Pronestyl) 500 mg four times per day for the past 8 months. Which symptom if experienced by the client would the nurse recognize as needing immediate investigation?
    1. Constipation
    2. Dizziness
    3. Shivering
    4. Diarrhea

70. The nurse is conducting an interview with a client who has bouts of paroxysmal atrial tachycardia and is placed on procainamide (Pronestyl) 500 mg qid. Which statement if made by the client indicates that teaching has been effective?
    1. "If I miss taking my medication, I should discontinue it and call the doctor."
    2. "This medication will have to be changed over time because of my body sensitivity."
    3. "I should report any bruising or bleeding to my physician immediately."
    4. "I should report any dizziness when rising from a sitting position to the nurse."

71. The client is transferred to the recovery room following pacemaker installation. The nurse caring for the client detects cardiac problems and calls a code. The physician responding to the code orders the nurse to defibrillate the client. The most appropriate action by the nurse is to:
    1. Defibrillate, placing the paddles over the pacemaker.
    2. Defibrillate, placing the paddles anteriorly and posteriorly.
    3. Defibrillate, placing the paddles laterally over the chest.
    4. Inform the physician that the client has a pacemaker.

72. The nurse is preparing the client for discharge after pacemaker implantation. Which of the following instructions should be started before surgery and continue throughout the hospital stay concerning potential problems?
    1. The need for strict adherence to dietary regimen
    2. The need for strict adherence to exercise regimen
    3. The need to watch for infection at the implant site
    4. The need to check the pacemaker battery carefully monthly

73. The client with a pacemaker is ambulating in the room with the assistance of the nurse. The client reports feeling dizzy and short of breath. The nurse recognizes these symptoms are caused by:
    1. Fatigue caused by prolonged bed rest
    2. Fear of pacemaker failure
    3. Drop in cardiac output
    4. Need for individualized attention

74. The client with a pacemaker is ambulating in the room with the assistance of the nurse. The client reports feeling dizzy and short of breath. The initial action by the nurse should be:
    1. Reassure the client that you will stay with him.
    2. Have him rest in bed immediately.
    3. Monitor his vital signs every hour.
    4. Do nothing because this is normal following surgery.

75. The client with a pacemaker is discharged home and is being followed by a home health nurse. The client reports to the nurse that he and his spouse enjoy traveling and have spent the last several years in Europe. The client questions the nurse regarding whether the pacemaker will interfer with their travels. Which instruction given by the nurse is most appropriate based on the needs for this client?
    1. "You will need to have monthly follow-up evaluations, so your travel will be limited."
    2. "You will need to show your pacemaker identification card to airport security."
    3. "You will need to discuss your travel plans with your cardiologist before travel."
    4. "You will be unable to travel for the first 3 years as your pacemaker is tested."

76. The client with a permanent pacemaker has returned home and is being seen by the home health nurse. The nurse notes an apical pulse rate of 50 and the rhythm is irregular. The client pacemaker code is set on 60. The client has no other symptoms and is not short of breath. The most appropriate action by the nurse is to:
    1. Inform the hospital
    2. Inform his physician
    3. Obtain a 12-lead electrocardiogram
    4. Do nothing because pulse rate is within normal limits.

77. A 79-year-old client is admitted to the hospital with a diagnosis of bacterial pneumonia. She has a temperature of 102.4°F, is coughing up tenacious purulent sputum, and is experiencing difficulty breathing. Which of the following nursing measures is most important in helping to liquefy these viscous secretions?
    1. Postural drainage
    2. Breathing humidified air
    3. Clapping and percussion over the affected lung
    4. Coughing and deep breathing exercises

78. The home health nurse visits a 98-year-old client who lives alone. The client is experiencing periods of forgetfulness and poor visual acuity. The client is currently taking the following medications: digoxin (Lanoxin) 0.125 mg bid; potassium chloride (K-Dur) 20 mEq daily; furosemide (Lasix) 40 mg daily; enalapril (Vasotec) 120 mg bid. The most appropriate nursing intervention for this client based on knowledge of pharmacology and drug interactions is:
    1. Monitor for hypernatremia.
    2. Monitor for hyperkalemia.
    3. Monitor for postural hypotension.
    4. Monitor for weight loss.

79. The home health nurse continues to visit with the client who is living alone and experiencing periods of

forgetfulness and decreased visual acuity. The physician orders indicate that the client is to remain on his current medications until follow-up in 3 months. The most appropriate nursing action by the nurse to increase compliance with the medical regimen is:

1. Teach the client the importance of follow-up medical appointments.
2. Teach the client about each medication and the need for compliance.
3. Prepare a prefilled medicine organizer each week with his medications.
4. Prepare a color-coded medication bottle for each medication prescribed.

80. A 70-year-old client is diagnosed with sleep apnea. The nurse begins teaching the client about this condition and therapeutic approaches to dealing with sleep apnea. The nurse correctly teaches the client to:

1. Drink a small glass of sherry before retiring for bed.
2. Avoid any alcoholic beverage during the daytime.
3. Take an over-the-counter stimulant during the daytime.
4. Eat a high-calorie, protein-rich food right before a bedtime.

81. A 66-year-old client was seen by the home health nurse. She reported insomnia with periods of hyperactivity accompanied by sluggishness, depression, cold intolerance, decreased appetite, and generalized aching all over. The physician notes that the client is receiving the following prescribed medications: paroxetine (Paxil) 20 mg bedtime (HS); multiple vitamin with ginseng bid; and lorazepam (Ativan) 10 mg prn insomnia. The client questions why she is experiencing hyperactivity when she feels depressed. The most appropriate response by the nurse is:

1. "Many times depression is accompanied by anxiety."
2. "Paroxetine may cause sluggishness and anxiety in some people."
3. "Insomnia can be caused by depression and anxiety."
4. "The may be caused by your medication or by hypothryoidism."

82. An 85-year-old client is attending a senior citizen center where the nurse is conducting blood pressure screening. The client tells the nurse that she has recently had problems with constipation. The nurse knows that the client has a history of colon cancer about 14 years ago and had surgery but no metastasis. The most appropriate nursing action at this time is:

1. Tell the client to increase fruits, fiber, and fluids in the diet.
2. Tell the client that constipation is to be expected sometimes.
3. Tell the client to take an over-the-counter stool softener.
4. Tell the client to see her physician for an evaluation.

83. The home health nurse is admitting a 66-year-old who is newly diagnosed as having insulin-dependent diabetes mellitus. The client lives alone in a low-income apartment. The nurse notes that the client

has no cognitive impairment but does have some difficulty learning. The primary nursing goal for this client is:

1. Encourage family involvement to promote compliance.
2. Refer to social services to gain financial assistance.
3. Provide educational materials to decrease knowledge deficit.
4. Assist with lifestyle change to adjust to current health concerns.

84. A 67-year-old adult is admitted to an acute care unit with the diagnosis of intestinal obstruction. Routine laboratory tests and radiographs were ordered. On reviewing laboratory results, the nurse noted a blood sugar of 200. The nurse questions the client, who indicates to the nurse that he ate approximately 2 hours prior to blood being drawn for laboratory work. The initial action by the nurse is:

1. Order the client a regular diet immediately.
2. Do nothing but continue to monitor the client status.
3. Inform the physician of the client's elevated blood sugar.
4. Call the laboratory and ask for a reevaluation of the results.

85. A nurse is evaluating a client for conductive hearing loss. If experienced by the client, which of the manifestations would the nurse correctly identify as associated with conductive hearing loss?

1. The client speaks in an excessively loud voice in many situations.
2. The client speaks in a relatively quiet voice that is difficult to hear.
3. The client may be sensitive to loud intensities of sound.
4. The client has scarring and sclerotic changes in the middle ear.

86. A 74-year-old client has been evaluated for hearing loss and is being fitted for a hearing aid. The nurse correctly instructs the client that the hearing aid:

1. Can be ordered for a 2- to 4-week trial period.
2. Can be purchased and reimbursed by Medicare.
3. Can only be purchased by his physician.
4. Cannot be returned to the vendor.

87. The nurse is instructing the client on the wearing of the new hearing aid. The nurse correctly informs the client to:

1. Wear the hearing aid 24 hours a day for the first week.
2. Wear the hearing aid during the day and remove at night.
3. Wear the hearing aid 4 hours a day at first and progress.
4. Wear the hearing aid when watching television or visiting.

88. If made by the client, which statement would indicate to the nurse that teaching related to hearing aid care has been effective?

1. "I will clean the ear mold with an alcohol and water solution."
2. "I should not be concerned if I don't hear a whistle set at loud volume."
3. "I should have to change the batteries every 10–14 days."
4. "I should have the hearing aid checked yearly for maintenance."

89. The nurse is teaching a client about the hearing aid. Which statement by the nurse might be most important to assist the client in adapting to wearing a hearing aid?
    1. "You might feel tense and nervous initially because of the sudden noise."
    2. "You may need to ask for assistance from friends when adjusting your aid."
    3. "You will be able to change your batteries after a few practice sessions."
    4. "You will be able to hear the voices of persons speaking to you."

90. A 65-year-old client was being prepared for an exploratory laparotomy. To prepare the client for surgery, the physician ordered cefazolin (Ancef) 250 mg prophylactically. Using a 1–g/mL vial, how many milliliters did the nurse administer?

_____

91. A 75-year-old client was seen in the local ER with severe ventricular tachycardia. The physician ordered amiodarone (Cordarone) 1000 mg PO. In stock were 200-mg tablets. How many tablets did the nurse administer?

_____

92. A 78-year-old was admitted with severe flatulence and dyspepsia. The physician ordered activated charcoal (Charcotabs) 975 mg after meals. On hand were 325 mg tablets. How many tablets did the nurse adminiser?

_____

93. A 54-year-old client developed an adrenocortical carcinoma. The physician ordered mitotane (Lysodren) 3 g tid. The pharmacist dispensed 500-mg tablets. The nurse instructed the client to take how many tablets?

_____

94. A 70-year-old client developed cutaneous larva migrans (creeping eruptions) on the skin. The client weighed 68 kg. The physician ordered thiabendazole (Mintezol) 25 mg/kg (1700 mg). Using a 500–mg/5 mL elixir, how many milliliters did the nurse administer?

_____

95. A 77-year-old client was diagnosed with pernicious anemia. The physician ordered 12 injection, 150 μg IM every day times 2 weeks. Using a 120–μg/mL vial, how many milliliters did the nurse administer IM?

_____

96. A 75-year-old home health client developed acute gouty arthritis. The physician ordered phenylbutazone (Butazolidin) 400 mg PO every 8 hours. The home health nurse instructed the client to take how many 100-mg tablets?

_____

97. A 70-year-old was admitted with congestive heart failure. The physician ordered hydrochlorothiazide (Esidrex) 75 mg daily IM. Using a 100–mg/mL vial, how many milliliters did the nurse administer?

_____

98. Your client, age 68, is a newly diagnosed non–insulin dependent diabetic. The physician ordered chlorpropamide (Diabinese) 150 mg PO bid. The pharmacy sent Diabinese 0.1-g tablets. The nurse will administer how many tablets to the client?

_____

99. The nurse had to administer lactulose 20 g via a gastric tube. On hand is lactulose syrup 10 g/15 mL. How much will the nurse give?

_____

100. The 60-year-old client was admitted for peptic ulcer. The physician ordered Maalox Plus 30 mL 30 minutes after meals and hour of sleep. How many containers will be needed from the pharmacy for a 24-hour schedule? (Each container holds 30 mL.)

_____

ANSWERS

1. **(1)** Integrated processes: nursing process — data collection; client need: physiological integrity; content area: older adult.

   RATIONALE

   (1) Although AIDS dementia and DAT have similar presenting symptoms, aphasia often accompanies DAT, but is rarely seen in AIDS dementia. Neurological findings such as ataxia, leg weakness, tremors, and peripheral neuropathies may be present with AIDS dementia. **(2)** Lethargy and a pronounced loss of weight are symptoms of AIDS dementia and are not seen until the later stages of DAT. **(3)** Peripheral neuropathies are not usually seen in DAT until the later stages, although they may be present in early AIDS dementia. **(4)** Leg weakness and tremors may be present in AIDS dementia, but are rarely seen in DAT until the later stages.

2. **(4)** Integrated processes: nursing process — implementation; communication and documentation; client need: safe, effective care environment; coordinated care; content area: older adult.

   RATIONALE

   (1) Moving one client to another section of the nursing home facility will not assist with the behavior being noted in these two cognitively aware individuals. **(2)** Calling family members is not warranted because both of the clients are cognitively aware and have the right to make decisions related to expressions of sexuality and intimacy. **(3)** Performing a thorough sexual assessment on both clients including tests for sexually transmitted disease is appropriate nursing action; however, it is not the most important action for the director to take at this time. **(4)** The feelings, attitudes, and concerns of the staff must be known before appropriate nursing interventions can be implemented. Calling a nursing conference will give the staff an opportunity to verbalize any concerns and to plan for the intimacy needs of these two individuals.

3. **(2)** Integrated processes: nursing process — data collection; client need: physiological integrity; physiological adaptation; content area: older adult.

   RATIONALE

   (1) Malignant brain tumors are sometimes experienced by older adults, but are primarily seen in younger clients. **(2)** Cardiovascular accidents (CVA) are the most common cause of aphasia in the older adult. **(3)** Head trauma may cause aphasia in older adults, but is not the most likely cause of aphasia. **(4)** Major depressive disorder may interfere with the ability of the older adult to communicate, but does not cause aphasia.

4. **(2)** Integrated processes: nursing process — data collection; client need: physiological integrity; physiological adaptation; content area: older adult.

   RATIONALE

   (1) Many postmenopausal women have voiding difficulty; however, stress incontinence is not due to stress brought on by menopause. **(2)** Stress incontinence is due to loss of structural support to the bladder neck and is caused by pelvic floor relaxation. **(3)** Urinary tract infections may bring about a feeling of need to urinate frequently, but do not usually bring about an involuntary loss of urine from the bladder. **(4)** Incontinence is not a normal aging change.

5. **(3)** Integrated processes: nursing process — implementation; teaching/learning; client need: physiological integrity; basic care and comfort; content area: older adult.

   RATIONALE

   (1) Behavior modification and psychological counseling may be implemented to treat sensory incontinence, but do not assist with incontinence that occurs as a result of pelvic floor relaxation. **(2)** Although this recommendation to the client may be made, this is not the only treatment for stress incontinence. Frequent change of pads and bathing twice a day may not be feasible for this client, who is experiencing embarrassment due to the incontinence. **(3)** All treatment for stress is elective and depends upon the severity of symptoms and the degree of concern and interference with lifestyle. **(4)** Surgical procedures are used as a form of treatment for stress incontinence, but may not be complex. Surgical procedures are not used for all clients with stress incontinence.

6. **(1)** Integrated processes: nursing process — data collection; client need: physiological integrity; pharmacological therapies; content area: older adult.

   RATIONALE

   (1) Propantheline (Pro-Banthine) should be used with caution in clients with urinary retention. **(2)** Propantheline (Pro-Banthine) should be used with caution in clients with heart disease, kidney disease, liver disease, and lung disease, but is not contraindicated in clients with diabetes mellitus. **(3)** Propantheline (Pro-Banthine) should be used with caution in clients with heart disease, kidney disease, liver disease, and lung disease, but is not contraindicated in clients with urinary tract infection. **(4)** Propantheline (Pro-Banthine) should be used with caution with drugs with anticholinergic effects, but is not contraindicated with antibiotics.

7. **(2)** Integrated processes: nursing process — implementation; teaching/learning; client need: physiological integrity; pharmacological therapies; content area: older adult.

   RATIONALE

   (1) Enlarged lymph nodes may be a result of an infectious process but are not related to the side effects of propantheline (Pro-Banthine). It is doubtful that the client would experience nasal drainage due to the drying properties of propantheline. **(2)** Side effects of propantheline (Pro-Banthine) include dry mouth, dry eyes, blurred vision, increased intraocular pressure, and constipation. **(3)** Orthostatic hypotension is a side effect of propantheline (Pro-Banthine) but is not life threatening or indicative of a more serious problem. **(4)** Presbyopia, the inability to focus on near objects, is a normal aging change and is expected to be found in older adults.

8. **(2)** Integrated processes: nursing process — implementation; teaching/learning; client need: physiological integrity; pharmacological therapies; content area: older adult.

   RATIONALE

   (1) Even though constipation may be a side effect of propantheline (Pro-Banthine) and eating green vegetables is encouraged to increase fiber in the diet, the anticholinergic action of the drug may decrease sweat and heat release from the body, and working in the garden on a very hot day could be more problematic for the client. **(2)** The anticholinergic action of the drug may decrease sweat and heat release from the body, and working in the garden on a very hot day could be more problematic for the client. **(3)** The anticholinergic action of the drug may decrease sweat and heat release from the body, and working in the garden on a very hot day could be more problematic for the client. **(4)** Caffeine, red wine, and aged cheese are to be avoided with monoamine oxidase (MAO) inhibitors, not with propantheline (Pro-Banthine).

9. **(3)** Integrated processes: nursing process — implementation; teaching/learning; client need: physiological integrity; reduction of risk potential.
   RATIONALE
   (1) A cystometrogram (CMG) is a graphic representation of bladder pressure and provides assessment information regarding the ability of the bladder to fill and store urine. **(2)** A cystometrogram (CMG) is a graphic representation of bladder pressure and provides assessment information regarding the ability of the bladder to fill and store urine. **(3)** A cystometrogram (CMG) is a graphic representation of bladder pressure and provides assessment information regarding the ability of the bladder to fill and store urine. **(4)** A cystometrogram (CMG) is a graphic representation of bladder pressure and provides assessment information regarding the ability of the bladder to fill and store urine.

10. **(1)** Integrated processes: nursing process — data collection; client need: physiological integrity; basic care and comfort; content area: older adult.
    RATIONALE
    (1) Functional incontinence is urinary leakage caused by environmental or functional factors. It is not associated with any pathological condition of the urinary system or voiding mechanism and is usually associated with cognitive deficits or motivational disorders. **(2)** A peripheral field deficit may cause the client not to be able to discriminate heights and to impair vision from the side view but is not a likely cause of functional incontinence. **(3)** While CVA may bring about incontinence because of immobility changes, this would likely be associated with a pathological condition. **(4)** Functional incontinence is urinary leakage caused by environmental or functional factors. It is not associated with any pathological condition of the urinary system or voiding mechanism and is usually associated with cognitive deficits or motivational disorders.

11. **(1)** Integrated processes: nursing process — data collection; client need: physiological integrity; basic care and comfort; content area: older adult.
    RATIONALE
    (1) Cognitive impairment is a cause of incontinence but does not prevent the client from discussing the problem of incontinence. **(2)** While incontinence does bring about feelings of embarrassment and distress, research studies indicate that the majority of individuals (particularly females) believe that incontinence is a normal result of aging. **(3)** Research studies indicate that the majority of individuals (particularly females) believe that incontinence is a normal result of aging. **(4)** Incontinence is a major factor in making a decision for long-term care; however, this does not prevent the client from discussing incontinence as a problem.

12. **(3)** Integrated processes: nursing process — implementation; teaching/learning; client need: physiological integrity; basic care and comfort; content area: older adult.
    RATIONALE
    (1) Clients on CAPD need to increase potassium intake by eating a wide variety of fruits and vegetables each day. **(2)** Sodium restriction is not necessary with CAPD clients, and both kale and collard greens contain potassium, which should be

increased. **(3)** Nutritionists recommend a dietary regimen that limits phosphorus intake to 1200 mg/day. Foods such as nuts and legumes are phosphorus-rich. **(4)** Protein intake is increased to provide 1.2–1.5 g/kg body weight.

13. **(2)** Integrated processes: nursing process — data collection; client need: physiological integrity; basic care and comfort; content area: older adult.
    RATIONALE
    (1) The early stage of cognitive impairment is not characterized by numerous complaints of constipation, and there is no evidence to suggest that this client is experiencing impaired cognition. **(2)** Sensory neurogenic dysfunction is damage to the sensory components of the rectal reflex arc or the sensory components of the central nervous system that takes the message of the stool in the rectum to the cerebral cortex. The motor components are intact, but the individual is not aware of stool in the rectum. **(3)** Motor neurogenic dysfunction is damage to the motor components of the central nervous system or the motor components of the rectal reflex arc. The individual feels the stool in the rectum, but is unable to evacuate the stool. **(4)** Constipation is a common adverse drug reaction; however, in this situation, there is nothing to suggest that this client is receiving a medication.

14. **(4)** Integrated processes: nursing process — data collection; client need: physiological integrity; pharmacological therapies; content area: older adult.
    RATIONALE
    (1) This is an example of a saline laxative. Saline laxatives act by retaining and increasing water content of feces by osmotic qualities. **(2)** This is an example of a bulk laxative. Bulk laxatives act by absorbing water and increasing the volume of intestinal contents. **(3)** This is an example of a hyperosmotic agent. Hyperosmotic agents act by retaining and increasing water content of feces by osmotic qualities. **(4)** Ducosate sodium (Colace) is an emollient or feces-softening agent. It acts by dispersing wetting agents, facilitating a mixture of water and fatty substances within the fecal mass; when a homogeneous mixture is produced, the feces becomes soft.

15. **(3)** Integrated processes: nursing process — implementation; communication and documentation; client need: physiological integrity; pharmacological therapies; content area: older adult.
    RATIONALE
    (1) Milk of magnesia is contraindicated in cardiac clients or those with renal impairments. It is a laxative of choice for fecal impaction if these conditions are not present. **(2)** Milk of magnesia is contraindicated in cardiac clients or those with renal impairments. It is a laxative of choice for fecal impaction if these conditions are not present. **(3)** Milk of magnesia is contraindicated in cardiac clients or those with renal impairments. It is a laxative of choice for fecal impaction if these conditions are not present. **(4)** Milk of magnesia is contraindicated in cardiac clients or those with renal impairments. It is a laxative of choice for fecal impaction if these conditions are not present.

16. **(1)** Integrated processes: nursing process —evaluation; client need: physiological integrity; pharmacological therapies; content area: older adult.
    RATIONALE
    (1) The goal of a bowel management program is soft, well-formed stools that are regular on the planned day and within 1 hour of the planned time. **(2)** The goal of a bowel management program is soft, well-formed stools that are regular on the planned day and within 1 hour of the planned time. **(3)** The goal of a bowel management program is soft, well-formed stools

that are regular on the planned day and within 1 hour of the planned time. (**4**) Skin integrity is not an appropriate evaluation criterion for a bowel management program.

17. (**2**) Integrated processes: nursing process — data collection; client need: physiological integrity; physiological adaptation; content area: older adult.

RATIONALE

(**1**) Injuries caused by surgical damage may result in disruption of the sphincter musculature or pudendal or sacral nerve branches, but are not neurogenic in nature. (**2**) Fecal incontinence caused by neurological disorders such as multiple sclerosis or spinal cord lesions are classified as neurological incontinence. (**3**) Psychiatric or behavioral disorders rarely cause fecal incontinence in older adults. (**4**) Fecal incontinence may be a result of habitual use of laxatives or enemas, but this would diminish muscle tone and would not be neurogenic in nature.

18. (**3**) Integrated processes: nursing process — implementation; client need: safe, effective care environment; coordinated care; content area: older adult.

RATIONALE

(**1**) Some auto insurance companies provide premium reductions to graduates of the American Association of Retired Persons (AARP) Mature Driver/55 Alive Program. (**2**) The local highway patrol does not usually have a driving program geared to older adults. (**3**) The AARP Mature Driver/55 Alive Program helps older drivers improve their skills and prevent traffic accidents by covering age-related physical changes, declining perceptual skills, rules of the road, and local driving problems. (**4**) The American Blindness Federation is a resource for audiovisual material for visually impaired persons.

19. (**2**) Integrated processes: nursing process — data collection; client need: physiological integrity; pharmacological therapies; content area: older adult.

RATIONALE

(**1**) Confusion is not a normal aging change. (**2**) Drugs prescribed by the physician or purchased over the counter are among the most common causes of confusional states in the older adult. Arthroplasty clients should receive narcotic analgesics during the first 48 hours postoperatively on a regular basis. (**3**) Although clients with dementia do have confusion, confusion is most likely reversible in this situation and does not indicate early signs of dementia. (**4**) Separation from a familiar environment is a possible cause, but because the client has been hospitalized for at least 4 days in this situation, it is less likely than drug therapy.

20. (**2**) Integrated processes: nursing process — planning; communication and documentation; client need: physiological integrity; reduction of risk potential; content area: older adult.

RATIONALE

(**1**) Pain is not of primary concern at this time because the client is several days postoperative and pain should be diminishing. (**2**) The skin is the first line of defense in the prevention of infection. The defense is broken due to an opening from the operative site and provides a medium for the entry of bacteria. Infection is a primary concern because this could be dangerous to the client. (**3**) A supportive environment is an important consideration of care, but the matter is not life threatening. (**4**) Explanation of the procedures is an important component of care, but the matter is not life threatening.

21. (**4**) Integrated processes: nursing process — data collection; client need: physiological integrity; reduction of risk potential; content area: older adult.

RATIONALE

(**1**) The ability to take medications as prescribed is an important assessment item, but is not as important in terms of safety and prevention of injury in ambulating. (**2**) The ability to manage activities of daily living is an important assessment item, but is not as important in terms of safety and prevention of injury in ambulating. (**3**) Support from family and friends is an important assessment item, but is not as important in terms of safety and prevention of injury in ambulating. (**4**) Prosthetic implants require strict adherence to partial weight bearing for at least 2 months. The older adult usually begins with a walker to achieve the partial weight bearing and then progresses to a cane. Weight bearing can cause injury to the joint and require hospitalization to repair.

22. (**1**) Integrated processes: nursing process — planning; client need: physiological integrity; basic care and comfort; content area: older adult.

RATIONALE

(**1**) Diet plans for the elderly should focus on increasing vitamins and minerals and decreasing caloric intake. Boiled pork chop is high in the B vitamins and reduces the fat through the boiling process. Cantaloupe is higher in vitamin C than orange slices or strawberries. (**2**) Ham is high in sodium, and both spinach and banana are lower in vitamins and minerals, particularly vitamins B and C, that the older adult requires. (**3**) Liver as a menu choice may not be the best selection because many people do not like the taste of liver, and unless prepared properly, it may be difficult for an older adult to chew. Both carrots and orange slices are lower in vitamins B and C, which the older adult requires. (**4**) Fried foods are not recommended for older adults because these increase calories and fats.

23. (**3**) Integrated processes: nursing process — planning; client need: physiological integrity; reduction of risk potential; content area: older adult.

RATIONALE

(**1**) There is no information given that indicates the client is unable to prepare food. (**2**) Sensory perceptual alteration is an appropriate nursing diagnosis for a client with glaucoma. Glaucoma, however, results in decreased peripheral vision, not an increase. (**3**) Clients with glaucoma will be on lifelong medications that must be instilled into the eye daily. For this reason, a nursing diagnosis of potential eye infection related to eye drop instillation must be a priority in planning care. (**4**) Body image is important, but a sight-threatening infection is a priority.

24. (**4**) Integrated processes: nursing process — planning; client need: physiological integrity; basic care and comfort; content area: older adult.

RATIONALE

(**1**) A protein-rich snack before bedtime would be filling, but the fullness might interfere with sleep. (**2**) There is no evidence at this time that a comprehensive physical examination is warranted, and, unless the client verbalizes additional complaints, it should not be done. (**3**) Milk is an effective sedative source at bedtime; however, sleeping pills are not recommended for the elderly. (**4**) Sleep problems are common in older adults, who report spending time in bed not sleeping, frequent nocturnal arousals, shortened nocturnal sleep time, and prolonged time falling asleep.

25. (**2**) Integrated processes: nursing process — data collection; client need: physiological integrity; reduction of risk potential; content area: older adult.

RATIONALE

(**1**) Although assessment of the ability to use unaffected extremities is important, passive therapy can be given to strengthen unaffected extremities if the client is unable to do so initially. **(2)** For rehabilitation to be effective for an older adult, active participation is necessary. If a client is unable to follow directions, active participation is not possible. **(3)** Although assessment of support systems may enhance rehabilitation in an older adult, it is not necessary for rehabilitation to be effective. **(4)** Clients may benefit from rehabilitation even if not returning to the community or home setting. Often, long-term care is necessary for rehabilitation to continue.

26. **(4)** Integrated processes: nursing process — implementation; client need: physiological integrity; reduction of risk potential; content area: older adult.

    RATIONALE

    (1) Talking with the client about past experiences, unless therapeutic communication is utilized, does little to help increase the psychological adjustment to the loss of the limb. **(2)** Delaying the use of a prosthesis until phantom pain diminishes or disappears hampers the rehabilitation of the client and may promote phantom sensations. **(3)** The liberal use of analgesics is usually not helpful in phantom pain and may impair rehabilitation due to side effects, confusion, or sedation. **(4)** Increased stimuli to the stump area relieves phantom pain. Wearing the prosthesis provides stimulation and decreases pain.

27. **(3)** Integrated processes: nursing process — planning; client need: physiological integrity; reduction of risk potential; content area: older adult.

    RATIONALE

    (1) Walking with crutches would consume more energy because the client would have to manipulate the crutches and his body. **(2)** Walking with a walker requires energy to pick up the appliance and to move it forward. Both feet must be brought forward, requiring more energy consumption. **(3)** Encouraging walking with the prosthesis more frequently for shorter periods of time will require less energy and will allow the client to increase endurance. **(4)** Strict bed rest is not warranted in this situation, and would actually interfere with rehabilitation and return to homeostasis.

28. **(3)** Integrated processes: nursing process — data collection; client need: physiological integrity; pharmacological therapies; content area: older adult.

    RATIONALE

    (1) Listening to the client is therapeutic, but should follow data collection that is to assist in finding the cause. **(2)** Impotence is related to physiological or psychological causes and is not a normal aging change. **(3)** A sexual history, with emphasis on current sexual function, should be part of the general medical evaluation of an older person. When a problem exists, evaluation of drugs being taken, psychological testing, and surgery may be necessary. **(4)** Although the nurse might refer the client to the physician, this would not be done until the nurse has completed assessment data to identify the problem. These data will guide the nurse and client mutually to seek the most effective solution.

29. **(2)** Integrated processes: nursing process — data collection; client need: physiological integrity; reduction of risk potential; content area: older adult.

    RATIONALE

    (1) Incontinence is caused by neurological or muscular impairments and is not a normal aging change. **(2)** Functional incontinence is observed in clients with normal bladder and urethral function. Too often, the diagnosis of functional incontinence is made inappropriately when the real problem is due to the client's restricted mobility and failure to get to the bathroom in time. **(3)** Stress incontinence is the involuntary loss of urine during physical exertion. **(4)** There is no evidence to suggest that there is pressure causing the incontinence.

30. **(3)** Integrated processes: nursing process — implementation; communication and documentation; client need: physiological integrity; pharmacological therapies; content area: older adult.

    RATIONALE

    (1) Gentamicin is excreted by the kidneys. Continuing to give the gentamicin could result in accumulation and untoward pharmacological effects. **(2)** Normal creatinine clearance ranges from 85 to 125 mL/min; values of 70 mL/min indicate decreased renal function. **(3)** Gentamicin is excreted by the kidneys. Continuing to give the gentamicin could result in accumulation and untoward pharmacological effects. **(4)** Calling the laboratory to see if this is in error is not an appropriate answer in terms of safety in medication administration.

31. **(3)** Integrated processes: nursing process — implementation; communication and documentation; client need: physiological integrity; reduction of risk potential; content area: older adult.

    RATIONALE

    (1) Creatinine clearance is not an indicator of respiratory function. **(2)** Creatinine clearance is not an indicator of cardiovascular function. **(3)** An excellent diagnostic indicator of renal function, the creatinine clearance test determines how efficiently the kidneys are clearing creatinine from the blood. **(4)** Creatinine clearance is not an indicator of gastrointestinal function.

32. **(1)** Integrated processes: nursing process — implementation; client need: physiological integrity; pharmacological therapies; content area: older adult.

    RATIONALE

    (1) Tegretol is slowly and incompletely absorbed from the gastrointestinal tract. Therapeutic serum levels are between 4 and 12 μgmL. This is within the therapeutic level, and the medication should be given as prescribed. **(2)** Therapeutic serum levels are between 4 and 12 μg/mL. This is within the therapeutic level, and there is no reason to call the physician. **(3)** Therapeutic serum levels are between 4 and 12 μg/mL. This is within the therapeutic level, and the medication should be given as prescribed. **(4)** Therapeutic serum levels are between 4 and 12 μgmL. This is within the therapeutic level, and the medication should be given as prescribed.

33. **(4)** Integrated processes: nursing process — planning; client need: physiological integrity; physiological adaptation; content area: older adult.

    RATIONALE

    (1) Making decisions about care is important to emotional health, but does not demonstrate knowledge specific to care of the cerebrovascular accident client. **(2)** The use of clock and calendar for orientation purposes is important, but there is no evidence that the client is experiencing disorientation. **(3)** Attending unit functions is important in social isolation diagnosis, but there is no evidence to suggest that the client is socially isolated. **(4)** Both left and right hemiplegic clients cope better in a structured, consistent environment.

34. **(4)** Integrated processes: nursing process — data collection; client need: physiological integrity; physiological adaptation; content area: older adult.

    RATIONALE

    (1) Brown pigmentation is not a characteristic symptom of earlier elder abuse. **(2)** Brown pigmentation is not a characteristic skin change in normal aging. **(3)** Brown pigmentation around the eyes and nose, not the ankles, is characteristic of lymphatic disease. (4) Chronic venous insufficiency is common in the elderly and is evidenced by distended tortuous veins, hair loss, brown pigmentation around the ankles, cool skin, and pedal edema that worsens during the day.

35. (2) Integrated processes: nursing process — implementation; communication and documentation; client need: psychosocial integrity; content area: older adult.

RATIONALE

(1) Leaving the room is appropriate only when the anxiety level is escalating quickly and allows the client to regain control. (2) The nurse should use a calm voice to aid in decreasing the anxiety level while encouraging verbalization of feelings. The nurse should try to identify the cause of the anxiety and to find measures to help the client cope more effectively with the anxiety. (3) Telling him there is nothing to worry about is false assurance, which is nontherapeutic. (4) Telling the client that the doctor knows best does little to assist in managing the anxiety or finding its source.

36. (4) Integrated processes: nursing process — data collection; client need: physiological integrity; physiological adaptation; content area: older adult.

RATIONALE

(1) Tachypnea is a symptom of left-sided congestive failure. (2) Pink frothy sputum indicates pulmonary edema. (3) Korotkoff's sounds are a symptom of left-sided congestive failure. (4) Symptoms of right-sided congestive heart failure include orthostatic hypotension, edema, distended jugular veins, liver enlargement, and S3 gallop.

37. (3) Integrated processes: nursing process — data collection; client need: physiological integrity; pharmacological therapies; content area: older adult.

RATIONALE

(1) Holding onto the wall may indicate dizziness, which is not a sign of digoxin toxicity in older adults. (2) Ringing of the ears is usually a sign of aspirin toxicity, not digoxin. (3) The clinical manifestations of digitalis toxicity are different for the elderly. Gastrointestinal disturbances, disorientation, agitation, hallucinations, color vision changes such as halos around lights, and changes in behavior are frequently seen. (4) Itching can be an adverse reaction to a medication, but is not a symptom of digoxin toxicity.

38. (4) Integrated processes: nursing process — implementation; client need: physiological integrity; reduction of risk potential; content area: older adult.

RATIONALE

(1) Normal serum digoxin level is 0.5–2.0 mg/mL. Giving an additional dose of digoxin is not a nursing decision, and the client could quickly become digoxin toxic. (2) The value given is above the normal serum digoxin level of 0.5–2.0 mg/mL. (3) Giving one-half the dose of digoxin is not a nursing decision, and the client could quickly become digoxin toxic. (4) Hypokalemia further disposes the client to digoxin toxicity, and the physician should be notified.

39. (1) Integrated processes: nursing process — implementation; teaching/learning; client need: physiological integrity; basic care and comfort; content area: older adult.

RATIONALE

(1) Chicken is higher in potassium than beef products. The baked potato and figs are both higher in potassium than any of the other menu selections. (2) Chicken is higher in potassium than beef products. The baked potato and figs are both higher in potassium than any of the other menu selections. (3)

Chicken is higher in potassium than beef products. The baked potato and figs are both higher in potassium than any of the other menu selections. (4) Fried foods are not appropriate for the cardiovascular client.

40. (1) Integrated processes: nursing process — planning; client need: physiological integrity; physiological adaptation; content area: older adult.

RATIONALE

(1) Weakness, muscle fatigue, decreased muscle tone, and weak irregular pulse are early symptoms of hypokalemia. (2) Diminished deep tendon reflexes indicate hypermagnesemia. (3) A positive Trousseau's sign is a symptom of hypocalcemia. (4) A positive Chvostek's sign is a symptom of hypocalcemia.

41. (1) Integrated processes: nursing process — planning; client need: physiological integrity; basic care and comfort; content area: older adult.

RATIONALE

(1) A quiet environment with no more than one or two people is necessary to reduce distraction and allow the client to complete a task. (2) The dining room will be filled with distractions that will further increase the client's frustration and irritability. (3) Offering a choice of items may produce frustration because the client may be unable to make decisions. (4) Hot foods may produce a burn if dropped or thrown.

42. (2) Integrated processes: nursing process — data collection; client need: physiological integrity; physiological adaptation; content area: older adult.

RATIONALE

(1) Parkinson's disease is a progressive, degenerative process affecting the nerve cells in the extrapyramidal system. Although many persons over the age of 65 years are affected, it is not a normal aging change. (2) Parkinson's disease is a progressive, degenerative process affecting the nerve cells in the extrapyramidal system, neurological in nature, and irreversible. (3) Although the musculoskeletal system is affected, the cause is neurological. (4) Parkinson's disease is progressive and is not reversible.

43. (4) Integrated processes: nursing process — implementation; teaching/learning; client need: physiological integrity; pharmacological therapies; content area: older adult.

RATIONALE

(1) Caffeine products may not be a therapeutic dietary need in the older adult, but they do not affect the drug therapy. (2) Foods high in fat are not recommended for the older adult, but they do not affect the drug therapy. (3) Foods high in calories are not recommended for the older adult, but do not affect the drug therapy. (4) Vitamin B_6 encourages the conversion of levodopa to dopamine, thereby inhibiting the effects of levodopa. Even with increased calories, the client with Parkinson's disease may lose weight, so extra calories are not a problem.

44. (4) Integrated processes: nursing process — data collection; client need: physiological integrity; pharmacological therapies; content area: older adult.

RATIONALE

(1) These behaviors are extrapyramidal symptoms and are not the result of carbidopa/levodopa. (2) These behaviors are extrapyramidal symptoms and are not the result of digoxin. (3) These behaviors are extrapyramidal symptoms and are not the result of Restoril. (4) These behaviors are extrapyramidal and are not the result of haloperidol.

45. (3) Integrated processes: nursing process — planning; client need: physiological integrity; basic care and comfort; content area: older adult.

RATIONALE

(1) Adding liquids while chewing might cause the client to aspirate. (2) Allowing the client to feed himself may increase the desire to eat and contribute to psychological well-being, but does little for the difficulty in swallowing experienced by the Parkinson's disease client. (3) Placing the client in a upright position minimizes facial and pharyngeal muscle rigidity. (4) Having the family bring favorite foods from home may stimulate the appetite and taste better than institutionally prepared menus, but does little for the difficulty in swallowing experienced by the client with Parkinson's disease.

46. **(3)** Integrated processes: nursing process — planning; client need: psychosocial integrity; content area: older adult.

RATIONALE

(1) Encouraging the client to perform activities of daily living for himself is important, but is not the most important action in keeping the client in his home. (2) Finding ways for the client to communicate his needs may decrease some frustration, but communication is not essential for the client to remain at home. (3) Attending to the physical and emotional needs of the caregiver is the most important nursing intervention in keeping the client at home. Providing for those needs decreases frustration, burnout, and feelings of social isolation, all of which contribute to physical illness of the caregiver and may make it necessary for institutionalization of the client. (4) Keeping the client active may not be possible as the disease progresses and is not a key factor in his remaining in the home.

47. **(1)** Integrated processes: nursing process — implementation; teaching/learning; client need: physiological integrity; basic care and comfort; content area: older adult.

RATIONALE

(1) Recommended calcium intake for premenopausal women is 1000 mg per day. Each glass of milk contains about 300 mg of calcium. (2) Vitamin D, not vitamin C, is necessary for calcium absorption. (3) Dietary calcium intake is utilized by the body; however, the average dietary intake of calcium is less than half what is recommended. (4) Oral phosphate has not been proven to reduce constipation.

48. **(3)** Integrated processes: nursing process — data collection; client need: physiological integrity; physiological adaptation; content area: older adult.

RATIONALE

(1) Psychotropic drug therapy may cause dizziness, but is not associated as a general rule with vision disturbance. (2) There is no evidence to suggest that the client is using visual disturbance as an excuse to avoid exercise. (3) An early symptom of posterior subcapsular cataracts is the complaint of glare from bright lights during the day or at night as a result of rays of light being scattered by the opacities. (4) Diuretic therapy may cause dizziness, but is not associated as a general rule with vision disturbance.

49. **(1)** Integrated processes: nursing process — data collection; client need: physiological integrity; physiological adaptation; content area: older adult.

RATIONALE

(1) A stage 2 decubitus ulcer appears as a superficial ulcer that may be a blister, abrasion, or shallow crater. (2) A stage 1 decubitus ulcer is a nonblanching erythema. (3) A stage 3 decubitus ulcer formation extends into the deeper subcutaneous tissue. (4) A stage 4 decubitus ulcer extends into the deep subcutaneous tissue and ends in full-thickness skin loss.

50. **(4)** Integrated processes: Nursing process — planning; client need: Psychosocial integrity; Content area: older adult.

RATIONALE

(1) A complete medical history is important, but the symptoms being expressed, even the somatic symptoms of feeling physically ill, are indicators of depression in older adults. The nurse should conduct a mental status exam first, before following up with a medical history and physical exam. (2) The nurse should conduct a mental status exam first, before following up with a medical history and physical exam and before accurate referral can be made. (3) A complete physical exam is not warranted until the mental status examination and a medical history are completed. (4) The client is presenting signs and symptoms of depression. Conducting a complete mental status exam will assist the nurse to intervene appropriately.

51. **(1)** Integrated processes: nursing process — planning; client need: psychosocial integrity; content area: older adult.

RATIONALE

(1) Unipolar depression is characterized only by episodes of depression with no manic or hypomanic episodes. (2) Depression associated with mania is a bipolar disorder. (3) Unipolar depression may occur more than one time. (4) Altered neurotransmission, not brain side, is one of the biological theories of depression.

52. **(2)** Integrated processes: nursing process — planning; client need: psychosocial integrity; reduction of risk potential; content area: older adult.

RATIONALE

(1) Thyroid function studies, serum thyroxine, and thyroid-stimulating hormone (TSH) should be elevated at baseline because lithium may predispose the older adult to hypothyroidism, but measurement of renal function also is essential before beginning lithium therapy. (2) Renal insufficiency may delay excretion of lithium and lead to toxicity. Blood urea nitrogen, serum creatinine, and urinalysis must be performed prior to beginning lithium therapy to determine hydration status, renal flow, and presence of renal defects. (3) Checking serum electrolytes is recommended prior to initiating lithium therapy but is not an essential nursing action. (4) White blood cell counts, total and differential, not red blood cell studies, are checked prior to administering lithium.

53. **(3)** Integrated processes: nursing process — data collection; client need: psychosocial integrity; content area: older adult.

RATIONALE

(1) This response does little to assist the client to verbalize feelings and may prevent further communication. (2) This response minimizes the feelings of the client and puts focus on the past rather than the here and now. (3) Feelings of worthlessness are common in major depression and may lead to suicidal ideation. Observation for behaviors or statements that may be indicators of self-harm may signal suicidal thoughts or intent and should be assessed. (4) "Why" questions are not considered therapeutic responses. This response does little to explore the feelings being expressed and may change the focus of the conversation.

54. **(1)** Integrated processes: nursing process — evaluation; client need: physiological integrity; pharmacological therapies; content area: older adult.

RATIONALE

(1) Significant therapeutic results occur after 2 weeks of therapy in 75% of clients receiving the medication, but may require 2–4 weeks before noticeable improvement is seen. (2) Requesting a new antidepressant at this time would hinder the therapeutic regimen and could result in prolonging depressive symptoms. (3) Discontinuing the medication unless there are adverse effects noted is not warranted. (4) There is nothing to suggest

that the client is throwing the medication away. Although the nurse may monitor for this, it is not the most appropriate action at 12 days.

55. **(1)** Integrated processes: nursing process — implementation; teaching/learning; client need: physiological integrity; pharmacological therapies; content area: older adult.

RATIONALE

(1) The client is taking nadolol (Corgard), a β-adrenergic blocker, which may cause impotence or other sexual problems. Instructing the client to report any sexual problems to the physician is important for the nursing diagnosis of altered sexual patterns. **(2)** Use of condoms for protection during sexual activity is important for older adults, but is not appropriate for this client because there is nothing in the assessment information to suggest fear of pregnancy or of acquiring a sexually transmitted disease. **(3)** Instructing the client to rise slowly from a sitting or lying position is important for this client due to the orthostatic hypotension potential. This instruction does not fit the nursing diagnosis for potential altered sexuality pattern. **(4)** This information may be given to a client who is resuming sexual activity following myocardial infarction, but there is nothing to support the need for nitroglycerin with this client.

56. **(1)** Integrated processes: nursing process — planning; client need: safe, effective care environment; safety and infection control; content area: older adult.

RATIONALE

(1) Biofeedback is most effective in stress and urge incontinence, both of which are caused by structural problems of the bladder of sphincter musculature. **(2)** Biofeedback is not effective with incontinence brought about by physical causes such as spinal cord injuries or head trauma. **(3)** Biofeedback requires that the client be cognitively intact and have a motivation to learn bladder inhibition and sphincter contraction activities. Clients with major depression may not have the energy or the desire to participate in biofeedback treatment modalities. **(4)** Biofeedback requires that the client be cognitively intact and have a motivation to learn bladder inhibition and sphincter contraction activities. Clients with cognitive impairment may not have the cognition required to participate in biofeedback treatment modalities.

57. **(4)** Integrated processes: nursing process — implementation; communication and documentation; client need: physiological integrity; physiological adaptation; content area: older adult.

RATIONALE

(1) The inability to speak or write is expressive aphasia or Broca's aphasia. **(2)** Cachexia is manifested by emaciation, loss of subcutaneous fat and lean body mass, brittleness of the hair, ridged or banded nails, and dermatosis of the lower legs. **(3)** Involuntary muscular movements of the arms and legs is an extrapyramidal symptoms known as dystonia. **(4)** Cachexia is manifested by emaciation, loss of subcutaneous fat and lean body mass, brittleness of the hair, ridged or banded nails, and dermatosis of the lower legs.

58. **(3)** Integrated processes: nursing process — data collection; client need: physiological integrity; physiological adaptation; content area: older adult.

RATIONALE

(1) Constipation is not known to inhibit participation in recreational or social events. **(2)** Pain can influence participation in recreational and social events, ambulation, posture, appetite, memory, dressing, grooming, and sleep patterns. **(3)** Depression may inhibit participation in recreational and social events, but the client is engaging in conversation that would make depres-

sion a less likely cause of this behavior. **(4)** There is nothing to suggest that this client has a cognitive impairment.

59. **(2)** Integrated processes: nursing process — implementation; communication and documentation; client need: physiological integrity; physiological adaptation; Content area: older adult.

RATIONALE

(1) Administering the prescribed antipyretic medication is not warranted with a temperature of 99°F. **(2)** These are symptoms of osteomyelitis, and it is necessary for this condition to be diagnosed and treated early. If the condition progresses to the sepsis stage, prognosis is poor. **(3)** There is nothing to indicate a need for the change in the decubitus care treatment regimen. **(4)** These are symptoms of osteomyelitis, and it is necessary for this condition to be diagnosed and treated early.

60. **(4)** Integrated processes: nursing process — data collection; client need: safe, effective care environment; safety and infection control; content area: older adult.

RATIONALE

(1) Assessment of knowledge of prescription medications is important, but at this point, the nurse has no evidence to suggest that the client is on medication. **(2)** Older adults need to be given instruction in small units. The nurse must continuously assess the client's knowledge of hospital procedures. **(3)** Assessment of baseline cognitive status is important and must be completed on the client shortly after admission. A priority at the beginning of every hospital admission for the older adult is the assessment of baseline functional status in order to develop an individual plan of care within the acute-care setting. **(4)** A priority at the beginning of every hospital admission for the older adult is the assessment of baseline functional status in order to develop an individual plan of care within the acute-care setting.

61. **(3)** Integrated processes: nursing process — implementation; teaching/learning; client need: physiological integrity; physiological adaptation; content area: older adult.

RATIONALE

(1) Type I diabetes is characterized by ketosis, signifying a lack of effective insulin. **(2)** Type II diabetes is distinguished by the absence of ketosis, signifying the presence of at least some effective insulin. **(3)** Type I diabetes is characterized by ketosis, signifying a lack of effective insulin. **(4)** Type II diabetes is distinguished by the absence of ketosis, signifying the presence of at least some effective insulin.

62. **(1)** Integrated processes: nursing process — implementation; teaching/learning client need: physiological integrity; physiological adaptation; content area: older adult.

RATIONALE

(1) The elderly person with a viral infection is very susceptible to dehydration. It is important that clients maintain their fluid and carbohydrate intake. Toast and crackers can be used to maintain energy levels. **(2)** Nutritional supplements may make the client nauseated and encourage vomiting. **(3)** The elderly person should contact the physician and ask about adjustments in type or amount of insulin that may be indicated based on blood and urine sugar levels. **(4)** While the physician may need to be notified of this condition and asked about adjustments in type or amount of insulin that may be indicated based on blood or urine sugar levels, there is nothing to suggest that emergency room care is needed immediately.

63. **(2)** Integrated processes: nursing process — implementation; teaching/learning; client need: health promotion and maintenance; content area: older adult.

RATIONALE

(1) While the client's usual dietary habits are important, in diabetic teaching, the first step is to determine the client's ideal body weight. (2) The first step in teaching diabetic dietary needs is to determine the client's ideal body weight. (3) While the client's compliance ability is important to assess, the first step in teaching diabetic dietary needs is to determine the client's ideal body weight. (4) Once the food plan is agreed on, the insulin dosage is adjusted to the prescribed diet, not vice versa.

64. **(4)** Integrated processes: nursing process — data collection; client need: physiological integrity; reduction of risk potential; content area: older adult.

RATIONALE

(1) Lipohypertrophy is an accumulation of subcutaneous fat, which occurs with repeated injections at the same site. Rotation of the injection site must be encouraged. (2) Lipohypertrophy is an accumulation of subcutaneous fat, which occurs with repeated injections at the same site. Rotation of the injection site must be encouraged. (3) Lipohypertrophy is an accumulation of subcutaneous fat, which occurs with repeated injections at the same site. Injections in these sites may be less uncomfortable and, therefore, rotation of the injection site must be encouraged. (4) Lipohypertrophy is an accumulation of subcutaneous fat, which occurs with repeated injections at the same site. Injections in these sites may be less uncomfortable and, therefore, rotation of the injection site must be encouraged.

65. **(2)** Integrated processes: nursing process — implementation; teaching/learning; client need: physiological integrity; pharmacological therapies; content area: older adult.

RATIONALE

(1) Drugs frequently used by the elderly that either intensify or weaken the effects of sulfonamide are glucocorticoid, thiazine, furosemide, nicotinic acid, alcohol, β blockers (propranolol), and the salicylates. (2) When taken as prescribed, acetaminophen is not known to have any potential drug interactions. (3) Drugs frequently used by the elderly that either intensify or weaken the effects of sulfonamide are glucocorticoid, thiazine, furosemide, nicotinic acid, alcohol, β blockers (propranolol), and the salicylates. (4) Drugs frequently used by the elderly that either intensify or weaken the effects of sulfonamide are glucocorticoid, thiazine, furosemide, nicotinic acid, alcohol, β blockers (propranolol), and the salicylates.

66. **(4)** Integrated processes: nursing process — evaluating; teaching/learning; client need: psychosocial integrity; content area: older adult.

RATIONALE

(1) While medical factors and family support are important in the assessment of incontinence, biofeedback requires that the client be cognitively intact and motivated to learn bladder inhibition and sphincter contraction. (2) While medical factors and family support are important in the assessment of incontinence, biofeedback requires that the client be cognitively intact and motivated to learn bladder inhibition and sphincter contraction. (3) While medical factors and family support are important in the assessment of incontinence, biofeedback requires that the client be cognitively intact and motivated to learn bladder inhibition and sphincter contraction. (4) Biofeedback requires that the client be cognitively intact and motivated to learn bladder inhibition and sphincter contraction.

67. **(4)** Integrated processes: nursing process — implementation; teaching/learning; client need: psychosocial integrity; content area: older adult.

RATIONALE

(1) Placing the mother in a nearby nursing home will do little to correct the problem experienced by the client and is not warranted based on the information. (2) There is no evidence to suggest that the client is not coping with the situations being presented, so mental health center services are not warranted until other causes have been ruled out. (3) From the situation presented, the nurse may ascertain that the change in sexual frequency may be the cause of the symptoms being described by the client. Referral is appropriate following a complete assessment by the nurse. (4) These symptoms are less likely if intercourse continues on a regular basis because periods of abstinence are more likely to be associated with these symptoms.

68. **(2)** Integrated processes: nursing process — implementation; client need: physiological integrity; reduction of risk potential; content area: older adult.

RATIONALE

(1) It is very common to experience muscle aches throughout the chest, upper back, shoulders, and neck. There is no reason to call the physician for this occurrence. (2) An ice pack can be placed on the muscle for 15 minutes and reapplied three times a day as necessary. (3) Medication is not recommended unless the spasms persist. (4) While muscle aches are common, they are uncomfortable, so the nurse should suggest placing an ice pack on the area for 15 minutes three times a day as necessary.

69. **(3)** Integrated processes: nursing process — data collection; client need: physiological integrity; pharmacological therapies; content area: older adult.

RATIONALE

(1) Constipation may occur with procainamide, but is not life threatening. (2) Dizziness may occur with procainamide, especially with older adults, but is not life threatening. (3) Investigate even a vague change such as shivering or fever because these may signal agranulocytosis. (4) Procainamide produces gastrointestinal irritation in some individuals. To lessen the irritation, the drug may be taken with or after meals. This side effect is not life threatening.

70. **(3)** Integrated processes: nursing process — evaluation; teaching/learning; client need: physiological integrity; pharmacological therapies; content area: older adult.

RATIONALE

(1) The client should not take a missed dose of medication, but should be cautioned to take the next regularly prescribed dose at the appropriate time. (2) Procainamide can be given as a long-term therapy as long as the client does not have adverse drug reactions or inappropriate blood values. Sensitivity to this drug is not suggested. (3) Any symptoms of unusual bleeding or bruising should be reported immediately. (4) Dizziness is an expected side effect of procainamide, and the client should be taught to be careful when rising from a sitting to a standing position. This side effect is not as crucial as bleeding.

71. **(4)** Integrated processes: nursing process — implementation; communication and documentation; client need: physiological integrity; physiological adaptation; Content area: older adult.

RATIONALE

(1) Legally, the nurse needs to make the physician know that the client has a pacemaker. (2) Legally, the nurse needs to make the physician know that the client has a pacemaker. (3) Legally, the nurse needs to make the physician know that the client has a pacemaker. (4) Legally, the nurse needs to make the physician know that the client has a pacemaker.

72. **(3)** Integrated processes: nursing process — planning; teaching/learning; client need: physiological integrity; reduction of risk potential; content area: older adult.

   RATIONALE

   (1) There is little need for adherence to a dietary regimen following pacemaker implant. **(2)** While exercise is important, there is little need for adherence to a strict exercise regimen following pacemaker implant. **(3)** Client should be instructed early on to watch for and monitor signs of infection at the implant site, including pain or tenderness, local heat or erythema, drainage, or wound dehiscence. **(4)** Follow-up checks are important, but the client is not able to check pacemaker batteries. Follow-up examinations are usually at 3-month intervals.

73. **(3)** Integrated processes: nursing process — data collection; client need: physiological integrity; physiological adaptation; content area: older adult.

   RATIONALE

   (1) Pacemaker implant does not result in prolonged bed rest. Undue fatigue, dizziness, syncope, and dyspnea may signal a drop in cardiac output. **(2)** The client may have a fear of pacemaker failure; however, undue fatigue, dizziness, syncope, and dyspnea may signal a drop in cardiac output. **(3)** Undue fatigue, dizziness, syncope, and dyspnea may signal a drop in cardiac output. **(4)** There is nothing to suggest that these symptoms are psychosomatic or that the client needs individualized attention from the nurse.

74. **(2)** Integrated processes: nursing process — implementation; client need: physiological integrity; physiological adaptation; content area: older adult.

   RATIONALE

   (1) Undue fatigue, dizziness, syncope, and dyspnea may signal a drop in cardiac output. The initial action by the nurse should be to place the client in bed and have him rest immediately to reduce the need for more cardiac output. Reassurance may assist the client emotionally, but does little to decrease the need for cardiac output. **(2)** The initial action by the nurse should be to place the client in bed and have him rest immediately to reduce the need for more cardiac output. **(3)** After placing the client in bed, the vital signs should be monitored every 15 minutes, not hourly. **(4)** The initial action by the nurse should be to place the client in bed and have him rest immediately to reduce the need for more cardiac output.

75. **(2)** Integrated processes: nursing process — implementation; teaching/learning; client need: physiological integrity; physiological adaptation; content area: older adult.

   RATIONALE

   (1) There will be follow-up examinations, but these can be done by phone every 3 months or so using a telephone transmitter supplied by the physician. **(2)** Because pacemakers will trigger alarms in metal detectors, the client should be advised to show his pacemaker identification card to airport security personnel before passing through the detector. **(3)** Once the client is dismissed from the hospital, the client is free to resume regular activities of daily living and is encouraged to do so. **(4)** Once the client is dismissed from the hospital, the client is free to resume regular activities of daily living and is encouraged to do so.

76. **(2)** Integrated processes: nursing process — implementation; client need: physiological integrity; reduction of risk potential; content area: older adult.

   RATIONALE

   (1) Informing the hospital is not appropriate because the client is in need of supervision from the cardiologist. **(2)** Significant pulse deficits are often the first indication that the pacemaker is

not working correctly. Reporting this to the physician is the most appropriate action the nurse must take. **(3)** The initial action by the nurse is to call the physician, who in turn may want an electrocardiogram (ECG) run to determine the amount of pacing and capturing. **(4)** Significant pulse deficits are often the first indication that the pacemaker is not working correctly. Reporting this to the physician is the most appropriate action the nurse must take.

77. **(2)** Integrated processes: nursing process — implementation; client need: physiological integrity; basic care and comfort; content area: older adult.

   RATIONALE

   (1) Postural drainage assists the client in expectorating the secretions, not liquefying them. **(2)** Breathing humidified air helps to liquefy secretions for easy removal. **(3)** This intervention helps loosen secretions for expectoration, not liquefy them. **(4)** These exercises help the client to expectorate secretions and expand the lungs, not liquefy secretions.

78. **(2)** Integrated processes: nursing process — implementation; client need: physiological integrity; pharmacological therapies; content area: older adult.

   RATIONALE

   (1) While furosemide does place the client at high risk for postural hypotension, the client is getting a potassium supplement in combination with enalapril, an angiotensin converting enzyme inhibitor (ACE). ACE inhibitors may increase potassium levels, and even though this has been prescribed by the physician, the nurse must be aware of the potential for a drug interaction. **(2)** The client is getting a potassium supplement in combination with enalapril, an angiotensin converting enzyme inhibitor (ACE). ACE inhibitors may increase potassium levels, and even though this has been prescribed by the physician, the nurse must be aware of the potential for a drug interaction. **(3)** While postural hypotension is an important aspect of care and should be included in client teaching, the potential for hyperkalemia is more serious and, therefore, is essential for the nurse to monitor. **(4)** The medications prescribed for this client are not associated with anorexia or decreased appetite and weight loss should not occur.

79. **(3)** Integrated processes: nursing process — implementation; client need: physiological integrity; reduction of risk potential; content area: older adult.

   RATIONALE

   (1) While this action is important, the client has 3 months before being seen by the physician; however, medications present a daily problem for the client with decreased visual acuity and forgetfulness. **(2)** The client is experiencing periods of forgetfulness. Teaching about the need for compliance does not assure it, nor does it deal with the problems that the client has—forgetfulness, decreased visual acuity, and medications. **(3)** Preparing a prefilled medication organizer weekly will assist the client to know if the medication has been taken and allows the nurse to monitor compliance. **(4)** Color coding the medication bottles may not be the best action for a client who has decreased visual acuity.

80. **(2)** Integrated processes: nursing process — implementation; teaching/learning; client need: physiological integrity; reduction of risk potential; content area: older adult.

   RATIONALE

   (1) Alcohol interferes with rapid eye movement (REM) sleep and should be avoided when possible. **(2)** Alcohol interferes with rapid eye movement (REM) sleep and should be avoided when possible. **(3)** The client with sleep apnea is encouraged to avoid any medication that interferes with sleep, including stimulants, sedatives, or hypnotics. **(4)** Clients with sleep apnea are encouraged to join in weight-loss programs. A high-calorie, protein-rich food right before bedtime is not appropriate for weight loss.

81. **(4)** Integrated processes: nursing process — implementation; teaching/learning; client need: physiological integrity; physiological adaptation; content area: older adult.

    RATIONALE

    (1) While a depressed client may experience anxiety, this is not the rationale for the hyperactivity experienced by the client. **(2)** Paroxetine may cause somnolence, sweating, tremors, and fatigue, but anxiety is not associated with paroxetine. **(3)** Insomnia can be caused by anxiety and depression, but this response by the nurse does not answer the question of the hyperactivity by the client. **(4)** The client does have symptoms of hypothyroidism and drug interaction, so this should be assessed by the physician and the nurse.

82. **(4)** Integrated processes: nursing process — implementation; teaching/learning; client need: physiological integrity; basic care and comfort; content area: older adult.

    RATIONALE

    (1) While increasing fruits, fiber, and fluids is an appropriate nursing action with the client history of previous cancer of the colon and the recent change in bowel habit, this should be evaluated by the physician. **(2)** Any recent change in bowel habit should be carefully assessed. Constipation is not a normal aging change. **(3)** Taking an over-the-counter stool softener may mask the symptoms exhibited by the client and make diagnosis difficult. **(4)** With the client's history of previous cancer of the colon and the recent change in bowel habit, this should be evaluated by the physician.

83. **(4)** Integrated processes: nursing process — planning; client need: health promotion and maintenance; content area: older adult.

    RATIONALE

    (1) There is nothing noted in this situation that the client has family or that the family would be willing or able to assist. Also, there is no assurance that with family involvement, compliance would be the outcome. **(2)** While the client lives in low-income housing, there is nothing to suggest that this client has a need for financial assistance. **(3)** If the client has some difficulty with learning, the educational level might be such that educational reading materials would be helpful to the client. **(4)** A newly diagnosed older adult with diabetes will have to learn new lifestyle behaviors. The nurse should prepare a carefully structured individualized plan to assist the client to learn new lifestyle behaviors and to implement these changes in daily living.

84. **(2)** Integrated processes: nursing process — implementation; client need: physiological integrity; reduction of risk potential; content area: older adult.

    RATIONALE

    (1) This may be important, but the client has a normal blood sugar for an older adult. **(2)** A 2-hour blood glucose of 200 is normal and requires only to be monitored by the nurse. **(3)** This is not a priority because this is normal for older adults. **(4)** A 2-hour blood glucose of 200 is normal and requires only to be monitored by the nurse.

85. **(2)** Integrated processes: nursing process — data collection; client need: physiological integrity; physiological adaptation; content area: older adult.

    RATIONALE

    (1) A client with sensorineural hearing loss may speak in an excessively loud voice in many situations where a loud voice is inappropriate. **(2)** The client with a conductive hearing loss usually speaks in a relatively quiet voice, making it difficult to hear him. **(3)** A client with a sensorineural hearing loss may be sensitive to loud intensities of sound and hear better in a quiet environment. **(4)** While the typmanic membrane may appear sclerotic and scarred in the older adult, these changes do not usually affect hearing.

86. **(1)** Integrated processes: nursing process — implementation; teaching/learning; client need: health promotion and maintenance; content area: older adult.

    RATIONALE

    (1) A hearing aid can be ordered from the hearing aid vendor for a 2- to 4-week trial. If for any reason the client cannot adjust to amplification, the hearing aid can be returned to the vendor within 4 weeks, which is allowed by law. **(2)** Medicare reimbursement does not include hearing aids. **(3)** The Food and Drug Administration requires an examination by a physician prior to dispensing a hearing aid, but does not require the physician to purchase the aid. **(4)** A hearing aid can be ordered from the hearing aid vendor for a 2- to 4-week trial. If for any reason the client cannot adjust to amplification, the hearing aid can be returned to the vendor within 4 weeks, which is allowed by law.

87. **(3)** Integrated processes: nursing process — implementation; teaching/learning; client need: health promotion and maintenance; content area: older adult.

    RATIONALE

    (1) The client should be instructed to wear the hearing aid 4–5 hours at first and for a longer period of time each day, removing the aid for bed, bathing, or showering. **(2)** The client should be instructed to wear the hearing aid 4–5 hours at first and for a longer period of time each day, removing the aid for bed, bathing, or showering. **(3)** The client should be instructed to wear the hearing aid 4–5 hours at first and for a longer period of time each day, removing the aid for bed, bathing, or showering. **(4)** The client should be instructed to wear the hearing aid 4–5 hours at first and for a longer period of time each day, removing the aid for bed, bathing, or showering.

88. **(3)** Integrated processes: nursing process — evaluation; teaching/learning; client need: psychosocial integrity; content area: older adult.

    RATIONALE

    (1) The ear mold should be cleaned once a week with a cloth dampened with mild, soapy water. **(2)** If a whistle (feedback) is not heard when the volume control is fully on, change the battery and the whistle should be heard; if not, there is a problem with the aid. **(3)** Hearing aid batteries are changed every 10 days to 2 weeks. **(4)** There is no set maintenance schedule for a hearing aid.

89. **(1)** Integrated processes: nursing process — implementation; teaching/learning; client need: psychosocial integrity; content area: older adult.

    RATIONALE

    (1) After living in a quiet world, suddenly hearing loud voices and noises can cause the client to become tense and nervous. Informing the client of this will assist the client in adapting to the hearing aid. **(2)** Adjusting the hearing aid in public or asking for assistance can be traumatic and embarrassing to the client. **(3)** Some clients may have physical impairments that make manipulation of the hearing aid batteries difficult or impossible, so the assistance of family members may be needed. **(4)** The hearing aid not only makes the speaker's voice louder, but it also amplifies everyone's speech and other noises in the room.

90. **(0.25 mL)** Integrated processes: nursing process — implementation; client need: physiological integrity; pharmacological therapies; content area: older adult.
   RATIONALE
   1000 mg : 1 mL = 250 mg : x = .025 mL

91. **(5 tablets)** Integrated processes: nursing process — implementation; communication and documentation; client need: physiological integrity; pharmacological therapies; content area: older adult.
   RATIONALE
   200 mg : 1 tablet = 1000 mg : x = 5 tablets

92. **(3 tablets)** Integrated processes: nursing process — implementation; communication and documentation; client need: physiological integrity; pharmacological therapies; content area: older adult.
   RATIONALE
   325 mg : 1 tablet = 975 mg : x = 3 tablets

93. **(6 tablets)** Integrated processes: nursing process — implementation; communication and documentation; client need: physiological integrity; pharmacological therapies; content area: older adult.
   RATIONALE
   500 mg : 1 tablet = 3000 mg : x = 6 tablets

94. **(17 mL)** Integrated processes: nursing process — implementation; communication and documentation; client need: physiological integrity; pharmacological therapies; content area: older adult.
   RATIONALE
   500 mg : 5 mL = 1700 mg : x = 17 mL

95. **(1.25 mL)** Integrated processes: nursing process — implementation; communication and documentation; client need: physiological integrity; pharmacological therapies; content area: older adult.

RATIONALE
120 μg : 1 mL = 150 μg : x = 1.25 mL

96. **(4 tablets)** integrated processes: nursing process — implementation; teaching/learning; client need: physiological integrity; pharmacological therapies; content area: older adult.
   RATIONALE
   100 mg : 1 tablet = 400 mg : x = 4 tablets

97. **(0.75 mL)** Integrated processes: nursing process — implementation; communication and documentation; client need: physiological integrity; pharmacological therapies; content area: older adult.
   RATIONALE
   100 mg : 1 mL = 75 mg : x = 0.75 mL

98. **(1.5 tablets)** integrated processes: nursing process — implementation; communication and documentation; client need: physiological integrity; pharmacological therapies; content area: older adult.
   RATIONALE
   150 mg divided by 100 mg × 1 tablet = 1.5 tablets

99. **(30 mL)** Integrated processes: nursing process — implementation; client need: physiological integrity; pharmacological therapies; content area: older adult.
   RATIONALE
   20 g divided by 10 g × 15 mL = 30 mL

100. **(4 containers)** Integrated processes: nursing process — implementation; communication and documentation; client need: physiological integrity; pharmacological therapies; content area: older adult.
   RATIONALE
   A dose after each meal = 3 doses, plus 1 dose at bedtime makes a total of 4 containers needed.

CHAPTER 7

Psychiatric–Mental Health Nursing: Content Review and Test

Eileen W. Keefe, RN.C, MS
Golden Tradewell, RN, PhD

Nursing Care of Psychiatric–Mental Health Clients

The psychiatric nurse promotes health through caring for and about the client. The health promotion is accomplished through understanding, observing, teaching, and physical care skills.

I. Care of physiological needs: Psychiatric clients are often unable to complete activities of daily living (ADLs) independently. The nurse monitors and supervises their performance.
  A. Feeding: Quantity and quality of food intake are observed and recorded. Calorie counts are recorded. Intake and output (I&O) of fluids are monitored. Confused, severely depressed, and severely retarded clients are fed by the nurse. Appetite is observed and documented.
  B. Sleep: Amount and quality of sleep are observed and recorded. Clients are checked every 30 minutes throughout the night. Sleep charts are recorded. Often clients are not allowed to sleep in the daytime to stabilize sleep patterns.
  C. Vital signs: Psychiatric medications may cause wide fluctuations in blood pressure and temperature. Vital signs are checked and recorded as the physician orders, usually four times daily. Orthostatic blood pressure measurements (checking the blood pressure with the client lying down and 1 minute later with the client standing) give physicians information about how medication is being metabolized in the client. A high temperature is a side effect of neuroleptic (antipsychotic) medication.
  D. Hygiene: Psychiatric clients, particularly those who are very confused, depressed, or withdrawn, need assistance with bathing, bed making, and dental care. Encourage the client to complete as many of the hygiene tasks as possible. The nurse assists the client in completing daily hygiene.
  E. Elimination: Psychiatric medications may alter elimination habits. Information about bowel and urinary function is gathered and documented by the nurse daily.
  F. Activity: The client's energy level is observed. Clients are encouraged to attend therapeutic activities (e.g., art therapy, music therapy). Mobility, gait, and coordination are observed. The nurse assists clients who cannot ambulate independently.

II. Safety: Psychiatric clients' safety is the responsibility of the nurse. Specific psychiatric nursing procedures include
  A. Admission: The nurse ensures the client's safety by removing guns, knives, sharp instruments, glass objects, and medications on admission. Often, very confused or disturbed clients are dressed in pajamas on admission. Most clients are allowed to wear street clothes, but belts and sharp jewelry are removed from the client to ensure safety.
  B. Restraints: When clients are assessed to be harmful to themselves or others, the physician may order restraints. All other measures must be exhausted before restraints are used. An order for restraints is *written* for a specified period not to exceed 12 hours (differs from state to state). The health-care team organizes the procedure before approaching the client. A *minimum* of five people is needed to restrain a client. Each team member is assigned a limb (arm or leg) to restrain. The team leader explains the procedure to the client and directs the team. With very violent clients, a waist restraint may be added.

A client in restraints is monitored constantly by a nurse to provide a calm and safe environment, to attend to physiological needs, and to observe reactions. Restraints are removed each hour to ensure circulation.

C. Seclusion: Clients who are assessed to be harmful to themselves or others are sometimes placed in seclusion (a bare room with a mattress) to decrease environmental stimuli. Seclusion allows the client to retain or regain control of behavior. The team escorts the client to seclusion (a minimum of three personnel) *after* a physician's order is obtained. Sharp objects, belts, and jewelry are removed from the client to ensure safety. Clients may be placed in various forms of seclusion.

1. Locked-door seclusion: The door is locked and the client and the mattress remain in the room. The client is constantly observed.
2. Open-door seclusion: The client remains in the room with the door unlocked and open. The client is observed constantly or every 5 minutes.
3. Room program: The client remains in the room 30 minutes but is allowed out of the room 30 minutes each hour. The client's reaction and behavior are observed. If the client resumes control of his or her behavior, the in-and-out time is altered accordingly (e.g., 45 minutes out, 15 minutes in).

D. Mobility: Psychiatric medication may cause dizziness (vertigo). All psychiatric clients are checked frequently (e.g., at 15, 30, or 60 minutes) to assess their safety.

E. Environmental: No cords over pathways, sharp corners on furniture, loose rugs, or items that are hard and can be thrown to cause harm are permitted. The nurse is responsible for the safety of the clients and staff. The psychiatric nurse observes client-client, client-family, and client-staff interactions to prevent outbursts.

III. Interaction/Communication: The psychiatric nurse encourages and assists clients to interact and communicate with others. The nurse observes

A. Emotional reactions: Does the client laugh or cry inappropriately? Does the client talk with clients and staff? Can he or she carry on a social conversation? Does the client react appropriately? Does he or she smile? Can the client demonstrate caring for others? Does he or she participate in activities? Can the client enjoy himself or herself?

B. Communication: What are the client's nonverbal and verbal communication skills? Is the client's behavior similar to the communication skills? Does he or she sound and look pleasant or sound happy *and* look angry?

C. Family: What are the interactions of the client with the family, spouse, and/or children? What pattern have they developed (are they sullen, silent, happy, fighting)?

IV. Self-esteem: The psychiatric nurse promotes the maintenance and development of a client's self-esteem.

A. Self-relationship: Assess for client self-worth, strengths, goals, problem-solving ability, motivation, state of independence, ability to participate in daily care, and discharge planning.

The Health-Care Team

I. A psychiatrist is a physician who specializes in the care of clients having mental disorders.

II. A psychiatric nurse is a nurse who specializes by experience and/or education in the care of psychiatric clients. A psychiatric clinical specialist has a master's degree in nursing or doctoral degree in nursing.

III. A psychologist specializes in psychological testing, counseling, and therapy.

IV. An occupational therapist specializes in teaching leisure, occupational, or daily skills to clients (e.g., cooking, art, typing).

V. A recreational therapist teaches clients recreational and leisure skills (e.g., painting, needlework, model cars).

VI. A social worker specializes in working with the family, in community resources, and in counseling and therapy.

VII. A molecular psychiatrist specializes in biochemical aspects of the brain, a neurophysiologist specializes in the physiology of the body's nervous systems, and a neuropsychiatrist specializes in the neurological system and behavior.

VIII. A psychopharmacologist specializes in psychotropic medications and drugs that affect behavior.

Psychiatric Terminology

Affect: Refers to mood or emotion; seen on one's face and described as blunted, flat, inappropriate, or bland

Ambivalence: Two feelings together (love-hate, pleasure-pain, like-dislike) toward a person, object, or idea

Behavior: Any observable, recordable act, movement, or response of an individual

Blocking: Interruption of flow of speech owing to distracting thoughts

Body language: Transmission of a message by body movements

Catatonia: State of immobilized stupor that can quickly swing to extreme agitation

Catharsis: Release that occurs when clients talk openly

Cathexis: Freud's term for attachment to an object or idea; when one connects to a person or idea, there is a strong bond

Circumstantial: Digression of thought into unnecessary details (e.g., explaining pain, but talking about one's mother's surgery)

Claustrophobia: Fear of closed places

Compulsion: Irresistible urge to perform some act (e.g., handwashing)

Congruent: Verbal communication that matches nonverbal communication

Delirium: Medical diagnostic term that describes rapidly occurring onset of confusion

Delusion: Fixed false belief (e.g., one believes that he is Christ)

Depression: Can be a sign, symptom, disease, or reaction of sadness or grief

Dissociation: Separation of mental processes from a person's consciousness

Diurnal mood: Changes in mood because of time of day

Echolalia: Imitation of another's words

Echopraxia: Imitation of another's body position

Ego boundaries: Person's perception of the boundaries between self and environment

Endogenous: Occurring within; refers to a type of depression

Environment: Circumstances, people, objects, and conditions that surround and have an impact on one's life

Ethnocentrism: Imposing of one's beliefs and values on other cultural groups

Fantasy: Daydreaming

Flight of ideas: Rapid shift of ideas while speaking (e.g., speaking of weather, to mother, to pain with no connection between subjects)

Grandiose: Ideas of fame, wealth, or importance that are unfounded or untrue (e.g., a woman thinking that she is Elizabeth Taylor)

Hallucination: Seeing, hearing, smelling, or feeling something that is not a result of external stimuli (e.g., seeing or feeling bugs crawl on the skin)

Hostility: An attitude of negativity or anger

Hypochondriasis: Belief that one is ill with no organic cause, such as pain with no cause

Hypomania: An older clinical term that refers to "less than severe manic" behavior (generally, behavior that is unfocused or hyperactive is called "manic"; if the client is excited and exhausted it is called "full-blown mania")

Illusion: Misinterpretation of sensory—usually visual—input (e.g., seeing water in the desert that is really sand)

Insight: Awareness and understanding of behavior

Institutionalized syndrome: Characterized by apathy, withdrawal, and submission to authority

Labile: Frequent and rapid change of emotions

Limit setting: Communicating the rights, responsibilities, and expectations to a person so that expected normal limits and rules can be identified

Manic-depressive illness (MDI): A psychotic state characterized by excited or severely depressed behavior; bipolar disorder

Neologism: Invention of a new word (e.g., "alzopra" instead of "chair")

Neurotic: Behavior or dysfunction that is characterized by anxiety but no distortion of reality

Nihilism: False belief that part of one's self is dead

Obsession: Recurring, unstoppable thought

Orientation: Knowing correctly the time, place, and person

Panic: Extreme anxiety that involves dread and loss of rational thought

Phobia: Extreme persistent fear that is out of proportion to reality

Psychosis: Severely dysfunctional behavior characterized by anxiety, reduced functioning, limited awareness, and personality distintegration; out of touch with reality

Reminiscence: Systematic review of life experiences

Repression: Involuntary exclusion of painful memories

Self-disclosure: Revealing information about one's ideals, feelings, and values in the context of a therapeutic or specific goal

Somnambulism: Sleepwalking

Transference: Response of a client to a nurse that was originally associated with an important figure in early life (e.g., a client treating a nurse like his or her mother)

Word salad: Jumbled disconnected words (e.g., down far black strip grass)

Types of Treatment Distinctive to Psychiatric Settings

The psychiatric nurse promotes a therapeutic environment for the client by assisting in the different types of treatment.

I. Somatic therapy
   A. Antipsychotic drugs
      1. Action: Stopping or diminishing disabling symptoms such as aggression, hallucinations, irritability, delusions
      2. Use: Psychotic disorders such as organic disorders, affective disorders, and schizophrenia
      3. Agents: Chlorpromazine (Thorazine), haloperidol (Haldol), loxapine (Loxitane), fluphenazine (Prolixin), molindone (Moban)
      4. Major side effects: Extrapyramidal side effects such as restlessness, shuffling gait, muscle rigidity, urinary retention, low blood pressure, sedation, and high temperature
      5. Nursing care: Reporting of observations of high temperature or movements; checking frequency of elimination patterns; monitoring vital signs lying down and standing
   B. Antidepressants
      1. Action: Stimulating the limbic system (tricyclics and heterocyclics) or inhibiting the oxidase enzyme (monamine oxidase inhibitors, or MAOIs); mood elevated
      2. Use: Clinical depression; depressive cycle of MDI
      3. Agents: Isocarboxazid (Marplan [MAOI]), tranylcypromine (Parnate [MAOI]), amitriptyline (Elavil), desipramine (Norpramin), imipramine (Tofranil)
      4. Nursing care: Intramuscular (IM) administration not recommended as absorption is slow and erratic; quickly absorbed sublinguinally. Observe for inhibition and excitement after multiple doses. Observe for withdrawal symptoms after long-term use. Monitor vital signs. Teach client not to consume alcohol while taking anxiolytics.
II. Electroconvulsive therapy: ECT is a series of controlled electrical currents applied to the brain to produce grand mal seizures; it is given under anesthesia. Nursing care of the client undergoing ECT includes
   A. Provide preoperative care (keep client on nothing by mouth [NPO], remove dentures, empty bladder).
   B. Give preoperative muscle relaxer IM.
   C. Complete preoperative checklist.
   D. Accompany client to ECT room.
   E. Monitor vital signs.
   F. Prevent aspiration as needed.
   G. Observe for complications of fractures.
   H. Assist in recovery, anticipate confusion; help to reorient.
   I. Document recovery.
   J. ECT is now used only as a last resort when all other treatments of certain depressions do not help the client.
   K. Provide safety measures and reorientation if client is confused.
III. Milieu therapy: The environment can promote recovery and health.

A. Manage physical and psychological aspects of the client's environment to promote behavioral changes.
B. Increase or decrease environmental stimuli to promote client's interactions, monitor activity, protect the client, enhance the client's personality.
C. Assist with adjunct therapies
   1. Occupational therapy
   2. Recreational therapy
   3. Group therapy
   4. Client education groups
   5. Discharge groups
   6. Family therapy groups
   7. Music therapy
   8. Dance therapy
   9. Pet therapy
   10. Movement therapy
   11. Psychodrama
   12. Reminiscence therapy

The Nurse-Client Relationship

I. The psychiatric nurse uses self as a tool to assist the client in healing. Nursing care includes:
   A. Understanding of self, needs, and feelings
   B. Awareness of personal strengths and limitations
   C. Respect for the client
   D. Ability to listen
   E. Being authentic
   F. Offering support, reassurance
   G. Maintaining a calm attitude
   H. Using empathy (understanding), which is more effective than sympathy (pity)
   I. Understanding of the client's cultural beliefs
   J. Understanding that the nurse-client relationship is goal oriented, time limited, and composed of three phases (introduction, working, ending)
II. Mental health nursing occurs in the following environments
   A. Inpatient hospital
   B. Outpatient clinic
   C. Day (or night) care
   D. Assisted living
   E. Homeless shelter
   F. Nursing home

Communication

Communication is a process of sending and receiving verbal (spoken) and nonverbal (body language) messages. The nurse uses communication to gather information, establish a relationship with the client, and provide nursing care.

I. Effective communication between the nurse and client is encouraged by
   A. Finding a private place to talk
   B. Making sure the client is comfortable
   C. Reducing distractions (television, radio, noise)
   D. Stating sentences clearly
   E. Listening to the client's words
   F. Listening to what the client means
   G. Maintaining eye contact with the client
   H. Sitting no farther than 3 feet away from the client
   I. Treating the client like a person
   J. Smiling; looking concerned
   K. Behaving in a caring manner
   L. Using language the client will understand
II. Nurses communicate in many ways
   A. Verbal (spoken or written) communication, including voice tone, vocabulary, speed of speech
   B. Nonverbal communication, including the body and facial expression (kinesis), how close or far the nurse sits to the client (proxemics)
III. Effective communication is
   A. Efficient and clear
   B. Consistent (say and mean the same thing)
   C. Open, friendly
   D. Purposeful
IV. Communication may be blocked by
   A. Giving advice ("Mr. Jones, I think you *should*... .")
   B. Changing topics quickly
   C. Blaming the client ("You know it's bad to smoke.")
   D. False reassurance ("Don't worry, it'll be OK.")
   E. Saying something that is not true (lying)
   F. Judging the client ("You're stupid to eat sweets.")
   G. Asking "why" too often
   H. Asking too many questions
   I. Being angry with the client
   J. Arguing with the client
V. Therapeutic communication techniques include
   A. Open-ended statements: Saying, "Tell me more about that."
   B. Reflection: When the client feels depressed, the nurse reflects, "You feel depressed."
   C. Finding the meaning: When the client says, "I feel depressed," the nurse says, "And 'depressed' means what to you?"
   D. Silence.
   E. Listening.
   F. Identifying themes: Helping the client see a pattern of thought and feeling ("You're talking about death a lot.").
   G. Accepting: Allowing the client to speak freely.
   H. Attentiveness: Calling client by name; responding nonverbally.
   I. Clarifying: "You mean... ."
   J. Restating: Rearranging words in a different order to clarify meaning.
   K. Focusing: Assisting client to stick to the topic.
   L. Giving information: Giving the client, e.g., facts about a diagnostic test.
   M. Providing feedback: "You have been speaking of anger against your Mom."
   N. Making observations: "You look happy."
VI. Therapeutic communication methods require the nurse to
   A. Become aware of and monitor own verbal and nonverbal communication patterns.
   B. Recognize that his or her own cultural and subcultural values and customs influence perception and interpretation of another's behavior.
   C. Check on his or her interpretations of client behavior with client or with other professionals.
   D. Operate on facts, not assumptions:
   E. State observations ("You are talking about funerals. Are you thinking of death?").
   F. Demonstrate acceptance of client.

G. Remain objective in assessing client's behavior.
H. Demonstrate concern, understanding, and respect.
I. Remain genuine and nonjudgmental.
J. Allow sufficient time and avoid a hurried approach.
K. Focus on strengths of client.
L. Use therapeutic communication techniques.
M. Communicate openness and willingness to trust client and to share a nurse-client relationship.
N. Select an environment that provides privacy, comfort, and minimal distraction.
O. Express empathy by accurately understanding client's feelings. The nurse's answers should reflect an awareness of and sensitivity to the client's culture, values, and life experiences.
P. Use resources of information (chart, family, physician).
Q. Assist the client to become more aware of an aspect of his or her behavior or problem.

Development of Self

I. The self may include
A. Self-concept: How one *thinks* of oneself
B. Self-ideal: One's ideal notion of who one should be
C. Self-esteem: How one feels about oneself
D. Spiritual self: Allows one the opportunity to connect with a higher being and to find meaning and purpose in one's experiences

E. Identity: A general sense of who one is
F. Character: A person's pattern of discipline, moral constitution, and reputation
G. Personality: Behaviors specific to each individual (e.g., a general pattern of self-centeredness, kindness, suspiciousness, and so on)
H. Role: One's perception of how one fits into social settings (e.g., role of aunt, employee, sister)

II. The self is the sum total of thoughts, feelings, physical characteristics, socioeconomic status, ethnicity, and family-cultural factors. Self is affected by
A. Heredity: Genetic impact on neurological system that influences behavior
B. Environment: External factors that influence behavior (family, culture, and so on)
C. Developmental norms: Level of development of self described by several theorists

Table 7–1 is an overview of three theories of development at each stage of life.

Nursing Care of Problem Behaviors

Anxiety

Anxiety is a generalized vague feeling of psychic pain that is associated with feelings of uncertainty and helplessness. It occurs as a result of a threat to a person's ideals, being, or self-esteem.

Table 7–1. Overview of Three Developmental Theories

Approximate Age	Freud	Erikson	Piaget
Infant (0–1 yr)	Oral stage: Characterized by dependence and narcissism; exploration using mouth especially when area stimulated	Trust versus mistrust: Characterized by establishing a trusting relationship with another	Sensorimotor: Learning to recognize object permanence
Toddler (1–3 yr)	Anal: Defiant behavior, socialization control established	Autonomy versus shame: Characterized by negativism and exertion of self-will	Preoperational: Learning to think in terms of past, present, and future
Preschooler (3–5 yr)	Phallic: Beginning socialization, faculty, sexual identity, sexual deviations	Initiative versus guilt: Imitation of adults, development of a conscience	
School Age (6–11 yr)	Latency: Group identification, intellectual growth	Industry versus inferiority: Intellectual curiosity, learning rules and regulations	Concrete operations: Ability to classify, order, and sort facts
Adolescent (12–18 yr)	Genital: Sexual maturity, heterosexual relations	Identity versus role confusion: Establishment of identity, development of heterosexual relationships	Formal operations: Ability to think abstractly and logically
Young Adult (19–34 yr)		Intimacy versus isolation: Close personal relationships with adults and with both sexes	
Middle Adult (35–60 yr)		Generativity versus stagnation: Creativity and productivity, development of lasting, fulfilling relationships	
Older Adult (>60 yr)		Ego integrity versus despair: Accepting of death, adjustment to changes in body image	

I. Data collection
   A. Mild anxiety is associated with day-to-day living. Person is alert, motivated, creative, productive, and aware.
   B. Moderate anxiety narrows the awareness of environment. Symptoms include tension in neck and shoulders, urinary frequency, headaches, perspiration, sleep disturbances, restlessness, being overly critical of self and others, and an inability to concentrate.
   C. Severe anxiety is very uncomfortable. The person is unable to focus on anything but obtaining relief. Observe for clinical symptoms of chest pain, angry outbursts, mood swings, helplessness, physical complaints, and inability to complete activities of daily living (ADLs).
   D. Panic is a feeling of terror, pain, or helplessness. Individuals experience a loss of control of increased motor activity, loss of rational thought, and an inability to function as an organized human being. Darting eyes, dilated pupils, fixed stare, hypertension, and flushed face are common symptoms.
II. Planning and implementation
   A. Keep client safe.
   B. Establish a trusting relationship.
   C. Administer medications (lorazepam [Ativan], alprazolam [Xanax]).
   D. Provide calm environment.
   E. Use short, simple sentences.
   F. Assist client to verbalize anxiety.
   G. Encourage client to identify acceptable methods of coping.
III. Evaluation
   A. Client remains free of anxiety symptoms.
   B. Client is able to verbalize source of anxiety.

Loss (Grief)

Loss is a life event experienced by everyone, regardless of age, sex, race, or economic status. Loss is defined as any change in an individual's situation. One can experience loss of others (through death, divorce, or separation); loss of objects; loss of abstractions of self (pride, self-esteem); or loss of self (amputation, suicide, death).

I. Data collection
   A. Stages of dying (Kübler-Ross) include
      1. Shock and denial: Person cannot believe that he or she will die; seeks second opinions, ignores facts, and is unable to accept own demise.
      2. Anger: Person realizes the truth and is enraged at this impending death; becomes demanding, dependent, or aggressive.
      3. Bargaining: Person bargains with God or authority for more time.
      4. Depression: Person feels sad, alone, and helpless to change fate; withdraws, cries, and ponders.
      5. Acceptance: Person is tranquil and ready for death; has made peace with the inevitable.
   B. States of grief (Engel): Loss of self (dying) is only one manifestation of loss. Loss of others, objects, or abstractions can produce a grief response. These states of grief are also seen in surviving significant others.
      1. Shock and disbelief: Person refuses to acknowledge or believe the loss.
      2. Developing awareness: Person experiences physical symptoms such as nausea, diarrhea, crying, and anger.
      3. Restitution: Person accepts that the loss has occurred; total resolution may take 1–2 years to adapt to new situation.
II. Planning and implementation
   A. Be empathetic and kind.
   B. Offer support, listening, presence.
   C. Use the techniques of life review and reminiscence.
   D. Attend to physical needs.
   E. Include family in process.
   F. Use resources that client may need (priest, spiritual counselor, lawyer, social worker, and so on).
III. Evaluation
   A. Client resolves loss and verbalizes meaning of experience.

Anger and Aggression

Anger is a *feeling* of resentment that occurs when a person feels a threat. Hostility is an *attitude* associated with anger. Aggression is a *behavior* aimed at hurting another psychologically or physically. Anger may be positive in that anger energizes people, encourages expression, increases self-esteem, protects the self, gives one a sense of control, and alerts one to the need for coping mechanisms. Aggression and rage are most often viewed as negative.

I. Data collection
   A. Observe what stimulates anger in the client; determine what threatens the client (husband or wife, job loss, boss, bankruptcy, pain).
   B. Aggressive acts range from attacks on objects to homicide; assess the client's level of self-control, own safety, and the safety of others.
   C. Diminished capacity to think and speak may be evident.
   D. Physiological responses (tight jaw, clenched fist, hypertension) should be documented.
II. Planning and implementation
   A. Observe and document physical and verbal symptoms.
   B. Keep client and staff safe.
   C. Stay calm.
   D. Set limits ("I understand your anger, but you may not throw the chair at me.").
   E. State expectations in a positive way.
   F. Help client to explore meaning of anger.
   G. Help client to explore spiritual needs.
   H. Teach client to express anger in appropriate way.
   I. Medicate, if necessary.
   J. *Never* see potentially violent client alone.
   K. *Never* block your escape route.
III. Evaluation
   A. Feelings are expressed without violence.
   B. Client discovers source of anger and identifies coping mechanisms for future.

Self-Destruction and Suicidal Behavior

Suicide is self-inflicted death. A suicidal gesture is a suicide attempt that is planned to be discovered. A suicidal threat is a nonverbal or verbal warning of an individual's plan to attempt suicide (e.g., "Will you remember me when I'm gone?"). Suicidal thoughts are thoughts about killing oneself. Confused, alcoholic, chronic pain, insomniac, and severely depressed persons have a suicide potential. *All* types of suicidal behaviors (both threats and gestures) should be considered serious by the nurse.

I. Data collection
   A. Symptoms of severe depression with suicide potential include
      1. Sleep disorders, appetite change, weight loss
      2. Despondency (severe sadness)
      3. Helplessness, hopeless feelings
      4. Poor impulse control
      5. Feelings of rage
      6. History of suicide threats
      7. Guilt, agitation
   B. Behaviors that suggest suicide potential include
      1. Giving away personal articles
      2. Early morning awakening (3 AM to 5 AM)
      3. Sudden changes in energy (depression to gaiety)
      4. Self-preoccupation
      5. Withdrawal from communication
      6. Putting things "in order" (will, personal files)
II. Planning and implementation
   A. Safety is the nurse's highest priority
      1. Remove all sharp objects, matches, and belts.
      2. Ensure that medications are swallowed (*never* leave the medications in the room, and *do* check the client's mouth after giving medications).
      3. Keep eyes *on* the client, but remain sensitive to privacy.
      4. Temperature, level of bath water, and the client's bathing should be monitored by nurse.
      5. Temperature is taken rectally or by axillary means (not orally).
      6. Client's poor impulse control (e.g., head-banging) may require seclusion or restraint.
      7. Supervise smoking.
      8. Stairwells and windows must be kept locked.
   B. Communication with suicidal clients includes
      1. Face your own feelings about suicide.
      2. Display understanding ("I understand that you feel like hurting yourself.").
      3. Tell the client that you intend to protect him or her by making statements such as "I am here to make sure that you are safe."
      4. Encourage the client to talk, but do not probe.
      5. Ask directly if the client has a plan ("Do you have a plan to hurt yourself?").
      6. Report and document the client's suicidal statements.
      7. Report and document client's mood change (e.g., depression to gaiety).
      8. Inform charge nurse when you are going to be with a suicidal client (charge nurse is responsible for safety of staff and client).
      9. Call for help if client becomes impulsive (e.g., if client begins to head-bang, get help).
III. Evaluation
   A. Client expresses feelings of safety and remains safe.

Withdrawal

Clients who demonstrate withdrawn behavior may be psychotic, depressed, confused, or angry. Withdrawal may be seen as seclusive or isolative. Extreme withdrawal is a break from reality (psychosis). Withdrawal may be physical, psychological, and/or social.

I. Data collection
   A. Symptoms of withdrawal include
      1. Lack of attention to personal hygiene
      2. Inability to experience pleasure (anhedonia)
      3. Talking to self (or imaginary persons)
      4. Suspicion of others; lack of trust
      5. Poor eye contact
      6. Lack of interest in surroundings
      7. Lack of appetite
      8. Preoccupation
      9. Blank expression on face (flat affect)
      10. Inability to make decisions
      11. Fear of others
      12. Thinking about one topic constantly (rumination)
      13. Unwillingness or inability to communicate
      14. Indifference, aloofness
      15. Lack of interest in others' feelings
II. Planning and implementation
   A. Demonstrate a quiet, warm, accepting presence with the client.
   B. Establish rapport through shared time and supportive companionship.
   C. Offer assistance with activities.
   D. Intervene when necessary to ensure client's physical health and safety.
   E. Be cognizant of maintaining appropriate physical distance and using touch cautiously.
   F. In an acute situation, reassure client and remain with him or her in a quiet setting.
III. Evaluation
   A. Client responds appropriately and is able to interact with people and within the environment.

Psychosis

Psychosis occurs when the client loses contact with reality. Often the thought content and form, as well as the client's affect and relationships, are severely disturbed. Psychotic clients require accurate and constant observation.

I. Data collection
   A. Symptoms of psychosis include
      1. Delusions
      2. Hallucinations
      3. Fear of staff
      4. Loose thinking
      5. Suspiciousness
      6. Aggressive behavior
      7. Blank stare on face

8. Rigid movement
9. Regressed, childlike behavior
II. Planning and implementation
A. Provide safe environment (remove sharp objects).
B. Stay with client.
C. Provide reassurance.
D. Monitor hygiene and food intake.
E. Stay calm.
F. Do not support delusions ("I know you believe that, but I do not.").
G. Do not support hallucinations ("I know you're frightened, but I see nothing.").
H. Do not argue with the client.
I. Document sleep pattern.
J. Involve client in structured activity.
K. Provide reassurance.
L. Protect other clients from intrusion.
M. Administer medications (lithium or antidepressants such as Elavil, or both).
N. Be firm but kind.
O. Assist with diagnostic studies.
P. Obtain family history of mood disorder.
Q. Document client's behavior.
R. Encourage family support.
III. Evaluation
A. Psychotic episodes have a cyclic pattern; improvement rather than cure is the goal.
B. Client remains safe, in a stable mood.
C. Client is able to return to work.

Personality Disorders

Manipulation is a hallmark of personality disorders. Personality disorders are diagnosed when personal traits are maladaptive and cause significant functional impairments or subjective distress.

Types of personality disorders include
A. Paranoid: Essential feature of suspicion
B. Schizoid: Pervasive pattern of strange thoughts, dress, and relationship deficits
C. Antisocial: Impulsive, self-centered pattern of behavior that concludes in frequent conflicts with society
D. Passive-aggressive: Characterized by passive resistance to demands in occupational and social settings
E. Borderline: Marked by instability of interpersonal behavior, mood, and self-esteem. (Instability "borders" between psychosis and neurosis.)
II. Data collection
A. Chronic, maladaptive social responses according to the *Diagnostic and Statistical Manual of Mental Disorders*, 4th edtion (DSM-IV) category:
1. Cluster A (paranoid, schizoid): aloofness, anger, anxiety in social situations
2. Cluster B (social, borderline, histrionic, narcissistic): suicidal tendency, irritability, poor frustration tolerance, impulsiveness, controlling behavior, dramatization, erratic behavior
3. Cluster C (disorders of anxiety or of a fearful nature): isolation, compulsive work habits, extreme criticism of others
III. Planning and implementation
A. Provide consistency of care, set limits, and teach self-responsibility for control.
B. Provide physical and psychosocial accessibility.
C. Include significant others in care.
D. Teach relaxation and alternative responses to anxiety-producing situations.
E. Protect client from, and prevent, serious physical harm.
F. Focus on client's strengths.
G. Develop behavioral contracts.
IV. Evaluation
A. Client returns to adequate social functioning, although personality disorders frequently show only marginal improvement.

Psychiatric Illness

Thought Disorders

Thought disorders are a cluster of disorders that compose a syndrome in which thought content, thought form, affect, and relationships are severely impaired. Schizophrenia is one thought disorder. Types of schizophrenia include:
1. Disorganized type: Regressed childlike behavior, inappropriate affect
2. Catatonic type: Disturbed psychomotor behavior alternating between withdrawal and excitement and accompanied by hallucinations, delusions, rigidity, and posturing
3. Paranoid type: Delusions, grandiosity, suspiciousness, and hallucinations
I. Data collection
A. Includes observations of
1. Delusions
2. Hallucinations
3. Tangential thought
4. Negativism
5. Aggressive behavior
6. Diminished thinking ability
7. Diminished self-care activities
8. Inappropriate emotional response
9. Spiritual distress
II. Nursing diagnosis: alteration in thought, self-care deficit
III. Planning and implementation
A. Provide safe environment.
B. Administer neuroleptic (haloperidol, chlorpromazine).
C. Assist client to decrease anxiety.
D. Provide reassurance.
E. Assist client to decrease hallucinations.
F. Monitor self-care patterns.
G. Monitor spiritual concerns.
H. Encourage family support.
I. Document behavior.
IV. Evaluation
A. Psychotic episodes have a pattern; improvement rather than cure is the goal.

Affective Disorders

Affective disorders are disorders of mood, thought, and affect (feelings). Affective disorders have a distinctive pattern. Types include
1. Bipolar disorders (manic, depressive, or mixed): mood swings from euphoria to profound depression

2. Major depression (dysthymic disorder): persistent despondency and withdrawal

I. Data collection
   A. Includes observations of
      1. Inappropriate dress
      2. Inexhaustible energy or lack of energy
      3. Grandiosity; spending money freely
      4. Arrogance
      5. Lack of self-care activities
      6. Self-doubt
      7. Sleep disturbances
      8. Weight loss
      9. Spending sprees or delusions of poverty
      10. Suicidal ideation

II. Nursing diagnosis: potential for injury, self-care deficit, alteration in thought, sleep pattern disturbance

III. Planning and implementation
   A. Provide safe environment.
   B. Monitor self-care activities.
   C. Structure time.
   D. Document sleep pattern.
   E. Provide reassurance.
   F. Administer medications (lithium or antidepressants such as Elavil, or both).
   G. Assist with diagnostic studies (magnetic resonance imaging, stress test).
   H. Obtain family history of mood disorder.
   I. Document client's behavior.
   J. Encourage family support.
   K. Provide for spiritual well-being.

IV. Evaluation
   A. Absence of mood alteration
   B. Structuring time
   C. Encouragement of activities
   D. Short, frequent visits
   E. Frequent documentation

Abuse Disorders

In our society, use of certain substances without a prescription to modify mood or behavior is generally regarded as abuse. Commonly abused substances include coffee, tea, and nicotine. A pathological dependence on or aversion to food is called an eating disorder. Dependence on psychoactive substances (alcohol, marijuana, phencyclidine piperidine [PCP], lysergic acid diethylamide [LSD], cocaine) is considered a mental disorder called psychoactive substance abuse.

Characteristics of Psychoactive Substance Abuser

1. Client recognizes that substance use is excessive.
2. A great deal of time is spent to produce substance.
3. Client suffers withdrawal symptoms when substance is not used.
4. Despite psychological, social, and physical problems, client continues to abuse substance.
5. Significant tolerance occurs.

I. Data collection
   A. Symptoms of substance abuse include
      1. Dilated or contracted pupils depending on drug involved
      2. Slurred speech
      3. Convulsions
      4. Restlessness, tremors
      5. Occupational difficulties
      6. Odor of alcohol
      7. Inappropriate behavior
      8. Little tolerance for frustration
      9. Marital problems
      10. Tendency to develop infections
      11. History of blackouts
      12. Poor attention span

II. Planning and implementation
   A. Provide emergency management for acute substance abuse.
   B. Assess vital signs, output, and mental alertness.
   C. Administer emergency drugs.
   D. Assist in diagnostic studies.
   E. Place in quiet environment.
   F. Provide safe environment.
   G. Assess pattern of substance abuse.
   H. Teach new coping behavior.
   I. Provide for spiritual well-being.

III. Evaluation
   A. Client experiences withdrawal without physical complications.
   B. Client seeks rehabilitation.

Eating Disorders

Eating disorders, characterized by a gross disturbance in eating behaviors, include anorexia nervosa and bulimia. Eating disorders can be thought of as a fear of obesity or an addiction to or drive toward thinness.

I. Data collection
   A. In anorexia, clients are 15% below normal weight in absence of organic disease.
   B. Symptoms of anorexia
      1. Bradycardia
      2. Electrolyte imbalance
      3. Malnourished appearance
   C. In bulimia, clients are usually of normal weight but purge (vomit) after overeating.
   D. Both anorexics and bulimics:
      1. Restrict food
      2. Exercise vigorously
      3. May have gastric ruptures or esophageal tears
      4. May have black teeth (from stomach acid)
      5. May use laxatives excessively

II. Planning and implementation
   A. Assess during meals.
   B. Lock bathroom to prevent purging (for bulimia).
   C. Remove wastebaskets.
   D. Assess closely to prevent overvigorous exercising.
   E. Teach about nutrition.
   F. Administer antianxiety medication before meals as prescribed.
   G. Weigh three times weekly.
   H. Assess for suicidal gestures.
   I. Assess for spiritual well-being.
   J. Refer client to formal eating disorder program.
   K. Assess hoarding of food and use of laxatives.
   L. Assess elimination practices.
   M. Involve family in therapy.

III. Evaluation
   A. Client maintains goal of a certain weight.
   B. Purging (frequent self-induced vomiting) and binge-ing (eating huge quantities of food in small amount of time) are absent.

Confusion

Organic mental syndrome refers to a group of psychological or behavioral signs and symptoms without reference to etiol-ogy, such as organic anxiety syndrome and dementia organic brain syndrome. *Organic mental disorder* designates a particu-lar mental syndrome in which the cause is known (e.g., Parkinson's disease, Huntington's chorea, multi-infarct dementia). Causes of organic mental disorders include

1. Central nervous system infection
2. Head trauma
3. Intracranial lesions
4. Hepatic disease
5. Subarachnoid hemorrhage
6. Cerebral hypoxia
7. Thyroid, parathyroid, or adrenal dysfunction
8. Genetic (e.g., Down's syndrome predisposes client to Alzheimer's disease)

I. Data collection
   A. Symptoms
      1. Weakness of limbs
      2. Unstable shuffling gait
      3. Tremors, slow speech
      4. Seizures
      5. Personality changes
      6. Anxiety
      7. Persistent hallucinations
      8. Impaired memory; making up stories to fill in memory gaps
      9. Rage reactions
      10. Impaired social judgment, apathy
      11. Tangential, circumstantial speech
      12. Inability for self-care
      13. Frequent falls, mobility impairment
      14. Mental confusion
      15. Repetitive movements
II. Planning and implementation
   A. Remove dangerous objects.
   B. Pad siderails.
   C. Administer neuroleptics as prescribed for agitation.
   D. Reorient client frequently; provide external signs of orientation (calendars, clocks).
   E. Attend to ADLs.
   F. Prevent complications.
   G. Provide calm, well-lighted, simple environment.
   H. Limit number of people caring for client.
III. Evaluation
   A. Client remains safe (impairment may be reversible or chronic).

Disorders of Youth (Children and Adolescents)

Although children and adolescents may suffer from thought disorders (schizophrenia), affective disorders (depression), and other psychiatric disorders commonly diagnosed in adults, some illnesses are specifically characteristic of these groups. These include mental retardation, learning and motor skill disorders, disruptive behavior and attention deficit dis-orders, feeding and eating disorders, and separation-anxiety disorders.

Mental Retardation

I. Characteristics
   A. Measured IQ level 70 or below
   B. Failure of developmental functioning
   C. Types: mild (IQ 55–70), moderate (IQ 40–55), severe (IQ 20–40), and profound (IQ <20)
   D. Social, sensimotor, or communication skills limited
II. Data collection
   A. Motor development
   B. Self-care abilities
   C. Communication abilities
   D. Family resources
   E. Family genogram
   F. Physiological function
   G. Spiritual development
III. Planning and implementation
   A. Maintain a consistent, caring approach.
   B. Strive to develop potential of client.
   C. Use community resources.
   D. Meet client at own level.
   E. Assess self-care needs.
   F. Provide for spiritual well-being.
   G. Develop and enhance strengths.
IV. Evaluation
   A. Client performs self-care activities.
   B. Client engages in a living pattern reflective of his or her potential.
   C. Community resources are used.

Coping Mechanisms and Defense Mechanisms

To deal with anxiety, loss, and anger, each individual uses a set of behaviors learned at an early stage of development to relieve tension. Coping mechanisms are action-oriented activities to increase one's ability to cope; defense mechanisms are unconscious reactions to protect oneself from feeling inadequate.

Coping Mechanisms

1. Seek out another person to gain comfort.
2. Use food to relax.
3. Express feelings (cry, scream, and so on).
4. Withdraw (become "couch potato").
5. "Talk it out."
6. "Think it out."
7. "Work it off" (walk, run, scrub floors).
8. Use symbolic comfort (religion).
9. Compromise (negotiate verbally).

Defense Mechanisms

I. Suppression
   A. Suppression is voluntary and involuntary exclusion from conscious level of ideas and feelings.

B. For example, a student who receives a poor report card forgets to show it to his or her parents.

II. Sublimation
   A. Sublimation is replacement of an unacceptable need, attitude, or emotion with one that is more acceptable.
   B. For example, a woman who feels unattractive puts her energy into competitive sport.

III. Rationalization
   A. Rationalization is an attempt to make unacceptable feelings and behaviors acceptable.
   B. For example, a student fails an exam and complains that the lectures were disorganized.

IV. Identification
   A. An attempt to change oneself to resemble an admired person is called identification.
   B. For example, a 6-year-old dresses like her mother.

V. Introjection
   A. Intense identification in which one incorporates values of another into self is known as introjection.
   B. For example, a child scolds her doll for spilling milk.

VI. Displacement
   A. Rejection of an emotional feeling from one idea, person, or objective to another is displacement.
   B. For example, a frustrated nurse goes home and screams at the cat.

VII. Projection
   A. Projection is attributing one's own thoughts or impulses to another.
   B. For example, a female physician denies her sexual feelings about a male nurse and accuses him of flirting with her.

VIII. Regression
   A. Regression is retreating to an earlier stage of development.

B. For example, a 6-year-old girl begins wetting her pants when her new baby brother comes into the family.

IX. Repression
   A. Repression is the involuntary exclusion of a painful thought, impulse, or memory.
   B. For example, after the loss of his spouse, a man cannot remember his marriage date.

X. Reaction formation
   A. Development of conscious attitudes and behaviors opposite to those one really feels is called reaction formation.
   B. For example, a male professor attracted to a female student treats her harshly.

XI. Intellectualization
   A. Intellectualization is excessive reasoning to avoid feeling.
   B. For example, a battered wife talks about how her husband beats her and says that she should leave for own her safety, but remains with her husband.

XII. Conversion
   A. Conversion is the expression of intrapsychic conflict through physical symptoms.
   B. For example, an unprepared student develops abdominal pain before a test.

XIII. Compensation
   A. The process by which a person makes up for his or her perceived deficiency is compensation.
   B. For example, a 5-foot-tall male neurosurgeon becomes aggressive, forceful, and controlling at work.

XIV. Denial
   A. Denial is disowning consciously intolerable thoughts and impulses.
   B. For example, a terminal cancer client tells her husband that the results of the biopsy were negative.

QUESTIONS

Eileen W. Keefe, RN.C, MS, and Golden M. Tradewell, RN, PhD

1. A 21-year-old secretary with a history of anxiety reactions is admitted to the emergency room. The nurse should know that the most common symptoms of an anxiety reaction are:

   1. Hypotension, pain
   2. Lethargy, flat affect
   3. Confusion, hunger
   4. Increased pulse, tightness in the chest

2. An initial care plan for a client with a diagnosis of anxiety would include which of the following interventions?

   1. Monitoring vital signs, offering reassurance
   2. Monitoring I&O, obtaining weight
   3. Observation of nailbed color
   4. History of drug use, offering high-carbohydrate food

3. To help a client modify an anxiety reaction, the nurse should speak slowly and softly, asking the client if there is anything in his or her life that is upsetting. The client responds, "Nothing is wrong; everything is perfect." This may be an example of:

   1. Introjection
   2. Sublimation
   3. Denial
   4. Displacement

4. Which of the following pharmacological agents is prescribed to reduce anxiety?

   1. Imipramine (Tofranil)
   2. Lorazepam (Ativan)
   3. Lithium (Lithane)
   4. Amitriptyline (Elavil)

5. After administering an anxiolytic to an emergency room client, the nurse checks to see if the siderails are secure. The nurse realizes that one of the common side effects of anxiolytics is:

   1. Drowsiness
   2. Convulsions
   3. Blurred vision
   4. Fear of falling

6. A client is given a prescription for lorazepam. It is the nurse's responsibility to inform the client that anyone taking lorazepam should not:

   1. Work
   2. Consume herring
   3. Consume alcohol
   4. Spend prolonged time in the sun

7. After a client suffering from an anxiety reaction was safely discharged from the emergency room, the nurse documented that the client experienced a rapid pulse, tightness of the chest, discomfort, and an inability to focus on anything but obtaining relief. The nursing diagnosis may conclude:

   1. Panic-level anxiety
   2. Mild anxiety
   3. Moderate anxiety
   4. Severe anxiety

8. A 59-year-old man is admitted to a medical unit with symptoms of lethargy and withdrawal. He was forced into early retirement because of his company's merger with a larger sister company. On admission, the nurse observes that the client will not make eye contact with any member of the staff. Poor eye contact is an example of:

   1. Verbal communication
   2. Therapeutic communication
   3. Nonverbal communication
   4. Mass communication

9. A nurse observes that a client has poor eye contact, complains of nausea and diarrhea, and is crying about the death of his wife. The nurse realizes that this cluster of symptoms is common in:

   1. Anxiety disorders
   2. Grief reactions
   3. Panic attacks
   4. Eating disorders

10. In planning initial care for a newly admitted client, the nurse realizes that one establishes a therapeutic relationship by:

    1. Assessing the client, remaining subjective
    2. Judging the client, offering advice
    3. Respecting the client, offering presence
    4. Confronting the client, displaying sympathy

11. A client informs the nurse that his wife died 2 days ago. The nurse replies, "Tell me more about that." This is an example of the therapeutic communication technique of:

    1. Restating
    2. Providing feedback
    3. Identifying themes
    4. Open-ended statement

12. During a conversation between a client and the nurse, the physician enters the room accompanied by seven medical students. The nurse and the client end their discussion because:

    1. Physicians are important in status.
    2. The physician's entry changed the context and psychosocial setting.
    3. The content of the communication between the nurse and the client should remain private.

4. The type, quality, and purpose of nurses' and physicians' communication are totally different.

13. A student nurse says to a client who has been grieving over the death of a spouse, "I think you should get on with life and stop mourning over the death." This is an example of communication called:
    1. Omission of content
    2. Offering personal opinion
    3. Rejection
    4. Faulty reassurance

14. In assessing a 61-year-old client, the nurse should know that the developmental stage is:
    1. Industry versus inferiority
    2. Intimacy versus isolation
    3. Ego integrity versus despair
    4. Generativity versus stagnation

15. A 60-year-old client becomes very upset after his sister visits. He throws a tray at the wall. The nurse's most effective response would be:
    1. Maintain a calm and supportive manner.
    2. Administer neuroleptic drugs.
    3. Encourage the client to call his sister.
    4. Report the incident to the hospital administrator.

16. A 75-year-old client tells the nurse that he wishes to see a priest because "it will help." The nurse realizes that this would be an example of:
    1. A coping mechanism
    2. A defense mechanism
    3. Reaction formation
    4. Intellectualization

17. A 39-year-old client has a diagnosis of depression. The physician prescribes ECT. The nurse must know that ECT:
    1. Requires preoperative nursing care
    2. Causes excessive weight gain
    3. Is administered in conjunction with neuroleptics
    4. Will result in mood suppression

18. A 14-year-old girl who displays symptoms of anorexia nervosa was brought to the clinic for an evaluation. She has a 15-year-old sister and lives with her parents, who are physicians. The client achieves well in school and is very active in sports activities. During the initial interview with the nurse, the client states that she is "just normal." Which of the following would suggest to the nurse that the client displays symptoms of anorexia nervosa?
    1. She expresses a desire to gain weight.
    2. She has episodes of overeating.
    3. She has had severe weight loss due to dieting.
    4. She uses large amounts of food to relax.

19. The nurse would know that the development stage of a 14-year-old adolescent is:
    1. Trust versus mistrust
    2. Autonomy versus shame and doubt
    3. Initiative versus guilt
    4. Identity versus role diffusion

20. The nurse should know that it is important to assess for which one of the following characteristics of anorexia nervosa?
    1. Vigorous exercise
    2. Increased libido
    3. Average intelligence
    4. Tachycardia

21. A 21-year-old client denies that she ever feels anxious, but the nurse observes her biting her fingernails. One component of nursing care for the client would be for the nurse to:
    1. Administer neuroleptic medication.
    2. Assess the client's coping mechanisms.
    3. Encourage vigorous exercise.
    4. Make arrangements for sculptured nails.

22. A client tells the nurse that when she gets upset, she kicks the cat. This is an example of which one of the following defense mechanisms?
    1. Rationalization
    2. Projection
    3. Displacement
    4. Regression

23. While interacting with a client with a diagnosis of anorexia nervosa, the client changes the conversation from talking about self to talking about the weather. The nurse must use which of the following communication techniques?
    1. Refocusing
    2. Restating
    3. Silence
    4. Summarizing

24. A 15-year-old female client with a diagnosis of anorexia is scheduled for an electrocardiogram (ECG). The nurse will:
    1. Teach the client about the procedure
    2. Tell the client that she has a heart problem
    3. Explain that persons with anorexia nervosa suffer from tachycardia
    4. Ask a male aide to accompany the client

25. An 18-year-old male client has serious problems with substance abuse. He has had difficulty with his school work and with school authority figures. He has come to the clinic for help. The nurse observes that the client is restless and pacing. Other physical characteristics of substance abusers that the nurse should pay special attention to include:
    1. Dilated pupils
    2. Increased concentration
    3. Euphoria
    4. Pale nailbeds

26. A 22-year-old client admitted to the emergency room stated that 1 month previously he had been brought to the emergency room for an overdose of cocaine. What

nursing actions in the emergency room would be most important in treating a client who has overdosed?

1. Monitoring vital signs and output
2. Obtaining weight and temperature
3. Inducing client to vomit
4. Obtaining a psychiatric evaluation

27. A client is admitted to an inpatient detoxification unit. During the acute phase of detoxification from drug abuse, which of the following would be the most important nursing action?

1. Monitoring manipulative behavior
2. Monitoring family dynamics
3. Evaluating vocational abilities
4. Monitoring vital signs frequently

28. A client in a substance abuse program tells the nurse during the first week of treatment that he has no drug problem. The nurse identifies this behavior as an example of the defense mechanism:

1. Denial
2. Projection
3. Displacement
4. Sublimation

29. When a client explains to the nurse that he does not have a drug abuse problem, the nurse replies, "What do you mean when you say you have no drug problem?" This communication technique is an example of:

1. Focusing
2. Clarifying
3. Providing feedback
4. Making an observation

30. Which of the following behaviors would the nurse expect to observe from a client who has successfully completed a substance abuse treatment program?

1. Identifying positive ways to cope with anxiety
2. Identifying ways to decrease but not discontinue drug use
3. Identifying the family members responsible for the drug abuse
4. Identifying methods of social isolation

31. A 48-year-old man is admitted to a surgical unit with the diagnosis of chronic cholecystitis. The client's chart reveals that he is scheduled for surgery the following morning and that he has lived in a sheltered residence home for 10 years and suffers from schizophrenia. As a nurse reads the chart, he or she should know that schizophrenia is:

1. A thought disorder
2. An affective disorder
3. A personality disorder
4. An adjustment disorder

32. With the diagnosis of schizophrenia, the nurse may anticipate which of the following cluster of symptoms?

1. Stuttering, cluttering, passive behavior
2. Delusions, tangential thought, hallucinations
3. Hyperactivity, crying, violence

4. Inexhaustible energy, absence of mood, altered sleep pattern

33. Clients who suffer from schizophrenia are most likely to be given a prescription for which of the following?

1. Anxiolytic medications
2. Antidepressant medications
3. Antipsychotic medications
4. Antiseizure medications

34. The nurse who cares for clients taking antipsychotic medication knows that:

1. The nurse must monitor temperature closely
2. The nurse must monitor vital signs
3. The nurse must monitor diet closely
4. The nurse must monitor blood levels

35. A hospitalized client recovering from surgery tells the nurse that "men from Mars are fixing get-well food to be put in my veins." The nurse knows that this is an example of:

1. A delusion
2. A hallucination
3. Anxiety
4. Tangential thought

36. As a 25-year-old male client suffering from schizophrenia recovers from surgery, he becomes more disorganized in his thinking, and his behavior becomes more inappropriate. The nurse's best nursing action is to:

1. Tell the client he is psychotic
2. Alter medications as needed
3. Tolerate the client's behavior
4. Document the client's behavior

37. A 40-year-old woman is admitted to the emergency room. Her husband states that she has not slept in 48 hours, is irritable and uncooperative, and has made comments about ending her life. When the nurse attempts to take the client's vital signs, she strikes the nurse's hand. The thermometer breaks and the client bursts into tears. The nurse's first response is to:

1. Comfort the client and hold her hand
2. Tell the client to act appropriately
3. Call for assistance
4. Obtain vital signs

38. A client is given a diagnosis of bipolar disorder. Bipolar disorder is:

1. A disorder of mood, affect, and thought
2. A disorder of personality and self-care
3. A disorder of interpersonal deficits
4. A disorder of intelligence and ideation

39. Clients with the medical diagnosis of bipolar disorder are often placed on lithium. Before administering this medication, the nurse is aware of:

1. The diet of the client
2. The sleep pattern of the client
3. The lithium blood level of the client
4. The activity level of the client

40. A client who has been taking lithium for a number of months and has a lithium blood level meq/L >1.2 may experience lithium toxicity. Lithium toxicity is characterized by:

1. Painful eyes, nausea, vomiting
2. Diarrhea, nausea, vomiting, tremors
3. Hypertension, swollen joints, fever
4. Hypotension, thirst, nausea, vomiting

41. A 90-year-old man who resides in a nursing home has been given a diagnosis of Alzheimer's disease. The nurse caring for this client would anticipate which of the following behaviors?

1. Overeating, overspending
2. Mood stability
3. Self-care deficits, impaired memory
4. Limb pain

42. In caring for clients with Alzheimer's disease, the nurse should:

1. Provide external signs of orientation.
2. Provide increased environmental stimulation.
3. Encourage frequent change.
4. Encourage group therapy.

43. A 75-year-old male client diagnosed with Alzheimer's disease becomes very agitated at night and begins tearing off the bed sheets. He tells the nurse that his suitcase is in the bed and he must catch a train to the office. The nurse's most appropriate response is to:

1. Restrain the client.
2. Reorient and reassure the client.
3. Provide a well-lighted environment.
4. Observe the client.

44. The nurse knows that a person in his 90th year is in the developmental stage of:

1. Trust versus mistrust
2. Ego integrity versus despair
3. Identity versus identity diffusion
4. Generativity versus stagnation

45. In caring for clients with Alzheimer's disease, the nurse's priority is:

1. Physiological care
2. Psychological care
3. Safety
4. Spiritual care

46. A 7-year-old girl is admitted to the pediatric unit. She is severely mentally retarded and is admitted for cellulitis. When admitting a retarded child, the nurse first assesses for:

1. Communication ability
2. Reading ability
3. Hobbies
4. Moral development

47. In caring for mentally retarded children, the nurse must:

1. Be aware of his or her own feelings.
2. Minimize family contact.
3. Interview the child extensively.
4. Teach the child to cope with anxiety.

48. The mother of a 10-year-old girl reports to the clinic nurse that her daughter has been acting "jumpy" lately. If the client is experiencing anxiety, the most important symptom that the nurse would likely observe is:

1. Withdrawal
2. Lethargy
3. Hunger
4. An increased heart rate

49. A 32-year-old client is receiving treatment for obsessive-compulsive disorder (OCD). Obsessive-compulsive behaviors manifest themselves as:

1. Reality orientation
2. Rigid perfectionism
3. A wide range of emotions
4. Ritualistic thoughts

50. A hospitalized client misses breakfast in the cafeteria three times in 1 week because of his ritualistic handwashing. His handwashing ritual may go on for 30 minutes. Which of the following nursing actions would be most appropriate for the client with an OCD?

1. Document the behavior, and work with the treatment team to design a treatment program to extinguish the behavior.
2. Tell the client to stop washing his hands and design a care plan to decrease anxiety.
3. Ask the client why he feels he must wash his hands and ask the physician for an order for an antianxiety agent.
4. Plan to bring a breakfast to the client's room and schedule three periods a day for handwashing activity.

51. A 14-year-old girl has been hospitalized by the court for psychiatric evaluation after running away from home repeatedly. The nurse finds the client in her room during school hours and asks why she is not in class. The client responds by stating that another nurse said she could miss class if she did not feel like going. The nurse knows the client's response is an example of:

1. Avoidance behavior
2. Manipulation
3. Rebellion
4. Projection

52. A 16-year-old girl who is hospitalized for running away from home refuses to attend class, stating that yesterday the other nurse told her she did not have to go to class if she did not want to. The nurse's best response would be:

1. "I know that you are lying."
2. "Missing class is against the rules."
3. "Why do you fight the system?"
4. "Fine, but you're confined to your room."

53. Acting-out behavior is exemplified by which one of the following?

    1. Discussing sexual feelings
    2. Attempting suicide
    3. Attending treatment activities
    4. Contracting for safety

54. Two 15-year-old boys are being treated on the psychiatric unit. During a card game in the recreation room, they begin fist-fighting. Nursing interventions for this incident would include: (**Select all that apply.**)

    1. Remove the boys to separate areas and set limits.
    2. Obtain an order for seclusion.
    3. Share observations with the boys.
    4. Restrain each boy as punishment for fighting.
    5. Call juvenile detention to have children detained
    6. Punish each boy with phone call restrictions.

55. A 17-year-old male client is readmitted to the hospital for leukemia. He is angry and refuses to talk with staff. The nurse should know that:

    1. Adolescents may find it difficult to talk about death
    2. Adolescents see death as temporary
    3. Adolescents feel that death is a punishment
    4. Adolescents are looking forward to the future

56. A client is being discharged from the hospital after a below-the-knee amputation. Which statement by the client would indicate that the client is getting in touch with the loss?

    1. "What is the use of going home with one leg?"
    2. "Why me, God? If only I had changed my ways!"
    3. "Are there support groups that help people like me?"
    4. "Please leave me alone until my friend comes to take me home."

57. A 13-year-old client's history reveals that his cultural orientation discourages him from verbalizing his spiritual issues. Which one of the following is the best nursing intervention?

    1. Reassure the client that it is all right to verbalize spiritual issues.
    2. Question the client about his religious orientation needs.
    3. Refer the client to a nondenominational group.
    4. Discuss immortality with the client.

58. Which of the following concepts should the nurse be aware of when interacting with survivors of victims of sudden death?

    1. Survivors have time to engage in anticipatory grief.
    2. Survivors may feel guilty for not engaging in special activities with the deceased.
    3. Survivors feel immediate detachment.
    4. Survivors may experience an uncomplicated grief response.

59. During an interview, an 83-year-old male client confides in the nurse that his spiritual needs are not being met. Which one of the following is most important for the nurse to explore?

    1. Source of strength and hope
    2. Purpose and meaning in living
    3. Spiritual orientation
    4. Religious affiliation

60. A 55-year-old male client who has been a heavy drinker for 20 years presents at the emergency room in a state of agitation, delirium, and diaphoresis. It is reported that the client has not consumed any alcohol during the past 72 hours. The nurse should know that the client is suffering from:

    1. Delirium tremens
    2. Korsakoff's syndrome
    3. Alcoholic hepatitis
    4. Alcoholic hallucinosis

61. A 16-year-old boy was brought to the emergency room by his parents because he was abusing cocaine and out of control. The nurse should know that one of the signs of cocaine intoxication is:

    1. Dry, cool skin
    2. Hypotension
    3. Bradycardia
    4. Psychomotor agitation

62. Which one of the following drugs is used to inhibit impulsive abuse of alcohol?

    1. Chlordiazepoxide (Librium)
    2. Disulfiram (Antabuse)
    3. Diazepam (Valium)
    4. Lithium

63. Which one of the following is a contributing factor in the development of codependency?

    1. Effective family dynamics
    2. Difficulty in negotiating boundaries
    3. Balanced internal ego states
    4. Positive aspects of self

64. What is the nurse's greatest responsibility when intervening with an alcoholic family?

    1. Instill hope in the family's future.
    2. Maintain homeostatic balance.
    3. Encourage cross-generational clinging.
    4. Promote the use of defense mechanisms.

65. A woman is admitted to a psychiatric unit for evaluation after displaying recurring bizarre behavior. The nurse explains to the client's family that:

    1. The mentally ill person has often learned inappropriate behaviors that must be unlearned or replaced with acceptable behaviors
    2. Treatment is aimed at complete recovery, which can occur at any time during the therapy
    3. Part of the mental illness is insensitivity of the person to how others react to him or her
    4. Evaluation is based on known criteria from which the mentally ill rarely deviate

66. The family of a newly admitted client is concerned about the client's rights should commitment be necessary. It is important to remember that:

1. Initially commitment implies custodial care and therefore a client's rights are not compromised
2. A client has the right to therapeutic treatment, informed consent, and to refuse treatment
3. Although a client retains all right to participate in his treatment, the facility cannot be held liable if treatment is not provided
4. Treatment will not be initiated until the client and the legal guardian consent

67. A mother received a call from her daughter's teacher. The 7-year-old child seems withdrawn, does not interact with other children, and does not participate in class. The concern of the mother and the teacher is based on the fact that:

1. Children progress through the stages of development at a similar rate and react to school with predictable behaviors.
2. This developmental period is psychologically stormy and changes in behaviors are considered significant.
3. Seven-year-old children rely on peer approval rather than positive reinforcement from parents.
4. This is usually a period during which the child makes great social and intellectual strides.

68. An individual's personality and perception of self are key factors in determining behavior. The nurse recognizes that:

1. Events occurring throughout life affect emotional adjustment
2. It is not necessary to complete one developmental stage before the individual can progress to the next stage
3. Withdrawn behavior illustrates a person's inability to move from one developmental stage to the next
4. The most psychologically significant stage of development is birth to 12 months

69. A 70-year-old severely dehydrated woman was admitted to a medical unit. Her husband died a month ago and she lives alone. Her only child lives 200 miles away with his wife and son. The nurse notes that the client always gazes downward and does not respond to questions. This behavior is an example of:

1. Conversion reaction
2. Suppression
3. Depression
4. Reaction formation

70. The developmental stage for a 70-year-old client is:

1. Industry versus inferiority
2. Intimacy versus isolation
3. Integrity versus despair
4. Generativity versus stagnation

71. In trying to reassure a recently widowed client, the nurse says, "Don't worry, everything is going to be fine." According to the principles of therapeutic communication, this statement communicates:

1. Empathy and understanding
2. Clarification of a client's feelings

3. Devaluation of a client's own perception
4. Caring and concern

72. During his monthly therapy session, a 48-year-old father of an adolescent son tells you that his son is "impossible" and cannot make decisions. On the basis of your knowledge of adolescent behavior, you know that:

1. All adolescents are difficult to control and cannot make sound decisions.
2. A hallmark of adolescence is ambivalence related to dependence and independence.
3. Adolescents want to be dependent and rely on others to make decisions.
4. At this developmental stage, the adolescent is primarily seeking parental approval.

73. Sex education during adolescence is important because:

1. Adolescents are unaware of the physical and emotional changes that are occurring.
2. The love object of an adolescent is primarily the parent of the same sex.
3. Adolescents are more concerned about self than others, and this is the focus of their attention.
4. As bodily changes occur, the adolescent has to feel comfortable discussing these changes.

74. In response to failing courses in school, an adolescent boy says, "Well, if I were all brains and nothing else, I would make As in all of my courses." This is an example of which defense mechanism?

1. Repression
2. Compensation
3. Denial of reality
4. Rationalization

75. At the conclusion of a therapy session, a client says to the therapist, "I'm really grateful for your time; you're a great listener. You know, you remind me of my wife." An appropriate response by the therapist would be:

1. "She must be a great listener too."
2. "That's because she and I are both concerned about you and your son."
3. "What about me reminds you of your wife?"
4. "Do you want to talk about this some time?"

76. The major clinical use of antipsychotics (or neuroleptics) is in the treatment of psychoses. When used in the treatment of schizophrenia, neuroleptics:

1. Eliminate the need for psychotherapy by effectively curing social withdrawal and apathy.
2. Provide symptomatic control by blocking the activity of dopamine.
3. Heighten the sex drive and require weekly titers to assess peak and trough.
4. Alter the client's response to reality and decrease paranoia.

77. The nurse's plan of care for the client taking neuroleptics must include observing for side effects, which include:

1. Nausea, vomiting, diarrhea, weight loss
2. Heartburn, hypoglycemia, edema
3. Nasal congestion, seizures, urinary retention
4. Insomnia, drooling, agranulocytopenia

78. A 3- to 4-month-old infant who is allowed to cry for hours or who is neglected:

    1. Will instinctively continue to cry until his or her needs are met and he or she no longer feels neglected
    2. Begins to mistrust people and surroundings even though the infant is too young to distinguish himself or herself from others
    3. Will withdraw from the world of reality to the world of fantasy, which feels less threatening
    4. Will develop alternate ways to feel good about himself or herself and about the world

79. A nurse is teaching parenting classes. When teaching growth and development, the nurse states, "The gradual realization in a child that neither the child nor his or her parent is omnipotent leads to …

    1. Sadness and withdrawal."
    2. Anger and displacement."
    3. Mastery of more skills."
    4. Developmental regression."

80. When the nurse is teaching the growth and development of a 2-year-old child, the nurse identifies that the child:

    1. Begins to develop a sense of autonomy
    2. Becomes dependent and less self-reliant
    3. Generally cannot master new challenges
    4. Cannot socialize and demonstrates fear of the environment

81. When teaching the growth and development of 3- to 5-year-old children, the nurse identifies:

    1. Little or no need for discipline
    2. Lack of concern for parental approval
    3. Increasing motor and intellectual skills
    4. Lack of social skills

82. A client who was raped 10 years ago is now unable to have a satisfying sexual relationship with her husband. The nurse identifies that the client may be exhibiting which defense mechanism?

    1. Reaction formation
    2. Displacement
    3. Repression
    4. Suppression

83. A man who was paralyzed from his waist down after an accident is asked what effect his paralysis will have on his previously active life. His response is, "no effect." The nurse identifies this as an example of:

    1. Denial of reality
    2. Compensation
    3. Fantasy
    4. Introjection

84. A 3- or 4-year-old child who has been toilet trained begins to have incontinent episodes and "talk baby talk" when her newborn sister is brought home from the hospital. This behavior demonstrates which defense mechanism?

    1. Displacement
    2. Regression
    3. Sublimation
    4. Reaction formation

85. A client experiences free-floating anxiety that has worsened since his recent divorce. He is taking a nonbarbiturate benzodiazepine agent. The nurse recognizes that this classification of drug:

    1. Is recommended because of its low potential for abuse, toxicity, and lethal overdose
    2. Works selectively on the limbic system of the brain, which is responsible for emotions such as rage and anxiety
    3. Has a tranquilizing effect without numbing emotions and produces reversible amnesia in the treatment of post-traumatic stress disorder (PTSD)
    4. Acts primarily by enhancing normal coping mechanisms, is well tolerated, and is nonaddictive

86. Antidepressants are used in the treatment of depressive disorders caused by emotional, physical, chemical, and/or environmental stressors. Regarding the classifications of antidepressants, the nurse knows that:

    1. Tricyclic antidepressants decrease the level of neurotransmitters in cases in which an increase in neurotransmitters causes depression
    2. MAOIs are effective when administered over a short period; they are less toxic than other classifications
    3. Tricyclic antidepressants are contraindicated in the treatment of depression associated with physiological symptoms such as insomnia, fatigue, and irritability
    4. Hypertensive crisis may result if MAOIs are taken with tyramine-rich foods, such as aged cheese, avocados, and chicken livers

87. Personality disorders are maladaptive patterns of seeing, relating to, and thinking about one's environment. Nursing care for clients with personality disorders should include:

    1. Reinforcing limits to counteract manipulative behavior
    2. Allowing hostile exchanges that foster open expression
    3. Assisting the client to focus by limiting diversional activities
    4. Helping the client to build self-esteem by ignoring inappropriate behaviors

88. During a therapeutic session, the client tells the nurse, "You're just like my mother, and you're never going to change. First you tell me to talk about how I feel, then when I talk, you cut me off and don't let me finish a sentence." This is an example of:

    1. Conversion reaction
    2. Blatant hostility
    3. Displacement
    4. Transference

89. A 40-year-old client with chronic schizophrenia and a history of multiple hospitalizations is readmitted for noncompliance with medication therapy. The most common reason for noncompliance with antipsychotic medications is:

1. Neuroleptics tend to produce unpleasant side effects and adverse reactions.
2. The medications are too expensive to purchase.
3. The client improves and believes that he no longer requires medication.
4. Neuroleptics are designed for short-term use only.

90. The nurse on the unit presents the client's medication in a pill cup already opened. The client refuses to take the medication, stating, "I don't know what that is." A nursing intervention to educate the client and promote compliance would be to:

1. Tell the client what the medication is and encourage him or her to take it.
2. Obtain an unopened labeled dose and show the client the medication.
3. Reassure the client that it is the right medication and that it is important that it be taken.
4. Tell the client if he or she refuses to take the medication orally, it will be administered intramuscularly.

91. During dinner a client refuses to eat, stating, "You are serving me dog flesh." The best response for the nurse would be:

1. "Don't be silly, we don't eat dog meat here."
2. "What makes you think this is dog flesh?"
3. "Don't worry, I'll get you something else."
4. "If you don't want to eat, it's up to you."

92. For the client with a history of noncompliance with medication therapy, the physician has decided to prescribe decanoate neuroleptics. Client and family teaching for this medication should include the following:

1. These neuroleptic medications have few side effects.
2. A special diet is required while on this medication.
3. Blood levels to assess effectiveness must be drawn monthly.
4. The medication is given IM every 2–4 weeks.

93. A 23-year-old female client has been admitted to the inpatient psychiatric unit with a diagnosis of catatonic schizophrenia. She appears weak and pale. The nurse would expect to observe which behaviors in this client?

1. Scratching and catlike motions of the extremities
2. Exaggerated suspiciousness and excessive food intake
3. Stuporous withdrawal, hallucinations, and delusions
4. Sexual preoccupation and word salad

94. A 28-year-old male client with a history of antisocial personality disorder is admitted to the psychiatric unit because of a suicide attempt while in jail awaiting trial for assault. The client acts very disinterested in treatment and has developed a rapport with several clients whom he is influencing in negative ways. In evaluating his progress, the nurse recognizes that he:

1. Could make behavioral changes within a short time if motivated.
2. May not be motivated to change his behavior or lifestyle.
3. Manipulates others but does not manipulate family members.
4. Usually requires intensive psychotropic drug therapy, which he refuses.

95. A 15-year-old girl is admitted with a diagnosis of anorexia. She is an honor student and participates in school activities. She is 40% below expected weight, states that she is fat, and demonstrates uncooperative behavior during the admission process. In anorexia, the client has a distorted view of:

1. Self-esteem and self-worth
2. Ability to control
3. Self-image and intellect
4. Need to mature

96. A 7-year-old boy is admitted for evaluation. His history reveals multiple reports by teachers that he is unable to sit still in class, is aggressive with the other children, and cannot concentrate on a task more than 5 minutes. An appropriate nursing intervention for the first few days includes:

1. Set clear, concise behavior expectations with consistent limits.
2. Put him in time-out if he does not follow the rules.
3. Observe his behavior and assess for patterns.
4. Ask him why he is acting as he is.

97. A physician prescribes lithium for a client who was recently admitted to a unit. The nurse knows the following to be true of this medication:

1. Onset of therapeutic effect is 7–14 days; side effects include fine tremors and blurred vision.
2. Nausea and vomiting are common side effects that are treated symptomatically with daily low doses of antiemetics.
3. Therapeutic effect is minimal, and noncompliance is difficult to detect; blood levels are therefore drawn weekly.
4. IM administration results in immediate relief of symptoms, and effects usually last 27–48 hours.

98. Three weeks after beginning lithium therapy, a client appears lethargic and ataxic and has a decreased level of consciousness. These symptoms indicate:

1. A decrease in therapeutic levels
2. Toxic ranges of lithium
3. Maximum therapeutic effectiveness of lithium
4. Expected side effects of lithium

99. In the case of suspected lithium toxicity, the best intervention for the nurse is to:

1. Assess the most current laboratory values and force fluids
2. Hold the next dose and draw a serum level
3. Notify the physican and wait for instructions
4. Give the medication and assess for further side effects

100. In the United States, older adults are more frequently the recipients of health care than are other age groups because:

1. They are prone to chronic illness and depression and require long-term therapy
2. Single-adult households are more common among older people, and this often means that family resources are less available
3. They are lonely, and health-care providers traditionally provide understanding and comfort
4. Physiological changes in older adults are irreversible and require planned health-care interventions.

101. During an assessment of a client admitted for anxiety disorder, the nurse determines that the client has been using addictive substances as a means of coping. When managing patient care, which one of the following would be considered a long-term goal?

1. Client will demonstrate ability to cope without exhibiting dependency behavior by the time of discharge.
2. Client will participate in decision-making regarding addictive substance use within 3 days.
3. Client will willingly attend therapy activities.
4. Client will verbalize desire to control the use of addictive substances within 7 days.

102. In psychosocial terms, the consequences are grave for a pregnant client admitted for bipolar disorder and opiate addiction. Which of the following should be part of the initial management regimen?

1. Physiological crisis
2. Symptomatically assessed
3. Psychological crisis
4. Promotion of abstinence

103. During the nursing management phase with a client diagnosed as having an eating disorder, which one of the following may indicate that the client has a need for providing relief from a negative emotional state?

1. Forming close and intimate relationships.
2. Exhibiting impulse control problems and self-mutilation.
3. Experiencing modest overt conflict.
4. Requesting frequent periods of dependency.

104. The nurse is caring for a client who admits to abusing marijuana and alcohol. After assessing the following risk factors for substance abuse, which one factor should the nurse initially manage?

1. Loss of social role
2. Co-occurring psychiatric diagnoses
3. Poor sense of self-worth
4. Codependency

105. When a client is alcohol dependent, which of the following is the medication of choice used for detoxification?

1. Benzodiazepines
2. Barbituates

3. Methadone
4. Clozapine

106. Which of the following methods may the nurse use for managing the symptoms of stress when helping a client improve his/her well being? (**Select all that apply.**)

1. Therapeutic touch
2. Exercise
3. Imagery
4. Acupuncture
5. Medication
6. Counseling sessions

107. When managing agitated and aggressive clients, which of the following disorders would most likely be a source of concern for the psychiatric nurse? (**Select all that apply.**)

1. Major depressive disorders
2. Organic brain disorder
3. Psychotic conditions
4. Personality disorders
5. Transient ischemic attacks
6. Vegetative state

108. When assisting a client in the management of stress reduction, select all of the listed feelings that the client experiences during periods of anxiety.

1. "I find it difficult to concentrate because of distracting thoughts."
2. "My stomach gets tied in knots."
3. "I get constipation."
4. "I pace up and down nervously."
5. "I cannot urinate very well."
6. "I feel so peaceful."

109. The nurse is aware that _____,_____, and _____may trigger a grief reaction.

110. When the nurse manages a client's psychotherapeutic medication regimen, which of the following factors may affect medication compliance? (**Select all that apply.**)

1. Positive side effects of the medication
2. Feelings of loss of personal control.
3. Fear of dependence and addiction.
4. Comorbidity
5. Acceptance of the disease process
6. Delegating medication administration to a family member

111. When working with family members of a mentally ill client, which of the following behaviors/attitudes may the nurse observe toward the mentally ill member? (**Select all that apply.**)

1. Recurrent grief
2. Feelings of guilt
3. Happiness
4. Powerlessness and fear
5. Gratitude and thanksgiving
6. Denial that a problem exists

112. A client admitted to the emergency room states that she has been sexually abused. Which of the following nurse managed interventions would initially be implemented?

1. Recommend a battered women's shelter.
2. Create a support system.
3. Collect and document vital evidence.
4. Respond judgmentally to the episodic nature of the abuse.

113. Which of the following are outcomes related to the patient advocacy role? **(Select all that apply.)**

1. Meet the patient's needs.
2. Provide value for services rendered.
3. Focus on the discharge needs of the patient.
4. Prepare nurse to meet self-care needs.
5. Meet family's needs.
6. Prepare physician to meet hospital's needs.

114. When communicating with a client who is actively psychotic, the nurse should be aware of which factors that negatively affect the interaction? **(Select all that apply.)**

1. Hallucinations and delusions
2. Consistent adherence to psychotropic medications
3. Motivation and grooming skills
4. Disorganized behavior
5. Client's acceptance of disease
6. Family's acceptance of disease

115. When managing client care, which professional ethical obligations are important for the nurse to implement? **(Select all that apply.)**

1. Improve standards of client care.
2. Provide services with respect to human dignity.
3. Safeguard the nurse's rights.
4. Evaluate necessity, appropriateness of health care services.
5. Negate client's privacy.
6. Require client to accept all treatments.

116. Which of the following barriers within the health care system hinder the development of the nurse-client relationship?

1. Profusion of value placed on caring.
2. Conflicting professional commitments
3. Client anxiety
4. Communication conflict with other health professionals

117. The most common form of violence in the workplace is against health-care providers. Which one of the following situations puts health-care workers at risk?

1. The use of brutal force to disable a violent client.
2. Adequate staffing patterns.
3. Educational programs on workplace violence.
4. Identification of potential areas for violence.

118. Which one of the following should the nurse keep in mind when managing a verbally hostile client?

1. Maintain a threatening body posture.
2. Disrespect the buffer zone.
3. Provide the client with multiple choices.
4. Maintain a staring eye contact.

119. When managing and maintaining a safe and secure therapeutic milieu, which one of the following goals is a nursing responsibiltiy?

1. Control or set limits on threats and aggressive acts.
2. Condone violent and/or aggressive behavior.
3. Screen all visitors for weapons.
4. Limit psychosocial skills.

120. There are several issues pertinent to managing triage of mental health clients during emergency care. Which one of the following is a critical strategy?

1. Medical screening as described by the federal regulations.
2. Client's condition should determine the type of screening that is requried.
3. Reimbursement is required prior to screening.
4. Immediate transfer to an inpatient setting.

121. Milieu therapy is important for mental health clients. Which of the following processes would provide the best possible environment? **(Select all that apply.)**

1. Family and/or significant other support.
2. Care by unlicensed personnel (UP).
3. Limited use of ancillary therapies.
4. Structured interaction.
5. Excessive stimuli
6. Deny family support

122. The Decade of the Brain saw trememdous growth in:

1. New highly effective medications.
2. Models of treatment that focus on biopsychosocial orientation.
3. Resources for follow-up care.
4. Inpatient education.

123. When managing the care of the chronically mentally ill, which of the following should the nurse address? **(Select all that apply.)**

1. Meet the physical and psychological needs of the client across the health care continuum.
2. Recognize that the client's needs stay constant.
3. Recognize that illness preventions are important in all stages of illness.
4. Acquire more information about the effects of managed health care.
5. Recognize that the family's needs stay constant.
6. Recognize that prevention is not as important as illness treatment.

124. A client exhibits positive symptoms of schizophrenia. The nurse knows that the three most pronounced outward signs of the disorder are: _____, _____, and _____.

125. The nurse would expect to administer _____ for a client who has been diagnosed with generalized anxiety disorder.

126. The client says to the nurse, "I'm physically and emotionally healthy." Which response by the nurse would support the client's thinking?

1. "That statement is cause for concern."
2. "I have observed that you accept yourself as a person."
3. "That statement is not based on sound judgment."
4. "What makes you think that you are emotionally healthy?"

127. A hostile client is admitted with very little insight, disorganized speech, poor contact with reality, and severe personality decompensation. This behavior is most suggestive of which of the following disorders?

1. Personality disorder
2. Psychosis
3. Neurosis
4. Psychophysiological disorder

128. A nurse on the obstetrical unit was preparing a client for discharge after the birth of a son. The client suddenly developed blindness. After an intensive workup, no physical problems were evident. Which of the following defense mechanism was the client using?

1. Regression
2. Repression
3. Reaction formation
4. Conversion formation

129. A salesman hoards all personal receipts, junk mail, news clippings, and restaurant napkins. He tells the nurse that he has no control over his behavior. What is the most appropriate nursing intervention?

1. Form a therapeutic alliance with the client.
2. Assist the client to prevent the ritualistic behaviors.
3. Encourage the client to rationalize his irrational behaviors.
4. Refer the client to hypnosis

130. The nurse is assessing a client who is a substance abuser. During the interview, the client minimizes the problem when he says to the nurse, "I use every day, but it rarely interferes with my work." The client is using which defense mechanism?

1. Projection
2. Displacement
3. Reaction formation
4. Denial

131. A 30-year-old client was given 5 mg of haloperidol (Haldol) for agitation. The client's chart was clearly stamped "Allergic: HALDOL." The client suffered anaphylactic shock and died. The family sued for:

1. Intentional tort
2. Negligence
3. An overdose of Haldol
4. Assault

132. A 27-year-old female client, who slashed both wrists, was admitted to the psychiatric unit under a physician's emergency certificate (PEC). She requested an immediate discharge. Which is the best response by the nurse?

1. "I understand that you are self-destructive. I cannot let you leave."
2. "You must sign this legal document, which indicates that you are leaving the hospital against medical advice (American Medical Association)."
3. "Discuss the issue with your physician."
4. "I will notify your minister."

133. A 27-year-old client diagnosed as having borderline personality disorder called her attorney, reporting client abuse and that the institution was holding her hostage. The nurse is aware that this is an example of:

1. Breach of confidentiality
2. Right of confidentiality
3. Failure to provide communication
4. Failure to comply with telephone rules

134. The activity therapist informs the nurse that she will be helping supervise a 15-person outing scheduled for early afternoon. The nurse would be correct in telling the therapist that:

1. "It's a good idea for the clients to participate in an outing."
2. "That is not a safe practice. A 2:15 ratio is too many clients."
3. "I will be glad to participate."
4. "Have you requested additional help?"

135. A 32-year-old client lost control of her behavior. She threatened staff and other clients and broke several windows. She was escorted to the seclusion room and put in four-point restraints. Which statement is most correct when explaining the situation to the client?

1. "This is a form of punishment for losing control."
2. "This is a means of providing safety for you and everyone else on the unit."
3. "The length of time is undetermined."
4. "The staff will do periodic checks."

136. Which of the following ethical guidelines do not relate to client rights?

1. Informed consent
2. Treatment
3. Refusal of treatment
4. Judicial commitment

137. A 34-year-old female client suffering from numbness of the extremities, trembling, and dyspnea is admitted with a diagnosis of severe anxiety disorder. An initial nursing intervention should be to:

1. Discuss functional coping measures.
2. Determine the source of the problem.
3. Quickly administer an anxiolytic medication.
4. Provide safety and comfort.

138. A 42-year-old male client experienced a severe psychic trauma 1 month ago. He developed paralysis of the lower extremities. Which of the following is the best nursing intervention?

1. Encourage the client to talk about his feelings.
2. Assess the client for organic causes of paralysis.
3. Provide range-of-motion (ROM) to the lower extremities.
4. Encourage discussion of future goals.

139. Which of the following foods would be most appropriate for a client in the manic phase?

1. Finger sandwiches, orange slices, and a banana
2. Pasta, meatballs, and a salad
3. Chicken fried steak with sauce and a salad
4. Beef stew, mashed potatoes, and a banana

140. A female client accused her roommate of stealing her comb and began biting, clawing, and scratching. Which of the following would be the best nursing intervention?

1. Provide a safe environment for both clients.
2. Notify the lawyer advocate.
3. Isolate the aggressor and place in restraints.
4. Discuss the angry behavior and available consequences.

141. A 23-year-old client physically attacks another person on the psychiatric unit and accuses the person of stealing. The nurse is aware that his behavior is an example of:

1. Displacement
2. Impulsive behavior
3. Identification
4. Impulse gratification

142. In a conversation between the nurse and a 50-year-old female client, the client tells the nurse that the hospital staff poisoned her meal and she refuses to eat. The most appropriate nursing intervention is to:

1. Focus on the delusion.
2. Focus on the fears and insecurities.
3. Agree with the client's decision.
4. Challenge the client's delusional system.

143. The emergency room nurse encounters a 20-year-old female wandering around and exhibiting extreme hyperactivity and bizarre behavior. She laughs, giggles, and is annoying to staff and other clients. Her thoughts are poorly organized. The main focus on nursing care for this client would be to:

1. Provide a safe environment.
2. Encourage social interaction.
3. Discuss the bizarre behavior.
4. Provide information regarding illness.

144. A 70-year-old was admitted to a psychiatric unit because he physically abused his wife. He said to the nurse, "My wife is having an affair with an 18-year-old and I want it investigated." The best response by the nurse is:

1. "That remark is absolutely ridiculous."
2. "I understand that you are upset. We will talk about it."
3. "That seems rather doubtful."

4. "An 18-year-old is too young. He does not want your wife."

145. In planning care for a delusional, paranoid person, it is important for the nurse to consider which one of the following characteristics?

1. Bright affect and extreme suspiciousness
2. Motor immobility
3. Regressive and primitive behaviors
4. Anger and aggressive acts

146. A 28-year-old client, diagnosed as having borderline personality disorder, presented at the mental health clinic and demanded to see a counselor immediately. Which one of the following is the best nursing strategy?

1. Instruct the client to leave the clinic.
2. Confront demanding behaviors.
3. Explain the rules and set limits.
4. Help the client problem-solve.

147. A 15-year-old girl tells the nurse that she wants to talk with her mother. The nurse is aware that the girl's mother does not want any further contact with her daughter. The client asks permission to use the telephone. What is the nurse's best response?

1. "Why do you want to call your mother?"
2. "No, not at this time. Tell me more about how you feel toward your mother."
3. "I don't believe it will be healthy to call her."
4. "Tell me how you feel, now that your mother has abandoned you."

148. In assessing a client with borderline personality disorder, the nurse should be aware of which one of the following traits?

1. Predictability
2. Controlled anger
3. Primitive dissociation
4. Stable and friendly relationships

149. A long-term goal for the nurse in planning care for a depressed, suicidal client would be to:

1. Provide him with a safe and structured environment.
2. Assist him to develop more effective coping mechanisms.
3. Have him sign a "no-suicide" contract.
4. Isolate him from stressful situations that may precipitate a depressive episode.

150. A 21-year-old female client tells the nurse that she finds it necessary to occasionally masturbate and asks for a professional opinion. The best statement by the nurse is:

1. "Only men masturbate to relieve tension."
2. "There is a possibility that masturbation causes voyeurism."
3. "Masturbation causes an orgasmic disorder in both males and females."
4. "Masturbation releases tension that is sexual in nature."

ANSWERS

1. **(4)** Integrated processes: nursing process — data collection; client need: physiological integrity; physiological adaptation; content area: psychiatric-mental health.
   RATIONALE
   (1) Hypotension and pain may be possible symptoms of anxiety but are not typical of a generalized anxiety reaction. **(2)** Lethargy and flat affect are not typical symptoms of anxiety. **(3)** Confusion and hunger are possible symptoms but not common features of an anxiety reaction. **(4)** Increased heart rate and tightness in the chest are common characteristics of anxiety.

2. **(1)** Integrated processes: nursing process — implementation; client need: physiological integrity; reduction of risk potential; content area: psychiatric-mental health.
   RATIONALE
   (1) The initial care plan would include monitoring vital signs and providing support and reassurance. The initial priority is to deal with the current anxiety reaction. **(2)** There is no reason to measure I&O or obtain weight for an anxiety reaction. **(3)** Nail bed color would not change during an anxiety reaction. **(4)** The nurse might later explore a history of drug use and offer high-carbohydrate foods, but not as an initial plan.

3. **(3)** Integrated processes: nursing process — data collection; caring; client need: psychosocial integrity; content area: psychiatric-mental health.
   RATIONALE
   (1) Introjection is identifying with another. **(2)** Sublimation is replacing an unacceptable need with one more acceptable. **(3)** The client is using denial. **(4)** Displacement is transferring feelings about one person onto another.

4. **(2)** Integrated processes: nursing process — implementation; client need: physiological integrity; pharmacological therapies; content area: psychiatric-mental health.
   RATIONALE
   (1) Imipramine is an antidepressant. **(2)** Lorazepam is an anxiolytic. **(3)** Lithium is a mood stabilizer. **(4)** Amitriptyline is an antidepressant.

5. **(1)** Integrated processes: nursing process — data collection; client need: physiological integrity; pharmacological therapies; content area: psychiatric-mental health.
   RATIONALE
   (1) Anxiolytics often have the side effect of drowsiness. **(2)** Some clients could experience convulsions; however, it is a more common side effect of an antipsychotic drug. **(3)** Although blurred vision may be experienced by some clients, it is not a common side effect of anxiolytics. **(4)** Fear of falling is not a common side effect of medications.

6. **(3)** Integrated processes: nursing process —implementation; teaching/learning; client need: physiological integrity; reduction of risk potential; Content area: psychiatric-mental health
   RATIONALE
   (1) Many persons work while taking psychiatric medications. **(2)** Persons taking antidepressants such as MAOIs should not consume herring. **(3)** A person taking lorazepam, an anxiolytic, should not consume alcohol. **(4)** Persons taking some antipsy-

chotics such as phenothiazine should be cautious in the sun because of the possibility of sunburn.

7. **(4)** Integrated processes: nursing process — data collection; communication and documentation; client need: physiological integrity; physiological adaptation; content area: psychiatric-mental health.
   RATIONALE
   (1) In panic-level anxiety, the person has dilated pupils, a feeling of terror, and loss of rational thought. **(2)** Mild anxiety is associated with day-to-day living. **(3)** Moderate anxiety manifests as tension in neck, headaches, hypercriticism, and inability to concentrate. **(4)** Severe anxiety is associated with the stated symptoms.

8. **(3)** Integrated processes: nursing process — data collection; communication and documentation; client need: psychosocial integrity; content area: psychiatric-mental health.
   RATIONALE
   (1) The medium of verbal communication is speech. **(2)** Therapeutic communication is a process of using specific techniques. **(3)** Poor eye contact is an example of nonverbal communication. **(4)** Mass communication is a component of journalism or marketing.

9. **(2)** Integrated processes: nursing process — data collection; client need: physiological integrity; physiological adaptation; content area: psychiatric-mental health.
   RATIONALE
   (1) Anxiety disorders manifest themselves with a different cluster of symptoms. **(2)** The cluster of symptoms is common in grief reactions, specifically the stage of developing awareness. **(3)** Panic attacks typically are characterized by a sudden onset of intense discomfort and often resemble symptoms of a heart attack. **(4)** The stated symptoms are not typical of eating disorders.

10. **(3)** Integrated processes: nursing process — implementation; caring; client need: psychosocial integrity; content area: psychiatric-mental health.
    RATIONALE
    (1) The nurse does not want to remain subjective, but rather objective. **(2)** The nurse does not want to judge the client or offer advice. **(3)** Therapeutic communication requires that the nurse respect the client and offer presence. **(4)** Empathy, rather than sympathy, is a therapeutic technique.

11. **(4)** Integrated processes: nursing process — implementation; communication and documentation; client need: psychosocial integrity; content area: psychiatric-mental health.
    RATIONALE
    (1) Restating is repeating the client's message using different words. **(2)** Providing feedback is making observations about the client's behavior. **(3)** Identifying a theme is helping the client see a pattern of thought. **(4)** The nurse is giving the client an opportunity to verbalize by using an open-ended statement.

12. **(2)** Integrated processes: nursing process — implementation; communication and documentation; client need: psychosocial integrity; content area: psychiatric-mental health.

RATIONALE

(1) Obviously, the nurse does not stop communicating simply because physicians have status. (2) A one-to-one communication is altered when physical (e.g., noise) or psychosocial (e.g., visitors, physicians) factors change. (3) There is no overriding reason that the communication between nurse and client should be private. Usually, the content of the communication is charted and shared with the team. (4) The purpose of other health team members' communication with the client is generally similar. All health-care disciplines are concerned with caring and communicating with the client.

13. **(2)** Integrated processes: nursing process — implementation; communication and documentation; client need: psychosocial integrity; content area: psychiatric-mental health.

RATIONALE

(1) Omission of content means failing to consider the entire conversation between the student and client. (2) The student offered personal advice, which stops open, effective communication. (3) The student is not rejecting the client; she is offering personal advice. (4) There is no indication that the student is offering faulty reassurances by offering a personal opinion.

14. **(2)** Integrated processes: nursing process — data collection; client need: health promotion and maintenance; content area: psychiatric-mental health.

RATIONALE

(1) According to Erikson's theory, industry versus inferiority occurs between 6 and 11 years. (2) Intimacy versus isolation occurs between 19 and 34 years. (3) The developmental stage of a 61-year-old is ego integrity versus despair. (4) The generativity versus stagnation developmental stage occurs between 35 and 60 years.

15. **(1)** Integrated processes: nursing process — implementation; caring; client need: psychosocial integrity; content area: psychiatric-mental health.

RATIONALE

(1) The nurse must offer calm support to maintain a relationship with the client and assess the situation. (2) Neuroleptic drugs are used to treat acute and chronic psychosis. (3) It is more important to help the client develop self-direction than to give advice. (4) Notifying the hospital administrator is inappropriate until more data are collected.

16. **(1)** Integrated processes: nursing process — data collection; client need: psychosocial integrity; content area: psychiatric-mental health.

RATIONALE

(1) Coping mechanisms are task-oriented behaviors to increase one's ability to cope. (2) Defense mechanisms are unconscious ego-oriented reactions for self-protection. (3) Reaction formation is a defense mechanism. (4) Intellectualization is also a defense mechanism.

17. **(1)** Integrated processes: nursing process — planning; client need: physiological integrity; reduction of risk potential; content area: psychiatric-mental health.

RATIONALE

(1) ECT is administered to depressed clients and requires all the nursing care that an operative procedure requires (e.g., NPO, preoperative permit, denture removal). (2) ECT does not cause weight gain. (3) ECT is not usually given in conjunction with neuroleptics. (4) ECT usually increases rather than decreases mood.

18. **(2)** Integrated processes: nursing process — data collection; client need: health promotion and maintenance; content area: psychiatric-mental health.

RATIONALE

(1) Clients with a diagnosis of anorexia are frightened of being fat. (2) Clients with a diagnosis of anorexia do not eat large amounts of food. (3) Clients with anorexia are very thin because of starvation. (4) Clients with a diagnosis of anorexia do not perceive food as comforting or relaxing.

19. **(4)** Integrated processes: nursing process — data collection; client need: health promotion and maintenance; content area: psychiatric-mental health.

RATIONALE

(1) The trust versus mistrust stage of development occurs in infancy, according to Erikson. (2) The autonomy versus shame and doubt stage of development occurs in a 2-year-old child, according to Erikson. (3) The initiative versus guilt stage of development occurs during the preschool years, according to Erikson. (4) A 14-year-old struggles with identity versus role diffusion, according to Erikson.

20. **(1)** Integrated processes: nursing process — data collection; client need: health promotion and maintenance; content area: psychiatric-mental health.

RATIONALE

(1) Individuals with anorexia nervosa often exercise 3–4 hours daily. (2) Individuals with anorexia nervosa have decreased libido. (3) Individuals with anorexia nervosa usually are of above-average intelligence. (4) Individuals with anorexia nervosa suffer from bradycardia.

21. **(2)** Integrated processes: nursing process — planning; client need: psychosocial integrity; content area: psychiatric-mental health.

RATIONALE

(1) Neuroleptic drugs are used to treat thought disorders. (2) Coping mechanisms should be assessed to determine the client's pattern of coping with anxiety. (3) Vigorous exercise should be discouraged. (4) Nurses do not "prescribe" fingernail treatment.

22. **(3)** Integrated processes: nursing process — data collection; client need: psychosocial integrity; content area: psychiatric-mental health.

RATIONALE

(1) Rationalization is an attempt to make unacceptable feelings acceptable. (2) Projection is attributing one's own thoughts to another. (3) This is a classic case of displacement. (4) Regression is retreating to an earlier stage of life.

23. **(1)** Integrated processes: nursing process — implementation; client need: psychosocial integrity; content area: psychiatric-mental health.

RATIONALE

(1) The nurse must help the client stick to a theme of therapeutic value. (2) Restating talk about self when the topic is weather is less than useful. (3) Silence would be inappropriate in this case. (4) Summarizing may be used to link themes and feelings and to review important points in the interaction. Summarizing would be an inappropriate communication technique in this case.

24. **(1)** Integrated processes: nursing process — planning; teaching/learning; client need: physiological integrity; reduction of risk potential; content area: psychiatric-mental health.

RATIONALE

(1) Clients should receive information regarding procedures. (2) The implications of the procedure should not be exaggerated or overexplained. (3) This response does not meet the client at her level of understanding. (4) A male aide should not accompany a teenage girl suffering from anorexia nervosa for an ECG because of the client's development stage.

25. (1) Integrated processes: nursing process — data collection; client need: physiological integrity; physiological adaptation; content area: psychiatric-mental health.

    RATIONALE

    (1) Clients suffering from substance abuse often have dilated pupils. (2) Substance abusers have poor concentration and low tolerance for frustration. (3) Euphoria is a psychological characteristic. (4) The color of nail beds is not generally affected by substance abuse.

26. (1) Integrated processes: nursing process — implementation; client need: physiological integrity; reduction of risk potential; content area: psychiatric-mental health.

    RATIONALE

    (1) Drug overdose can lead to unstable vital signs and diminished urine output. (2) Obtaining weight and temperature is not an immediate concern. (3) Some drug overdoses would preclude inducing vomiting. (4) A psychiatric consultation may be obtained after the threatening situation is resolved.

27. (4) Integrated processes: nursing process — implementation; client need: physiological integrity; reduction of risk potentia; content area: psychiatric-mental health.

    RATIONALE

    (1) The nurse may consider monitoring manipulative behavior but not during the acute phase of detoxification. (2) Intervening in family dynamics is not an important issue during the acute phase of detoxification. (3) Evaluating vocational skills during the acute phase of detoxification is not an appropriate nursing action. (4) Monitoring a client's vital signs is an important nursing task during the acute phase of withdrawal.

28. (1) Integrated processes: nursing process — data collection; client need: psychosocial integrity; content area: psychiatric-mental health.

    RATIONALE

    (1) Denial is consciously disowning intolerable compulsions and thoughts. Denial is extremely common in substance abuse clients. (2) Projection is attributing one's own thoughts to another. (3) Displacement is shifting your emotions to another person or object. (4) Sublimation is substituting a socially acceptable goal for an unwanted drive.

29. (2) Integrated processes: nursing process — implementation; communication and documentation; client need: psychosocial integrity; content area: psychiatric-mental health.

    RATIONALE

    (1) Focusing provides statements that help the client expand on the topic. (2) Clarifying is a communication technique that is effective in seeking consensual validation of the client's perception of reality and its significance and meaning to his or her life. (3) Providing feedback promotes exchange with the sender and the receiver. (4) Making an observation is the receiver telling the sender what he or she sees and thinks.

30. (1) Integrated processes: nursing process — evaluation; client need: psychosocial integrity; content area: psychiatric-mental health.

RATIONALE

(1) At the termination of therapy, the client will identify new modes of coping. (2) Clients must discontinue all drug use. (3) Clients must accept responsibility for their lives and actions. (4) Clients must find new ways of social interaction.

31. (1) Integrated processes: nursing process — data collection; client need: psychosocial integrity; content area: psychiatric-mental health.

    RATIONALE

    (1) Schizophrenia is a thought disorder characterized by disturbances of thought content, form, affect, and relationship. (2) Affective disorders are disorders of feeling or mood. (3) Personality disorders are disorders of personality traits that are inflexible and maladaptive. (4) An adjustment disorder is one in which psychological factors affect physical conditions; it is usually short lived and related to stress.

32. (2) Integrated processes: nursing process — data collection; client need: psychosocial integrity; content area: psychiatric-mental health.

    RATIONALE

    (1) Stuttering, cluttering, and passive behavior are not symptoms characteristic of schizophrenia. (2) Schizophrenia is characterized by delusions, hallucinations, grandiosity, suspiciousness, disorganized behavior, tangential thought, negativism, diminished self-care, and inappropriate emotional responses. (3) Hyperactivity, crying, and violence are symptoms of mood disorders. (4) These symptoms are characteristic of other mood disorders or thought disorders but not of schizophrenia.

33. (3) Integrated processes: nursing process — planning; client need: physiological integrity; pharmacological therapies; content area: psychiatric-mental health.

    RATIONALE

    (1) Anxiolytic medications are used for anxiety disorders. (2) Antidepressant medications are used for mood disorders. (3) Schizophrenia is a thought disorder that generally responds to antipsychotic medications such as haloperidol, trifluoperazine (Stelazine), or fluphenazine. (4) Antiseizure medications are used for various types of seizures (e.g., epilepsy).

34. (2) Integrated processes: nursing process — planning; client need: physiological integrity; reduction of risk potential; content area: psychiatric-mental health.

    RATIONALE

    (1) Less frequently, antipsychotic medications may cause neuroleptic malignant syndrome (NMS) in which the client experiences high temperatures (105°F [40.5°C]). (2) Antipsychotic medications frequently result in orthostatic hypotension, and therefore blood pressure measurements are taken lying and standing before the medication is administered. Although NMS is less common than orthostatic hypotension, it is important to monitor vital signs such as blood pressure and temperature. (3) There is no indication that antipsychotic medications have complex interactions with various foods in a client's diet. (4) Blood samples should be ordered by the physician at frequent intervals to determine the therapeutic level of the medication. The nurse should notify the physician of abnormal laboratory results.

35. (1) Integrated processes: nursing process — data collection; client need: psychosocial integrity; content area: psychiatric-mental health.

    RATIONALE

    (1) This is an example of a delusion or a faulty thought process or belief. (2) A hallucination is a sensory response to something

or someone not present. **(3)** Anxiety is a feeling of vague uneasiness that may cause physiological arousal. **(4)** Tangential thought is skipping from one topic to another.

36. **(4)** Integrated processes: nursing process — implementation; communication and documentation; client need: safe, effective care environment; coordinated care; content area: psychiatric-mental health.

RATIONALE

(1) Telling the client that he is psychotic is not an acceptable nursing action. **(2)** Medications are altered by physician's orders, not by the nurse. **(3)** Tolerating the behavioral change is not an accountable action. **(4)** When a client's behavior changes, the nurse must document the assessment.

37. **(3)** Integrated processes: nursing process — implementation; client need: safe, effective care environment; coordinated care; content area: psychiatric-mental health.

RATIONALE

(1) The nurse must demonstrate respect for the client's personal space. An invasion of the client's space will likely escalate the agitated behavior. **(2)** Telling the client to act appropriately may lead to a communication barrier between nurse and client. Avoid giving advice. **(3)** When a client strikes a nurse, the client is displaying poor impulse control. Safety of self, the client, and the staff is a priority. Impulsive clients should not be managed alone. The nurse should call for assistance before any other nursing actions are planned. **(4)** Obtaining vital signs is important information but inappropriate at this time.

38. **(1)** Integrated processes: nursing process — data collection; client need: psychosocial integrity; content area: psychiatric-mental health.

RATIONALE

(1) In bipolar disorder, client behavior ranges from excitability to depression. Bipolar disorder is an alteration of mood, affect, and thought. **(2)** Many clients have personality problems and self-care deficits, but the central issue of the disorder is altered mood. **(3)** Interpersonal functioning may contribute to altered mood episodes. **(4)** Intelligence and ideation are not relevant.

39. **(3)** Integrated processes: nursing process — planning; client need: physiological integrity; pharmacological therapies; content area: psychiatric-mental health.

RATIONALE

(1) The nurse might monitor the diet but not specifically for administration of lithium. **(2)** The sleep pattern may also be monitored but not specifically for administration of lithium. **(3)** Lithium is a salt; its blood level must be monitored. The range of normal blood levels is 1.0–1.2 mEq/L. If the lithium blood level is >1.2, the nurse will hold the medication and notify the physician. **(4)** The nurse might monitor the activity level as part of overall care but not specifically for administration of lithium.

40. **(2)** Integrated processes: nursing process — data collection; client need: physiological integrity; pharmacological therapies; content area: psychiatric-mental health.

RATIONALE

(1) Lithium toxicity usually does not cause painful eyes, nausea, or vomiting. **(2)** Lithium toxicity is a serious disorder characterized by diarrhea, tremors, nausea, and vomiting. Generally, toxicity is reversed by intravenous infusion. **(3)** These symptoms are not typical of lithium toxicity. **(4)** Hypotension, thirst, nausea, and vomiting usually are not common symptoms of lithium toxicity.

41. **(3)** Integrated processes: nursing process — data collection; client need: physiological integrity; physiological adaptation; content area: psychiatric-mental health.

RATIONALE

(1) Overeating and overspending are not characteristics of Alzheimer's disease. **(2)** Labile mood rather than mood stability is characteristic of Alzheimer's disease. **(3)** Alzheimer's disease is characterized by impaired memory, self-care deficits, anxiety, impaired judgment, rage reactions, and weakness of limbs. **(4)** Limb pain is not a characteristic of Alzheimer's disease.

42. **(1)** Integrated processes: nursing process — planning; client need: psychosocial integrity; content area: psychiatric-mental health.

RATIONALE

(1) Clients with Alzheimer's disease are frequently confused and disoriented. Clocks, calendars, and open drapes help the client to know time, place, and person. **(2)** These clients need a stable environment and decreased environmental stimuli when they no longer can tolerate the sensory level. **(3)** Clients with Alzheimer's disease need a consistent care routine. **(4)** Because of the narrowed communication ability, these clients usually are unable to work in group situations.

43. **(2)** Integrated processes: nursing process — implementation; caring; client need: psychosocial integrity; content area: psychiatric-mental health.

RATIONALE

Restraints and medication may be necessary, but these are not the first line of intervention. **(2)** Clients with Alzheimer's disease often become confused at night. This is called "sundowning." The nurse should first reorient the client and offer reassurance. **(3)** Controlling the light is an important environmental factor and may enhance the client's ability to maintain orientation, but reassurance is most important. **(4)** Safety issues are the responsibility of the caregiver, and observation of all clients serves to eliminate unsafe conditions.

44. **(2)** Integrated processes: nursing process — data collection; client need: health promotion and maintenance; content area: psychiatric-mental health.

RATIONALE

(1) The development stage of trust versus mistrust occurs between 0 and 12 months of age. **(2)** The aged client's developmental stage is ego integrity versus despair. The wisdom, experience, and purpose of one's life should synthesize in old age to create an integration of the self or ego. **(3)** Identity versus identity confusion occurs in the teen years. **(4)** Generativity versus stagnation occurs in the middle years.

45. **(3)** Integrated processes: nursing process — planning; client need: safe, effective care environment; safety and infection control; content area: psychiatric-mental health.

RATIONALE

(1) Nursing care must be planned to meet the physiological needs of the person if the client is unable to meet these needs. Impaired cognition usually involves sensory and perceptual disorders that may endanger the client's safety. Meeting the client's safety need is the number one priority. **(2)** Alzheimer's disease is a progressive deterioration that robs the person of intellectual functioning with possible emotional changes. Falls become a safety concern in clients with Alzheimer's disease. **(3)** A safe environment allows for both simple activities and security. Attention span and the ability to concentrate may be impaired as a result of neurological brain disease. To promote and maintain optimal health, the nurse must attend to the client's safety. If priorities must be set, safety is of extreme importance to the care of the client with Alzheimer's disease. **(4)** Spiritual care must be appropriate for the client and should be included as part of holistic nursing interventions, but safety is the number one priority.

46. **(1)** Integrated processes: nursing process — data collection; communication and documentation; client need: physiological integrity; physiological adaptation; content area: psychiatric-mental health.

    RATIONALE

    (1) Although severely retarded children usually have an IQ between 20 and 40, it is important to assess for communication abilities so that their needs can be understood. **(2)** Severely retarded children usually do not read. **(3)** Children who are severely retarded do not usually participate in hobbies. **(4)** These children may not know right from wrong.

47. **(1)** Integrated processes: nursing process — planning; client need: safe, effective care environment; coordinated care; content area: psychiatric-mental health.

    RATIONALE

    (1) Mentally retarded children are exceptional and need a great deal of care. Their handicaps often elicit feelings within nurses that should be recognized and processed. **(2)** It is important to have family contact. **(3)** The child's mental development precludes extensive interviewing. **(4)** Teaching coping skills may be attempted but may prove to be futile.

48. **(4)** Integrated processes: nursing process — data collection; client need: physiological integrity; physiological adaptation; content area: psychiatric-mental health.

    RATIONALE

    (1) Withdrawal is not typical of anxiety reactions. **(2)** Lethargy may exist without anxiety. **(3)** Hunger is not related to an anxiety reaction. **(4)** The nurse may see an increased heart rate, hypervigilance, a startled response, or irritability in children with anxiety.

49. **(2)** Integrated processes: nursing process — data collection; client need: psychosocial integrity; content area: psychiatric-mental health.

    RATIONALE

    (1) Reality orientation is not associated with OCD. **(2)** Persons with a diagnosis of obsessive-compulsive behavior disorder exhibit a preoccupation with rules, lack spontaneity, and are perfectionistic. **(3)** A wide range of emotions is not associated with OCD. **(4)** Ritualistic thought is the obsessive part of the disorder. Compulsion describes the action.

50. **(1)** Integrated processes: nursing process — implementation; client need: psychosocial integrity; content area: psychiatric-mental health.

    RATIONALE

    (1) The most appropriate nursing intervention would be to document the behavior and work with the treatment team to design a consistent treatment program. The treatment of OCD requires an interdisciplinary approach that addresses the anxiety, dread, and guilt of the client; extinguishes the behavior; allows a safe environment; and assists the client to understand his or her feelings and actions. Rituals are extinguished in a systematic time-step fashion over a period of weeks. **(2)** Asking the client to stop the ritualistic behavior may produce anxiety that the client is unable to manage. **(3)** Asking a "why" question is unrealistic and may cause the client to become defensive. **(4)** Reinforcing the behavior is ineffective.

51. **(2)** Integrated processes: nursing process — data collection; client need: psychosocial integrity; content area: psychiatric-mental health.

    RATIONALE

    (1) Avoidance is a conscious or unconscious defense mechanism used to manage anxiety-laden experiences through evasive behaviors. There is no indication that the client is exhibiting avoidance behavior. **(2)** The client is trying to manipulate the nurse by playing one staff member against the other (commonly called "splitting"). Manipulation is characterized by (a) having a conflict of goals, (b) consciously and intentionally trying to influence others, (c) practicing deception, and (d) feeling good about the act of manipulation. **(3)** The client is not opposing or resisting authority. She is playing one staff member against the other. **(4)** The client is not using the unconscious defense mechanism of projection. Projection is attributing one's own thoughts to another.

52. **(2)** Integrated processes: nursing process — implementation; client need: psychosocial integrity; content area: psychiatric-mental health.

    RATIONALE

    (1) Accusatory statements do not facilitate constructive communication. **(2)** Missing class is against the rules. Reinforcing the rule avoids a power struggle with the client. The client needs to understand rules and limitations, and that these rules and limitations will be reinforced consistently. **(3)** The question is inappropriate at this stage of the illness. **(4)** Closed-ended comments inhibit communication between the nurse and the client.

53. **(2)** Integrated processes: nursing process — data collection; client need: psychsocial integrity; content area: psychiatric-mental health.

    RATIONALE

    (1) A discussion of sexual feelings can increase knowledge and may decrease anxiety and facilitate problem solving. **(2)** Attempted suicide is an extreme form of acting out. Acting-out behavior is limit testing. Limits are challenged in an attempt to communicate feelings of fear or anger, which the client is unable to communicate directly. **(3)** Attending activities is not a form of acting-out behavior. **(4)** Contracting for safety suggests that the client is seeking security in the environment.

54. **(1, 3)** Nursing process phase: Implementation; client need: psychosocial integrity.

    RATIONALE

    (1) To defuse the situation, the nurse should provide a safe, nonthreatening environment and remove the stimulus reinforcement. Limits are clearly reinforced in conversation. **(2)** Seclusion is viewed as control over personal freedom. **(3)** Sharing observations assists the client to problem solve (e.g., "Fighting is against the rules. It doesn't solve the conflict. What happened to start the fight? How could it be handled differently?"). **(4)** Restraints should not be used as punishment. Clients are restrained if they are possibly harmful to themselves or others. **(5)** Behavior modification works better than calling in the legal authorities. **(6)** To defuse the situation, the nurse should provide a safe, nonthreatening environment and remove the stimulus reinforcement.

55. **(1)** Integrated processes: nursing process — data collection; client need: health promotion and maintenance; content area: psychiatric-mental health.

    RATIONALE

    (1) Adolescents find it difficult to engage in a discussion related to death. **(2)** It is the child who sees death as temporary. **(3)** School-age children feel that death is a punishment. **(4)** Adolescents are thinking about the future and realize that they might not participate.

56. **(3)** Integrated processes: nursing process — data collection; client need: psychosocial integrity; content area: psychiatric-mental health.

    RATIONALE
    (1) The client is angry and feels helpless and hopeless. **(2)** The client is in the bargaining stage of the grief process. **(3)** The client indicates that she is willing to move on with her life. **(4)** The client sounds depressed and continues to mourn over the loss.

57. **(1)** Integrated processes: nursing process — planning; client need: psychosocial integrity; content area: psychiatric-mental health.

    RATIONALE
    (1) Spiritual development is an important aspect of the personality. A holistic approach to nursing care is provided within the framework of the nurse-client relationship and includes spiritual health. **(2)** Questioning may sort out the religious preoccupation, but the client may use it as a barrier for any further communication. **(3)** Because it is impossible to be informed about all religious traditions, it is important to discuss the client's spiritual issues with informed members of the health-care team before referring him to any group. **(4)** A discussion about immortality would be inappropriate.

58. **(2)** Integrated processes: nursing process — planning; client need: psychosocial integrity; content area: psychiatric-mental health.

    RATIONALE
    (1) Survivors do not have time to engage in anticipatory grief, the progression through the phases of grief before the death. **(2)** Many survivors feel guilty for not having given something special or extra to the deceased. **(3)** Survivors' immediate responses to a sudden death are feelings of shock, disbelief, guilt, despair, desertion, or betrayal. Detachment takes place over time and is the process of "letting go." **(4)** An uncomplicated grief reaction is an essential emotional process that is a normal response to a loss. Survivors of victims of sudden death do not have time to prepare for the loss.

59. **(2)** Integrated processes: nursing process — data collection; caring; client need: psychosocial integrity; content area: psychiatric-mental health.

    RATIONALE
    (1) Significant others and religious beliefs may serve as a source of help and strength, but often do not. Clients need to experience hope and support for the beliefs that give them strength. **(2)** Spirituality concerns, especially among elderly persons, cause them to question the meaning and purpose in living. Persons experiencing spiritual distress question their own existence and the reasons for suffering. **(3)** Information about the client's spiritual component is hard to obtain because it does not always lend itself to direct observation. **(4)** Religious affiliation may be most meaningful for the client, and it is an outlet for the expression of spirituality, but it is not the issue here.

60. **(1)** Integrated processes: nursing process — data collection; client need: physiological integrity; physiological adaptation; content area: psychiatric-mental health.

    RATIONALE
    (1) The symptoms indicated are associated with delirium tremens and usually develop 72 hours after the last drink. **(2)** Korsakoff's syndrome is a disturbance of short-term memory possibly related to thiamine deficiency. **(3)** Alcoholic hepatitis is

a physical effect of chronic alcoholism. There is no observable evidence of hepatitis at this time. **(4)** Alcoholic hallucinosis refers to auditory hallucinations. The client did not present with hallucinations.

61. **(4)** Integrated processes: nursing process — data collection; client need: physiological integrity; physiological adaptation; content area: psychiatric-mental health.

    RATIONALE
    (1) A sign of cocaine intoxication is diaphoresis, not dry, cool skin. **(2)** Clients suffering from cocaine intoxication experience elevated blood pressure. **(3)** A common effect of cocaine detoxification on the body is a demand for oxygen and an increase in the heart rate. **(4)** A common sign of cocaine intoxication is psychomotor agitation.

62. **(2)** Integrated processes: nursing process — planning; client need: physiological integrity; pharmacological therapies; content area: psychiatric-mental health.

    RATIONALE
    (1) Librium is commonly used in the treatment of alcohol withdrawal. **(2)** Disulfiram is used as a deterrent to drinking if the client wishes to stop drinking alcohol. Ingestion of alcohol while Antabuse is in the body results in an unpleasant physical reaction. **(3)** Valium is used to reduce the symptoms of alcohol withdrawal. **(4)** Lithium is the drug of choice for clients suffering from mood disorders.

63. **(2)** Integrated processes: nursing process — data collection; client need: psychosocial integrity; content area: psychiatric-mental health.

    RATIONALE
    (1) The harboring of family secrets and the inability to express true feelings are dysfunctional behaviors that may contribute to ineffective family dynamics rather than effective family dynamics. **(2)** A person who is codependent has difficulty with establishing a separate identity. Ego boundaries are weak and the diffuseness of boundaries inhibits the development of autonomy. **(3)** Codependency involves an imbalance in internal ego states. **(4)** Codependency involves negative messages about self that came from childhood experiences.

64. **(1)** Integrated processes: nursing process — implementation; caring; client need: psychosocial integrity; content area: psychiatric-mental health.

    RATIONALE
    (1) Instilling hope in the family's future is one of the nurse's greatest responsibilities. **(2)** Alcoholic families are dysfunctional and lack homeostatic balance. **(3)** Cross-generational clinging is dysfunctional and should be discouraged. **(4)** Promoting defense mechanisms such as rationalization or blaming others for behaviors associated with alcohol abuse serves only to prolong the denial.

65. **(1)** Integrated processes: nursing process — implementation; teaching/learning; client need: psychosocial integrity; content area: psychiatric-mental health.

    RATIONALE
    (1) Behavior modification therapy can be effective in facilitating coping skills and adaptive behaviors in certain mental illnesses. **(2)** Although complete recovery may be possible, the aim of treatment is to facilitate the client's ability to function more effectively. **(3)** Mentally ill persons are sensitive about how others will react to them. **(4)** Evaluation is based on observation of the individual's behavior. Diagnostic criteria are delineated in the *Diagnostic and Statistical Manual of Mental Disorders,* 4th edition (DSM-IV). This may not be significant to the family.

66. **(2)** Integrated processes: nursing process — planning; client need: safe, effective care environment; coordinated care; content area: psychiatric-mental health.

RATIONALE

(1) Clients have a right to therapeutic, not custodial, care. **(2)** A client's Bill of Rights ensures that a client has the right to therapeutic treatment, informed consent, and to refuse treatment. **(3)** Court cases have found in behalf of clients who did not receive therapeutic treatment and/or who were not treated humanely. The facility was held liable, and the client was released. **(4)** The courts can look at competency versus incompetency of the person. Competency is defined as the capability of making a decision. At times, the courts have appointed a guardian, but not always. Therefore, a client may not even have a guardian.

67. **(4)** Integrated processes: nursing process — data collection; client need: health promotion and maintenance; content area: psychiatric-mental health.

RATIONALE

(1) Individuals develop at their own rate, although, in any stage, most individuals accomplish certain tasks within that stage. **(2)** This school-age period (6–16 years) is psychologically the quiet years. **(3)** During this developmental period, children usually get a sense of approval from positive reinforcement from the parent. **(4)** Sexual curiosity is replaced by intellectual curiosity; great social and intellectual strides are accomplished; group activities become more important.

68. **(1)** Integrated processes: nursing process — data collection; client need: health promotion and maintenance; content area: psychiatric-mental health.

RATIONALE

(1) Events occurring throughout life may affect emotional adjustment; most experts believe that events which occur in the first 20 years have the greatest impact; some believe the first 6 years are the most significant. **(2)** Every developmental stage is the foundation for the next. If a stage is completed successfully, the foundation is firm; if not, the personality structure may be weakened. **(3)** Inability to progress through a developmental stage does not always result in withdrawn behavior, and it is not the primary cause of withdrawn behavior. **(4)** Events occurring during the first 12 months of life primarily affect the development of trust versus mistrust, but this period is not the most psychologically significant.

69. **(3)** Integrated processes: nursing process — data collection; client need: psychosocial integrity; content area: psychiatric-mental health.

RATIONALE

(1) Conversion reaction occurs when unacceptable feelings disguised by repression manifest as physical symptoms. **(2)** Suppression is consciously keeping unacceptable feelings and thoughts out of awareness. **(3)** Symptoms of depression can include withdrawal, poor eye contact, and failure to perform ADLs such as eating and hygiene. **(4)** Reaction formation occurs when unacceptable feelings are disguised by repression of the true feelings and reinforcement of the opposite feelings.

70. **(3)** Integrated processes: nursing process — data collection; client need: health promotion and maintenance; content area: psychiatric-mental health.

RATIONALE

(1) This is the developmental stage for ages 6–12 years. **(2)** This is the developmental stage for ages 18–25 years. **(3)** This is the developmental stage for ages 65 years to death. **(4)** This is the developmental stage for ages 30–45 years.

71. **(3)** Integrated processes: nursing process — implementation; communication and documentation; client need: psychosocial integrity; content area: psychiatric-mental health.

RATIONALE

(1) Empathy is the ability to feel the feelings of others so that one can relate to the situation in their terms. **(2)** The client is aware that everything will not be fine; she is alone and her spouse is deceased. **(3)** This communication block does not acknowledge the client's own perception of her situation. **(4)** Superficial reassurance denies the client's feelings and her grief.

72. **(3)** Integrated processes: nursing process — data collection; client need: health promotion and maintenance; content area: psychiatric-mental health.

RATIONALE

(1) This statement is all-inclusive; therefore, "all-or-none" cannot be correct. **(2)** Adolescents want independence without responsibility, and this accounts for ambivalent feelings. **(3)** The dependence versus independence conflict accounts for much of adolescents' irritable and erratic behavior; they long to be independent and self-sufficient. **(4)** Peer approval is very important to adolescents; they are deeply involved in their own feelings of self-worth and self-identity.

73. **(4)** Integrated processes: nursing process — planning; client need: health promotion and maintenance; content area: psychiatric-mental health.

RATIONALE

(1) Adolescents are aware of physical and emotional changes as well as of the sexual changes equated with maturity and the need to belong. **(2)** "Love" relationships are likely to be based on what the "loved" person does to strengthen the adolescent's own self-esteem; these love objects are found among peers and others outside the home setting. **(3)** Adolescents have a need to be accepted by others, as is evident by the development of language or cues unique to the group and the creation of inclusive situations that readily make the members identifiable. **(4)** The adolescent is keenly aware of body changes and maturation and shows a readiness to learn about them. Sex education during this period is important to prevent pregnancy and sexually transmitted diseases.

74. **(4)** Integrated processes: nursing process — data collection; client need: psychosocial integrity; content area: psychiatric-mental health.

RATIONALE

(1) Repression is unconsciously keeping unacceptable feelings out of awareness. **(2)** Compensation is overachievement in one area because of feeling of inadequacy in another. **(3)** Denial of reality involves the repression of a reality as though it does not exist (e.g., an alcoholic who says he does not have a drinking problem). **(4)** Rationalization is the falsification of experience through the creation of a logical or socially acceptable explanation of the behavior.

75. **(3)** Integrated processes: nursing process — implementation; communication and documentation; client need: psychosocial integrity; content area: psychiatric-mental health.

RATIONALE

(1) This response makes assumptions about characteristics that may or may not be true or contribute to the client's perceptions. **(2)** This response makes inappropriate generalizations of emotions about family and/or significant others. **(3)** This response is an open-ended question that does not cue the client as to an expected response. **(4)** This response does not maintain the focus of the session or the direction of the interaction. In addition, the therapist is setting himself or herself up for a boundary violation.

76. **(2)** Integrated processes: nursing process — evaluation; client need: physiological integrity; pharmacological therapies; content area: psychiatric-mental health.
    RATIONALE
    (1) Neuroleptics do not cure social withdrawal and apathy; they treat brain chemistry to aid in the reintegration and reorganization of thoughts. **(2)** Increased levels of dopamine increase the neurotransmitter activity in the brain and result in erratic behavior associated with schizophrenia. **(3)** Neuroleptics do not increase sex drive; in men, they cause ejaculation dysfunction. **(4)** Alteration of reality is unclear in terms of how the client's perception of reality changes. Paranoia does not occur in all schizophrenia; it is a component or symptom of some mental illnesses.

77. **(3)** Integrated processes: nursing process — data collection; client need: physiological integrity; pharmacological therapies; content area: psychiatric-mental health.
    RATIONALE
    (1) Neuroleptics cause weight gain secondary to decreased metabolism and gastric motility. **(2)** Neuroleptics may precipitate a *hyperglycemic* response in individuals who are predisposed but are not associated with precipitating diabetes. **(3)** Nasal congestion, seizures, and urinary retention are serious side effects that are believed to occur because of the additive anticholinergic properties of phenothiazine. **(4)** A common side effect of neuroleptics is hypersomnia.

78. **(2)** Integrated processes: nursing process — data collection; client need: psychosocial integrity; content area: psychiatric-mental health.
    RATIONALE
    (1) Infants will withdraw and no longer cue their needs through crying. **(2)** The developmental stage for this age group is trust versus mistrust. The unrelenting frustration of not having needs met can result in the negative outcome of mistrust. **(3)** Infants do not possess the cognitive ability to create an alternate or fantasy world. **(4)** Infants lack the cognitive ability to accomplish this.

79. **(3)** Integrated processes: nursing process — implementation; teaching/learning; client need: health promotion and maintenance; content area: psychiatric-mental health.
    RATIONALE
    (1) This realization is a turning point in the infant's development of self and self-sufficiency. **(2)** The infant does not have the emotional ability to displace anger or frustration on others. **(3)** Gradually, the child begins to master more skills that allow him or her to feel more in control of the environment and more secure. **(4)** As skills are developed and mastered, the infant progresses developmentally.

80. **(1)** Integrated processes: nursing process — data collection; client need: health promotion and maintenance; content area: psychiatric-mental health.
    RATIONALE
    (1) A 2-year-old's exploration of the environment leads to conquests and feelings of autonomy. **(2)** The 2-year-old child is independent and self-reliant. **(3)** New challenges, for example, toilet training, are mastered. **(4)** Social skills are increased, usually secondary to a curiosity about the environment.

81. **(3)** Integrated processes: nursing process — data collection; teaching/learning; client need: health promotion and maintenance; content area: psychiatric-mental health.

RATIONALE
(1) Discipline is needed to provide the 3- to 5-year-old with structure and a sense of security. **(2)** Parental approval is important in the development of good self-esteem. **(3)** Motor and intellectual skills are increasing, and in 3- to 5-year-olds, accomplishments such as the ability to ride a tricycle, run with only a few falls, and dress themselves boost their self-esteem. **(4)** This age group is becoming more aware of peers and group activities; socialization skills improve.

82. **(3)** Integrated processes: nursing process — data collection; client need: psychosocial integrity; content area: psychiatric-mental health.
    RATIONALE
    (1) Reaction formation is denial of unacceptable feelings and the adoption of the opposite behavior. If this were the case, the client would be promiscuous. **(2)** Displacement occurs when the client transfers hostile or unacceptable behavior from one object to another. **(3)** Repression is unconsciously keeping unacceptable feelings out of awareness. This client has repressed her feelings about the catastrophic sexual experience earlier in life. **(4)** Suppression is the conscious keeping of unacceptable feelings out of awareness.

83. **(1)** Integrated processes: nursing process — data collection; client need: psychosocial integrity; content area: psychiatric-mental health.
    RATIONALE
    (1) The reality in this situation is the paralysis. To deny that paralysis will change his previously active life is to deny its reality. **(2)** Compensation allows the individual to cover up a perceived area of inadequacy or weakness by overexcelling in another area. **(3)** Fantasy allows the temporary escape from a painful environment; it can also help the individual arrive at solutions to problems that he otherwise may not be able to solve. **(4)** Introjection occurs when the person incorporates into his own personality attributes of others, thus protecting him from threatening circumstances.

84. **(3)** Integrated processes: nursing process — data collection; client need: psychosocial integrity; content area: psychiatric-mental health.
    RATIONALE
    (1) Displacement occurs when a person transfers hostile and aggressive feelings from one object to another object or person. For example, a man who gets "chewed out" at work comes home and kicks the dog or yells at his wife and children. **(2)** Regression, displayed by this child, is a reaction against anxiety that allows the person to go back in development to a time when he or she felt more at ease and better able to cope with his environment. **(3)** Sublimation allows the person to divert unacceptable impulses and motives into socially acceptable ones. For example, persons with strong aggressive impulses participate in physically violent sports or other socially accepted activities. **(4)** Reaction formation occurs when one denies unacceptable feelings and impulses by adopting conscious behavior that appears (at least on the surface) to be contradictory to the feelings being denied.

85. **(2)** Integrated processes: nursing process — evaluation; client need: physiological integrity; pharmacological therapies; content area: psychiatric-mental health.
    RATIONALE
    (1) This classification of drugs, which includes chlordiazepoxide (Librium), diazepam (Valium), clorazepate (Tranxene), lorazepam (Ativan), and oxazepam (Serax), has a high potential for abuse, toxicity, and lethal overdose, and it is recommended

that these drugs be used for a short time only (1–2 weeks). **(2)** By binding with γ-aminobutyric acid, the benzodiazepine agent decreases anxiety and produces a sedative effect by blocking the release of γ-aminobutyric acid. **(3)** Although drugs in this classification have a tranquilizing effect without sedation, they may also numb emotions and decrease one's enthusiasm for life. **(4)** Benzodiazepines interfere with normal coping mechanisms and may cause an increase in irritability, aggression, hostility, and depression.

86. **(4)** Integrated processes: nursing process — evaluation; client need: physiological integrity; pharmacological therapies; content area: psychiatric-mental health.

RATIONALE

(1) Tricyclic antidepressants increase the level of the neurotransmitter serotonin or norepinephrine; a deficiency in neurotransmitters is thought to cause depression. **(2)** MAOIs prevent the metabolism of neurotransmitters; they must be given for long periods (2–6 weeks) and are more toxic. Those commonly used include isocarboxazid (Marplan), phenelzine (Nardil), and tranylcypromine (Parnate). **(3)** Tricyclic antidepressants are used to treat the symptoms of depression. In about 85% of the cases, individuals demonstrate an increase in mental alertness and physical activity within a few days of beginning treatment. **(4)** Hypertensive crisis may result if MAOIs are taken with tyramine-rich foods, such as aged cheese, avocados, bananas, and chicken livers. Clients should avoid drinking beer, red wine, and caffeine-containing beverages.

87. **(1)** Integrated processes: nursing process — planning; client need: psychosocial integrity; content area: psychiatric-mental health.

RATIONALE

(1) Many personality disorder clients are manipulative and do not have appropriate personal and social boundaries. Limits must therefore be reinforced. **(2)** Interventions should encourage relaxed rather than hostile exchanges. **(3)** Planned diversional activities are recommended in the care of clients with personality disorders. **(4)** Commonly occurring inappropriate behaviors include blaming, accusing, and intimidating. The nurse should directly and clearly identify inappropriate behaviors that alienate others.

88. **(4)** Integrated processes: nursing process — evaluation; client need: psychosocial integrity; content area: psychiatric-mental health.

RATIONALE

(1) In conversion reaction, unacceptable thoughts and feelings are repressed and manifest as physical symptoms. **(2)** The client is not demonstrating hostility toward the nurse. The object of any hostility in this exchange would have to be the client's mother. **(3)** In displacement, a client transfers hostile or unacceptable behavior from one object to another. **(4)** Transference is the result of unresolved childhood experiences with significant others; the client transfers unresolved feelings to present relationships in an attempt to resolve them.

89. **(1)** Integrated processes: nursing process — data collection; client need: physiological integrity; pharmacological therapies; content area: psychiatric-mental health.

RATIONALE

(1) The side effects include anticholinergic effects such as dry mouth, urinary retention, weight gain, and sexual dysfunction. **(2)** Neuroleptics are not considered cost prohibitive, and many clients are subsidized through mental health clinics. **(3)** In chronic mental illness, clients are usually aware of their need for medication therapy. **(4)** Neuroleptics are designed for long-term use in mental illness.

90. **(2)** Integrated processes: nursing process — implementation; teaching/learning; client need: physiological integrity; pharmacological therapies; content area: psychiatric-mental health.

RATIONALE

(1) The paranoid client is mistrustful; your explanations will not be accepted. **(2)** This action removes the stimulus on which this mistrust is based. **(3)** The paranoid client's feelings of mistrust are not helped by reassurance. **(4)** This is and will be perceived by the client as a threat and will further exacerbate the trust issues.

91. **(2)** Integrated processes: nursing process — implementation; client need: psychosocial integrity; content area: psychiatric-mental health.

RATIONALE

(1) This is a demeaning and superficial response that attacks the client's self-esteem. **(2)** This open-ended question allows the client to express his or her perception and provides an opportunity for intervention. **(3)** This response indicates that the nurse is contributing to the client's delusional structure. **(4)** This noninterventional response makes no attempt to assess the client's perception or to provide the client with the opportunity for reality orientation.

92. **(4)** Integrated processes: nursing process — planning; teaching/learning; client need: physiological integrity; pharmacological therapies; content area: psychiatric-mental health.

RATIONALE

(1) There are only two decanoate drugs: haloperidol (Haldol) and fluphenazine (Prolixin). Their delivery is different; both have side effects. **(2)** The client is not required to adhere to a special diet while taking neuroleptics. **(3)** Behavioral changes and improvement in thought reorganization are used to measure the effectiveness of neuroleptics. **(4)** The decanoate salt is slowly absorbed and has a sustained duration of action that decreases the need for frequent dosing. The dose amount and frequency are highly individualized and determined by the resolution of specific symptoms.

93. **(3)** Integrated processes: nursing process — data collection; client need: psychosocial integrity; content area: psychiatric-mental health.

RATIONALE

(1) This is not a characteristic of catatonic schizophrenia. **(2)** This is a characteristic of paranoid schizophrenia that is not generally seen in catatonic schizophrenia. The symptoms can result in an unwillingness or inability to eat. **(3)** Stuporous withdrawal, hallucinations, and delusions are characteristics of catatonic schizophrenia. **(4)** Sexual preoccupation is more a characteristic of sexual disorders and the manic phase of bipolar disorder. Word salad is a speech pattern in which words do not make sense, and is not characteristic of catatonic schizophrenia.

94. **(2)** Integrated processes: nursing process — evaluation; client need: psychosocial integrity; content area: psychiatric-mental health.

RATIONALE

(1) Clients with antisocial personality disorder reject social norms as limits and exhibit poor impulse control. This client cannot be expected to monitor his own behavior effectively. **(2)** Establishing clear, consistent limits on behavior will contribute to this client's ability to interact appropriately on the unit. **(3)** Peer interaction offers the opportunity for the client to receive feedback about his interactions with others. Encouraging peer interaction also helps model social norms. **(4)** Clients with antisocial personality disorder come from dysfunctional families and have poor, often volatile, interpersonal relationships. The nurse cannot expect these families and significant others to participate effectively with the client in treatment.

95. **(3)** Integrated processes: nursing process — data collection; client need: psychosocial integrity; content area: psychiatric-mental health.
RATIONALE
(1) Although therapy serves to reinforce self-esteem and self-worth, this is not at the basis of the deficit. **(2)** Exerting control over eating habits and weight provides positive reinforcement; the client feels in control and able to live in an otherwise out-of-control environment. **(3)** Although the client may "see" herself as "fat," this is a figurative distortion and does not include intellect. **(4)** The need to mature is not a part of this struggle and does not enter into the consideration of how to deal with her environment.

96. **(3)** Integrated processes: nursing process — planning; client need: psychosocial integrity; content area: psychiatric-mental health.
RATIONALE
(1) Behaviors that he is currently exhibiting are usually accompanied by low frustration level and easy distractibility. Initially he will not be able to meet concise behavioral expectations and will react with increased agitation. **(2)** Isolation will not provide him with the feedback he needs. He may see this only as another step in ritualistic behavior without recognizing its relationship to inappropriate behavior. **(3)** This intervention is most important at this time. Even though he has a short attention span and appears unable to concentrate, the sequence of behaviors may provide insight. **(4)** Initially, he will not know how to respond; at this point he lacks the insight to provide this information.

97. **(1)** Integrated processes: nursing process — planning; client need: physiological integrity; pharmacological therapies; content area: psychiatric-mental health.
RATIONALE
(1) To minimize side effects, therapeutic levels of lithium are reached over 7–14 days. **(2)** These are not "common" side effects of lithium therapy, and prophylactic treatment is not required. **(3)** Noncompliance results in the reappearance of symptoms and is therefore observable. **(4)** Lithium is not a short-onset, fast-acting drug. It is intended for use in long-term care.

98. **(2)** Integrated processes: nursing process — data collection; client need: physiological integrity; pharmacological therapies; content area: psychiatric-mental health.
RATIONALE
(1) Decrease in therapeutic levels results in agitated behavior. **(2)** Toxic ranges are possibly a result of self-administration error or noncompliance. **(3)** Lithium therapy is intended to control symptoms while allowing maximum level of functioning. **(4)** Lethargy and other emotional blunting symptoms are not expected side effects of lithium therapy.

99. **(3)** Integrated processes: nursing process — implementation; client need: physiological integrity; reduction of risk potential; content area: psychiatric-mental health.
RATIONALE
(1) Lithium levels would be the most significant laboratory value at this time. Forcing fluids would not be the priority intervention. **(2)** The concern is toxicity, which would require direct intervention to reverse, rather than passive intervention, such as withholding a dose of lithium. **(3)** This is the most appropriate and priority nursing intervention in this situation in which a

toxic level appears to have accumulated. **(4)** This intervention would result in further elevation of lithium levels and more critical symptoms as toxicity worsens.

100. **(2)** Integrated processes: nursing process — data collection; client need: health promotion and maintenance; content area: psychiatric-mental health.
RATIONALE
(1) This response is a prejudiced opinion that stereotypes older adults. Not all older adults are "prone" to depression, and not all require long-term care. **(2)** It is estimated that 20%–25% of all United States households are occupied by single adults. For the older adult, this means that there are fewer times when family members or significant others are in close enough proximity to respond to health-care needs. **(3)** This response is a stereotypical statement that is untrue. **(4)** Not all physiological changes in older adults are irreversible.

101. **(1)** Integrated processes: nursing process —planning; client need: psychosocial integrity; content area: psychiatric-mental health.
RATIONALE
(1) Long-term goals should focus on the client's ability to learn alternate coping skills. **(2)** Short-term goals are within a specific time frame. (2). Three days. **(3)** This goal has no time frame. **(4)** Although this is a long-term goal, it does not indicate a plan of action.

102. **(1)** Integrated processes: nursing process —planning; client need: physiological integrity; physiological adaptation; content area: psychiatric-mental health.
RATIONALE
(1) When an acute physical condition is present, the initial management of physiological care that supports homeostatic regulation takes priority over other health needs of the client. **(2)** Physiological care takes priority over other health needs of the client. **(3)** Physiological care takes priority over other health needs of the client. **(4)** Physiological care takes priority over other health needs of the client.

103. **(2)** Integrated processes: nursing process — data collection; client need: psychosocial integrity; content area: psychiatric-mental health.
RATIONALE
(1) The client will not likely have any close friends because of the secretive nature of the symptoms. **(2)** Self-mutilation, alcohol abuse, and shoplifting may be a means of providing relief and soothing from negative emotional state. **(3)** Clients with eating disorders come from families that exhibit overt conflict. **(4)** The onset of the eating disorder may coincide with periods of greater autonomy during which time the individual feels ill-equipped to manage independence.

104. **(2)** Integrated processes: nursing process — planning; client need: psychosocial integrity; content area: psychiatric-mental health.
RATIONALE
(1) Multiple social crises have contributed to the risk for drug abuse (loss of job opportunities, cultural, and social roles). **(2)** Substance use problems are common among psychiatric clients. Mental health nurses should routinely assess all clients for these problems. Substance use may be causing the psychopathology (a substance-induced mental disorder). Clients may use substances to self-medicate the symptoms of their mental disorder. **(3)** Substance abusers have low self-esteem and difficulty expressing emotions. **(4)** Codependency refers to a family member who alternately rescues and blames the person abusing substances.

105. **(1)** Integrated processes: nursing process — planning; client need: physiological integrity; pharmacological therapies; content area: psychiatric-mental health.

    RATIONALE

    (1) When a client is alcohol dependent, benzodiazepines are the medication of choice regardless of the other addictive properties used for the management of alcohol withdrawal. Benzodiazepines help prevent delirium tremens. **(2)** Barbituates, specifically phenobarbital, are used in a client who is addicted to alcohol and benzodiazepines. **(3)** Methadone is frequently used to treat heroin and morphine (opiate) addiction. **(4)** Clozapine is an antipsychotic medication used in the treatment of schizophrenia.

106. **(1, 2, 3)** Integrated processes: nursing process — implementation; client need: psychosocial integrity; content area: psychiatric-mental health.

    RATIONALE

    (1) Therapeutic touch includes relaxation techniques that promote comfort, reduce anxiety, and alleviate stress and may improve coping skills. **(2)** Exercise can reduce the emotional and behavioral responses to stress. **(3)** Imagery helps achieve relaxation and/or direct attention away from undesirable sensations. **(4)** Acupuncture is performed by a certified acupuncturist and not by a nurse. **(5)** Medication is given only with physician's order. **(6)** Counseling is done by licensed professional social worker, not the nurse.

107. **(2, 3, 4)** Integrated processes: nursing process — data collection; client need: psychosocial integrity; content area: psychiatric-mental health.

    RATIONALE

    (1) Clients diagnosed with a major depressive disorder report decreased energy, tiredness, fatigue, anxiety, irritability, hopelessness, despair, and impaired ability to think, concentrate, and make decisions. **(2)** Behavior changes of clients with organic brain disorder include frustration, irritability, verbal or physical aggression, and violence. **(3)** Clients who are psychotic/cognitively impaired exhibit common behavioral responses which include frustration, aggression, agitation, and the potential for violence and negativism. **(4)** Characteristics of personality disorders include tantrums, angry outbursts, impulsiveness, and unpredictable behavior that may be displayed as a physical attack toward another person. **(5)** Transient ischemic attacks (TIAs) do not create personality disorders. **(6)** A vegetative state implies that the individual has limited cognitive ability and does not act out with aggression and violence.

108. **(1, 2, 4)** Integrated processes: nursing process — planning; client need: psychosocial integrity; content area: psychiatric-mental health.

    RATIONALE

    (1) Client is expressing anxiety symptoms cognitively. **(2)** This is a physical response to stress and anxiety. **(3)** Diarrhea is usually the physical response to stress and anxiety. **(4)** Client's emotions are exhibited through behavioral symptoms. During periods of anxiety, clients present with physical, emotional, cognitive, and behavioral symptoms. **(5)** Urinary frequency is a physical response to stress and anxiety. **(6)** This is not a physical response to stress and anxiety.

109. **(Multiple losses, illusions of freedom and power, and illusions of safety)** Integrated processes: nursing process — data collection; client need: psychosocial integrity; content area: psychiatric-mental health.

    RATIONALE

    Multiple losses, illusions of freedom and power, and illusions of safety may trigger grief reactions. Grief is painful and a deeply felt subjective response to the loss of something highly valued or someone loved.

110. **(2, 3, 4)** Integrated processes: nursing process — evaluation; client need: physiological integrity; pharmacological therapies; content area: psychiatric-mental health.

    RATIONALE

    (1) Negative side effects of medications very often cause the client to feel worse from the treatment, including interference in decision-making ability. **(2)** Administering medications to clients places the nurse in a position of control which may result in the client feeling loss of personal control. **(3)** Studies have shown that clients fear addiction to prescribed psychotherapeutic medications. **(4)** Concurrent substance use is a risk factor for noncompliance. **(5)** Denial of the disease process affects the client's ability to comply with medication regimen. **(6)** Having family members administer medications results in the client feeling loss of personal control.

111. **(1, 2, 4)** Integrated processes: nursing process — data collection; client need: psychosocial integrity; content area: psychiatric-mental health.

    RATIONALE

    (1) Because mental illness is usually cyclical, grief tends to be recurrent. **(2)** Family members often feel guilty about the relative's illness and blame themselves. **(3)** Anger may be directed toward the mentally ill client but it is more often directed toward other family members and against mental health providers. **(4)** Family members feel powerlessness and frustrated when dealing with a long-term illness. **(5)** Family members often feel guilty about the relative's illness and blame themselves. **(6)** Family members often feel guilty about the relative's illness and blame themselves.

112. **(3)** Integrated processes: nursing process — implementation; communication and documentation; client need: safe, effective care environment; coordinated care; content area: psychiatric-mental health.

    RATIONALE

    (1) Recommending a shelter should not be the initial intervention. It may also communicate that the problem is too distasteful to handle. **(2)** Creating a support system is important, but not the initial intervention. **(3)** Because of the alleged recent attack, physical evidence and accurate documentation is needed for potential legal action. **(4)** An immediate response of nonjudgmental listening and psychological support is essential.

113. **(1, 2, 3)** Integrated processes: nursing process — evaluation; client need: safe, effective care environment; coordinated care; content area: psychiatric-mental health.

    RATIONALE

    (1) Mental health providers meet the physical and emotional needs of their patients. **(2)** Nurses and hospital/clinic providers assist clients with available health-care services, influence the quality of existing services, and develop new resources. **(3)** Discharge needs are determined during the assessment phase of the nursing process. **(4)** Health-care providers assist patients with improving self-care and the importance of living as independently as possible. **(5)** Mental health providers meet the physical and emotional needs of their patients. **(6)** Health-care providers assist patients with improving self-care and the importance of living as independently as possible.

114. **(1, 4)** Integrated processes: nursing process —evaluation; client need: psychosocial integrity; content area: psychiatric-mental health.

RATIONALE

(1) Hallucinations and delusions are overt symptoms of schizophrenia and may cause the nurse anxiety if he or she lacks knowledge about psychosis. (2) The nurse and the client may have been partners in medication-based planning to help the client take control over his or her medication regimen and would not negatively affect the interaction. (3) Motivation and grooming are reality based and should not necessarily interfere with the nurse-client interaction. (4) Disorganized speech and behavior presents as a distortion of normal functioning and does interfere with the communication process. (5) Client's acceptance of disease does not affect the nurse-client interaction in a negative manner. (6) Family's acceptance of the disease does not affect the nurse-client interaction in a negative manner.

115. **(1, 2, 4)** Integrated processes: nursing process — planning; client need: safe, effective care environment; coordinated care; content area: psychiatric-mental health.

RATIONALE

(1) Improving standards of client care is a critical ethical issue and is part of the principles in the ethical code for all nurses. (2) Providing services with respect to human dignity is a critical ethical issue and is part of the principles in the ethical code for all nurses. (3) Safeguarding the client's rights to privacy is a critical ethical issue and is part of the principles in the ethical code for all nurses. (4) Evaluating necessity and appropriateness of health care are critical ethical issues and are part of the principles in the ethical code for all nurses. (5) Safeguarding the client's rights to privacy is a critical ethical issue and is part of the principles in the ethical code for all nurses. (6) Providing services with respect to human dignity is a critical ethical issue and is part of the principles in the ethical code for all nurses. Client has the right to refuse treatments.

116. **(4)** Integrated processes: nursing process — evaluation; client need: safe, effective care environment; coordinated care; content area: psychiatric-mental health.

RATIONALE

(1) Rather than a profusion of value, within the health-care system, there is a lack of emphasis placed on the value of caring. (2) Within the nurse, there are conflicting professional commitments as the nurse strives to deliver quality care. (3) Within the client, there is a feeling of anxiety and lack of personal space. (4) Within the health-care system, a communication conflict with other health professionals has been identified as a barrier to nurse-client relationship.

117. **(1)** Integrated processes: nursing process — evaluation; client need: safe, effective care environment; safety and infection control; content area: psychiatric-mental health.

RATIONALE

(1) On a mental health unit, the degree of force considered necessary to deal with aggressive behavior is limited to those staff persons that are necessary to gain control of the client. The health-care provider is not justified in using brutal physical force to disable a client. (2) With adequate staffing, nurses involved in risk management may ensure client safety. (3) Educating employees on work place violence may ensure that staff assess potential risk situations before they develop in order to maintain milieu control and safety. (4) Potential areas for violence should be identified and corrective steps taken to reduce unreasonable risks to health-care workers.

118. **(3)** Integrated processes: nursing process — planning; client need: psychosocial integrity; content area: psychiatric-mental health

RATIONALE

(1) If the nurse's body posture suggests physical contact or physical aggression, this nonverbal behavior may provoke the client causing a violent reaction. (2) If the client's body language suggests imminent physical aggression, establishing a safe body zone is important. (3) Give the client choices and allow the client to understand that actions taken are directly related to the choices the client makes. (4) The nurse should not turn his or her back on the client. Maintaining unchallenging eye contact should help the nurse anticipate the client's next move.

119. **(1)** Integrated processes: nursing process — planning; client need: psychosocial integrity; content area: psychiatric-mental health.

RATIONALE

(1) It is the nurse's responsibility to set limits to ensure a safe and therapeutic milieu. Those who fail to control or set limits on aggressive acts are sanctioning violence. (2) Condoning or ignoring violent and/or aggressive behavior may be setting the stage for future violence in the milieu. (3) Weapon screening is not a nursing responsibility. It is the responsibility of the agency security system. (4) It is important and a nursing responsibility to assist clients with psychosocial skills.

120. **(2)** Integrated processes: nursing process — planning; client need: psychosocial integrity; content area: psychiatric-mental health.

RATIONALE

(1) Medical screening is not described by federal regulations. (2) Clearly, the physical and emotional condition of the client is a determinant in the screening that is necessary. (3) In an emergency situation, a client must be stabilized prior to requesting reimbursement. (4) A client must be screened and stabilized prior to transferring to an inpatient setting. Depending on the findings of the assessment, a transfer to an inpatient setting may not always be necessary or appropriate.

121. **(1, 4)** Integrated processes: nursing process — planning; client need: psychosocial integrity; content area: psychiatric-mental health.

RATIONALE

(1) Family is viewed as a part of the client's life and ties should be maintained if at all possible. (2) Nursing provides leadership, assumes responsibility in promoting therapeutic milieu, and is responsible for coordination of unit activities. (3) When therapies are limited, it is difficult to provide therapy using the total environment and to sustain a therapeutic community. (4) Structured interaction allows clients to interact with others and discuss daily chores, behavioral expectations, respect toward others, and unit rules and regulations. Leadership in this situation may be assumed by a client who is elected or volunteers. (5) Excessive stimuli reduces a therapeutic environment. (6) Family is viewed as a part of the client's life and ties should be maintained if at all possible.

122. **(1)** Integrated processes: nursing process — assessment; client need: physiological integrity; physiological adaptation; content area: psychiatric-mental health.

RATIONALE

(1) The Decade of the Brain saw a change in practice in mental health care through the development of new antipsychotic, antidepressant with fewer side effects. (2) Treatment approaches rely heavily on biological interventions rather than on biopsychosocial ones. There is a need to integrate the psychobiological component with the long-standing psychosocial perspective of nursing care. (3) During the deinstitutionalization period, there was a shift toward community resources for

follow-up care. (4) There is lack of sufficient time in inpatient settings to provide client education that will help them with compliance.

123. **(1, 3, 4)** Integrated processes: nursing process — planning; client need: psychosocial integrity; content area: psychiatric-mental health.

    RATIONALE

    (1) Chronically mentally ill clients require a health-care delivery system that meets all aspects of their health/illness continuum. (2) The nurse must recognize that the health-care needs of the chronically mentally ill fluctuate and do not remain constant. (3) Client's need for health promotion and disease and illness prevention are important in all stages of the client's illness. (4) When the nurse increases her or his knowledge about availability of care and quality of care, she or he can emphasize continuity of care, prevention and health promotion, and education in self-care management. (5) The nurse must recognize that the health-care needs of the family fluctuate and do not remain constant. (6) Client's need for health promotion and disease and illness prevention is important in all stages of the client's illness.

124. **(Hallucinations, delusions, and disorganized speech and behavior)** Integrated processes: nursing process — data collection; client need: psychosocial integrity; content area: psychiatric-mental health.

    RATIONALE

    Hallucinations are perceptual experiences that occur in absence of actual external sensory stimuli and the most common disturbance in schizophrenia. Delusions are erroneous fixed beliefs about the self, and involve misinterpretation of the environment that is held even in the face of disconfirming evidence. Disorganized speech and behavior are outward signs of disordered thoughts that include agitated, purposeless, repetition of words, or abnormal random movements and catatonia in which there are limited responses to the environment.

125. **(Venlafaxine)** Integrated processes: nursing process — planning; client need: physiological integrity; pharmacological therapies; content area: psychiatric-mental health.

    RATIONALE

    Venlafaxine (Effexor) is an antidepressant closely related to selective serotonin reuptake inhibitors (SSRIs). It is more widely recommended in the treatment of generalized anxiety disorders because benzodiazepines remain highly controversial.

126. **(2)** Integrated processes: nursing process — implementation; caring; client need: psychosocial integrity; content area: psychiatric-mental health.

    RATIONALE

    (1) This response negates the client's thinking. (2) This statement acknowledges the client's thinking and is nonaccusatory. (3) This response is judgmental and may put the client on the defensive. (4) This statement is seeking clarification that is not needed.

127. **(2)** Integrated processes: nursing process — data collection; client need: psychosocial integrity; content area: psychiatric-mental health.

    RATIONALE

    (1) Personality disorder patterns of behavior are inflexible and maladaptive, causing significant functional impairment. (2) A person suffering from psychosis may exhibit a disturbance in one or more major areas of functioning. (3) Neurosis is an

emotional disturbance of all kinds other than psychosis. (4) This is a group of disorders characterized by physical symptoms that are affected by emotional factors.

128. **(4)** Integrated processes: nursing process — data collection; client need: psychosocial integrity; content area: psychiatric-mental health.

    RATIONALE

    (1) Regression is a retreat to an earlier stage of development. (2) Repression banishes or excludes unacceptable impulses and thoughts from consciousness. (3) Reaction formation allows a person to adopt attitudes and behaviors that are opposite of his or her impulses. (4) The client was using conversion formation, which is the process of converting emotional stress into impaired physical functions.

129. **(1)** Integrated processes: nursing process — implementation; caring; client need: psychosocial integrity; content area: psychiatric-mental health.

    RATIONALE

    (1) Forming a therapeutic alliance with the client reduces the threat that the nurse may pose to the client. (2) The goal of therapy is to assist the client to reduce anxiety and learn to delay ritualistic behavior. (3) Clients use compulsive rituals to control anxiety. Rationalizing irrational behaviors is not an appropriate intervention because it may cause the anxiety level to increase. (4) Referring the client is not the most appropriate nursing intervention.

130. **(4)** Integrated processes: nursing process — data collection; client need: psychosocial integrity; content area: psychiatric-mental health.

    RATIONALE

    (1) Projection enables a person to justify his or her own unacceptable feelings and impulses by attributing the behaviors to others. (2) Displacement operates unconsciously and is used by an individual to transfer hostile and aggressive feelings from one object to another object or person. (3) Reaction formation enables a person to adopt attitudes and behaviors that are opposite to his or her own behaviors. (4) Denial is characterized by avoidance of disagreeable realities and unconscious refusal to acknowledge a thought, feeling, need, or desire. The client is denying that he has a substance abuse problem.

131. **(2)** Integrated processes: nursing process — implementation; client need: safe, effective care environment; safety and infection control; content area: psychiatric-mental health.

    RATIONALE

    (1) An intentional tort is a willful act that violates another person's rights. The nurse did not intentionally give Haldol to harm the client. (2) The nursing action was an unreasonable or careless act. The nurse is negligent and liable for the client's death. (3) The amount of Haldol given was within a therapeutic range. (4) An assault is a threatening act that causes another person to be afraid.

132. **(1)** Integrated processes: nursing process — implementation; client need: safe, effective care environment; safety and infection control; content area: psychiatric-mental health.

    RATIONALE

    (1) A client who is harmful to self may be detained until it has been determined that there are no further indications of self-destructive behavior. (2) A client may sign a legal document to be discharged (American Medical Association). However, because of self-destructive behavior, it is important to maintain a safe environment for all clients. (3) This is not the best response. This situation calls for a nursing intervention.

(4) Self-destructive behavior is confidential information and not available for public knowledge.

133. **(2)** Integrated processes: nursing process — evaluation; client need: safe, effective care environment; coordinated care; content area: psychiatric-mental health.

     RATIONALE

     (1) The client is disclosing information about herself. **(2)** Privileged communication is the right of all clients to discuss information with their attorney. **(3)** Information cannot be disclosed without a client's permission. **(4)** Psychiatric clients have the right to reasonable access to telephones.

134. **(2)** Integrated processes: nursing process — implementation; client need: safe, effective care environment; coordinated care; content area: psychiatric-mental health.

     RATIONALE

     (1) Clients need outside activity. However, having a safe ratio is essential. **(2)** To manage effectively, client groups should not be larger than 10 persons. **(3)** The response supports unsafe care practices. **(4)** This is an appropriate response. However, the therapist needs to be reminded that health-care practices must be delivered safely.

135. **(2)** Integrated processes: nursing process — implementation; communication and documentation; client need: safe, effective care environment; safety and infection control; Content area: psychiatric-mental health.

     RATIONALE

     (1) Restraints and seclusion are not a form of punishment. **(2)** It is important to provide safeguards in order to protect clients who are out of control. **(3)** It is against the law to leave a client in restraints and seclusion for an undetermined length of time. **(4)** Clients in restraints or seclusion must be checked on a routine basis according to the hospital policy.

136. **(4)** Integrated processes: nursing process — planning; client need: safe, effective care environment; coordinated care; content area: psychiatric-mental health.

     RATIONALE

     (1) Clients have the right to informed consent. **(2)** Clients have the right to treatment under the U.S. Constitution. **(3)** Clients have the right to refuse treatment under the U.S. Constitution. **(4)** Judicial commitment is not one of the eight ethical guidelines.

137. **(4)** Integrated processes: nursing process — implementation; caring; client need: safe, effective care environment; safety and infection control; content area: psychiatric-mental health.

     RATIONALE

     (1) In severe anxiety, the sensory perception is greatly reduced, lessening the capacity to problem solve. **(2)** The source of the problem should be probed only if the person is experiencing mild and well-controlled anxiety. **(3)** An anxiolytic medication may be ordered by the physician, but the initial intervention is to assure the client of safety and provide psychological support. **(4)** Clients exhibiting severe anxiety require immediate psychological and sometimes physical support.

138. **(2)** Integrated processes: nursing process — implementation; client need: psychosocial integrity; content area: psychiatric-mental health.

     RATIONALE

     (1) Verbalization of feelings is not the first priority. **(2)** The first priority is to rule out a neurological disorder. **(3)** Physical therapy should not be attempted until organic causes are ruled out.

(4) Assistance with future planning is important, but not this time.

139. **(1)** Integrated processes: nursing process — implementation; client need: physiological integrity; basic care and comfort; content area: psychiatric-mental health.

     RATIONALE

     (1) Provide preferred nutritious snacks. Making them accessible throughout the day will help replenish burned calories. **(2)** The client is too hyperactive to sit for a meal. **(3)** This is not a balanced meal. **(4)** This is a meal that requires the client to sit.

140. **(1)** Integrated processes: nursing process — implementation; client need: safe, effective care environment; safety and infection control; content area: psychiatric-mental health.

     RATIONALE

     (1) Client safety is the nurse's first priority. **(2)** If a client is dissatisfied with psychiatric or mental health care, the lawyer advocate may be contacted by the client. **(3)** Restraints dehumanize and interfere with a client's autonomy. It is important to use alternative strategies. **(4)** Because anger narrows the perceptual field, postpone discussion of anger and consequences until the client is in control.

141. **(2)** Integrated processes: nursing process — data collection; client need: psychosocial integrity; content area: psychiatric-mental health.

     RATIONALE

     (1) Displacement operates on an unconscious level. An emotion, idea, or wish is transferred from the original object to a more acceptable substitute. **(2)** Poor control of impulsive behavior shows limited insight and poor judgment. **(3)** Identification is an ego defense mechanism whereby a person tries to become like someone he or she admires. **(4)** Gratification or a source of satisfaction comes from getting needs met. This client has poor impulse control.

142. **(2)** Integrated processes: nursing process — implementation; caring; client need: psychosocial integrity; content area: psychiatric-mental health.

     RATIONALE

     (1) Focusing on the delusional content may increase anxiety. **(2)** Focusing on the fears and insecurities promotes the client's trust and willingness to be helped. **(3)** Agreeing with the client may reinforce the delusion. **(4)** Challenging the client's delusional system is not appropriate because it may increase tension and force the client to defend it.

143. **(1)** Integrated processes: nursing process — implementation; caring; client need: psychosocial integrity; content area: psychiatric-mental health.

     RATIONALE

     (1) The client is unable to control her mental state of health. Providing a safe environment with reduced external stimuli will provide feelings of security and safety. **(2)** Social interactions should not be encouraged until after the mood has been stabilized. **(3)** Discussion of the bizarre behavior may increase anxiety and cause anger and a defensive attitude. **(4)** With disorganized thoughts, the client may not be capable of processing the information.

144. **(2)** Integrated processes: nursing process — implementation; client need: psychosocial integrity; content area: psychiatric-mental health.

     RATIONALE

     (1) This response criticizes the client and may cause unnecessary anger and conflict. **(2)** This response gives recognition and acknowledgement of feelings. **(3)** Denying the belief serves no purpose, because delusional ideas are not eliminated by this approach. **(4)** This response rejects the client's belief and may cause the client to limit further interaction.

145. **(4)** Integrated processes: nursing process — planning; client need: psychosocial integrity; content area: psychiatric-mental health.

    RATIONALE

    (1) Paranoid clients exhibit a flat, dull affect and suspicious behaviors. **(2)** Abnormalities in motor behavior are characteristics of catatonic schizophrenia. **(3)** Regressive and primitive features are present in disorganized schizophrenia. **(4)** The paranoid client is often angry, aggressive, and guarded.

146. **(3)** Integrated processes: nursing process — implementation; caring; client need: psychosocial integrity; content area: psychiatric-mental health.

    RATIONALE

    (1) Instructing the client to leave without an explanation may cause anger and alienation. **(2)** Confrontation in an open setting may be perceived as punitive. **(3)** Clear boundaries and set limits will provide firm structure necessary for clients diagnosed with a personality disorder. **(4)** One of the health teachings of a person diagnosed with borderline personality disorder is problem solving, which is a long-term issue.

147. **(2)** Integrated processes: nursing process — implementation; client need: psychosocial integrity; content area: psychiatric-mental health.

    RATIONALE

    (1) Asking the client a "why" question can be intimidating and implies that the client must defend the request. **(2)** This response is direct and explores the relationship between mother and daughter that may provide relevant information. **(3)** This response is judgmental and opposes the client's request. **(4)** Probing for information that is difficult to answer may place the client on the defensive.

148. **(3)** Integrated processes: nursing process — data collection; client need: psychosocial integrity; content area: psychiatric-mental health.

    RATIONALE

    (1) These clients are unpredictable due to impulsiveness and lack of responsibility. **(2)** These persons demonstrate poorly controlled anger. **(3)** Clients diagnosed as having a borderline personality disorder use the defense mechanism of splitting. **(4)** One criterion for the borderline personality disorder is a pattern of unstable and intense interpersonal relationships.

149. **(2)** Integrated processes: nursing process — planning; client need: psychosocial integrity; content area: psychiatric-mental health.

    RATIONALE

    (1) This statement represents a short-term goal. **(2)** Long-term therapy should be directed toward assisting the client to cope effectively with stress. **(3)** Suicide contracts represent short-term interventions. **(4)** This statement represents an unrealistic goal. Stressful situations cannot be avoided in reality.

150. **(4)** Integrated processes: nursing process — implementation; teaching/learning; client need: psychosocial integrity; content area: psychiatric-mental health.

    RATIONALE

    (1) Masturbation is a common practice among both sexes. **(2)** There is no research that indicates masturbation causes voyeurism. **(3)** There is no evidence that masturbation causes any organic disorder. **(4)** Masturbation is used to release tension and frustration. Both sexes obtain sexual satisfaction.

Related Sciences
Reviews and Tests

CHAPTER 8

Procedures for the Licensed Practical Nurse: Content Review and Test

Cynthia Bowers Howard, RN, APRN, MSN, BC, CNS

A very important part of nursing is the ability to perform certain skills and procedures. No matter what type of procedure is done, certain standards must be met to obtain the highest level of health possible for the client. The purpose of this chapter is to assist the practical nurse (PN) in carrying out common procedures. A brief description and purpose of each procedure is given. The steps in each procedure, along with the reasons for each step, are provided. Each procedure also includes a section on the nursing implications. The entire procedure should be read carefully before actually carrying it out. When the PN knows what the procedure should include, there is less chance of forgetting important steps.

New information may require some changes in the way a procedure is carried out. Each hospital or other health-care facility should have a procedures manual on hand and revise it as necessary when new information is obtained. Certain procedures may differ from one health-care institution to another; for example, the number of times the temperature, pulse, respirations, and blood pressure are taken after a blood transfusion. The procedures presented in this chapter are based on current knowledge.

Procedure: Placing a Nasal Cannula

Description: A nasal cannula is used to give oxygen to the client. The nasal tips (prongs) come out from the center of a plastic tube and are placed into the nose openings. This allows the client to breathe through the nose or mouth.

Purpose: To deliver low to moderate amounts of oxygen to clients with certain types of pulmonary disease, heart surgical procedures, and other illnesses.

STEP	RATIONALE
1. Wash hands.	Washing hands decreases transfer of microorganisms.
2. Collect necessary equipment: • Wall or tank oxygen source • Plastic nasal cannula with a connecting tube • Humidifier filled with sterile water • Flowmeter	Having the required equipment on hand makes it safer and quicker to start. A humidifier is a special container that, when filled with sterile water, provides moisture to the lining of the nose and upper respiratory system.
3. Connect flowmeter to oxygen. Attach humidifier with nasal cannula tubing.	Humidification helps to prevent drying of mucous membranes, which makes the client more comfortable.

(Continued on following page)

STEP	RATIONALE
4. Check physician's order for the rate of flow and check to make sure that the flow rate is correct. The usual dose is 1–6 L/min. There should be bubbling in the humidifier container.	Giving oxygen to a client requires a physician's order. Rates of flow >6 L/min do not increase the amount of oxygen the client is receiving and may cause extreme dryness of the lining of the nose and throat, as well as increase gastric bloating.
5. Gently place the nasal prongs into the nasal openings.	Oxygen enters the upper respiratory system directly through the nasal cannula.
6. Adjust the tubing around the back of the ears so that the nasal prongs fit comfortably. Slide the plastic adjuster up under the chin until the fit is correct.	The client is likely to be more comfortable and cooperative in keeping the nasal cannula in place.
7. Observe and record how the client responds to the treatment by checking his or her breathing and mental orientation to time and place. Check ABGs.	Indicates how well client is responding to the treatment. Arterial blood gas (ABG) testing is the best way of determining that adequate amounts of oxygen are being delivered and of allowing the physician to determine if changes need to be made in the medical plan.

Nursing Implications: Make sure that the level of sterile distilled water in the humidifier container is correct. Check the physician's orders in regard to the oxygen administration as well as the setup at least once every 8 hours. Observe the client's nasal openings and the back of the ears for irritation and skin breakdown. If the client complains of pressure behind the ears, apply clean 2 × 2 or 4 × 4 dressings over the pressure area.

Record the amount of oxygen being administered and observations at the beginning and end of each shift. Note any changes in client's response resulting from oxygen administration, as well as any changes in the physician's orders. Any changes or abnormal reactions should be reported to the head nurse and physician immediately. Place "No Smoking" signs over client's bed and on the door.

Procedure: Inserting a Nasal Catheter

Description: In this procedure, a plastic nasal catheter is placed into the nose (one nostril) and into the nasopharynx. The nasal catheter is usually used for a short time.

Purpose: To give oxygen at flow rates of 1–6 L/min to decrease oxygen needs of the client.

STEP	RATIONALE
1. Wash hands.	Washing hands decreases the transfer of microorganisms.
2. Ask client to breathe through one naris while other naris is occluded.	Asking the client to breathe through nares determines patency of nasal passage.
3. Collect necessary equipment: • Wall or tank oxygen source • Flowmeter • Oxygen tubing • Nasal catheter (check for size) • Humidifer filled with sterile water.	The distance from nose to ear lobe approximately equals the distance that the catheter needs to be placed through the nose to the area called the oropharynx.
4. Repeat with other naris.	Asking the client to breath through nares determines patency of nasal passage.
5. Don clean gloves. Connect flowmeter with the wall or tank source of oxygen.	Donning clean gloves decreases the transfer of microorganims.
6. Measure the length of the nasal catheter from the client's nose to ear lobe. Mark this area with a small piece of tape.	Organizing necessary equipment allows quick and safe implementation. The oxygen catheter is a smooth, flexible tube with openings in the tip that allow the oxygen to pass through the nose into the lungs. The size of the catheter differs for children and adults.
7. Attach the humidifier with the nasal catheter and tubing.	Humidification helps to prevent drying of the lining of the nose and throat.
8. Use the lubricant on the tip of the catheter.	Lubricating the tip allows easier placement and decreases the possibility of injuring the lining of the nose and back of mouth.

(Continued on following page)

STEP	RATIONALE
9. Set flow rate at 2–3 L/min and gently place catheter into one nostril. The catheter should enter and proceed easily. Stop placement when taped area is reached. If the nostril is obstructed, do not force catheter.	Allows oxygen flow to decrease risk of obstructing catheter by secretions in the nose.
10. Inspect placement of catheter by observing oral cavity. The tip of the catheter should be visible. Gently pull the catheter back about 0.25 inch until the tip of the catheter can no longer be seen. Use a flashlight and a tongue depressor to help you see the nasal catheter tip.	Ensures that the catheter has been placed correctly and decreases chance of swallowing too much air.
11. Set flow rate according to the physician's orders. The usual rate is 1–6 L/min.	Giving oxygen to a client requires a physician's orders. Flow rates >6L/min may cause excessive dryness of the lining of the nose and throat as well as gastric bloating.
12. Attach catheter to nose with tape.	Tape prevents catheter from being moved out of place.
13. Discard gloves and wash hands.	Discarding gloves and washing hands decreases the transfer of microorganisms.
14. Observe and record how client responds to treatment by checking his or her breathing and mental orientation to time and place. Check ABG test results.	The client's breathing and orientation to time and place indicate the client's response to the treatment. ABG testing is the best way of determining whether adequate amounts of oxygen are delivered in needed amounts and of allowing the physician to determine if changes need to be made in the medical plan.

Nursing Implications: Change the nasal catheter at least once a day and transfer to opposite nostril. The catheter tip may become clogged with secretions, decreasing the amount of oxygen the client is receiving. Record the oxygen treatment, including the rate of flow, at the beginning and end of each shift. Note changes in the client's response to oxygen treatment or the physician's orders. Any abnormal reaction or changes in response should be reported to the head nurse and physician immediately. Keep sterile distilled water in the humidifer container at the correct level. Check the physician's orders and oxygen setup at least once every 8 hours. Place a "No Smoking" sign on the client's door and above the bed.

Procedure: Applying a Venturi Mask

Description: A Venturi mask is an oxygen mask that fits comfortably over the client's mouth and nose to make sure that the oxygen the client is receiving is in the correct amount and concentration. The openings can be adjusted to allow oxygen to be given at 24%–40% of concentration. Venturi masks are used for clients who retain more carbon dioxide in their system than normal (e.g., clients with chronic obstructive lung disease).

Purpose: To deliver a known depth of oxygen while delivering a high amount of moisture to the upper airway.

STEP	RATIONALE
1. Collect necessary equipment: • Wall or tank oxygen source • Venturi mask for correct mix of oxygen and air (24%, 28%, 31%, 35%, 40%) • Compressed air source (for high humidity) • Nebulizer with sterile water, if ordered	Organizing necessary equipment allows quick and safe implementation.
2. Connect Venturi mask with tubing to flow gauge and wall or tank oxygen source.	
3. Turn on oxygen flow gauge (meter) and adjust dial on mask opening (port) to the rate ordered by the physician. The proper setting and depth (concentration) of oxygen is usually noted on the side of the mask.	The correct mix of air to oxygen must be provided so that the correct amount of oxygen is delivered. The Venturi mask mixes a fixed flow of oxygen with different amounts of air. Oxygen enters through an opening at a high speed. The larger the opening, the lower the amount of room air drawn into the mask.
4. Place Venturi mask gently over client's nose and mouth. Adjust the placement of the elastic strap. Make sure that openings for the entry of room air are not blocked by client's bedding.	Any obstruction in air openings will interfere with the air-oxygen mixture.

(Continued on following page)

STEP	RATIONALE
5. Observe and record client's response to the procedure by checking his or her breathing and mental status.	Observation can assist in deciding the success of the oxygen delivery procedure. Checking the ABGs is the best means of judging if adequate oxygen is being delivered and provides a reason for changes in the medical plan by the physician.

Nursing Implications: Change mask, tubing, and nebulizer every day. Check water level in the nebulizer often for proper amount. Drain tubing often to remove extra amount of water that has formed. This extra water will interfere with the correct amount of oxygen being delivered to the client. Document procedure, including amount of oxygen delivered, at the beginning and end of each shift. Place "No Smoking" signs on client's door and above the bed. Wash hands before and after the procedure.

Procedure: Applying a Simple Face Mask, With or Without Aerosol

Description: A simple face mask is used to give oxygen in a low-flow system. The amount of oxygen the client gets depends on his or her breathing rate.

Purpose: To administer levels of oxygen at 35%–40% concentration; aerosol given to assist in removal of secretions.

STEP	RATIONALE
1. Collect necessary equipment: • Wall or tank oxygen source • Nebulizer with distilled water • Plastic aerosol mask with tubing • Flowmeter (gauge)	Organizing necessary equipment allows for quick and safe implementation.
2. Connect the flowmeter (gauge) with the wall or tank oxygen source and attach the nebulizer with aerosol mask and tubing.	The nebulizer helps to prevent extreme drying of the lining of the nose and upper airway of the client.
3. Set the correct amount of oxygen depth on the nebulizer bottle (check the physician's orders for the correct setting).	The percentage of oxygen to be inhaled by the client is 35%–40% and is determined by the setting on the nebulizer.
4. Set the flow rate until the right amount of mist is seen (usual rate is 10–12 L/min).	The flow rate must meet or exceed the highest amount of breath that the client can take in. The client must get a good enough flow of oxygen so that he or she gets the correct amount and depth of oxygen.
5. Place mask gently over the client's nose and mouth. Make sure elastic strap fits comfortably and mask is in right position.	Correct placement of mask is required so that the correct amount and depth of oxygen is delivered to the client.
6. Observe and record the client's response to the oxygen procedure. Observe and report the client's breathing and mental status. Check and report ABG values to the head nurse and physician.	Good observation can help the physician's decision in making changes in the medical plan. The best means of deciding whether oxygen delivery is correct for the client is to pay attention to the ABG reports.

Nursing Implications: Change mask, tubing, and nebulizer every day. Check the water level in the nebulizer often for the correct amount of water. Drain tubing often to remove extra water that has formed in the tubing. This extra water will interfere with the correct amount of oxygen being delivered to the client.

Record the procedure and amount of oxygen being delivered at the beginning and end of each shift. Place "No Smoking" signs on the client's door and above the bed. If heating equipment is used, check the temperature often to prevent the client's airway from being burned.

Procedure: Performing Postural Drainage

Description: Place the client in certain positions to assist in removal of secretions from the lung. Different positions help to drain certain areas of the lung (bronchial tree). Suctioning the trachea (windpipe) or having the client cough will help to remove secretions.

Purpose: To clear secretions from the tracheobronchi (windpipe and main divisions leading to the lung) in the client having difficulty (abnormality) clearing his or her airway.

STEP	RATIONALE
1. Examine the client to determine areas of congestion (excess fullness) in the lungs. Check information recorded on the chart, including radiographic reports. Check the lungs with a stethoscope to determine areas of congestion.	Each client must be examined to determine the best position for drainage.
2. Place client in position so that the congested lung is highest. Maintain comfort and proper position with pillows.	Placing the client in the correct position allows secretions to drain from the affected area of the lung.
3. Keep client in same position for 10–15 minutes for an adult and 3–5 minutes for a child. Observe breathing.	Some clients who have difficulty breathing are not able to stay in the same position for long.
4. After 10–15 minutes (adult) have client sit up and cough. If the client is unable to cough, suction trachea (windpipe).	Any secretions that collect because of the positioning should be expectorated (removed by coughing or suction) before placing the client in another position.
5. After client has rested for a short time, change the client's position as needed to drain other congested areas of the lung.	A short period of rest can help to prevent fatigue (exhaustion).

Nursing Implications: Do the positioning before meals. In some cases, secretions may not be present after positioning. Some clients with fractures or severe softening of the bones may not be able to stay in all the positions required. The time for the entire procedure should not exceed 30–60 minutes. Observe client for signs of difficulty in breathing or changes in pulse, respiratory rate, and blood pressure readings; evidence of chest pain; or complaints of discomfort, as well as any signs of not being able to stay in the position in which he or she has been placed. If any of these signs is present, stop the treatment. Have client cough secretions into a plastic container. Chart and record client's response to the procedure, including a description of the secretions. Postural drainage is often accompanied by chest percussion (clapping the chest with cupped hands).

Procedure: Performing Percussion and Vibration (Chest Physiotherapy)

Description: Percussion involves clapping the chest with cupped hands while the client is in a postural drainage position (position that assists the congested lung area in removing secretions). Vibration involves using the flat part of the hand on the chest during exhalation (breathing out) during postural drainage.

Purpose: To help in the removal of secretions in the tracheobronchi (windpipe and major divisions leading to the lung).

STEP	RATIONALE
1. Check client for areas of lung congestion (fullness). Use information from the recorded radiographic reports and listen to the breath sounds using a stethoscope to determine which areas of the lung are congested. Do not perform procedure if the client has fractures of the ribs or any bleeding problems.	Each client must be checked to determine his or her best position for drainage.
2. Place client so that the congested lung is in the highest position.	Helps the secretions to drain from the lung.
3. Ask the client to take long, deep breaths and not to hold his or her breath.	Helps the client to relax.
4. Percuss (clap chest with cupped hands) or vibrate (apply pressure on the affected lung area while the client is breathing out) for 5–7 minutes.	Helps to remove secretions from the affected areas of the lung.
5. After completion of each percussion or vibration, have client sit up and cough. If he or she is not able to cough, suctioning of the trachea (windpipe) may be required.	Helps to get rid of secretions that are a result of the treatment and helps to keep the client's airway open.

Nursing Implications: Always follow the way the ribs are moving when using vibration. Percussion (clapping) should not be painful; check with client if there is any feeling of discomfort. Observe client for any signs of breathing difficulty, changes in pulse and breathing rates, and changes in blood pressure readings. If any of these occurs, stop the treatment. Let client sit up and cough as needed.

Procedure: Bed Bath

Description: A total bath given to clients in bed who are unable to bathe themselves.

Purpose: To ensure personal cleanliness and make client comfortable; to remove secretions or excretions that have collected on the skin.

STEP	RATIONALE
1. Wash hands.	Prevents transfer of microorganisms to client's skin.
2. Collect necessary equipment:	Organizing necessary equipment allows for quick and safe implementation.
• Clean gloves	
• Washcloth	
• Face towel	
• Bath towel	
• Cotton balls	
• Clean gown	
• Bath blanket	
• Soap and soap dish	
• Wash basin	
• Bath thermometer	
3. Arrange bath articles on overbed table or on top of bedside stand.	
4. Draw the client's screen or curtain around bed.	Ensures privacy.
5. Don clean gloves and offer bedpan or urinal or assist client to commode or bathroom. Empty bedpan or help client back to bed.	Assists in making client comfortable during the bath procedure. Donning clean gloves prevents contact with body secretions.
6. Change gloves and wash hands as needed throughout the procedure.	Removes secretions, excretions, germ particles.
7. Remove spread and blanket. Discard in hamper or fold and place on chair.	Prepares bed for changing of linen after bath is given.
8. Remove top sheet while placing bath blanket over the client. A top sheet or spread may be used if bath blanket is not available.	Bath blanket keeps client warm and ensures privacy.
9. Check water with bath thermometer. Water temperature should be 115°–120°F. (46.1°–48°C).	Water tends to cool rapidly. Washcloth absorbs considerable amount of heat from water.
10. Fill wash basin two-thirds full of water.	Prevents spilling.
11. Place basin on overbed table.	This keeps basin in a comfortable position for bathing client.
12. Remove the client's gown while placing bath towel over chest. Put on disposable gloves.	Prepares client for bath.
13. Dip cotton ball into water and squeeze out excess water. Wipe the client's eye from the inner to the outer edge where the upper and lower eyelids meet. Repeat procedure for other eye, using a new cotton ball.	Bathes the eyes with clean water (may use clean washcloth).
14. Wrap washcloth around your hand, folding extra cloth into the palm of your hand.	Makes a wash mitt that prevents ends of cloth from hanging out.
15. Place washcloth and your hand in wash basin. Wring out washcloth to remove excess water. Gently wash the client's face, ears, and neck, using soap if requested. Pat skin dry using towel on the client's chest.	Soap may dry facial skin. Patting skin reduces chances of harming skin than if rubbed dry.
16. Place bath towel under arm opposite from where you are. Keep bath blanket over the client's body.	Puts towel in place for drying area and decreases chance of contamination of arm nearest work area by nurse leaning over to reach opposite side.
17. Wash arm from shoulder to fingertips.	Stimulates blood flow.
18. Rinse and dry each body part after washing. Cover with bath blanket.	Removing soap decreases drying of skin. Use of bath blanket keeps client warm.
19. Rinse washcloth and replenish soap periodically.	Cleans washcloth and provides more soap for bathing.

(Continued on following page)

STEP	RATIONALE
20. Wash, rinse, and dry axilla.	Cleanses remaining arm.
21. Place towel under arm nearest work area and repeat steps 17–20.	
22. If the client wishes to wash own hands, position over-bed table over the client's legs and place his or her hands in wash basin.	Lets client place hands in water for a refreshing handwash.
23. Gently wash and dry hands, especially between fingers. Check nails.	Stops moisture from collecting between fingers. Determines whether special care is needed.
24. Place towel over chest and abdomen. Fold bath blanket to just above pubic area.	Ensures warmth and privacy.
25. Wash chest and abdomen under towel. Dry, especially under the breasts of a female client. Bring bath blanket back over chest and abdomen. Remove towel.	Ensures warmth and privacy. Prevents moisture from collecting between skin surfaces, causing skin breakdown.
26. Remove bath blanket from leg and tuck blanket around pubic area.	Cleanses body part farthest from work area and decreases chance of communicating leg nearest work area by leaning over to reach opposite side. Tucking blanket around pubic area provides privacy.
27. Wash leg from hip to ankle using long, firm strokes. Dry and cover with bath blanket.	Stimulates blood flow.
28. Repeat steps 26 and 27 for leg nearest work area.	
29. Place bath towel on bed. Place basin on bath towel. Uncover foot farthest from work area, place in basin, hold basin firmly.	Provides foot bath. Soaking helps soften skin and nails of foot. Helps to remove skin secretions.
30. Gently wash and dry foot, especially between toes. Check feet and toenails.	Determines whether special attention is needed.
31. Repeat steps 29 and 30 for opposite foot.	
32. Empty wash basin; rinse and fill with clean, warm water.	Removes dirty water and provides fresh, warm water.
33. Help client into a side-lying position. Keep covered with bath blanket.	Gets client ready for back wash and back rub.
34. Place towel lenghtwise on bed next to the client's back. Fold bath blanket to just below buttocks.	Exposes back only; ensures privacy.
35. Wash back from shoulders to buttocks; include buttocks. Dry thoroughly; cover back, leaving buttocks uncovered.	
36. Rinse and apply soap on washcloth. Wash, rinse, and dry area between buttocks.	Cleanses area between buttocks. Decreases moisture collecting between skin surfaces; lessens chance of skin breakdown.
37. Help client lie on back (supine position).	Positions client for care of genital area.
38. Empty, rinse, and refill basin with clean warm water.	Provides clean warm water after bathing between buttocks.
39. If client is able to wash genital area, position head of bed to a comfortable position. Place wash basin within reach of client. Let client complete washing, rinsing, and drying of genital area.	Allows client to wash own genital area; lessens embarrassment to the client.
40. If client cannot or does not wish to complete bath, place towel over chest and abdomen, folding back bath blanket from pubic area. Gently wash the pubic area. Wash between the folds. Dry gently but thoroughly.	Reduces possible embarrassment and produces as little exposure as possible. Decreases moisture from collecting between skin surfaces, thus decreasing possible skin breakdown.
41. Reposition bath blanket over client's body. Remove towel and discard into laundry hamper.	Ensures warmth and privacy. Removes soiled towel.
42. Assist client in putting on gown.	
43. Make occupied bed.	
44. Proceed with hair, nail, and shaving needs.	See procedures for hair and nail care.
45. Raise side rails as necessary.	Ensures safety.
46. Remove soiled linens and place into laundry hamper. Remove basin; empty, rinse, replace.	Removes soiled articles from bedside.
47. Make sure call signal is within easy reach of client.	Enables client to call for assistance if necessary.
48. Open bedside curtain.	
49. Ensure comfort.	
50. Remove gloves and wash hands.	Prevents transfer of microorganisms.

(Continued on following page)

STEP	RATIONALE
Bag Bath System (addendum to bed bath)	
1. Wash hands	Prevents transfer of microorganisms to client's skin.
2. Collect necessary equipment:	Organizing necessary equipment allows quick and safe implementation.
• Commercial bag bath system	
• Disposable bag	
• Clean gloves	
• Bath blanket	
• Clean gown	
3. Heat package in microwave recommended time.	Makes bath procedure more comfortable for client.
4. Proceed in same manner used for conventional bed bath, removing one cloth at a time from package, using a new cloth for each section of the body. Rinsing is not required with disposable systems.	
5. Discard cloths in appropriate receptacle in room as they are used for bath.	Removes soiled cloths.

Nursing Implications: Clients who need help to bathe or must be bathed by the nurse feel exposed and vulnerable. The nurse needs to be aware of the client's feelings and approach the client with a caring attitude. The bath gives the nurse the opportunity to observe the skin and body parts for any potential problems. Examination of the color of the skin may help in assessing the vascular system. By moving the extremities, the nurse may gain information about the musculoskeletal system. This procedure also provides an opportunity to establish communication with the client, as well as the opportunity to teach the client the principles of good hygiene if necessary.

Procedure: Mouth Care

Description: Mouth care is given to clients who are unable to give themselves mouth care.

Purpose: To ensure personal cleanliness for clients who have ineffective mouth care; are malnourished or dehydrated; have not had fluids by mouth for longer than 24 hours; are continuously breathing through their mouths; have had contact with irritating chemicals; have injured the tissues in or around their mouth; or have an infection of the mouth.

STEP	RATIONALE
1. Wash hands.	Prevents transfer of microorganisms to client's skin.
2. Collect necessary equipment; place on bedside stand. (If client is up and about, place equipment near client's sink or on bedside within easy reach.)	Organizing necessary equipment allows quick and safe implementation.
• Fresh water or mouthwash	
• Cup	
• Emesis basin	
• Toothbrush	
• Toothpaste	
• Dental floss	
• Asepto bulb syringe	
• Gauze pad	
• Denture cup	
• Denture cream or powder	
• Water-soluble lubricant	
• Towel	
• Clean gloves	

Mouth Care for Conscious Client:

1. Explain procedure.	Informs client of procedure.
2. Wash hands; put on clean gloves.	Prevents transfer of microorganisms.
3. Raise head of bed to sitting position.	Decreases chances of getting water into lungs.
4. Raise bed to a comfortable working position.	Decreases chances of straining nurse's back.
5. Place towel under client's chest and tuck under chin.	Protects client and linens from spillage of water.

(Continued on following page)

Step	Rationale
6. Put fresh water into cup.	
7. Place toothpaste on toothbrush.	
8. Place emesis basin under chin.	Allows collection of rinse water and prevents spilling on bed linens.
9. Wrap moistened gauze pad around index finger and middle finger of hand not used in giving mouth care.	Allows gentle handling of tissues of the mouth cavity without slipping.
10. Instruct client to open mouth.	Prepares client for mouth care.

Mouth Care for Unconscious Client:

Step	Rationale
1. Explain procedure to the client.	If hearing is intact, the client may understand procedure.
2. Collect necessary equipment.	Organizing the equipment allows for safe and quick implementation.
3. Wash hands; put on gloves.	Decreases chances of contamination by germs.
4. Pour fresh water into cup. Fill Asepto bulb syringe with 30–50 mL of water. Place toothpaste on toothbrush. Attach suction catheter to suction source. Wrap gauze pads around tongue blade. Secure it with adhesive.	Allows for efficiency in giving care.
5. Place client on side, if not contraindicated, with head lowered.	Allows rinse water to drain from mouth to prevent swallowing or having water enter lungs.
6. Place towel under head and neck.	Protects bed linens.
7. Place suction tip under tongue or between cheek and lower jaw; if suction is unavailable, place emesis basin against cheek and neck under mouth.	Removes rinse water from mouth to prevent it from being swallowed or taken into lungs.
8. Wrap gauze pad moistened with water around index and middle fingers of hand to be used in giving mouth care.	Allows nurse to handle moist mouth tissues without slipping.
9. Insert tongue blade between upper and lower teeth; gently open jaws.	Opens jaws to let nurse examine inner surfaces of mouth and to allow insertion of toothbrush.
10. Squirt about 10 mL of water from Asepto bulb syringe into each side of the mouth. Allow rinse water to reach suction tip or drain into emesis basin.	Assists in removal of particles. Prevents water from being taken into the lungs.
11. Replace tongue blade; use moistened gauze pad around fingers and clean mouth tissues and tongue. (Special solutions may be ordered to clean the mouth. Check with team leader or head nurse.)	Removes remaining material from mouth when client is unable to eat or drink.
12. Use Asepto bulb syringe to rinse mouth as necessary.	Ensures removal of remaining particles and other materials from mouth.
13. Remove emesis basin; dry mouth and chin with towel.	Prevents potential skin breakdown.
14. Place water-soluble lubricant to the lips.	Adds moisture to tissues.
15. Remove towel from under head and neck.	
16. Place client in correct alignment with head and mouth facing toward the bed for at least 15 minutes.	Prevents any remaining water from being taken into the lungs.
17. Remove, clean, rinse, and replace equipment.	Makes equipment ready for future use.
18. Remove gloves and wash hands.	Prevents transfer of microorganisms.

Mouth Care Using Floss in Conscious Client:

After Completion of Mouth Care:

Step	Rationale
1. Wrap end of floss around the middle fingers of both hands. Tighten floss by stretching it with your thumbs.	Places the floss in the correct position.
2. Place the floss between upper teeth beginning at back of mouth. Slide floss back and forth between teeth from the tips of the teeth to the gum line. Continue around the mouth until all spaces between the teeth have been flossed.	Assists in removing plaque and food particles that have not been removed by brushing.
3. Use a new piece of floss and repeat steps 1 and 2 for the bottom teeth.	
4. Have client rinse mouth until returns are clear.	Completes removal of any particles.
5. Wipe face with washcloth.	Removes toothpaste and water.

(Continued on following page)

STEP	RATIONALE
6. Remove and discard rinse water. Clean and rinse emesis basin; store in proper place. Replace other equipment used.	Prepares equipment for future use. Tidies the area around the client.
7. Secure call signal within reach. Place client in comfortable position.	Ensures ability to call nurse when needed.
8. Remove gloves and wash hands.	Prevents transfer of microorganisms.

Denture Care:

STEP	RATIONALE
1. Explain procedure.	Informs client of procedure.
2. Collect necessary equipment and place on overbed table within reach of client.	Organizing necessary equipment allows quick and safe implementation.
If client is up and about, place equipment at client's sink if he or she has access to one.	Makes it convenient for the client to use.
3. Wash hands; put on gloves.	Prevents transfer of microorganisms.
4. Raise head of bed to a comfortable sitting position.	Makes it less likely for water to enter lungs.
5. Raise bed to a comfortable working position.	Decreases possibility of back strain for the nurse.
6. Place towel on chest and tuck under chin.	Protects client and bed linens from possible spillage of rinse water.
7. Position denture cup on overbed table within client's reach. Have him or her remove dentures.	Allows client to cleanse dentures. Checks for any abnormality.
8. If client needs assistance in removing dentures, hold upper denture with a gauze pad and gently move denture up and down until it is loose.	Gauze pad allows for a good grip on denture. Wiggling dentures helps break the suction between denture and gums.
9. Place denture in denture cup. Repeat step 8 for removal of lower denture.	Allows safety and security of denture.
10. Have client brush and rinse mouth in usual way.	Assists in removal of particles from mouth.
11. If client is unable to clean dentures, wrap gauze pad around fingers. Moisten with water or mouthwash.	Assists in cleaning inside the mouth.
12. Place emesis basin under client's chin.	Collects rinse water.
13. Wipe inside the mouth on all surfaces.	Removes particles. Sucks out excess water and stops the client from swallowing water or inhaling it into the lungs.
Or Gently brush gums, mouth, and tongue.	
14. If client cannot rinse mouth, place a suction tip under tongue and turn suction source on low.	Used to help rinse out mouth.
15. Using an Asepto bulb syringe, squirt 30–50 mL of water to rinse out both sides of the mouth.	
16. Wipe dry face and chin. Remove suction tip.	Removes any spillage and helps to prevent possible skin breakdown.
17. Take dentures in cup to a sink. Fill sink about one-third full of lukewarm water.	Helps to ensure safety of dentures; water acts as cushion in case dentures are dropped. Hot water may soften plastic denture material.
18. Place denture cleaning paste on toothbrush.	Denture cleaning paste is made especially for denture cleaning.
19. Remove denture from cup over water in sink. Rinse with lukewarm water.	Water in sink acts as cushion for denture if accidentally dropped.
20. Brush denture on all surfaces with toothbrush. Rinse and replace denture in cup.	Removes particles and used denture paste that may have collected on dentures.
21. Repeat steps 18–20 for remaining denture.	Encourages wearing of dentures.
22. Return dentures to client. Have client place dentures in his or her mouth.	
23. If client cannot replace dentures, place denture cream evenly over inner surface of denture.	Used to create a bond between inner surface of dentures and gums.
24. Have client open mouth, place denture on gum, and press gently to create bond between inner surface of denture and gums.	
25. Wipe and dry the client's face.	Removes any excess water and paste.
26. Place client in a comfortable position; place call signal within reach.	Leaves client comfortable and secure in knowledge that call signal can be used to call nurse if needed.
27. Clean and replace denture cup in proper place.	Denture cup is ready for next use.

Nursing Implications: Examination of the mouth helps in determining the type of mouth care to be done. If client is able to perform his or her own mouth care, then the procedure to be followed is that for a conscious client with the addition of flossing or denture care if required. Any complaints of pain, irritation, or other problems related to the oral cavity should be noted, reported, and documented. Further evaluation may be necessary. If the client does not drink or eat for more than 12–24 hours, the germs and other materials that build up could further damage the tissues in the mouth. Oil-soluble lubricants should never be used because these substances may be aspirated into the lungs, causing a specific type of pneumonia called lipid pneumonia. If the client is unconscious, a mouthwash such as hydrogen peroxide or potassium permanganate (weak antiseptics) may be used. These solutions are often part of commercially prepared mouthwashes. Check with the team leader or head nurse for specific mouth care lubricants and antiseptics.

Procedure: Nail Care

Description: Nail care includes cleaning and trimming.

Purpose: To ensure that nails are clean and trimmed and cuticles are smooth and without hangnails; to ensure that skin of hands and feet is smooth; and to examine condition of nails and surrounding skin of hands and feet.

STEP	RATIONALE
1. Wash hands and don clean gloves.	Prevents transfer of microorganisms.
2. Collect necessary equipment: • Nail clippers or scissors • Emery board or nail file • Orange stick • Tissues • Water and soap • Small basin • Towel • Nail polish remover	Organizing necessary equipment allows for quick and safe implementation.
3. Explain procedure.	Informs client of procedure.
4. Arrange necessary equipment on bedside table or overbed table.	Organizes work area.
5. Fill basin with water heated to about 105°F (40.5°C). For care of fingernails, place basin on overbed table; for toenails, place basin on floor covered with protective material or near client's feet on bed (cover sheet with protective material).	Temperature should be comfortable for client's hands and feet. Places basin in correct location for soaking hands and feet. Protects floor and linens from water spillage.
6. Have client soak hands or feet in basin for about 15–20 minutes. Exchange water if it becomes cool.	Softens and prepares nails for trimming and cleaning.
7. Remove hand or foot, dry thoroughly, especially between fingers and toes. Remove other hand or foot from basin and repeat drying.	Prevents moisture from collecting between fingers and toes.
8. Push cuticles back gently with towel. Use nonpointed end of orange stick until cuticles are pushed back.	Prevents drying of cuticles, which prevents potential hangnails and inflammation.
9. Using orange stick or nail file, remove material that has collected under nails, wipe stick or file on tissue. Repeat until all nails are cleaned.	Removes collection of materials from under nails.
10. Remove basin.	
11. Clip or trim nails straight across. Do not cut surrounding skin.	Prevents splitting of nail margins, which can cause injury to surrounding skin.
12. File or shape fingernails with emery board. Smooth cut edges of nails.	Smooths and evens the cut edges of nails; prevents injury to surrounding skin.
13. Apply lotion to dry areas of hands and feet.	Softens and moisturizes dry skin.
14. Place the client in a comfortable position. Place call signal in client's reach.	Ensures comfort and safety.
15. Empty and clean basin. Store in appropriate place.	Prepares equipment for next use.
16. Remove gloves and wash hands.	Prevents transfer of microorganisms.

Nursing Implications: Check hospital policy regarding cutting of toenails. Some health-care facilities require that only a podiatrist cut toenails. Record nail care. Report any unexpected problems to team leader or head nurse.

Procedure: Care of the Hair

Description: Combing or brushing the hair is considered part of the client's bath. The nurse is responsible for care of the client's hair if he or she is unable to care for it. Shampooing the hair is done by the nurse as needed.

Purpose: To keep the client's hair clean, fresh smelling, and arranged in a neat, attractive manner that is satisfying to the client.

STEP	RATIONALE
1. Collect necessary equipment for combing and brushing or shampooing hair: • Comb, brush, or pick • Shampoo, conditioner, moisturizer • Towels, washcloth • Mirror • Shampoo tray • Bath thermometer • Plastic sheet • Basin for discarding rinse water • Hairdryer, if available	Organizing necessary equipment allows for quick and safe implementation.

Combing and Brushing Hair:
1. Explain procedure.
2. Wash hands and don gloves.
3. Place client's bed in upright position or place client upright in chair. Place a mirror in front of client.
4. Put a clean towel around client's shoulders.
5. If hair is straight or slightly curly, comb hair from scalp to the ends of hair. Gently use the comb's teeth or brush bristles against the scalp.
6. For tangled hair, hold ends near scalp with hand and gently comb through tangled hair one section at a time.
7. Arrange hair the way the client likes it. Use combs or rubber bands for long hair.
8. If approved by client, braid hair, especially if client is bedbound.
9. If hair is tight and curly, remove tangles using fingers to free strands. Place fingers in hair and spread fingers apart.
10. Divide hair into sections. Use a wide-toothed comb or pick for freeing tangles, beginning at ends and working toward the scalp.
11. Brush hair from scalp to ends.
12. Apply hair products as client desires if not contraindicated by client's condition.
13. Remove towel; place in laundry hamper. Remove collected hair and hair products.
14. Clean comb, brush, or pick. Place in client's bedside stand.
15. Position client in a comfortable position. Secure call signal bell within easy reach.
16. Remove gloves and wash hands.

Shampooing the Hair:
1. Explain procedure.
2. Collect necessary equipment; wash hands.

Informs client of procedure; gains cooperation.
Prevents transfer of microorganisms.
Position is convenient for the nurse and prevents back strain.
Keeps stray hairs from falling on client's clothes.
Separates and smooths hair strands. Stimulates scalp.

Prevents pulling of hair follicles.

Makes the client comfortable with her or his appearance. Keeps long hair in place.
Prevents tangling.

Loosens tangle.

Makes it easier to free tangles close to scalp.

Makes client comfortable with his or her appearance.

Prepares equipment for future use. Tidies client's immediate area.
Makes client feel comfortable and secure in ability to call nurse if needed.
Decreases possibility of transfer of germs.

Informs client of procedure.
Organizing necessary equipment allows quick and safe implementation. Handwashing prevents transfer of microorganisms.

(Continued on following page)

STEP	RATIONALE
For Client in Bed:	
3. Place bed in a flat position. Raise bed to comfortable working position. Place client on back near working position.	Places client with head down and keeps water from the client's face while the hair is washed and rinsed. Raising the bed and positioning client on side of bed nearest working area help to prevent back strain in the nurse.
4. Place a plastic sheet covered with towel or sheet under client's head, neck, and shoulder.	Protects bed, linens, and client.
5. Position client's head on shampoo tray. Use folded washcloth or small towel between client's neck and rim of tray. Cover client's eyes with small towel.	Prepares client for shampoo. Protects neck muscles and underlying blood vessels and nerves from pressure against rim of tray. Protects eyes from water spillage and shampoo.
6. Place basin under tray drain.	Basin used for draining rinse water.
7. Fill pitcher with water at a temperature of about 105°F. (40.5°C).	Water temperature of 105°F (40.5°C) prevents potential injury to scalp.
8. Don gloves and wet hair with water. Distribute water through hair with fingers.	Allows for even distribution of water throughout hair.
9. Put small amount of shampoo in palm of hand. Make a lather by rubbing hands together.	Lather allows for even distribution of suds throughout hair.
10. Lather client's hair. Massage scalp lightly using tips of fingers in a circular motion.	Allows thorough distribution of suds throughout hair. Massage assists in circulation of blood to scalp and stimulates natural hair oils, which moisturize and aid hair growth.
11. Remove excess shampoo. Rinse with clean water, using pitcher.	Removes excess shampoo, dirt, and other particles. Any shampoo remaining on hair is potentially irritating and may cause dryness of the scalp.
NOTE: Use hand-held spray, if available.	
12. Repeat steps 9–11.	Ensures cleanliness of hair.
13. Wrap large bath towel around client's head. For clients in bed, remove shampoo tray. Dry hair by massaging with towel.	Removes excess moisture from hair. Prevents accidental spills.
14. Position another towel around client's shoulders. Remove towel from head. Place towel in laundry hamper.	Prepares client for completion of hair grooming.
15. Comb hair; be careful in removing tangles. If available, use hairdryer.	Hairdryer allows for speedier drying and prevents chilling.
16. Comb and arrange hair in manner requested by client.	Ensures comfort.
17. Remove towel, plastic sheet, and cover. Discard in an appropriate manner.	Keeps client's environment neat.
18. Remove gloves and wash hands.	Prevents transfer of microorganisms.
For Client in Tub or Shower:	
19. Repeat previous steps 1 and 2.	
20. Place washcloth or small towel over client's eyes.	Prevents water and shampoo from getting into eyes.
21. Test water temperature.	Ensures that water is not too hot or too cold.
22. Rinse hair with clean water after bath is completed. Use clean warm water at about 105°F (40.5°C) temperature. (If available, use hand-held spray instead of pitcher.)	Prepares hair for even distribution of shampoo. Prevents burning of scalp.
23. Repeat previous steps 9–18.	
For Client Sitting in Chair:	
24. Place chair so that it faces away from bathroom sink.	Places chair in best position for shampooig client's hair.
25. Assist client to sit in chair. Place towel around shoulders.	Protects client's bedclothes from accidental spilling of water.
26. Help client to hyperextend head and neck by putting head back as far as possible. Place folded washcloth or small towel between neck and rim of sink. Place washcloth or small towel over eyes.	Prevents pressure on neck muscles, blood vessels, and nerves, thereby decreasing potential for injury. Prevents water and shampoo from entering eyes.
27. Make sure that water temperature is about 105°F (40.5°C)	Decreases potential to burn scalp.
28. Wet hair thoroughly.	Wetting hair strands helps to distribute shampoo.
29. Repeat previous steps 9–18.	Completes procedure.

Nursing Implications: Examine condition of hair and scalp. Determine whether there is any irritation, injury, or dryness of scalp. Report and document any problems. If hair and scalp are dry, request physician's order for special hair preparation if necessary. Use dry hair formula shampoo and rinse with conditioner. Request that hair shampooing be done less frequently.

Use cream rinse or an oil preparation, if available, to loosen tangles and snarls. Do not cut hair unless permission is received to do so. If a regular shampooing is not possible, see if a dry shampoo is available for use.

Procedure: Eye Care

Description: Cleansing of the eyes of clients is part of the bath when eye pathology is present, and includes cleansing of eyeglasses or care of contact lenses.

Purpose: To remove foreign particles, including microorganisms, from the eye; to give proper care to eyeglasses and contact lenses.

STEP	RATIONALE
1. Collect necessary equipment: • Fresh tap water or sterile water or saline • Sterile cotton balls or gauze pad • Small clean or sterile basin • Tissue wipes • Clean towel • Sterile lubricant and preparation prescribed by physician • Eyedropper (optional) • Cleansing solution and papers for lens • Contact lens suction cup	Organizing necessary equipment allows for quick and safe implementation.

Eye Cleansing:

STEP	RATIONALE
1. As part of bath, encourage client to wash eyes. If client is not able, explain procedure.	Gives client a sense of independence for own care. Prepares client for procedure.
2. Place required equipment on bedside table. Place bedside table next to bed for easy access to equipment by nurse.	Prepares for procedure.
3. Wash hands. Put on disposable gloves.	Prevents transfer of microorganisms.
4. Raise the bed to a comfortable working position.	Prevents back strain.
5. Place client in sitting position. Place pillow behind shoulders to allow client's head to fall backward and eyes and face to lift upward (hyperextension of neck).	Ensures comfort.
6. Place towel over client's chest and under chin.	Prevents solution from dripping on bedclothes; towel is in position when needed.
7. Pour a small amount of water into basin.	Prepares client for cleansing.
8. Dip cotton ball or gauze into water and remove excess water.	Wets the cotton ball or gauze. Prevents excess water from dripping on client's clothes or bed linens.
9. Gently wipe eye from inner portion (inner canthus) of eye to outer portion (outer canthus) with cotton ball or sponge.	Prevents particles or secretions from entering lacrimal sac (tear duct), which is located in the inner canthus.
10. Repeat step 9 with other eye using clean cotton ball or sponge.	Prevents contamination from the first eye.
11. If crusts or secretions are present, moisten gauze pad and place over closed eyes.	Softens and loosens crust.
12. Leave gauze pads in place until crusts are softened. Remove and discard sponges.	Assists in removal of crusts.
13. If client is unconscious: • Lower side rails. • Raise eyelids; instill "artificial tears" if ordered. Gently pull lower eyelid downward to instill eyedrops in order not to injure the eyeball (cornea).	Moistens eyes. Unconscious clients lack the "blink reflex" and are unable to moisten eyeball.
14. Close eyelids. Place eyepad over eyes and tape in position.	Protects eye from foreign particles that may injure the eye. Taping pad in position prevents eyes from opening further, thus protecting the eyes from injury as the blink reflex is absent.

(Continued on following page)

STEP	RATIONALE
15. Lower bed. Place client in a comfortable position. Raise side rails as necessary.	Ensures safety and comfort.
16. Wash hands.	Decreases chances of transfer of microorganisms.

Care of Eyeglasses:

STEP	RATIONALE
1. Collect necessary equipment.	Organizing necessary equipment allows for quick and safe implementation.
2. Wash hands.	Prevents transfer of microorganisms.
3. Ask client to remove glasses. If client is unable to remove glasses, explain procedure. Take hold of both earpieces above ears. Lift eyeglass frame up and out from ears. Move glasses down and away from face.	Allows for feeling of independence. Avoids pulling at client's ears; prevents twisting or bending eyeglass frames.
4. Examine the eyeglass lenses for any scratches or damage.	Determines condition of lenses and the amount of cleansing needed.
5. Wash and rinse lenses with slightly warm (tepid) water or cleansing solution. (Never use warm or hot water.)	Removes smudges, body oils. Use of very warm or hot water may soften or distort plastic frames.
6. Hold glasses by earpieces without twisting frame. Be careful not to drop glasses.	Prevents damage to frames or lenses.
7. Dry lenses with clean tissue or lens tissue. (Do not use rough material in wiping glasses or touch lenses with fingers.)	
8. Fold frame and place in eyeglass case. Place in drawer of bedside table. If case not available, place eyeglasses between tissues; do not place glasses on any surface with lenses facing down.	Prevents accidental damage. Protects eyeglasses from smudging.
9. Cleanse eyes, if necessary, after eye-cleansing procedure (steps 1–16 under Eye Cleansing).	
10. Remove glasses from case or tissues; unfold frames.	
11. Hold eyeglass frames by both earpieces.	Prepares eyeglasses for placement over client's eyes.
12. Place earpieces just above each ear in correct position and nosepiece of frame over bridge of nose.	Prevents bending or twisting of frames.
13. Check to see whether glasses are in the correct position. Check with client as to whether glasses are in a comfortable position.	Prevents hitting client's face with earpieces.
14. Repeat steps 15 and 16 under Eye Cleansing.	Places frames correctly.

Care of Contact Lenses (may differ with type of contact lenses):

STEP	RATIONALE
1. Collect necessary equipment.	Organizing necessary equipment allows for quick and safe implementation.
2. Ask client to remove lenses.	Prevents possible injury to eye.
3. If client is unable to remove lenses, then wash hands and separate upper and lower eyelids with thumbs.	Makes contact lens visible.
4. Gently push upper eyelid to the top edge of the lens. Hold upper lid in place by pressing against upper bony portion under eyebrow. Press lower lid against contact lens. Or Use special lens suction cup. Attach cup on lens and remove lens.	Loosens lens from eye (cornea) by breaking the suction.
5. Catch lens in clean washcloth and store in correct lens container.	Prevents lens from falling out of view.
6. Repeat steps 3–5 for removal of remaining contact lens.	
7. Take lens container to sink. Close drain and fill with about 2 or 3 inches of water.	Provides cushion of water to catch lens if it accidentally falls.
8. Hold one lens between thumb and index finger over water. Squeeze a small amount of lens cleanser on each side of lens. Spread cleanser evenly over lens with finger.	Cleans and lubricates lens.
9. Rinse lens with commercially prepared rinsing and storing solution. Place in correct lens container.	Rinses cleanser from lens. Protects lens.
10. Repeat steps 8 and 9 for remaining lens.	
11. Cleanse client's eyes, if necessary.	See steps 1–16 under Eye Cleaning.

(Continued on following page)

STEP	RATIONALE
Reinsertion of Lenses:	
1. Remove one lens from container; hold between thumb and index finger.	Prepares lens for reinsertion.
2. Apply a drop of lens-wetting solution to inside of lens.	Moistens lens and creates correct amount of suction when lens is placed over the eyeball (cornea).
3. Hold outside of lens in tip of index finger and place it gently over iris (colored portion of eye) and pupil.	Positions lens correctly.
4. Repeat steps 1–3 for replacement of remaining contact lens.	
5. Repeat steps 15 and 16 under Eye Cleansing.	

Nursing Implications: Record procedure. Report any unusual observations such as inflammation, redness, tearing, and swelling. Check whether pupils respond normally to light. Check to see if eyes move together. Watch for excessive secretions and for crusts, and note color of secretions. Report any client complaints such as irritation, burning, pain, or dryness, as well as any problems with eyeglasses or contact lenses.

Procedure: Applying Restraints

Description: Special devices are used to immobilize client or extremities (arms or legs). A physician's order is necessary.

Purpose: To prevent unwanted movement when giving certain treatments, when client is restless or confused; to control client from harming himself or herself or others; and to assist the client to support posture.

Use of Jacket or Vest: Prevents client from falling out of bed or chair; secures client but allows some freedom of movement

Use of Mitt: Prevents client from scratching skin and allows greater freedom than use of wrist restraint

Use of Wrist or Ankle Restraint: Prevents client from moving arm or leg when intravenous (IV) line or other devices are in place

Use of Belt Restraint: Prevents client from falling out of bed or stretcher

Use of Infant Restraint: Immobilizes infant while a treatment procedure is being done

STEP	RATIONALE
1. Collect necessary equipment: • Restraints: vest or jacket; safety wrist or ankle mitt; belt; blanket or sheet • Safety pins • Foam or cotton padding • Rolled bandage	Organizing necessary equipment allows for quick and safe implementation.
Application of Vest or Jacket:	
1. Explain procedure.	Informs client of procedure and reason for restraint.
2. Using the vest, place client's arms through armholes. Check that overlapping vest pieces are to the front of client's body.	Places vest to allow for some movement but limits freedom.
3. Overlap front body pieces. Place ties through slots and loops on side of vest.	Secures vest restraint.
Applying Restraints:	
1. Criss-cross ties over front of vest.	Secures vest restraint.
For Client in Bed:	
2. Take ties and secure to the bed frame (movable part). Make a half-bow knot.	Secures vest restraint. Prevents tightness when bed is raised or lowered or when client moves. Half-bow knot makes it easier to untie vest from bed in an emergency.
3. Examine client and restraint.	Prevents injury and ensures client's safety.

(Continued on following page)

STEP	RATIONALE
For Client in Chair:	
4. Follow steps above up to and including step 1 under Applying Restraints.	
5. Cross vest straps behind chair seat and lower legs. Make sure that left strap is tied to right leg of chair, and right strap is tied to left leg of chair.	Secures client to chair.
6. Follow step 3.	
Applying a Mitt Restraint:	
1. Explain procedure.	Informs client of procedure and reason for restraint.
2. Using a rolled bandage, place client's fingers around bandage.	Places client's fingers in a natural position to prevent strain on muscles and joints.
3. Place the client's hand into the mitt. Tie wrist ties.	Secures mitt to hand and wrist.
4. Tie ends of ties to movable part of bed frame and complete by using a half-bow tie.	Prevents tightness when bed is raised or lowered. Half-bow tie makes it easier to release restraint in case of an emergency.
5. Check client and restraint.	Prevents possible injury and ensures client's safety.
Application of Wrist or Ankle Restraint:	
1. Explain procedure.	Informs client of procedure and reason for restraint.
2. Place cotton or foam padding around wrist or ankle.	Protects skin by decreasing pressure against skin and by decreasing potential for skin breakdown.
3. Place wrist or ankle restraint around padding.	
Application of Restraint:	
4. Pull tie through opening on side of restraint.	Secures restraint on body part.
5. Attach end of tie to movable part of bed frame and tie with half-bow.	Prevents tightness when bed is raised or lowered. Prevents possible injury. Half-bow tie allows for easy release of restraint when necessary.
6. Examine client and restraint carefully.	Ensures safety.
Belt Restraint:	
1. Explain procedure.	Informs client of procedure and reason for restraint.
2. Place client in supine position (lying on back).	Prepares client for application of restraint.
3. Position the long part of belt under the client. Tie ends of belt to movable part of bed.	Attachment of belt to frame before securing belt to client helps to prevent problems when attaching belt to client.
4. Take shorter part of belt and place it around client's waist. Secure ends of belt.	Secures restraint.
5. Examine client and restraint.	Ensures safety.
Infant Restraint:	
1. Explain procedure to family or significant others.	Informs family or significant others of procedure and reason for restraint.
2. Lay blanket or sheet on bed or other flat surface.	Prepares infant for restraint.
3. Fold down top corner of blanket, making sure tip is on the center of blanket.	Prepares restraint for infant's head.
4. Place infant on back (supine position) on blanket with head lying midway on the folded corner.	Prepares infant for restraint.
5. Fold one side corner of blanket over infant and tuck it under body just below axilla (armpit).	Restrains infant.
6. Repeat step 5 using remaining side corner of blanket.	
7. Raise the infant and fold bottom corner under body.	Completes restraint procedure.
8. Check infant and restraint.	Ensures safety.

Nursing Implications: Check client's behavior before, during, and after application of restraints. Record procedure and reasons for same. Indicate type of restraint, status of client, and any problems or complications that may have occurred. Report to team leader or head nurse.

Check the pulse, temperature, and skin color of extremities of restrained client. Check for ability of movement. If abnormal, may be sign of pressure on the nervous and vascular systems. Restraints must be loosened, and range of motion (ROM) performed, every 2 hours. Client must be checked every 30 minutes or per hospital policy.

Know the policies of the institution in regard to use of restraints. **The use of restraints requires a physician's order.** If client is confused or disoriented, use of restraints may be justified. However, use of inappropriate restraints or improper attachment of restraints may be considered imprisonment.

Procedure: Perineal Care

Description: In perineal care, the perineal area is cleansed in clients who are unable to bathe themselves.

Purpose: To ensure personal cleanliness, remove secretions from the urethra, vagina, and anus for clients who are unconscious or helpless or need special hygienic measures.

STEP	RATIONALE
1. Collect necessary equipment: • Bath blanket • Wash basin and water • Washcloth and towels • Soap • Bath thermometer • Plastic sheet • Toilet tissue • Clean gloves • Pitcher	Organizing necessary equipment allows for quick and safe implementation.
2. Explain procedure. State steps in a manner that does not embarrass client.	Informs client of procedure. Reassures client.
3. Obtain water; check temperature. Arrange equipment on overbed table. Have pitcher and wash basin with warm water.	Ensures warmth of water. Organizes work area.
4. Close curtains around client's bed. Close door to room.	Ensures privacy.
5. Wash hands; put on clean gloves before offering bedpan.	Prevents transfer of microorganisms.
6. If client is conscious, check whether bedpan is needed. Give bedpan if necessary; remove and discard urine appropriately; then clean and replace bedpan in proper place.	Ensures emptying of bladder before procedure.
7. Raise bed to proper working position using proper body mechanics.	Prevents back strain.
8. If side rail is up, lower it on working side of bed and help client to a supine (back-lying) position.	Places client in position for the procedure.
9. Remove top covers while placing bath blanket over client. Pull top covers to bottom of bed, leaving bath blanket over client. Fold bed covers and place on chair.	Covers client for privacy.
10. Place plastic sheet covered with bed linen under client.	Protects bottom sheet and mattress.
11. Fold bath towel and place under hips. Place bedpan under buttocks.	Raises hips slightly so that perineal area is in correct position.
12. Flex client's knees and hips. Have client move, or move client's legs, so that toes point outward and heels inward (rotate legs toward the outside).	Positions perineal area correctly for perineal care.
13. Move the bath blanket so that the corners form a diamond. (Top corner points toward head of bed; two side corners point down each side of bed; lower corner drapes over client's legs.)	Covers client's body and legs, provides warmth, and protects privacy.
14. Wrap two side corners around client's legs and place corner under hips.	Prepares client for perineal care.
15. Place washcloth into basin of warm water, apply soap, and wring out excess water.	Prepares client for bathing.
16. Raise corner of blanket from between client's legs and place corner toward client's head.	Exposes perineal area only.
17. Wash and rinse upper thighs. Dry thoroughly.	Removes secretions from area near perineal area.

(Continued on following page)

STEP	RATIONALE
For the Female Client:	
1. Follow steps 1–17.	
2. Rinse washcloth and reapply soap. Wash labia majora (top outer part of the perineal area), moving the washcloth from front to back (anus). Do not wash over area that has already been washed. Redo procedure, if necessary, using clean washcloth, soap, and water.	Bathes from the area of the least germs and secretions (the urethra, or opening from the bladder) to that of the most (the anus). Prevents contamination of urethra by germs from the anus. Decreases possibility of infection.
3. Rinse washcloth. Do not reapply soap. Spread labia majora (outer perineal area) with hand not being used to bathe perineal area.	Prevents irritation of sensitive tissues.
4. Wash the labia minora (inner perineal area) with a corner of washcloth, moving washcloth down toward the anus. Rinse. Use a fresh corner for each area. If client is menstruating or has a catheter in place, use cotton balls to clean the inner labia.	Prevents contamination of the labia with germs and secretions from other parts of perineal area.
5. Pour pitcher of warm water over perineal area. Remove bedpan when rinse is completed.	Rinses soap, water, germs, and secretions from perineum.
6. Dry perineal area gently but thoroughly. Apply dusting powder lightly.	Prevents moisture collection and growth of germs. Decreases possibility of infection. Use of powder (lightly) helps in absorbing moisture and prevents irritation caused by contact of two skin surfaces.
7. Remove towel pad from under hips. Position client on side with her back toward working area.	Prepares for bathing the anal area.
8. Inspect space between buttocks; remove any excretions with toilet tissue, if present.	Prevents possible contamination of wash water and surrounding skin.
9. Wash between buttocks, especially around the anus. Dry thoroughly. Apply powder lightly.	Decreases possibility of infection by removing secretions and germs.
10. Remove plastic sheet and cover. Place client in a comfortable position and replace top covers. Remove bath blanket. Place call signal in easy reach.	Disposes of used linens. Ensures comfort. Allows client to call the nurse if necessary.
11. Place used linens in laundry hamper. Wash, rinse, dry, and replace equipment in proper place.	Disposes of contaminated linen. Prepares equipment for future use.
12. Discard gloves and wash hands.	Limits transfer of germs.
For the Male Client:	
1. Follow steps 1–17.	
2. Raise and place towel under penis. Hold penis and move foreskin from tip of penis, if present, downward. Wash the area exposed, beginning with the tip of the penis and moving to the area to which the foreskin has been moved. Replace foreskin.	Protects scrotum and bed linens. Removes secretions and germs that may have collected under foreskin. Prevents contamination of the urethra with germs on the remainder of the penis.
3. Rinse and resoap washcloth; wash remainder of penis, using downward strokes.	Bathes remainder of penis.
4. Rinse, resoap, and wash the scrotum, especially between the folds of skin. Dry thoroughly.	Removes germs and moisture that may cause infection. Completes procedure.
5. Follow steps 5–11 under For the Female Client.	

Nursing Implications: Record procedure. Report and record any unusual findings or problems. Report and document any complaints of itching, pain, or discomfort. For female clients, check, report, and record any vaginal, urethral, or anal discharge or odor. Discharge, odor, or both may be signs of infection.

Report and record any signs of incontinence of urine or stool. If client has had perineal surgery, check for, report, and record amount, color, and odor of drainage if present. Such drainage requires frequent assessment and perineal care to prevent irritation and infection.

Procedure: Handwashing

Description: Hands are washed correctly before and after performing any procedure.

Purpose: To limit transfer of microorganisms.

STEP	RATIONALE
1. Collect necessary equipment: • Soap • Running water • Clean towel or sterile towel	Organizing necessary equipment allows for quick and safe implementation.
2. Check hands for any skin breaks. If present, use clean sterile gloves to prevent contamination.	Prevents contamination.
3. Remove all hand jewelry except smooth-surfaced rings.	Prevents microorganisms from collecting in and under jewelry.
4. Slide watchband up arm.	Wrists need to be washed to remove any germs that may have collected under watchband.
5. Stand in front of sink without touching sink surfaces.	Prevents back strain. Prevents contamination of uniform with organisms on sink surface.
6. Use a paper towel to turn on water faucet. Adjust flow and temperature. Use elbow, knee, or foot pedal, if available.	Prevents contamination of hands. Prevents hot water from injuring skin.
7. Wet lower arms, wrists, and hands, holding them under running water with fingers pointing downward.	Water flows from the area of least contamination (lower arms) to area of greatest contamination (fingertips).
8. Apply soap and produce a lather. If bar soap is used, rinse bar under running water before placing soap in soap dish.	Removes any microorganisms before use by another person.
9. Rub hands together using a back-and-forth and circular motion; cover all parts of hands, including fingers, area between fingers, palm, back of hand, and wrists. Continue procedure for about 3 minutes unless there is a potential for a greater risk of contamination; then continue washing hands for up to 3 minutes more.	Exposes hands and wrists to soap and water, including areas between fingers.
10. Rinse hands under running water with fingers pointing downward.	Soapy water flows downward from area of least contamination to area of greatest contamination.
11. Dry hands from fingers to wrist to lower arms with a paper towel. Use a clean, dry towel for each hand.	Dries skin from the cleanest area to the dirtiest. Removes moisture and prevents chapping.
12. Discard towel. Turn off water. Use a clean paper towel to close water flow if hand controls are used.	Prevents contamination of hands.

Nursing Implications: Routine handwashing is not usually recorded or reported. Check whether hands are dry or chapped; may need to use hand creams or other softening agents. Check for any cuts or abrasions or infection. Report same. Check whether client has any signs of infection. Report signs and symptoms to team leader or head nurse. Record same. Handwashing should be performed before and after caring for each client.

Procedure: Surgical Asepsis

Description: These methods establish and maintain sterility.

Purpose: To produce a relatively sterile field in order to remove harmful organisms from skin surfaces by washing, scrubbing, and disinfection; to create a sterile field using sterile protective clothing and sterile equipment, depending on type of sterile field required.

STEP	RATIONALE
1. Collect necessary supplies and equipment: • Antiseptic detergent • Scrub brushes • Orange stick • Sterile cap, gown, and mask • Sterile gloves • Sterile packages • Sterile solution	Organizing necessary supplies and equipment allows quick and safe implementation.

(Continued on following page)

STEP	RATIONALE
Surgical Hand Scrub:	
1. Remove all jewelry.	Prevents microorganisms from collecting on and under jewelry.
2. Examine hands for any skin breaks.	Check to see if other procedures may be necessary to protect nurse from possible exposure to harmful organisms.
3. Put on scrub clothes or make sure mid upper arms are not covered.	Prepares for procedure.
4. Put on face mask.	Prevents organisms from mouth and nose from contaminating sterile field.
5. Turn on and adjust water flow and temperature using foot or knee controls.	Prepares for hand scrub.
6. Wet one arm thoroughly from upper arm to fingertips. Repeat with other arm. Keep arms bent with hands above elbows. Point fingers downward.	Allows water to drip from dirtiest part (fingers).
7. Lather hands with antiseptic detergent to above elbows.	Covers hands and arms with lather.
8. Use orange stick to clean under fingernails; rinse stick and fingers under running water.	Removes collected material and organisms from under nails.
9. Rinse each arm from fingertips to above elbows.	Allows lather and organisms to drain.
10. Reapply detergent and repeat step 9.	
11. Scrub each hand with brush, using a back-and-forth motion for about 45 seconds.	Friction along with action of detergent loosens and removes material and microorganisms from skin.
12. Scrub upper arms above elbows for 15–20 seconds.	Moves from the dirtiest area (hands) to the cleanest (upper arm).
13. Scrub lower arm thoroughly for 45 seconds.	
14. Dispose of brush. Rinse arms and hands from upper arms to fingertips. Keep arms bent so fingertips are above elbow.	Allows for water to drain from cleanest area (hands) toward arm.
15. Use second brush and scrub each hand for 1 minute.	Extra scrubbing allows removal of remaining organisms.
16. Discard brush and repeat step 14.	
17. Using knee or foot control, turn off water. Keep fingertips above elbows.	Holding hands and fingers up decreases chances of touching any surfaces.
18. Keep arms elevated; dry one hand and arm with a sterile towel by patting it dry. Discard towel. Repeat step for other hand and arm.	Patting prevents unnecessary injury to skin surfaces that may be irritated by detergent and scrubbing action.
Putting on Sterile Cap	
1. Using the correct-size cap, separate elastic band with hands. Pull cap over back of head so that elastic band is below earlobes.	Allows good fit and complete coverage of hair.
2. Make sure that cap completely covers all hair.	Prevents contamination of sterile field by hairs.
Putting on a Face Mask:	
1. Choose a face mask. Locate top. Hold mask by the top two strings and place over face with nose strip over nose.	Keeps clean the part of the mask that covers nose and mouth.
2. Place top strings or loops over the top of ears. Tie strings behind head or slip loops over ears.	Prevents contamination of the mask; secures mask in place.
3. If mask has strings (not loops), tie bottom strings behind neck so that lower edge of mask is under chin.	Makes edges of mask fit against face. Helps prevent escape of organisms from mouth and nose.
4. Make sure plastic or metal bridge (if present) is placed over bridge of nose and that mouth and nose are completely covered.	Prevents escape of organisms from mouth and nose.
Putting on Sterile Gown:	
1. Pick up gown, hold inside of neck surface. Hold gown away from body.	Prevents contamination of outside of gown, keeping it sterile.
2. Lift gown so that it does not touch floor. Let gown unfold by holding inside neck surface with both hands. Do not touch outside of gown.	
3. Open gown so that inside shoulder seams are visible.	

(Continued on following page)

STEP	RATIONALE
4. Place one hand through armhole while holding inside neck surface with other hand. Place other hand through armhole.	
5. Raise arm upward; place arms into sleeves.	Allows placement of sleeves on arms without contaminating outside of gown.
6. Have another worker pull inside back of gown toward back so that back edges of gown overlap. Have worker tie neck ties.	Keeps outside of gown sterile, and secures gown in position. Prevents touching of outside of gown.
7. Have worker tie waistband securely.	

Putting on Sterile Gloves:

STEP	RATIONALE
1. Open glove package by pulling apart the sides of package.	
2. Remove inner package and place on clean surface.	
3. Open package by touching only the corners.	Prevents contamination of gloves and inside of package.
4. Check for right and left gloves; pick up inside cuff with the nondominant hand (the one you use less than the other).	Prevents touching of outside of sterile glove. Inside of glove now contaminated.
5. Slip the other hand inside glove, making sure that thumb and fingers are lined up with the glove thumb and fingers. Do not touch outside of glove.	
6. Push hand into glove, pulling the inside cuff with thumb and index finger of the nondominant hand. Make sure that only the inside of glove is touched.	
7. Using the gloved hand, slip fingers under cuff of remaining glove and slip nondominant hand inside glove.	Contamination of glove is prevented by using sterile gloved hand to put on second glove.
8. Push nondominant hand inside glove. With the gloved hand under the cuff, pull glove over nondominant hand.	Prevents contamination of outside of gloved hand.
9. Interlock fingers of hands (place fingers of one hand between fingers of other hand).	Allows free movement of fingers and thumb.

Opening a Sterile Package:

STEP	RATIONALE
1. Collect necessary equipment.	Organizing necessary equipment allows for quick and safe implementation.
2. Check label for contents, expiration date, and any instructions.	Checks sterility of package.
3. Place package on clean surface at waist level.	Places package in good working position.
4. Break seal, touching only edge of package. Open one flap away from you. Do not bend over package.	Prevents contamination of inside of package. Prevents airborne dust particles from contaminating inside of package.
5. Open side flap, let fall flat on surface. Repeat same with other side flap.	
6. Lift flap nearest you; open flap toward you and let it fall flat on surface.	

Pouring Sterile Liquid:

STEP	RATIONALE
1. Open sterile set. Locate empty sterile container.	
2. Open sterile solution bottle or package. Set cap or lid with the inside up on a clean surface.	Prevents inside of bottle or cap from contamination.
3. Pick up bottle, holding it with label inside palm of hand.	Protects label from drainage while pouring solution.
4. Pour a small amount of solution into a disposable receptacle. (Do not touch disposable receptacle with bottle lip.) Discard solution in disposable receptacle.	Washes bottle lip with solution that is to be discarded.
5. Pour appropriate amount of solution into sterile container. Do not touch lip of bottle to sterile container. Avoid splashing and dripping solution on sterile field.	Prevents contamination of sterile field.
6. Place solution bottle on clean surface and replace cap.	Prevents microorganisms in air from entering solution bottle.

Nursing Implications: Check to see whether client has signs or symptoms or diagnosis of an infection. Report and record any signs of redness, pain, swelling, drainage, increased temperature, or elevated white blood count. Such signs may indicate that both nurse and client require protection from contamination.

Any break in surgical asepsis is considered dangerous. Change protective clothing and equipment if they become contaminated.

Procedure: Protective Asepsis

Description: This method controls infection for the protection of the client, health-care personnel, and any other people who may be exposed to the infection.

Purpose: Depending on the way the infection enters the body, to provide protection for the person(s) who get the disease and for those who come in contact with one who has the disease.

Category-Specific Precautions

Strict Isolation: Provides methods to prevent transmission of highly contagious infectious diseases that are spread through air or by direct contact. Examples include smallpox, chickenpox, and measles.

Respiratory Isolation: Provides methods to prevent transmission of diseases that are spread over short distances, such as particles or droplets containing the disease agent that are transferred through the air. Examples include many of the childhood diseases.

Contact Isolation: Provides methods to prevent transmission of highly contagious diseases that are spread by close or direct contact but that do not require strict isolation. Examples include impetigo, burn infections, and acute respiratory infections in infants and children.

Tuberculosis (TB) Isolation: Provides methods to prevent transmission of the tubercle bacillus, which is the infectious agent of TB. Method of isolation is specific for clients who have pulmonary (lung) TB as diagnosed by sputum smear or chest radiograph.

Drainage or Secretion Precautions: Provide methods of preventing direct or indirect contact with infected material or fluid draining from an infected site in the body. Examples include abscesses, infected burns, wounds, and pressure sores.

Blood or Body Fluid Precautions: Provide methods to prevent direct or indirect transfer of infectious agents through contact with blood or other body fluids. Examples include acquired immunodeficiency syndrome (AIDS), hepatitis B, syphilis, and gonorrhea.

Enteric Isolation Precautions: Provide methods to prevent transfer of infectious agents that are spread through direct or indirect contact with feces. Examples include cholera, viral hepatitis A, and gastroenteritis.

Standard Precautions: All nurses should use standard precautions at all times when caring for clients.

STEP	RATIONALE
1. Collect necessary equipment: • Protective face mask • Protective gown and gloves • Disposable dishes and eating utensils • Isolation cart • Plastic or special disposable laundry or trash bags	Organizing necessary equipment allows for quick and safe implementation.
Isolation Room Preparation: 1. Explain procedure. Include significant others in discussion.	Informs client of procedure and reason for use. Gains cooperation.
2. Use private room for isolation, if available. Equipment in room should include: • Sink in room • Adjoining private bathroom • Rack to hang reusable gowns, if needed	Provides a unit with necessary equipment for isolation.
3. Collect supplies to be kept in room: • Single-use antiseptic soap • Laundry hamper (considered dirty) • Waste container lined with plastic bags • Fresh linen • Tissues, soap, wash basin, other toiletries, water container, disposable cup or glass	Prevents transfer of disease agent by decreasing the number of times room is entered for bringing in supplies. Allows for disposal of trash and equipment.
4. Collect and place supplies outside the room door, including: • Supply cart • Clean gowns, gloves, masks	Keeps protective clothing and equipment outside of infected or contaminated area.

(Continued on following page)

STEP	RATIONALE
• Large isolation laundry bags • Large plastic disposable trash bags • Specific disinfectants as required	
5. Place precaution sign on door.	Informs staff that protective measures are needed.
6. Move client into room.	
7. Place sign on room door requiring visitors to go to nurse's station for information.	Informs visitors of need of protective measures.
8. Show client the protective measures that need to be taken. Include family, if present. Answer questions.	Decreases anxiety and gains cooperation.

Putting on Protective Gown, Mask, and Gloves:

STEP	RATIONALE
1. Remove jewelry.	Prevents transfer of microorganisms in and out of room.
2. If watch is needed, place in a clear plastic bag.	Protects watch from contaminated items if touched.
3. Wash hands.	Prevents transfer of microorganisms.
4. Place mask on face.	See Surgical Asepsis procedure.
5. Take clean gown from supply cart.	
6. Hold gown up by inside neck surface and let gown unfold with open part of back facing nurse.	Protects uniform when in contact with client and contaminated materials.
7. Slip one arm into sleeve, touching only neck of gown. Slip other arm into sleeve.	Prevents hands from contacting outside gown.
8. Working inside the sleeve with hand covered by gown, pull sleeve up on one arm and shoulder. Repeat with other arm.	
9. Place fingers inside neck of gown at the back and fix gown so that it fits well over shoulders.	
10. Tie neck ties. Do not touch hair.	Prevents contamination of hands with hair.
11. Draw gown edges together at back so that edges overlap and entire back is covered.	Provides total coverage of nurse's uniform.
12. Tie waist ties securely.	Secures gown in place.
13. Put on clean or sterile gloves. See Surgical Asepsis procedure.	Protects hands from contact by infectious agent.
14. Collect necessary supplies and enter room.	Prepares client for procedure.
15. Place watch (in plastic bag) near work area.	Prevents contamination of watch.

Removal of Gown, Mask, and Gloves:

STEP	RATIONALE
1. Remove gloves by bringing gloves down from wrist so that gloves are inside out when removed.	Prevents outside of gloves (contaminated side) from touching clean areas.
2. Remove mask by untying ties. Do not touch face part of mask.	Face part of mask may contain organisms spread through air.
3. Untie waist ties.	
4. Wash hands.	Prevents transfer of microorganisms that may have come in contact with hands during removal of mask and gloves and in untying waist ties.
5. Untie neck ties. Do not touch outside of gown.	Prevents transfer of microorganisms that may be on gown.
6. Place index finger under cuff of one sleeve. Pull sleeve over hand without touching outside gown.	Begins removal of contaminated gown.
7. Using the hand covered by gown sleeve, pull other sleeve off the arm.	
8. Remove gown without touching the outside gown or having gown touch uniform.	
9. Fold gown inside out. Do not shake gown.	
10. Roll up gown and discard it into dirty laundry bag.	Prevents transfer of microorganisms on gown into air.
11. Wash hands.	Removes any organisms that hands may have come in contact with during removal of gown.
12. Slip hand into plastic bag and get watch. Do not touch outside of bag. Keep hand in plastic bag and discard plastic bag.	
13. Open door with paper towel when leaving room.	Prevents transfer of disease agent that might be present on inside of door.

(Continued on following page)

STEP	RATIONALE
Taking Supplies and Equipment into Room:	
1. Collect necessary disposable equipment.	Prevents transfer of disease agents.
2. Place equipment and supplies on cart outside room.	
3. Put on protective clothing.	See procedure of Putting on Protective Gown, Mask, and Gloves.
4. Hold supplies or equipment in gloved hands. Push room door open with arms or back.	
5. When care of client is completed, discard contaminated disposable equipment and supplies into trash container. Empty liquids into toilet and flush.	Prevents transfer of disease agent.
6. Remove protective clothing and leave room.	See procedure for Removal of Gown, Mask, and Gloves.
Double Bagging for Removal of Discarded Supplies and Trash:	
1. Put on protective clothing and enter room.	See procedure for Putting on Protective Gown, Mask, and Gloves.
2. Empty waste materials into special bag in room. Seal bag. Place new bag in position.	Prevents transfer of microorganisms by closing bag tightly. Organizes supply for next time that it is needed.
3. Have a second person outside room hold a clean bag open with the top of the bag cuffed over her or his hands.	Protects second worker's hands from contamination.
4. Place sealed bag inside clean bag. Do not touch the outside clean bag.	
5. Have the second worker close, seal, and label outside bag for special disposal.	Prevents transfer of germs by placing contaminated items in two bags. Label identifies material as being contaminated.
6. Leave isolation room.	
7. Remove double-bagged container to appropriate place for disposal.	Prevents microorganism growth in contaminated items.
8. Wash hands.	
Removing a Specimen from the Room:	
1. Bring labeled specimen container and plastic bag into room when entering.	Prepares for efficient performance of procedure.
2. Collect specimen, close container, and place in plastic bag.	Allows specimen container to be seen by laboratory personnel.
3. Have another person outside room hold a large, clear plastic bag cuffed over hands.	Prevents transfer of disease agent.
4. Place bag containing specimen into bag held by second person. Do not touch outside bag held by second person.	
5. Have second person close, secure, and label bag with client's name, room number, and type of isolation precautions.	Protects worker who receives specimen.
6. Remove protective clothing; leave room.	See procedure for leaving (step 13 under Removal of Gown, Mask, and Gloves.)
7. Take double-bagged specimen to laboratory.	
Transporting Client Who Is Isolated:	
1. Explain procedure and reason for leaving room to client.	Informs client of procedure.
2. Cover wheelchair or stretcher with a clean sheet before taking it into room.	Protects vehicle from contamination.
3. Help client to put on isolation gown, mask, and cap if required (strict or respiratory isolation).	Protects other persons outside isolation room.
4. Help client into wheelchair or onto stretcher.	
5. Place a clean sheet or bath blanket over client's body, including shoulders and feet.	
6. Leave room with client.	
7. Make sure that personnel receiving client know what isolation precautions are necessary.	Prepares personnel in other departments.

Nursing Implications: The type of protective isolation depends on how the microorganisms are transmitted. Check with institutional policy and team leader or head nurse. Each procedure is done to prevent the transfer of the microorganism responsible for the onset of the disease to others.

For Strict Isolation Procedures: The room should be private and the door kept closed. All persons entering the room must wear a protective gown, gloves, and mask. All contaminated articles need to be bagged and labeled before being discarded.

For Respiratory Isolation Procedures: A private room is usually designated for this type of isolation; however, room may be shared if both clients have the same respiratory condition. Check with team leader or head nurse and institutional policies. Gowns and gloves are not indicated. A mask should be worn.

For Contact Isolation Procedures: Usually the client is placed in a private room, although some institutions allow the room to be shared if both clients have the same infectious disease. If there is a possibility of soiling uniform, then a protective gown should be worn. Gloves should be worn if the nurse is in contact with infective material. Masks should be worn if there is close contact with the client. Contaminated articles that are to be discarded should be bagged and labeled.

TB Isolation Procedures: A private room is usually designated but may be shared if both clients have TB. The room should be specially ventilated and the door kept closed. Gowns are worn to prevent contamination of clothing. Gloves are not indicated but a mask should be used, particularly if the client is coughing.

Drainage or Secretions Precautions: Room may be shared. A gown and gloves are required if infective material is to be touched. A mask is usually not indicated.

Blood or Body Fluid Precautions: A private room may be used if necessary, especially if the client does not have good hygienic habits. A gown and gloves are indicated if infective material is to be touched. A mask is usually not indicated.

Enteric Isolation Precautions: The same precautions are taken as for blood and body fluid precautions.

Procedure: Chart Recording

Description: Care given to the client from admission to discharge is recorded.

Purpose: To describe accurately and completely objective and subjective information as it relates to client care, including mental and physical assessment of the client's condition, all treatments prescribed and given, and any treatments refused by the client or any care not given with the reason for same; to communicate information that is correct and important for health-care personnel to use in continuing effective client care.

STEP	RATIONALE
On Admission:	
1. Interview client.	Helps to determine client's understanding of his or her condition and complaints.
2. Ask client for information about pain, type, location, and changes in severity; other physical symptoms such as weakness, fever, chills, dizziness, fear, and mood changes; and onset of such symptoms.	Obtains subjective complaints.
3. Ask client for information on any changes in eating, swallowing, bowel habits, voiding, sleeping, walking, standing, hearing, vision, taste, and smell.	Helps to identify any changes that may show worsening of or improvement in the client's condition.
On Examination:	
1. Check level of consciousness.	Changes in level of consciousness may indicate changes in brain function.
2. Check on whether client displays any evidence of pain, anxiety, weakness, and the like.	Checks on client's statements made during interview.
3. Check for any signs of sweating, changes in skin color, temperature of skin, spasms.	Obtains physical evidence of problems.
4. Check vital signs (temperature, pulse, respiration, blood pressure).	Obtains information that may indicate changes occurring in body.
5. Check for the following signs: • Bleeding • Tenderness and location • Stiffness in joints and deformities • Drainage location, type, amount, odor (describe in detail) • Difficulty in moving about • Problems in communication	Obtains information of changes that may be occurring in body functions. Type of drainage or excretions that are usual (urine or feces may show presence of bleeding, changes in color, and so on). Other drainage may be abnormal, for example, drainage from wounds.
6. Assess each body system for signs and symptoms indicating a problem.	Obtains systematic information from physical assessment.

(Continued on following page)

STEP	RATIONALE

Entering Information on Chart:

To Ensure Legality of Notes:

1. Write date and time of entry of information in ink (check with policy in regard to color of ink).
2. Do not leave blank spaces.
3. Do not erase any information.

4. Do not add more information after notations have been signed.

5. End notation with signature and abbreviated title (LVN or LPN).

Legal requirement. Prevents changing of information in chart.

Prevents new information from being added at a later time.

Prevents questions about information being changed or deleted. If error occurs, draw line through error and write in "error" with your initials.

New information should be noted with time and labeled as a "late notation" and signed. For information that has been written earlier and incorrect, begin new notation with corrected statement.

Identifies notation by name and title of person doing the recording.

To Ensure Accuracy and Completeness of Charted Information:

1. Record all important information.
2. Record any critical information immediately.
3. Use institution's policy in regard to medical terms and abbreviations.
4. Use proper grammar, spelling, and punctuation.
5. Record data obtained from assessment of client. Include:
   • Any changes in condition
   • Changes in behavior
   • New symptoms and signs
   • Information on drainage (type, amount, location, character, and so on)
   • Response to treatments
   • Decreases in or absence of earlier signs or symptoms
6. Write information from your assessment in a logical, organized fashion.
7. Do not use terms such as "little" or "small." If exact size is unknown, use phrases such as "reddened area the size of a half-dollar noted on sacrum."
8. Make sure that body locations are correctly recorded.
9. Write notations in chart at regular intervals.
10. Record the following information with correct date and time:
    • Initial assessment
    • Changes in condition
    • Nursing care given such as treatments, helping with activities of daily living (ADLs), teaching
11. Record visits of physician and other health professionals.
12. Record specific information, including laboratory data, vital signs, changes in client's condition, and physician's response.
13. Record medications given after they have been given.

Ensures completeness.

Ensures promptness.

Prevents misunderstanding by reader.

Demonstrates professionalism.

Ensures completeness of information, including any observations in regard to changes in client's physical and/or mental status.

Makes it easier to follow and ensures completeness.

Such terms have different meanings to different people.

Ensures accurate information.

Provides accurate information on a continuous basis.

Provides accurate written information of client's progress. Keeps a record of treatment regimen and client's responses.

Reports on visits that are necessary to obtain reimbursement funds from special outside agencies such as Medicare.

Ensures accuracy and completeness.

Flow Sheet Recording:

1. Obtain necessary information requested on flow sheet.
2. Enter date and time of information.
3. Write information in correct location.
4. Sign signature or initials in correct spot (check institutional policy).

Ensures information requested is obtained.

Ensures time sequence.

Ensures accuracy of information.

Identifies person recording information.

Nursing Implications: Written records are used to communicate accurate and complete data regarding care received by the client and must follow the policy in terms of the institutional and legal requirements. The Joint Commission on Accreditation of Healthcare Organizations (JCAHO) requires evidence of the nursing process. Information on charts is used in lawsuits and in reimbursement of funds from outside agencies and therefore must be accurate and complete. Charts are used by other health-care personnel to determine client's condition, treatment effects, and so on.

Procedure: Taking Vital Signs

Description: This is the procedure for taking the body temperature, pulse, respirations, and blood pressure measurements.

Purpose: To assess the vital signs in an accurate manner to determine the amount of heat stored in the body.

The temperature is taken on admission and as ordered by the physician, as well as when the client shows signs of a fever such as feeling cold, hot, or thirsty, or is shivering or perspiring.

The pulse is taken to obtain information about the function of the heart, the circulatory system, and the client's general physical state.

The respirations are taken to determine the rate per minute and its depth, quality, and pattern of respiration, and to assess if any changes occur over time.

The blood pressure is measured as systolic (upper figure) and diastolic (lower figure). It is taken to determine the relationship between the cardiac output (the amount of blood pumped out of the heart) and the resistance to the blood flow by the blood vessels outside the heart. The assessment of blood pressure assists health-care personnel in determining if the client is within the normotensive (normal), hypertensive (high blood pressure), or hypotensive (low blood pressure) state.

Step	Rationale
1. Collect necessary equipment for taking the temperature: • Thermometer (glass or electronic) • Probe cover, tissues, lubricant • Paper towel and disposable gloves	Organizing necessary equipment allows quick and safe implementation.
Oral Temperature: 1. Explain procedure. 2. Wash hands.	Informs client of procedure. Prevents transfer of microorganisms.
When Using a Glass Thermometer: 3. Hold at end opposite bulb part and rinse in cold water.	Avoids touching the bulb part that will be placed in client's mouth. Rinsing removes disinfectant and other material on thermometer. Hot water expands the chemical and may break the thermometer.
4. Wipe thermometer from fingers to bulb part with a clean tissue.	Removes water from area of greatest contamination (part not stored in disinfectant solution and touched by nurse's fingers) to area of least contamination (bulb part of disinfectant solution).
5. Hold thermometer lengthwise at eye level, turn until measuring scale can be seen, and read the number at the end of the chemical level.	Allows ease in viewing scale to make sure that the chemical level is below body temperature. Mercury thermometers have been removed from health care institutions, but some chemical thermometers are still used.
6. Hold end opposite bulb and shake thermometer downward with a flick of the wrist until the chemical reads 95°F (35°C).	Lowers the chemical level so that it is below expected body temperature.
7. Before inserting an electronic thermometer, remove the portable unit from base. Check to make sure that the unit is charged.	Prepares thermometer for use.
8. When using either thermometer: Instruct client to open mouth and hold tongue against upper teeth.	
9. Insert thermometer tip or probe gently under tongue.	Positions the chemical tip or probe in heat area of mouth.
10. Ask client to close mouth and hold tip or probe in place between his or her lips. Ask client not to bite down on glass thermometer.	Keeps thermometer in place until temperature is recorded. Prevents possible injury of mouth if thermometer breaks.
11. When using a glass thermometer, leave thermometer in place for 3–11 minutes, depending on your institution's guidelines. (At this time check other vital signs.)	Ensures adequate time for accurate temperature reading.

(Continued on following page)

STEP	RATIONALE
12. Once time interval is completed, hold the end of the thermometer and ask client to open his or her mouth.	Reduces possibility of dropping thermometer.
13. Remove thermometer; wipe with a tissue moving from end held in your fingers to bulb part.	Removes germs and other materials from area of least contamination to area of most contamination.
14. Read the thermometer and record.	Ensures accurate notation.
15. Wash thermometer with cool soapy water; rinse with cool water. Dry with tissue or clean paper towel. Replace in container.	Removes microorganisms and other material.
16. When using an electronic thermometer, check digital panel until a signal is heard indicating that the maximum temperature has been reached.	Provides evidence that indicates the thermometer is recording the temperature.
17. Hold end of probe and ask client to open his or her mouth. Remove probe.	Prevents probe from falling out of client's mouth.
18. Read the temperature on digital panel and record immediately.	Ensures accurate notation.
19. Eject probe cover into waste receptacle.	Discarding of probe cover prevents contamination of other clients.
20. After use of either thermometer, inform client of his or her temperature if allowed.	Decreases anxiety.
21. Wash hands.	Prevents transfer of microorganisms.

Rectal Temperature:

STEP	RATIONALE
1. Explain procedure.	Decreases anxiety; gains cooperation.
2. Follow steps 1–7 for taking an oral temperature.	
3. When using a rectal glass thermometer or electronic thermometer, put on clean disposable gloves.	Protects hands from becoming contaminated with client's body excreta.
4. Place lubricant on bulb end of glass thermometer or on probe of electronic thermometer.	Allows for easier insertion of thermometer into the rectum.
5. Pull curtains around client's bed or close room door.	Ensures privacy.
6. Ask or assist client to lie on his or her side with upper leg bent.	Places client in position so that rectal area is visible.
7. Lower pajama bottom, if worn, and place bed linens so that only buttocks are visible.	Ensures privacy.
8. Separate buttocks gently with one hand.	Exposes the anus to view.
9. Touch tip of probe or bulb end of glass thermometer to anus, explaining what is being done. Ask client to take a deep breath.	Client feels the position of thermometer. Placing thermometer tip against the anal area relaxes the anal muscles. Deep breathing helps to relax the client.
10. Place probe or tip gently into anus and point tip toward umbilicus (belly button) and guide it along rectal wall. Insert tip up to about 3 inches in the adult and about 1/2 inch in infants.	Placement of bulb against wall of rectum places tip close to blood vessels. Placing thermometer carefully in the proper area of the rectum helps to prevent injury to the rectal tissues.

When Using a Glass Thermometer:

STEP	RATIONALE
11. Hold thermometer in place for 2–4 minutes. Check institutional policies.	Gives enough time for correct reading.
12. Remove thermometer gently. Wipe the thermometer from fingers to bulb with clean tissue, turning the tissue around the thermometer.	Decreases discomfort. Removes germs and other material from thermometer from the area of least contamination to the area of most contamination. Turning the tissue allows for removal of fecal material.
13. Read thermometer; place it aside. Inform client of temperature if not contraindicated by institutional policy.	Decreases anxiety.
14. Record temperature.	Allows prompt and accurate reading.
15. Remove any remaining lubricant from anal area with tissue. Client may wish to clean area himself or herself. Give client tissue.	Ensures personal hygiene.
16. Replace pajama bottoms, if worn, and replace bed linens. Place client in comfortable position. Raise side rails if required.	Ensures comfort.

(Continued on following page)

STEP	RATIONALE
17. Wash thermometer with cool soapy water and rinse with cool water; dry with paper towel or tissue. Replace in storage container.	Removes remaining material and other organisms from thermometer before replacing in container.
18. Discard gloves; wash hands.	Prevents transfer of microorganisms.
19. Open curtains or doors to room.	

When Using an Electronic Thermometer:

STEP	RATIONALE
20. Watch digital panel until unit signals that the maximum temperature has been reached.	Indicates that thermometer is recording the temperature.
21. Remove thermometer gently. Check the temperature readout on the digital panel of the thermometer.	Decreases discomfort. Obtains accurate reading.
22. Eject the probe cover into waste receptacle.	Prevents contamination of other clients.
23. Follow steps 14–19 for taking a rectal temperature with a glass thermometer.	

Axillary Temperature:

STEP	RATIONALE
1. Explain procedure.	Informs client of procedure. Decreases anxiety; gains cooperation.
2. Wash hands.	Decreases transfer of microorganisms.

When Using a Glass Thermometer or Electronic Probe:

STEP	RATIONALE
3. Follow steps 1–7 for taking an oral temperature.	
4. Draw curtain around bed or close room door.	Ensures privacy.
5. Place client on back or in sitting position.	Places client in best position for placement of thermometer.
6. Assist client to remove gown or other top clothing.	Prepares for exposing area under arm (axilla).
7. Raise client's arm or ask him or her to raise the arm; gently dry axilla.	Dries any moisture under arm that may lower the temperature readout because of evaporation.
8. Place bulb or probe tip into the center of the axilla. Hold in place.	Places thermometer near blood vessel supply.
9. Lower client's arm over thermometer and position his or her arm across chest.	Keeps thermometer in place.
10. Hold glass thermometer in place for 10 minutes; hold electronic thermometer in place until signal is heard.	Ensures accurate reading.
11. Raise client's arm, remove probe or glass thermometer. Replace gown or clothing.	
12. Wipe thermometer with a tissue, using a twisting motion toward bulb end.	Removes contaminants from thermometer from area of least contamination to area of greatest contamination.
13. Read and record temperature.	
14. Wash thermometer with cool soapy water and rinse with cool water. Dry with clean paper towel or tissue; replace in storage container.	Ensures accurate information.
15. Inform client of temperature unless contraindicated.	Decreases anxiety.
16. Place client in a comfortable position. Open curtains or door.	Ensures comfort.
17. Wash hands.	Decreases transfer of microorganisms.

When Using an Electronic Thermometer:

STEP	RATIONALE
18. Remove portable unit from base. Check to ensure that unit is charged.	Prepares thermometer for use. A maximally charged unit produces an accurate temperature recording.
19. Place a probe cover over probe.	Prepares the thermometer.
20. Follow steps 4–17.	

Nursing Implications: Report any changes in temperature to team leader or head nurse. Document temperature on chart and flow sheet. Report elevated or subnormal temperature immediately. Such readings may signify an imbalance between heat produced and heat lost. Extremely low or high temperatures may cause damage to body cells and even death if these temperatures remain over a prolonged period of time. The body temperature may be measured in different sites depending on the client's condition. The decision of the site depends on the client's condition, the order of the physician, and the decision of the team leader or head nurse. Such decisions are made based on the following:

- Nearness of major arteries, because arterial blood temperature is the closest measure of total body temperature
- Amount of accuracy required based on client's condition
- Age of client (e.g., infants and very young children cannot hold a thermometer in their mouths for the required time)
- Presence of inflammation (e.g., inflamed tissue having higher temperature than normal tissue)
- Client's overall condition (e.g., unconscious, paralyzed clients may not be able to have temperatures taken by mouth; in burned clients, location of temperature reading requires special decisions)

Temperature may be taken rectally instead of orally if client has recently eaten, drunk, or smoked. These conditions may raise or lower the temperature under the tongue, resulting in an incorrect temperature reading.

Procedure: Taking the Pulse

Description: Methods of measuring the pulse rate include radial, apical, and apical-radial measurements.

Purpose: To obtain information about the functioning of the heart, the circulatory system, and client's general physical state; to measure client's emotional state and body responses to stress, exercise, blood loss, fatigue, and injury to tissues; and to evaluate response to trauma, surgery, medications, and other treatments (including rate, rhythm, and depth).

STEP	RATIONALE
1. Collect necessary equipment: • Stethoscope • Antiseptic swabs • Watch with second hand or digital panel	Organizing necessary equipment allows quick and safe implementation.

Radial Pulse:

STEP	RATIONALE
1. Explain procedure.	Informs client of procedure. Decreases anxiety; gains cooperation.
2. Wash hands.	Prevents transfer of microorganisms.
3. For clients lying on their backs, place client's arm across chest, palm down. For those who are sitting, place arm on his or her lap, palm down.	Places wrist in a resting position.
4. Place first three fingers of your hand on client's radial artery, located just below client's thumb on his or her wrist.	Positions fingers over artery. *Never* use thumb to take a pulse. The pulse in your thumb may be felt instead of the client's pulse.
5. Feel for pulse sensations. Note rhythm and strength of pulse.	Check quality and rhythm of pulse.
6. Look at watch. Note location of second hand and wait until 15, 30, or 60 seconds have passed.	If taking routine pulse rate, a 15-second count is usually sufficient unless institutional policy differs. If any abnormalities are present, count for a full 60 seconds.
7. Multiply the count by 4 if pulse was taken for 15 seconds, by 2 if taken for 30 seconds.	Determines pulse rate for a full minute.
8. Inform client of pulse unless contraindicated.	Relieves anxiety.
9. Record pulse rate, rhythm, and quality.	Ensures accurate documentation.
10. Wash hands.	Prevents transfer of microorganisms.

Apical Pulse:

STEP	RATIONALE
1. Follow previous steps 1 and 2.	
2. Clean earpieces and diaphragm of stethoscope with an antiseptic swab.	Prevents transfer of possibly dangerous organisms from previous use.
3. Help client to a back-lying position or a low-Fowler's (sitting) position.	Places client in comfortable position. Prevents possible changes in heart rate by decreasing strain on the client.
4. Close room door or draw curtains around bed.	Ensures privacy.
5. Expose left chest by placing bed linens away from left chest and removing gown from left chest area.	Removes clothing and linens that may interfere with hearing heart sounds.
6. Rub bell or diaphragm of stethoscope with palm of hand.	Warms diaphragm before placement on chest wall.
7. Place earpieces in your ears. Place stethoscope bell or diaphragm on the fourth or fifth rib space (intercostal space) on left chest.	Prepares to take apical pulse. Positions stethoscope near apex of heart.

(Continued on following page)

STEP	RATIONALE
8. Listen for a "lub-dup" sound. Move bell or diaphragm until sound is heard.	This sound identifies two normal heart sounds: S1 (closure of semilunar valves of heart) and S2 (closure of atrioventricular valves).
9. Check the rhythm of heart sound.	Evaluates rhythm.
10. Time the heart rate, rhythm, and quality using the second hand of watch or digital readout.	A full-minute count should be taken so that any abnormalities may be noted.
11. Remove stethoscope; replace gown and bed linens. Place client in a comfortable position.	Ensures comfort.
12. Record apical pulse.	Ensures accurate and prompt documentation.
13. Wash hands. Clean stethoscope earpieces, diaphragm, or bell with antiseptic swabs.	Prevents transfer of microorganisms.

Apical-Radial Pulse:

STEP	RATIONALE
1. Explain procedure: "One nurse will be counting heartbeats; a second nurse will count radial pulse to compare the rates." Answer any questions.	Informs client of procedure; decreases anxiety.
2. Prepare for measuring apical pulse; follow steps 1–9 for taking apical pulse.	
3. Have second nurse take the radial pulse after procedure for taking apical pulse.	
4. Watching the second hand or digital dial, let second nurse know when to begin counting radial pulse. Begin counting the radial and apical pulses at the same time.	Coordinates the count. This verifies if any differences exist between the apical and radial pulse counts.
5. Both nurses count the heart rate for 1 full minute.	Ensure accuracy.
6. Tell second nurse to stop when 1 minute has passed.	Ensures accuracy.
7. Place client in comfortable position. Record apical and radial pulse. Note and report any differences between apical and radial pulse rates.	Ensures comfort. Ensures prompt and accurate reading.
8. Wash hands; clean stethoscope earpieces, diaphragm, or bell with antiseptic swabs.	Prevents transfer of microorganisms.

Nursing Implications: Document pulse, report any changes in pulse rate, depth, rhythm, and quality to team leader or head nurse. Checking the pulse rate provides how many times the heart beats every minute, as well as the rhythm and the quality of heartbeats. Remember that many different factors can affect pulse rate. Age of the client affects pulse rate. For example, a newborn infant's pulse rate is normally between 120 and 140 bpm. A child of 6 or 7 years has a pulse rate of about 100, whereas the adult female pulse rate ranges from 55 to 90. The male pulse rate may range from 50 to 85. Other factors affecting pulse rate include exercise, emotions, body chemicals, body temperature, and diseases involving the heart and other body organs.

The quality of the pulse is affected by the function of the heart and the circulatory system. Conditions such as dehydration cause blood volume to decrease, thereby producing a weak, thready pulse.

Sites where the pulse rate may be measured, other than the apical and radial sites, include the temporal pulse, located between the outside of the eye and the hairline. This site is often used in infants and children and when other sites are not accessible, as in the presence of severe body burns, body casts, and so on.

The pulse may also be measured at the carotid artery (carotid pulse), located just below the angle of the jaw. This location is often used in times of emergencies. Because the carotid artery is located near the heart, the pulse may often be detected even when blood volume is low and other pulses cannot be felt.

The brachial pulse is taken over the brachial artery, which runs down the arm and is measured just below the inner side of the antecubital fossa. This pulse site is used to listen to sounds reflective of the arterial blood pressure.

Another site for monitoring the pulse is close to the pubis bone near the upper inner thigh. This site is often used to check the circulation of the lower extremities or to perform special circulatory tests.

The popliteal pulse is found under the knee. The knee needs to be flexed (bent) to locate the pulse. This site is used to check the circulation of the lower extremity and may be used to check the arterial blood pressure in the leg.

Another site that is used to check the circulation in the feet is the dorsalis pedis pulse. It is located on the top of the foot, a little toward the tendon of the big toe. It should be noted that this artery does not exist in a small percentage of individuals.

One final site is located on the inside of the ankle. It is at this site that the posterior tibial pulse may be monitored. This site is used to check the circulation of the lower extremities. It should be noted that this pulse is often difficult to find, especially if the individual is edematous or obese, and even may not be found in some instances.

Procedure: Taking the Respirations

Description: This measures the respiratory rate of clients.

Purpose: To measure the respiratory rate in order to obtain information reflecting the process of oxygen delivery to the cells and the return of oxygen to the outside air; to determine the client's usual pattern, rate, quality of respirations, and any changes that have occurred; to assist in the evaluation of pathological conditions that are reflected by abnormal rates.

STEP	RATIONALE
1. Collect necessary equipment: wristwatch with second hand or digital readout. **NOTE:** This procedure is done immediately after taking the radial pulse.	Organizing necessary equipment allows for quick and safe implementation.
2. Keep client's wrist over chest after taking radial pulse.	This position allows nurse to watch rise and fall of wrist and count respirations without having client control his or her respirations and in turn change rate.
3. Note rhythm, depth, quality, and pattern of respirations.	Checks for abnormality.
4. Using watch, count respirations for 1 full minute.	Ensures accuracy of rate.
5. Record respiratory rate.	Ensures accurate and prompt recording.
6. Wash hands.	Prevents transfer of microorganisms.

Nursing Implications: Record findings. Report any unusual findings immediately to team leader or head nurse.

When Client's Respirations Are Slower Than Usual: If client is conscious, have him or her take deep breaths at about 10–12/min. Check other vital signs and report findings immediately to team leader or head nurse. Check if client has received depressant medication. Be prepared to assist in giving artificial respiration if required.

When Client's Respirations Are Faster Than Usual: Report to team leader or head nurse. If pain or fever is present, check with team leader about prescribed medications. If client is under emotional stress and consequently is hyperventilating, talk quietly to client for reassurance. If hyperventilation is caused by anxiety, try placing a paper bag over client's mouth and nose and ask him or her to breathe into it. The client rebreathes the exhaled carbon dioxide, thus decreasing the depth of the respiration and slowing its rate. If hyperventilation is a result of respiratory or nervous system disorders, report to team leader or head nurse immediately if it is a change from previous measurements of the respirations.

If client has stopped breathing, begin respiratory resuscitation immediately: 12 respirations per minute for adults and 20 respirations per minute for children. Call or have someone call for a respiratory arrest team.

The respiratory rate varies depending on age, exercise, disease or disorders, certain metabolic changes, medications, and emotions.

Age: Newborn infant's respirations are about 35/min; adult's are 14–20/min.

Exercise: When exercising, the body cells require more oxygen. To supply the need, respirations increase. Resting lowers the respiratory rate. It should be noted that respiratory rates in individuals who have been immobilized for a long time may be increased because of factors affecting the respiratory and circulatory systems.

Disease or Disorders: Certain diseases or disorders may cause a mild decrease of oxygen in the arterial blood circulation (hypoxic state) that will increase respiratory rates. If the hypoxic state is severe, the usual body mechanisms that control respirations may be affected and so increase the respiratory rates.

Certain Metabolic Changes: An example of metabolic changes is increases or decreases in thyroid hormones that regulate metabolism in the body. If these hormones decrease or increase, respiratory rates also decrease or increase.

Medications: Medicines that depress the central nervous system (brain) may decrease respiratory rates.

Emotions: Anger, anxiety, and fear induce a response from the autonomic nervous system causing an increase in respiratory rates.

Procedure: Measuring Blood Pressure

Description: This measures the compression against the brachial artery by an inflated cuff (part of sphygmomanometer) and the auscultation (listening to the first and last sounds of the blood flow through the artery when the cuff is slowly deflated, causing a decompression against the brachial artery).

Purpose: To assess the blood pressure reading of a client as a part of vital sign measurement; to determine any changes from the normal range or usual range for the client, which may indicate need for further treatment.

Step	Rationale

1. Collect necessary equipment:
  • Sphygmomanometer: mercury or aneroid with inflation cuff
  • Stethoscope
  • Antiseptic swabs
	Organizing necessary equipment allows for quick and safe implementation.

2. Explain procedure.	Informs client of procedure; decreases anxiety.
3. Wash hands.	Prevents transfer of microorganisms.
4. Place bedridden client in back-lying or side-lying position with arm resting at side, with upper arm at heart level with palm up. *Or* Place sitting client's arm on his or her lap or armrest of chair, with upper arm at heart level with palm up.	Arm elevated above heart may cause ineffective compression or artery.
5. Make sure that mercury level or dial needle is at 0.	Ensures proper reading.
6. Measure cuff width against client's arms to check for accurate fit.	False reading may occur if cuff is too small because of ineffective compression over artery.
7. Make sure that the mercury meniscus is at eye level or aneroid dial is directly in front of eyes.	Prevents false readings by having accurate visualization of scale.
8. Palpate (feel) the brachial artery pulse.	Locates artery for correct placement of arm cuff.
9. Release valve lock to remove any air in inflation bladder located in the cuff.	Uneven inflation may give inaccurate readings.
10. Center the arrow on cuff over artery with lower edge of cuff about 1 inch above the antecubital fossa.	Ensures inflation bladder is over artery. Makes sure that lower edge of cuff does not cover brachial site where stethoscope will be placed.
11. Wrap cuff evenly around client's upper arm, making sure of a snug fit.	
12. Fasten Velcro or tuck end under cuff.	Secures cuff in correct position for inflation.
13. Wipe stethoscope earpieces and diaphragm or bell with antiseptic swabs.	Prevents transfer of microorganisms.
14. Place earpieces of stethoscope in ears and feel for the brachial artery pulse.	Prepares for taking blood pressure reading.
15. Hold hand pump in one hand and tighten valve lock with thumb.	Prevents air from leaking out. Ensures effective compression of artery.
16. Inflate cuff with a brisk pumping motion. Palpate artery and watch mercury level or needle of dial.	Ensures adequate amount of blood in artery during compression.
17. When brachial pulse disappears, remove fingers from artery area and place diaphragm or bell over brachial artery.	Indicates sufficient compression to stop blood flow through artery and time to begin listening (auscultating) for return of blood flow.
18. Stop inflating cuff when mercury level increases to 30 mm above the point where pulse disappeared.	Indicates that sufficient compression has occurred and prevents false readings if compression stops during ausculatory gap.
19. Loosen valve lock slowly and deflate cuff at a rate of 2–3 mm Hg per heartbeat.	Begins to decompress artery, allowing blood flow to restart. Decompressing the artery too fast makes it difficult to read the scale accurately. Decompressing too slowly may cause falsely high measurements and increase discomfort for client.
20. Listen carefully for the first "tap-tap" sounds (Korotkoff's sounds). Note the mercury level and read the measurement scale.	Indicates systolic reading.
21. Listen for changes in the sounds.	
22. When sounds disappear, note the measurement reading.	Indicates diastolic reading.
23. Open valve cock completely. Note diastolic sound; rapidly deflate and remove cuff.	Removes compression and discomfort.
24. Inform client of reading unless contraindicated.	Decreases anxiety.
25. Place client in comfortable position. Record reading immediately.	Ensures comfort. Ensures prompt and accurate recording.
26. Wash hands; cleanse stethoscope earpieces and diaphragm or bell with antiseptic swabs.	Decreases potential for transfer of microorganisms.

Nursing Implications: The most common method of taking the blood pressure is by auscultation (listening for sounds of blood flow with a stethoscope). Note usual blood pressure. Check and report any changes. Factors that control blood pressure include the amount of circulating blood. More blood flow increases blood pressure, whereas less blood volume circulation decreases blood pressure. If the heart muscle becomes damaged, the output from the heart chambers decreases and blood pressure decreases. The greater the resistance by the vessels outside of the heart, the higher the blood pressure. The greater the width of the blood vessel, the lower the pressure. Dilation (widening) of blood vessels decreases blood pressure. Narrowing of blood vessels, such as that caused by atherosclerosis, lessens the elasticity of the blood vessel walls and so increases resistance to blood flow, thereby increasing blood pressure. The viscosity (thickness or thinness) of blood affects blood pressure in that when the blood is thicker, blood flow slows down. If the tone of the smooth muscles of the blood vessels becomes impaired, the blood vessels lose their elasticity and become overdistended. This process affects the diastolic pressure.

Certain receptors found at several points in the arterial system send impulses to the vasomotor section of the brain in response to changes in blood volume and chemical composition. The brain, in turn, responds by causing either dilation or constriction of blood vessels.

Certain body chemicals, such as epinephrine, antidiuretic hormone, and histamine, cause vasodilation (widening) of blood vessels.

Output from the heart is affected by exertion, exercise, stress, and other emotions that raise blood pressure. Other factors that affect blood pressure include age (gradual increase in blood pressure with aging); gender (women have lower blood pressures than men between the beginning and end of menstruation and higher pressures after menopause); weight (obesity tends to raise blood pressure); and race (blacks have higher blood pressure than whites).

Generally, blood pressure is lowest in the morning and highest in the late afternoon or early evening in individuals who normally sleep at night. The average normal adult blood pressure reading is 120/80. A systolic blood pressure of 140 and a diastolic pressure of 90 are considered the upper limits of the range, according to the American Heart Association, although normal range may be up to 160/90. To determine that blood pressure is higher or lower than the normal range for individuals, one must have prior blood pressure readings for comparison.

If blood pressure reading is 20–30 mm Hg or more lower than previous readings, retake the blood pressure to make sure that the reading was accurate. If pressure is still low, recheck blood pressure in opposite arm.

Check client for other signs and symptoms such as changes in pulse rate, respiration, and temperature. Check for changes in skin color, skin temperature, chest pain, confusion, lethargy, or unconsciousness. If there is no evidence of other signs and symptoms, place client in a back-lying position, report findings immediately, and continue taking the blood pressure at regular intervals.

In cases when the blood pressure measurement is 20–30 mm Hg higher than the client's usual range, retake blood pressure and check findings using the correct techniques including an accurate cuff size for the client's arm. Retake blood pressure in opposite arm if findings still indicate a higher pressure than usual.

Check the client for other signs and symptoms suggestive of high blood pressure, such as changes in other vital signs, chest pain, difficulty breathing, and skin color and temperature changes.

If any of these signs and symptoms are present, report finding immediately. If no other signs and symptoms are present, retake the blood pressure in 15–20 minutes and recheck at regular intervals. Document and report all findings.

In cases when the sounds heard through the stethoscope are faint or absent, check all vital signs. Check equipment for proper working order. Have client raise arm above shoulder and rapidly inflate cuff. Lower arm and take reading. If difficulty still persists, inform team leader or head nurse immediately.

If other noises interfere with ability to hear Korotkoff's sounds, check to see that the stethoscope or blood pressure monitor tubings are not hitting against each other or against other objects. If sounds are caused by others making noise, such as loud talking or television or radio interference, request that such noise interference be muted until the procedure is completed.

Procedure: Intake and Output

Description: This is the process of measuring, recording, and reporting the intake of oral fluids, IV fluids, blood or blood products, total parenteral nutrition, and enteral nutrition. Measurement of output including urinary output (with or without indwelling catheter), vomitus, liquid stools, and drainage from nasogastric tube and other tubes such as chest tubes and T-tubes.

Purpose: To assess for signs of imbalance of both fluids and electrolytes (normally fluid intake is approximately equal to fluid output of the body; an imbalance suggests unusual or abnormal processes).

STEP	RATIONALE
1. Put intake and output (I&O) record in place, as indicated in institutional policies.	Alerts staff to necessity for measuring I&O.
2. Place I&O sign near client's bedside.	Alerts staff and client that I&O is to be measured.

(Continued on following page)

STEP	RATIONALE
3. Check, measure, and record intake from: • IV fluids • Blood and blood products • Total parenteral nutrition • Oral fluid intake, including liquid supplements and semiliquid food such as sherbet, ice cream, gelatin.	Records all applicable fluid intake.
4. Check, measure, and record output from: • Urinary output (including indwelling catheter) • Vomitus • Liquid stools • Nasogastric tube drainage • Drainage from wounds (including bedsores) or other tubes	Records all applicable fluid output.
5. Explain that urine is measured as output.	Informs client of procedure.
6. Show client where urinary collection receptacle is and demonstrate method of collection.	Prepares client for measuring output.
7. Show client how to measure and record urinary output.	Demonstrates how to measure and record output.
8. Ask client to demonstrate how to measure and record urinary output.	Checks on client's ability to measure and record output accurately.
9. Explain to family and visitors reasons for monitoring I&O. Ask them to assist client if needed.	Ensures understanding and possible assistance in measuring and recording fluid I&O.
10. Check on client's I&O recording periodically.	Ensures accuracy of recording.
11. Place completed I&O sheet in client's record according to policy.	Ensures completeness of record.
12. Report any unusual findings, such as blood in urine, very small (<30 mL/hr) or excessive amount of urine output.	Ensures immediate response.

Nursing Implications: Record I&O, reporting any unusual finding such as decreased or increased urine output, concentrated urine, weight loss, increased pulse, increased body temperature, decreased fluid intake, dry skin or mucous membranes, complaints of thirst or weakness, and confusion. These symptoms indicate an imbalance in fluid and electrolytes and suggest a fluid volume deficit.

Report any signs of edema, tightness of skin, weight gain, and increased blood pressure. These signs may indicate an imbalance in fluid and electrolytes suggestive of fluid volume excess.

Procedure: Assisting with IV Fluid Administration (LPN role varies according to state law).

Description: The practical nurse assists in the procedure of starting an IV solution.

Purpose: Allows for the replacement of fluids and electrolytes resulting from decreased fluid volume, concentration, and makeup of electrolytes in the body; allows for potential replacement of lost fluids and electrolytes during surgical or other treatments.

STEP	RATIONALE
1. Obtain necessary supplies and equipment: • IV solution ordered by physician • IV administration set and tubing • Infusion tray • Clean gloves • Correct needle and catheter • Tourniquet • IV pole • Adhesive tape • Antiseptic swabs or other preparation equipment • Sterile 2 × 2 gauze pads • Armboard	Organizing necessary equipment allows quick and safe implementation.

(Continued on following page)

STEP	RATIONALE
• Disposable razor	
• Label	
2. Wash hands.	Prevents transfer of microorganisms.
3. Double check IV solution for correct solution and expiration date with registered nurse (RN).	Ensures that client is receiving correct solution.
4. May shave excessive body hair from chosen site if requested.	Prepares site for IV needle and catheter insertion.
5. Hand tourniquet to RN if requested.	Tourniquet will be used to compress vein and distend venipuncture site.
6. Hand antiseptic swab or other prep material to RN when ready to disinfect skin surface.	Prepares site for IV needle and catheter insertion.
7. If requested, may attach sterile needle to tip of tubing; run fluid through needle, and reclamp tubing. Replace sterile cap over needle.	Primes needle.
8. Hand tubing with needle (remove needle cap using aseptic technique) to RN.	Keeps needle tip sterile.
9. Open clamp on tubing on request, after correct insertion of needle into vein and removal of tourniquet.	Allows IV fluid to enter vein.
10. Hand adhesive strips to RN.	Ensures placement of needle.

When a Venous Catheter Is to Be Used:
11. Follow previous steps 1–6.
12. Hand needle and catheter to RN, who will remove cover.
13. Follow previous steps 9 and 10.

For Both Needle and Catheter Insertion:

14. Provide RN with iodine preparation or other authorized preparation.	Placement of prep at puncture site limits possible contamination of needle or catheter and the blood.
15. After completion of procedure, check site for swelling or return of blood in the tubing.	Checks for infiltration.
16. Discard used equipment; return unused supplies to proper place.	
17. Wash hands.	

Managing a Continuous Intravenous Infusion:

1. Check that correct amount and rate of flow of IV solution is being used. (Refer to physician's orders and nursing care plan.)	Ensures that correct solutions is being administered within prescribed time.
2. Examine IV equipment and flow sheet at regular times (hourly checks are recommended) to check the following: • Presence of correct drip rate • Correct IV solution • Amount of IV fluid infused (compare with prescribed amount) • Intact IV system	Checks for accuracy.
3. Check site of IV needle or catheter for evidence of infiltration: • Swelling at site • Redness, warmth at site • Redness along vein path • Complaint of burning pain along venous pathway	Ensures immediate response in removal and/or replacement.
4. If solution is not dripping: • Check to see if clamp on tubing is too tight. • Check whether tubing is kinked or lying under client. • Inspect IV site for infiltration. • Check height of IV solution container. • Check to see if drip chamber is half full. • Check tape over puncture site. • Check that tubing stays above puncture site.	Catching problem early can make it easier to continue IV infusion at prescribed rate. Raising height increases gravity flow. Allows for ability to see the dripping solution. A tape that is too tight interferes with IV fluid entering vein. Gravity assists in IV flow.

(Continued on following page)

STEP	RATIONALE
5. Check for signs of dyspnea; edema; weak, rapid pulse; rapid and shallow respirations occurring on a regular basis.	Assessment of complications caused by overload of IV fluid.
6. Report any unusual problems to RN immediately.	Ensures continuation of IV infusion.

Changing Intravenous Solution Container (Based on Institutional Policy):

STEP	RATIONALE
1. Check amount of IV fluid infused until less than 50 mL remains in container.	Keeps some IV solution in tubing. Traps any microorganisms that may be present on the surface of the solution (which may occur when using glass bottle containers).
2. Check physician's orders and nursing care plan for correct IV solution rate of flow and amount to be infused.	Ensures correctness of order.
3. Obtain new correct IV container and take to client's bedside. Explain procedure.	Decreases anxiety.
4. Wash hands.	Prevents transfer of microorganisms.
5. Remove protective cover from new solution. Make sure that sterility is maintained.	Prevents contamination of solution.
6. Take used IV container from IV standard; clamp tubing; invert container (turn container so that top of container is opposite to what it was when infusing). Remove spike of tubing from container (maintain sterility of spike).	Removes used container.
7. Insert spike into stopper or top of the container without twisting tubing.	Attaches new IV container to IV tubing.
8. Hang the new container on the IV standard immediately.	Ensures gravity force to start flow rate.
9. Open clamp and check rate of solution flow.	
10. Check system on a regular basis.	Ensures proper functioning.

Discontinuing an Intravenous Infusion:

STEP	RATIONALE
1. Explain procedure.	Informs client of procedure.
2. Wash hands; put on gloves.	Prevents transfer of microorganisms.
3. Clamp IV tubing.	Stops IV flow.
4. Hold needle and catheter steady and loosen tape from IV site.	Decreases possibility of injury to vein.
5. Place antiseptic swab above IV site.	Prevents contamination.
6. Remove needle and catheter by gently pulling needle out.	Decreases possibility of injury to vein.
7. Press swab and gauze against site for 2–3 minutes or until bleeding stops.	Presses down on the vein so bleeding stops. *Do not rub IV site!* Rubbing may cause bleeding into tissues.
8. Apply bandage or dressing to site.	Prevents contamination.
9. Record the amount of solution infused on IV record.	Documents accurate amount infused.
10. Discard used solution container and tubing set.	
11. Leave client in comfortable position. Make sure call signal is within easy reach.	Ensures comfort.
12. Remove gloves; wash hands.	Prevents transfer of microorganisms.

Nursing Implications: Document site of infusion every 8 hours. Record any signs and symptoms of infection (e.g., warmth to the site, streaking up the vein). Record any signs and symptoms of an infiltration (e.g., site cool to touch, swelling around the infusion site). Change IV dressing site every 8 hours as outlined in the agency's policies. Change IV tubing every 24–48 hours as outlined in the agency's policies.

Procedure: Applying an External Catheter

Description: Application of an external catheter (Texas or condom catheter) is for the incontinent or paralyzed or unconscious male client (physician's order required).

Purpose: Allows urine to empty into a bag attached to client's leg or a collecting bag attached to the bed frame.

STEP	RATIONALE

1. Collect necessary equipment:
  • Condom catheter with drainage tube
  • Adhesive strip
  • Leg or collecting bag
  • Alcohol wipes
  • Soap, water
  • Washcloth, towel
  • Disposable gloves
	Organizing necessary equipment allows for quick and safe implementation.

2. Explain procedure.	Informs client of procedure.
3. Close curtains around bed or close room door.	Ensures privacy.
4. Place equipment on bedside table or overbed table.	Prepares for procedure.
5. Wash hands; put on clean gloves.	Prevents transfer of microorganisms.
6. Raise bed to a comfortable working position.	Prevents back strain.
7. Lower covers to expose genital area.	Prepares for procedure.
8. Using the soap and water, clean around penis with a circular movement. Rinse and dry. Wipe area with alcohol wipe. Allow to dry.	Removes material around penis. Helps in keeping condom catheter adhered in place.
9. Attach collection bag to bed frame or client's leg as appropriate.	Prepares bag for use.
10. Hold penis along shaft with one hand.	Places the sheath of penis in a secure manner.
11. Place rolled condom catheter at tip of penis with other hand. Gently unroll condom sheath onto shaft of penis.	
12. Allow about 1 inch between tip of penis and end of condom catheter that empties into collecting bag.	Provides a space (reservoir) for urine to pass into before draining into tubing.
13. Position end of sheath of catheter and anchor it by placing the adhesive strip around the penis so that the adhesive does not touch skin or make the catheter too tight around the penis.	Provides a tight fit of the catheter to the penis and prevents the leakage of urine around the opening.
14. Attach catheter end to the drainage tubing.	Provides for drainage into the collecting bag.
15. Make a coil of excess tubing and attach to bottom bed sheet.	Allows straight drainage of urine.
16. Replace bed covers; place client in a comfortable position. Make sure call signal is within reach. Open curtains or room door.	Ensures comfort.
17. Discard washcloth and towel. Remove gloves; wash hands.	Prevents transfer of microorganisms.

Nursing Implications: Record procedure. Document reason for external catheter application. Record and report response of client to procedure. Report and record any skin irritation from urine. Check for presence of edema. Check and report any unusual urinary problems, including color and odor of urine collected. Watch for any signs of skin impairment. Be aware of potential embarrassment involving the procedure. Act professionally.

If catheter sheath is too tight, remove and replace sheath. Reapply adhesive strip and ensure that it is not too tight.

If urine leaks from upper part of catheter, remove catheter, wash penis. Dry with alcohol and replace catheter. Wrap adhesive firmly but not too tightly around base of penis, without allowing adhesive to touch skin. If the catheter sheath falls off, wash penis as previously indicated, and reapply catheter.

Procedure: Giving Enema Using Disposable Enema Equipment

Description: Enemas introduce a solution into the rectum.

Purpose: To stimulate peristalsis (intestinal mobility), to remove flatus (gas) or feces, or to instill prescribed medications.

STEP	RATIONALE

1. Collect necessary equipment:
  • Enema administration package or equipment
  • Clean pitcher
	Organizing necessary equipment allows quick and safe implementation.

(Continued on following page)

STEP	RATIONALE
• Protective covered plastic sheet or protective padding • Enema solution and prescribed solution • Bath thermometer • Lubricant • IV pole (standard) • Clean gloves • Toilet tissue • Bedpan • Disposable gloves	
2. Wash hands.	Prevents transfer of microorganisms.
3. Open enema package; remove items.	Prepares for procedure.
4. Pour appropriate amount of warmed solution (water or saline) into enema administration container.	Prepares solution before placement into enema administration container.
5. Check solution with bath thermometer: 105–110°F (40.5–43.3°C). If saline is used, warm by placing saline container in basin of hot water.	Prevents cramping that may occur if solution is too cool. Decreases chances of tissue injury if temperature is too hot.
6. Add soap (for soapsuds enema) and mix into water.	Allows soap to dissolve evenly in solution. Addition of soap after water is prepared decreases bubbles in solution. The absence of bubbles decreases flatus in the bowel.
7. Clamp enema administration tubing.	Prevents solution from passing through tubing when solution is placed in enema container.
8. Pour enema solution into enema bag.	Prepares for enema administration.
9. Close top of container.	
10. Explain procedure. Determine the amount of solution he or she can tolerate.	Informs client of procedure.
11. Bring prepared enema to bedside. Hang bag or container on IV pole next to client.	Places enema administration near client.
12. Draw curtain around bed and/or close room door.	Ensures privacy.
13. Raise bed to comfortable working position.	Prevents back strain.
14. Assist client into a left Sims' (side-lying) position to expose buttocks.	Permits solution to flow into the rectum by gravity.
15. Place protective pad or covered plastic sheet under buttocks and thighs.	Prevents soiling bed linens.
16. Position bedpan next to client.	Bedpan will be within easy reach if client cannot retain enema.
17. Put on disposable gloves.	Protects nurse's hands from possible soiling by feces.
18. Remove protective cap from enema tip or nozzle. Open clamp on tubing; let solution flow through tubing into bedpan.	Fills tubing with solution. Air is removed from tubing. Prevents air from entering rectum.
19. Lubricate 3–4 inches of rectal tube or nozzle.	Allows easier insertion.
20. Remove enema container from IV pole and hold at the same height as the client's rectum.	Decreases the pressure of the solution entering rectum and allows the solution to enter rectum slowly, thereby increasing retention of solution.
21. Separate buttocks and visualize anus.	Prepares for procedure.
22. Ask client to take a deep breath and at the same time insert nozzle or rectal tube into anus; point tip of tube or nozzle toward umbilicus for about 3–4 inches.	Relaxes the anus. Placing the nozzle or rectal tube into rectum and pointing same toward umbilicus allows the nozzle or rectal tube to stay inside the rectum without injuring the rectal mucosa (tissue).
23. Unclamp tubing; raise container until solution flows into rectum.	Gradual increase of pressure in enema tubing prevents injury to rectal tissue. If the container is too high, there will be increased pressure and rapid instillation, which can cause painful distention of rectum and early evacuation.
24. Tell client that the solution is being instilled. Ask him or her to let you know if there is any pain or cramping. If so, clamp tubing briefly until pain or cramping stops.	Informs client of procedure. Allows the client to let the nurse know if pain or cramping occurs.
25. Clamp tubing, remove rectal tube and nozzle when all solution is used or client is no longer able to hold solution.	Prevents accidental spilling of any remaining solution in container.

(Continued on following page)

STEP	RATIONALE
26. Wipe anal area with toilet tissue; remove gloves inside out and discard.	Removes any feces and solution from buttocks and surrounding area; decreases chances of irritating skin.
27. Set aside enema equipment. Place client on bedpan or assist to commode or bathroom when ready (if client uses bathroom, ask him or her not to flush toilet).	Readies client for evacuation of solution, flatus, and feces. Allows nurse to check results of enema procedure.
28. Place call signal within easy reach; ask client to use call signal when finished.	Ensures privacy and comfort.
29. Assist client to clean perianal area with soap and water after donning clean gloves; dry perianal area.	Decreases potential irritation of skin around anal area.
30. Assist client to a comfortable position in bed. Leave protective pad in place unless soiled. If soiled, replace with a clean protective pad.	Ensures comfort. Decreases chances of further soiling of bed linens.
31. Check the enema return before emptying bedpan or commode or flushing toilet.	Evaluates results of enema.
32. Remove gloves and wash hands.	Prevents transfer of microorganisms.
33. Wash, rinse, and hang enema equipment to dry.	Readies the equipment for later use by the same client.
34. Record results of enema in terms of amount, color, and odor of feces and of solution.	Ensures accurate recording of results.

Prepackaged Enema Administration:

1. Follow previous steps 10–18.	
2. Inspect nozzle for lubricant (add lubricant if needed).	Allows easier insertion of nozzle into rectum.
3. Squeeze container gently.	Expels air before insertion.
4. Separate buttocks and locate anus.	Prepares for insertion of nozzle.
5. Follow previous steps 24–27.	
6. Record results of enema.	Ensures accurate recording of procedure and results.

Nursing Implications: Record and report any unusual problems, such as fresh blood in the returned enema solution and feces, inability to insert nozzle or rectal tube because of fecal impaction, client complaints of severe cramping, and distention with rigidity of the abdomen as noted during or following an enema. This last symptom may indicate perforation of the bowel. If this occurs, remove the tube immediately and check vital signs. If vital signs are within normal range and symptoms disappear, check with RN regarding reinsertion of rectal tube. If discomfort continues and vital signs indicate a problem, notify the RN in charge immediately.

If the client begins to expel the enema solution before the procedure is completed, place the client on a bedpan, reinsert rectal tube or nozzle, and *slowly* instill the remaining solution. This tends to stimulate peristalsis and assist in removal of feces and flatus (gas).

If the client does not expel the enema solution or feces after a small enema has been given, the enema may have been given to soften fecal material, as is the case with an oil-retention enema. If so, the client is expected to expel feces within 12–24 hours. If the purpose of the enema was to stimulate peristalsis and the enema has not been expelled, the solution may have been absorbed in the stool without stimulating the walls of the rectum (peristalsis).

Report these findings to the RN or team leader to determine if another enema should be given. Document all findings.

Procedure: Inserting Rectal Tube

Description: A rectal tube is inserted into the rectum.

Purpose: Assists in the removal of feces or flatus (gas); must be ordered by the physician.

STEP	RATIONALE
1. Collect necessary equipment: • Disposable rectal tube • Plastic bag or plastic specimen container • Protective pad • Rubber band • Lubricant • Adhesive tape • Clean gloves	Organizing necessary equipment allows for quick and safe implementation.

(Continued on following page)

STEP	RATIONALE
2. Explain procedure.	Informs client of procedure.
3. Place rectal tube, end opposite the tip, into plastic bag or plastic specimen container.	Provides a container for liquid feces expelled.
4. Place within reach two pieces of tape, each about 6 inches long.	Prepares for later use.
5. Wash hands.	Prevents transfer of microorganisms.
6. Close curtains around bed or close room door.	Ensures privacy.
7. Assist client into a left-lying position.	Allows inserted tube to follow anatomic curve without injury to rectal tissue.
8. Put protective pad under buttocks and thighs.	Prevents soiling of bed linens.
9. Put on clean gloves.	Helps to keep hands from becoming contaminated with feces.
10. Lubricate the tip of rectal tube.	Allows easier insertion into rectum and decreases potential for injury to rectal tissue.
11. Ask client to take a deep breath and at the same time insert rectal tube about 4–6 inches into rectum. Point tube toward umbilicus while inserting.	Relaxes the anal musculature; decreases chances of injuring rectal tissues.
12. Place tapes in position to secure tube in rectal area.	Fixes the tube so that it stays in place.
13. If plastic bag is used, tape the plastic bag tightly around bag and rectal tube.	Decreases chances of accidental soiling of bed linen.
14. If specimen container is used, place tape around rectal tube near slit and anchor tape to container.	
15. Remove and discard gloves.	
16. Replace client's bed linens. Make sure call signal is within easy reach.	Leaves client comfortable.
17. Leave rectal tube in place for 20–30 minutes.	Allows sufficient time to expel flatus.
18. Ask client if he or she has expelled flatus. Put on gloves; remove rectal tube and set aside.	Determines results of procedure.
19. Remove protective pad. Wash, rinse, and dry anal and surrounding skin area.	Removes fecal material from perianal area.
20. Take rectal tube and container to bathroom; examine contents.	Evaluates results of procedure.
21. Discard rectal tube and container.	
22. Remove gloves; wash hands.	Prevents transfer of microorganisms.

Nursing Implications: Document procedure and results. If the rectal tube cannot be inserted because of fecal impaction, notify the RN or team leader for instructions. Any complaints of severe cramping with obvious signs of distention and rigidity of the abdomen upon insertion of the rectal tube demand immediate attention; report to RN or team leader immediately. This situation may indicate a perforation of the bowel. If the symptoms disappear and vital signs are within normal range, check with RN or team leader about reinsertion of rectal tube. If vital signs are abnormal and symptoms remain, notify RN or team leader.
    Document procedure and all findings.

Procedure: Managing Wounds

Description: Wound management includes the assessment, cleaning, and protection of wounds.

Purpose: To prevent infection so that healing can take place.

STEP	RATIONALE
Application of a Dry Dressing:	
1. Obtain necessary supplies and equipment:	Organizing necessary supplies and equipment allows for quick and safe implementation.
• Sterile gloves	
• Sterile dressing set	
• Sterile drape	
• Gauze pads	
• Abdominal pads	

(Continued on following page)

STEP	RATIONALE

- Cotton balls and swabs
- Scissors
- Forceps and hemostat
- Small basin
- Dressing materials (nonadherent or transparent dressings)
- Ointment or powder if prescribed
- Waterproof pad
- Tape, ties, elastic bandages, Montgomery straps, butterflies
- Bath blanket
- Waterproof disposal bag

STEP	RATIONALE
2. Explain procedure.	Informs client of procedure. Decreases anxiety.
3. Check whether client has pain; check with RN regarding administration of pain medication.	
4. Bring supplies and equipment to bedside. Ask client not to touch any of the supplies during the procedure.	Prepares for procedure.
5. Pull curtains around bed or close room door.	Ensures privacy.
6. Position client so that wound can be accessed. Make client as comfortable as possible.	Allows care of wound.
7. Lower bedclothes; drape around wound area with sheet or bath blanket.	Ensures privacy.
8. Wash hands.	Prevents transfer of microorganisms.
9. Fold top of waterproof bag over back of straight chair or in easy reach.	Provides a container for disposal of used materials.
10. Remove dressing binder or untie Montgomery straps if used.	Prepares for procedure.
11. Loosen tape (if used). Hold skin and peel the edges of the tape.	Prevents injury to upper thin layers of skin.
12. Remove tape by pulling in a line with wound.	Prevents injury (peeling of upper layers of skin).
13. Put on clean gloves. Hold a corner of dressing at edge away from client's face; roll it off wound and remove old dressing.	Protects hands from contamination with microorganisms. Keeps contamination of airborne microorganismss from client's mouth and nose.
14. Check the amount, odor, color, and thickness of any drainage on dressing.	May indicate possible infection or excess drainage.
15. Fold the edges of the dressing inward and dispose of in waterproof container.	Prevents contamination.
16. Remove gloves and discard in bag.	Prevents transfer of microorganisms.
17. Wash hands.	Prevents transfer of microorganisms.
18. Place sterile dressing tray on overbed table; open tray using aseptic technique and add necessary supplies.	Prepares for wound management.
19. Fill sterile basin with sterile solution.	Prepares for wound cleansing.
20. Use sterile forceps to remove any remaining contact dressing over wound.	Prevents contamination of hands that may be present on dressing.
21. If dressing is stuck to wound, pour a small amount of solution from basin directly over dressing.	Prevents injury to skin and helps to loosen dressing from wound.
22. Check the odor, consistency, color, and amount of drainage. Check wound for signs of healing or complications.	Evaluates the condition of the wound.
23. Discard forceps.	
24. Put on sterile gloves.	Maintains sterility.
25. Using new forceps, pick up gauze or cotton balls; keep tips of forceps pointed downward.	Prevents potential contaminants from traveling up forceps.
26. Clean wound. Clean first over incisional area and then next to incision, using a circular motion.	Moves from area of least contaminantion to area of greatest contamination.
27. Discard cotton ball or gauze after one use.	Use of clean gauze or cotton balls prevents spread of microorganisms.
28. Dry wound in the same way, using dry cotton balls or gauze.	

(Continued on following page)

STEP	RATIONALE
29. Discard forceps.	
30. Apply prescribed ointment or solution using aseptic technique.	
31. Place enough sterile gauze directly over wound to absorb drainage.	Decreases the amount of drainage on surrounding skin areas or bandages.
32. Remove and discard disposable sterile gloves in bag.	Prevents transfer of microorganisms.
33. Touching only outside pad, place abdominal pad over dressing.	Absorbs drainage and prevents airborne microorganisms from contaminating wound.
34. Place tape, Montgomery straps, or binder over dressing.	Secures dressing.
35. Discard remaining materials and supplies.	
36. Remove drape and place the client in a comfortable position. Place call signal within easy reach.	Ensures comfort.
37. Wash hands.	Prevents transfer of microorganisms.

Nursing Implications: Document procedure and amount, color, odor, and viscosity of drainage. Report any unusual findings immediately to RN or team leader. Indicate location of wound and record drainage or moisture on outside of the dressing that was removed. Such findings may indicate excessive wound secretions, which will need more absorbent dressing materials. Check for any fresh blood on dressing, including amount in documentation. This may indicate hemorrhage, which will need immediate attention. A pressure dressing may be required. Determine if client is in pain, and check with RN or team leader regarding pain medication before dressing application is started.

Procedure: Performing Passive Range-of-Motion Exercises

Description: Exercises of the joints are performed by the health-care worker three to four times a day to maintain joint function.

Purpose: To maintain joint function and prevent contractures of muscular groups of those joints that a client is unable to move or has restricted movement of.

STEP	RATIONALE
1. Explain procedure.	Informs client of procedure; gains cooperation.
2. Wash hands.	Prevents transfer of microorganisms.
3. Pull curtains around client's bed or close room door.	Ensures privacy.
4. Raise bed to a comfortable working position. Place bed in a flat position.	Prevents back strain. Places client in correct position for the procedure.
5. Remove top bed linens and any clothing that may restrict movement. Cover with bath blanket.	Makes it easier to do the exercises. Ensures privacy.
6. Lower side rails on one side of bed and move client's body toward that side of the bed.	Assist nurse in using good body mechanics and permits closer proximity to client.
7. Place hands under client's neck and back of head. Raise head, move chin toward chest, flexing (bending) the neck. Lower head so neck is in a resting position.	ROM exercise for neck. Repeat each step two times.
8. Lower client's head and turn head to one side. Repeat in other direction. Move head to normal resting position.	
9. Rotate head slowly three times. Put client's head in a normal resting position when neck exercises are completed.	
10. Explain steps and reason for exercise to client or significant other.	Teaches client and/or significant other.
11. Hold client's arm farthest away from you by the elbow and hand. Flex (bend) shoulder by raising his or her arm in an arc (circular motion) from bed to above his or her head. Extend (straighten) shoulder and lower arm to client's side of bed.	ROM exercise for shoulder. Repeat each shoulder exercise slowly two times.
12. Abduct (move away from midline of body) shoulder; hold wrist and elbow and move client's arm away from his or her side.	

(Continued on following page)

STEP	RATIONALE
13. Adduct (move toward midline of body) shoulder; return arm over client's body toward opposite side.	
14. Hold upper arm away and out from body at the level of the shoulder; hold elbow and grasp client's palm. Raise his or her hand above head level. Internally rotate shoulder by turning client's palm above his or her head toward the body.	
15. Externally rotate shoulder by moving client's palm (hand) away from the body. Keep hand over client's head during this step.	
16. Flex (bend) elbow by grasping client's palm; place other hand under client's elbow. Move client's forearm toward his or her upper arm.	Exercises elbow through its normal ROM. Repeat each step two times.
17. Extend elbow (straighten arm).	
18. Supinate forearm by holding palm and elbow upward.	Exercises wrist through its normal ROM. Repeat each step slowly two times.
19. Pronate forearm by moving forearm so that palm faces downward.	
20. Flex (bend) wrist by turning hand toward inner part of forearm.	
21. Extend (straighten) wrist.	
22. Hyperextend wrist by moving hand toward the back of arm.	
23. Rotate (turn) thumb toward the thumb (radial) side of hand. Then turn the opposite side of palm toward the little finger.	Exercises finger joints through their normal ROM. Repeat each step slowly two times.
24. Close your hand and fingers around the back of the client's hand while holding his or her wrist; flex (bend) client's finger joints.	
25. Extend (straighten) joints by opening client's hand.	
26. Move client's thumb toward his or her little finger and back again.	
27. Repeat steps 11–26 for arm closest to you.	
28. Place one of your hands under knee and one hand under heel of leg farthest from you.	Exercise knee and hip through their normal ROM. Repeat steps slowly two times.
29. Raise lower leg, making sure that both hip and knee are flexed (bent). Lower leg and straighten (extend) hip and knee.	
30. Keeping one hand under knee and other hand under heel, abduct client's hip by moving leg away from midline of body. Adduct hip by moving leg toward the midline of body and over opposite leg.	
31. Holding the client's heel, rotate (turn) the entire leg internally (inward) and externally (outward).	
32. Put your hand under client's heel, and forearm against bottom of his or her foot. Bend (dorsiflex) the ankle so that toes point upward toward client's knee.	Exercise ankle through its normal ROM. Repeat steps 30–32 two times.
33. Plantar flex (straighten) ankle so that toes point downward, away from knee.	
34. Hold client's heel with one hand and turn (invert) foot inward.	
35. Turn (evert) foot outward with other hand.	
36. Hold bottom of foot over arch with hand, flex (bend) toes forward. Extend (straighten) toes.	
37. Move each toe separately by separating and placing them together.	Exercise toe joints through their normal ROM. Repeat steps three times.
38. Repeat steps 28–37 for opposite leg.	
39. Remove drapes; replace client's clothing and bed linens. Place client in a comfortable position. Replace side rails, if required. Lower bed. Place call signal within easy reach.	Ensures comfort.
40. Open curtains and room door.	
41. Wash hands.	

(Continued on following page)

Nursing Implications: Document procedure and level of ROM. Record and report any unusual signs and symptoms such as complaints of pain. If client complains of severe pain, check with RN or team leader about the possibility of administering pain medication and postpone exercises until client is more comfortable. Note limits of ROM for each joint.

In the presence of risk factors for potential contractures, as in clients who have had a stroke, ROM exercises are essential to prevent development of such contractures.

Check to see if any joints appear swollen or inflamed. On exercising specific joints, report and record any unusual sound or movement. Check muscles of extremities to determine if there is less or more muscle mass in one extremity than in the other. Report all findings to RN or team leader.

Teach joint exercises so that client, if able, may do his or her own active ROM exercises or may participate actively in the exercise as it is given by the nurse.

Procedure: Care of Decubitus Ulcer

Description: Management of stages I–IV decubitus ulcers.

Purpose: To decrease the potential for further breakdown of decubitus ulcers once they have occurred.

Stage I: Reddening of skin. Skin is pinkish-red and mottled. These signs disappear in about 5 minutes once pressure is relieved over the part. Black clients have purplish or darker discoloration. Skin is not broken. There is usually no remaining tissue damage if ulcer is taken care of properly.

Stage II: Superficial (outside) skin damage including superficial blood vessels. Reddening of skin does not disappear with release of pressure. The area is edematous, showing blistered, cracked, or broken skin. Damage to skin may be shallow or include destruction to skin layers (dermis and epidermis).

Stage III: Deep tissue involvement. Skin is broken, drainage is present. Area may be necrotic (black), draining (yellow), or granulating (red). Infection is more likely to occur in ulcers at this stage.

Stage IV: Advanced destruction of capillaries under skin layers and muscle. Large ulcerated areas penetrate to muscle and bone. Dead (necrotic) tissue is visible in the ulcerated area and extensive drainage is present. Infection at this stage is common.

STEP	RATIONALE
Management of Stage I Decubitus Ulcer:	
1. Obtain necessary supplies and equipment:	Organizing necessary supplies and equipment allows for quick and safe implementation.
• Extra pillows	
• Air mattress, egg-crate or foam mattress, sheepskin, alternating-pressure mattress, or water bed	
• Turning sheet	
• Sterile culture tubes	
• Heating lamp (if ordered under supervision of RN)	
• Sterile culture tubes	
• Wound care supplies	
• Irrigating solution	
• Dressings	
• Asepto bulb syringe	
• Basin	
• Disposable gloves	
2. Place client on protective mattress used in your institution.	Distributes body weight evenly to decrease amount of pressure over bony parts of the body.
3. Apply sheepskin heel or elbow protectors.	Protects bony areas against too much pressure over capillaries. These areas have very little fat or muscle.
4. Turn client every 2 hours or less. Use lift or turning sheet; ambulate; exercise as able. Get client up in chair, if ordered, but for not more than 1 hour.	Changes pressure areas.
5. Do not place client on affected area until signs of stage I bedsores disappear.	Decreases pressure on developing decubitus.
6. Check bony parts of body every 2–4 hours.	Checks for early signs.
7. Keep skin dry and free of excretions and secretions.	Excretions and secretions may help in developing bedsores.
8. Do not use soaps, perfumed lotions, or other products with an alcohol base.	Use of such products increases excess drying of skin surfaces.
9. Encourage fluid intake (240 mL every 2 hours unless restricted). Monitor I&O.	Ensures sufficient fluids to maintain body fluid balance.

(Continued on following page)

STEP	RATIONALE
10. Encourage a well-balanced diet, especially with high-protein foods.	Ensures protein intake required for tissue rebuilding.
11. Do not massage the decubitus area.	Massage of decubitus area interferes with protective mechanism of hyperemia.
12. Place pillows to cushion bony areas when sitting in chair or wheelchair.	Protects skin from pressure over time.

Management of Stage II Decubitus Ulcer:

STEP	RATIONALE
1. Use same measures as in stage I. Apply gloves.	Ensures continuation of care.
2. Clean the affected area using sterile technique with sterile saline or other agent prescribed by the physician.	Helps to remove harmful microorganisms or other materials.
3. Rinse area with normal saline.	Removes cleansing agents and other materials.
4. Be careful not to further injure the area of decubitus or surrounding skin area.	Broken skin encourages further breakdown of skin.
5. Apply prescribed medication to decubitus as prescribed by physician or institutional policy.	
6. Apply a sterile dressing (4 × 4 gauze pads) over broken skin area and about 2 inches around area. Secure with paper tape.	Protects open area from micoorganisms; paper tape is less likely to injure skin than other types of tape.
7. Change dressing per hospital protocol or physician's order.	

Management of Stage III Decubitus Ulcers:

STEP	RATIONALE
1. Use the same processes as in stages I and II.	
2. Send a culture specimen of the wound secretions to laboratory.	Identifies organisms responsible for infection.
3. Use medications and treatment as ordered by the physician.	Provides comprehensive care.
4. Encourage diet with increased amount of proteins and vitamin C.	Adds extra protein and vitamin C to assist in tissue rebuilding.
5. Assess client's age and weight, and check about increasing fluid intake.	Lubricates body cells and tissues.
6. Cleanse wound as described in stage II management.	Removes wound secretions, microorganisms, and other waste material.
7. Irrigate ulcer with sterile saline or other solution prescribed by physician. Use sterile technique.	Loosens dead (necrotic) tissue and scabs. Stimulates new tissue growth.
8. Have RN debride necrotic tissue and scabs (eschar) using irrigation and cleansing with saturated gauze pads (sterile technique).	Removes necrotic tissue and other materials.
9. Apply sterile wet to dry dressing for continued debridement.	Helps to continue removal of dead tissue.
10. Apply medication to area as prescribed by physician.	
11. Remove gloves and wash hands.	Decreases spread of microorganisms.

Management of Stage IV Decubitus Ulcers:

STEP	RATIONALE
1. Use same measures as in stages I–III.	
2. RN will consult with physician with regard to medical and/or surgical treatment.	Provides comprehensive treatment. If ulcerated areas are very deep and penetrate to muscle and bone, surgical closure may be necessary. The wound must first be free of infection before surgical treatment is attempted.

Nursing Implications: Assess client for risk of developing decubitus ulcers (e.g., low serum albumin, immobility, incontinence, anemia). Document findings and record measures taken to treat the decubitus ulcer. Report to RN any findings that may indicate the formation of new ulcers. Check to see if the decubitus has progressed from one stage to another; report such findings. Check to see if healing is taking place by determining whether wound secretions and size are decreasing and whether granulation is taking place at the edges of the wound.

Check with RN regarding pain medications if client complains of pain. Check vital signs. A temperature increase may suggest an increase in the decubitus size and development to a further stage.

Be careful when sitting the client up in bed. A shearing force occurs when the client's skin sticks to the bed linen as he or she slides down to the foot of the bed. The tissues underlying the outer skin surface slide simultaneously in the opposite direction, injuring the tissue.

Clients who are poorly nourished may lose muscle mass and subcutaneous tissue. This results in less padding between skin and bone. Fluid and electrolyte imbalances and loss of protein inhibit wound healing. Clients with impaired circulation or anemia and elderly clients are at high risk for development of decubitus ulcers.

Incontinence leads to continuous moisture on the skin and allows growth of bacteria that thrive in a moist, warm, dark environment. This environment is conducive to infection. Infection also increases body temperature, which in turn increases moisture on the skin.

Clients who are immobilized in bed, chair, or wheelchair are susceptible to pressure and the development of decubitus ulcers. Clients in traction or immobilized in a cast may develop decubitus ulcers from pressure from the equipment or cast. Note that pressure sores can also develop from pressure exerted by an improperly secured nasogastric tube or other catheters if present for prolonged periods.

Procedure: Performing Cardiopulmonary Resuscitation

Description: Cardiopulmonary resuscitation (CPR) is the basic emergency procedure for cardiopulmonary arrest and consists of artificial ventilation and manual external cardiac massage.

Purpose: To restore cardiac and respiratory function.

STEP	RATIONALE
1. Assess to determine responsiveness by gently tapping or shaking client's shoulder.	Confirms unconsciousness.
2. If client is unresponsive, call for help and access emergency medical system (EMS).	Assistance may be needed to notify the emergency system.
3. Position the victim by turning on back as a unit, supporting head and neck.	For CPR to be effective, the person must be supine and on a firm, flat surface.
4. Determine breathlessness by opening or maintaining the airway. Use head-tilt/chin-lift maneuver. Place ear over the person's mouth and observe the chest—look, listen, and feel for breathing. In infants (younger than 1 year), do not hyperextend the neck.	The most important action in successful resuscitation is immediate opening of the airway. Hyperextending the neck in infants blocks off the airway.
5. If no respirations are noted, deliver two ventilations at 1.0–1.5 seconds per inspiration. Observe chest rise and fall before delivering the second ventilation. Maintain head-tilt/chin-lift position during ventilations; pinch nose with one hand and seal mouth completely. Deliver only as much volume as needed to expand the chest.	An excess of air volume and fast inspiratory flow rates are likely to cause gastric distention.
6. Assess to determine pulselessness. Adult: Feel for carotid pulse for 5–10 seconds while maintaining head-tilt with the other hand. Child (1–8 years): Check carotid pulse 5–10 seconds. Infant: Check brachial pulse 5–10 seconds.	Chest compressions should not be performed on a person with a pulse. Time should be allowed for correct assessment of pulselessness.
7. If pulseless, begin chest compressions and repeat call for help: a. Kneel by victim's shoulders. b. Locate proper hand position and begin compressions. Adults: Compress 1.5–2.0 inches with a rate of 80–100 per minute. Child: Compress 1.0–1.5 inches with a rate of 80–100 per minute. Infant: Compress 0.5–1.0 inches with a rate of 100 per minute.	b. Proper hand position reduces risk of injury. Proper hand position and compression depth ensure adequate circulation of blood volume.
8. Compression-to-ventilation rate: Adult—one-person CPR: 15 compressions to two ventilations at 1.5–2.0 seconds per inspiration. Adult—two-person CPR: five compressions to one ventilation. Child: Five compressions to one ventilation. Infant: Five compressions to one ventilation.	

(Continued on following page)

STEP	RATIONALE
9. Assessment for pulse after: Adult—one-person CPR: Four cycles of 15 compressions to two ventilations (or 1 minute). Adult—two-person CPR: After 1 minute and at intervals thereafter. Child: 10 cycles of five compressions to one ventilation. Infant: 10 cycles of five compressions to one ventilation.	
10. Determine pulselessness by assessing for 5 seconds. If pulse and ventilations are absent, continue CPR. If pulse but no respiration is present, perform rescue breathing: Adult: 12 times per minute Child: 15 times per minute Infant: 20 times per minute	
11. If pulse and respirations are present, monitor the person and contact emergency medical personnel. Place in recovery position. Client lies on right side, with upper leg slightly drawn up and left arm crooked. Hand is under head.	All persons who undergo CPR need to be seen by the physician.

Nursing Implications: All nursing personnel need to be certified annually for basic life support (BLS). Support CPR efforts for as long as possible or until emergency personnel are on the scene. Do not interrupt CPR for more than 7 seconds except in special circumstances.

Procedure: Care of Client with Skeletal Traction

Description: Metal pins or nails are inserted into the tissue structure and attached to traction devices.

Purpose: To immobilize, position, or align a fractured bone and facilitate healing; to provide supportive care and safety measures.

STEP	RATIONALE
1. Examine traction for proper body alignment and weight. Check knots, ropes, and pulleys.	Ensures proper traction. Make sure that weights are free swinging.
2. Assess client's response: note presence of pain, spasm, or sense of comfort.	Relief of pain or muscle spasms may not be immediate.
3. Administer narcotics or relaxants as ordered and needed.	Decreases anxiety and ensures comfort.
4. Check affected extremity for temperature, pulses, color, movement (of fingers or toes) and sensation every 1–2 degrees × 24 hours, then as ordered.	Provides information on neurovascular status.
5. Wash hands and don sterile gloves. Perform pin care using sterile technique by cleansing area around pin insertion site with prescribed cleansing agent.	Reduces microorganisms at insertion sites. Check with physician before performing site care.
6. Observe insertion sites for signs of redness, swelling, or drainage.	Indicates presence of inflammation or infection.
7. Remove gloves and wash hands.	Decreases spread of microorganisms.

Nursing Implications: Be alert for signs and symptoms of fat embolism: restlessness, mental status alterations, tachycardia, tachypnea, hypotension, dyspnea, and petechial rash over upper chest and neck. Clients at risk are those with long bone fractures. Fat embolism usually occurs within the first 72 hours.

Report any signs of swelling (edema), increased pain, or inability to move joints, which could indicate compartment syndrome. This leads to decreased perfusion and tissue anoxia.

Procedure: Applying an Abdominal Binder

Description: A snugly fitting wrap is secured across an abdominal incision.

Purpose: To provide support of the operative incision site and underlying musculature; to provide comfort and security with movement.

STEP	RATIONALE
1. Obtain abdominal binder of appropriate size. The binder should be large enough to wrap around abdomen and overlap for safe securing of Velcro closure. Measure abdomen with tape measure, if necessary.	Abdominal binder must be of appropriate size for fit and comfort.
2. Position client lying on side. Fold one end of binder and place against back toward midline.	This position is more comfortable for placement of binder.
3. Roll client in the other direction over the folded end of the binder. Pull out folded section and smoothe.	Lessens the pull on abdominal incision and muscles.
4. Roll client on back over center of binder and position so that lower edge of binder is at level of symphysis pubis.	Centering ensures proper placement and support of underlying structures.
5. Pull distal end over abdomen and maintain tension while pulling proximal portion over. Secure with Velcro closure.	
6. Ask client whether binder feels secure and comfortable.	

Nursing Implications: A binder that is too tight may hinder breathing and limit circulation. A binder that is positioned incorrectly may pull on incision line and cause separation and bleeding. Assess respirations with binder on and readjust if necessary.

Procedure: Applying a Sling

Description: A triangular cloth is applied to securely hold the affected arm in a bent position across chest. Manufactured slings with Velcro closures are also used.

Purpose: To immobilize the affected arm, providing support and decreasing muscle strain.

STEP	RATIONALE
1. Obtain triangular bandage or commercial sling. Position open sling with binder center under arm, pointed end at wrist, and base of triangle at elbow.	Provides support at elbow.
2. Pull ends up, encasing arm in sling, bent at elbow. Position arm across chest.	Reduces strain on shoulder and neck muscles.
3. Bring top of binder point over neck on unaffected side.	
4. Bring other binder point over neck on affected side.	
5. Position arm with wrist above elbow. Tie ends behind neck in square knot.	Enhances circulation. Prevents dependent edema of wrist and hand.
6. Place gauze squares between neck and sling knot to pad the area.	Enhances comfort.
7. Fold remaining bandage around elbow for support and fasten with safety pin.	

Nursing Implications: Assess circulation (color, pulses, warmth), mobility, and sensation of extremities. Assess skin daily for signs of pressure or breakdown. Provide padding or readjust sling as necessary.

Procedure: Assisting with a Sitz Bath

Description: A specially designed tub allows the client to sit in warm water without immersing legs or upper trunk.

Purpose: To promote circulation, relaxation, and comfort to incisional areas, wounds, or hemorrhoids.

STEP	RATIONALE
1. Fill sitz tub or bathtub with warm water. Add medications, if ordered.	Excessively warm water can damage tissue and cause burns.
2. Assist client into sitting position in tub. Adjust water temperature if necessary.	Water should feel comfortably warm to client.
3. Place bath blanket around client's shoulders, if desired. Place a call signal next to client.	Prevents chilling.
4. After 15 minutes, assist client out of tub and dry skin gently.	Ensures safety.

Nursing Implications: Instruct client not to attempt to get out of tub alone if he or she is weak or unsteady. For bedridden clients, a plastic sitz basin can be used. Have client notify nurse if symptoms such as dizziness arise. Be prepared to check blood pressure and discontinue sitz bath if hypotension occurs. Properly clean bath basin between uses.

Procedure: Applying Warm Soaks

Description: Affected body part is immersed in warm water or warmed solutions for a prescribed period of time.

Purpose: To debride wounds and improve circulation; to apply medicated solutions that facilitate healing.

STEP	RATIONALE
1. Fill basin with warmed water or solution. Test for proper temperature.	Excessively high temperature may damage tissues or cause burns.
2. Place waterproof pad under client if soiling of linen is likely.	
3. Immerse affected body part in basin.	
4. Cover client with a bath blanket to prevent chilling.	
5. Allow to soak for 15–20 minutes. Remove and gently pat dry.	Ensures comfort.

Nursing Implications: If it is not possible to soak a body area in a basin, towels may be soaked in the warmed solution and applied. Wrap toweled area in waterproof pad and leave in place for approximately 15 minutes.

If continuous warm soaks are ordered, wrap a heating pad around the moist towel or sterile saline dressings and waterproof pad; keep on low warming temperature. Wet towel or dressings with solution every 1–2 hours. Check to be sure that temperature is not too warm. Assess skin and wound condition and document.

Procedure: Using a Heat Lamp

Description: An application of dry heat using 40- to 75-watt infrared or regular household bulb situated at a safe distance from the client's skin.

Purpose: To promote circulation and healing without risk of injury from the heat source.

STEP	RATIONALE
1. Provide privacy for client.	
2. Assist client into a comfortable position that exposes the area to be treated. Pad with pillows, if necessary.	Because client will have to maintain position for 15–20 minutes, ensure that position is comfortable.
3. Make sure that skin to be exposed is dry.	Moisture may act as a conductor of heat.
4. Place heat lamp about 24 inches away for 40–60 watts and about 30 inches away for 75 watts. Turn on lamp.	Protects skin from burning.
5. Adjust light for direct effect on area to be treated. Position call bell and instruct client to ring for nurse if experiencing any discomfort.	Ensures that the correct area is treated with heat. Ensures safety.
6. While heat lamp treatment is in progress, check client every 5 minutes. Assess skin and position of lamp.	Some clients may have decreased sensation. Assess any changes in skin condition.

(Continued on following page)

STEP	RATIONALE
7. After 20 minutes, discontinue the treatment. Assess skin condition and redress wound, if required. Position for comfort.	Some clients may not be able to tolerate the heat treatment for the entire period.

Nursing Implications: Document procedure, including the amount of heat, distance of source from skin, length of treatment, area treated, and client's response.

Procedure: Teaching Controlled Coughing Techniques

Description: When the cough reflex is diminished because of central nervous system depression, anesthesia, pain, or sedation, the potential for atelectasis (collapsed lung) and infection increases.

Purpose: To clear airway of secretions; to prevent pneumonia, atelectasis, and airway infections.

STEP	RATIONALE
1. Identify clients at risk for ineffective cough: those with lung diseases, profound weakness, immobility, postoperative states, central nervous system diseases, depression, lung cancer, or an artificial airway.	Certain conditions predispose client for the nursing diagnosis of ineffective airway clearance.
2. Place client in best position for cough effectiveness. Usually sitting up and leaning forward is most beneficial.	Allows lung expansion and expiratory effort.
3. Deep breathing and coughing: Position client upright. Have client take two or three deep breaths, hold last breath for count of three, then cough twice forcefully while pulling in abdominal muscles. If client is recovering from surgery, splint incisional area with hands or a pillow.	Taking deep breaths expands the lung, moving air behind mucous secretions. Two consecutive coughs help to remove secretions and dislodge mucus. Splinting reduces the pain of coughing by decreasing incisional pulling.
4. Cascade cough: Have client take slow, deep breaths and hold second breath for count of two. Instruct client to open mouth and cough several times in succession while contracting expiratory muscles. The client should cough until all the air is expelled. After each cascade cough, have client breathe slowly and quietly, allowing a period of rest.	The cascade cough helps to clear large and small airways. Rest prevents paroxysms of coughing.
5. Huff cough: Have client take two slow, deep breaths and hold second breath for a count of two. Instead of a series of coughs, have the client say "huff."	Clients with lung disease may not be able to perform cascade cough. Huff cough may be effective in producing natural cough reflex.
6. Quad cough: Have client take two slow, deep breaths and hold second breath for count of two. Have client exhale forcefully while nurse or client presses upward and inward against diaphragm.	External pressure assists the muscular efforts of the cough and assists in expelling secretions.

Nursing Implications: Observe and record effectiveness of coughing techniques. Support and encourage client efforts. For clients with copious or tenacious secretions, coughing techniques may need to be performed every hour. For the routine postoperative client, coughing techniques should be performed every 2 hours.

Procedure: Nasal and Oral Pharyngeal Suctioning

Description: These two procedures involve inserting a plastic suction tube into the nasal or oral pharynx and then applying suction to remove secretions.

Purpose: To remove excess oral and nasal secretions and prevent aspiration of secretions or body fluids; to provide a patent airway.

STEP	RATIONALE

1. Obtain necessary equipment:
  • Suction source
  • Suction catheter kit with sterile gloves
  • Sterile distilled water
  • Sterile water-soluble lubricant
  • Connecting tubing
  • Towel
	Organizing necessary equipment allows quick and safe implementation.

2. Have client assume semi-Fowler's position, if allowed, and place towel across the chest.	This position is generally comfortable for the client and accessible for the nurse. The towel protects the client and bed linen from secretions.
3. Turn on suction source and adjust setting. Start with 100–150 mm Hg and increase as necessary.	Excessive suction pressures may cause trauma to tissues. Pressure needed for suctioning may vary depending on catheter size and amount and consistency of secretion.
4. Attach connecting tubing to suction.	
5. Unwrap suction kit package. Open inner suction package and carefully remove sterile basin. Open basin and pour in sterile water. Do not touch inside of sterile basin or any part of the inner suction kit package.	Prevents contamination of equipment.
6. Open lubrication jelly and carefully expel contents onto sterile section of the inner suction package.	Use water-soluble lubricant. Lubrication decreases trauma to tissues and allows easier insertion of suction catheter.
7. Apply sterile gloves.	
8. Pick up suction catheter wrapped in plastic bag with nondominant hand. With dominant hand, remove suction catheter and attach to connecting tubing. Be sure to keep sterile hand and sterile catheter tip from becoming contaminated.	Prepares for suctioning while preventing the spread of microorganisms.
9. Check suction by suctioning a small amount of sterile water from prepared basin.	Checks suction before beginning procedure.
10. Coat suction catheter tip with lubricant.	
11. Insert catheter into naris using dominant hand and pass gently into the pharynx using a downward slant. If resistance is met, do not force.	
12. Apply suction by placing nondominant thumb over vent in catheter tubing. Use an intermittent suction rather than continuous suction, pulling back catheter slowly.	Limit suction time to 10 seconds or less. Intermittent suction reduces trauma to tissues.
13. Rinse catheter in sterile water, using continuous suctioning until catheter is clear of secretions.	
14. Repeat steps 12 and 13 until secretions are cleared. Allow rest time between suctioning.	

Nursing Implications: If oxygen is in use, remove before suctioning and replace after suctioning. Observe client's respiratory and cardiac status; suctioning can cause hypoxia, arrhythmias, and bronchospasm.

Document client's response to suctioning, including respiratory status before and after. Note and chart the color, amount, and consistency of secretions. If client requires frequent nasal pharyngeal suctioning, a nasal airway may be required to limit trauma to tissues. In clients with bleeding disorders, nasal pharyngeal suctioning is generally contraindicated.

Procedure: Nasal and Oral Tracheal Suctioning

Description: This procedure involves inserting a suction catheter through the nasal or oral passage into the trachea to clear the airway.

Purpose: To remove secretions and maintain airway clearance; to stimulate deep cough reflex.

STEP	RATIONALE
1. Follow steps 1–9 of the procedure for nasal and oral pharyngeal suctioning.	

(Continued on following page)

STEP	RATIONALE
2. Insert lubricated catheter gently into naris with dominant hand. Angle catheter tip downward to pass it through to the pharynx. Do not apply suction. Have client take a breath and pass catheter quickly into trachea. Apply intermittent suction with nondominant thumb over vent in catheter tubing. Limit suction time to 10 seconds. Rotate catheter back and forth while removing slowly. Client usually coughs when trachea entered.	Suctioning during insertion of catheter increases hypoxia. Intermittent suctioning prevents undue trauma to tissues.
3. Rinse catheter in sterile water until catheter is clear of secretions.	
4. Repeat steps 2 and 3, if necessary, allowing a short period of rest between suctioning.	Rest reduces risk of impaired oxygenation.

Nursing Implications: If oxygen is in use, remove before suctioning and replace immediately after. The depth required for proper nasal tracheal suctioning in the adult is approximately 20 cm. To verify correct length, measure from nose to ear and ear to mid sternum. If resistance is met during suctioning, release suction pressure. If resistance is met passing the catheter, do not force.

Document client response to suctioning, including respiratory status before and after. Note and chart the color, amount, and consistency of secretions. If client requires frequent nasal tracheal suctioning, a nasal airway may be required.

Procedure: Endotracheal or Tracheostomy Tube Suctioning

Description: Involves passing a suction catheter through an endotracheal or tracheostomy tube to remove secretions.

Purpose: To remove secretions and maintain a patent airway; to stimulate cough reflex.

STEP	RATIONALE
1. Collect necessary equipment: • Suction source • Suction catheter kit with sterile gloves • Sterile distilled water • Sterile water-soluble lubricant • Connecting tubing • Ambu bag with reservoir tubing and tracheostomy adaptor • Oxygen supply with appropriate tubing to connect to Ambu bag • Sterile gauze • Sterile saline for suctioning (optional) • Towel	Organizing necessary equipment allows for safe and quick implementation.
2. Connect Ambu bag to oxygen source and turn flowmeter to 15 L. Attach connecting tubing to suction device.	
3. Have client assume semi-Fowler's position, if allowed, and place towel across chest.	This position is generally comfortable for the client and accessible for the nurse. The towel protects the client and bed linen from secretions.
4. Turn on suction source and adjust setting. Start with 100–150 mm Hg and increase as necessary.	Excessive suction pressures may cause trauma to tissues. Pressure needed for suctioning may vary depending on catheter size and/or amount and consistency of secretions.
5. Unwrap suction kit package. Open inner suction package and carefully remove sterile basin. Open basin and pour in sterile water. Do not touch inside of sterile basin or any part of the inner suction kit package.	Avoids contamination of equipment.
6. Apply sterile gloves.	
7. Pick up suction catheter, wrapped in plastic bag, with nondominant hand. With dominant hand, remove suction	Prepares for suctioning while preventing the spread of microorganisms.

(Continued on following page)

STEP	RATIONALE
catheter and attach to connecting tubing. Be sure to keep sterile glove and sterile catheter tip from becoming contaminated.	
8. Check suction by aspirating a small amount of sterile water from prepared basin.	
9. Remove oxygen delivery device or humidity source from endotracheal or tracheostomy tube with nondominant hand. Using Ambu bag, deliver two to three hyperinflated breaths.	Preoxygenation reduces risk of altered oxygenation during suctioning procedure.
10. With dominant hand, insert suction catheter into endotracheal or tracheostomy tube and pass gently but quickly into trachea. Do not activate suction during insertion of catheter.	Suctioning during catheter insertion will increase hypoxia.
11. Insert catheter until resistance is met. Recent research indicates that a premeasured depth of insertion decreases trauma. Pull back about 1 cm and activate suction using the nondominant thumb over the vent of the suction tubing. Suction intermittently while pulling back slowly on the catheter, using a rotating movement.	Limit suction time to 10 seconds to prevent hypoxia. Intermittent suctioning reduces trauma to the tissues.
12. Hyperoxygenate client using Ambu bag. Give two to three breaths.	
13. Rinse catheter in sterile water using continuous suctioning until catheter is clear of secretions.	
14. Repeat steps 12 and 13 if necessary. Replace oxygen delivery device after completion of procedure.	

Nursing Implications: Document client response to suctioning, including respiratory status before and after. Note and chart color, amount, and consistency of secretions. Observe respiratory and cardiac status; suctioning can cause hypoxia, arrhythmias, and bronchospasm.

   NOTE: If secretions are particularly thick and difficult to remove, sterile saline (about 5–10 mL) may be instilled before hyperoxygenation with Ambu bag. It takes practice to perform endotracheal or tracheostomy tube suctioning alone. The procedure is easier with two nurses, one to operate the Ambu bag and one to suction.

Procedure: Care of the Artificial Eye

Description: Cleansing the artificial eye is performed with soap and water.

Purpose: To provide integrity of the eye socket, prevent infection, and maintain client's self-image.

STEP	RATIONALE
1. Collect necessary equipment: • Washcloth • Wash basin with warm water • Mild soap • Rubber bulb syringe • Saline	Organizing necessary equipment allows safe and quick implementation.
2. Wash hands thoroughly before proceeding with intervention.	Prevents transfer of microorganisms to the eye tissues.
3. To remove prosthesis, gently pull back lower eyelid and press lightly against lower orbital ridge below eyelid.	This breaks the suction within the eye socket and allows the artificial eye to slide out.
4. Clean prosthesis with mild soap and warm water. Handle with care. Rinse well and dry with washcloth or tissue.	Removes microorganisms that may cause infection.
5. Clean eyelid and eye socket with washcloth or gauze moistened with saline. Dry with gauze.	Cleansing without soap is necessary, as soap is difficult to remove and may cause irritation.
6. To replace prosthesis, expose eye socket with thumb and index finger of nondominant hand. Place moistened	Careful and correct insertion of prosthesis allows proper fit.

(Continued on following page)

STEP	RATIONALE
artificial eye into socket with notched edge toward nose. Depress lower lid to allow artificial eye to slip into place. Make sure eyelashes are turned away from prosthesis.	
7. Observe the position of the artificial eye and ask the client if proper fit has been achieved.	Ensures proper position of prosthesis.

Nursing Implications: If artificial eye is not replaced in client, store in water in covered plastic case. Observe and report any changes in tissue surrounding the eye, particularly signs of infection. Remove artificial eye and store appropriately before sending client to surgery. Avoid demonstrating any signs of revulsion about the procedure. The procedure for cleansing the artificial eye need not be sterile. Maintain client's dignity and privacy during procedure.

Procedure: Administering Eyedrops and Ointment

Description: Eyedrops and ointment must be instilled correctly.

Purpose: To treat infection and combat irritation; to supply moisture and lubrication to the cornea; to dilate or constrict the pupil.

STEP	RATIONALE
1. Wash hands well and don disposable gloves before instilling medication.	Prevents transfer of microorganisms.
2. Using forefinger of nondominant hand, pull lower eyelid down by placing finger over cheek bone and pulling down gently. Instruct client to look upward.	Exposes inner surface of lid.
3. Drop eyedrop medication into center of lower lid. If instilling ointment, squeeze tube gently to deposit a ribbon of medication along lower lid.	Medication should not be instilled directly onto cornea. Take care not to touch the eye with the dropper or ointment tube tip. Prevents contamination of medication.
4. Instruct client to slowly close eyes and slowly open.	If medication can cause systemic effects, apply gentle pressure with gloved finger to client's nasolacrimal duct for 30–60 seconds. Allows medication to be distributed evenly. Prevents systemic distribution of drugs, which could cause adverse side effects.
5. Wipe off excess medication with a tissue and instruct client not to rub the eye.	
6. Remove gloves and wash hands after procedure.	Prevents transfer of microorganisms.

Nursing Implications: Observe and record appearance of the eye and response to treatment. If client is to be discharged home with eye medication, teach proper administration to client and family. Medications stored in refrigerator should be warmed to room temperature before use. Provide safety measures if client has blurred vision after instillation of eye medication.

Procedure: Administering Eardrops

Description: Eardrops must be instilled correctly.

Purpose: To treat infection and relieve discomfort; to loosen cerumen for removal.

STEP	RATIONALE
1. Have client lie on side, with affected ear up.	
2. Pull pinna upward and outward to expose ear canal. In children, pull pinna down and back.	Provides easier acccess to ear canal structures.
3. Instill the prescribed medication. Hold dropper 0.5 inch above ear canal.	
4. Have client lie on side for several minutes. Apply gentle massage to tragus of ear.	Allows even distribution of medication.

Nursing Implications: Do not force eardrops into an occluded ear canal. If cerumen or drainage is present, wipe gently with a cotton-tipped applicator. Do not force cerumen inward. Eardrops should be warmed to room temperature before use.

Record condition of the ear and response to medication. If the client is to be discharged home with eardrops, teach client and family proper procedure. Gloves should be worn if any drainage from client's ear is present.

Procedure: Administering Nasal Medications

Description: Nasal spray and drops must be instilled correctly.

Purpose: To relieve nasal congestion, inflammation, and irritation.

STEP	RATIONALE
Instilling Nasal Spray:	
1. Wash hands and don clean gloves. Place client in supine position.	Gloves should be worn to decrease spread of microorganisms.
2. Ask client to occlude one nostril. Spray required amount in other nostril and ask client to inhale simultaneously.	
3. Repeat step 2 for opposite nostril.	
4. Client may blot nose but should not blow nose for several minutes.	Allows time for medication to be absorbed.
5. Remove gloves and wash hands.	Decreases spread of microorganisms.
Instilling Nasal Drops:	
1. Wash hands and don clean gloves. Place client in supine position.	Gloves should be worn to decrease spread of microorganisms.
2. Tilt head backward. Use a small pillow or rolled towel under neck for support.	This position allows for medication to reach sinus area.
3. Have client breathe through mouth.	Decreases risk of aspiration of medication.
4. Instill nasal drops by holding dropper 0.5 inch above nares. Instill medication midline toward the ethmoid bone.	Allows proper distribution of medication.
5. Have client remain in same position for 5 minutes.	
6. Client may blot nose but should not blow nose for several minutes.	Allows medication to be absorbed.
7. Remove gloves and wash hands.	Decreases spread of microorganisms.

Nursing Implications: Nasal decongestants may cause rebound effect and should only be used as directed for 3–5 days. Dropper or applicator need not be sterile; rinse in hot water after each use.

Record effect on breathing. Record color of secretions.

Procedure: Administering Medications Intramuscularly via Z-Track Method

Description: The Z-track method of injection deposits the medication into the muscle without tracking residual medication.

Purpose: To protect the skin and subcutaneous tissues from irritating medications.

STEP	RATIONALE
1. Wash hands thoroughly before preparing medication for injection.	Prevents transfer of microorganisms.
2. Prepare medication for administration as directed. Draw medication into the syringe.	
3. Apply a new needle to the syringe:	Ensures that no solution remains on the needle shaft.

(Continued on following page)

STEP	RATIONALE
• 23 gauge 1.0–1.5 inches for adults • 25–27 gauge 0.5–1.0 inch for children	
4. Draw up 0.2–0.3 mL of air to create an air lock.	An air lock prevents tracking medication into subcutaneous tissue.
5. Select an intramuscular site, preferably dorsal gluteal or ventrogluteal, and prepare with an antiseptic swab.	
6. Pull the skin and subcutaneous tissues 1.0–1.5 inches laterally.	
7. Holding skin taut with nondominant hand, inject needle at a 90-degree angle deep into muscle tissue.	
8. Aspirate on syringe; then inject medication if no blood return is noted.	Aspirate to ensure that needle is not in blood vessel.
9. After withdrawing needle, release the skin immediately.	This method leaves a zigzag path that seals the medication within the muscle tissue.

Nursing Implications: Medications such as iron should be given via the Z-track method. Record location of injection and method of medication record. Observe site for any signs of tissue irritation.

Procedure: Mixing Medications from Two Vials

Description: Two medications for intramuscular injection are drawn up into one syringe.

Purpose: To reduce the number of injections administered to the client.

STEP	RATIONALE
Mixing Medication from a Single and Multidose Vial:	
1. Check compatibility of medications with pharmacy or their reference. In a syringe, pull back a volume of air equal to the amount of solution needed from the single-dose vial.	
2. Inject the air from the syringe into the single-dose vial.	Creates positive pressure needed to withdraw solution.
3. Using the same syringe, aspirate a volume of air equal to the amount of solution needed from the multidose vial.	
4. Inject air into multidose vial and withdraw desired amount. Withdraw syringe carefully.	
5. Insert needle into single-dose vial and pull back desired dosage.	The positive pressure in single-dose vial allows for easier withdrawal.
6. Discard needle in proper receptacle and place a new needle on syringe.	Decreases potential for transfer of microorganisms. Placing a new needle on the syringe assures that the needle is sharp, especially if injection is to be given intramuscularly. Makes injection less painful.

Nursing Implications: Be certain that medications mixed in the same syringe are compatible. A cloudy appearance noted in the syringe after mixing may indicate incompatibility. Care must be taken not to contaminate the multidose vial. When the volume of the air is injected into the single-dose vial, be careful not to allow the needle to touch the solution.

Some medications may be saved if entire bottle is not used. Other medications should be discarded (e.g., those without a preservative). Narcotics that are wasted must be witnessed by an RN.

Procedure: Administering Blood Products (check with institutional policy and state LPN law)

Description: Procedure involves initiating blood therapy and monitoring client for adverse reactions.

Purpose: To replace blood volume lost as a result of surgery, trauma, or disease process.

STEP	RATIONALE
1. Obtain blood component consent form if applicable.	Required by some agencies.
2. Assess IV site for inflammation. Note size of IV catheter. If smaller than 20 gauge, a new IV infusion must be started.	IV catheters smaller than 20 gauge may cause damage to red blood cells and clotting in the catheter. Make sure that IV catheter is patent and of appropriate size before picking up unit from blood bank. The unit must be hung within 30 minutes.
3. According to agency protocol, obtain blood product from blood bank.	
4. Verify blood component with RN. Check and compare the following information: a. Client's name and hospital identification number with the prepared unit b. Client's blood group and Rh type with those of the donor unit c. Crossmatch compatibility of donor unit to client's blood d. Blood expiration date e. Hospital unit number on blood bag and blood slip f. All information, to ensure correctness g. Blood for abnormal appearance (e.g., clots or color changes)	Strict verification procedure must be followed to protect client from incompatible blood.
5. Check client's arm band with blood product information. *Do not* administer if any information (name, hospital number) does not match.	
6. Obtain and record baseline vital signs (including temperature).	Important to note pretransfusion status.
7. Using a Y-tubing blood administration set, spike a 0.9 normal-saline IV administration bag. Flush tubing with normal saline solution and prime the filter chamber. Close all roller clamps after tubing is flushed. Some agencies also require a microaggregate filter.	Normal saline solution is isotonic and reduces hemolysis. Do not administer with dextrose solutions or any medications. Filters remove large aggregates or microaggregates that may form in stored units of whole blood or packed red blood cells.
8. Attach end of flushed Y-tubing to the hub of an 18- or 20-gauge (or larger) IV catheter. Securely tape tubing in place.	A large-bore catheter prevents hemolysis.
9. Spike blood bag with second tubing of blood administration set. Open clamp below blood component bag and regulate flow with roller clamp below filter.	
10. Infuse blood slowly (2–5 mL/min), remaining with client during first 15–20 minutes.	Most blood reactions occur in the first 15–20 minutes.
11. Document client's vital signs according to institutional policy.	Changes in vital signs may be an indication of transfusion reaction.
12. Regulate infusion according to physician's orders. Rotate blood bag periodically.	Infusion rate should be based on age, cardiac status, and rate of blood loss. Rotation mixes and maintains infusion, reducing risk of clotting.
13. Observe client for signs of transfusion reaction such as chills, fever, flushing, rash, dyspnea, chest pain, or itching. Stop infusion and notify physician of any signs of reaction. Start infusion of normal saline at a keep-open rate to maintain IV patency. Follow institutional policy for transfusion reaction, which usually involves sending remaining blood and tubing to the laboratory along with a urine specimen. The physician may order medications such as antihistamines.	
14. After blood is administered, close roller clamp of tubing connected to saline and flush tubing.	Infuses remainder of blood in tubing and filter chamber. Keeps vein open between units.
15. Note and record vital signs 1 hour after infusion.	Blood reactions can occur up to 1 hour after transfusion.

Nursing Implications: If an 18- to 20-gauge or large-bore IV catheter is needed, begin before obtaining the blood from the blood bank. Blood components should not hang for longer than 4–5 hours because of risk for bacterial growth, destruction of red blood cells, and clotting in tubing. Only one unit at a time should be obtained from the blood bank. For rapid infusion, a pressure bag may be used around the unit of blood. Pressure should not exceed 300 mm Hg. *Do not* use infusion machines unless specifically designed for blood; other machines will damage cells. Blood warmers may be required if rapid administration of blood products will be detrimental or if the client has cold agglutinins.

Procedure: Bottle-Feeding an Infant

Description: Nutritional feeding is provided via a nippled bottle.

Purpose: To provide proper nutritional intake for growth and development; to maintain fluid balance; to provide nurturing and bonding.

STEP	RATIONALE
1. Prepare formula according to instructions. Prepare the bottle with sterile nipple.	
2. Check infant's armband to ensure correct identification and correct formula.	Eliminates chance of giving the wrong formula to the infant.
3. Position infant for bottle feeding. Sit comfortably in chair. Cradle infant in one arm, while supporting against chest or lap.	Ensures comfort, safety, and security.
4. Touch corner of mouth with tip of nipple.	Stimulates rooting reflex, causing infant to turn toward nipple.
5. Hold bottle inverted with nipple down and insert filled nipple into infant's mouth.	Holding bottle upright prevents infant from sucking air.
6. Burp infant once during feeding and after feeding is completed. Some infants require more burping than others.	Releases swallowed air. Helps absorption of feeding.
7. Allow baby to feed until satisfied, around 10–25 minutes.	
8. Place infant on back after feeding.	Prevents regurgitation.

Nursing Implications: Assess infant for signs of allergic reaction to formula: rash, flushing, diarrhea, increased crying. Infant should gain weight and demonstrate tolerance to formula. Warm formula to room temperature; do not allow to sit out on counter. Some prepared formulas require refrigeration; others do not.

Procedure: Administering Enteral Nutrition via Nasogastric or Gastrostomy Tube

Description: The procedure involves instilling easily digestible nutrients into the stomach, allowing delivery of partially digested nutrients to the bowel at a slow rate. Enteral feedings are administered via nasogastric or gastrostomy tube.

Purpose: To maintain or promote nutritional status.

STEP	RATIONALE
1. Collect necessary equipment: • 60-mL syringe • Enteral tube-feeding formula • Enteral feeding bag and tubing • Enteral feeding pump	Organizing necessary equipment allows quick and safe implementation.
2. Connect tubing to bag and add proper formula in ordered strength. Some agencies add blue dye (usually food coloring) to formula to detect aspiration in clients with a tracheostomy.	
3. Prime tubing with formula and set up infusion pump.	An infusion pump helps to regulate continuous feeding.
4. Place client in high-Fowler's position. If client is to receive continuous tube feeding, position client with head elevated at least 30 degrees.	Elevation of head prevents aspiration.
5. Assess for presence of bowel sounds.	Indicates peristalsis.

(Continued on following page)

STEP	RATIONALE
6. Check placement of nasogastric or gastrostomy tube by instilling a small amount of air (10 mL) via 60-mL syringe into tube. Auscultate simultaneously over epigastrium. Air will be heard entering the stomach.	Verifies correct placement of tube, ensuring that tube is not displaced.
7. Aspirate gastric contents to check residual. If greater than 50–100 mL, notify physician and hold feeding. **NOTE:** Small, soft feeding tubes usually collapse on aspiration and no residual is obtained. Flush with water after aspirating gastric contents.	Indicates delayed gastric emptying.
8. Connect tube feeding and begin at prescribed rate. Check for gastric residual at least every 8 hours.	Checking for residual allows assessment of gastric motility and absorption of forumula.

Nursing Implications: If client is receiving continuous tube feedings, hang only enough formula to last 3–4 hours. (Some formulas may hang longer at room temperature.) Formulas hanging longer are susceptible to bacterial growth. Change tubing and bag every 24 hours. Check to see if the tape is securely in place.

If pulmonary aspiration occurs, notify physician, suction client to remove gastric contents from lungs, and obtain a chest radiograph. Hold feedings until client is evaluated by physician.

If feeding tube is occluded, remove it and insert a new tube. Follow guidelines for insertion.

If intermittent or bolus feedings are ordered, attach 60-mL syringe, without plunger, to fit the end of tube. Add amount of formula ordered by physician and allow to infuse by gravity. Flush tubing with 30–60 mL of water after bolus feeding. To administer medications, prepare according to hospital policy (crushing tablets or obtaining elixir forms) and give as bolus feedings. Flush tubing with water (30–60 mL) after giving medications.

Check for tube placement at least once every 8 hours and before administering medications.

Note and record residuals every 8 hours. Note and record abdominal assessment, daily weights, electrolytes, and bowel status each day. Clients may develop diarrhea, which requires reducing the strength of the enteral formula or addition of an antidiarrheal agent. To prevent the development of diarrhea, the tube feeding is often started at one-half strength and then increased to full strength over a period of a few days.

If gastrostomy tube is in place, wash area daily with soap and water. A clean gauze dressing may be placed over the site.

Procedure: Administering Enteral Feeding via a Jejunostomy or Nasojejunal Feeding Tube

Description: The procedure involves giving tube feedings via the jejunal route, bypassing the stomach, and is indicated for clients with gastric resection, gastric cancer, or chronic nausea and vomiting.

Purpose: To provide and maintain nutritional status; to reduce risk of aspiration.

STEP	RATIONALE
1. Collect necessary equipment: • 60-mL syringe • Enteral tube-feeding formula • Enteral feeding bag and tubing • Enteral feeding pump	Organizing necessary equipment ensures quick and safe implementation.
2. Connect tubing to bag containing formula in ordered strength.	Initiation of feeding usually involves administering diluted formula and increasing strength as tolerated.
3. Prime tubing with formula and set up infusion pump.	An infusion pump helps to regulate continuous feeding.
4. Elevate client's head at least 30 degrees.	Elevating the head of bed prevents aspiration, although risk is reduced with the feeding tube in the jejunum.
5. Assess for presence of bowel sounds.	Indicates peristalsis.
6. Check placement of jejunostomy tube by aspirating with syringe. Return of intestinal secretions should be observed.	Indicates proper placement of feeding tube. However, some small or soft tubes collapse during aspiration.
7. Connect feeding tube and begin at prescribed rate. Check for residual at least every 8 hours.	Checking for residual allows for assessment of intestinal motility and absorption of formula.

Nursing Implications: If client is receiving continuous feedings, change formula every 8–12 hours. Formulas hanging longer are susceptible to bacterial growth. Change tubing and bag every 24 hours.

Note and record residuals every 8 hours and abdominal assessment, weight, electrolytes, and bowel status each day. Clients may develop diarrhea, which requires reducing the strength of the enteral formula or feeding rate or addition of an antidiarrheal agent.

The site around the jejunostomy tube should be cleansed with soap and water daily. A gauze dressing may be applied to the site.

If jejunostomy tube is to be clamped intermittently, turn off formula infusion and disconnect tubing. Flush jejunostomy tube with water (30 mL) and place a catheter plug on the end of the tube (a C clamp can be used for this purpose).

If medications are to be administered, prepare according to hospital policy and give via gravity flow through a 60-mL syringe (with appropriate tip to fit jejunostomy tube) with plunger removed. Flush with water to keep tube patent and to deliver all of the medication.

Procedure: Administering Hyperalimentation via Peripheral Vein

Description: This involves infusing total parenteral nutrition (TPN) by way of a peripheral vein. TPN is the infusion of an IV solution and amino acids, glucose, vitamins, electrolytes, minerals, and trace elements.

Purpose: To provide short-term nutritional support.

STEP	RATIONALE
1. Compare peripheral TPN solution prepared by pharmacy with physician's order. Check expiration date and time.	Ensures infusion of proper solution. Peripheral TPN has less glucose than central TPN.
2. Check armband for client's name.	Ensures correct identification.
3. Connect tubing with inline filter. Use macrodrip tubing for rates >100 mL/hr.	Inline filter prevents infusion of microorganisms. TPN solution is a good medium for bacterial growth.
4. Prime tubing and thread it through infusion device.	Tubing is primed to prevent infusion of air.
5. Attach tubing to hub of IV catheter; tape securely.	
6. Set correct rate on infusion device and check once every hour for proper delivery.	The infusion pump regulates flow, but nurse must check to ensure correct delivery.

Nursing Implications: Observe IV site for redness, swelling, or signs of infiltration. Restart IV infusion if necessary. Change tubing and filter every 24 hours. Change IV site every 3 days to prevent infection. Before administering TPN, inspect bag for any particles or signs of contamination. Store TPN in refrigerator; remove 1 hour before hanging to allow solution to warm to room temperature.

Check blood glucose levels as ordered and report any abnormal values. Assess lung fields at least once each shift for presence of crackles, indicating fluid overload.

If other IV piggyback fluids are needed, consider using a heparin lock at a second IV site to avoid possible compatibility problems.

Procedure: Administering Fat Emulsions

Description: An emulsified fat solution containing linoleic acid is infused simultaneously with hyperalimentation or separately. Linoleic acid is an essential fatty acid that prevents fatty-acid deficiency.

Purpose: To prevent fatty-acid deficiency; to provide a high caloric count and energy supply; to provide and maintain nutritional status.

STEP	RATIONALE
1. Obtain fat emulsion bottle from pharmacy or central supply. Check the order for correct concentration (usually 10%–20%). Observe bottle for separation of emulsion. If separated, return to source.	
2. Spike bottle with vented tubing and flush the line. In some cases, special tubing accompanies the solution and should be used for the infusion.	Air vent allows for infusion via IV tubing by allowing air to displace the fat emulsion draining from the bottle.
3. Attach needle to end tubing. Swab primary IV tubing of the TPN solution at an injection site below the filter.	Infusing fat emulsion through filter causes occlusion of tubing.

(Continued on following page)

STEP	RATIONALE
4. Using an infusion device, set rate appropriately. For the first 30 minutes, infusion should run no faster than 1 mL/min. Check for adverse reactions. Continue at a 4–6 hour rate for 250–500 mL fat emulsion.	Reduces risk of adverse reactions such as chills, fever, flushing, diaphoresis, dyspnea, and chest and back pain.

Nursing Implications: The signs and symptoms of fatty-acid deficiency are dry scaly skin, sparse hair growth, impaired wound healing, decreased resistance to stress, increased susceptibility to respiratory infections, and anemia.

Fat emulsions are contraindicated in clients with abnormal fat metabolism, as in pancreatitis. Inform physician of abnormal liver function tests. Client may not be able to metabolize lipids. Fat emulsion may be piggybacked into peripheral hyperalimentation but should not be mixed with other medications. The emulsion may separate. Phlebitis often occurs when fat emulsions are given.

Procedure: Administering Hyperalimentation via Central Vein

Description: Hyperosmolar TPN is administered into the central circulation.

Purpose: To provide and maintain nutritional support when enteral nutrition is contraindicated, not appropriate, or inadequate to meet needs.

STEP	RATIONALE
1. If refrigerated, remove bag 0.5–1.0 hour before use. Check central TPN with physician's orders. Inspect bag for floating particles or signs of contamination. Confirm placement of central line with a chest radiograph if not done previously (if this is the first bag).	Ensures proper solution mixture. If contamination observed, return bag to pharmacy.
2. Check central IV site for redness, swelling, or signs of infiltration. If present, have physician restart line.	Infected central lines can lead to sepsis, a major complication.
3. Compare client armband identification with that on TPN bag.	Correct identification is essential in preventing drug errors.
4. Spike TPN bag with macrodrip tubing with inline filter.	Inline filters help to prevent infusion of microorganisms.
5. Prime tubing and insert in infusion device.	Prevents introduction of air. The infusion device regulates flow rate; it is critical for central TPN because a bolus dose of hyperosmolar glucose solution can produce rapid cellular dehydration.
6. Set desired rate. Check infusion every hour.	The infusion pump regulates flow, but nurse must check to ensure correct delivery.

Nursing Implications: Change tubing and filter every 24 hours. Solution should be changed at least once every 24 hours. Store central TPN in refrigerator; remove 1 hour before hanging to allow solution to warm to room temperature.

Check blood glucose levels as ordered and report any abnormal values. Assess lung fields at least once each shift for presence of crackles, indicating fluid overload. Notify physician of abnormal electrolyte levels or blood glucose. Client may need to be on insulin while on central TPN.

Initial rate is usually 50 mL/hr, and it is then increased daily as tolerated. The client should be weaned from central TPN gradually. Watch for hypoglycemia at this time. Carefully monitor I&O. Osmotic diuresis can occur.

Do not play "catch-up"—i.e., accelerate administration—if central TPN is behind schedule. Site care should be performed using aseptic technique with masks. If available, use ever-lock connections to prevent air embolus. Do not piggyback other drugs into central TPN, except for lipid emulsions.

Procedure: Catheterizing Bladder Using Indwelling or Intermittent Catheter

Description: A sterile rubber or silicone tube is introduced through the urethra and into the bladder, providing continuous or intermittent outflow of urine.

Purpose: To relieve bladder distention and maintain urinary tract patency; to obtain accurate urine output measures.

STEP	RATIONALE
1. Obtain catheter insertion kit with urine drainage bag or intermittent catheter kit. Bring an extra pair of sterile gloves in case of contamination. If catheterizing a woman, bring an extra catheter.	Kits contain the necessary supplies for quick and safe implementation.
2. Explain procedure and ensure privacy.	
3. Place bed at comfortable working level.	Decreases anxiety and embarrassment and increases cooperation.
4. Position client: a. Woman: Supine with knees flexed and thighs relaxed in external rotation b. Man: Supine with legs slightly abducted, with client draped for comfort	Provides proper visualization of urethral opening.
5. Apply clean latex gloves. Wash perineal area with warm water and mild soap; rinse and dry.	Decreases risk of introduction of microorganisms during catherization.
6. Identify urethral meatus, which in the woman is forward of vagina, and in the man at the tip of the penis.	Identifying structures before proceeding promotes accurate placement of catheter.
7. Using bed or bedside table, open catheter insertion kit. Place moisture-proof pad under the buttocks. Do not touch any part of kit while removing pad.	Protects bed linen and client. Prevents contamination of sterile kit.
8. Put on sterile gloves. Place fenestrated sterile drape with opening over perineal area, exposing structures. Care must be taken to avoid touching contaminated areas. Restless, confused, or weak clients are best draped after setting up the supplies in the kit. If necessary, an assistant can restrain the client.	
9. Open packet containing antiseptic cleaning solution and pour evenly over the cotton balls. (If client is allergic to povidone-iodine [Betadine], use hexachlorophene [pHisoHex].)	
10. Examine catheter and check to see that it is securely connected to urine drainage bag. Tip of catheter is surrounded by a balloon. Attach syringe with sterile water to injection port of catheter. Do not inject water into balloon at this point in the procedure.	Equipment should be in good condition and without tears. Prepares catheter for insertion and keeps syringe handy.
11. Open lubricant packet and apply along catheter tip.	Lubrication assists in ease of insertion and promotes client's comfort.
12. Place kit between legs of women or on thighs of men.	
13. Cleanse urethral meatus and surrounding area: a. Woman: (1) With nondominant hand, pull back labia with thumb and forefinger to expose urethral opening. Maintain position with this hand throughout procedure. (2) With dominant hand, use forceps to grasp a cotton ball soaked in antiseptic solution. Using a downward motion, cleanse the urethral opening by starting above the structure and wiping down past the vaginal area. Drop cotton ball (not on sterile field) and grasp another. Use one cotton ball per wipe. Also cleanse area to the sides of the meatus.	Maintains visualization of urethral opening. Assistant's help may be needed to expose if client is contracted, restless, or obese. Additional light source such as flashlight may be needed. Maintains a sterile dominant hand and avoids contamination. Cleanses area of microorganisms. Reduces chance of bladder contamination.
b. Man: (1) Pull back foreskin, if present, with nondominant hand. Hold penis at shaft below glans and pull upward. Maintain this position throughout procedure.	Exposes meatus for catheterization.
(2) With dominant hand using forceps, grasp cotton ball soaked with antiseptic solution. Cleanse in circular motion from meatus to base of glans. Use a new cotton ball for each wipe.	Cleanses area of microorganisms. Reduces chance of bladder contamination.

(Continued on following page)

STEP	RATIONALE
14. Pick up catheter with dominant hand and insert lubricated tip into urethra. Ask client to take a deep breath and exhale slowly. For men, hold penis perpendicular to body. If resistance is felt, pull back slightly and attempt passage again. Rotating catheter slightly may help. If lubricant in kit is in a syringe, some may be placed directly into the meatus.	Relaxes sphincter muscles and aids in passing catheter. Forcing catheter may damage urethral lining. Some resistance may normally be felt in prostate area.
15. Advance catheter 2–3 inches in women and 7–8 inches in men until urine is noted. Then advance further to ensure that balloon is in bladder.	Ensures placement of catheter in bladder.
16. a. Indwelling catheter: Inject 10 mL sterile water into injection port of catheter. Pull gently until resistance is met.	Positions catheter in bladder and prevents dislodging.
16. b. Intermittent catheterization: Drain urine into receptacle provided in the kit. Allow urine to drain until bladder is empty. Remove catheter, cleanse client, and dry well.	
17. Place catheter drainage bag below level of bladder. Attach to bed.	Prevents urine from backing up into bladder.
18. Tape catheter to inner side of thigh. Make sure that system drains urine freely without obstruction.	Reduces trauma to meatus and urethra during movement. Maintains patent urine flow.
19. Measure and document amount of urine output. Send urine specimen to laboratory, if ordered. Do not disconnect catheter from tubing to obtain specimens.	
20. Discard used supplies in proper receptacle.	

Nursing Implications: When repositioning client, make sure catheter and tubing are not obstructing flow of urine. Instruct client not to pull on catheter.

In women, if no urine is obtained when inserting catheter, check position: the catheter may be in vagina. If so, insert new sterile catheter into urethra, leaving first catheter in place to avoid repeating error. Remove and discard original catheter. If tube is definitely in bladder but no urine is obtained, notify physician.

Report and record size of catheter placed (use smallest size possible), amount of water used to inflate the balloon, color and character of urine, and amount obtained. Document type of drainage in use.

If intermittent catheterization is ordered, document the amount and character of urine and the time. If client voided before intermittent catheterization, note time and amount.

Procedure: Routine Catheter Care

Description: Perineal hygiene is performed for clients with an indwelling catheter.

Purpose: To reduce risk of bladder infection; to provide complete perineal hygiene.

STEP	RATIONALE
1. Collect necessary supplies: • Clean latex gloves • Mild soap and warm water • Povidone-iodine solution (if ordered) • Povidone-iodine ointment (if ordered) • Sterile swabs • Tape NOTE: Some studies have shown soap and water to be as effective as povidone-iodine.	Organizing necessary supplies allows for quick and safe implementation.
2. Ensure privacy. Position client as in catheterization procedure. Drape client with bath blanket.	Provides comfort and lessens embarrassment.
3. Using the gloves, wash perineal area with soap and water. Rinse and dry.	Gloves protect the nurse from transmission of microorganisms. Cleansing reduces possible contaminants.

(Continued on following page)

STEP	RATIONALE
4. With nondominant hand, pull back labia or foreskin to expose meatus.	Meatus must be visualized for proper cleansing.
5. If ordered, cleanse area around meatus with sterile swabs soaked in antiseptic solution. Cleanse along catheter with solution.	Prevents transfer of microorganisms.
6. If ordered, apply antiseptic ointment with sterile swab to base of catheter near meatus.	Reduces risk of introduction of microorganisms into urethra.
7. Replace tape anchoring catheter to thigh. Replace drainage bag, if needed, maintaining a sterile connection.	Changing bag when signs of leakage or sediment buildup are noted reduces risk of infection.

Nursing Implications: Document catheter care after performing procedure. Care should be performed daily or more often if area becomes contaminated with stool. Observe and report condition of meatus. Note character of urine and report foul odor or cloudy appearance. Empty catheter drainage bag every 8 hours or when full. Empty bag before transporting client to a diagnostic procedure.

Procedure: Irrigating a Colostomy

Description: This process involves instilling 500–1000 mL of tepid water through colostomy stoma, then allowing the water and stool to drain into a collection bag.

Purpose: To remove stool, prevent continuous oozing of stool; to regulate bowel movements to a routine time; to cleanse the bowel before a diagnostic procedure.

STEP	RATIONALE
1. Collect necessary supplies and equipment: • Irrigator with tubing • Irrigation sleeve with belt • Water-soluble lubricant • Clamps • Irrigation cone	Organizing necessary supplies and equipment allows for quick and safe implementation.
2. If client is ambulatory, position client sitting on toilet. If client is on bedrest, position on side. Provide privacy.	Sitting position is generally comfortable for bowel evacuation.
3. Put on clean gloves. Remove appliance and wash area with soap and water; dry.	
4. Apply irrigation sleeve with belt. Let sleeve hang so that it touches water in toilet.	Allows for direct flow of water and stool into toilet.
5. If client is lying in bed, clamp end of sleeve.	Prevents possibility of spilling contents and controls odor.
6. Fill irrigator with 500–1000 mL of tepid water, and flush tubing.	Sufficient amount of solution to stimulate colon emptying. Flushing tubing prevents air from entering colon.
7. Attach cone to irrigation tubing and apply lubricant to cone tip.	
8. Insert cone into stoma through top of sleeve. Insert carefully without force. May need to dilate stoma before insertion, using gloved lubricated finger. Insert cone in direction of bowel lumen.	Protects stoma from trauma.
9. Begin flow of irrigation solution, clamping tube if cramping occurs. Release clamp as cramping subsides. Hang bag so that bottom is at level of client's shoulder or slightly higher.	If solution enters bowel rapidly, cramping results, reducing ability to hold sufficient volume of solution.
10. Clamp tubing when irrigation completed.	Prevents backflow of irrigation solution.
11. Remove cone carefully so that sleeve covers stoma.	Protects client and area.
12. A gush of fluid return should occur in spurts.	
13. Clamp top of sleeve and allow solution and stool to return.	About 1 hour may be required for complete return. May clamp end of sleeve if client wishes to walk around.
14. When all fecal material has been irrigated from bowel, remove sleeve and belt.	

(Continued on following page)

STEP	RATIONALE
15. Wash and prepare skin around stoma. Apply new pouch.	Allows pouch to stick firmly without leaks.
16. Wash out sleeve, cone, and irrigator tubing. Store articles in proper place for reuse.	Keeps articles clean for reuse.

Nursing Implications: Avoid frequent irrigation of colostomy with water, which can cause loss of electrolytes and fluid imbalance. To regulate the bowel, irrigation should be performed around the same time each day, preferably an hour after a meal.

Record amount of irrigation instilled and amount returned, if possible. Examine client's abdomen every shift, noting bowel sounds and any areas of tenderness. Record amount and character of returned stool.

Procedure: Collecting a Midstream Urine Specimen

Description: Urine is collected during midstream in a sterile container.

Purpose: To collect urine for culture and sensitivity test in order to determine the presence of bacteria or other organisms.

STEP	RATIONALE
1. Instruct client to wash perineal area with soap and water and rinse well. Provide privacy in bathroom, if possible.	Cleanses perineal area of fecal and other contaminants.
2. Obtain midstream urine kit. Remove antiseptic swab or towelette and have client wipe perineal area front to back in one wipe.	Removes bacteria.
3. Rinse with one wipe of sterile water front to back.	Antiseptic may contaminate specimen and alter results.
4. Instruct client to start to void and stop midstream. Place sterile collection cup under client and instruct to complete voiding.	Initial stream of urine flushes urethra of microorganisms that may give false-positive reading.
5. Screw lid on cup securely. Be careful not to contaminate inside cup.	Ensures an accurate culture test.

Nursing Implications: Label container with name, hospital number, date and time of voiding, and method of collection. Send or take specimen to laboratory as soon as possible. Document procedure in nurse's notes. Obtain culture before administration of antibiotics, if possible. If client is already receiving antibiotics, list drug(s) on laboratory request form.

Procedure: Checking Urine for Glucose and Ketones

Description: This involves measuring glucose and ketones by dipping a chemically prepared strip into clean urine or adding drops of urine to chemically prepared tablets.

Purpose: To identify the presence of glucose and ketones in a urine sample; to quickly assess diabetic status.

STEP	RATIONALE
1. Obtain double voided specimen in clean container. (With children, second voided specimens have not been found to be more accurate.)	Urine that has been in the bladder for a long time does not reflect accurate amount of glucose and ketones.
2. Test urine with glucose reagent tablet:	
a. With a medicine dropper (supplied with kit) place 10 drops of urine into test tube.	
b. Rinse dropper; place 10 drops of water into test tube.	
c. Place test tube in holder and add reagent tablet without touching tablet.	The combination results in a chemical reaction that produces heat.
d. Allow to "boil." Do not hold tube, which becomes quite hot.	

(Continued on following page)

STEP	RATIONALE
e. After 15 seconds, shake test tube and check color against chart provided. Watch for rapid change.	Glucose reagent test tablets measure 0%–2% glucose. If solution is allowed to remain in test tube too long, the test results will be inaccurate.
3. Test urine with glucose and ketone reagent strip: a. Insert reagent strip into clean urine and gently shake off excess. b. Follow directions on reagent container for time interval allowed before reading results; use watch to time. c. Compare color change on reagent strip to color chart on container. d. Close reagent-strip bottle tightly. 4. Test urine with acetone tablet: a. Place tablet on paper towel. b. Add one drop of urine to tablet. Wait 30 seconds. c. Compare color change with chart.	Each brand of reagent strips requires a specific time for accurate results. Moisture may alter accuracy of test strips. Measures presence of ketone bodies.

Nursing Implications: Keep supplies clean and ready for next testing. Discard urine appropriately. Record in nurses' notes or diabetic record and continue with prescribed therapy. Depending on brand of tablet used, be aware of possible false-positive test results that occur with some medications.

Procedure: Collecting a Stool Specimen

Description: A small amount of stool is obtained for laboratory testing.

Purpose: To detect presence of blood, bile, fat, urobilinogen, nitrogen content, ova, parasites, protozoa, or bacteria in the stool.

STEP	RATIONALE
1. Collect stool specimen appropriately for purpose of test.	Stool specimen may have to be collected by a certain method. Check with laboratory if uncertain.
2. Place clean specimen hat in toilet, if client is able to use it.	Prevents stool from falling into toilet water.
3. Explain to client that stool must be free of urine, water, and toilet tissue.	Urine inhibits bacterial growth and may conflict with results.
4. Using clean gloves and tongue blade, place stool specimen in plastic container that has client's label on outside.	Maintains cleanliness and prevents transfer of microorganisms.
5. Place specimen in plastic bag and send to laboratory as soon as possible.	Fresh samples produce more accurate results.

Nursing Implications: Clean all equipment immediately and dispose of tongue blade and gloves in trash receptacle. Document in nurses' notes the color and character of stool and method of collection.

Procedure: Testing for Occult Blood in Stool

Description: This simple laboratory test can quickly assess presence of blood in the stool.

Purpose: To determine presence of GI bleeding.

STEP	RATIONALE
1. Obtain Hemoccult cardboard slide, two wooden sticks, Hemoccult developing agent, and clean stool specimen.	Hemoccult slides are the most commonly used guaiac tests.
2. Put on clean gloves. With wooden stick, obtain small amount of stool. Open flap of cardboard slide and place a smear of stool in circle A. Discard stick.	

(Continued on following page)

STEP	RATIONALE
3. With second wooden stick, obtain a small smear of stool from a different area of the stool specimen and place on circle B. Close flap.	The results of Hemoccult testing are more conclusive if positive results are obtained from both samples.
4. Turn cardboard slide over and open the other flap. Place 2 drops of Hemoccult developing solution on each circle. Put a drop on monitor circle. Positive one should turn blue and negative one stays white.	Filter paper on slide is prepared with guaiac, which will turn blue if blood loss exceeds 5 mL/day. Ensures that guaiac slide is working properly.
5. Wait 30–60 seconds before reading test results. Bluish color indicates presence of occult blood.	Accurate timing is important for accurate results.
6. Discard cardboard slide, used wooden sticks, and gloves in trash receptacle. Discard stool specimen appropriately.	Prevents transfer of microorganisms.

Nursing Implications: Send to laboratory immediately. Label specimen with name, date, and time. False-positive results may occur if the client has a diet high in meat, bananas, drugs (aspirin), iron preparations, anticoagulants, and corticotropin. Black stools are associated with upper GI bleeding, and bright-red stools with lower GI problems such as hemorrhoids and carcinomas.

Procedure: Collecting Nose and Throat Cultures

Description: A swab of mucosal membranes is performed to be used as a testing specimen for bacterial or fungal growth on a culture medium.

Purpose: To determine the presence of pathogenic organisms and the antibiotics that are effective in treatment.

STEP	RATIONALE
For Throat Culture: 1. Obtain two culturette tubes with sterile swabs. Label each tube with client's name and information.	
2. Position client sitting up comfortably with head tilted back.	
3. Using tongue blade, visualize the pharynx. Insert swab without touching teeth or gums, and gently swab tonsillar areas and areas of redness or drainage.	Touching gums or teeth may result in contamination with resident bacteria.
4. Carefully withdraw swab without contaminating. Insert swab into culture tube and press tip to crush ampule.	The culture medium maintains the presence of bacteria until testing.
For Nose Culture: 5. Use the second culturette for the nasal specimen. Use penlight to visualize nostrils. Choose nostril with greatest patency. (Client may have to blow nose to open obstruction.)	
6. Insert culture swab and swab areas inside nostril that appear red or inflamed. Try not to touch sides of nostril. (A nasal speculum may be used.)	Prevents contamination with resident bacteria.
7. Carefully remove swab and place inside culture tube. Press tip of culture tube to break ampule.	Culture medium maintains the presence of bacteria until testing. Crushing ampule releases medium so that it is in contact with tip of swab.

Nursing Implications: Send to laboratory immediately. Label specimens with name, time, and date. Document procedure in nurses' notes, describing color and character of secretions. Indicate any antibiotics the client is taking.

Procedure: Care of the Client with a T-Tube

Description: During a cholecystectomy, a T-tube is placed in the common bile duct and connected to a drainage bag.

Purpose: To drain bile after a cholecystectomy and bile-duct exploration; to prevent contracture and stenosis of the duct during healing.

STEP	RATIONALE
1. Place client in low-Fowler's to semi-Fowler's position.	Facilitates draining.
2. Check T-tube for kinks of obstruction of drainage.	Prevents possible obstruction of drainage.
3. Measure output and record every 8 hours. With gloved hands, open bottom port of drainage bag and allow bile to drain into graduated container for measuring. Close drainage bag securely.	It is important to record output; record is used to determine when to remove tube.
4. Cleanse and dry area around tube and place sterile dry dressing around insertion site daily.	

Nursing Implications: Assess sclera for yellowish color, which may indicate biliary obstruction. Record stools, noting color and character. The T-tube drain may be removed in 1–2 weeks. Usually, T-tube is clamped at intervals before removing. Be aware of potential for nausea and vomiting or signs of biliary obstruction. Stools will be clay colored if tube is *unclamped.*

QUESTIONS
Cynthia Bowers Howard, RN, APRN, MSN, BC, CNS, and Golden M. Tradewell, RN, PhD

1. The LPN/LVN demonstrates awareness of the single most important infection control method when the nurse does which of the following?
   1. Uses gloves when administering nose drops.
   2. Uses sterile gloves when giving a bed bath.
   3. Uses sterile technique for changing surgical dressings.
   4. Washes hands before and after every client contact.

2. To maintain standard precautions, a nurse working with a hospitalized client would do which of the following? Select all that apply.
   1. Use protective equipment, such as masks and gloves, when serving the client's meals.
   2. Conduct proper hand washing before and after all client care.
   3. Dispose of used syringes and needles in an appropriate biohazard container.
   4. Follow the institution's protective procedures when a potential for exposure to body fluids or blood exists.
   5. Place all clients in protective isolation.
   6. Dispose used syringes and needles in wastebasket.

3. An order is written for the nurse to obtain a urine sample from a client with an indwelling urinary catheter. The nurse avoids contaminating the specimen by doing which of the following?
   1. Wiping the port on the drainage bag with an alcohol wipe before obtaining the sample.
   2. Obtaining the sample from the urinary drainage bag.
   3. Aspirating a sample from the port on the drainage bag.
   4. Clamping the tubing of the drainage bag.

4. Supplies needed by a licensed practical nurse to suction a client safely with a diagnosis of AIDS (acquired immunodeficiency syndrome) include which of the following?
   1. Gloves, gown, protective eyewear
   2. Gloves, gown, mask
   3. Gloves, mask, and protective eyewear
   4. Gown, mask, and protective eyewear

5. When suctioning a client's tracheostomy, the nurse should position the client in which position to promote deep breathing and coughing?
   1. Supine position
   2. Semi-Fowler's position
   3. Lateral position
   4. High-Fowler's position

6. The nurse is inserting an indwelling urinary catheter in a male client. How far should the catheter be inserted before inflating the balloon?
   1. 2–3 inches
   2. 4–5 inches

3. 7–9 inches
4. 10–12 inches

7. The nurse is suctioning the airway of a client with a tracheostomy. To perform this procedure safely, the nurse should do which of the following? (**Select all that apply.**)
   1. Turn the wall suction to 80 mm Hg.
   2. Use sterile water to lubricate and flush the suction catheter.
   3. Use clean gloves for all steps of the procedure.
   4. Insert the catheter until the client coughs or resistance is felt.
   5. Use unsterile water to lubricate and flush the suction catheter.
   6. Use sterile gloves for all steps of the procedure.

8. After administering an injection to a client, the nurse accidentally drops the syringe on the floor. The most appropriate action for the nurse to take is:
   1. Call the housekeeping department to pick up the syringe.
   2. Pick up the syringe with hemostats and discard.
   3. Carefully pick up the syringe and dispose in a sharps container.
   4. Carefully pick up the syringe and recap the needle.

9. While administering medication to a client via a nasogastric tube, the nurse suspects that the tube has become clogged. The first action the nurse should take is:
   1. Aspirate the tube.
   2. Remove and replace the tube.
   3. Flush with warm water.
   4. Flush with carbonated beverage.

10. The nurse is administering 5000 units of heparin to a 45-year-old client. Correct steps to take in performing this task include: (**Select all that apply.**)
    1. Wiping the injection site with an alcohol wipe before the injection.
    2. Insuring that the correct medication, dose, route, and client are identified.
    3. Aspirating before giving the heparin.
    4. Massaging the site after the injection.
    5. Using a sterile gauze to clean the injection site before the injection.
    6. Using the Z-track method to give heparin.

11. A client has no bowel sounds and has been vomiting for the last hour. The nurse places a nasogastric tube (as ordered by the physician). In order to estimate the distance to the beginning of the esophagus, this nurse will measure the distance from the tip of the nose to the:
    1. Lower tip of the ear lobe.
    2. Xiphoid process

3. Thyroid gland
4. Cricoid cartilage

12. A client is ready to have the nasogastric tube removed. As the nurse removes the tube, the client is asked to:

1. Cough
2. Breathe deeply
3. Turn her head to the side
4. Perform the Valsalva maneuver

13. A client has a nasogastric tube in place for continuous tube feedings. The nurse will:

1. Irrigate the tube with normal saline every 4 hours.
2. Insert the tube another inch every 2 hours.
3. Check the tube for placement every shift.
4. Remove the tape and check the nostril every shift.

14. A client was admitted for evaluation of melena. Today, the client returns to the hospital room following a barium enema. The nurse will be sure to:

1. Obtain an order for a laxative.
2. Check the vital signs frequently.
3. Maintain NPO status until barium is passed.
4. Evaluate lower extremities for neurovascular signs.

15. A client is receiving continuous tube feedings through a jejunostomy via a Keofeed tube. The nurse makes certain that:

1. The container for the feeding does not run dry.
2. The container for the feeding is never below the jejunum.
3. The client is in High Fowler's position.
4. The head of the bed remains elevated at 30 to 45 degrees.

16. A client is receiving continuous tube feedings through a Keofeed tube. The flow of the feeding is being controlled by a pump. The nurse should:

1. Check the tube for kinks and dependent loops.
2. Aspirate and flush the tube every 4 hours.
3. Administer about 100 mL of water every 4 hours.
4. Administer medications through the tube as needed.

17. A client with amyotrophic lateral sclerosis (ALS) is receiving tube feedings and medications through a gastrotomy tube. The nurse initiates a feeding by aspirating stomach contents (for placement of the tube and for residual). Sixty milliliters are obtained. What should the nurse do with these gastric contents?

1. Discard it.
2. Return it to the stomach.
3. Send it to the laboratory.
4. Add it to the feeding.

18. A 12-month-old returns to his hospital room following surgical repair of his hypospadias. He has an IV infusion and both a ureteral and a suprapubic catheter in place. The nurse tells the parents that the primary purpose of the suprapubic catheter is to provide:

1. An entry port for bladder irrigation.
2. An alternate urinary elimination route.

3. Accurate measurement of urinary output.
4. An opportunity to observe the color of the urine.

19. The father of a toddler who is eating a hot dog suddenly yells, "Help!" He's choking to death!" Which of the following signs would indicate that lifesaving measures are necessary?

1. Gagging
2. Coughing
3. Pulse over 100
4. Inability to speak

20. Which of the following reflects recommended procedure for cardiopulmonary resuscitation of the pediatric patient?

1. To check for a pulse in an infant under 1 year of age, the brachial artery is palpated.
2. The compression-to-ventilation ratio for children under the age of 8 years is 15:2.
3. If an infant is not breathing, give four quick breaths followed by a pause to allow for exhalation.
4. The cardiac compression rate for children between the ages of 1 and 8 years should be 120 per minute.

21. A child has been admitted to your unit with a tentative diagnosis of immune suppression. One nursing action you will initiate is to:

1. Establish strict isolation to limit the spread of infections.
2. Screen visitors to prevent exposure to known cases of influenza and varicella.
3. Offer a diet high in raw fruits and vegetables to promote good nutrition.
4. Ask her parents to bring her stuffed animals in from home to establish a sense of normalcy.

22. In administering oxygen therapy to a child in respiratory difficulty, a preventive measure to be taken by the nurse in regard to the untoward effects of oxygen therapy is:

1. Padding elastic bands of the face mask
2. Taking the apical pulse before starting therapy
3. Humidifying the gas before delivery
4. Placing the client in the orthopneic position

23. Countertraction to support a child's position and alignments in bed is primarily supplied by:

1. Weights, pulleys, and ropes
2. Elevation of the foot of the bed
3. Gravity and body weight
4. Elevation of the knee gatch

24. Regardless of age, children with congestive heart failure should be placed in which position to maximize cardiac function?

1. Semi-Fowler's
2. Prone
3. Supine
4. Trendelenburg's

25. A 21-year-old man is admitted with suspected appendicitis. He is scheduled the next morning for an

exploratory laparotomy. On his preoperative orders, the nurse notes an order for a Fleets Enema X1 in the morning. Which of the following would be an appropriate action for the nurse?

1. Administer the Fleets enema the night before surgery to allow more time for it to work.
2. Call the physician and verify the order.
3. Administer the Fleets enema in the morning as ordered.
4. Ask the client if he has had a bowel movement today and hold the enema if he has.

26. A 22-year-old client is diagnosed with HIV. In the laboratory of the physician's office, the nurse is asked to draw blood. Which of the following approaches is best by the nurse?

1. Use universal precautions.
2. Isolate the patient.
3. Wear a gown to draw the blood.
4. Wear a face shield to draw the blood.

27. When caring for clients undergoing chemotherapy, the nurse identifies the most effective way to prevent infection in a neutropenic client is:

1. Meticulous hand-washing prior to client contact.
2. Monitoring oral temperature every 4 hours.
3. A sitz bath after each bowel movement
4. Encouraging a high-calorie, high-protein diet

28. Health-care professionals including nurses are constantly exposed to hepatitis B. The best way to avoid contracting hepatitis B is to:

1. Double-bag soiled tissues.
2. Avoid needle stick injuries.
3. Obtain the appropriate immunization.
4. Protect clothing by wearing a gown.

29. A 24-hour urine collection for 17-hydrocycortico-steroid (17-OHCS) and ketosteroids is to be collected from 8 AM Monday to 8 AM Tuesday. What should the nurse do with the specimen voided at 8 AM Tuesday?

1. Put it in the 24-hour specimen container.
2. Put it in a separate urinary container.
3. Send it to the laboratory for culture.
4. Measure the urine and then discard it.

30. When teaching clients about infection control, the nurse reinforces that currently the Centers for Disease Control recommends which of the following disinfectants in a 1:10 dilution for cleaning surfaces contaminated with blood or body fluids?

1. Bleach
2. Alcohol
3. Phenols
4. Peroxide

31. The development of acquired immune deficiency syndrome (AIDS) resulting from infection with the human immunodeficiency virus (HIV) has changed health-care practices. Universal blood and body fluid precautions are recommended for use with:

1. All clients cared for by health-care workers
2. All untested clients from high-risk population
3. All clients in high-risk categories for AIDS
4. All clients who are positive for HIV antibodies

32. Surgical wound infections are the second most frequent type of nosocomial infection found in most hospitals. The nurse knows that she can best reduce these infections by:

1. Strictly adhering to the principles of effective hand washing.
2. Always cleansing incisions from bottom to top—from the most contaminated to the least contaminated area.
3. Leaving incisions open to air to promote healing.
4. Using clean gloves as the protective barrier when chaning dressings.

33. A 57-year-old client has been experiencing anorexia, weight loss, and diarrhea and is admitted to the general surgery unit for diagnostic purposes. He has an order for enemas in preparation for a barium enema the next day. Which is the best nursing action related to correct enema administration procedure?

1. Insert tubing 1–2 inches with client lying in the left lateral position with right leg flexed.
2. Expel air from tubing and then lubricate and insert tip of tubing into the anus until resistance is felt. The client should be lying in the right lateral position with left leg flexed.
3. Insert tubing and open clamp to allow solution to flow moderately fast with container 20 inches above the client's anus.
4. Once tubing is inserted, allow the solution to flow slowly until the container is empty or until the client is unable to take anymore, then clamp the tubing and remove from anus.

34. After a cholecystectomy, a 50-year-old client has an incision site with a Penrose drain. When cleansing her wound, the best action by the nurse would be to:

1. Go over the wound several times with the same swab.
2. Use antiseptic solution followed by a normal saline rinse.
3. Cleanse from the outer regions of the wound toward the middle.
4. Start cleansing at the drain site and move outward.

35. When irrigating a wound, the nurse recognizes that the client should be positioned so that the solution will flow from one end of the wound toward the other end. The rationale for this action is to:

1. Direct the flow of liquid from least contaminated to most contaminated area.
2. Assist the nurse in proceeding in an organized fashion to complete the procedure.
3. Facilitate irrigating the wound as quickly as possible.
4. Enhance client comfort.

36. The nurse recognizes that a frequent site and cause of a nosocomial infection is:

1. The urinary tract, related to placing the drainage bag above the bladder.

2. The incision, related to use of aseptic technique when changing the dressing.
3. The bloodstream, related to self-administration of insulin.
4. The respiratory system, related to clients coughing without covering their mouth.

37. A client has a feeding tube in place. Before beginning the intermittent tube feeding, the best action by the nurse will be to:
    1. Auscultate the bowel sounds with the instillation of 100 mL of air.
    2. Auscultate the bowel sounds with the instillation of 10 mL of tap water.
    3. Submerge the end of this tube in a glass of water.
    4. Aspirate and reinstall his stomach contents.

38. When instructing a client to obtain a urine specimen at the clinic today, the best explanation by the nurse would be:
    1. Clean the area, start to urinate, and then catch the last few drops in the container.
    2. Clean the area and catch the entire amount of urine in the container.
    3. Clean the area and then catch the first 50 mL of urine in the container.
    4. Clean the area, start to urinate, catch the middle of the stream of urine in the container, and then finish urinating.

39. Handwashing is crucial in preventing the spread of infection. The nurse recognizes that this practice is aimed at breaking the "chain of infection" during which phase of the cycle?
    1. Portal of entry to host
    2. Reservoir
    3. Method of transmission
    4. Portal of exit from source

40. As the nurse caring for a client in isolation to prevent transmission of infection related to feces, you recognize that this type of isolation is called:
    1. Blood and body fluids
    2. Contact
    3. Drainage and secretion
    4. Enteric

41. The nurse knows that a specimen of urine for a routine urinalysis should be:
    1. Sent to the laboratory as a stat procedure.
    2. At least 60 mL.
    3. Put in a sterile container.
    4. An early morning specimen.

42. The surgical team approaches the sterile field for surgery. Which area of the scrubbed team's gowns is considered sterile?
    1. 4 inches above front waist
    2. 8 inches below front waist
    3. 6 inches above the elbow
    4. 4 inches above posterior chest

43. An elderly client is admitted to the long-term care unit following a feeding tube placement. After the tube has been cleared by the physician for use, the nurse begins to administer the medication through the tube. Which type of medication should the nurse administer through the feeding tube?
    1. Enteric-coated tablets
    2. Time-released compounds
    3. Compressed tablets
    4. Sublingual tablets

44. For the nurse to correctly take a child's blood pressure, the blood pressure cuff should cover what percentage of the child's upper arm when taking the child's blood pressure?
    1. 25%
    2. 33%
    3. 50%
    4. 75%

45. A newly admitted 4-month-old baby has an order for a blood sugar. The nurse knows a proper location for the puncture site is which of the following locations?
    1. Femoral artery
    2. Center of the dorsal heel
    3. Center of the finger pad of the index finger
    4. Outer aspects of the heel

46. A 5-year-old child is found unresponsive, not breathing, and without a pulse. The nurse begins CPR. The proper depth for chest compressions is which of the following?
    1. 0.5–1.0 inch
    2. 1.0–1.5 inches
    3. 1.5–2 inches
    4. 2.0–2.5 inches

47. A 3-month-old infant is found in the crib and appears to be cyanotic and unresponsive. The nurse begins CPR. The nurse will check for circulation by assessing which of the following?
    1. Carotid pulse
    2. Brachial pulse
    3. Femoral pulse
    4. Radial pulse

48. When performing the proper technique for chest compression on a 5-month-old infant, the nurse would use:
    1. The heel of one hand with the other hand on top
    2. The heel of one hand
    3. The index, middle, and ring fingers
    4. The index and middle fingers

49. A 2-year-old child was sucking on a piece of peppermint candy. He begins to choke. He is conscious, coughing, and making a high-pitched sound. The appropriate nursing action would be which of the following?
    1. Open the child's mouth and look for a foreign object.
    2. Perform the Heimlich maneuver.

3. Stay with the child, but do not perform any intervention.
4. Perform a combination of back blows and chest thrusts.

50. The client develops a stage II decubitus ulcer. What documentation, if made by the nurse correctly, reflects the diagnosis of a stage II decubitus ulcer?

1. A lesion appearing as a blister, which appears as a shallow crater.
2. A lesion appearing as a large nonblanching erythema.
3. A lesion that extends into the deeper subcutaneous tissue.
4. A lesion that extends into the subcutaneous tissue with skin loss.

ANSWERS

1. **(4)** Integrated processes: nursing process — implementation; client need: safe, effective care environment; safety and infection control; content area: procedures

RATIONALE

(1) The most important infection control method is the washing of hands before and after every client contact. **(2)** Sterile gloves are not necessary when giving a client a bed bath. **(3)** The most important infection control method is the washing of hands before and after every client contact. **(4)** The most important infection control method is the washing of hands before and after every client contact.

2. **(2, 3, 4)** Integrated processes: nursing process — implementation; client need: safe, effective care environment; safety and infection control; content area: procedures.

RATIONALE

(1) Gloves and masks are not necessary when routinely serving meals to clients. **(2)** Hand washing should be done before and after all client care, regardless of the use of gloves. **(3)** Used syringes and needles should always be disposed of in appropriate puncture-proof biohazard containers. **(4)** Institution's protective procedures should be followed when there is any potential for exposure to blood or body fluids. **(5)** Universal precautions need to be practiced with all clients; not placing clients in protective isolation. **(6)** Used syringes and needles should always be disposed of in appropriate puncture-proof biohazard containers.

3. **(1)** Integrated processes: nursing process — implementation; communication and documentation; client need: safe, effective care environment; safety and infection control; content area: procedures.

RATIONALE

(1) Wiping the port on the drainage bag with an alcohol wipe before obtaining the sample is the best way to avoid contamination of the specimen. **(2)** A urine specimen should not be taken from the drainage bag because changes occur to urine while sitting in the bag. **(3)** The correct technique for obtaining a sterile specimen requires wiping the port on the drainage bag with an alcohol wipe before obtaining the sample. **(4)** Clamping the tubing on the drainage bag is necessary prior to obtaining a sample but does not prevent contamination of the aspirated sample.

4. **(3)** Integrated processes: nursing process — implementation; client need: safe, effective care environment; safety and infection control; content area: procedures.

RATIONALE

(1) Universal precautions include the use of gloves whenever there is any actual or potential contact with blood or body fluids. **(2)** Gloves, mask, and protective eyewear are the supplies needed by the nurse to safely suction a client with AIDS. **(3)** Gloves, mask, and protective eyewear are the supplies needed by the nurse to safely suction a client with AIDS. **(4)** During suctioning, the nurse should wear gloves, mask, and protective eyewear.

5. **(2)** Integrated processes: nursing process — implementation; client need: physiological integrity; reduction of risk potential; content area: procedures.

RATIONALE

(1) Supine and lateral positions would not allow for maximum lung expansion. **(2)** Semi-Fowler's position is the optimum posi-

tion to promote deep breathing and coughing and allow for optimum visualization of the tracheostomy. **(3)** Supine and lateral positions would not allow for maximum lung expansion. **(4)** High-Fowler's position would not allow for adequate visualization of the tracheostomy.

6. **(3)** Integrated processes: nursing process — implementation; client need: physiological integrity; basic care and comfort; content area: procedures.

RATIONALE

(1) The correct choice is 7–9 inches since the male urethra is 6–8 inches long. **(2)** The correct choice is 7–9 inches since the male urethra is 6–8 inches long. **(3)** The procedure for inserting an indwelling catheter in a male client is to insert the catheter until urine begins to flow and then advance the catheter another 1–2 inches before attempting to inflate the balloon. The correct choice is 7–9 inches since the male urethra is 6–8 inches long. **(4)** The correct choice is 7–9 inches since the male urethra is 6–8 inches long.

7. **(2, 4, 6)** Integrated processes: nursing process — implementation; client need: physiological integrity; reduction for risk potential; content area: procedures.

RATIONALE

(1) Wall suction is normally set to 100–120 mm Hg for suctioning an adult. **(2)** Sterile saline or water is used to lubricate and flush the suction catheter. **(3)** Sterile gloves are needed to hold the suction catheter. **(4)** The catheter is inserted in the client until coughing or resistance is felt, then it is removed using intermittent suction. **(5)** Sterile saline or water is used to lubricate and flush the suction catheter. **(6)** Sterile gloves are needed to hold the suction catheter.

8. **(3)** Integrated processes: nursing process — implementation; client need: safe, effective care environment; safety and infection control; content area: procedures.

RATIONALE

(1) It is not appropriate to contact the housekeeping department to pick up the syringe. **(2)** Hemostats are not needed to safely pick up a syringe. **(3)** Used syringes should always promptly be placed in a sharps container. **(4)** Needles should never be recapped in order to prevent being stuck with a contaminated needle.

9. **(3)** Integrated processes: nursing process — implementation; client need: safe, effective care environment; safety and infection control; content area: procedures.

RATIONALE

(1) If the sterile field is contaminated in any way, the safest action for the nurse to take is to discard all supplies and prepare a new sterile field. **(2)** Changing gloves does not prevent contamination of objects on a sterile field if a nonsterile object has been touched. **(3)** If the sterile field is contaminated in any way, the safest action for the nurse to take is to discard all supplies and prepare a new sterile field. **(4)** If the sterile field is contaminated in any way, the safest action for the nurse to take is to discard all supplies and prepare a new sterile field.

10. **(1, 2)** Integrated processes: nursing process —implementation; client need: physiological integrity; pharmacological therapies; content area: procedures.

RATIONALE

(**1**) Alcohol should always be used to cleanse the injection site. (**2**) Medication, dose, route, and client should always be verified before administering any medication. (**3 and 4**) Aspirating and massaging the site are not recommended for administering heparin. (**5**) Alcohol should always be used to cleanse the injection site. (**6**) Heparin is given subcutaneously, not by Z-track method.

11. (**1**) Integrated processes: nursing process — implementation; client need: physiological integrity; reduction of risk potential; content area: procedures.

RATIONALE

(**1**) The distance from the tip of the nose to the lower tip of the ear lobe is equivalent to the distance from the nose to the area where the epiglottis covers the respiratory tract and the esophagus begins. (**2**) The distance from the tip of the nose to the xiphoid process would not be a good estimate. (**3**) The distance from the tip of the nose to the lower tip of the ear lobe is equivalent to the distance from the nose to the area where the epiglottis covers the respiratory tract and the esophagus begins. (**4**) The distance from the tip of the nose to the lower tip of the ear lobe is equivalent to the distance from the nose to the area where the epiglottis covers the respiratory tract and the esophagus begins.

12. (**4**) Integrated processes: nursing process — implementation; communication and documentation; client need: physiological integrity; reduction of risk potential; content area: procedures.

RATIONALE

(**1**) The epiglottis would be open with coughing. (**2**) The opening into the respiratory tract would be open, and aspiration would occur. (**3**) Removal of the tube would be more complicated. (**4**) The Valsalva maneuver would close the epiglottis and prevent aspiration.

13. (**3**) Integrated processes: nursing process — implementation; client need: physiological integrity; reduction of risk potential; content area: procedures.

RATIONALE

(**1**) Too much irrigation would wash out electrolytes. (**2**) The tube should stay in position unless otherwise ordered by the physician. (**3**) Placement is checked each shift to be sure it is not in the respiratory tract. (**4**) The tape should be removed only as necessary.

14. (**1**) Integrated processes: nursing process — planning; communication and documentation; client need: physiological integrity; reduction of risk potential; content area: procedures.

RATIONALE

(**1**) A laxative is needed to clean the barium out of the gastrointestinal tract. (**2**) A frequent check of vital signs will not be necessary. (**3**) Fluids should be forced to help eliminate the barium, and the client should eat. (**4**) Evaluation of lower extremities for neurovascular signs would not be necessary.

15. (**4**) Integrated processes: nursing process — implementation; client need: physiological integrity; basic care and comfort; content area: procedures.

RATIONALE

(**1**) It is not necessary to keep the container filled at all times. (**2**) No damage would be done if the container for the feeding were below the jejunum. (**3**) The client might be uncomfortable in high-Fowler's position. (**4**) The head of the bed must remain elevated 30–40 degrees at all times to prevent aspiration.

16. (**3**) Integrated processes: nursing process — implementation; client need: physiological integrity; reduction of risk potential; content area: procedures.

RATIONALE

(**1**) The pump would alarm if occlusion occurred. (**2**) Aspirating and flushing a Keofeed tube would be difficult because of the size of the bore. (**3**) Water is necessary to prevent dehydration caused by osmotic diuresis. Most tube feedings have a high osmolarity. (**4**) Unless medications were in liquid form, they would probably clog the tube.

17. (**2**) Integrated processes: nursing process — implementation; client need: physiological integrity; reduction of risk potential; content area: procedures.

RATIONALE

(**1**) The aspirate should not be discarded because electrolytes would be wasted. (**2**) The aspirate should be returned to the stomach to preserve electrolyte balance. (**3**) The data do not indicate that a specimen should be sent to the laboratory. (**4**) The aspirate should not be added to the feeding because bacterial growth would be enhanced.

18. (**2**) Integrated processes: nursing process — implemenation; teaching/learning; client need: physiological integrity; basic care and comfort; content area: procedures.

RATIONALE

(**1**) Bladder irrigation will not be performed after hypospadias repair. (**2**) The suprapubic catheter is placed as an alternate urinary elimination route following the reconstruction of the meatus. This ensures that the bladder will not become distended if the primary urinary catheter should become blocked. (**3**) While a suprapubic catheter would allow for accurate urine measurement, this is not the reason it is placed following hypospadias repair. (**4**) While this is true, this is not the reason a suprapubic catheter is placed following hypospadias repair.

19. (**4**) Integrated processes: nursing process — implementation; client need: physiological integrity; physiological adaptation; content area: procedures.

RATIONALE

(**1**) Gagging indicates that the toddler still has a patent airway. The toddler should be watched carefully to see that he can still speak. No lifesaving measures are necessary at this time. (**2**) Coughing indicates that the toddler can exchange air. The toddler should be watched to make sure that he can clear the food from his throat by coughing. Should he suddenly not be able to speak, lifesaving measures are indicated. (**3**) A pulse over 100 bpm is appropriate for a toddler and does not indicate the need for lifesaving measures. The key parameter to observe with choking is the ability to speak. (**4**) Inability to speak indicates an obstructed airway. Lifesaving measures are indicated at this time to clear the obstruction from the airway.

20. (**1**) Integrated processes: nursing process — implementation; client need: physiological integrity; physiological adapation; content area: procedures.

RATIONALE

(**1**) The brachial pulse is felt for infants under 1 year of age. The carotid pulse is difficult to palpate in infants. (**2**) The compression to ventilation ratio for children under the age of 8 years is one breath to every five compressions. (**3**) If an infant is not breathing, give two slow breaths (1.0–1.5 sec each). Observe chest rise and allow lung deflation between breaths. (**4**) The cardiac compression rate for children between the ages of 1 and 8 years should be 100 per minute.

21. (**2**) Integrated processes: nursing process — planning; client need: safe, effective care environment; safety and infection control; content area: procedures.

RATIONALE

(1) Strict isolation is not indicated at this time for the client. (2) All visitors should be screened for symptoms of influenza and varicella, because these are highly contagious and could present significant risk to the client. Visitors should also observe careful handwashing. (3) Raw fruits and vegetables may transmit disease organisms to the client. All fruits and vegetables should be canned or cooked. (4) Stuffed animals can harbor infectious organisms. Toys that can be easily disinfected should be encouraged.

22. **(3)** Integrated processes: nursing process — implementation; client need: physiological integrity; reduction of risk potential; content area: procedures.

RATIONALE

(1) Padding the elastic bands is not usually done because the bands need to fit snugly and can be adjusted to prevent skin irritation. (2) The nurse may take the pulse before starting therapy but this is not a preventive measure. (3) Humidifying the oxygen gas before administration is a protective measure of oxygen administration because it helps to prevent drying fo the nose and mouth mucosa. (4) If client is experiencing severe difficulty with breathing, placing the client in the orthopneic position may faciliate easier breathing, but this is not a protective measure of oxygen therapy.

23. **(1)** Integrated processes: nursing process — evaluation; client need: safe, effective care environment; safety and infection control; content area: procedures.

RATIONALE

(1) Weights, pulleys, and ropes help maintain countertraction to support position and alignment of a fracture. (2) Elevation of the foot of the bed will not maintain position or alignment. (3) Gravity and body weight alone do not support position and alignment of a fracture. (4) Elevation of the knee gatch will not support position and alignment of a fracture.

24. **(1)** Integrated processes: nursing process — implementation; client need: physiological integrity; basic care and comfort; content area: procedures.

RATIONALE

(1) This position will facilitate respirations and decrease cardiac workload. (2) A prone position will not facilitate respiratory effort and may increase cardiac workload. (3) A supine position will not faciliate respirations and may increase cardiac workload. (4) Trendelenburg's position, although useful in cases of shock, will not assist the child in congestive heart failure and may worsen respirations and cardiac function.

25. **(2)** Integrated processes: nursing process — implementation; communication and documentation; client need: safe, effective care environment; safety and infection control; content area: procedures.

RATIONALE

(1) Administering an enema to a client with suspected appendicitis is contraindicated and could produce injury. (2) You would call and question the physician about this order. Administering an enema to a client with suspected appendicitis is contraindicated and could produce injury. (3) Administering an enema to a client with suspected appendicitis is contraindicated and could produce injury. (4) The purpose of the enema is to clear the intestines of any matter prior to surgery. Whether or not the client has had any bowel movements, in this situation, is not relevant.

26. **(1)** Integrated processes: nursing process — implementation; client need: safe, effective care environment; safety and infection control; content area: procedures.

RATIONALE

(1) Universal precautions, which include gloving and correct disposal of sharps, would be used with all patients. (2) Isolation of the patient would not be necessary for blood drawing. (3) Drawing a routine blood sample would not require gowning. (4) Wearing a face shield would not be necessary during routine blood drawing.

27. **(1)** Integrated processes: nursing process — implementation; client need: safe, effective care environment; safety and infection control; content area: procedures.

RATIONALE

(1) Meticulous handwashing prior to client contact is the best way to prevent infection. (2) Measuring temperature does not prevent infection; it indicates presence of infection. (3) Meticulous handwashing prior to client contact is the best way to prevent infection. (4) Meticulous handwashing prior to client contact is the best way to prevent infection.

28. **(3)** Integrated processes: nursing process — implementation; client need: safe, effective care environment; safety and infection control; content area: procedures.

RATIONALE

(1) Immunization with the hepatitis B vaccine is the best way to prevent infection with the hepatitis B virus. (2) Immunization with the hepatitis B vaccine is the best way to prevent infection with the hepatitis B virus. (3) Immunization with the hepatitis B vaccine is the best way to prevent infection with the hepatitis B virus. (4) Immunization with the hepatitis B vaccine is the best way to prevent infection with the hepatitis B virus.

29. **(1)** Integrated processes: nursing process — implementation; client need: physiological integrity; reduction of risk potential; content area: procedures.

RATIONALE

(1) The first specimen collected at 8 AM Monday is discarded; all urine voided until 8 AM Tuesday is collected. (2) It is not necessary to place the urine in a separate container. (3) A culture was not ordered. (4) Discarding the urine would invalidate the results of the test.

30. **(1)** Integrated processes: nursing process — implementation; teaching/learning; client need: safe, effective care environment; safety and infection control; content area: procedures.

RATIONALE

(1) Freshly prepared solutions of sodium hypochlorite (bleach) in a 1:10 dilution are effective disinfectants. (2) Bleach is the most effective disinfectant for cleaning up blood and body fluid spills. (3) Bleach is the most effective disinfectant for cleaning up blood and body fluid spills. (4) Bleach is the most effective disinfectant for cleaning up blood and body fluid spills.

31. **(1)** Integrated processes: nursing process — implementation; client need: safe, effective care environment; safety and infection control; content area: procedures.

RATIONALE

(1) When the health-care worker is at risk of being directly exposed to any client's blood or body secretions, universal precautions are mandated. (2) The health-care worker often has no way of knowing which clients have been tested or are at risk for HIV infections. (3) The health-care worker often does not know which clients are members of high-risk groups; therefore, universal precautions are necessary for all client contact where risk is involved. (4) Universal precautions are necessary for all client contact where risk of blood/body fluid exposure is possible.

32. **(1)** Integrated processes: nursing process — implementation; client need: safe, effective care environment; safety and infection control; content area: procedures.

RATIONALE

(1) Handwashing is considered one of the most effective ways to prevent the spread of infection because of the constant contact of nurses with infectious materials. (2) Incisions are cleansed from top to bottom, which includes cleaning from the least contaminated to the most contaminated area. (3) Although this intervention would help prevent wound infection in some cases, it is not the best action by the nurse in this situation. (4) Although this practice may help prevent the transmission of infections, handwashing before and after is the safest and most effective method of preventing the spread of infection.

33. **(2)** Integrated processes: nursing process — implementation; client need: physiological integrity; reduction of risk potential; content area: procedures.

RATIONALE

(1) The tip of the tubing has to be lubricated for easier insertion and must be inserted approximately 3–4 inches into the rectum past the internal sphincter. (2) The client needs to be in the left lateral position with the right leg flexed to promote comfort while the solution is introduced into the intestine. (3) The solution should be introduced slowly over a period of 5–10 minutes to prevent rapid distention of the intestine and a desire to defecate. The container should not be higher than 18 inches above the anus, or this will increase the rate and cause rapid bowel distention. (4) Fluid should flow slowly. The client should take as much as possible of the amount ordered. The tubing should be clamped before removing it from the anus to prevent leakage. The tip is lubricated, and the left lateral position with the right leg flexed facilitates accurate fluid distribution in the intestine and minimizes discomfort from cramping.

34. **(4)** Integrated processes: nursing process — implementation; client need: safe, effective care environment; safety and infection control; content area: procedures.

RATIONALE

(1) Once a swab or gauze has been used, it is considered contaminated and should be discarded, and then a new one should be used. (2) Wound care with an antiseptic solution requires a physician's order. (3) This method introduces organisms back into the wound for recontamination. (4) The wound or incision should be cleansed from the area of least contamination to the area of greater contamination.

35. **(1)** Integrated processes: nursing process — implementation; client need: safe, effective care environment; safety and infection control; content area: procedures.

RATIONALE

(1) This method prevents further contamination of the wound and reduces the chance of infection. (2) This does not describe the correct rationale for irrigating a wound and does not guarantee organization by the nurse to complete the procedure. (3) This is not the correct rationale for the direction of fluid flow to irrigate a wound. (4) Irrigation of a wound with the client in various positions does not always enhance comfort.

36. **(1)** Integrated processes: nursing process — implementation; client need: safe, effective care environment; safety and infection control; content area: procedures.

RATIONALE

(1) A nosocomial infection is one that results from the delivery of health services in a health-care facility. The urinary tract is a prime site; placing the urinary drainage bag above the level of the bladder allows a reflux of urine in the catheter or bag (which could be contaminated) to reenter the bladder and become a source of infection. (2) Aseptic technique would help prevent an infection at the incision site, but a urinary tract infection is the most common nosocomial infection. (3) Self-administration

of insulin would not cause a nosocomial infection. (4) Spreading germs by not covering the mouth is not an example of a nosocomial infection.

37. **(4)** Integrated processes: nursing process — data collection; client need: safe, effective care environment; safety and infection control; content area: procedures.

RATIONALE

(1) Although instillation of air assists in placement assessment, it does not provide the nurse with residual volume data. (2) Auscultating the bowel sounds with the use of 10 mL of tap water is not a safe intervention because the fluid can be aspirated into the lungs and only air should be instilled to ensure accurate tube placement. (3) Although submerging the end of a feeding tube in a glass of water can indicate correct tube placement, aspirating the contents is the safest and most accurate nursing intervention in this situation. (4) It is best for the nurse to aspirate the stomach contents in order to ascertain tube position as well as the client's absorption of the tube feedings. The gastric contents are reinstilled to prevent electrolyte imbalance.

38. **(4)** Integrated processes: nursing process — data collection; client need: physiological integrity; reduction of risk potential; content area: procedures.

RATIONALE

(1) Catching the midstream of urine will provide the most accurate urinalysis. Also, the laboratory needs at least 10 mL of urine for proper analysis. (2) If all urine is collected in the container, there is a greater chance of contamination of the urine from bacteria and cleaning solution collected with the specimen. (3) The first 50 mL of urine may be contaminated with bacteria and cleansing solution. The midstream provides the most accurate urinalysis. (4) The midstream of urine provides minimal or no contamination by bacteria or cleansing solution and therefore, provides the best specimen for an accurate urinalysis.

39. **(3)** Integrated processes: nursing process — implementation; client need: safe, effective care environment; safety and infection control; content area: procedures.

RATIONALE

(1) The portal of entry to host is a source of acquiring an infection — not a practice to break the "chain of infection." (2) The reservoir is a host for infection — not a method to transfer infection from one source to another and therefore not a practice to break the "chain of infection." (3) The method of transmission of infection is the phase in which hand washing before and after various tasks can break the "chain of infection" and lead to safe, effective client care. (4) The portal of exit from host refers to blood, wound drainage, feces, and urine, which can transmit disease because of improper handling and improper handwashing technique.

40. **(4)** Integrated processes: nursing process — implementation; client need: safe, effective care environment; safety and infection control; content area: procedures.

RATIONALE

(1) Isolation specific to preventing transmission of infection related to feces is not blood and body fluids. (2) Isolation specific to preventing transmission of infection related to feces is not contact isolation. (3) Drainage and secretion isolation is used with clients for protection of wound drainage, not specifically for infection related to feces. (4) Enteric isolation is specifically used to prevent the transmission of infection related to feces.

41. **(4)** Integrated processes: nursing process — implementation; client need: physiological integrity; reduction of risk potential; content area: procedures.

RATIONALE

(1) A routine urinalysis is not considered a stat procedure unless specifically ordered by the physician. The urine specimen needs to be sent to the laboratory to be examined within 2 hours, otherwise it will become alkaline unless refrigerated. (2) For a routine analysis, the laboratory needs at least 10 ml of urine. (3) A routine urinalysis does not require being in a sterile container. Any small clean container is appropriate. A sterile container is required for a urine culture and sensitivity. (4) The first voided specimen in the morning is best for a routine urinalysis because the urine is concentrated and any abnormalities will become more evident in the screening procedure.

42. **(1)** Integrated processes: nursing process — implementation; client need: safe, effective care environment; safety and infection control; content area: procedures.

RATIONALE

(1) Only a small part of the scrubbed person's body is considered sterile: from the waist to the shoulder area, forearm, and gloves. (2) The scrub gown below the waist is not considered sterile. (3) The scrub gown above the elbow is not considered sterile. (4) The back of one's scrub gown is not considered sterile.

43. **(3)** Integrated processes: nursing process — implementation; client need: physiological integrity; pharmacological therapies.

RATIONALE

(1) Enteric pills should never be crushed, and if the medication arrives with this type of coating, the nurse should call the pharmacy to try to get a liquid form of the medication for administration down the feeding tube. (2) Time-released compounds should never be crushed to place down a feeding tube. The pills are made to be released slowly into the system, and crushing the medication will negate this effect. (3) Compressed tablets are the only type of pill medication that should be crushed for administration into a feeding tube. (4) Sublingual medication, such as nitroglycerin, is meant to be placed under the tongue for slow absorption. This type of medication is not to be crushed and placed into a feeding tube.

44. **(4)** Integrated processes: nursing process — implementation; client need: physiological integrity; reduction of risk potential; content area: procedures.

RATIONALE

(1) The most important factor in accurately measuring the BP is the use of an appropriate cuff size. The BP cuff should cover 75% of the child's upper arm to obtain an accurate measurement. (2, 3, and 4) The BP cuff should cover 75% of the child's upper arm to obtain an accurate measurement.

45. **(4)** Integrated processes: nursing process — implementation; client need: physiological integrity; reduction of risk potential; content area: procedures.

RATIONALE

(1) Arterial blood sampling is painful and unnecessary for accurate blood sugars. (2) The center of the heel is not appropriate because more nerve endings are located there. (3) In infants, the heel is recommended. Also, a finger stick site is to the side of the finger pad because there are more blood vessels and fewer nerves lateral to the finger pad. (4) The boundaries for a heel puncture can be marked by an imaginary line extending posteriorly from a point between the fourth and fifth toes running parallel to the lateral aspect of the heel and another line extending posteriorly from the middle of the great toe and running parallel to the medial aspect of the heel. The puncture sites are the outer aspects of the heel defined by the identified lines.

46. **(2)** Integrated processes: nursing process — implementation; client need: physiological integrity; physiological adaptation; content area: procedures.

RATIONALE

(1) This is the proper depth to use with infants under the age of 1 year. (2) This is the proper depth for a child from 1 year through 8 years of age. (3) This is the proper depth from 8 years of age through adulthood. (4) This is too deep and not advocated for any age person.

47. **(2)** Integrated processes: nursing process — implementation; client need: physiological integrity; physiological adaptation; content area: procedures.

RATIONALE

(1) The carotid pulse is assessed in children over the age of 1 year. (2) The brachial pulse is used to assess circulation in infants from birth to 1 year of age. (3) The femoral pulse is not used in CPR. (4) The radial pulse is not used in CPR.

48. **(4)** Integrated processes: nursing process — implementation; Client need: Physiological integrity; physiological adaptation; Content area: procedures.

RATIONALE

(1) The use of both hands is done from 8 years of age through adulthood. (2) The heel of one hand is used in children from 1 to 8 years of age. (3) Three fingers are never used. (4) The index and middle fingers are used on newborns to the age of 1 year.

49. **(3)** Integrated processes: nursing process — implementation; client need: physiological integrity; physiological adaptation; content area: procedures.

RATIONALE

(1) This would be appropriate if the child becomes unconscious. (2) This would be appropriate if the child is conscious, but unable to cough, talk, or make sounds. (3) This is appropriate because the child is conscious and can still cough and make sounds. The airway is not completely obstructed. (4) These actions would be appropriate for an infant whose airway is obstructed.

50. **(1)** Integrated processes: Nursing process — data collection; client need: physiological integrity; physiological adaptation; content area: procedures.

RATIONALE

(1) A stage II decubitus ulcer appears as a superficial ulcer that may be a blister, abrasion, or shallow crater. (2) A stage one decubitus ulcer is a nonblanching erythema. (3) A stage III decubitus ulcer formation extends into the deeper subcutaneous tissue. (4) A stage IV decubitus ulcer extends into the deep subcutaneous tissue and ends in full-thickness skin loss.

REFERENCES

Potter, P and Perry, A: Fundamentals of Nursing, ed 5. CV Mosby, St. Louis, 2001.

Smith, S, Duell, D, and Martin, B: Clinical Nursing Skills: Basic to Advanced Skill. Prentice-Hall, Upper Saddle River, NJ, 2004.

Smith-Temple, J and Johnson, J: Nurse's Guide to Clinical Procedures, ed 4. Lippincott Williams & Wilkins, Philadelphia, 2002.

CHAPTER 9

Leadership, Management, and Delegation: Content Review and Test

Valecia Carter-Vaughn, RN, MSN
Jerry Denny, RN, MS, MSN
Golden M. Tradewell, RN, PhD

I. Nurse Practice Act
   A. Regulated by licensing authorities within each jurisdiction
   B. Each jurisdiction requires candidates to meet requirements
      1. Completion of program of study
      2. Passing an examination that measures competencies
   C. Beliefs about nursing
      1. People are finite beings
      2. People have varying capacities of function in society
      3. Unique individuals with defined systems of daily living
      4. Individuals are influenced by values, cultures, motives, and lifestyle
      5. Individuals have the right to make decisions regarding their health-care needs
   D. Beliefs about nursing practice
      1. Profession helps client to achieve optimal level of health
      2. Profession contributes in a variety of settings.
      3. Profession based on understanding of human condition across the life span
      4. Founded on professional body of knowledge
      5. Integrates concepts from biological, behavioral, and social sciences.
      6. Goal is to promote comfort and quality health care.
      7. Assists individuals by responding to their needs, conditions and events that result from actual or potential health problems.
   E. Beliefs about practical/vocational nursing
      1. Specialized knowledge and skills which meet the health needs of people
      2. Knowledge and skills practiced under the direction of qualified health professionals.
      3. Using clinical problem-solving process (the nursing process) to collect and organize relevant health-care data
      4. Assists in the identification of the health needs/problems with predictable outcomes.
      5. Contributes to the interdisciplinary team in a variety of settings.

II. Client Needs
   A. Four major Client Needs categories
      1. Safe and effective care environment
         a. Coordinated care
         b. Safety and infection control
      2. Health promotion and maintenance
      3. Psychosocial integrity
      4. Physiological integrity
         a. Basic care and comfort
         b. Pharmacological therapies
         c. Reduction of risk potential
         d. Physiological adaptation
   B. Framework of Client Needs
      1. Universal structure for defining nursing actions and competencies
      2. Universal structure for a variety of clients across all settings
      3. Is congruent with state law/rules

III. Safe, Effective Care Environment
   A. Coordinated care
      1. Incident/Irregular Occurrence/Variance Reports
         a. The purpose of an incident report, irregular occurrence report, and variance report is the same. These reports are written and filed as a means of recording an unusual event that

involves the patient, family members of the patient, friends or visitors of the patient, health-care employees, vendors, or anyone visiting the facility.

b. The report allows the facility to keep a written record of the incident, thereby providing the facility with factual information.

c. The report can also serve as a tool in providing statistical information that provides support for organizational or institutional changes that are needed to enhance functioning and/or increase safety in the healthcare facility.

d. Information to be included in the report
   1) The report identifies the person involved in the unusual event or accident. The individual's name and hospital or identification number is listed as appropriate.
   2) The location of the incident, time of the occurrence and date of the occurrence is also provided.
   3) A description of the event, as witnessed is given.
   4) All witnesses are identified.
   5) Any equipment or unusual circumstance is also recorded.

B. Informed consent
1. The client must receive full disclosure of risks, benefits, alternative treatments or consequences of lack of treatment in order to give informed consent. When informed consent is given, a form is signed by the client to document this event. The nurse witnesses the client's signing of the informed consent. If the nurse is aware that the client is not clear on information given, it is the nurse's responsibility to report this to the physician immediately.
2. It is the physician's responsibility to obtain informed consent for surgical and medical treatment.
3. It is the nurse's responsibility to obtain informed consent for nursing procedures.
4. Criteria necessary to obtain informed consent
   a. Must be voluntary.
   b. Client must have the capacity and competence for understanding the information.
   c. Client must be given enough of the correct information regarding the procedure.
5. Types of informed consent
   a. Express consent can be written or oral.
   b. Implied consent is given by nonverbal behavior: During an emergency, during surgery when further treatment consistent with present treatment is needed, and when the client continues with ongoing treatment without recanting or rescinding previous consent.
6. Exceptions to informed consent
   a. A parent or guardian can give consent for minors or for adults with the mental functioning of a minor.
   b. Consent can be given by the closest adult relative or by the law when a client is unconscious or injured to a degree that prevents consenting.

c. Consent can be given by the closest adult relative or by the law when the client is incompetent due to mental illness.

IV. Legal Responsibilities
A. Legal responsibilities for the practical nurse (PN) are set by the State Board of Nursing through the Nurse Practice Act.
B. Responsibilities of the State Board of Nursing include
   1. Giving accreditation to nursing schools when they meet the criteria established by the Board
   2. Setting minimum standards of nursing practice
   3. Governing PN licensure
   4. Investigating suspected violations of the Nurse Practice Act
   5. Interpreting the Nurse Practice Act
C. Legal management duties of the PN are set by each individual State Board of Nursing. Each PN must be familiar with the Nurse Practice Act of the state in which practice occurs. PN duties include assessment, planning, implementation, and evaluation of patient care. They also include administration of certain medications and supervision of unlicensed assistive personnel.

V. Referral Processes
A. The referral process is an approach to problem solving that helps clients reach their individual goals, psychosocial and health-care needs. In order to refer adequately, the nurse must have at least a basic knowledge of resources available.
   1. Referrals should contain as much information about the client and the client's needs as possible.
   2. For reimbursement purposes, referrals require a physician's written order.

VI. Resource Management
A. Resource management involves the responsible use of available resources. Proper management of resources helps to keep health-care costs down for the client and aid in the client's prolonged accessibility to quality care.

VII. Advocacy
A. Patient care involvement to improve health care by bringing about change.
B. Patient advocate role is to inform, support, and mediate to ensure patient access to health-care services according to the patient's needs.
C. An essential part of nursing leadership in which the leader/advocate works toward certain desired changes to produce quality of care.
   1. Protecting patient's rights to be informed and participate in decision making as it relates to the patient's care
   2. Assisting in identifying health-care risks through risk management
   3. Lobbying for safe nursing practice standards

Patient's Rights
D. Moral rights to determine care and outcome of care of one's own body
E. Right to information to make an informed decision
F. Right to information regarding actual and potential effects of care

G. Right to accept, refuse, or terminate treatment

H. American Hospital Association Statement on a Patient's Bill of Rights (revised 1992, nos. 1–12) incorporates patient responsibilities and obligations

VIII. Ethical Practice

A. Nursing decisions and actions based and guided by a code of ethics

B. A set of rules having higher requirements than legal standards which define right and wrong conduct relating to patient care

C. Concerned with relationships which go beyond personal references

D. Based on professional agreement regarding:
1. Responsibility
2. Accountability
3. Advocacy
4. Confidentiality
5. Veracity

E. The ethical decision made in various situations, may be compromised or not made due to client circumstances and laws.

IX. Advance Directives

A. Documents stating patient's wishes in the event of health conditions deeming the patient's inability to make own health-care decisions.
1. Living Will (patient chooses wishes)
2. Durable Power of Attorney (patient delegated person to make medical decisions if patient is unable to do so)

B. The Patient Self-Determination Act, 1991 (PSDA)
1. Health-care facilities receiving Medicare and Medicaid reimbursement are required to:
a. Recognize advance directives.
b. Ask patient if he/she has an advance directive.
c. Provide educational materials regarding advance directives.
2. Nurses must know the state law regarding PSDA.
3. Nurses must know institution policy and procedures for implementation of PSDA.

X. Establishing Priorities

A. Determine importance and establish an order within a time frame.

B. Time constraints.
1. STAT: must be done within established time frame to prevent harm, usually within minutes. STAT medication, physician orders for lab work are done within minutes.
2. Immediate: must be done as soon as possible to prevent harm and within short time period.
3. Time frame for tasks to be completed may be within 1 hour, within 2–4 hours, within an undesignated time during the work shift, or delegated to the on-coming shift.
4. Nurses must decide what is to be done.
a. RN-only responsibilities
b. LPN responsibilities
c. Unlicensed staff member responsibilities
d. Referred to other members of the health-care team
5. Nurses manage by
a. Planning

b. Completing the most important task to be done first
c. Completing one task before starting another
d. Evaluating plan and relating new information to reprioritize as indicated.

C. Maslow Hiearchy of Needs (1954) provides the nurse with a priority of client care needs organized to provide care directed toward preventing harm.
a. Physiological (necessary for life)
b. Safety (safe, effective environment)
c. Love
d. Esteem
e. Self-actualization

XI. Patient Care Assignments

A. Be aware of job descriptions, level of education, and proficiency of skill.

B. Be aware of available resources.

C. Be available to assist.

D. Verify completion of tasks is according to the standards of care.

E. Delegation is a management tool that improves productivity.
1. Five Rights of Delegation (National Council of State Boards of Nursing, 1995)
a. Right task specific to patient's needs.
b. Right circumstances—patient setting and available resources
c. Right person—qualified delegation to qualified person for specific patient care
d. Right direction—Communication-clarity in task description including expectations
e. Right supervision—appropriate monitoring, assistance, and evaluation
2. Delegation involves having the authority to perform the task.
a. Accountability cannot be delegated.
b. Responsibility can be delegated.
c. Legally, an individual is accountable for his/her own actions.

XII. Concepts of Management and Supervision

A. The nurse uses knowledge of management and supervision concepts to learn how to work with people in the work environment, to understand the work of the nurse and to control situations in the work environment.

B. Effective management is directed toward achieving organizational goals

C. Effective supervision is directed toward
1. Providing guidance or direction
2. Performance evaluation

D. Directed toward follow-up on the completion of an assigned task

E. Effective leadership
1. Behavior directed toward influencing others
2. Purpose is to achieve goals of a group, unit, or organization

F. Role of the nurse
1. Works as an individual
2. Works as a member of a team
3. Works within groups
4. Works to accomplish the work of the nurse

5. Works to meet the objectives of the health-care organization
G. Role of the nurse manager
1. Management functions and roles
2. Supervisor responsibilities and accountability
3. Leader and follower role
4. Leadership behaviors and styles
5. Nursing roles, functions, and job descriptions

XIII. Confidentiality
A. The nurse is responsible for maintaining client confidentiality through the following agency policies, standards, and guidelines. The Health Insurance Portability and Accountability Act (HIPPA) provided information on patient rights and expectations of employers to protect patient rights.
B. HIPPA directives and consequences of failure of nurses to comply with directives.
C. Patient Rights and nurse's responsibilities
1. Written documentation
2. Verbal communication among nursing personnel

XIV. Consultation with members of the health-care team
A. Problem solving and decision making
1. Client care
a. Use of knowledge and experience to make decisions
b. Consults with various members of the health-care team
2. Work environment
a. RN and LPN roles and responsibilities
b. LPN and physician communication
c. LPN and other health-care team member communication
d. Chain of command and communication expectations
e. Job expectations of LPN in acute care hospitals
f. Job expectations of LPN in community agencies.

XV. Continuity of Care
A. Nursing Standards of Practice
1. Based on written standards, protocols, and guidelines.

2. Continuity of care provided by practicing according to established nursing practice standards
3. Continuity of care provided by following community agency policies and procedures
B. Nursing Care Plans/Critical Pathways and Protocols
1. A policy is a written guide for making decisions about client care or work situations.
2. A procedure is a step-by-step guide to follow when implementing specific tasks related to client care.
3. A protocol is a written client care planning document that may contain physician orders, nursing care orders, orders from physical therapy, dietary, or social services.
4. Written documents such as "Advanced Directives" or a "Living Will" are examples of forms that directly impact client care.

XVI. Continuous Quality Improvement
A. Nurses act as individuals, as members of a health-care team, and in consultation with others to provide quality care and positive client outcomes.
1. Quality of health care can depend on the client's expectation and outcome of having health needs met at a manageable cost.
2. Continuous quality improvement (CQI) is an ongoing process of review and improvement
3. Nurses participate in CQI activities at a unit level by collecting data, auditing records, observations, and participating in focus groups.
a. Teamwork
b. Patient's perspective of care
c. Measurement of standards set for staff, actions, and results or outcome of care provided.
d. Resources
4. Nurses monitor nursing practices, identify problems, and participate in taking actions to improve health care by:
a. Reporting problems using an Incident/Variance Report
b. Participating in continuing education and in-service education as ways to promote quality client care outcomes.

QUESTIONS

Valecia Carter-Vaughn, RN, MSN, Jerry Denny, RN, MS, MSN, and Golden M. Tradewell, RN, PhD

1. The purpose of the incident report is to
   1. Provide documentation on the client's chart regarding an unusual incident.
   2. Provide written documentation regarding an unusual event.
   3. Place blame on the client for any accidents or injuries that occur during hospitalization.
   4. Document that you are not responsible for the unusual occurrence.

2. The incident report
   1. Identifies the person(s) involved in the incident.
   2. Gives a subjective, nonfactual description of the event and witnesses present.
   3. Protects the institution from lawsuits.
   4. Cannot be viewed by hospital personnel.

3. If an employee is injured due to inadequately functioning equipment, the employee should
   1. File a workmen's compensation form in place of an incident report.
   2. Fill out an incident report leaving out information regarding the malfunctioning equipment.
   3. Expect risk management to decide if an incident report should be filed.
   4. Fill out an incident report including information regarding the malfunctioning equipment.

4. What are the exceptions to obtaining informed consent from the patient?

   _____

5. In order to obtain informed consent, it must be
   1. Voluntary
   2. Coerced
   3. Given after the physician performs the procedure.
   4. Only written

6. Expressed consent
   1. Must be written to be valid.
   2. Can be written or verbalized orally.
   3. Can be verbalized only if the patient is unable to write.
   4. Does not exist.

7. Implied consent
   1. Must be written to be valid.
   2. Can be written or verbalized orally.
   3. Is given by nonverbal behavior.
   4. Must be given by parents.

8. The nurse is in the patient's room before a scheduled angiogram. The client signed the consent earlier that morning. The client informs the nurse that she had taken her diazepam (Valium) 40 minutes before signing the consent and really does not understand what the physician will be doing. She further states she will have the procedure done anyway. What should the nurse do?
   1. Nothing, the patient has verbalized that she does not object to the procedure.
   2. Explain the procedure, risks, benefits and alternatives.
   3. Notify the physician immediately.
   4. Have client re-sign another consent form.

9. Legal responsibilities for the practical nurse are set by

   _____ .

10. Legally, the practical nurse's duties include
    1. Patient assessment, planning, implementation, and evaluation of patient care
    2. Dispensing of all ordered medications
    3. Investigating suspected violations of the nurse practice act
    4. Supervision of licensed personnel

11. The practical nurse can legally
    1. Dispense any type of medication.
    2. Delegate duties to unlicensed assistive personnel.
    3. Order treatments for the client
    4. Delegate duties to licensed personnel

12. The nurse is referring her patient to the hospital social worker. The nurse is aware that referrals
    1. Should be concise and contain the least information possible.
    2. Are an independent nursing function and do not require a physician's signature.
    3. Should contain as much information about the patient as possible.
    4. Should only take place outside of the hospital setting.

13. The referral process helps the patient
    1. Reach individual goals, psychosocial and health-care needs
    2. Receive full reimbursement for all health-care administered
    3. Depend on the health-care facility for his or her needs
    4. Understand the restriction of resources

14. Resource management
    1. Involves the responsible use of available resources
    2. Is the responsibility of hospital administration and managers only
    3. Helps to increase health-care costs
    4. Restricts accessibility to health-care resources.

15. The charge nurse on a nursing unit makes decisions concerning the management of the nursing unit without staff input. The leadership style of the charge nurse is:

1. Autocratic
2. Democratic
3. Laissez-faire
4. Transformational

16. An LPN has been assigned four clients. A nurse's aide is assigned to assist the LPN caring for the clients. Which of the following assignments may be done by the nurse's aide without direct supervision by the LPN? **(Select all that apply.)**

   1. Accompany a client being discharged home.
   2. Collect a urine specimen from a 75-year-old client.
   3. Feed a severely disabled teenage client breakfast.
   4. Offer sips of water to a postoperative client.
   5. Catheterize an elderly client.
   6. Administer oral medications.

17. The RN team leader has a newly graduated PN and a nurse's aide on the team. There are six clients assigned to these individuals. The RN assigns the PN to give medications to all six clients. The PN needs to be aware of the following when accepting an assignment from the RN. **(Select all that apply.)**

   1. The charge nurse's lunch assignment schedule
   2. The hospital's job description for LPNs
   3. The head nurse's unit plan of care
   4. The State Nurse Practice Act
   5. The job description of the unlicensed assistive personnel (UAP)
   6. The job description of the physician

18. The nurse and the nurse's aide are listening to report when the nurse's aide makes the following comment on the client's family circumstances. "My mother lives next door to her and she said they all use drugs." The nurse's response is:

   1. "If you can only say harmful things, be quiet."
   2. "Please stop talking about the client's family."
   3. "That is interesting, but not needed here."
   4. "What is the purpose of sharing that information?"

19. A client's visitor is talking with the family members in the hallway outside the client's room. As the visitor is leaving, he stops at the desk and comments to the nurse, "I didn't want to bother the family with too many questions, but I just want to know … what is wrong with him, so I can tell his other church friends about how he is doing?" Which response is evidence of the nurse's accountability for client confidentiality?

   1. "He is not my client."
   2. "On this unit, only the head nurse gives out that information."
   3. "Only the client determines who has access to any information about his medical condition."
   4. "The hospital's policy prevents nurses from providing client information to friends."

20. As the nurse in the Obstetrical Clinic is assisting a female teen-age client in changing clothing, the nurse observes several dark bruised areas on the client's back. The client becomes extremely upset and asks the nurse not to tell anyone about her bruises. The nurse's response is:

   1. "I have to report what I see to the physician."
   2. "I won't say anything, but you need to get help."
   3. "I won't say anything, but if it does happen again, you should call the police."
   4. "You have possible internal injuries that could be harmful to your health."

21. During a home health visit, the PN asked the 83-year-old client about her medications when the client comments, "Well, I took my blood pressure yesterday morning and it was too low so I didn't take my medicine." The nurse's responses to the client include which of the following? **(Select all that apply.)**

   1. "Did you talk with your physician about your blood pressure before you decided not to take your medication?"
   2. "I need to report the changes in your blood pressure to the physician."
   3. "Let's check your blood pressure now."
   4. "That is probably a good thing to do since your blood pressure was low."
   5. "I have to call into the office and report this to my supervisor."
   6. "Are you sure you took your blood pressure correctly?"

22. The physician has requested the nurse teach the family to begin home care for an elderly client. The nurse is talking with the daughter about preparing and feeding the client formula through a PEG (percutaneous endoscopic gastrostomy) tube. The daughter is anxious and tells the nurse, "I never want to be kept alive on tubes and machines and I told the doctor I was not going to do this!" The nurse should:

   1. Ask someone else in the family to learn the procedure.
   2. Offer to sit with the daughter until she is calmer.
   3. Report the daughter's feelings and comments to the nursing supervisor.
   4. Terminate the discussion and leave.

23. During a home health visit, the elderly client complains of "back pain again, and every time I have therapy, my back hurts so much." The nurse's responsibilities include which of the following actions? **(Select all that apply.)**

   1. Ask the client if she would like pain medication.
   2. Gather data concerning the location, duration, and intensity of the pain.
   3. Inform the client to make an appointment with her physician about the back pain.
   4. Report the client's complaint to the nursing supervisor for further assessment.
   5. Report the client's complaint to the physical therapist.
   6. Report the client's complaint to the physician.

24. A client with the diagnosis of chest pain is admitted to the unit. The nurse received a verbal report via telephone from the nurse in the emergency room. The order for aspirin was not documented on the critical pathway documentation record as being given. The nurse's first action is to:

1. Ask the client if he was given any aspirin in the emergency room.
2. Administer the dosage of aspirin ordered on the critical pathway.
3. Notify the charge nurse of the problem.
4. Phone the emergency room nurse to verify client care and medications administered to the client.

25. A nurse is caring for a client with severe congestive heart failure. The client has been hospitalized three times within the past 6 months with cardiac problems related to congestive heart failure. The client states, "This is the last time I am going to let them do heart massage on me." The most appropriate action for the nurse is to:

    1. Offer the client a copy of the hospital's Living Will form.
    2. Tell the client to discuss his feelings with the family.
    3. Tell the client that his physician must be notified of his request.
    4. Tell the client that his request would be reported to the nurse supervisor.

26. A nurse is caring for a client diagnosed with acute renal failure. The nurse instructs the nurse's aide to do which of the following actions for the client first?

    1. Ambulate the client.
    2. Assist the client with breakfast.
    3. Monitor the client's level of consciousness every hour.
    4. Remove the water pitcher from the bedside.

27. The nurse discovers a medication error was made on the previous shift. Her responsibility is to:

    1. Tell the charge nurse on the shift the incident occurred and let her pursue the problem.
    2. Complete an incident report.
    3. Call the nurse who made the error and inform her that she made an error and she has to complete an incident report.
    4. Write a note in the patient's chart that an incident report was completed.

28. A client had been receiving a medication by injection for a number of weeks. You are preparing to give the client the injection when the client objects by stating, "My doctor changed this to a pill and I am not going to take that shot again." Your first action is to:

    1. Go back to the chart and check for the order.
    2. Check the order sheet for the changed order and then speak with the patient's physician concerning the order.
    3. Talk with the nurse who had taken care of the client while he or she was off duty.
    4. Talk with the charge nurse about the advisability of giving an oral rather than injectable medication.

29. The PN on the unit has an assignment of four clients. One of the clients needs to have an ostomy bag changed. The PN tells the RN that she did attend the education program and had been checked off on the procedure, and that she has not actually performed the procedure on a client. The most appropriate action of the PN is to:

    1. Request that another PN observe the procedure being performed.
    2. Request that the RN call the staff education nurse to observe the procedure being performed.
    3. Request the ostomy nurse to perform the procedure.
    4. Request to perform the procedure with the RN.

30. While drawing up medication through the new computerized medication administration system, you notice that the nurse ahead of you had signed out for a narcotic that was to be given to your client for pain control. In checking the chart, there was no record of the narcotic being given. Your client denied receiving anything for pain since the previous night. Which action should the nurse take first?

    1. Approach the nurse who had signed out the narcotic to seek clarification about the missing drug.
    2. Notify the pharmacist that a narcotic is missing.
    3. Notify the charge nurse/supervisor that the client did not receive the prescribed pain medication.
    4. Notify the client that someone else received his pain medication.

31. A client's husband plans to accompany his wife into the delivery room. When should the nurse plan to have him change into scrub attire?

    1. During the latent phase of labor
    2. Once active labor is established
    3. When complete dilation occurs
    4. When the fetal head is visible

32. A client at 32 weeks' gestation is admitted for possible preterm labor. The health-care provider performs an amniocentesis. Which nursing actions should occur immediately following the procedure?

    1. Monitor the needle entry site for signs and symptoms of infection.
    2. Monitor fetal heart tones and for uterine contractions.
    3. Explain the purpose of the amniocentesis to the client.
    4. Encourage the client to verbalize her concerns regarding the procedure.

33. A breast-feeding client who is 1-week postpartum calls the obstetrical clinic with a report of a hard lump and localized tenderness in the upper outer quadrant of the left breast. She also reports a temperature of 102°F (38.8°C), headache, and malaise. Considering these symptoms, which of the following instructions by the nurse would be most appropriate?

    1. "You should come into the clinic for a breast examination and maybe a biopsy. A painful lump could indicate cancer."
    2. "You should be admitted to the hospital right away. You have a serious breast infection and need to be started on IV antibiotics."
    3. "It is normal to have tender, lumpy breasts when you are breast-feeding. It will go away when you wean the baby."
    4. "Go to bed with your baby. Nurse every chance you get. Take acetaminophen (Tylenol) and drink lots of water."

34. The nurse is caring for a client whose baseline blood pressure (BP) was 110/60 mm Hg. Her blood pressure in the latent stage of labor is 146/76 mm Hg. What is the appropriate nursing action?
   1. The client's BP is still within an acceptable range. The nurse should continue routine monitoring of the BP.
   2. The client's BP is expected to increase in this stage of labor. The nurse should consider this a normal finding.
   3. If the client has no other complaints, the nurse should continue to observe her.
   4. The nurse should consider this reason for concern and notify the primary health-care provider.

35. You are orienting a new nurse to the newborn nursery. As she begins to assess a baby, you note that she listens to the apical heart rate for a full minute. How should you intervene in this situation?
   1. Tell her that it is a lot quicker if she listens for 15 seconds and multiplies that by four to get the heart rate.
   2. Instruct her to do a brachial pulse instead of listening to the apical heart rate.
   3. Give her positive feedback for performing this skill correctly.
   4. Tell her that as she gets more experience, this skill will become easier.

36. The nurse notices that one of the clients is unable to eat without assistance. Which action is most appropriate?
   1. Stop and assist the client with his meal.
   2. Ask the team leader to assist the client with his meal.
   3. Ask the nursing assistant to help the client with his meal.
   4. Notify dietary that the client cannot eat.

37. During the job evaluation, the nurse states that which of the following is one of her strengths on the job?
   1. She handles all of the problems herself.
   2. She can delegate nonskilled tasks to unlicensed personnel.
   3. She spends too much time in the client's room visiting with family members.
   4. She plans her day poorly.

38. Ethical issues in community-based nursing practice center on the rights of the client. Which of the following is a client right?
   1. Right not to be told of the prognosis
   2. Right to be restricted in type of treatment
   3. Right to confidentiality
   4. Right to have nurse disclose information regarding disease

39. In addition to honoring the client's rights, the nurse must fulfill her own responsibilities. Which of the following is considered the nurse's responsibility?
   1. Openly discussing the client's condition with nonprofessionals.
   2. Encourage the client to accept all treatment regardless of how it affects the quality of life.

   3. Be honest with the client about the care and treatment he or she is receiving.
   4. It is okay to lie to the client about his or her illness and prognosis.

40. The failure to adhere to one's legal duty is called:
   1. Statutes
   2. Common law
   3. Breach of duty
   4. Liability

41. Malpractice is:
   1. Failure to meet the standard of care
   2. Omission of a duty
   3. Professional conduct
   4. Duty to harm the client

42. An example of failing to meet the standard of care is:
   1. Properly administering insulin injections
   2. Providing instructions to a diabetic client
   3. Administering the wrong medication
   4. Instructions to the caregiver on how to administer medications

43. What type of nurse's behavior is appropriate to help avoid a malpractice lawsuit?
   1. Use aggressive communication with client and family members.
   2. If a mistake occurs, do not tell anyone.
   3. Document only what the client says.
   4. Communicate with the physician and supervisors when changes occur in the client's condition.

44. A standard of care is:
   1. Required by the American Medical Association
   2. Required by state licensing statutes
   3. Required by the Council on Aging
   4. Required by the President of the State Nurses' Association

45. What would be considered a deviation from the standard of care in community-based nursing?
   1. Analyzing data collected from client and family
   2. Identifying potential problems
   3. Identifying inappropriate nursing diagnoses
   4. Planning health promotion activities

46. What is the major cause of injury to clients in their homes?
   1. Poor electrical outlets
   2. Poor drainage in their yard
   3. Electric heaters
   4. Cluttered rooms with inaccessible walkway

47. What kind of client is at risk for falls?
   1. 45-year-old on IV antibiotic therapy
   2. 78-year-old with total knee replacement
   3. 65-year-old with congestive heart failure
   4. 70-year-old with diabetes

48. A nursing care plan for clients who are at high risk for falls includes:

1. Restrain the client to the bed.
2. Keep side rails down.
3. Remove throw rugs and clutter.
4. Have family member check on client weekly.

49. What action would predispose the nurse to a lawsuit?

1. Documenting an assessment on the client
2. Documenting communications with physician
3. Documenting telephone and verbal orders
4. Failing to document client instruction in wound care

50. Which of the following is considered to be an advanced directive?

1. Family member can choose to have cardiopulmonary resuscitation (CPR) performed on client without permission from the client. .
2. Family member can choose to have client placed on respirator as needed.
3. Client can refuse intravenous fluids.
4. Family member can choose to have a feeding tube inserted into client without permission.

51. Who is responsible for documenting client's advanced directives?

1. Unit secretary
2. Nursing assistant
3. Licensed practical nurse/licensed vocational nurse (LPN/LVN)
4. Physician

52. A home-care client with a terminal illness asks you directly if he is dying. The physician has left instructions that the client is not to be told about his status as it might cause too much anxiety. What should you do?

1. Encourage the client to ask his physician about his prognosis.
2. Tell the client that he is dying.
3. Inform the physician that he is wrong in not telling the client about his prognosis.
4. Tell the family the truth about his illness.

53. A prenatal client, 32 weeks' gestation, has uncontrolled premature labor. A regimen of antenatal corticosteroids is recommended by her physician. After the physician leaves the room, the client asks the nurse to clarify how corticosteroids work. The best response by the nurse is:

1. "Let me get the physician to answer that question for you."
2. "The mechanism of action is unknown but produces consistently good results."
3. "At this time in your baby's development, she does not have surfactant in her lungs. Without surfactant the air sacs collapse and cause lung damage. This medication stimulates the lungs to produce the needed surfactant."
4. "Corticosteroids suppress the inflammatory response mechanism of the immune system. This suppression activates the trigger for surfactant production in the fetal lung."

54. Concerning children's legal rights and ethical considerations for their care, which of the following statements is true?

1. Children are regarded as possessions of their parents and therefore under total parental control.
2. Children do not have the right of confidentiality or access to their medical records.
3. Children over 13 years of age are considered "mature minors."
4. Most states allow minors to obtain birth control and treatment for sexually transmitted disease (STD) without parental consent.

55. A 14-year-old Quaker girl comes to the emergency room with an asthma exacerbation. What beliefs about medical care may impact on her treatment in the hospital?

1. No special rites or restrictions exist in the Quaker religion regarding medical care.
2. Illness or injury is thought to be a result of sins committed in a previous life.
3. Quakers are opposed to the use of blood and blood products in illness treatment.
4. Quakers believe in divine healing through church leaders.

56. A 14-year-old client was admitted with a fracture to the left leg related to a sports injury. The coach of the soccer team brought the teen to the emergency room. In this case, from whom is it most appropriate to obtain the consent to perform the surgical procedure?

1. The teen himself
2. The client's soccer coach
3. The emergency room physician
4. The client's parents

57. An elderly client told his daughter that he had prepared an advance directive directing health-care providers not to perform heroic measures on him in the event he would become unconscious. During his most recent hospitalization, he became unconscious. Which nursing action is most appropriate?

1. Have him transferred to intensive care unit.
2. Perform CPR on him.
3. Notify his attending physician.
4. Call his immediate next of kin.

58. The nurse is responsible for charting the administration of a narcotic on the client's medication administration record (MAR) and in which other area?

1. Pharmacy's note
2. Computer database
3. Flow sheet
4. Narcotic control log

59. In preparing a client preoperatively, the nurse read the physician's order. "Give atropine sulfate 5 mg IM and Demerol 25 mg IM." The nurse knows that the usual preoperative dose of atropine is 0.4–0.6 mg. What is the nurse's responsibility?

1. Give the usual preoperative dose of atropine.
2. Administer just the Demerol at this time.
3. Hold all the medication and notify the physician.
4. Consult the pharmacist on the action to take.

60. In caring for a client scheduled for a modified radical mastectomy, the nurse listened to the client express her fears about the surgery. She stated, "I would like to have a second opinion about the results of the biopsy." What action should the nurse take?

   1. Explain that most biopsies are accurate.
   2. Help advocate for her choice of treatment.
   3. Discourage her from opposing the physician.
   4. Recommend that she seek a second opinion.

61. While working in an adolescent behavioral unit, the nurse witnesses an adolescent hitting a nursing assistant. The nurse documents the event. Which example of documentation is best?

   1. Became angry for no reason and an assault occurred.
   2. Hit caregiver unexpectedly even though not provoked.
   3. Struck nursing assistant when being helped from bed.
   4. Attacked nursing assistant without prior warning.

62. The ward clerk informed the nurse that the teenager's mother was on the phone requesting information about her daughter. The nurse responds by saying:

   1. "The clinic cannot release that information."
   2. "Inform her mother that her daughter will call her shortly."
   3. "Inform her mother that her daughter cannot receive calls."
   4. "Inform her mother that her daughter came to clinic because of drug abuse."

63. When visiting a client, the pastor asked to read the chart. Which is the best nursing response?

   1. "You will have to obtain permission from the client."
   2. "Are you a certified hospital chaplain?"
   3. "The chart is a confidential record."
   4. "I will have to check with the physician."

64. While working at a local rural health clinic, a young woman informed the nurse that she is engaged to be married to one of the clients. The nurse knows that this client is HIV positive. The nurse is legally obligated to:

   1. Inform the young woman of the fiancé's HIV infectious status.
   2. Recommend that the friend be tested for HIV antibodies.
   3. Advise the friend to postpone the marriage indefinitely.
   4. Safeguard information in the fiancé's health history.

65. An older adult was admitted to the intensive care unit because of a severe stroke. He did not have an advance directive. The family asked that life-support measures be discontinued. What is the nurse's responsibility?

   1. Consider the cost of continued life-support measures.
   2. Check the client's insurance to see how long the insurance will pay.
   3. Validate that all immediate family members agree on this decision.
   4. Consult with a hospital chaplain.

66. While working in a drug treatment center, the nurse encountered a client who became angry and refused his medication. Legally, the nurse:

   1. Should respect the client's right to refuse the ordered medication.
   2. Can administer the medication to protect the safety of self and others.
   3. Must get permission from a probate court judge to administer the medication.
   4. Should ask the hospital's attorney about the client's rights to refuse.

67. A nurse was supervising the home health aide giving a bed bath to a client. The home health aide gave the bed bath without gloves. The nurse responded:

   1. "Tell me your understanding of Universal Precautions."
   2. "I think I will need to report you to the nursing director."
   3. "Are you sure that you have been careful?"
   4. "Did the client give you permission to bathe him without gloves?"

68. The nurse was called in to work due to excessive staffing absences. Among the following four clients, prioritize the order in which that the nurse would care for them.

   1. A client with suspected ruptured appendix.
   2. A client receiving blood and requiring 30-minute vital signs.
   3. An Alzheimer's client who keeps getting out of bed.
   4. A postoperative surgical client ready for discharge.

69. While the charge nurse was making rounds, the physician asked the LPN to remove the client's sutures. The charge nurse's response is:

   1. "LPNs cannot legally remove sutures."
   2. "I will remove them right away."
   3. "It is your responsibility to remove the sutures."
   4. "Please write the order and we will take care of it."

70. The LPN assigned the nurse's aide to monitor vital signs on an oncologic client receiving chemotherapy. Upon entering the client's room, the LPN saw the nurse's aide adjusting the rate of the chemotherapy infusion. What action should the LPN take first?

   1. Report the incident to the charge nurse.
   2. Reprimand the nurse's aide because this is not within the aide's realm of practice.
   3. Fill out an incident report.
   4. Have nurse's aide meet with you and the charge nurse to discuss the aide's inappropriate action.

71. An LVN was assigned to a rehabilitation unit. The nurse had two UAP to care for 15 clients. When dele-

gating care, what is the most important concept for the nurse to keep in mind?

1. The skill level of the UAP.
2. The knowledge level of the UAP.
3. The knowledge level of the LVN.
4. The acuity level of the clients.

72. On a busy medical-surgical unit, the following clients were being cared for by one RN, two LVNs, and 3 UAPs. Which of the following is the most appropriate to care for the critically ill clients?

1. Physician
2. RN
3. UAP
4. LVN

73. Which of the following is best able to care for a terminally ill client?

1. Social worker
2. RN
3. UAP
4. LVN

74. Which of the following is best able to care for a client getting ready for discharge with discharge instructions?

1. Certified nursing assistant (CNA)
2. RN
3. UAP
4. LVN

75. A 52-year-old woman admitted herself to an alcoholic treatment unit. She lives alone, is a heavy smoker, and has a history of end-stage cirrhosis of the liver. In planning for her care, the priority nursing action is to:

1. Instruct on adequate nutrition.
2. Observe for withdrawal symptoms.
3. Insert a Foley catheter.
4. Measure abdominal girth daily.

76. An elderly client who underwent a total knee replacement was assigned to a rehabilitation unit. Which of the following duties can the LPN delegate to the UAP?

1. Go to physical therapy with the client.
2. Change dressings on surgical wound.
3. Make rounds with the physician.
4. Perform range-of-motion (ROM) exercises on knee with the replacement.

77. The LVN had a full workload and must reassign some of her patients to a UAP. Which of the following clients could the UAP care for?

1. Newly admitted total knee replacement
2. Cerebral vascular accident (CVA) client who was being transferred to a skilled nursing floor
3. Terminally ill client with continuous morphine infusing
4. Preoperative client with suspected cancer of the colon

78. The LVN assigns a client with severe eczema to the UAP. The client continues to scratch and complain of severe itching. Which of the following actions can be delegated to the UAP?

1. Wash with mild soap and water, and then apply lotion.
2. Use oatmeal in the water.
3. Use a weak vinegar solution with no soap.
4. Use water only and then apply lotion.

79. A client on a telemetry floor needs to be monitored by which of the following staff?

1. Nurse's aide
2. UAP
3. RN
4. LVN

80. In preparing for practice, the LVN must understand that which of the following agencies determine her or his scope of practice?

1. American Medical Association
2. National Council of State Boards
3. American Nurses' Association
4. Individual agency policies employing the LVN

81. At the end of the shift, the LVN notices that the UAP had charted the wrong vital signs on a chart. The appropriate action is to:

1. Draw a single line over the error, write "error," and then initial the document.
2. Write an incident report about the error.
3. Discard the notes and ask the UAP to rewrite the vital signs.
4. Scratch out the incorrect entry using a black ink pen.

82. You have been offered the job of nurse manager for a 40-bed unit in a nursing home. You are a novice leader and manager and want to be sure the position is right for you. What aspects of the position are you going to examine before deciding if the job is right for you?

1. Determine the leadership style of the UAP.
2. Determine the leadership style of the physician.
3. Determine the leadership style of the administrator.
4. Take a leadership and management course for college credit.

83. Which of the following is defined as "the personal traits necessary to establish vision and goals for an organization and the ability to execute them?"

1. Management
2. Delegation
3. Leadership
4. Case management

84. Which of the following is defined as "the personal traits necessary to plan, organize, motivate, and manage the personnel and material resources of an organization?"

1. Management
2. Delegation
3. Leadership
4. Case management

85. The RN on the floor explained her rationale for the patient care assignments. She then asked the LVN, "Please repeat to me what you understand from what I have told you." This is a form of:

    1. Hostile communication
    2. Aggressive communication
    3. Feedback
    4. Communication block

86. The LVN called the physician to report to him that the client did not understand the procedure and did not sign the informed consent form. The physician angrily told the LVN that she "was stupid." Which is the best response by the LVN?

    1. "You can't call me stupid and get by with it."
    2. "Oh, I am sorry to bother you."
    3. "Would you like to tell me that in person?"
    4. "I feel disrespected with that comment."

87. Which of the following statements concerning nursing liability is true?

    1. The RN may assume personal liability for the negligent acts of the LVN.
    2. The LVN is responsible for her own negligent acts.
    3. The hospital will always cover the actions by the LVN.
    4. Malpractice insurance will always cover the damages assessed against the LVN.

88. Which of the following might negate liability on the part of the nurse in a negligent action?

    1. The family consented to the act.
    2. The harm was not reasonably foreseeable.
    3. The nurse had not knowledge of how to do the procedure.
    4. The nurse had not verified with the nursing supervisor on how to do the procedure.

89. The decision as to whether or not a nurse can lawfully restrain a client in a long-term care facility is made by the:

    1. Nurse
    2. Family
    3. Physician
    4. Client

90. A physician in a long-term care facility wrote a medication order that was incorrect. The LVN gave the medication without questioning the physician. The client died from the overdose. Who is liable?

    1. The physician and the LVN
    2. The LVN who gave the medication
    3. The long-term care facility
    4. The pharmacist

91. The LVN was trying to decipher the physician's medication orders. Whom should the nurse consult for clarification about the order?

    1. The pharmacist.
    2. The nursing supervisor

    3. The physician
    4. Another nurse on the floor

92. The Patient's Bill of Rights is defined as:

    1. Rights supported by criminal law
    2. Rights specifically written into many laws
    3. A declaration by the United Nations
    4. A position paper developed by the American Hospital Association

93. The LVN had to cosign the chart after the UAP documented the intake and output and vital signs. Which of the following would aid in decreasing legal liability?

    1. Discuss the information with the UAP before cosigning.
    2. Make sure the information is accurate.
    3. Double check with another nurse before signing.
    4. Review the UAP's flow sheet for accuracy.

94. One of the elements of negligence is breach of standard of care. "Standard of care" may be defined as:

    1. Health services as prescribed by governmental agencies
    2. Giving care to clients in good faith to the best of one's ability
    3. Avoiding all possible harm to the client
    4. Degree of judgment and skill in nursing care given by a reasonable and prudent professional nurse under similar circumstances

95. The terminally ill client asked the LVN about her terminal condition. The LVN explained the disease process. The LVN was functioning under which ethical principle?

    1. Beneficence
    2. Nonmaleficence
    3. Justice
    4. Veracity

96. Understanding ethical decision making helps the nurse to:

    1. Prevent risks and benefits of all actions
    2. Act as better advocates for clients
    3. Make decisions for the clients
    4. Prevent family members from participating in the client's care

97. Health-care professionals have traditionally favored which ethical principle in providing care for a client?

    1. Autonomy
    2. Maleficence
    3. Paternalism
    4. Justice

98. As the nursing manager of the floor in the long-term care facility, which of the following actions is considered your responsibility?

    1. Checking the chart to ensure that UAP document that they loosened and reapplied the restraints.

2. Making rounds to ensure the UAP loosen and reapply restraints carefully.
3. You have no responsibility for the UAP actions.
4. Use a buddy-system when assigning UAP to loosen and reapply restraints.

99. The LVN found the UAP pinning up a racist cartoon in the client's room. Which is the best nursing action?

1. Report it to the nursing supervisor.
2. Ignore it.
3. Take it down.
4. Laugh with the UAP at the cartoon.

100. The nurse manager is responsible for which of the following actions?

1. Cleaning out the stock room.
2. Mopping the client's room.
3. Supervising the workplace environment.
4. Reporting neglectful actions to a client's family members.

1. **(2)** Integrated processes: nursing process — data collection; communication and documentation; client need: safe, effective care environment; safety and infection control; content area: leadership/management/delegation.

RATIONALE

(1) Incident reports are not placed on the client's chart. **(2)** The report is used as a written record kept by the institution regarding unusual events. They are used to review incidents, provide statistical data regarding occurrences, and as written support for changes in procedure or practice. **(3)** Reports are not written for blame, but as learning tools to improve processes and practices, and to monitor for potential safety issues. **(4)** Incident reports are written to document an incident even if you are responsible for the occurrence.

2. **(1)** Integrated processes: nursing process — implementation; communication and documentation; client need: safe, effective care environment; safety and infection control; content area: leadership/management/delegation.

RATIONALE

(1) The incident report identifies the person(s) involved in the incident. **(2)** The incident report must give a factual description of the event and witnesses present. **(3)** The incident report does not protect the institution from lawsuits. If discovered, they may even serve as evidence to enhance a lawsuit. **(4)** Incident reports are not part of the permanent record; however, they can be viewed by hospital personnel upon request.

3. **(4)** Integrated processes: nursing process — data collection; communication and documentation; client need: safe, effective care environment; safety and infection control; content area: leadership/management/delegation.

RATIONALE

(1) An incident report should always be filed when an unusual occurrence takes place. **(2)** The incident report should contain information regarding the defective equipment. **(3)** Risk management does not decide if an unusual occurrence should be reported; it is standard practice to provide this report. **(4)** The employee should fill out the incident report, including information regarding the defective equipment.

4. **(A minor or adult with the mental functioning of a child)** Integrated processes: nursing process — data collection; communication and documentation; client need: safe, effective care environment; coordinated care; content area: leadership/management/delegation.

RATIONALE

Exceptions to obtaining informed consent from the patient include an unconscious patient, one injured to the degree that prevents consenting, and a patient incompetent due to mental illness.

5. **(1)** Integrated processes: nursing process — implementation; communication and documentation; client need: safe, effective care environment; coordinated care; content area: leadership/management/delegation

RATIONALE

(1) Informed consent must be voluntary. **(2)** Informed consent cannot be coerced; coercion implies involuntary action. **(3)**

Informed consent must be given before the procedure is implemented. **(4)** Informed consent can be implied or expressed.

6. **(2)** Integrated processes: nursing process — implementation; communication and documentation; client need: safe, effective care environment; coordinated care; content area: leadership/management/delegation.

RATIONALE

(1) Expressed consent can be verbal or written. **(2)** Expressed consent can be verbal or written. **(3)** A patient capable of writing can give expressed consent verbally. **(4)** Expressed consent can be verbal or written.

7. **(3)** Integrated processes: nursing process — implementation; communication and documentation; client need: safe, effective care environment; coordinated care; content area: leadership/management/delegation.

RATIONALE

(1) Implied consent is given by nonverbal behavior. It need not be written to be valid. **(2)** Implied consent is neither written nor verbal; it is given by nonverbal behavior. **(3)** Implied consent is given by nonverbal behavior. **(4)** Implied consent is given by nonverbal behavior.

8. **(3)** Integrated processes: nursing process — implementation; communication and documentation; client need: safe, effective care environment; coordinated care; content area: leadership/management/delegation.

RATIONALE

(1) It is the nurse's responsibility to notify the physician when a client has consented while incompetent; an informed consent is not legal when signed by an incompetent client. **(2)** It is the physician's responsibility to provide information for medical and surgical procedures. **(3)** The nurse must notify the physician when an informed consent has been signed and the client does not understand the information given. **(4)** The nurse must notify the physician when an informed consent has been signed and the client does not understand the information given.

9. **(The State Board of Nursing)** Integrated processes: nursing process — evaluation; client need: safe, effective care environment; coordinated care; content area: leadership/management/delegation.

RATIONALE

Each State Board of Nursing is responsible for determining legal responsibilities of the nurse practicing in each individual state.

10. **(1)** Integrated processes: nursing process — implementation; client need: safe, effective care environment; coordinated care; content area: leadership/management/delegation.

RATIONALE

(1) It is the nurse's legal responsibility to assess, plan, implement, and evaluate patient care. **(2)** Dispensing medications is the function of the pharmacy, not the practical nurse. **(3)** It is the State Board of Nursing responsibility to investigate suspected violations of the Nurse Practice Act. **(4)** Practical nurses can supervise unlicensed assistive personnel, not licensed personnel.

11. **(2)** Integrated processes: nursing process — implementation; client need: safe, effective care environment; coordinated care; content area: leadership/management/delegation.

    RATIONALE

    (1) The practical nurse cannot dispense medications; that is a function of the pharmacy. **(2)** Legally, the practical nurse can delegate duties to unlicensed assistive personnel. **(3)** A physician or licensed advanced practice nurse can order treatments for a client. **(4)** Legally, the practical nurse cannot delegate duties to licensed personnel.

12. **(3)** Integrated processes: nursing process — implementation; communication and documentation; client need: safe, effective care environment; coordinated care; content area: leadership/management/delegation.

    RATIONALE

    (1) Referrals should contain as much information as possible about the client. **(2)** A physician's signature is required for reimbursement purposes. **(3)** Providing as much information as possible helps to ensure that all client needs are met. **(4)** Client referrals should be made whenever and wherever there is a need.

13. **(1)** Integrated processes: nursing process — implementation; communication and documentation; client need: safe, effective care environment; coordinated care; content area: leadership/management/delegation.

    RATIONALE

    (1) The referral process helps the client reach individual goals, psychosocial needs, and health-care needs. **(2)** Referrals do not guarantee monetary reimbursement. **(3)** The referral process helps the client reach individual goals, psychosocial needs, and health-care needs. **(4)** The referral process helps the client reach individual goals, psychosocial needs, and health-care needs.

14. **(1)** Integrated processes: nursing process — implementation; communication and documentation; client need: safe, effective care environment; coordinated care; content area: leadership/management/delegation.

    RATIONALE

    (1) Resource management involves the responsible use of available resources. **(2)** Resource management is everyone's responsibility, including the nurse. **(3)** Resource management helps to keep health-care costs down. **(4)** Resource management involves the use of available resources.

15. **(1)** Integrated processes: nursing process — implementation; client need: safe, effective care environment; coordinated care; content area: leadership/management/delegation

    RATIONALE

    (1) Autocratic leadership style is directive and focuses on task completion. Position power and personal power are used in making decisions to meet organizational goals. **(2)** Democratic leadership style is cooperative and focuses on group work and individual growth through feedback. **(3)** Laissez-faire leadership is permissive, providing no direction or feedback. **(4)** Transformational leadership focuses on purposeful group task accomplishment through mutual trust between leader and follower.

16. **(1, 2, 4)** Integrated processes: nursing process — implementation; client need: safe, effective care environment; coordinated care; content area: leadership/management/delegation

    RATIONALE

    (1) Accompanying a client being discharged home is within the scope of practice of the nurse's aide. **(2)** Collecting a urine specimen is within the scope of practice of the nurse's aide. **(3)** Feeding a client with disabilities is a nonroutine task with potential client harm. **(4)** Offering sips of water to a postoperative client is within the scope of practice of the nurse's aide. **(5)** Catheterizing an elderly client is not within the scope of practice of the nurse's aide. **(6)** Administering oral medications is not within the scope of practice of the nurse's aide.

17. **(2, 4)** Integrated processes: nursing process — implementation; client need: safe, effective care environment; coordinated care; content area: leadership/management/delegation

    RATIONALE

    (1) The charge nurse's lunch assignment schedule is a time management tool. **(2)** Understanding the hospital's job description for LPNs is essential related to making client care direct care assignments for staff members. **(3)** The head nurse's Unit Plan of Care is a unit staffing management tool. **(4)** Understanding the State Nurse Practice Act is essential related to making client care direct care assignments for staff members. **(5)** Understanding the hospital's job description for LPNs is essential related to making client care direct care assignments for staff members. **(6)** Understanding the hospital's job description for LPNs is essential related to making client care direct care assignments for staff members.

18. **(4)** Integrated processes: nursing process — implementation; communication and documentation; client need: safe, effective care environment; coordinated care; content area: leadership/management/delegation.

    RATIONALE

    (1) This statement is a form of aggressive communication and does not address client confidentiality. **(2)** This statement is directed toward ending the interaction and possibly initiates defensive behavior by the nurse's aide, but does not address client confidentiality. **(3)** This statement does not address client confidentiality. **(4)** This statement addresses the inappropriate behavior of the nurse's aide and initiates clarification of accountability for confidentiality of client information.

19. **(3)** Integrated processes: nursing process — implementation; communication and documentation; client need: safe, effective care environment; coordinated care; content area: leadership/management/delegation.

    RATIONALE

    (1) This statement does not relate to protecting client privacy. **(2)** This statement fails to address the client's right to privacy and reflects lack of accountability. **(3)** This statement reflects knowledge of Health Insurance Portability and Accountability Act (HIPAA) directives concerning protecting the client's right to privacy. **(4)** This statement fails to address the client's right to privacy from anyone other than specifically identified individuals as mandated by HIPAA guidelines.

20. **(1)** Integrated processes: nursing process — implementation; communication and documentation; client need: safe, effective care environment; coordinated care; content area: leadership/management/delegation.

    RATIONALE

    (1) This statement reflects the nurse's knowledge of client confidentiality except in situations of child or elderly abuse. **(2)** This statement does not address the need for intervention nor does it indicate that the nurse would follow the law. **(3)** This statement does not address the need for intervention nor does it indicate that the nurse would follow the law. **(4)** This statement is beyond the scope of practice.

21. **(2, 3)** Integrated processes: nursing process — data collection; communication and documentation; client need: safe,

effective care environment; coordinated care; content area: leadership/management/delegation.

RATIONALE

(1) This statement will make the client feel inadequate and place communication barriers between the nurse, physician, and client. (2) As a member of the health-care team, the nurse must gather information and report client changes in health status to the physician in order to provide safe care. (3) As a member of the health-care team, the nurse must gather information and report client changes in health status to the physician in order to provide safe care. (4) This statement reinforces unsafe client decision making and is a barrier to client teaching. (5) As a member of the health-care team, the nurse must gather information and report client changes in health status to the physician in order to provide safe care. (6) This statement will make the client feel inadequate and place communication barriers between the nurse, physician, and client.

22. **(3)** Integrated processes: nursing process — implementation; communication and documentation; client need: safe, effective care environment; coordinated care; content area: leadership/management/delegation.

RATIONALE

(1) The nurse needs further data for safe, effective care to be provided. (2) The client's needs are not addressed. (3) The nurse is aware of the need for further information and the potential risk of the situation for the client and the family. (4) The client's needs are not addressed.

23. **(2, 4, 5, 6)** Integrated processes: nursing process — data collection and implementation; communication and documentation; client need: safe, effective care environment; coordinated care; content area: leadership/management/delegation.

RATIONALE

(1) Further data need to be collected to meet the client's need before medication is administered. (2) This action focuses on the client's needs and involves members of the health team who can address the client's needs through a multidisciplinary approach. (3) This action does not address the client's needs. (4) This action focuses on the client's needs and involves members of the health team who can address the client's needs through a multidisciplinary approach. (5) This action focuses on the client's needs and involves members of the health team who can address the client's needs through a multidisciplinary approach. (6) This action focuses on the client's needs and involves members of the health team who can address the client's needs through a multidisciplinary approach.

24. **(4)** Integrated processes: nursing process — implementation; communication and documentation; client need: safe, effective care environment; coordinated care; content area: leadership/management/delegation.

RATIONALE

(1) This is a high-risk action that may result in increased anxiety and harm for the client. (2) Administering the dosage of aspirin without finding out if the aspirin had been administered previously is a high-risk action and could result in an overdose. (3) Notifying the charge nurse is appropriate, but not the first action to be taken by the nurse to address the situation. (4) The nurse's first action to solve the problem is to clarify actions and verify documentation.

25. **(3)** Integrated processes: nursing process — implementation; communication and documentation; client need: safe, effective care environment; coordinated care; content area: leadership/management/delegation.

RATIONALE

(1) This action does not address the need for a physician's order for "Do Not Resuscitate" (DNR). (2) This action does not meet the client's needs. (3) The client has the right to refuse external cardiac massage. The physician must be notified so that an order of "Do Not Resuscitate" (DNR) can be placed in the client's medical record. (4) This action does not address the client's needs.

26. **(4)** Integrated processes: nursing process — implementation; client need: safe, effective care environment; safety and infection control; content area: leadership/management/delegation.

RATIONALE

(1) Although this is within the scope of practice for the nurse's aide, this is not a priority action. (2) Although this is within the scope of practice for the nurse's aide, this is not a priority action. (3) This is not within the scope of practice for the nurse's aide. (4) Monitoring fluid intake is the responsibility of all team members caring for a client with acute renal failure.

27. **(2)** Integrated processes: nursing process — implementation; communication and documentation; client need: safe, effective care environment; safety and infection control; content area: leadership/management/delegation.

RATIONALE

(1) Reporting the error is required; however, the nurse who finds the error follows the hospital's standard of practice regarding documentation. (2) The nurse who identifies an error completes the incident report form to protect the client, the nurse, and the hospital. (3) This is not in the scope of practice for the staff nurse. (4) This does not follow the hospital's standard of practice.

28. **(1)** Integrated processes: nursing process — implementation; communication and documentation; client need: safe, effective care environment; safety and infection control; content area: leadership/management/delegation.

RATIONALE

(1) This action is taken to prevent an error and harm to the client, the nurse, and the hospital. (2) The nurse is responsible for following procedures regarding medication administration. (3) The staff is not responsible for actions of other staff members. (4) This action does not follow the standard of practice regarding safe medication administration.

29. **(4)** Integrated processes: nursing process — implementation; communication and documentation; client need: safe, effective care environment; safety and infection control; content area: leadership/management/delegation.

RATIONALE

(1) Quality assurance through verification of safe performance is within the scope of practice of the RN delegating the assignment to the LPN. (2) This request may reflect a lack of knowledge regarding LPN and RN delegation of responsibilities, hospital and nursing standards of practice, and protocol. (3) This request may reflect a lack of knowledge regarding LPN and RN delegation of responsibilities, hospital and nursing standards of practice, and protocol. (4) This action prevents harm to the client, the nurse, and the hospital and follows nursing standards of practice regarding work responsibilities of staff nurses.

30. **(1)** Integrated processes: nursing process — implementation; communication and documentation; client need: safe, effective care environment; coordinated care; content area: leadership/management/delegation.

RATIONALE
(1) Approaching the nurse who had signed out the narcotic would be the first action taken by the PN. (2) Notifying the pharmacist is appropriate; however, it is not the first action taken by the PN. (3) The charge nurse/supervisor needs to be notified after the nurse has been approached. (4) It is not appropriate that the client be told that someone else received his pain medication.

31. **(2)** Integrated processes: nursing process — implementation; communication and documentation; client need: safe, effective care environment; coordinated care; content area: leadership/management/delegation.
RATIONALE
(1) To avoid a last minute rush and to ensure the husband's presence, an early change to scrub attire is recommended. (2) To avoid a last minute rush and to ensure the husband's presence, an early change to scrub attire is recommended. (3) To avoid a last minute rush and to ensure the husband's presence, an early change to scrub attire is recommended. (4) To avoid a last minute rush and to ensure the husband's presence, an early change to scrub attire is recommended.

32. **(2)** Integrated processes: nursing process — implementation; client need: safe, effective care environment; coordinated care; content area: leadership/management/delegation.
RATIONALE
(1) Amniocentesis is done under sterile conditions. In addition, signs and symptoms of infection usually take 12–24 hours to manifest after an invasive procedure. (2) There is a risk for precipitation of uterine contractions and compromised fetal well-being. (3) Informed consent is required before this invasive procedure. Any explanations should occur before the amniocentesis is performed. (4) Although encouraging the client to verbalize concerns is always appropriate, physiological needs have priority over psychological needs.

33. **(4)** Integrated processes: nursing process — implementation; communication and documentation; client need: physiological integrity; physiological adaptation; content area: leadership/management/delegation.
RATIONALE
(1) These are symptoms of early mastitis. A biopsy is not indicated. (2) Hospitalization and IV antibiotics are reserved for severe cases of breast infection. (3) As lactation is established, a lump may be felt. However, a filled milk duct will shift position from one day to the next. It is not normal for pain to persist for as long as a week postpartum. (4) Mastitis is an infection of a milk duct. Early mastitis can be effectively treated with rest, fluid, acetaminophen, and thorough emptying of the plugged milk duct.

34. **(4)** Integrated processes: nursing process — implementation; client need: physiological integrity; reduction of risk potential; content area: leadership/management/delegation.
RATIONALE
(1) The client's BP is not within an acceptable range. She has experienced an increase of 36 mm Hg above her systolic and 16 mm Hg above her diastolic BP. This is one of the defining characteristics of preeclampsia and should be evaluated further. (2) The client's BP may increase slightly with contractions in the active phase of labor. In the latent phase of labor, contractions are usually mild and very well tolerated; a BP increase is not expected. (3) Client complaints should not be used as a basis for further assessment. The nurse must decide to further evaluate the client based on the objective findings. (4) The client's BP is not within an acceptable range. She has experienced an increase of 36 mm Hg above her systolic and 16 mm Hg above her diastolic BP. This is one of the defining characteristics of preeclampsia and should be evaluated further.

35. **(3)** Integrated processes: nursing process — implementation; client need: physiological integrity; reduction of risk potential; content area: leadership/management/delegation.
RATIONALE
(1) Listening to the apical heart rate for a full minute is the correct technique. (2) Listening to the apical heart rate for a full minute is the correct technique. (3) Listening to the apical heart rate for a full minute is the correct technique. (4) Listening to the apical heart rate for a full minute is the correct technique.

36. **(3)** Integrated processes: nursing process — implementation; client need: safe, effective care environment; coordinated care; content area: leadership/management/delegation.
RATIONALE
(1) Delegating the feeding of the client to the nursing assistant is appropriate. (2) Delegating the feeding of the client to the nursing assistant is appropriate. (3) Delegating the feeding of the client to the nursing assistant is appropriate. (4) Delegating the feeding of the client to the nursing assistant is appropriate.

37. **(2)** Integrated processes: nursing process — implementation; client need: safe, effective care environment; coordinated care; content area: leadership/management/delegation.
RATIONALE
(1) Handling all of the problems alone is not a strength. (2) Delegating nonskilled tasks to unlicensed personnel is a strength. (3) Spending time in the client's room visiting with family members is a strength. (4) Planning and time management are strengths.

38. **(3)** Integrated processes: nursing process — implementation; client need: safe, effective care environment; coordinated care; content area: leadership/management/delegation.
RATIONALE
(1) Clients have the right to be told of the prognosis. (2) Clients have the right to refuse treatment. (3) Clients have the right to confidentiality. (4) Clients have the right to confidentiality.

39. **(3)** Integrated processes: nursing process — implementation; communication and documentation; client need: safe, effective care environment; coordinated care; content area: leadership/management/delegation.
RATIONALE
(1) Openly discussing the client's condition with nonprofessionals is a breach of confidentiality. (2) It is not the nurse's responsibility to encourage the client to accept all treatment regardless of how it affects the quality of life. (3) It is the nurse's responsibility to be honest with the client about the care and treatment he or she is receiving. (4) It is not appropriate to lie to the client about his illness and prognosis.

40. **(3)** Integrated processes: nursing process — implementation; client need: safe, effective care environment; coordinated care; content area: leadership/management/delegation.
RATIONALE
(1) The failure to adhere to one's legal duty is called a breach of duty. (2) The failure to adhere to one's legal duty is called a breach of duty. (3) The failure to adhere to one's legal duty is called a breach of duty. (4) A breach of duty results in liability.

41. **(1)** Integrated processes: nursing process — implementation; client need: safe, effective care environment; coordinated care; content area: leadership/management/delegation.

RATIONALE

(1) Malpractice is the failure to meet the standard of care. (2) Omission of a duty results in liability. (3) Malpractice is the failure to meet the standard of care. (4) It is the nurse's responsibility to protect the client from harm.

42. (3) Integrated processes: nursing process — implementation; client need: safe, effective care environment; coordinated care; content area: leadership/management/delegation.

RATIONALE

(1) Properly administering insulin injections is a standard of care. (2) Providing instructions to a diabetic client is a standard of care. (3) Administering the wrong medication is a violation of the standard of care. (4) Instructing the caregiver on how to administer medications is a standard of care.

43. (4) Integrated processes: nursing process — implementation; communication and documentation; client need: safe, effective care environment; coordinated care; content area: leadership/management/delegation.

RATIONALE

(1) Nurses are to be respectful at all times to family members. (2) If a mistake occurs, it is important to notify the charge nurse or supervisor. (3) Documentation includes factual data surrounding an event. (4) Communication with the physician and supervisors when changes occur in the client's condition will help to avoid a malpractice lawsuit.

44. (2) Integrated processes: nursing process — implementation; communication and documentation; client need: safe, effective care environment; coordinated care; content area: leadership/management/delegation.

RATIONALE

(1) Standards of care are required by state licensing statutes. (2) Standards of care are required by state licensing statutes. (3) Standards of care are required by state licensing statutes. (4) Standards of care are required by state licensing statutes.

45. (3) Integrated processes: nursing process — implementation; client need: safe, effective care environment; coordinated care; content area: leadership/management/delegation.

RATIONALE

(1) Analyzing data collected from client and family is an appropriate standard of care in community-based nursing. (2) Identifying potential problems is an appropriate standard of care in community-based nursing. (3) Identifying appropriate nursing diagnoses is an appropriate standard of care. (4) Planning health-promotion activities is an appropriate standard of care.

46. (4) Integrated processes: nursing process — data collection; client need: safe, effective care environment; safety and infection control; content area: leadership/management/delegation.

RATIONALE

(1) Falling is the major cause of injury to clients in their homes. (2) Falling is the major cause of injury to clients in their homes. (3) Falling is the major cause of injury to clients in their homes. (4) Cluttered rooms with inaccessible walkways place a client at high risk for falling. Falling is the major cause of injury to clients in their homes.

47. (2) Integrated processes: nursing process — data collection; client need: safe, effective care environment; safety and infection control; content area: leadership/management/delegation.

RATIONALE

(1) An older client with a total knee replacement is at higher risk for falling. (2) An older client with a total knee replacement is at higher risk for falling. (3) An older client with a total knee replacement is at higher risk for falling. (4) An older client with a total knee replacement is at higher risk for falling.

48. (3) Integrated processes: nursing process — implementation; client need: safe, effective care environment; safety and infection control; content area: leadership/management/delegation.

RATIONALE

(1) Clients who are at high risk for falling should not be restrained to the bed. (2) Side rails need to be up if the client is at high risk for falling. (3) Removing throw rugs and clutter will help to reduce the risk for falling. (4) Family members should check *daily* on clients who are at high risk for falling.

49. (4) Integrated processes: nursing process — implementation; communication and documentation; client need: safe, effective care environment; safety and infection control; content area: leadership/management/delegation.

RATIONALE

(1) Documenting an assessment on the client would not predispose the nurse to a lawsuit. (2) Documenting communication with the physician would not predispose the nurse to a lawsuit. (3) Documenting telephone and verbal orders would not predispose the nurse to a lawsuit. (4) Failing to document client instruction in wound care would predispose the nurse to a lawsuit.

50. (3) Integrated processes: nursing process — implementation; communication and documentation; client need: safe, effective care environment; coordinated care; content area: leadership/management/delegation.

RATIONALE

(1) With an advance directive, the client determines whether CPR can be performed, not the family members. (2) With an advance directive, the client determines whether to be placed on a respirator or not. (3) With an advance directive, the client can refuse intravenous fluids. (4) With an advance directive, the client determines whether a feeding tube will be inserted or not.

51. (3) Integrated processes: nursing process — implementation; communication and documentation; client need: safe, effective care environment; coordinated care; content area: leadership/management/delegation.

RATIONALE

(1) Nurses, not the unit secretary, are required to document the client's advance directives. (2) Nurses, not the nursing assistant, are required to document the client's advance directives. (3) Nurses are required to document the client's advance directives. (4) Nurses, not the physician, are required to document the client's advance directives.

52. (1) Integrated processes: nursing process — implementation; communication and documentation; client need: safe, effective care environment; coordinated care; content area: leadership/management/delegation.

RATIONALE

(1) The nurse cannot legally tell the client about his illness; it is the physician's responsibility. Encourage the client to ask his physician about his prognosis. (2) Telling the client that he is dying is a breach of duty. (3) It would be inappropriate for the nurse to tell the physician he was wrong in not telling the client about his prognosis. (4) It is the physician's responsibility to tell the family the truth about the client's illness.

53. (3) Integrated processes: nursing process — implementation; teaching/learning; client need: safe, effective care environ-

ment; coordinated care; content area: leadership/management/delegation.

RATIONALE

(1) This response does not address the client's concerns. (2) The mechanism is known. (3) This is an accurate response communicated in such a way that promotes the client's understanding and ability to participate actively in decision making regarding her health care. (4) Although corticosteroids suppress the inflammatory response, this suppression does not activate the development of surfactant.

54. (4) Integrated processes: nursing process — implementation; client need: safe, effective care environment; coordinated care; content area: leadership/management/delegation.

RATIONALE

(1) Children are not regarded as possessions of their parents and legally may be given emancipation rights or placed under the guardianship of another adult. (2) All clients have the right of confidentiality and access to their medical records, preferably under the supervision of a health-care professional who can clarify and answer questions appropriate for the client. (3) Children over the age of 15 years, if deemed able to understand medical interventions and risks, may be considered mature minors. (4) Most states allow minors to obtain birth control and treatment for STDs without parental consent.

55. (1) Integrated processes: nursing process — implementation; client need: safe, effective care environment; coordinated care; content area: leadership/management/delegation.

RATIONALE

(1) This child's religious beliefs will not impact her medical treatment. (2) The Hindu religion embraces this belief. (3) The Jehovah's Witnesses faith strongly opposes the use of transfusions. (4) Devout Mormons believe that divine healing is possible.

56. (4) Integrated processes: nursing process — implementation; client need: safe, effective care environment; coordinated care; content area: leadership/management/delegation.

RATIONALE

(1) A 14-year-old is not considered a mature minor; therefore, his parents would need to sign the consent for the surgical procedure. (2) The teen's parents, not the soccer coach, would need to sign the consent for the surgical procedure. (3) The teen's parents, not the emergency room physician, would need to sign the consent for the surgical procedure. (4) The teen's parents would need to sign the consent for the surgical procedure.

57. (3) Integrated processes: nursing process — implementation; communication and documentation; client need: safe, effective care environment; coordinated care; content area: leadership/management/delegation.

RATIONALE

(1) If a client who has an advanced directive becomes unconscious, notify the attending physician for further orders. (2) If a client who has an advanced directive becomes unconscious, it is not appropriate to perform CPR on him. (3) Notify the attending physician. (4) Notify the attending physician and then call the next of kin.

58. (4) Integrated processes: nursing process — implementation; communication and documentation; client need: safe, effective care environment; coordinated care; content area: leadership/management/delegation.

RATIONALE

(1) The nurse is responsible for charting the administration of a narcotic on the client's MAR and the narcotic control log. (2) The nurse is responsible for charting the administration of a narcotic on the client's MAR and the narcotic control log. (3) The nurse is responsible for charting the administration of a narcotic on the client's MAR and the narcotic control log. (4) The nurse is responsible for charting the administration of a narcotic on the client's MAR and the narcotic control log.

59. (3) Integrated processes: nursing process — implementation; communication and documentation; client need: safe, effective care environment; coordinated care; content area: leadership/management/delegation.

RATIONALE

(1) The nurse never administers a different dose until consulting with a physician. (2) The physician wrote the order as a combined preoperative medication; therefore, giving the Demerol alone is not appropriate. (3) Hold all the medication and notify the physician are the most appropriate actions. (4) The physician is the only one who can change the order.

60. (2) Integrated processes: nursing process — implementation; communication and documentation; client need: safe, effective care environment; coordinated care; content area: leadership/management/delegation.

RATIONALE

(1) Competent adults have the right to make decisions about their care once they receive all of the information. (2) Helping the client to advocate for her choice of treatment is an appropriate action. (3) To discourage the client from opposing the physician promotes passivity. (4) Helping the client to advocate for her choice of treatment is an appropriate action.

61. (3) Integrated processes: nursing process — implementation; communication and documentation; client need: safe, effective care environment; coordinated care; content area: leadership/management/delegation.

RATIONALE

(1) This statement is a value statement. The nurse needs to document factual information. The nurse does not know if the adolescent is angry. (2) The nurse does not know if the event was provoked or not. (3) This is an example of factual documentation about the event. (4) This statement is an emotionally charged term that suggests more violence than what may have actually occurred.

62. (1) Integrated processes: nursing process — implementation; communication and documentation; client need: safe, effective care environment; coordinated care; content area: leadership/management/delegation.

RATIONALE

(1) Releasing information without the adolescent's consent is a breach of confidentiality. (2) Neither the nurse nor any clinic personnel can reveal the client's identity or reason for treatment without the client's consent. (3) Releasing information without the adolescent's consent is a breach of confidentiality. (4) Releasing information without the adolescent's consent is a breach of confidentiality.

63. (3) Integrated processes: nursing process — implementation; communication and documentation; client need: safe, effective care environment; coordinated care; content area: leadership/management/delegation.

RATIONALE

(1) Information on a chart belongs to the client, the physician, and the hospital. (2) It is a breach of confidentiality to provide the medical record to anyone besides the client, the physician, and the hospital. (3) This is the best response for the nurse. (4) Information on a chart belongs to the client, the physician, and the hospital.

64. **(4)** Integrated processes: nursing process — implementation; communication and documentation; client need: safe, effective care environment; coordinated care; content area: leadership/management/delegation.
RATIONALE
(1) The nurse is responsible for safeguarding the information in the fiancé's health history. **(2)** The nurse is responsible for safeguarding the information in the fiancé's health history. **(3)** The nurse is responsible for safeguarding the information in the fiancé's health history. **(4)** The nurse is responsible for safeguarding the information in the fiancé's health history.

65. **(3)** Integrated processes: nursing process — implementation; communication and documentation; client need: safe, effective care environment; coordinated care; content area: leadership/management/delegation.
RATIONALE
(1) The nurse needs to validate that all immediate family members agree on this decision. **(2)** The nurse needs to validate that all immediate family members agree on this decision. **(3)** The nurse needs to validate that all immediate family members agree on this decision. **(4)** The nurse needs to validate that all immediate family members agree on this decision.

66. **(2)** Integrated processes: nursing process — implementation; client need: safe, effective care environment; coordinated care; content area: leadership/management/delegation.
RATIONALE
(1) Legally, the nurse can administer the medication against a client's will when there appears to be a danger to either the client or to others. **(2)** Legally, the nurse can administer the medication against a client's will when there appears to be a danger to either the client or to others. **(3)** Legally, the nurse can administer the medication against a client's will when there appears to be a danger to either the client or to others. **(4)** Legally, the nurse can administer the medication against a client's will when there appears to be a danger to either the client or to others.

67. **(1)** Integrated processes: nursing process — implementation; communication and documentation; client need: safe, effective care environment; coordinated care; content area: leadership/management/delegation.
RATIONALE
(1) This statement will help the nurse evaluate whether the home health aide has an understanding of Universal Precautions. **(2)** The nurse needs to evaluate whether the home health aide has an understanding of Universal Precautions. **(3)** The nurse needs to evaluate whether the home health aide has an understanding of Universal Precautions. **(4)** The nurse needs to evaluate whether the home health aide has an understanding of Universal Precautions.

68. **(1, 2, 3, 4)** Integrated processes: nursing process — implementation; client need: safe, effective care environment; coordinated care; content area: leadership/management/delegation.
RATIONALE
(1) A client receiving blood would require monitoring by the nurse as the first priority. **(2)** A client with suspected ruptured appendix would have to be ready for surgery. This client can be delegated to the LPN to give the preoperative medication. **(3)** The nurse could delegate the care of an Alzheimer's client who keeps getting out of bed to an UAP. **(4)** A postoperative surgical client ready for discharge would be the least priority.

69. **(4)** Integrated processes: nursing process — implementation; communication and documentation; client need: safe, effec-

tive care environment; coordinated care; content area: leadership/management/delegation.
RATIONALE
(1) LPNs can legally remove sutures; however, the physician must write the order. **(2)** Both the RN and the LPN can legally remove sutures; however, the physician must write the order. **(3)** Both the RN and the LPN can legally remove sutures; however, the physician must write the order. **(4)** Both the RN and the LPN can legally remove sutures; however, the physician must write the order.

70. **(1)** Integrated processes: nursing process — implementation; client need: safe, effective care environment; coordinated care; content area: leadership/management/delegation.
RATIONALE
(1) The first priority would be to report the nurse's aides action to the charge nurse. **(2)** Reprimanding the aide in front of the client is not appropriate. The first action would be to report the behavior to the charge nurse. **(3)** Unless too much medication had been given, an incident report need not be filled out. **(4)** After the charge nurse has been notified of the event, the nurse's aide, the LPN, and the charge nurse need to meet to discuss the actions of the nurse's aide.

71. **(1)** Integrated processes: nursing process — planning; client need: safe, effective care environment; coordinated care; content area: leadership/management/delegation.
RATIONALE
(1) The skill level of the UAP is the most important concept for the nurse to keep in mind while delegating to the UAP. **(2)** The skill level of the UAP is the most important concept for the nurse to keep in mind while delegating to the UAP. **(3)** The skill level of the UAP is the most important concept for the nurse to keep in mind while delegating to the UAP. **(4)** The skill level of the UAP is the most important concept for the nurse to keep in mind while delegating to the UAP.

72. **(2)** Integrated processes: nursing process — implementation; client need: safe, effective care environment; coordinated care; content area: leadership/management/delegation.
RATIONALE
(1) The knowledge level of the RN is necessary to care for the critically ill clients. **(2)** The knowledge level of the RN is necessary to care for the critically ill clients. **(3)** The knowledge level of the RN is necessary to care for the critically ill clients. **(4)** The knowledge level of the RN is necessary to care for the critically ill clients.

73. **(2)** Integrated processes: nursing process — implementation; client need: safe, effective care environment; coordinated care; content area: leadership/management/delegation.
RATIONALE
(1) The knowledge level of the RN is necessary in caring for a terminally ill client. **(2)** The knowledge level of the RN is necessary in caring for a terminally ill client. **(3)** The knowledge level of the RN is necessary in caring for a terminally ill client. **(4)** The knowledge level of the RN is necessary in caring for a terminally ill client.

74. **(4)** Integrated processes: nursing process — implementation; client need: safe, effective care environment; coordinated care; content area: leadership/management/delegation.
RATIONALE
(1) Discharge teaching can be delegated to the LPN/LVN. **(2)** Discharge teaching can be delegated to the LPN/LVN. **(3)** Discharge teaching can be delegated to the LPN/LVN. **(4)** Discharge teaching can be delegated to the LPN/LVN.

75. **(2)** Integrated processes: nursing process — planning; client need: safe, effective care environment; coordinated care; content area: leadership/management/delegation.
RATIONALE
(1) Observing for withdrawal symptoms is the first nursing priority. Instructing on adequate nutrition would come later. **(2)** Observing for withdrawal symptoms is the first nursing priority. **(3)** Observing for withdrawal symptoms is the first nursing priority. **(4)** Observing for withdrawal symptoms is the first nursing priority.

76. **(1)** Integrated processes: nursing process — implementation; client need: safe, effective care environment; coordinated care; content area: leadership/management/delegation.
RATIONALE
(1) The LPN/LVN can delegate to the UAP to go with the client to physical therapy. **(2)** Changing dressings on a surgical wound is not within the scope of practice for an UAP; therefore, the LPN/LVN cannot delegate this task. **(3)** Making rounds is not within the scope of practice for an UAP; therefore, the LPN/LVN cannot delegate this task. **(4)** Performing ROM exercises on a client with a total knee replacement is not within the scope of practice for an UAP; therefore, the LPN/LVN cannot delegate this task.

77. **(2)** Integrated processes: nursing process — planning; client need: safe, effective care environment; coordinated care; content area: leadership/management/delegation.
RATIONALE
(1) A newly admitted client with a total knee replacement would require supervision by licensed nursing personnel. **(2)** A CVA client being transferred to a skilled nursing floor can be assisted by the UAP. **(3)** A terminally ill client with continuous morphine infusion would require supervision by licensed nursing personnel. **(4)** A preoperative client with suspected cancer of the colon would require supervision by licensed nursing personnel.

78. **(1)** Integrated processes: nursing process — implementation; client need: safe, effective care environment; coordinated care; content area: leadership/management/delegation.
RATIONALE
(1) Washing with mild soap and application of lotion to a client with severe eczema can be delegated to the UAP. **(2)** Research does not indicate that oatmeal in the water helps eczema. **(3)** Vinegar would be painful to skin that is sensitive due to excessive scratching. **(4)** Water would only dry the skin. The best method of treating eczema is to wash with a mild soap and apply lotion to the sensitive skin.

79. **(3)** Integrated processes: nursing process — implementation; client need: safe, effective care environment; coordinated care; content area: leadership/management/delegation.
RATIONALE
(1) Due to the instability of a cardiac client, the RN needs to monitor the client. **(2)** Due to the instability of a cardiac client, the RN needs to monitor the client. **(3)** Due to the instability of a cardiac client, the RN needs to monitor the client. **(4)** Due to the instability of a cardiac client, the RN needs to monitor the client.

80. **(2)** Integrated processes: nursing process — planning; client need: safe, effective care environment; coordinated care; content area: leadership/management/delegation.
RATIONALE
(1) The State Board of Nursing in each state determines the scope of practice by formulating the Nurse Practice Act for licensed personnel within that state. The Nurse Practice Act specifies the rules and regulations for practice and licensure for LPN/LVNs. **(2)** The State Board of Nursing in each state determines the scope of practice by formulating the Nurse Practice Act for licensed personnel within that state. The Nurse Practice Act specifies the rules and regulations for practice and licensure for LPN/LVNs. **(3)** The State Board of Nursing in each state determines the scope of practice by formulating the Nurse Practice Act for licensed personnel within that state. The Nurse Practice Act specifies the rules and regulations for practice and licensure for LPN/LVNs. **(4)** The State Board of Nursing in each state determines the scope of practice by formulating the Nurse Practice Act for licensed personnel within that state. The Nurse Practice Act specifies the rules and regulations for practice and licensure for LPN/LVNs.

81. **(1)** Integrated processes: nursing process — implementation; communication and documentation; client need: safe, effective care environment; coordinated care; content area: leadership/management/delegation.
RATIONALE
(1) The most appropriate way to correct an incorrect documentation is to draw a single line over the error, write "error," and then initial the documentation. Then proceed to document the correct entry. **(2)** It is not necessary to write an incident report about the error. **(3)** The most appropriate way to correct an incorrect documentation is to draw a single line over the error, write "error," and then initial the documentation. Then proceed to document the correct entry. **(4)** It is inappropriate to scratch out the incorrect entry using a black ink pen.

82. **(3)** Integrated processes: nursing process — planning; client need: safe, effective care environment; coordinated care; content area: leadership/management/delegation.
RATIONALE
(1) Determining the leadership style of the administrator will help you to adjust to the new role of nurse manager. **(2)** Determining the leadership style of the administrator will help you to adjust to the new role of nurse manager. **(3)** Determining the leadership style of the administrator will help you to adjust to the new role of nurse manager. **(4)** Determining the leadership style of the administrator will help you to adjust to the new role of nurse manager.

83. **(3)** Integrated processes: nursing process — planning; client need: safe, effective care environment; coordinated care; content area: leadership/management/delegation.
RATIONALE
(1) Management is defined as "the personal traits necessary to plan, organize, motivate, and manage the personnel and material resources of an organization." **(2)** Delegation means you are transferring to another person the authority to perform a select nursing act on a select patient for that moment. **(3)** Leadership is defined as "the personal traits necessary to establish vision and goals for an organization and the ability to execute them." **(4)** Case management is defined as "an approach that coordinates and links health-care services to clients and their families."

84. **(1)** Integrated processes: nursing process — planning; client need: safe, effective care environment; coordinated care; content area: leadership/management/delegation.
RATIONALE
(1) Management is defined as "the personal traits necessary to plan, organize, motivate, and manage the personnel and material resources of an organization." **(2)** Delegation means you are transferring to another person the authority to perform a select

nursing act on a select patient for that moment. **(3)** Leadership is defined as "the personal traits necessary to establish vision and goals for an organization and the ability to execute them." **(4)** Case management is defined as "an approach that coordinates and links health-care services to clients and their families.

85. **(3)** Integrated processes: nursing process — planning; communication and documentation; client need: safe, effective care environment; coordinated care; content area: leadership/management/delegation.

    RATIONALE
    (1) Hostile communication is when nurses talk about each other or to each other in passive-aggressive ways. **(2)** Aggressive communication is the same as hostile communication. **(3)** Feedback is part of every communication to verify that the message you wanted to give was received by the listener. Feedback requires acknowledgment of what has been said. **(4)** Communication block is an interaction where the communication that was planned or anticipated did not occur.

86. **(4)** Integrated processes: nursing process — planning; communication and documentation; client need: safe, effective care environment; coordinated care; content area: leadership/management/delegation.

    RATIONALE
    (1) This statement is a form of hostile communication. **(2)** This statement is a form of passive communication. **(3)** This statement is a form of passive-aggressive communication. **(4)** This statement is a form of assertive communication.

87. **(2)** Integrated processes: nursing process — planning; client need: safe, effective care environment; coordinated care; content area: leadership/management/delegation.

    RATIONALE
    (1) The RN is held accountable for all actions taken by the staff; however, each licensed nurse is responsible for their own actions as outlined by their Nurse Practice Act. **(2)** Licensed nurses are responsible for their own actions as outlined by their Nurse Practice Act. **(3)** The hospital does have coverage for their employees; however, they may not always cover the actions by the LPN/LVN. **(4)** Malpractice may not always cover the damages assessed against licensed personnel.

88. **(2)** Integrated processes: nursing process — planning; client need: safe, effective care environment; coordinated care; content area: leadership/management/delegation.

    RATIONALE
    (1) Liability does not exist if basic rules of human conduct are not violated. Therefore, the harm was not reasonably foreseen. **(2)** Liability does not exist if basic rules of human conduct are not violated. Therefore, the harm was not reasonably foreseen. **(3)** Liability does not exist if basic rules of human conduct are not violated. Therefore, the harm was not reasonably foreseen. **(4)** Liability does not exist if basic rules of human conduct are not violated. Therefore, the harm was not reasonably foreseen.

89. **(3)** Integrated processes: nursing process — planning; communication and documentation; client need: safe, effective care environment; coordinated care; content area: leadership/management/delegation.

    RATIONALE
    (1) The physician must write the order for restraints in any health-care setting. **(2)** The physician must write the order for restraints in any health-care setting. **(3)** The physician must write the order for restraints in any health-care setting. **(4)** The physician must write the order for restraints in any health-care setting.

90. **(1)** Integrated processes: nursing process — implementation; client need: safe, effective care environment; coordinated care; content area: leadership/management/delegation.

    RATIONALE
    (1) Both physician and licensed nurse are held liable for their actions for harm resulting from their negligence. **(2)** Both physician and licensed nurse are held liable for their actions for harm resulting from their negligence. **(3)** Both physician and licensed nurse are held liable for their actions for harm resulting from their negligence. **(4)** Both physician and licensed nurse are held liable for their actions for harm resulting from their negligence.

91. **(3)** Integrated processes: nursing process — implementation; client need: safe, effective care environment; coordinated care; content area: leadership/management/delegation.

    RATIONALE
    (1) Nurses need to clarify and verify unclear orders with the physicians. **(2)** Nurses need to clarify and verify unclear orders with the physicians. **(3)** Nurses need to clarify and verify unclear orders with the physicians. **(4)** Nurses need to clarify and verify unclear orders with the physicians.

92. **(2)** Integrated processes: nursing process — planning; client need: safe, effective care environment; coordinated care; content area: leadership/management/delegation.

    RATIONALE
    (1) Many states have provision for the rights of patients written into their statutory laws. These laws can be enforced by the law. **(2)** Many states have provision for the rights of patients written into their statutory laws. These laws can be enforced by the law. **(3)** Many states have provision for the rights of patients written into their statutory laws. These laws can be enforced by the law. **(4)** Many states have provision for the rights of patients written into their statutory laws. These laws can be enforced by the law.

93. **(2)** Integrated processes: nursing process — implementation; communication and documentation; client need: safe, effective care environment; coordinated care; content area: leadership/management/delegation.

    RATIONALE
    (1) The LPN/LVN needs to make sure the information is accurate before cosigning with another individual. **(2)** The LPN/LVN needs to make sure the information is accurate before cosigning with another individual. **(3)** The LPN/LVN needs to make sure the information is accurate before cosigning with another individual. **(4)** The LPN/LVN needs to make sure the information is accurate before cosigning with another individual.

94. **(4)** Integrated processes: nursing process — implementation; client need: safe, effective care environment; coordinated care; content area: leadership/management/delegation.

    RATIONALE
    (1) Standard of care is defined as the degree of judgment and skill in nursing care given by a reasonable and prudent professional nurse under similar circumstances. **(2)** Standard of care is defined as the degree of judgment and skill in nursing care given by a reasonable and prudent professional nurse under similar circumstances. **(3)** Standard of care is defined as the degree of judgment and skill in nursing care given by a reasonable and prudent professional nurse under similar circumstances. **(4)** Standard of care is defined as the degree of judgment and skill in nursing care given by a reasonable and prudent professional nurse under similar circumstances.

95. **(4)** Integrated processes: nursing process — implementation; client need: safe, effective care environment; coordinated care; content area: leadership/management/delegation.

    RATIONALE

    (1) Beneficence is the principle of doing good. **(2)** Nonmaleficence is the principle of doing no harm. **(3)** Justice is the obligation to be fair. **(4)** Veracity is the obligation to tell the truth.

96. **(2)** Integrated processes: nursing process — implementation; client need: safe, effective care environment; coordinated care; content area: leadership/management/delegation.

    RATIONALE

    (1) Understanding ethical decision making helps the nurse to see that there are risks and benefits to all actions. **(2)** Understanding ethical decision making helps the nurse act as a better advocate for clients. **(3)** Understanding ethical decision making helps the nurse understand that clients may not necessarily see ethical matters in the same way that we see them. **(4)** Understanding ethical decision making helps the nurse act as a better advocate for clients.

97. **(3)** Integrated processes: nursing process — implementation; client need: safe, effective care environment; coordinated care; content area: leadership/management/delegation.

    RATIONALE

    (1) Autonomy is the principle of personal liberty, of acting for one's self, and making one's own decisions. **(2)** Maleficence is doing harm to another. **(3)** Paternalism occurs when a person, like a physician or a nurse, makes a decision for someone else, like a patient, in the belief that the decision maker knows more about the situation and knows what is best for the other person. **(4)** Justice is the obligation to be fair.

98. **(2)** Integrated processes: nursing process — implementation; client need: safe, effective care environment; coordinated care; content area: leadership/management/delegation.

    RATIONALE

    (1) As the nursing manager of the floor in the long-term care facility, it is your responsibility to make rounds to ensure the UAPs loosen and reapply restraints carefully. **(3)** As the nursing manager of the floor in the long-term care facility, it is your responsibility to make rounds to ensure the UAPs loosen and reapply restraints carefully. **(3)** As the nursing manager of the floor in the long-term care facility, it is your responsibility to make rounds to ensure the UAPs loosen and reapply restraints carefully. **(4)** As the nursing manager of the floor in the long-term care facility, it is your responsibility to make rounds to ensure the UAPs loosen and reapply restraints carefully.

99. **(3)** Integrated processes: nursing process — implementation; client need: safe, effective care environment; coordinated care; content area: leadership/management/delegation.

    RATIONALE

    (1) The best nursing action is to take down the cartoon. The second action would be to report it to the nursing supervisor. **(2)** The best nursing action is to take down the cartoon. **(3)** Nursing managers are accountable for the characteristics of a workplace. **(4)** The best nursing action is to take down the cartoon.

100. **(3)** Integrated processes: nursing process — implementation; client need: safe, effective care environment; coordinated care; content area: leadership/management/delegation.

    RATIONALE

    (1) The nurse manager can delegate the cleaning out of the stock room. **(2)** The nurse manager can delegate mopping the client's room. **(3)** It is the nurse manager's responsibility to supervise the workplace environment. **(4)** Reporting neglectful actions to a client's family members against another member of the health-care team is inappropriate.

REFERENCES

Davis, A., & Aroskar, M. (1991). Ethical Dilemmas and Nursing Practice (3rd edition). Appleton & Lange: Norwalk, Conneticut, 1991.

Kozier, B., Erb, G., Berman, A., & Burke, K. Fundamentals of Nursing: Concepts, Process, and Practice, (6th edition). Prentice Hall Health: Upper Saddle River, New Jersey, 2001.

Potter, P. & Perry, A. (2001). Fundamentals of Nursing (5th edition). Mosby: St. Louis, Missouri.

Robbins, S., & Decenzo, D. (2001). Fundamentals of Management (3rd edition). Prentice Hall: Upper Saddle River, New Jersey.

CHAPTER 10

Administration of Pharmacological Agents: Content Review and Tests

Danny Willis, RN, DNSc
Larry D. Purnell, RN, PhD
Demetrius J. Porche, RN, CCRN, DNS
Golden Tradewell, RN, PhD

Medication Errors

I. Causes
  A. Failed communication
    1. Poorly handwritten or verbal orders
    2. Drugs with similar-sounding or similar-looking names
    3. Misuse of zeros in decimal numbers
    4. Use of apothecary measures (grains, drams) on
    5. Use of package units (amps, vials, tablets) instead of metric measures (grams, milligrams, milliequivalents)
    6. Misinterpreted abbreviations
    7. Ambiguous or incomplete orders
  B. Poor distribution practices
  C. Dose miscalculations
  D. Drug packaging and drug delivery systems
  E. Incorrect drug administration
  F. Lack of patient education
II. Prevention Strategies
  A. Professional responsibilities include
    1. Clarify any orders that are not obviously and clearly legible.
    2. Clarify the dosage and ask the prescriber to write out the word "units."
    3. Clarify any abbreviated drug name or the abbreviated dosing frequencies.
    4. Do not accept dosages expressed in package units or volume instead of metric weight.
    5. Suspect a missed decimal point and clarify any order if the dose requires more than three dosing units.
    6. If dose ordered requires use of multiple dosage units or very small fractions of a dose unit, review the dosage, have another health-care provider check the original order and recalculate formulas, and confirm the dosage with the prescriber.
    7. If taking a verbal order, ask prescriber to spell out the drug name and dosage to avoid sound-alike confusion.
    8. Clarify any order that does not include metric weight, dosing frequency, or route of administration.
    9. Check the nurse's/clerk's trascription against the original order.
    10. Do not start a patient on new medication by borrowing medications from another patient.
    11. Always check the patient's name band before administering medications.
    12. Use the facility's standard drug administration times to reduce the chance of an omission error.
    13. Be sure to understand fully any drug administration device before using it.
    14. Have a second practitioner independently check original order, dosage calculations, and infusion pump settings for any high-alert medications.
    15. Realize that the printing on packaging boxes, vials, ampules, prefilled syringes, or any container in which a medication is stored can be misleading.
    16. Educate patients about the medications they take.

Detecting and Managing Adverse Drug Reactions (ADRs)

I. Types of ADRs
  A. Dose-related reactions (toxic reactions)
  B. Drug-drug interactions

C. Idiosyncratic reactions

D. Hypersensitivity reactions

II. Recognizing an ADR

    A. Suspect ADR when there is a negative change in a patient's condition, particularly when a new drug has been introduced.

    B. Patient findings

        1. Rash

        2. Change in respiratory rate, heart rate, blood pressure, or mental state

        3. Seizure

        4. Anaphylaxis

        5. Diarrhea

        6. Fever

    C. Additional steps to recognize ADRs

        1. Determine that the drug ordered was the drug given and intended.

        2. Determine that the drug was given in the correct dosage by the correct route.

        3. Establish the chronology of events: time drug was taken and onset of symptoms.

        4. Stop the drug and monitor patient status for improvement

        5. Restart the drug, if appropriate, and monitor closely for adverse reactions.

Special Dosing Considerations

I. Pediatric patient

    A. Main reason for adjustment is body size

    B. Weight-based pediatric drug dosages are expressed in number of milligrams per kilogram of body weight (mg/kg)

    C. Dosages calculated on body surface area are expressed in milligrams per meter squared (mg/m^2).

II. Geriatric patient

    A. Absorption, distribution, metabolism, and excretion altered in adults over 55 years of age.

    B. Pharmacokinetic properties are affected by

        1. Percentage of body fat, lean muscle mass, and total body water

        2. Decreased plasma proteins, especially in the malnourished patient

        3. Diminished gastrointestinal (GI) motility and blood flow, which delays absorption

        4. Slower hepatic and renal function, which delays excretion

    C. Older adults need the lowest possible effective dose at the initiation of therapy followed by careful titration of doses as needed.

    D. Many elderly patients are taking prescribed multiple drugs, thus increasing risk for ADRs.

III. Patient of reproductive age

    A. Both mother and fetus must be considered

    B. Fetus is vulnerable during the first and the last trimesters of pregnancy.

        1. First trimester: fetal organs are forming and ingestion of tertogenic drugs may lead to fetal malformation or miscarriage.

        2. Third trimester: drugs administered to mother are transferred to fetus.

    C. Male patients need to be informed about the possibility of a medication altering sperm quality and quantity.

IV. Renal disease

    A. Kidneys are major organs of drug elimination.

    B. Failure to account for decreased renal function is a preventable source of ADRs.

    C. Renal function measured by creatinine clearance.

    D. Dosages in renally impaired patient can be optimized by measuring medication blood levels.

V. Liver disease

    A. Liver is major organ of drug metabolism

    B. Changes a drug from fat-soluble compound to a water-soluble substance, thus being able to be excreted by the kidneys.

    C. Patient severely jaundiced is at risk for ADRs.

    D. Patient with a very low serum protein is at risk for ADRs.

VI. Congestive heart failure

    A. Results in passive congestion of blood vessels to the GI tract, which impairs drug absorption.

    B. Also slows drug delivery to the liver, delaying metabolism

VII. Body size

    A. Drug dosing based on total body weight

    B. Some drugs selectively penetrate fatty tissues

    C. If drug does not permeate fatty tissues, dosages for the obese patient should be determined by ideal body weight or estimated body lean mass.

    D. Ideal body weight may be determined from tables of desired weights or may be estimated using formulas for lean body mass.

    E. Elderly patients, chronic alcoholics, patients with acquired immunodeficiency disease (AIDS), and patients with terminal cancer or debilitating illnesses need careful attention to dosing.

    F. Drug dosing in patients with a limb amputated needs to be readjusted because of alterations in body size.

VIII. Drug interactions

    A. Use of multiple drugs, especially those known to interact with other drugs, may necessitate dosage adjustments.

    B. Some drugs decrease the liver's ability to metabolize other drugs.

    C. Drugs that significantly alter urine pH can affect excretion of drugs for which the excretory process is pH dependent.

    D. Some drugs compete for enzyme systems with other drugs.

    E. There are no general guidelines for nutritional factors. It is prudent to check for GI problems and make the necessary dosage adjustments.

    F. Herbal supplements may interact with prescribed medications.

Educating Patients About Safe Medication Use

I. Patients should know both the brand and generic names of each medication.

II. Patients have a right to know what the therapeutic benefit of the medication will be.

III. Patients have a right to know the consequences of not taking the prescribed medication.

IV. Patient must know dosage and how to take the medication.

V. Always explain to patients what to do if a dose is missed.

VI. Patients need to take medication for the duration of therapy.

VII. Inform the patient that all medications have potential side effects.

VIII. Inform the patient of the possibility of serious side effects.

IX. Patient and family need to know which other medications, including which over-the-counter medications, to avoid.

X. Food-drug interactions are not uncommon and can have effects similar to drug-drug interactions.

XI. Medications must be stored properly to maintain potency.

XII. Anyone taking medication requires ongoing care to assess effectiveness and appropriateness of medications.

XIII. Inform patients not to take expired medications or someone else's medication.

XIV. Stress the importance of concurrent therapy.

XV. Provide written instructions in a simple and easy-to-read format.

Cultural Considerations: Variations in Drug Metabolism

I. People of African American heritage
   A. Research indicates that African Americans do not always respond to drugs in the same manner as European Americans.
   B. Drugs include: alcohol, antihypertensives, beta blockers, psychotropic drugs, and caffeine.
   C. Side effects of psychotropic and antidepressant drugs vary.
   D. Psychiatric clients experience a higher incidence of extrapyramidial effects with haloperidol (Haldol).
   E. More susceptible to tricyclic antidepressant (TCA) delirium.
   F. For a given dose of TCA, African Americans show higher blood levels and a faster therapeutic response, thus increasing toxic effects.
   G. Research indicates that African Americans are twice as likely to develop tardive dyskinesia than their white counterparts.
   H. Observation for side effects related to tricyclics and other psychotropic medications.
   I. African Americans are at a higher risk of misdiagnosis for psychiatric disorders; thus may be treated inappropriately with drugs.
   J. Eye color of African Americans creates a different response to mydriatic drugs.
   K. Causes of death include: homicide, cirrhosis, malnutrition, chemical dependency, and diabetes.
   L. Leading causes of death in African American women are cancer, stroke, chronic obstructive pulmonary disease, pneumonia, unintentional injuries, diabetes, suicide, and human immodeficiency virus (HIV)/AIDS.
   M. Alcohol, illicit drug use, and depression are also leading causes of death for African American women.
   N. Genetic diseases include: sickle cell anemia, glucose-6-phosphate dehydrogenase deficiency.

II. People of Amish heritage
   A. No drug studies specifically related to the Amish has been conducted.
   B. Genetic disorders in the Amish include
      1. Dwarfism
      2. Cartilage hair hypoplasia
      3. Pyruvate kinase anemia
      4. Hemophilia B
      5. High prevalence of phenylketonuria
      6. Glutaric aciduria
      7. Bipolar disorders

III. People of Appalachian heritage
   A. No drug studies specifically related to Appalachian heritage
   B. Diseases and health conditions include:
      1. Respiratory diseases
      2. Hypochromic anemia
      3. Otitis media
      4. Cardiovascular diseases
      5. Female obesity
      6. Non–insulin-dependent diabetes mellitus
      7. Parasitic infections
      8. Children are at greater risk for sudden infant death syndrome, congenital malformations, and infections.

IV. People of Arab heritage
   A. Research indicates that 1.0% to 1.4% of Arabs have difficulty metabolizing substances such as antiarrhythmics, antidepressants, beta blockers, neuroleptics, and opioid agents.
   B. Small number of Arab Americans experience elevated blood levels and adverse effects when customary dosages of antidepressants are prescribed.
   C. Codeine dosages may prove inadequate because some individuals cannot metabolize codeine to morphine to promote optimal analgesic effect.
   D. Incidence of infectious diseases, such as tuberculosis, malaria, trachoma, typhus, hepatitis, typhoid fever, dysentery, and parasitic infestations varies.
   E. Glucose-6-phosphate dehydrogenase (G-6-PD) deficiency, sickle cell anemia, and the thalassemias are common in Arabs.
   F. High consanguinity (marrying first cousins) and bearing children up to menopause contribute to the prevalence of genetically determined disorders.
   G. Cardiovascular disease is major cause of death.

V. People of Chinese heritage
   A. Research indicates a poor metabolism of mephenytoin; sensitivity to beta blockers, such as propranolol, as evidenced by a decrease in the overall blood levels accompanied by a seemingly more profound response; atropine sensitivity, as evidenced by an increased heart rate; and increased responses to antidepressants and neuroleptics given at lower doses.
   B. Analgesics have been found to cause increased gastrointestinal side effects.

C. Increased sensitivity to the effects of alcohol.

D. Common health conditions include: heart disease, other circulatory diseases, and cancers.

E. Genetic diseases include: thalassemia, glucose-6-phosphate dehydrogenase deficiency, increased incidence of lactose intolerance.

F. Increased incidence of hepatitis B and tuberculosis.

G. Chinese American women have a 20% higher rate of pancreatic cancer and higher rates of suicide after the age of 45 years.

H. All Chinese have higher death rates due to diabetes.

VI. People of Cuban heritage

A. Little or no drug data are available specific to Cuban Americans.

B. Common health conditions include: overweight, diabetes mellitus, hypertension, nonalcoholic cirrhosis, chronic bronchitis, total tooth loss, gingival inflammation, and periodontitis.

VII. People of Filipino heritage

A. Compared to the white American population, Asians require lower doses of central nervous depressants such as Haldol.

B. Lower tolerance for alcohol, and are more sensitive to adverse effects of alcohol.

C. May have adverse effects of anti-infectives.

D. Health-care providers need to assess Filipino clients individually when administering and monitoring medications.

E. Ten leading causes of morbidity include: diarrhea, bronchitis/bronchiolitis, pneumonia, influenza, hypertension, respiratory tuberculosis, malaria, heart disease, chickenpox, typhoid/parathyroid fever.

F. Ten leading causes of mortality include: heart disease, vascular system disease, pneumonia, accidents, malignancy, tuberculosis (TB), chronic obstructive pulmonary disease, other respiratory diseases, diabetes mellitus, and renal disease.

G. Breast, cervical, prostatic thyroid, lung, and liver cancers are major threats to this population.

H. Liver cancer tends to be diagnosed in the late stages and appears to be associated with the presence of hepatitis B virus.

VIII. People of Irish heritage

A. No reported studies on drug responses are specific to the Irish.

B. Most studies of pharmacological responses have used data aggregated under the category of whites.

C. Heart disease and cancer are the leading causes of premature mortality in Ireland compared with the U.S. Irish.

D. Irish Americans had the highest mortality rates for coronary artery disease.

E. Cancer is second to coronary heart disease as a major cause of mortality in Ireland.

F. The risk of coronary heart disease, a silent killer of women, increases after the age of 65 years.

G. Osteoporosis is another significant health problem affecting older women.

H. Major cause of infant mortality in Ireland is congential abnormalities, such as phenylketonuria, neural tube defects, and fetal alcohol syndrome.

IX. People of Italian heritage

A. No specific reports on drug metabolism or interactions specific to Italians or Italian Americans.

B. Health conditions such as Mediterranean-type G-6-PD deficiency and thalassemia have a profound effect on drug metabolism.

C. Conditions such as hypoxemia and acidosis, ingestion of fava beans, and the administration of sulfonamides, antimalarial agents, salicylates, and naphthaquinolones can exacerbate health conditions.

D. In addition to genetic diseases, Italian Americans have a high incidence of hypertension and coronary artery disease related to smoking and their type A behavior.

E. Research indicates Italian Americans have significantly higher risks of nasopharyngeal, stomach, liver, and gallbladder tumors.

F. An increased incidence of ventricular septal defects in children of Italian heritage and that congenital heart disease in infants is associated with older maternal age at conception.

G. Italian Americans are also at increased risk for multiple sclerosis (MS).

X. People of Japanese heritage

A. Drug dosages need to be adjusted for the physical stature of Japanese adults.

B. More Asians than whites are poor metabolizers of mephenytoin and related medications, potentially leading to increased intensity and duration of the drug's effects.

C. Asians tend to be more sensitive to the effects of some beta blockers, many psychotropic drugs, and alcohol.

D. Japanese people rapidly metabolize acetylate substances, which has an impact on metabolism of tranquilizers, tuberculosis drugs, caffeine, and some cardiovascular agents.

E. Asians require lower doses of some benzodiazepines and neuroleptics.

F. Opiates may be less effective than analgesics, but GI side effects may be greater.

G. The leading causes of death in Japan include: cancers, heart disease, stroke, pneumonia, accidents, motor vehicle accidents, suicide, renal disease, liver disease, diabetes, hypertension (related to the high sodium in their diet), and tuberculosis.

XI. People of Jewish heritage

A. Twenty percent of Jewish clients taking clozapine developed agranulocytosis.

B. Genetic disorders include: Tay-Sachs disease, Gaucher disease, Canavan disease, familial dysautonomia, torsion dystonia, Niemann-Pick disease, Bloom syndrome, Fanconi anemia, and mucolipidosis.

C. Other health conditions include: inflammatory bowel disease, colorectal cancer, increased risk to develop breast cancer.

XII. People of Korean heritage

A. Studies show that Asian populations require lower dosages of psychotropic drugs.

B. Other studies have shown variations in drug metabolism and interaction with propranolol, isoniazid, and diazepam among Asians.

C. Common health conditions include schistosomiasis and other parasitic diseases endemic to certain regions of Korea; Korean immigrants need to be assessed for asbestos-related health problems.

D. High prevalence of stomach and liver cancer, tuberculosis, hepatitis, and hypertension in South Korea predispose immigrants to these conditions.

E. As with other Asians, there is a high occurrence of lactose intolerance among people of Korean ancestry.

F. High incidence of gum diseases and oral problems exist.

XIII. People of Mexican heritage

A. Because of mixed heritage of many Mexican Americans, it may be more difficult to determine a therapeutic dose of selected drugs.

B. Several studies report differences in absorption, distribution, metabolism, and excretion of drugs in Hispanic populations.

C. Hispanics require lower doses of antidepressants and experience greater side effects than non-Hispanic whites.

D. Common health problems in Mexico are malnutrition, malaria, cancer, alcoholism, drug abuse, obesity, hypertension, diabetes, heart disease, adolescent pregnancy, dental disease, and HIV/AIDS.

E. In Mexican American migrant worker populations, infectious, communicable, and parasitic diseases continue to be major health risks.

F. Research has revealed increased incidence of malaria in the border towns of the southwestern part of the United States.

G. Cardiovascular disease is the leading cause of death and disability in Mexican American communities.

H. Mexican Americans have five times the rate of diabetes mellitus.

XIV. Navajo Indians

A. Lidocaine reactions occur in 29% of the Navajo population as compared with 11% to 15% of European Americans.

B. Water on Navajo reservations is impure and unchlorinated resulting in injestion of waterborne bacteria.

C. *Salmonella* infection is common because lack of refrigeration.

D. Higher death rates in Navajo Indians include: alcoholism, tuberculosis, diabetes mellitus type II, unintentional injuries, suicide, pneumonia, influenza, homicide, gastrointestinal diseases, infant mortality, and heart disease.

E. Studies with the Navajo have identified a high incidence of severe combined immunodeficiency syndrome (SCIDS), an immunodeficiency syndrome unrelated to AIDS, that results in a failure of the antibody response and cell-mediated immunity.

F. Navajo neuropathy is unique to this population. Symptoms include: poor weight gain, short stature, sexual infantilism, serious systemic infections, and liver derangement.

G. Genetic disorders include: albinism and genetically prone blindness.

XV. People of Polish heritage

A. No report of any pharmacological studies specific to people of Polish descent.

B. Common health problems include heart disease, respiratory disease, and cancer, especially leukemia.

XVI. People of Puerto Rican heritage

A. Because of the African heritage of many Puerto Ricans, drug absorption, metabolism, and excretion differences experienced by African Americans and Native Americans may hold true for Puerto Ricans.

B. Puerto Ricans are short in stature and have higher subscapular and triceps skin folds, long trunks, and short legs; therapeutic dosages need to be recalculated.

C. Common health conditions include: heart disease, malignant neoplasm, diabetes mellitus, unintentional injuries, and AIDS.

D. Puerto Ricans in the United States have higher incidence of chronic conditions such as mental illness among younger adults and cardiopulmonary and osteomuscular diseases among the elderly.

E. Puerto Rican women in the United States have a high incidence of being overweight.

F. Dengue, a mosquito-transmitted disease, is an endemic disease that migrants may bring to the United States.

G. Puerto Rico has a higher HIV infection rate than any U.S. state. In some states, AIDS is the leading cause of death for Puerto Rican women aged 25–44 years.

XVII. People of Vietnamese heritage

A. Variations in drug metabolism are the same as for other Asian groups.

B. Vietnamese women have the highest rate of cervical cancer.

C. Cancer and other problems common to Vietnamese people may also be associated with the widespread application of chemical agents during the Vietnam War.

D. Mental health research indicates that Vietnamese refugees have higher rates of depression, generalized anxiety disorders, and post-traumatic stress experiences.

E. Vietnamese people have a higher rate of tuberculosis, leprosy, hepatitis B, high levels of parasitism, syphilis, and moderate to severe dental problems.

Classifications of Drugs

The following drug classifications are taken from *Davis's Drug Guide for Nurses*, ed 9. Philadelphia, F.A. Davis Company, 2005. Please see that book for a full presentation on each drug classification.

1. Anti-Alzheimer's agents
2. Antianemics
3. Antianginals
4. Antianxiety agents
5. Antiarrhythmics
6. Antiasthmatics

7. Anticholinergics
8. Anticoagulants
9. Anticonvulsants
10. Antidepressants
11. Antidiabetics
12. Antidiarrheals
13. Antiemetics
14. Antifungals
15. Antihistamines
16. Antihypertensives
17. Anti-infectives
18. Antineoplastics
19. Antiparkinson agents
20. Antiplatelet agents
21. Antipsychotic agents
22. Antipyretics
23. Antiretrovirals
24. Antirheumatics
25. Antituberculars
26. Antiulcer agents
27. Antivirals
28. Beta blockers

29. Bone resorption inhibitors
30. Bronchodilators
31. Calcium channel blockers
32. Central nervous stimulants
33. Cortiocsteroids
34. Diuretics
35. Hormones
36. Immunosuppressants
37. Laxatives
38. Lipid-lowering agents
39. Minerals/electrolytes/pH modifiers
40. Natural/herbal products
41. Nonopiod analgesics
42. Nonsteroidal anti-inflammatory agents
43. Opiod analgesics
44. Sedative/hypnotics
45. Skeletal muscle relaxants
46. Thrombolytics
47. Vaccines/immunizing agents
48. Vascular headache suppressants
49. Vitamins
50. Weight-control agents

QUESTIONS

Danny Willis, RN, DNSc, Larry D. Purnell, RN, PhD, Demetrius J. Porche, RN, CCRN, DNS, and Golden Tradewell, RN, PhD

Test 1: Pharmacological Principles

1. Meperidine (Demerol) is classified as:
   1. Psychotropic
   2. Antibiotic
   3. Analgesic
   4. Cardiotonic

2. Polycillin is classified as:
   1. Psychotropic
   2. Analgesic
   3. Antibiotic
   4. Diuretic

3. Hydrochlorothiazide (HydroDIURIL) is classified as:
   1. Antibiotic
   2. Analgesic
   3. Cardiotonic
   4. Diuretic

4. Diazepam (Valium) is classified as:
   1. Antibiotic
   2. Psychotropic
   3. Cardiotonic
   4. Diuretic

5. Digoxin (Lanoxin) is classified as:
   1. Antibiotic
   2. Cardiotonic
   3. Diuretic
   4. Psychotropic

6. A drug that is absorbed into the bloodstream and carried to specific organs is said to have:
   1. A systemic effect
   2. A local effect
   3. An untoward effect
   4. An indirect effect

7. A drug has an idiosyncratic effect when:
   1. The drug is absorbed into the body and carried to all cells.
   2. Psychological dependence occurs when the drug is injected.
   3. Unusual, unpredictable, unexpected reactions occur.
   4. All of the drug's intended effects occur.

8. A medication that consists of a suspension of fat globules and water is classified as:
   1. An emulsion
   2. An ointment
   3. A tincture
   4. An elixir

9. The action of antibiotics is that:
   1. They allow the body to build up its defenses to fight infection.
   2. They increase the number of phagocytes to ingest bacteria.
   3. They break down the bacterial cell wall and inhibit growth of microorganisms.
   4. They destroy microorganisms.

10. The goal of antihypertensive therapy is to:
    1. Cure the client of high blood pressure
    2. Control the blood pressure and prevent complications
    3. Make the client hypotensive and prevent congestive heart failure
    4. Prevent the left ventricle from pumping blood

11. The word *antiseptic* means:
    1. Increasing body activities
    2. Inhibiting the growth of bacteria
    3. Slowing down bodily activities
    4. Destroying bacteria

12. The most rapid route of administration of a drug is:
    1. Subcutaneous (SC)
    2. Intramuscular (IM)
    3. Intravenous (IV)
    4. Oral (PO)

13. The single most important organ that detoxifies drugs is the:
    1. Lung
    2. Stomach
    3. Liver
    4. Bone marrow

14. Anaphylactic shock can occur as a result of drug allergy. Some of the signs of this reaction are:
    1. Flushed skin, dyspnea, hypertension
    2. Bradycardia, pallor, edema of the extremities
    3. Hypotension, dyspnea, diaphoresis
    4. Fever, rash, bradycardia

15. Clients who are receiving antineoplastic agents that depress bone marrow function may require reverse isolation or placement in a pathogen-free environment because:
    1. The client has an infection that could be transmitted to others.
    2. Bacteria normally found in the air could prove fatal.
    3. Exposure to pathogens might cause hyponatremia.
    4. Anemia might result.

16. Female clients who are receiving androgens for treatment of a neoplasm may develop:

1. Endometrial carcinoma
2. Alopecia
3. Mild to moderate masculinization
4. Ulcerations of the mouth

17. Promethazine (Phenergan), when combined with a narcotic:

    1. Causes central nervous system (CNS) stimulation.
    2. Produces a triple response.
    3. Potentiates the effect of the narcotic.
    4. Increases the need for narcotics.

18. Chronic use of mineral oil

    1. Can cause dysphagia.
    2. Hinders the absorption of fat-soluble vitamins.
    3. Chemically interacts with water-soluble vitamins.
    4. Leads to dumping syndrome.

19. Tricyclic drugs are considered to be in which of the following categories of drugs?

    1. Antidepressants
    2. Antidiarrheals
    3. Antiemetics
    4. Hypnotics

20. An example of a central nervous system (CNS) stimulant is:

    1. Thyroxine
    2. Diazepam
    3. Amphetamine
    4. Alcohol

21. Which of the following procedures is recommended if it becomes necessary for a nurse to discard a narcotic?

    1. Have another person witness you discarding the drug.
    2. Report discarding the narcotic to the physician who prescribed it.
    3. Have the pharmacy director issue an identical amount of drug to replace what you had to discard.
    4. Save the discarded amount and return it to the pharmacy.

22. A client asks a physician for a specific medication, but the nurse has trouble reading the physician's order. Which of the following persons should the nurse consult in order to clarify the order?

    1. The unit clerk who transcribed the order
    2. The physician who wrote the order
    3. The pharmacist who will fill the order
    4. The client who has been taking the medication on a regular basis over the last 2 years.

23. To verify an alert client's identity, the nurse checks the client's identification band before giving medications. It is also recommended that:

    1. The nurse call the client by name
    2. The client be asked to state his or her name
    3. A relative be asked to verify the client's identification
    4. A second nurse be asked to verify the client's identity

24. A nurse notes an error about 0.5 hour after giving a medication to a client. The nurse's first action in this situation should be to:

    1. Prepare an incident report
    2. Call the physician
    3. Notify the client that an error has been made
    4. Check the client's condition

25. The "five rights" for drug administration are:

    1. Right time, dose, route, room, client
    2. Right dose, route, client, room, medication
    3. Right route, dose, client, physician, room
    4. Right time, dose, drug, client, route

26. One of the problems encountered in the use of antineoplastic drugs is that:

    1. Surgery or radiation cannot be used concomitantly to treat the malignancy.
    2. The tumor may be too small or too large to treat with drugs.
    3. These drugs also affect normal cells.
    4. Only a few types of malignancies can be treated with these drugs.

27. A client, aged 66 years, had exploratory surgery for possible cancer of the colon. Because the tumor had spread and was inoperable, the physician decided to administer 5-fluorouracil (5-FU) for palliative management of the tumor. The client began to develop adverse drug effects. As a nurse you know that:

    1. Drug therapy will have to be discontinued.
    2. This outcome is a sign that the drug is ineffective and another must be tried.
    3. There are times when some of these effects must be tolerated in order to obtain optimum therapeutic results.
    4. No other type of drug can be given to lessen adverse drug effects.

28. After several weeks of chemotherapy treatment, an oncology client begins to develop alopecia and is very upset. What might a nurse suggest to the client or the family about this problem?

    1. Limit visitors to the immediate family, and include only those who are understanding.
    2. Move the client to a private room.
    3. Suggest that client purchase a wig.
    4. Tell the client not to worry because the hair always grows back.

29. An oncology client develops leukopenia, which is manifested by:

    1. Fatigue and shortness of breath
    2. Nausea and vomiting
    3. Easy bruising
    4. Lesions in the buccal cavity

30. A client develops thrombocytopenia, which is manifested by:

    1. Fatigue
    2. Easy bruising

3. Shortness of breath on exertion
4. Decreased resistance to infection

31. When a client has a new diagnosis of a convulsive disorder, the nurse should first:

1. Obtain a thorough history from the client or the family.
2. Explain what epilepsy is to the family.
3. Assure the family that drugs will control the seizures.
4. Never leave the client's bedside.

32. Close observation of a client with a convulsive disorder is most important because:

1. The nurse will ultimately have to describe the seizures to the client's family.
2. Drug therapy cannot begin until the client has another seizure that has been observed by nursing personnel.
3. It may help the physician to diagnose the type of convulsive disorder.
4. The nurse will be in charge of protecting the client from injury during a seizure.

33. Phenytoin has been selected to treat a client with a convulsive disorder. Now that drug therapy has been instituted:

1. It is no longer necessary to describe the seizures that may occur because the diagnosis has been established.
2. Ongoing nursing observations often help the physician to evaluate the effectiveness of drug therapy.
3. The client will have no more seizures.
4. There is no longer any need to describe the seizure.

34. A client complains of nausea, which appears to be drug related. GI discomfort may be prevented by giving a drug:

1. Early in the morning
2. Late in the evening
3. With two or more glasses of water
4. With or immediately after meals

35. Ibuprofen (Motrin):

1. Has only analgesic activity
2. Provides analgesic and anti-inflammatory activity
3. Has no known adverse effects
4. Should always be taken on an empty stomach for best results

36. A tranquilizer that is also used as a muscle relaxant is:

1. Phenobarbital
2. Chlorpromazine
3. Perphenazine
4. Diazepam

37. You are instructed to give a client 5 mL of an expectorant. The client refuses it. You should:

1. Leave it by the bedside so that the client can take it later.
2. Discard the medication and report it to the physician.
3. Return the medication to the bottle and report it to the physician,

4. Get somebody to help you force the client to take the medicine.

38. A client is taking furosemide (Lasix) 80 mg bid. A nursing action before administering the drug is to check the client's:

1. History of allergies to penicillins
2. Red-green discrimination
3. Optic nerve damage
4. Potassium level

39. A client is receiving digoxin 0.25 mg PO qd. Before administration of the drug, the nurse would take the client's:

1. Apical pulse for 30 seconds
2. Apical pulse for 60 seconds
3. Radial pulse for 30 seconds
4. Radial pulse for 60 seconds

40. A client is taking the antacid aluminum hydroxide. The nurse would encourage the client to also:

1. Take milk of magnesia nightly
2. Decrease fluid intake
3. Increase bulk in the diet
4. Decrease bulk in the diet

41. Drugs that initiate a response are called:

1. Antagonists
2. Agonists
3. Depressants
4. Antiseptics

42. The serum half-life of a drug is:

1. The time required after absorption for half of the drug to be eliminated
2. The time required for half of a drug dose to be absorbed
3. The time required for a drug to exert half of its total effect
4. Half of the time required for a drug to be completely metabolized

43. Knowledge of drug potency does not enable us to predict whether a potent drug is more or less toxic. The valid indicator that measures the safety of the drug is:

1. Side effect profile
2. Therapeutic range
3. Duration of action
4. Biological half-life

44. A large initial dose to achieve minimum effective concentration is known as:

1. Threshold dose
2. Therapeutic range
3. Loading dose
4. Free (unbound) drug

45. A common side effect of many anti-inflammatory agents (e.g., aspirin, indomethacin, ibuprofen) is:

1. Urinary retention
2. Increased pulse rate

3. Behavioral changes
4. GI disturbances

46. Ibuprofen is one of the newest drugs in the group of nonsteroidal anti-inflammatory drugs (NSAIDs). Ibuprofen agents should be administered:
   1. With food or large glass of water
   2. On an empty stomach
   3. Before breakfast, lunch, and dinner, and at bedtime
   4. With aspirin or other NSAIDs

47. The nurse is instructed to give an IM injection in the vastus lateralis. The location of the vastus lateralis for the site for administration is:
   1. At the lateral portion of the thigh with one hand's breadth above the knee and one hand's breadth below the greater trochanter
   2. At the lateral portion of the thigh with one hand's breadth below the knee and one hand's breadth above the greater trochanter
   3. At the lower edge of the acromion to the middle third of the front part of the thigh
   4. At the middle third of the front part of the thigh to above the knee

48. When mixing neutral protamine Hagedorn (NPH) and regular insulin, the best sequence is:
   1. Air into NPH, then air into the regular and draw it up, followed by drawing up the NPH
   2. Air into NPH and draw up, then air into the regular and draw up
   3. Air into regular, then air into NPH and draw up, followed by drawing up regular
   4. Giving two separate injections; do not mix insulin

49. An unconscious client is in shock with metabolic acidosis. The nurse should be sure to have which of the following drugs on hand?
   1. Dobutamine
   2. Sodium nitroprusside
   3. Sodium bicarbonate
   4. Calcium gluconate

50. Drugs can be given IV, intradermally, IM, and SC. Aspiration is contraindicated in which method?
   1. IV
   2. Intradermally
   3. SC
   4. IM

51. A client was seen in the emergency department with digitalis toxicity. Which lab results would the nurse expect to see?
   1. Elevated hematocrit
   2. Elevated hemoglobin
   3. Elevated potassium
   4. Decreased potassium

52. The client told the nurse that she takes a herbal treatment "to help her remember." Which of the following herbs is contraindicated with the usage of Lanoxin (digoxin)?

1. Verapamil
2. Calcium
3. Erthromycin
4. Ginseng

53. Which of the following drugs has a prolonged effect on blood clotting?
   1. Heparin
   2. Coumadin
   3. Digoxin
   4. Ginseng

54. Which of the following herbal therapies enhances the effectiveness of warfarin (Coumadin)?
   1. Acetaminophen
   2. Echinacea
   3. Ginseng
   4. Ibuprofen

55. Which of the following herbal therapies decrease the effectiveness of Coumadin?
   1. Acetaminophen
   2. Echinacea
   3. Ginseng
   4. Ibuprofen

56. Which of the following lab values need to be monitored for an elevation when the client is taking Lasix (furosemide)?
   1. Calcium
   2. Magnesium
   3. Potassium
   4. Cholesterol

57. At what age group is the usage of Lasix contraindicated?
   1. Less than 12 months of age
   2. Teenage
   3. Middle age
   4. Adulthood

58. The purpose for use of nitroglycerin is to:
   1. Manage angina pectoris
   2. Elevate blood pressure during surgical procedures
   3. Produce hypertension
   4. Increase work load of the heart

59. Nitroglycerin is available in various forms such as: (**Select all that apply.**)
   1. Oral
   2. Transdermal
   3. Subcutaneous
   4. Suppository
   5. Intravenous
   6. Intramuscular

60. Which of the following is given to a postoperative cataract client to reduce corneal swelling?
   1. Ibuprofen
   2. Acetaminophen
   3. Lasix
   4. Dexamethasone

61. A client arrived to the emergency department in a status epilepticus condition. Which drug of choice is used to treat this condition?

1. Ibuprofen
2. Dexamethasone
3. Diazepam
4. Elavil

62. The abbreviation qid means:

1. Every 4 days
2. Every 4 hours
3. Four times each day
4. Every day

63. The term *ac* means:

1. Before meals
2. After meals
3. At mealtime
4. At once

64. One fluid ounce is equivalent to:

1. 15 mL
2. 30 mL
3. 2 tsp
4. 3 tsp

65. The physician orders Maalox 15 mL. How many tablespoons would you give?

1. 3 tsp
2. 2 tsp
3. 1 tsp
4. 1 tbsp

66. One gram is equivalent to:

1. 10 mg
2. 100 mg
3. 1000 mg
4. 10,000 mg

67. The physician ordered 100 units of salmon calcitonin to be given to an elderly woman with osteoporosis. Which method of adminstration would the nurse use?

1. IV
2. IM
3. Oral
4. Suppository

68. The client has been using a calcium replacement in a nasal spray. What might a nurse suggest to the client or the family about this type of drug administration:

1. Spray both nostrils for one full dose.
2. Use the same nostril for each dose.
3. Spray every 4 hours.
4. If your nose starts to bleed, discontinue the drug.

69. The pediatrician ordered cefaclor 250 mg tid. This drug is most commonly used for:

1. Gonorrhea
2. Spastic colon
3. Otitis media
4. Cellulitis

70. What might the nurse suggest to the client or the family about taking cefaclor?

1. Stop medication if diarrhea begins.
2. Obtain stool culture if diarrhea begins.
3. Take medication until fever has subsided.
4. Eat yogurt daily to restore intestinal flora.

71. The physican ordered cefazolin (Ancef) postoperatively. The nurse is preparing the powder to give an intramuscular injection. What solution does the nurse mix the powder to reconstitute it?

1. 10% normal saline
2. Sterile water
3. Unsterile water
4. 10% dextrose in water

72. What might the nurse suggest to the client or the family about taking celecoxib (Celebrex)?

1. It is safe to use during pregnancy.
2. Report any unexplained weight gain.
3. Report any unexplained weight loss.
4. Periodically monitor the calcium level.

73. A client undergoing a surgical procedure was experiencing severe anxiety. The physician ordered chlorpromazine (Thorazine) 50 mg IM. Before the nurse administers the drug, what information is important to know about the client?

1. If the client is schizophrenic
2. If the client is diabetic
3. If the client is nauseated
4. If the client has the hiccups

74. What might the nurse suggest to the client or the family about taking a drug with codeine?

1. Refrain from taking herbal treatments
2. May cause diarrhea
3. May cause diuresis
4. It is safe to take with alcohol

75. What might the nurse suggest to the client or the family about taking over-the-counter Robitussin DM?

1. Can be given to all age groups.
2. Can be used in males with enlarged prostates.
3. Can cause excitability in children.
4. Acts similar to morphine.

76. A 33-year-old client with type I insulin-dependent diabetes is a businessman with a very active lifestyle. He has maintained control of his diabetes until recently. His insulin routine is 5 units of regular insulin plus 20 units of NPH insulin every morning before breakfast at 7 AM. Because the client takes NPH insulin, he should have a snack at which time of the day?

1. After breakfast (10 AM)
2. Midafternoon (2 PM)
3. Early evening (7 PM)
4. Before bedtime (9 PM)

77. Which type of insulin can be given intravenously (IV)?

1. Regular
2. NPH

3. Lente
4. Humulin N

78. What would be the correct technique to administer regular insulin and NPH insulin with one injection?

1. NPH insulin should never be mixed with any other form of insulin.
2. Using aseptic technique, first withdraw the proper dose of regular insulin; then withdraw the proper dose of NPH insulin.
3. Using aseptic technique, first withdraw the proper dose of NPH insulin; then withdraw the proper dose of regular insulin.
4. Regular insulin should never be mixed with any other form of insulin.

79. Intravenous fluids containing potassium are administered slowly and cautiously to prevent:

1. Metabolic acidosis
2. Fluid overload
3. Cardiac arrest
4. Infiltration

80. Digoxin (Lanoxin) 0.125 mg IV has been ordered for a cardiac client. The ampule is labeled "digoxin 0.5 mg/2 mL." The nurse should:

1. Administer 0.5 mL
2. Administer 0.25 mL
3. Administer 1.0 mL
4. Call the physician to verify the order

81. The physician orders 10 mL of a medication. The medicine is available only to be administered in minims. What is the correct amount to administer?

1. 30 minims
2. 35 minims
3. 80 minims
4. 160 minims

82. After administration of morphine 10 mg IM for pain relief, which of the following data has lowest priority?

1. Urine output
2. Blood pressure
3. Respiratory status
4. Pain relief

83. There are "five rights" of medication administration to avoid medication errors. Which of the rights is related to reading the armband of a client?

1. Right client
2. Right medication
3. Right dose
4. Right route

84. Which of the following is most important before administering any medication?

1. Check the input and output (I&O) records.
2. Assess for symptoms.
3. Check the admitting diagnosis.
4. Check the client's identification band.

85. An order reads: "Tylenol (acetaminophen) gr X suppository PRN every 4 hours for temperature greater than 100°F." The nurse should administer:

1. 325 mg
2. 650 mg
3. 900 mg
4. 1200 mg

86. Which finding would indicate a therapeutic response to levodopa therapy?

1. Increased tremors
2. Increased rigidity
3. Decreased tremors
4. Twitching

87. A client has a diagnosis of *Pneumocystis carinii* pneumonia. The client is receiving pentamidine in a 300-mg aerosolized treatment every day during the acute illness. What is the correct position for pentamidine aerosolized treatment?

1. Lying supine
2. Lying prone
3. Sitting upright
4. Turning from side to side every 3–5 minutes

88. Mannitol has been administered to a client for cerebral edema. The nurse can evaluate mannitol's effectiveness by assessing:

1. Increased potassium level
2. Decreased potassium level
3. Increased urine output
4. Increased respiratory rate

89. Which of the following is an indication for a decrease in the dosage of nitroglycerin?

1. An increase in chest pain
2. Lightheadedness and dizziness
3. Increased blood pressure
4. A pulse rate of 80 bpm

90. Correct heparin administration involves:

1. Never rotating injection sites
2. Aspirating to assess for blood vessel entry
3. Always giving heparin by deep IM injection
4. Never rubbing the area after the injection

91. A 74-year-old female client with a history of cardiac disease is admitted to the hospital for congestive heart failure (CHF). Her condition is stable. She is receiving furosemide (Lasix) 20 mg bid and digoxin 0.25 mg every morning. Before the digoxin is given, which of the vital signs should be assessed and documented?

1. Temperature
2. Apical pulse
3. Blood pressure
4. Respiratory rate

92. A client in CHF is placed on digoxin and furosemide therapy; the nurse can evaluate the effectiveness of digoxin and furosemide by:

1. Increased pupillary reaction
2. Increased respiratory rate

3. Increased urine output
4. Increased edema

93. A 35-year-old male client on a telemetry unit begins to have more than 10 unifocal premature ventricular contractions (PVCs) per minute. The nurse should prepare to administer:
   1. Digoxin
   2. Lidocaine
   3. Propranolol (Inderal)
   4. Atropine

94. A postoperative IV fluid order reads: "Lactated Ringer's 1000 mL to be infused over 8 hours." The infusion set delivers 15 gtt/mL. The nurse should regulate the rate of flow at:
   1. 15 gtt/min
   2. 31 gtt/min
   3. 60 gtt/min
   4. 90 gtt/min

95. A client has begun having grand mal seizures. He is now in stable condition. The physician orders 2 g of $MgSO_4$ in 100 mL D_5W over 30 minutes. The infusion set delivers 10 gtt/mL. When this infusion is monitored, the rate of flow should be:
   1. 15 gtt/min
   2. 33 gtt/min
   3. 66 gtt/min
   4. 99 gtt/min

96. During the $MgSO_4$ infusion, the nurse should assess for signs of toxicity every 15 minutes. Which of the following is not a sign of $MgSO_4$ toxicity?
   1. Depressed knee jerk
   2. Increased knee jerk
   3. Confusion
   4. Respiratory distress

97. Which of the following statements made by a client about the potential side effects of aminoglycosides indicates the need for further teaching?
   1. "Ototoxicity can be a side effect."
   2. "Nephrotoxicity can be a side effect."
   3. "Neurotoxicity can be a side effect."
   4. "Photosensitivity can be a side effect."

98. While monitoring a client with histoplasmosis who has been placed on amphotericin B therapy, the nurse identifies:
   1. Afebrile reaction
   2. Hyperkalemia
   3. Hypokalemia
   4. Elevated blood pressure

99. Which statement about antineoplastic medication is incorrect?
   1. Drug combinations increase effectiveness.
   2. Antineoplastic drugs may be used with radiation therapy.
   3. Antineoplastic drugs kill only neoplastic cells.
   4. Common side effects are stomatitis, GI distress, alopecia, and bone marrow suppression.

100. A client is being discharged home on thyroid USP. Which statement made by the client indicates the need for further teaching?
   1. "Weight loss is a potential side effect of thyroid USP."
   2. "Insomnia is a potential side effect of thyroid USP."
   3. "Bradycardia is a potential side effect of thyroid USP."
   4. "Tachycardia is a potential side effect of thyroid USP."

101. Aspirin can be given for which of the following reasons?
   1. To decrease platelet aggregation
   2. To decrease carbon dioxide retention
   3. To inhibit peptic ulcer disease
   4. To reduce emphysema

102. When a client is receiving heparin therapy, the nurse should do which of the following?
   1. Shave the client with a straight razor daily.
   2. Assess for irritability.
   3. Assess for ecchymosis or signs of bleeding.
   4. Encourage a full-liquid diet.

103. A new client admitted to the unit has a diagnosis of asthma. Breath sounds exhibit wheezes and rhonchi in all lobes. The client is receiving aminophylline (which contains theophylline) 250 mg q6h. Which of the following indicates that the medication is effective?
   1. Increased wheezes
   2. Decreased wheezes
   3. Increased rhonchi
   4. Decreased rhonchi

104. An 85-year-old client recovering from a cerebrovascular accident (CVA) resides in a skilled nursing facility. There are minimal sequelae from the CVA. The client is able to walk and perform activities of daily living with minimal assistance. However, he is unable to swallow whole pills. Four pills are to be taken at 12 noon. Which of the following would be the most appropriate method of administering the pills?
   1. Give one pill at a time every 5 minutes.
   2. Break pills into pieces, giving one at a time every 5 minutes.
   3. Crush pills and place in applesauce.
   4. Give one pill whole every 15 minutes.

105. The client has received diazepam (Valium) 10 mg PO for anxiety. What would be the most appropriate nursing function?
   1. Encourage client to ambulate independently.
   2. Assist with ambulation.
   3. Counsel client on chemical dependency.
   4. Place in bed with siderail raised and soft restraints on both arms.

106. A client is receiving diphenhydramine (Benadryl) 50 mg tid. An appropriate nursing action would be to inform the client that:
   1. Drowsiness may occur
   2. Tinnitus usually occurs

3. Alcohol has no effect on diphenhydramine
4. Diphenhydramine increases mental alertness

107. Which of the following is important to tell a client receiving phenazopyridine (Pyridium)?

1. Appetite may increase.
2. Urine may change color to red-orange.
3. Urine may change color to blue-purple.
4. Pain will occur with voiding.

108. Which client statement about rifampin is true?

1. "Rifampin is usually given with other antituberculosis drugs."
2. "Rifampin is usually given with other antimalaria drugs."
3. "My urine and feces may be colored red-orange."
4. "My saliva, sputum, sweat, and tears may be colored red-orange."

109. Which of the following statements by the client about nitroglycerin's administration indicates that further teaching is needed?

1. "I will need to assess my blood pressure before administration."
2. "I will need to assess my blood pressure after administration."
3. "I will need to change positions rapidly."
4. "The sublingual nitroglycerin may sting when taken."

110. In caring for an elderly adult who is taking NSAIDs for osteoarthritis pain, what instructions must the nurse give?

1. Do not take NSAIDs with food.
2. Take NSAIDs with food.
3. Alternate NSAIDs with acetaminophen.
4. Take the maximum dose of NSAIDs.

Test 2: Calculation of Dosages

FILL IN THE BLANK:

111. You are instructed to give nitroglycerin 0.4 mg. The drug label reads "1/150-grain tablet." How many tablets would you give?

_____

112. You are instructed to give cephalexin monohydrate (Keflex) 0.5 g. The drug comes as 250 mg per capsule. How many capsules would you give?

_____

113. You are instructed to give penicillin V potassium (Pen-Vee K suspension) 0.75 g. The drug is available as 250 mg per 5 mL. How many milliliters would you give?

_____

114. You are instructed to give cyclophosphamide (Cytoxan) 4 mg/kg per day PO. The client weighs 154 lb. How much Cytoxan would you give each day?

_____

115. You are instructed to give cephalexin monohydrate 3 g over the next 24 hours, divided into six equally spaced doses. How much would you give for each dose?

_____

116. Aspirin is available in 5-gr tablet. The physician orders aspirin 300 mg. The amount of drug to be administered is:

_____

117. Vitamin K is available in 1 mg per 0.5 mL. The physician orders vitamin K 0.5 mg. The amount of vitamin K to be administered is:

_____

118. Digoxin is available in 0.125 mg per tablet. The physician orders digoxin 0.25 mg. The amount of drug to be administered is:

_____

119. Meperidine is available in 75 mg/mL. The physician orders Demerol 0.50 mg. The amount of drug to be administered is:

_____

120. Codeine is available in 1-gr tablet. The physician orders codeine 30 mg. The amount of drug to be administered is:

_____

121. Hydroxyzine (Vistaril) is available in 25 mg/mL. The physician orders 100 mg q4–6h PRN. How many milliliters would you give per as-needed dose?

_____

122. The amount of solution and amount of IV aminophylline received by a client each hour when there is 500 mg aminophylline in 250 mL solution given every 24 hours is:

_____

123. The amount of solution and amount of IV aminophylline received by the client each minute when there is 250 mg aminophylline in 250 mL solution given over 16 hours is:

_____

124. The amount of solution and amount of IV aminophylline received by a client each hour when there is 500 mg aminophylline in 500 mL solution over 12 hours is:

_____

125. The amount of solution and amount of IV dopamine received by a client each hour when there is 400 mg dopamine in 500 mL solution over 24 hours is:

_____

126. If the client is to receive insulin at 3 units/hr with a solution of 50 units per 100 mL in normal saline (NS), the rate of infusion in milliliters would be:

_____

127. The correct formula for converting total volume and hours of infusion into rate of drops (guttae, abbreviated gtt) per minute using calibration of IV tubing is:

_____

128. You are instructed to give morphine sulfate 10 mg SC. The drug label reads "15 mg/mL." How many milliliters would you give?

_____

129. Hydroxyzine 25 mg IM has been ordered. Vial reads "100 mg in 2 mL." How many milliliters would you give?

_____

130. The order reads "5000 units heparin SC every 6 hours." Vial reads "20,000 units/mL." How many milliliters would you give?

_____

131. The physician orders lactated Ringer's solution 1000 mL to be infused over 8 hours. Drops per milliliter equals 15. How many drops per minute would you give?

_____

132. You are instructed to infuse 150 mL of D_5W over 1 hour. Drops per milliliter equals 10. How many drops per minute would you give?

_____

133. A hypertonic solution of 10% dextrose in water is to be infused over 10 hours via a 16-gauge IV needle. The total amount of fluid is 1000 mL, and the drop factor is 10. How many drops per minute would you give?

_____

134. You are instructed to infuse 100 mL of solution in 2 hours. The set calibration is 60 gtt/mL. How many drops per minute would you give?

_____

135. You are instructed to infuse 900 mL of solution in 2 hours. The set calibration is 20 gtt/mL. How many drops per minute would you give?

_____

136. You are instructed to infuse 1000 mL of solution in 8 hours. The set calibration is 10 gtt/mL. How many drops per minute would you give?

_____

137. You are instructed to administer a solution IV at 150 mL/hr. The set calibration is 60 gtt/mL. How many drops per minute would you give?

_____

138. You are instructed to infuse 50 mL of antibiotic in 30 minutes. The set calibration is 60 gtt/mL. How many drops per minute would you give?

_____

139. You are instructed to infuse 15 mL of medication over 15 minutes. The set calibration is 60 gtt/mL. How many drops per minute would you give?

_____

140. You are instructed to infuse 600 mL of IV fat emulsion (Intralipid) over 8 hours. The set calibration is 10 gtt/mL. How many drops per minute would you give?

_____

141. You are instructed to infuse 150 mL of fluid over 2 hours using minidrip (minidrip equals 60 gtt/mL). How many drops per minute would you give?

_____

142. A client is to receive 1000 mL D_5 in one-half NS with 20 mEq potassium chloride over 10 hours. Drip factor is 15 gtt/mL. How many drops per minute would you give?

_____

143. The physician orders 100 mL lactated Ringer's solution to be infused over 2 hours. The set calibration is 10 gtt/mL. How many drops per minute would you give?

_____

144. You are instructed to infuse 15 mL of fluid over 30 minutes. The set calibration is 60 gtt/mL. How many drops per minute would you give?

_____

145. A client is to receive 1800 mL of fluid over 10 hours. The set calibration is 10 gtt/mL. How many drops per minute would you give?

_____

146. The physician orders lactated Ringer's solution 1000 mL to be infused over 6 hours. Drops per milliliter equals 15. How many drops per minute would you give?

_____

147. You are instructed to infuse D_5W 250 mL over 1 hour. Drops per milliliter equals 15. How many drops per minute would you give?

_____

148. A hypertonic solution of 10% dextrose and water is to be infused over 12 hours. The total amount of fluid is 1000 mL and the drop factor 15. How many drops per minute would you give?

_____

149. You are instructed to infuse 300 mL of solution in 2 hours. The set calibration is 60 gtt/mL. How many drops per minute would you give?

_____

150. You are instructed to infuse 900 mL of fluid in 2 hours. The set calibration is 10 gtt/mL. How many drops per minute would you give?

_____

151. You are instructed to infuse 1500 mL of fluid in 8 hours. The set calibration is 10 gtt/mL. How many drops per minute would you give?

_____

152. You are instructed to administer an IV infusion of 250 mL of D_5W at 100 mL/hr. The set calibration is 60 gtt/mL. How many drops per minute would you give?

_____

153. You are instructed to infuse 60 mL of antibiotic in 15 minutes. The set calibration is 10 gtt/mL. How many drops per minute would you give?

_____

154. You are instructed to infuse 20 mL of medication over 30 minutes. The set calibration is 60 gtt/mL set. How many drops per minute would you give?

_____

155. You are instructed to infuse 800 mL of IV fat emulsion over 6 hours. The set calibration is 20 gtt/mL. How many drops per minute would you give?

_____

156. You are instructed to infuse 105 mL of fluid over 2 hours using a minidrip of 60 gtt/min. How many drops per minute would you give?

_____

157. The client is to receive 1000 mL D_5W in one-half NS with 20 mEq potassium chloride over 8 hours. Drip factor is 10 gtt/mL. How many drops per minute would you give?

_____

158. The physician orders 100 mL lactated Ringer's solution to be infused over 2 hours. The set calibration is 10 gtt/mL. How many drops per minute would you give?

_____

159. You are instructed to infuse 30 mL over 30 minutes. The set calibration is 60 gtt/mL. How many drops per minute would you give?

_____

160. The client is to receive 1000 mL of fluid over 10 hours. The set calibration is 15 gtt/mL. How many drops per minute would you give?

_____

ANSWERS

Test 1

1. **(3)** Integrated processes: nursing process — evaluation; client need: physiological integrity; pharmacological therapies; content area: pharmacology.
   RATIONALE
   (1) Psychotropics alter the mood. **(2)** Antibiotics inhibit the growth of bacteria. **(3)** Analgesics relieve pain. Meperidine is given to relieve pain. **(4)** Cardiotonics make the heart pump more efficiently.

2. **(3)** Integrated processes: nursing process — evaluation; client need: physiological integrity; pharmacological therapies; content area: pharmacology.
   RATIONALE
   (1) Psychotropics alter the mood. **(2)** Analgesics relieve pain. **(3)** Antibiotics inhibit the growth of bacteria. Polycillin is given to inhibit the growth of bacteria. **(4)** Diuretics promote fluid excretion.

3. **(4)** Integrated processes: nursing process — evaluation; client need: physiological integrity; pharmacological therapies; content area: pharmacology.
   RATIONALE
   (1) Antibiotics inhibit the growth of bacteria. **(2)** Analgesics relieve pain. **(3)** Cardiotonics make the heart pump more efficiently. **(4)** Diuretics promote fluid excretion. Hydrochlorothiazide is given to promote fluid excretion.

4. **(2)** Integrated processes: nursing process — evaluation; client need: physiological integrity; pharmacological therapies; content area: pharmacology.
   RATIONALE
   (1) Antibiotics inhibit the growth of bacteria. **(2)** Psychotropics alter the mood. Diazepam is given to alter the mood. **(3)** Cardiotonics make the heart pump more efficiently. **(4)** Diuretics promote fluid excretion.

5. **(2)** Integrated processes: nursing process — evaluation; client need: physiological integrity; pharmacological therapies; content area: pharmacology.
   RATIONALE
   (1) Antibiotics inhibit the growth of bacteria. **(2)** Cardiotonics make the heart beat more efficiently. Digoxin is given to make the heart beat more efficiently. **(3)** Diuretics promote fluid excretion. **(4)** Psychotropics alter the mood.

6. **(1)** Integrated processes: nursing process — evaluation; client need: physiological integrity; pharmacological therapies; content area: pharmacology.
   RATIONALE
   (1) Drugs that affect the entire body are described as having a systemic effect. **(2)** A drug with a local effect affects only a targeted local area. **(3)** An untoward effect is one that is undesirable. **(4)** An indirect effect occurs as an unplanned consequence and is not the primary effect.

7. **(3)** Integrated processes: nursing process — evaluation; client need: physiological integrity; pharmacological therapies; content area: pharmacology.
   RATIONALE
   (1) A drug that is carried to all cells has a systemic effect. **(2)** In psychological dependence, the client has an incapacitating need for a drug. **(3)** An idiosyncratic effect is an unusual, unpredictable, unexpected reaction. **(4)** An effective drug is one that produces all of its intended effects.

8. **(1)** Integrated processes: nursing process — evaluation; client need: physiological integrity; pharmacological therapies; content area: pharmacology.
   RATIONALE
   (1) An emulsion is a mixture of two insoluble liquids, such as fat and water. **(2)** An ointment is a topical semisolid. **(3)** A tincture is an alcohol extract liquid. **(4)** An elixir is a sweetened, aromatic liquid form of a drug.

9. **(4)** Integrated processes: nursing process — evaluation; client need: physiological integrity; pharmacological therapies; content area: pharmacology.
   RATIONALE
   (1) Building up the body's defenses to fight infection is not the direct action of antibiotics. **(2)** Antibiotics do not increase the number of phagocytes. **(3)** Antibiotics do not break down the cell wall. They have no action on growth of new cells. **(4)** By definition, antibiotics inhibit the growth of or destroy microorganisms.

10. **(2)** Integrated processes: nursing process — planning; client need: physiological integrity; pharmacological therapies; content area: pharmacology.
    RATIONALE
    (1) Antihypertensive drugs help to control high blood pressure, but they do not cure the disease. **(2)** Hypertension is a chronic disease. The goals are to control the blood pressure and to prevent complications. **(3)** Hypotension can be a side effect of antihypertensive therapy, but it is not the goal. **(4)** Antihypertensive drugs allow the heart to pump under reduced pressure. The left ventricle should not be prevented from pumping blood.

11. **(2)** Integrated processes: nursing process — evaluation; client need: physiological integrity; pharmacological therapies; content area: pharmacology.
    RATIONALE
    (1) Catabolic refers to increasing body activities. **(2)** Antiseptic means inhibiting the growth of bacteria. **(3)** Anabolic refers to decreasing body activities. **(4)** Sterilization refers to destroying bacteria.

12. **(3)** Integrated processes: nursing process — evaluation; client need: physiological integrity; pharmacological therapies; content area: pharmacology.
    RATIONALE
    (1) The SC route is faster than the oral route but slower than IM and IV. **(2)** The IM route is faster than SC route but slower than IV. **(3)** The IV route is a direct route for administration of a drug that does not require absorption of the drug from the tissues. **(4)** The slowest route for absorption is the oral form.

13. **(3)** Integrated processes: nursing process — evaluation; client need: physiological integrity; pharmacological therapies; content area: pharmacology.

RATIONALE
(1) The lungs help excrete drugs but do not detoxify. (2) The stomach absorbs drugs. (3) The liver is the main organ for detoxification. (4) The bone marrow helps to absorb and store drugs but does not detoxify.

14. (3) Integrated processes: nursing process — data collection; client need: physiological integrity; pharmacological therapies; content area: pharmacology.
RATIONALE
(1) Shock produces hypotension, not hypertension. (2) Shock produces tachycardia, not bradycardia. (3) Hypotension, dyspnea, and diaphoresis are classic signs of anaphylaxis, which is a life-threatening, acute allergic reaction. (4) Shock produces tachycardia, not bradycardia.

15. (2) Integrated processes: nursing process — implementation; client need: physiological integrity; pharmacological therapies; content area: pharmacology.
RATIONALE
(1) The client may have an infection that can be transmitted, but reverse isolation is used to protect the compromised client. (2) These clients have decreased reserves to fight normal flora. (3) Exposure to pathogens does not cause hyponatremia. (4) The client may be anemic, but reverse isolation is not used for anemia, a condition with reduced red blood cells (RBCs).

16. (3) Integrated processes: nursing process — data collection; client need: physiological integrity; pharmacological therapies; content area: pharmacology.
RATIONALE
(1) Androgens do not cause endometrial cancer. (2) Alopecia is a side effect of antineoplastic agents. (3) Mild to moderate masculinization can result from the administration of male hormones (androgens). (4) Ulcerations of the mouth are a side effect of antineoplastic agents.

17. (3) Integrated processes: nursing process — data collection; client need: physiological integrity; pharmacological therapies; content area: pharmacology.
RATIONALE
(1) Promethazine decreases stimulation of the CNS. (2) There is no triple response. (3) The action of promethazine is to potentiate the effect of the narcotic. (4) Phenergan decreases the need for narcotics.

18. (2) Integrated processes: nursing process — evaluation; client need: physiological integrity; pharmacological therapies; content area: pharmacology.
RATIONALE
(1) There is no evidence that mineral oil causes dysphagia (difficulty swallowing). (2) A side effect of mineral oil is that it hinders the absorption of fat-soluble vitamins. (3) Mineral oil does not mix with water-soluble vitamins. (4) Dumping syndrome is caused by increased emptying time of the stomach. Mineral oil works on the lower gastrointestinal (GI) tract.

19. (1) Integrated processes: nursing process — evaluation; client need: physiological integrity; pharmacological therapies; content area: pharmacology.
RATIONALE
(1) Tricyclics affect the mood and are in the category of antidepressants. (2) Antidiarrheal drugs help to prevent or reduce diarrhea. (3) Antiemetics help to prevent nausea and vomiting. (4) Hypnotics induce a clinical state resembling sleep.

20. (3) Integrated processes: nursing process — evaluation; client need: physiological integrity; pharmacological therapies; content area: pharmacology.

RATIONALE
(1) Thyroxine is a thyroid hormone and increases metabolism, but it is not a CNS stimulant. (2) Diazepam is a tranquilizer and decreases CNS stimulation. (3) An amphetamine is a CNS stimulant. (4) Alcohol is a depressant, not a stimulant.

21. (1) Integrated processes: nursing process — implementation; communication and documentation; client need: physiological integrity; pharmacological therapies; content area: pharmacology.
RATIONALE
(1) Narcotics are included under federal controlled substances regulations. Federal regulations recommend having another person witness you discarding the drug. (2) There is no need to notify the physician. (3) You may inform the pharmacy about the discard, but not to replace it with an identical amount. (4) There is no need to return the discard to the pharmacy; the pharmacy can neither verify the drug nor reissue it.

22. (2) Integrated processes: nursing process — evaluation; communication and documentation; client need: physiological integrity; pharmacological therapies; content area: pharmacology.
RATIONALE
(1) Consulting the unit clerk is not the safest option. The unit clerk did not write the order. (2) The only person who really knows the desired order is the physician, and this is the safest option. (3) Consulting the pharmacist is not the safest option. The pharmacist did not write the order. (4) Consulting the client is not the safest option. The client did not write the order.

23. (2) Integrated processes: nursing process — planning; communication and documentation; client need: physiological integrity; pharmacological therapies; content area: pharmacology.
RATIONALE
(1) A confused client may respond to other than his or her own name, or there may be two persons with the same name. (2) The most accurate way is to have the client state his or her name. (3) A relative could be asked for verification, but a relative is not the most direct source in this situation. (4) A second nurse is not the most direct or accurate way to verify the client's identity in this situation.

24. (4) Integrated processes: nursing process — implementation; client need: physiological integrity; pharmacological therapies; content area: pharmacology.
RATIONALE
(1) Preparing an incident report is recommended but is not the highest priority in this situation. (2) Calling the physician is recommended but is not the highest priority in this situation. (3) Notifying the client is a possible action but is not the highest priority in this situation. (4) The highest priority is to check the client first to assess the response to the drug.

25. (4) Integrated processes: nursing process — implementation; client need: physiological integrity; pharmacological therapies; content area: pharmacology.
RATIONALE
(1) Room is not one of the five rights. (2) Room is not one of the five rights. (3) Room is not one of the five rights. (4) These are the five rights. Memorization of them is standard practice.

26. (3) Integrated processes: nursing process — evaluation; client need: physiological integrity; pharmacological therapies; content area: pharmacology.

RATIONALE
(1) Surgery and radiation are both used to treat malignancy. (2) The size of the tumor has no relationship to its treatment with antineoplastic drugs. (3) A side effect of antineoplastic agents is that they also affect normal cells. (4) Antineoplastic drugs are used to treat a wide variety of malignancies.

27. (3) Integrated processes: nursing process — planning; client need: physiological integrity; pharmacological therapies; content area: pharmacology.

RATIONALE
(1) Drugs are discontinued for allergic reactions but not necessarily for adverse effects. (2) Side effects do not mean that the drug is ineffective; all drugs have some side effects. (3) Beneficial effects must be weighed against adverse effects. (4) When side effects occur, another drug may be given at the same time to decrease the side effects (e.g., an antiemetic may be given to decrease the side effects of nausea created by an antibiotic).

28. (3) Integrated processes: nursing process — planning; teaching/learning; client need: physiological integrity; pharmacological therapies; content area: pharmacology.

RATIONALE
(1) Limiting visitors will not help with self-esteem and may cause an increased feeling of isolation. (2) Moving the client to a private room may create a further feeling of isolation. (3) Alopecia is loss of hair. A wig might help this client's self-esteem. (4) The hair does not always grow back, so this response may be false reassurance.

29. (4) Integrated processes: nursing process — evaluation; client need: physiological integrity; pharmacological therapies; content area: pharmacology.

RATIONALE
(1) Anemia may cause fatigue and shortness of breath. (2) Nausea and vomiting are side effects of many drugs. (3) Easy bruising is not caused by a decreased number of white cells. (4) Lesions in the buccal cavity are a side effect of leukopenia.

30. (2) Integrated processes: nursing process — evaluation; client need: physiological integrity; pharmacological therapies; content area: pharmacology.

RATIONALE
(1) A decrease in RBCs produces fatigue. (2) Thrombocytopenia, or a decrease in platelets, affects the clotting of the blood, resulting in easy bruising. (3) Shortness of breath results from anemia. (4) A reduction in white blood cells (WBCs) decreases resistance to infection.

31. (1) Integrated processes: nursing process — data collection; client need: physiological integrity; pharmacological therapies; content area: pharmacology.

RATIONALE
(1) The first step in assessment is obtaining a history. (2) There is no evidence that the client's specific disorder is epilepsy. (3) One cannot assure the family that drugs will control the seizures at this point. (4) The client does not require constant attention, only close observation.

32. (4) Integrated processes: nursing process — planning; client need: physiological integrity; pharmacological therapies; content area: pharmacology.

RATIONALE
(1) Describing the seizures to the family is not as important as protecting the client from injury. (2) Drug therapy is important but not the most important reason for close observation of the client. (3) Diagnosing the specific type of convulsive disorder is helpful but not the most important reason for close observation of the client. (4) It would be most important for the nurse to protect the client from injury.

33. (2) Integrated processes: nursing process — planning; client need: physiological integrity; pharmacological therapies; content area: pharmacology.

RATIONALE
(1) Describing the seizures is necessary. (2) The nurse is still responsible for ongoing assessment. (3) Seizures may still occur after treatment is started. (4) Describing the seizures is necessary.

34. (4) Integrated processes: nursing process — implementation; client need: physiological integrity; pharmacological therapies; content area: pharmacology.

RATIONALE
(1) Time of day is less important than food in preventing discomfort. (2) Time of day is less important than food in preventing discomfort. (3) Water is less important than food in preventing discomfort. (4) Manufacturers recommend giving drugs with food to help relieve nausea.

35. (2) Integrated processes: nursing process — evaluation; client need: physiological integrity; pharmacological therapies; content area: pharmacology.

RATIONALE
(1) Ibuprofen also has an anti-inflammatory effect. (2) Ibuprofen is a nonsteroidal anti-inflammatory drug (NSAID) with antipyretic and analgesic properties. (3) All drugs have some side effects. (4) It is best to take ibuprofen with food to help prevent mucosal irritation.

36. (4) Integrated processes: nursing process — evaluation; client need: physiological integrity; pharmacological therapies; content area: pharmacology.

RATIONALE
(1) Phenobarbital is not used as a muscle relaxant. (2) Chlorpromazine is an antipsychotic. (3) Perphenazine is an antiemetic and antipsychotic. (4) Diazepam is a muscle relaxant that also has antianxiety effects.

37. (2) Integrated processes: nursing process — implementation; communication and documentation; client need: physiological integrity; pharmacological therapies; content area: pharmacology.

RATIONALE
(1) The nurse should never leave medicine at the bedside. (2) Discarding the medication is safer than risking returning the medication to the wrong bottle. The physician should be notified if the client is not taking medication. (3) The nurse should never return the medication to the bottle. (4) The nurse should never force a client to take a medicine.

38. (4) Integrated processes: nursing process — evaluation; client need: physiological integrity; pharmacological therapies; content area: pharmacology.

RATIONALE
(1) Furosemide is a sulfonamide derivative. Check the client for allergies to sulfa drugs. (2) Furosemide has no effect on red-green discrimination. (3) Furosemide does not cause optic nerve damage, but may cause loss of hearing. (4) Furosemide is a potassium-wasting diuretic, so it is important to check potassium levels before its administration. It also increases excretion of chloride and sodium.

39. **(2)** Integrated processes: nursing process — implementation; client need: physiological integrity; pharmacological therapies; content area: pharmacology.
    RATIONALE
    (1) Taking the apical pulse for 30 seconds is not the recommended length of time for the most accurate measurement. **(2)** With all cardiotonics, the only acceptable method to determine pulse rate is to take an apical pulse for a full minute. **(3)** An apical pulse is heard over the apex of the heart and is more accurate than a radial pulse. **(4)** An apical pulse is heard over the apex of the heart and is more accurate than a radial pulse.

40. **(3)** Integrated processes: nursing process — implementation; teaching/learning; client need: physiological integrity; pharmacological therapies; content area: pharmacology.
    RATIONALE
    (1) Laxatives are not a first defense. **(2)** Decreasing fluid intake increases the chances of constipation. **(3)** Aluminum hydroxide causes constipation; thus, increasing bulk in the diet will help to prevent constipation. **(4)** Decreasing bulk increases the chances for constipation.

41. **(2)** Integrated processes: nursing process — evaluation; client need: physiological integrity; pharmacological therapies; content area: pharmacology.
    RATIONALE
    (1) An antagonist is a drug that makes another drug less effective. **(2)** By definition, an agonist stimulates receptors to initiate a response. **(3)** A depressant is a drug that slows a vital process. **(4)** Antiseptics inhibit the growth of bacteria.

42. **(1)** Integrated processes: nursing process — evaluation; client need: physiological integrity; pharmacological therapies; content area: pharmacology.
    RATIONALE
    (1) The time it takes for eliminating processes to reduce the blood concentration of the drug by half is called the drug half-life. **(2)** Half-life is measured by elimination, not absorption. **(3)** The time for a drug to exert half of its total effect cannot be measured. **(4)** The time required for a drug to be completely metabolized cannot be measured.

43. **(2)** Integrated processes: nursing process — evaluation; client need: physiological integrity; pharmacological therapies; content area: pharmacology.
    RATIONALE
    (1) All drugs have common side effects. **(2)** By definition, therapeutic range is the ratio between the lethal dose and the mean effective dose. **(3)** Duration of action is how long the drug is circulating in the body. **(4)** Biological half-life is the time it takes for half of the drug to disappear from the serum.

44. **(3)** Integrated processes: nursing process — evaluation; client need: physiological integrity; pharmacological therapies; content area: pharmacology.
    RATIONALE
    (1) The threshold dose of a drug is barely sufficient to produce desired effects. **(2)** Therapeutic range is the ratio between lethal dose and the mean effective dose. **(3)** A loading dose is a large initial dose to achieve minimum effective concentration. **(4)** Free drug is the amount in the serum that is ineffective in its purpose.

45. **(4)** Integrated processes: nursing process — evaluation; client need: physiological integrity; pharmacological integrity; content area: pharmacology.

RATIONALE
(1) Anti-inflammatory drugs do not cause urinary retention. **(2)** Anti-inflammatory drugs do not commonly cause increased pulse rate. **(3)** Anti-inflammatory drugs do not commonly cause behavioral changes. **(4)** Many anti-inflammatory agents irritate the lining of the stomach. These should not be used in clients with a history of ulcers.

46. **(1)** Integrated processes: nursing process — planning; client need: physiological integrity; pharmacological therapies; content area: pharmacology.
    RATIONALE
    (1) Administering ibuprofen with food or a large glass of water helps to prevent gastric irritation. **(2)** Administering NSAIDs on an empty stomach increases the chances for gastric irritation. **(3)** Administering NSAIDs before meals or at bedtime does not provide protection against gastric irritation. **(4)** Administering NSAIDs with aspirin or other NSAIDs increases the chance of gastric irritation.

47. **(1)** Integrated processes: nursing process — data collection; client need: physiological integrity; pharmacological therapies; content area: pharmacology.
    RATIONALE
    (1) These are landmarks for location of the vastus lateralis. The vastus lateralis is the preferred injection site for children because it is well developed and has few major nerves present that could be injured. **(2)** This is not a landmark for an injection of any kind. **(3)** This is not a landmark for an injection of any kind. **(4)** This is not a landmark for an injection of any kind.

48. **(1)** Integrated processes: nursing process — implementation; client need: physiological integrity; pharmacological therapies; content area: pharmacology.
    RATIONALE
    (1) Regular insulin is pure and NPH a mixture; so if contamination does occur, it would be best to contaminate the NPH. **(2)** This sequence may cause contamination of NPH into the pure regular insulin. **(3)** This sequence may cause contamination of NPH into the pure regular insulin. **(4)** You should not give the client two injections if one injection can suffice.

49. **(3)** Integrated processes: nursing process — implementation; client need: physiological integrity; pharmacological therapies; content area: pharmacology.
    RATIONALE
    (1) Dobutamine does not combat metabolic acidosis. **(2)** Sodium nitroprusside does not combat metabolic acidosis. **(3)** Sodium bicarbonate is the only drug listed that helps to reverse acidosis. **(4)** Calcium gluconate does not combat metabolic acidosis.

50. **(2)** Integrated processes: nursing process — evaluation; client need: physiological integrity; pharmacological therapies; content area: pharmacology.
    RATIONALE
    (1) With an IV injection, the nurse must aspirate to make sure the needle is in the vein and not in the tissue. **(2)** Intradermal injection is just under the skin; no danger exists of injection into a blood vessel. **(3)** Aspiration is needed in SC injections to make sure that the needle is not in a blood vessel. **(4)** Aspiration is needed in IM injections to make sure that the needle is not in a blood vessel.

51. **(3)** Integrated processes: nursing process — data collection; client need: physiological integrity; reduction of risk potential; content area: pharmacology.

RATIONALE

(1) A client with digitalis toxicity would have an elevated potassium, not an elevated hematocrit. (2) A client with digitalis toxicity would have an elevated potassium, not an elevated hemoglobin. (3) A client with digitalis toxicity would have an elevated potassium. (4) A client with digitalis toxicity would have an elevated potassium, not a decreased potassium.

52. **(4)** Integrated processes: nursing process — data collection; client need: physiological integrity; pharmacological therapies; content area: pharmacology.

RATIONALE

(1) Verapamil is not a herbal treatment. (2) Calcium is a mineral, not a herbal treatment. (3) Erythromycin is an antibiotic, not a herbal treatment. (4) Ginseng is considered a herbal treatment used to enhance memory.

53. **(2)** Integrated processes: nursing process — evaluation; client need: physiological integrity; pharmacological therapies; content area: pharmacology.

RATIONALE

(1) Heparin has a fast-acting effect on blood clotting. (2) Coumadin has a prolonged effect on blood clotting. (3) Digoxin has no effect on blood clotting. (4) Ginseng has no effect on blood clotting.

54. **(2)** Integrated processes: nursing process — evaluation; client need: physiological integrity; reduction of risk potential; content area: pharmacology.

RATIONALE

(1) Acetaminophen is not a herbal therapy, but does enhance the effectiveness of Coumadin. (2) Echinacea is a herbal therapy that enhances the effectiveness of Coumadin. (3) Ginseng is a herbal therapy, but does not enhance the effectiveness of Coumadin. (4) Ibuprofen is not a herbal therapy, but does enhance the effectiveness of Coumadin.

55. **(3)** Integrated processes: nursing process — evaluation; client need: physiological integrity; reduction of risk potential; content area: pharmacology.

RATIONALE

(1) Acetaminophen is not a herbal therapy, but does enhance the effectiveness of Coumadin. (2) Echinacea is a herbal therapy that enhances the effectiveness of Coumadin. (3) Ginseng, a herbal therapy, decreases the effectiveness of Coumadin. (4) Ibuprofen is not a herbal therapy, but does enhance the effectiveness of Coumadin.

56. **(4)** Integrated processes: nursing process — evaluation; client need: physiological integrity; reduction of risk potential; content area: pharmacology.

RATIONALE

(1) Cholesterol levels may become elevated when a client is taking Lasix and must be monitored. (2) Magnesium levels are not affected if a client is taking Lasix. (3) Potassium levels drop when a client is taking Lasix. (4) Cholesterol levels may become elevated when a client is taking Lasix and must be monitored.

57. **(1)** Integrated processes: nursing process — evaluation; client need: physiological integrity; reduction of risk potential; content area: pharmacology.

RATIONALE

(1) The usage of Lasix is contraindicated in infants less than 12 months of age. (2) Lasix can be used in teenagers. (3) Lasix can be used in adults. (4) Lasix can be used in adults.

58. **(1)** Integrated processes: nursing process — evaluation; client need: physiological integrity; pharmacological therapies; content area: pharmacology.

RATIONALE

(1) Nitroglycerin is used to manage angina pectoris. (2) Nitroglycerin is also used to decrease blood pressure during surgical procedures. (3) Nitroglycerin produces hypotension. (4) Nitroglycerin reduces the work load of the heart.

59. **(1, 2)** Integrated processes: nursing process — evaluation; client need: physiological integrity; pharmacological therapies; content area: pharmacology.

RATIONALE

(1) Nitroglycerin is available in oral and transdermal forms. (2) Nitroglycerin is available in oral and transdermal forms. (3) Nitroglycerin is available in oral and transdermal forms, not in a subcutaneous form. (4) Nitroglycerin is available in oral and transdermal forms, not in a suppository form. (5) Nitroglycerin is available in oral and transdermal forms, not in an intravenous form. (6) Nitroglycerin is available in oral and transdermal forms, not an intramuscular form.

60. **(4)** Integrated processes: nursing process — implementation; client need: physiological integrity; pharmacological therapies; content area: pharmacology.

RATIONALE

(1) Dexamethasone eye drops are used to reduce corneal swelling. Ibuprofen may be used if the client experiences pain. (2) Acetaminophen may be used if the client experiences pain. (3) Lasix is not used to reduce corneal swelling. (4) Dexamethasone eye drops are used to reduce corneal swelling.

61. **(3)** Integrated processes: nursing process — implementation; client need: physiological integrity; pharmacological therapies; content area: pharmacology.

RATIONALE

(1) Diazepam (Valium) is used to treat status epilepticus. (2) Dexamethasone is used to treat cerebral edema, not to treat status epilepticus. (3) Diazepam (Valium) is used to treat status epilepticus. (4) Elavil is a tranquilizer; however, it is not used to treat status epilepticus.

62. **(3)** Integrated processes: nursing process — evaluation; client need: physiological integrity; pharmacological therapies; content area: pharmacology.

RATIONALE

(1) Every 4 days is q4d. (2) Every 4 hours is q4h. (3) Four times each day is qid. (4) Every day is qd.

63. **(1)** Integrated processes: nursing process — evaluation; client need: physiological integrity; pharmacological therapies; content area: pharmacology.

RATIONALE

(1) Before meals is ac. (2) After meals is pc. (3) At meals is cc. (4) At once is stat.

64. **(2)** Integrated processes: nursing process — evaluation; client need: physiological integrity; pharmacological therapies; content area: pharmacology.

RATIONALE

(1) Fifteen milliliters is 0.5 oz. (2) Thirty milliliters is 1 oz. (3) Two teaspoons is 10 mL. (4) Three teaspoons is 15 mL.

65. **(4)** Integrated processes: nursing process — evaluation; client need: physiological integrity; pharmacological therapies; content area: pharmacology.

RATIONALE

(1) Three teaspoons is 15 mL, but the question asks for tablespoons. (2) Two teaspoons is 10 mL, but the question asks for tablespoons. (3) One teaspoon is 5 mL, but the question asks for tablespoons. (4) One tablespoon is 15 mL.

66. **(3)** Integrated processes: nursing process — evaluation; client need: physiological integrity; pharmacological therapies; content area: pharmacology.
RATIONALE
(1) Ten milligrams is equivalent to 1/100 g. **(2)** One hundred milligrams is equivalent to 1/10 g. **(3)** One thousand milligrams is equivalent to 1 g. **(4)** Ten thousand milligrams is equivalent to 10 g.

67. **(2)** Integrated processes: nursing process — evaluation; client need: physiological integrity; pharmacological therapies; content area: pharmacology.
RATIONALE
(1) Salmon calcitonin is to given IM, not IV. **(2)** Salmon calcitonin is to be given IM. **(3)** Salmon calcitonin is to be given IM, not orally. **(4)** Salmon calcitonin is to be given IM, not in suppository form.

68. **(4)** Integrated processes: nursing process — evaluation; teaching/learning; client need: physiological integrity; pharmacological therapies; content area: pharmacology.
RATIONALE
(1) Use only one nostril to give a dose of nasal calcium replacement. **(2)** Alternate nostrils when giving a dose of nasal calcium replacement. **(3)** Spray once daily. **(4)** Nasal bleeding is an indication to discontinue the drug.

69. **(3)** Integrated processes: nursing process — evaluation; client need: physiological integrity; pharmacological therapies; content area: pharmacology.
RATIONALE
(1) Cefaclor is a broad-spectrum antibiotic used to treat otitis media. It is not effective in treating gonorrhea. **(2)** Cefaclor is a broad-spectrum antibiotic used to treat otitis media. It is not effective with spastic colon. **(3)** Cefaclor is a broad-spectrum antibiotic used to treat otitis media. **(4)** Cefaclor is a broad-spectrum antibiotic used to treat otitis media, not cellulitis.

70. **(4)** Integrated processes: nursing process — implementation; teaching/learning; client need: physiological integrity; pharmacological therapies; content area: pharmacology.
RATIONALE
(1) Diarrhea is a common side effect of Cefaclor. **(2)** Stool cultures are not necessary, since diarrhea is a common side effect of Cefaclor. **(3)** Take all the medication as ordered. **(4)** Eat yogurt daily to restore intestinal flora.

71. **(2)** Integrated processes: nursing process — implementation; client need: physiological integrity; pharmacological therapies; content area: pharmacology.
RATIONALE
(1, 2, 3, 4) Ancef needs to be reconstituted with bacteriostatic normal saline or sterile water.

72. **(2)** Integrated processes: nursing process — implementation; teaching/learning; client need: physiological integrity; pharmacological therapies; content area: pharmacology.
RATIONALE
(1) Celebrex is not safe to use during pregnancy. **(2)** It is necessary to report any unexplained weight gain. **(3)** It is necessary to report any unexplained weight gain. **(4)** It is necessary to monitor liver function tests.

73. **(2)** Integrated processes: nursing process — data collection; client need: physiological integrity; reduction of risk potential; content area: pharmacology.
RATIONALE
(1) This low dose of Thorazine is not used to treat schizophrenia. **(2)** Thorazine is contraindicated if a client has diabetes. **(3)**

Phenergan is the drug of choice to treat nausea. **(4)** Thorazine can be used to treat hiccups.

74. **(1)** Integrated processes: nursing process — implementation; teaching/learning; client need: physiological integrity; pharmacological therapies; content area: pharmacology.
RATIONALE
(1) Refrain from using codeine if taking herbal treatments. **(2)** Codeine may cause constipation. **(3)** Codeine may cause urinary retention. **(4)** Codeine is not to be taken with alcohol.

75. **(3)** Integrated processes: nursing process phase: implementation; teaching/learning; client need: physiological integrity; pharmacological therapies; content area: pharmacology.
RATIONALE
(1) Robitussin DM is not safe with infants less than 2 years of age. **(2)** Robitussin DM is contraindicated for males with enlarged prostates. **(3)** Robitussin DM can cause excitability in children. **(4)** Robitussin DM is chemically related to morphine, but without central hypnotic or analgesic effect.

76. **(2)** Integrated processes; nursing process — implementation; self-care; client need: physiological integrity; pharmacological therapies; content area: pharmacology.
RATIONALE
(1) After breakfast is too early for action of NPH insulin. **(2)** The peak action of NPH insulin occurs 6–8 hours after administration. **(3)** Early evening is too late for the peak action of NPH insulin. **(4)** Before bedtime is too late for the peak action of NPH insulin.

77. **(1)** Integrated processes; nursing process — implementation; client need: physiological integrity; pharmacological therapies; content area: pharmacology.
RATIONALE
(1) Only regular insulin can be administered IV. **(2)** NPH insulin is cloudy. Only clear insulin can be given IV. **(3)** Lente insulin is cloudy. Only clear insulin can be given IV. **(4)** Humulin N insulin is cloudy. Only clear insulin can be given IV.

78. **(2)** Integrated processes: nursing process — implementation; client need: physiological integrity; pharmacological therapies; content area: pharmacology.
RATIONALE
(1) NPH can be mixed with regular insulin. **(2)** Regular insulin is drawn first to avoid contaminating it with NPH. NPH cannot be given IV, which could be a problem if the regular insulin was contaminated with NPH insulin. **(3)** Do not contaminate regular insulin with NPH insulin. **(4)** Regular insulin can be mixed with other types of insulin.

79. **(3)** Integrated processes: nursing process — implementation; client need: physiological integrity; pharmacological therapies; content area: pharmacology.
RATIONALE
(1) Metabolic acidosis can cause hyperkalemia but not the reverse. **(2)** Rapid infusion of IV fluids can cause fluid overload. Rapid infusion of potassium does not. **(3)** Potassium chloride should be administered slowly and cautiously to prevent fatal hyperkalemia resulting in cardiac arrest. **(4)** Infiltration can occur regardless of the type of fluid.

80. **(1)** Integrated processes: nursing process — implementation; client need: physiological integrity; pharmacological therapies; content area: pharmacology
RATIONALE
(1) If 2 mL equals 0.5 mg, then 1 mL equals 0.25 mg, and 0.5 mL equals 0.125 mg. **(2)** Math calculation for the correct

answer explains incorrect answers. (3) Math calculation for the correct answer explains incorrect answers. (4) Calling the physician to verify the order is not necessary in this situation.

81. (4) Integrated processes: nursing process — implementation; client need: physiological integrity; pharmacological therapies; content area: pharmacology.
RATIONALE
(1) Math calculation for the correct answer explains incorrect answers. (2) Math calculation for the correct answer explains incorrect answers. (3) Math calculation for the correct answer explains incorrect answers. (4) 1 mL = 16.2 minims, 10 mL × 16.2 minims/mL = 160 minims.

82. (1) Integrated processes: nursing process — evaluation; client need: physiological integrity; pharmacological therapies; content area: pharmacology.
RATIONALE
(1) Urine output is not affected by morphine administration. (2) Morphine may lower the blood pressure. (3) Morphine may lower the respiratory rate. (4) Pain relief is the desired outcome.

83. (1) Integrated processes: nursing process — planning; client need: physiological integrity; pharmacological therapies; content area: pharmacology.
RATIONALE
(1) The five rights to correct medication administration are right client, right medication, right dose, right route, and right time. Reading the client's armband allows the nurse to validate the right client. (2) The five rights to correct medication administration are right client, right medication, right dose, right route, and right time. Reading the client's armband allows the nurse to validate the right client. (3) The five rights to correct medication administration are right client, right medication, right dose, right route, and right time. Reading the client's armband allows the nurse to validate the right client. (4) The five rights to correct medication administration are right client, right medication, right dose, right route, and right time. Reading the client's armband allows the nurse to validate the right client.

84. (4) Integrated processes: nursing process — data collection; client need: physiological integrity; pharmacological therapies; content area: pharmacology.
RATIONALE
(1) With specific medications, it is necessary to check I&O. (2) The nurse would check for symptoms. (3) The nurse would be aware of the diagnosis. (4) It is most important to check that you are administering the correct medicine to the correct client.

85. (2) Integrated processes: nursing process — evaluation; client need: physiological integrity; pharmacological therapies; content area: pharmacology.
RATIONALE
(1) Math calculation explains the incorrect answers. (2) 1 grain = 64.8 mg, 10 grains × 64.8 mg/grain = 648 mg. The nurse should administer the 650-mg suppository. (3) Math calculation explains the incorrect answers. (4) Math calculation explains the incorrect answers.

86. (3) Integrated processes: nursing process — evaluation; client need: physiological integrity; pharmacological therapies; content area: pharmacology.
RATIONALE
(1) This choice indicates an increase in symptoms. (2) This choice indicates an increase in symptoms. (3) Levodopa is the drug of choice for parkinsonism. Levodopa relieves the tremors, rigidity, and twitching associated with parkinsonism. (4) This choice indicates an increase in symptoms.

87. (3) Integrated processes: nursing process — implementation; client need: physiological integrity; pharmacological therapies; content area: pharmacology.
RATIONALE
(1) Position would not produce this effect. (2) Position would not produce this effect. (3) Lung scans after treatment showed that distribution was most uniform when clients were sitting upright, with more aerosol reaching the upper lung. (4) Position would not produce this effect.

88. (3) Integrated processes: nursing process — evaluation; client need: physiological integrity; pharmacological therapies; content area: pharmacology.
RATIONALE
(1) Mannitol increases potassium excretion. (2) Mannitol may decrease potassium as a side effect but not as a measure of effectiveness. (3) Mannitol is an osmotic diuretic used to promote diuresis. (4) Mannitol does not increase respirations.

89. (2) Integrated processes: nursing process — data collection; client need: physiological integrity; pharmacological therapies; content area: pharmacology.
RATIONALE
(1) Nitroglycerin is a vasodilator that is used to decrease blood pressure and to dilate coronary arteries. (2) Excessive dosage is characterized by headache, lightheadedness and dizziness, syncope, tachycardia, and low blood pressure. (3) Nitroglycerin is a vasodilator that is used to decrease blood pressure and to dilate coronary arteries. (4) A pulse rate of 80 bpm is considered normal.

90. (4) Integrated processes: nursing process — implementation; client need: physiological integrity; pharmacological therapies; content area: pharmacology.
RATIONALE
(1) One should always rotate injection sites. (2) One should not aspirate for heparin to decrease possibility of tissue trauma. (3) Heparin is given subcutaneously (SC), not IM. (4) Rubbing the area after heparin administration would increase the likelihood of bleeding.

91. (2) Integrated processes: nursing process — implementation; client need: physiological integrity; pharmacological therapies; content area: pharmacology.
RATIONALE
(1) Temperature is not specifically assessed for digitalis administration. (2) A fall in heart rate to 60 bpm in adults is a criterion used for withholding medication and notifying the physician. The apical pulse should be assessed for one full minute, noting rate, rhythm, and quality, before administering digoxin. (3) Blood pressure is not specifically assessed for digitalis administration. (4) Respiration is not specifically assessed for digitalis administration.

92. (3) Integrated processes: nursing process — evaluation; client need: physiological integrity; pharmacological therapies; content area: pharmacology.
RATIONALE
(1) These medications have no effect on pupillary responses. (2) These medications do not increase respiratory rate as a therapeutic effect. (3) Furosemide promotes diuresis. The effectiveness of both these drugs in CHF is evident from the increased urine output. (4) Furosemide decreases edema rather than producing it.

93. **(2)** Integrated processes: nursing process — planning; client need: physiological integrity; pharmacological therapies; content area: pharmacology.

RATIONALE

(1) Digoxin may be ordered as a cardiotonic but not as a first choice for PVCs. **(2)** Lidocaine is the first-line drug of choice for ventricular ectopy. **(3)** Propranolol may be ordered but not as a first choice for PVCs. **(4)** Atropine increases the heart rate but has no direct effect on PVCs.

94. **(2)** Integrated processes: nursing process — implementation; client need: physiological integrity; pharmacological therapies; content area: pharmacology.

RATIONALE

(1) Math calculation explains incorrect answers. **(2)** Amount to be infused × drop factor / time of infusion in minutes, 1000 mL × 15 gtt/min / 480 min = 31 gtt/min. **(3)** Math calculation explains incorrect answers. **(4)** Math calculation explains incorrect answers.

95. **(2)** Integrated processes: nursing process — implementation; client need: physiological integrity; pharmacological therapies; content area: pharmacology.

RATIONALE

(1) Math calculation explains incorrect answers. **(2)** Amount to be infused × drop factor / time of infusion in minutes, 100 mL × 10 gtt/mL / 30 min = 33 gtt/min. **(3)** Math calculation explains incorrect answers. **(4)** Math calculation explains incorrect answers.

96. **(2)** Integrated processes: nursing process — evaluation; client need: physiological integrity; pharmacological therapies; content area: pharmacology.

RATIONALE

(1) Signs of $MgSO_4$ toxicity are flushing, sweating, extreme thirst, hypotension, sedation, confusion, depressed or no reflexes, muscle weakness, depressed cardiac function, and respiratory paralysis. **(2)** Increased reflexes are not a sign of magnesium toxicity. **(3)** Signs of $MgSO_4$ toxicity are flushing, sweating, extreme thirst, hypotension, sedation, confusion, depressed or no reflexes, muscle weakness, depressed cardiac function, and respiratory paralysis. **(4)** Signs of $MgSO_4$ toxicity are flushing, sweating, extreme thirst, hypotension, sedation, confusion, depressed or no reflexes, muscle weakness, depressed cardiac function, and respiratory paralysis.

97. **(4)** Integrated processes: nursing process — evaluation; teaching/learning; client need: physiological integrity; pharmacological therapies; content area: pharmacology.

RATIONALE

(1) Potential side effects of aminoglycosides include ototoxicity. **(2)** Potential side effects of aminoglycosides include nephrotoxicity. **(3)** Potential side effects of aminoglycosides include neurotoxicity. **(4)** There is no documentation that aminoglycosides cause photosensitivity.

98. **(3)** Integrated processes: nursing process — evaluation; client need: physiological integrity; pharmacological therapies; content area: pharmacology.

RATIONALE

(1) Amphotericin B does not directly cause afebrile reactions, hyperkalemia, or elevated blood pressure. **(2)** Amphotericin B does not directly cause afebrile reactions, hyperkalemia, or elevated blood pressure. **(3)** Potential side effects of amphotericin B are anorexia, weight loss, nausea, vomiting, diarrhea, hypokalemia, muscle pain, chills, fever, anemia, and rash. **(4)** Amphotericin B does not elevate blood pressure.

99. **(3)** Integrated processes: nursing process — implementation; client need: physiological integrity; pharmacological therapies; content area: pharmacology.

RATIONALE

(1) Incorrect option is explained in rationale for correct answer. **(2)** Incorrect option is explained in rationale for correct answer. **(3)** The effects of antineoplastic drugs are usually not limited to neoplastic cells. Most antineoplastic drugs are damaging to dividing cells, thus preventing cell proliferation. **(4)** Incorrect option is explained in rationale for correct answer.

100. **(3)** Integrated processes: nursing process — evaluation; teaching/learning; client need: physiological integrity; pharmacological therapies; content area: pharmacology.

RATIONALE

(1) Potential side effects of thyroid USP are palpitations, arrhythmias, headache, tremors, insomnia, tachycardia, weight loss, nervousness, and anorexia. **(2)** Potential side effects of thyroid USP are palpitations, arrhythmias, headache, tremors, insomnia, tachycardia, weight loss, nervousness, and anorexia. **(3)** Bradycardia is not a side effect of thyroid replacement. **(4)** Potential side effects of thyroid USP are palpitations, arrhythmias, headache, tremors, insomnia, tachycardia, weight loss, nervousness, and anorexia.

101. **(1)** Integrated processes: nursing process — planning; client need: physiological integrity; pharmacological therapies; content area: pharmacology.

RATIONALE

(1) Aspirin may be prescribed to treat headache, arthritis, joint pain, dental pain, and antipyretic effects and to decrease platelet aggregation (clotting). **(2)** Aspirin has no effect on decreasing carbon dioxide retention. **(3)** Aspirin does not inhibit peptic ulcer disease and may exacerbate the condition. **(4)** Aspirin has no effect on SC emphysema.

102. **(3)** Integrated processes: nursing process — evaluation; client need: physiological integrity; pharmacological therapies; content area: pharmacology.

RATIONALE

(1) Shaving with a straight razor increases the chances for nicking the skin and bleeding. **(2)** Irritability has no effect on heparin administration. **(3)** Bleeding as evidenced by ecchymosis could be a sign of excessive anticoagulation. **(4)** A full-liquid diet has no effect on heparin administration.

103. **(2)** Integrated processes: nursing process — evaluation; client need: physiological integrity; pharmacological therapies; content area: pharmacology.

RATIONALE

(1) Aminophylline does not increase wheezing. **(2)** Aminophylline is prescribed for bronchospasms caused by bronchitis, asthma, and emphysema. Aminophylline should improve the quality and rate of respirations. Aminophylline decreases wheezing. **(3)** Aminophylline does not increase rhonchi. **(4)** Aminophylline does not increase rhonchi.

104. **(3)** Integrated processes: nursing process — implementation; client need: physiological integrity; pharmacological therapies; content area: pharmacology.

RATIONALE

(1) Spacing the time when giving the pills will not correct the problem with swallowing the pills. **(2)** Breaking pills will not correct the problem of not being able to swallow pills. **(3)** The pills should be crushed and placed in food with good consistency for ease of swallowing. (4) Spacing the time when giving the pills will not correct the problem with swallowing the pills.

105. (2) Integrated processes: nursing process — implementation; client need: physiological integrity; pharmacological therapies; content area: pharmacology.

RATIONALE

(1) Ambulation should be supervised. (2) Diazepam may cause CNS reactions such as drowsiness, fatigue, confusion, dizziness, and muscle weakness. Ambulation should be supervised. (3) There is nothing to indicate that the client needs counseling for chemical dependency. (4) There is no need for use of restraints.

106. (1) Integrated processes: nursing process — implementation; teaching/learning; client need: physiological integrity; pharmacological therapies; content area: pharmacology.

RATIONALE

(1) Drowsiness is the principal side effect of diphenhydramine. (2) There are no data to show that diphenhydramine causes tinnitus. (3) Alcohol potentiates the effects of diphenhydramine. (4) Diphenhydramine decreases alertness; it does not increase alertness.

107. (2) Integrated processes: nursing process — implementation; client need: physiological integrity; pharmacological therapies; content area: pharmacology.

RATIONALE

(1) Phenazopyridine has no direct effect on the appetite. (2) Phenazopyridine may color the urine orange to red. (3) Phenazopyridine may color the urine orange to red, not blue-purple. (4) Phenazopyridine may decrease rather than increase pain on urination.

108. (1) Integrated processes: nursing process — implementation; client need: physiological integrity; pharmacological therapies; content area: pharmacology.

RATIONALE

(1) Rifampin is an anti-infective and antibiotic active against tuberculosis and some gram-negative and gram-positive organisms. Rifampin is usually prescribed with other antituberculosis drugs for treating tuberculosis. (2) Rifampin has no effect on malaria. (3) Rifampin does not alter the color of body fluids. (4) Rifampin does not alter the color of body fluids.

109. (3) Integrated processes: nursing process — implementation; teaching/learning; client need: physiological integrity; pharmacological therapies; content area: pharmacology.

RATIONALE

(1) Assessing blood pressure before administration of nitroglycerin is routine. (2) Assessing blood pressure after administration of nitroglycerin is routine. (3) Dizziness, lightheadedness, and syncope occur because of postural hypotension. Advise the client to change positions slowly. (4) Sublingual nitroglycerin may sting when taken.

110. (2) Integrated processes: nursing process — implementation; teaching/learning; client need: physiological integrity; reduction of risk potential; content area: pharmacology.

RATIONALE

(1) NSAIDS need to be taken with food. (2) NSAIDS need to be taken with food. (3) The physician will recommend how NSAIDS are to be given in conjunction with other medications; this is not within the practical nurse's scope of practice. (4) The physician will order the dosage of medications; this is not within the practical nurse's scope of practice.

Test 2

111. (0.4 mg) Integrated processes: nursing process — implementation; client need: physiological integrity; pharmacological therapies; content area: pharmacology.

RATIONALE

$60 \text{ mg} / x = 1 \text{ gr} / 1/150$, $x = 0.4$ mg
0.4 mg = 1 Tablet

112. (2 capsules) Integrated processes: nursing process — evaluation; client need: physiological integrity; pharmacological therapies; content area: pharmacology.

RATIONALE

0.5 g = 500 mg, 500 mg : x : 250 mg : 1 capsule, $250x = 500$, $x = 2$ capsules.

113. (15 mL) Integrated processes: nursing process — evaluation; client need: physiological integrity; pharmacological therapies; content area: pharmacology.

RATIONALE

50 mg : 1 mL : : 750 mg : x, 750 mg : x : : 50 mg : 1 mL, $50x = 750$, $x = 15$ mL.

114. (280 mg) integrated processes: nursing process — evaluation; client need: physiological integrity; pharmacological therapies; content area: pharmacology.

RATIONALE

1 kg = 2.2 lb, 154 lb / 2.2 lb = 70 kg, 70 kg × 4 mg/kg = 280 mg.

115. (500 mg) Integrated processes: nursing process — evaluation; client need: physiological integrity; pharmacological therapies; content area: pharmacology.

RATIONALE

3 g = 3000 mg in 24 hours, 3000 mg / 6 doses = 500 mg.

116. (1 tablet) Integrated processes: nursing process — evaluation; client need: physiological integrity; pharmacological therapies; content area: pharmacology.

RATIONALE

1 grain = 60 mg, 60 mg × 5 grains = 1 tablet, 300 mg : 1 tablet : : 300 mg : x, $300x = 300$ mg, $x = 1$ tablet.

117. (0.25 mL) Integrated processes: nursing process — evaluation; client need: physiological integrity; pharmacological therapies; content area: pharmacology.

RATIONALE

1 mg : 0.5 mL : : 0.5 mg : x, $x = 0.25$ mL.

118. (2 tablets) Integrated processes: nursing process — evaluation; client need: physiological integrity; pharmacological therapies; content area: pharmacology.

RATIONALE

0.125 mg : 1 tablet : : 0.25 mg : x, $0.125x = 0.25$, $x = 2$.

119. (0.7 mL) Integrated processes: nursing process — evaluation; client need: physiological integrity; pharmacological therapies; content area: pharmacology.

RATIONALE

75 mg : 1 mL : : 50 mg : x, $75x = 50$, $x = 0.66$ or 0.7 mL.

120. (0.5 tablet) Integrated processes: nursing process — evaluation; client need: physiological integrity; pharmacological therapies; content area: pharmacology.

RATIONALE
1 grain = 60 mg, 60 mg : 1 tablet : : 30 mg : x, 60x = 30, x = 0.5 tablet.

121. (**4 mL**) Integrated processes: nursing process — evaluation; client need: physiological integrity; pharmacological therapies; content area: pharmacology.
RATIONALE
25 mg : 1 mL : : 100 mg : x, 25x = 100, x = 4 mL.

122. (**10 mL/hr**) Integrated processes: nursing process — evaluation; client need: physiological integrity; pharmacological therapies; content area: pharmacology.
RATIONALE
500 mg / 24 hr = 20.8 or 21 mg/hr, 250 mL / 24 hr = 10.4 or 10 mL/hr.

123. (**0.26 mL/min**) Integrated processes: nursing process — evaluation; client need: physiological integrity; pharmacological therapies; content area: pharmacology.
RATIONALE
250 mg / 16 hr = 15.6 mg/hr / 60 min/hr = 0.26 mg/min, 250 mL / 16 hr = 15.6 mL/hr / 60 min/hr = 0.26 mL/min.

124. (**42 mg/hr**) Integrated processes: nursing process — evaluation; client need: physiological integrity; pharmacological therapies; content area: pharmacology.
RATIONALE
500 mL / 12 hr = 41.6 or 42 mL/hr, 500 mg / 12 hrs = 41.6 or 42 mg/hr.

125. (**21 mL/hr**) Integrated processes: nursing process — evaluation; client need: physiological integrity; pharmacological therapies; content area: pharmacology.
RATIONALE
400 mg / 24 hr = 16.6 or 17 mg/hr, 500 mL / 24 hr = 20.8 or 21 mL/hr.

126. (**6 mL**) Integrated processes: nursing process — evaluation; client need: physiological integrity; pharmacological therapies; content area: pharmacology.
RATIONALE
50 units = 100 mL, 1 unit = 2 mL, 3 unit = 6 mL.

127. (**[mL/hr 3 gtt/mL]÷60 minutes**) Integrated processes: nursing process — evaluation; client need: physiological integrity; pharmacological therapies; content area: pharmacology.
RATIONALE
You must know formula.

128. (**0.7 mL**) Integrated processes: nursing process — evaluation; client need: physiological integrity; pharmacological therapies; content area: pharmacology.
RATIONALE
10 mg : x mL : : 15 mg : 1 mL, 15x = 10, x = 0.66 or 0.7 mL.

129. (**0.5 mL**) Integrated processes: nursing process — evaluation; client need: physiological integrity; pharmacological therapies; content area: pharmacology
RATIONALE
25 mg : : x : : 100 mg : : 2 mL, 100x = 50, x = 0.5 mL.

130. (**0.25 mL**) Integrated processes: nursing process — evaluation; client need: physiological integrity; pharmacological therapies; content area: pharmacology.
RATIONALE
20,000 : 1 mL : : 5000 : : x, 20,000 = 5000x, x = 0.25 mL.

131. (**31 gtt/min**) Integrated processes: nursing process — evaluation; client need: physiological integrity; pharmacological therapies; content area: pharmacology.
RATIONALE
1000 mL × X 15 gtt/mL / 60 min/hr × 8 hr = 15,000/480 = 31.2 or 31 gtt/min.

132. (**25 gtt/min**) Integrated processes: nursing process — evaluation; client need: physiological integrity; pharmacological therapies; content area: pharmacology.
RATIONALE
150 mL × 10 gtt/mL / 60 min/hr × 1 hr = 1500/60 = 25 gtt/min.

133. (**17 gtt/min**) Integrated processes: nursing process — evaluation; client need: physiological integrity; pharmacological therapies; content area: pharmacology.
RATIONALE
1000 mL × 10 gtt/mL / 10 hr × 60/min/hr = 10,000/600 = 16.6 or 17 gtt/min.

134. (**50 gtt/min**) Integrated processes: nursing process — evaluation; client need: physiological integrity; pharmacological therapies; content area: pharmacology.
RATIONALE
100 mL × 60 gtt/mL / 60 min/hr × 2 hr = 6000/120 = 50 gtt/min.

135. (**150 gtt/min**) Integrated processes: nursing process — evaluation; client need: physiological integrity; pharmacological therapies; content area: pharmacology.
RATIONALE
900 mL × 20 gtt/mL / 60 min/hr × 2 hr = 18,000/120 = 150 gtt/min.

136. (**21 gtt/min**) Integrated processes: nursing process — evaluation; client need: physiological integrity; pharmacological therapies; content area: pharmacology.
RATIONALE
1000 mL × 10 gtt/mL / 8 hr × 60 min/hr = 10,000/480 = 20.8 or 21 gtt/min.

137. (**150 gtt/min**) Integrated processes: nursing process — evaluation; client need: physiological integrity; pharmacological therapies; content area: pharmacology.
RATIONALE
150 mL × 60 gtt/mL / 60 mL = 9000/60 = 150 gtt/min.

138. (**100 gtt/min**) Integrated processes: nursing process — evaluation; client need: physiological integrity; pharmacological therapies; contents area: pharmacology.
RATIONALE
50 mL × 60 gtt/mL / 30 min = 3000/30 = 100 gtt/min.

139. (**60 gtt/min**) Integrated processes: nursing process — evaluation; client need: physiological integrity; pharmacological therapies; content area: pharmacology.
RATIONALE
15 mL × 60 gtt/mL / 15 min = 900/15 = 60 gtt/min.

140. (**13 gtt/min**) Integrated processes: nursing process — evaluation; client need: physiological integrity; pharmacological therapies; content area: pharmacology.
RATIONALE
600 mL × 10 gtt/mL / 60 min/hr = 6000/480 = 12.5 or 13 gtt/min.

141. **(75 gtt/min)** Integrated processes: nursing process — evaluation; client need: physiological integrity; pharmacological therapies; content area: pharmacology.
RATIONALE
150 mL × 60 gtt/mL / 60 min/hr × 2 hr = 9000/120 = 75 gtt/min.

142. **(25 gtt/min)** Integrated processes: nursing process — evaluation; client need: physiological integrity; pharmacological therapies; content area: pharmacology.
RATIONALE
1000 mL × 15 gtt/mL / 60 min/hr × 10 hr = 15,000/600 = 25 gtt/min.

143. **(8 gtt/min)** Integrated processes: nursing process — evaluation; client need: physiological integrity; pharmacological therapies; content area: pharmacology.
RATIONALE
100 mL × 10 gtt / 2 hr × 60 min/hr = 1000/120 = 8.3 or 8 gtt/min.

144. **(30 gtt/min)** Integrated processes: nursing process — evaluation; client need: physiological integrity; pharmacological therapies; content area: pharmacology.
RATIONALE
15 mL × 60 gtt/mL / 30 min = 900/30 = 30 gtt/min.

145. **(30 gtt/min)** Integrated processes: nursing process — evaluation; client need: physiological integrity; pharmacological therapies; content area: pharmacology.
RATIONALE
1800 mL × 10 gtt/mL / 60 min/hr × 10 hr = 18,000/600 = 30 gtt/min.

146. **(42 gtt/min)** Integrated processes: nursing process — evaluation; client need: physiological integrity; pharmacological therapies; content area: pharmacology.
RATIONALE
1000 mL × 15 gtt/mL / 60 min/hr × 6 hr = 15,000/360 = 41.6 or 42 gtt/min.

147. **(63 gtt/min)** Integrated processes: nursing process — evaluation; client need: physiological integrity; pharmacological therapies; content area: pharmacology.
RATIONALE
250 mL × 15 gtt/mL / 60 min/hr × 1 hr = 3750/60 = 62.5 or 63 gtt/min.

148. **(21 gtt/min)** Integrated processes: nursing process — evaluation; client need: physiological integrity; pharmacological therapies; content area: pharmacology.
RATIONALE
1000 mL × 15 gtt/mL / 12 hr × 60 min/hr = 15,000/720 = 20.8 or 21 gtt/min.

149. **(150 gtt/min)** Integrated processes: nursing process — evaluation; client need: physiological integrity; pharmacological therapies; content area: pharmacology.
RATIONALE
300 mL × 60 gtt/mL / 60 min/hr × 2 hr = 18,000/120 = 150 gtt/min.

150. **(75 gtt/min)** Integrated processes: nursing process — evaluation; client need: physiological integrity; pharmacological therapies; content area: pharmacology.
RATIONALE
900 mL × 10 gtt/mL / 60 min/hr × 2 hr = 9000/120 = 75 gtt/min.

151. **(31 gtt/min)** Integrated processes: nursing process — evaluation; client need: physiological integrity; pharmacological therapies; content area: pharmacology.
RATIONALE
1500 mL × 10 gtt/mL / 60 min/hr × 8 hr = 15,000/480 = 31.25 or 31 gtt/min.

152. **(100 gtt/min)** Integrated processes: nursing process — evaluation; client need: physiological integrity; pharmacological therapies; content area: pharmacology.
RATIONALE
100 mL × 60 gtt/mL / 60 min/hr × 1 hr = 6000/60 = 100 gtt/min.

153. **(40 gtt/min)** Integrated processes: nursing process — evaluation; client need: physiological integrity; pharmacological therapies; content area: pharmacology.
RATIONALE
60 mL × 10 gtt/mL / 15 min = 600/15 = 40 gtt/min.

154. **(40 gtt/min)** Integrated processes: nursing process — evaluation; client need: physiological integrity; pharmacological therapies; content area: pharmacology.
RATIONALE
20 mL × 60 gtt/mL /30 min = 1200/30 = 40 gtt/min.

155. **(44 gtt/min)** Integrated processes: nursing process — evaluation; client need: physiological integrity; pharmacological therapies; content area: pharmacology
RATIONALE
800 mL × 20 gtt/mL / 60 min/hr × hr = 16,000/360 = 44.4 or 44 gtt/min.

156. **(53 gtt/min)** Integrated processes: nursing process — evaluation; client need: physiological integrity; pharmacological therapies; content area: pharmacology
RATIONALE
105 mL × 60 gtt/mL / 60 min/hr × 2 hr = 6300/120 = 52.5 or 53 gtt/min.

157. **(21 gtt/min)** Integrated processes: nursing process — evaluation; client need: physiological integrity; pharmacological therapies; content area: pharmacology.
RATIONALE
1000 mL × 10 gtt/mL / 60 min/hr × 8 hr = 10,000/480 = 20.8 or 21 gtt/min.

158. **(8 gtt/min)** Integrated processes: nursing process — evaluation; client need: physiological integrity; pharmacological therapies; content area: pharmacology.
RATIONALE
100 mL × 10 gtt/mL / 60 min/hr × 2 hr = 1000/120 = 8.3 or 8 gtt/min.

159. **(60 gtt/min)** Integrated processes: nursing process — evaluation; client need: physiological integrity; pharmacological therapies; content area: pharmacology.
RATIONALE
30 mL × 60 gtt/mL / 30 min = 1800/30 = 60 gtt/min.

160. **(25 gtt/min)** Integrity processes: nursing process — evaluation; client need: physiological integrity; pharmacological therapies; content area: pharmacology.
RATIONALE
1000 mL × 15 gtt/mL / 60 min/hr × 10 hr = 15,000/600 = 25 gtt/min.

CHAPTER 11

Nutrition and Diet Therapy: Content Review and Test

Patricia Gauntlett Beare, RN, PhD
Demetrius J. Porche, RN, CCRN, DNS
Larry D. Purnell
Golden M. Tradewell, RN, PhD

I. Nutrients
  A. Chemical substances needed for growth, maintenance, and repair
  B. Divided into 6 groups
    1. Carbohydrates
    2. Fats
    3. Proteins
    4. Minerals
    5. Vitamins
    6. Water
  C. Functions
    1. Serve as energy source of heat
    2. Support the growth and maintenance of tissue
    3. Aid in the regulation of basic body processes

II. Types of nutrition disorders
  A. Malnutrition—occurs when body cells receive too much or too little of one or more nutrients.
  B. Undernutrition related to
    1. Inability to obtain foods that contain essential nutrients
    2. Failure to consume essential nutrients
    3. Inability to use nutrients in food
    4. Diseases that increase the body's need for nutrients
    5. Disease process that causes nutrients to be excreted too rapidly from the body
  C. Overnutrition— excessive intake of nutrients caused by
    1. Self-prescribed over-the-counter vitamin and mineral supplements
    2. Eating too much food

III. Basic nutritional parameters
  A. Height-weight tables
    1. Information used to calculate a person's percentage of healthy body weight
  B. Body mass index
    1. Designed to provide a measure of weight independent of height.
    2. Varies with gender, race, stage of maturation, and waist-to-hip ratio in 7 to 17 year olds.
  C. Waist-to-hip ratio (WHR)
    1. Waist measurement is divided by the hip measurement.
  D. Dietary guidelines for Americans
    1. Used to evaluate the dietary status of individuals and to educate clients about food choices.
    2. Guidelines target the healthy general population to assist in the prevention of chronic and degenerative diseases.
  E. The food pyramid
    1. Illustrates healthful diet choices
    2. Serving size is specified
  F. Tables of food composition
    1. List foods and the amounts of selected nutrients for a specified volume or weight of the food
  G. Computerized diet analysis
    1. Compares an individual's intake with the recommended daily allowance (RDA)

IV. Dietary guidelines for healthy living
  A. Eat a variety of foods.
  B. Balance the food you eat with physical activity; maintain or improve your weight.
  C. Choose a diet with plenty of grain products, vegetables, and fruits.
  D. Choose a diet low in fat, saturated fat, and cholesterol.
  E. Choose a diet moderate in sugars.
  F. Choose a diet moderate in salt and sodium.
  G. Drink alcoholic beverages in moderation.

V. Impact of culture on nutrition
  A. African Americans
    1. Cook with a lot of saturated fats
  B. Hispanic Americans
    1. Corn is the staple
    2. Foods are stewed or fried in oil

3. Sweet foods, such as yeast pastries, are common
4. Sugar is added to foods

C. Native Americans
1. Native Hawaiians consume taro, sweet potatoes, breadfruit, fruit, greens, and seaweed.
2. After arrival of Westerners, food consumed is high in fat and sugar.

D. Chinese Americans
1. Wheat is produced in northern China
2. Rice is produced in southern China

E. Jewish Americans
1. Kosher food preparations.
2. Only designated animals can be eaten.
3. Some animals can be ritually slaughered and dressed.
4. Dairy products and meats must not be eaten at the same meal.
5. If kosher meal is unavailable, a cottage cheese and fruit plate is a good choice for an orthodox Jew.

VI. Life cycle nutrition
A. Pregnancy
1. Protein required to build fetal tissue.
   a. 10 gm/day is needed. Can be achieved in one extra cup of milk and one additional ounce of meat
2. Vitamin needs
   a. Vitamin C is needed to convert folic acid to an active form, enhance the absorption of iron, and help to form connective tissues.
   b. Thiamin, riboflavin, niacin, and vitamin B_6 are coenzymes involved in the metabolism of the energy nutrients.
   c. 400 μg of synthetic folic acid is needed.
3. Fat-soluble vitamins
   a. Avoid vitamin A beyond RDA requirements (10,000 IU). It predisposes to fetal deformities.
   b. Diet provides vitamins D, E, and K.
4. Mineral needs
   a. Both mother and fetus require minerals to build new tissue.
5. Iron
   a. Total iron is estimated to be 0.8–1.0 g.
   b. During third trimester, 3–4 mg of iron per day is transferred to the fetus.
6. Calcium
   a. Intestinal absorption of calcium increases during pregnancy.
   b. Adequate intake (AI) for pregnant and lactating women over 19 years of age and older is 1000 mg.
   c. AI for women 18 years of age and younger is 1300 mg.
   d. 3.5–4.5 servings of milk or milk products is equivalent to AI calcium.
7. Phosphorus and magnesium
   a. Women 25 years of age and older need 1.5 times more phosphorus than the normal allowed for nonpregnant women.
8. Iodine
   a. Pregnant woman's usual need is met by using iodized salt.
9. Fluoride

a. Fetus develops teeth at 10–12 weeks of pregnancy.
b. Fewer dental caries are found in infants of mothers whose diets were supplemented with 1 mg of fluoride.

10. Zinc
   a. Deficiency increases risk of abnormally long labors and delivery of small and malformed infants.
   b. To provide for fetus, mother needs constant intake.
   c. Three servings of meat or meat substitute per day will provide adequate zinc for pregnant woman.

11. Substances to avoid
   a. Alcohol predisposes to fetal alcohol syndrome (FAS), which is major cause of mental retardation.
   b. Caffeine causes a change in fetal heart rate and breathing patterns.
   c. The causative agent of listeriosis (*Listeria monocytogenes*) is found in raw or contaminated milk, soft cheeses, contaminated vegetables, and ready-to-eat meats.
   d. Listeriosis infections can cause influenza-like symptoms with fever and chills.
   e. Listeriosis illness may not appear until 2–8 weeks after a person has eaten the contaminated food.
   f. Infection may result in abortion or in septicemia or meningitis in the newborn.
   g. Women who smoke one or more packs/day deliver infants weighing about 0.5 lb less than infants delivered by nonsmoking women.
   h. Infants of women who smoke have increased risk of perinatal mortality.
   i. Increases in abortions and preterm deliveries are related to smoking.
   j. Chronic cocaine addiction causes a weight deficit in the fetus of as much as 500 g.
   k. Infants of women with cocaine addiction suffer from immature mental development.

B. Breast-feeding mothers
1. Additional foods
   a. Two milk exchanges
   b. One meat exchange
   c. One fruit or vegetable high in vitamin C
   d. Increase fluid intake of 1 L/day
2. Human lactation is associated with alterations in calcium metabolism that are independent of dietary calcium intake and unresponsive to increase in calcium intake.

C. Infancy
1. Breast milk is natural food for human infants
2. Protein
   a. First 6 months, infants need 13 g/day.
   b. Second 6 months, infants need 14 g/day.
3. Carbohydrate
   a. Breast milk contains amylase that is 40–60 times more active than cow's milk.
   b. Lactose in milk provides galactose, which is necessary for brain cell formation.

    c. Honey should not be given to an infant until after the first birthday because it contains botulism spores.
    d. Feeding honey increases the risk of allergies.
4. Fat
    a. Infant needs 30%–55% of kilocalories from fat.
    b. Best indicator of adequate kilocaloric intake is a normal growth rate according to standard growth charts.
5. Vitamins
    a. Cow's milk contains nine times the vitamin B_{12} of breast milk.
    b. Human breast milk contains more vitamin C, but less vitamin D, than cow's milk.
    c. Cholesterol in breast milk functions as a precursor of vitamin D.
    d. Breast milk supports proliferation of *Lactobacillus* organisms rather than *Escherichia coli*, which contributes to infant mortality.
6. Minerals
    a. Breast milk contains one-third the sodium, potassium, and chloride and one-eighth the phosphorus of cow's milk.
    b. Breast milk also contains less iron than cow's milk.
    c. Breast milk contains one-sixth to one-twenty-fifth the calcium of cow's milk.
    d. Bioavailability of zinc in breast milk is 60%, compared to 43%–50% in cow's milk, and 27%–32% in infant formulas.
    e. Fluoride should not be administered until after 6 months of age.
D. Weaning the infant
    1. Schedule for infant foods
        a. 4 months—infant cereal mixed with formula
        b. 5–6 months—strained vegetables
        c. 6–7 months—strained fruits
        d. 6–8 months—finger foods
        e. 7–8 months—strained meats
        f. 10 months
            1) Strained or mashed egg yolk. Due to possible allergy, delay egg whites until 1 year.
            2) Bite-sized cooked foods.
        g. 12 months—foods from adult table
    2. Nutritional problems in infancy
        a. Iron-deficiency anemia caused by drinking too much milk, and is common in low-income families, or black or Mexican American children.
        b. Food allergies affect 1%–2% of the total population, but as many as 5%–8% of children under 3 years of age are affected.
        c. Foods that produce allergic reactions include milk, eggs and egg whites, nuts (e.g., peanuts and Brazil nuts), peanut butter, oranges and orange juice, wheat protein, and chocolate.
E. Nutrition in childhood
    1. Nutrition of the toddler
        a. Expected weight gain 4–6 lb.
        b. Needs all essential nutrients.
        c. Introduce unmodified cow's milk, egg white, wheat, citrus fruits, seafood, chocolate, and nut butters after first birthday.

    d. Small serving size is recommended (1 tbsp = 1 serving).
    e. Daily serving of vitamin C–rich fruit or vegetable and green leafy or yellow vegetable.
    f. Limit sugar consumption.
    g. Increase fiber.
    h. Offer three meals and three nutritious snacks.
    i. Discourage consumption of heavily salted foods.
    j. Limit milk to 24 oz/day.
2. Nutrition of the preschool child
    a. Expected weight gain 4–5 lb.
    b. Three-year-old may need 1300–1500 Kcal/day.
    c. Serving size for 4–6 year olds are same as adult.
    d. Needs three meals and three nutritious snacks.
    e. Wholesome snacks should be available.
    f. Concentrated sweets and soda pop should be strictly limited.
    g. Emphasize brushing teeth after meals.
    h. American Academy of Pediatrics recommends supplements only for children at nutritional risks.
3. Nutrition of the school-age child
    a. Adult balanced diet is good for school-age child.
    b. Provide variety, balance, and moderation.
    c. Breakfast is an important meal.
    d. Liberal intake of milk and milk products before age of 10 years is advantageous.
    e. Moderation of sodium intake is indicated for girls under 11 years of age.
    f. Eating dinner with family is associated with improved diet.
4. Nutrition in adolescence
    a. May require 60–80 Kcal/kg of body weight/day.
    b. Need for B vitamins for athletic teens.
    c. Two common nutritional problems in teens are overenthusiastic weight control and poor choices of food.
F. Nutrition in the mature adult
    1. Adult men have better diets than women.
    2. Women's diets parallel men's except that fewer than 50% of women consume the recommended serving of any food group.
    3. Aging affects all body systems, thus affecting nutrition.
VII. Complementary medicine and nutrition
    A. Potentially safe botanical products
        1. Asian ginseng (*Panax ginseng*)
            a. Used to combat lassitude, lack of energy, and decrease concentration
            b. Recommended not to be used by pregnant women, persons with hypertension, psychological imbalances, headaches, heart palpitations, insomnia, asthma, inflammation, or infections with high fever
            c. May exert an estrogen-like effect in postmenopausal women
            d. Avoid use with anticoagulants and nonsteroidal anti-inflammatory drugs

2. Echinacea (*Echinacea purpurea*)
   a. Used to bolster immune system especially for colds, flu, and chronic upper respiratory infections, and urinary tract infections
   b. Immunosuppression has been reported with long-term use
   c. Not recommended for longer than 8 weeks of use orally or 3 weeks parenterally
   d. May cause liver toxicity
   e. May decrease the effectiveness of corticosteroids
3. Feverfew (*Tanacetum parthenium*)
   a. Used to prevent migraine headaches.
   b. Should be avoided in pregnant and lactating women, children under 2 years of age, and allergies to plants in the daisy family.
   c. Side effects include GI ulcers or canker sores.
   d. Abrupt cessation may cause rebound headache.
   e. May interfere with anticoagulants.
   f. Potentiates the antiplatelet effect of aspirin.
4. Garlic (*Allium sativum*)
   a. Used to treat hyperlipoproteinemia and prevent arteriosclerosis
   b. Known to inhibit platelet function and to increase levels of two antioxidant enzymes
   c. Adverse effects: heartburn, flatulence, sweating, light headedness, and excessive menstrual flow
   d. May potentiate anticoagulant's effects
5. Ginger (*Zingiber officinale*)
   a. Used as a digestive aid and to treat motion sickness
   b. Improves gastroduodenal motility
   c. Being investigated as a cancer preventive agent
   d. Prolongs bleeding times; avoid use with anticoagulant drugs
   e. Side effects: heartburn and diarrhea
6. Ginkgo (*Ginkgo biloba*)
   a. Used for treatment of cerebral circulatory disturbances, dementia, and peripheral arterial insufficiency.
   b. Suggested use for glaucoma.
   c. May cause spontaneous bleeding.
   d. Taking aspirin, nonsteroidal anti-inflammatory, or anticoagulants with gingko is ill advised.
   e. May diminish effectiveness of anticonvulsant drugs.
   f. Potentiates the risk of seizures with medications known to decrease the seizure threshold.
   g. Side effects: gastric disturbances, headache, dizziness, and vertigo.
7. Saw palmetto (*Serenoa repens*)
   a. Used to decrease difficulties with urination associated with benign prostatic hypertrophy.
   b. Pregnant women and children should not take saw palmetto.
   c. Side effects: headache, nausea, and upset stomach.
   d. Use with caution with other hormonal therapies.
8. St. John's wort (*Hypercium perforatum*)
   a. Used for anxiety and depression.
   b. Avoid during pregnancy.

c. May cause allergies.
   d. Side effects: GI irritation, tiredness, and restlessness.
   e. Use with caution with warfarin and indinavir.
   f. Interferes with the metabolism of cyclosporine.
   g. Possiblity of interactions with serotonin reuptake inhibitors.
   h. May prolong the effects of anesthesia.
   i. Use with other drugs causing photosensitivity should be avoided.
9. Valerian (*Valeriana officinalis*)
   a. Used to manage restlessness and nervous disorders of sleep.
   b. Side effects: headache, hangovers, excitability, insomnia, uneasiness, cardiac disturbances, ataxia, decreased sensibility, hypothermia, hallucinations, and increased muscle relaxation.
   c. Avoid with use of barbituates.
VIII. Diet in diabetes mellitus and hypoglycemia
   A. Diabetes is directly related to how the body uses food.
   B. Nutrition is essential component of management for all persons with diabetes.
   C. Medical nutritional management
      1. Educate to make changes in food and exercise habits that lead to improve metabolic control.
      2. Meal spacing is more crucial in type 1 than in type 2 diabetes.
      3. Eat every 4–5 hours while awake.
      4. The Exchange Lists of the American Dietetic and American Diabetes Associations are used to calculate energy nutrient distribution.
      5. Acceptable blood glucose is 70–110 mg/dL before meals and less than 200 mg/dL 2 hours after meals.
      6. The food pyramid provides an initial acceptable dietary guide of what foods should be eaten.
      7. Foods chosen from the food pyramid guide should be divided into three or more equal feedings.
      8. Carbohydrate-containing foods are especially important to distribute evenly throughout the day.
      9. Eat at regular times each day, avoid skipping meals, and eat about the same amount each day.
      10. Limit fat, salt, sugar, and alcohol intake.
      11. Portion control is important.
      12. Increase intake of fruits, vegetables, and whole grains
      13. ADA recommends a fiber intake of between 20–35 g/day for clients with diabetes.
      14. Excessive amounts of dietary protein should be avoided in people with diabetes.
      15. 10% of fat should come from polyunsaturated fat, 10% from saturated fat, and 10% from monounsaturated fat.
      16. Cholesterol should ideally be kept below 300 mg/day.

IX. Diet in cardiovascular disease
   A. Dietary/Supplementary
      1. Higher intakes of folic acid and vitamins B_{12} and B_6 have been linked to lower risk of vascular disease.
   B. Hypertension
      1. High salt intake
         a. Age-related increases in blood pressure (BP) are related to salt intake.
         b. Intake goal of 6 g of sodium chloride is considered reasonable by the National Institutes of Health.
      2. Calcium
         a. Diets containing less than 600 mg of calcium daily are most clearly associated with hypertension.
      3. Potassium
         a. Increased potassium intake produces a greater reduction in BP in African Americans than in whites.
         b. Increased risk of stroke was associated with lower potassium, magnesium, and cereal fiber intakes.
   C. Elevated blood cholesterol
      1. Cholesterol is precursor of adrenal hormones and the sex hormones.
      2. Blood cholesterol levels are measured to promote health and prevent disease.
      3. Trans saturated fatty acids in vegetable oil products have been identified as more potent risk factors for cardiovascular disease than saturated fat.
      4. 63%–75% of the intake of trans fatty acids is derived from baked goods, fried fast foods, and other prepared foods rather than from margarines.
      5. Trans fat has been shown to raise low-density lipoprotein (LDL) levels and lower high-density lipoprotein (HDL) levels.
      6. The higher the LDL, the greater the risk of coronary artery disease (CHD).
      7. Excess body fat is a cause of hypertension and CHD.
      8. Omega-3 fatty acids help decrease serum triglycerides, while lowering total cholesterol and blood pressure.
      9. Fish that contain omega-3 fatty acids include herring, mackerel, rainbow trout, salmon, sardines, swordfish, and tuna.
      10. Consumption of greater amounts of fruits and vegetables was shown to be associated with lower risk of ischemic stroke.
      11. The Food and Drug Administration (FDA) approved a health claim stating that eating 25g of soy protein daily as part of a low-fat, low-cholesterol diet may reduce the risk of cardiovascular disease.
      12. Major differences between the basic Food Guide Pyramids and the DASH (Dietary Approaches to Stop Hypertension) diet are:
         a. An increase in one daily serving of vegetables
         b. An increase of one to two daily servings of fruits
         c. Inclusion of four to five servings per week of nuts, seeds, and beans
   D. Dietary modifications in cardiovascular disease
      1. Cholesterol-lowering diets
         a. Step I diet is a strict interpretation of the recommended dietary intake for Americans.
         b. Step II diet reduces saturated fat to 7% of Kcal and limits cholesterol to less than 200 mg/day.
         c. Reducing saturated fat intake decreases serum cholesterol more than reducing dietary cholesterol.
         d. Intake of trans fatty acids was directly related to the risk of CHD in women and risk of myocardial infarction (MI) in both men and women.
         e. Soluble fiber lowers serum cholesterol by binding with it, promoting fecal elimination.
         f. Examples of foods high in soluble fiber are legumes, oats, barley, broccoli, apples, and citrus fruits.
         g. A high sucrose intake further increases triglyceride levels.
         h. For best results, consult the clinical dietitian.
      2. Sodium-controlled diet
         a. As many as one third of mild hypertensive cases can be controlled with sodium restriction, usually a 2-g sodium diet.
         b. Unseen contributions to sodium intake may come from other beverages, over-the-counter medications, and drinking water.
         c. American Heart Association recommends a limit of 20 mg of sodium per liter of water as a standard for persons who require a restricted sodium diet.
         d. Clients who require a diet containing less than 2 g of sodium may use bottled, distilled, deionized, or demineralized water for drinking and cooking in order to consume preferred sodium-containing foods.
         e. Diet prescriptions should be written in milligrams of sodium to achieve the desired result.
      3. Other modifications
         a. Clients taking potassium-wasting diuretics may require dietary or supplemental potassium.
         b. As the client recovers from a MI, the diet usually progresses from a 1000-Kcal to a 1200-Kcal liquid diet to a soft diet of small, frequent meals.
         c. Foods need to be served at a moderate temperature.
         d. Clients should avoid caffeine after heart attacks.
         e. Hypertensive clients should use caffeine in moderation because it increases blood pressure.
         f. Foods for the client with CHF should be nutrient dense, easily eaten, and easily digested.
         g. An hour's rest before meals conserves energy for clients with CHF.
         h. Thicker rather than thinner liquids are easier for persons who have had a stroke due to difficulty in swallowing.
         i. Nurses feeding clients with hemiplegia should place the food on the unaffected side of the tongue.

j. Turning a hemiplegic client's head toward the weak side while sitting upright may help with swallowing.

X. Diet in renal disease
  A. Nutritional care of the renal client
    1. Common complaints include anorexia, nausea, and vomiting.
    2. Malnutrition caused by increased catabolism, metabolic derangement, decreased food intake, and low economic status.
    3. Oral supplements, tube feedings, IV feedings, and intradialytic parenteral nutrition have been used to treat protein-energy malnutrition.
  B. Goals of nutrition therapy
    1. Attain and maintain optimal nutritional status.
    2. Prevent net protein catabolism.
    3. Minimize uremic toxicity.
    4. Maintain adequate hydration status.
    5. Maintain normal serum potassium levels.
    6. Control the progression of renal osteodystrophy.
    7. Modify diet to meet other nutrition-related concerns (i.e., diabetes).
    8. Retard the progression of renal failure and postpone the initiation of dialysis.
  C. Dietary components
    1. Kilocalorie intake increased for clients with renal disease
      a. May require an alternate feeding route to attain and maintain optimal nutritional status
    2. Protein
      a. Primary goal is control of nitrogen intake.
      b. Diet of high biological value (HBV) protein is used when client has elevated BUN.
      c. Examples of HBV protein include eggs, meat, and dairy products.
      d. Studies indicate that vegetarian diets have proven to be beneficial.
      e. Hemodialysis clients require high-protein diets because hemodialysis results in a loss of 1–2 g of amino acids per hour of dialysis.
      f. A client on continuous ambulatory peritoneal dialysis (CAPD) has an even higher protein need because of continuous dialysis.
    3. Sodium
      a. Intake may be restricted to prevent sodium retention in the body resulting in generalized edema.
    4. Potassium
      a. Dietary potassium needs to be evaluated.
      b. Salt substitutes are high in potassium.
      c. Water softeners may be a source of dietary potassium.
    5. Phosphorus, vitamin D, and calcium
      a. In clients with kidney disease, vitamin D cannot be activated leading to a low serum calcium level.
      b. Phosphorus is found mainly in diary products, dried beans and peas, nuts, peanut butter, and beverages such as cocoa, beer, and cola soft drinks.
    6. Fluid
      a. Clients on hemodialysis are restricted to 500–1000 mL/24 hr.
      b. Predialysis clients are restricted to 500 mL plus output.
      c. In clients on CAPD, fluid restriction is "as tolerated" according to their daily weight fluctuations and BP.
    7. Saturated fat and cholesterol
      a. Significant hypertriglyceridemia is present in clients with a history of renal disease.
      b. Modified fat diet and a modification of carbohydrate intake is required.
      c. Restrict simple sugars and alcohol.
    8. Iron
      a. Treatment for iron deficiency anemia is oral or parenteral iron products and an increase in dietary sources of iron.
      b. Iron supplements of 210 mg of ferrous iron salts/day divided among three to four doses.
      c. Absorption is enhanced when iron supplements are taken on an empty stomach or with vitamin C.
    9. Vitamin and mineral supplementation
      a. Loss of water-soluble vitamins in dialysis.
      b. Supplementation of these nutrients is recommended.
      c. Fat-soluble vitamins are not lost in dialysate; therefore, supplementation is not recommended.
  D. National renal diet
    1. Dietary management is tailored to the stage of disease and treatment approach.
    2. Six types of diets
      a. Renal insufficiency without diabetes
      b. Renal insufficiency with diabetes
      c. Hemodialysis without diabetes
      d. Hemodialysis with diabetes
      e. Peritoneal dialysis without diabetes
      f. Peritoneal dialysis with diabetes
    3. National meal-planning system offers standardized guidelines for nutrition intervention and client education.
  E. Kidney stones
    1. Drink 3000 mL, or 13 cups, of water/day.
    2. Exclude foods high in oxalates, such as coffee, tea, blackberries, whole-wheat bread, and dry cocoa.
    3. If stone is high in calcium, a low-calcium diet is prescribed.
    4. Dietary purines cause stones to be high in uric acid. Restrict foods high in purines.
    5. Foods high in purine are: liver, kidney, organ meats, herring, sardines (in oil). Whole-grain cereals, asparagus, and spinach have moderate amounts of purine.

XI. Diet in gastrointestinal disease
  A. Dietary considerations in surgical clients
    1. Preoperative nutrition
      a. Obese clients are instructed to lose weight to reduce the risks of surgery.
      b. Bowel preparation requires a low-residue diet for 2–3 days to minimize feces left in the bowel.
    2. Postoperative nutrition
      a. Minimum replacement of IV fluids, such as 2 L of 5% dextrose in water (D_5W) in 24 hours.

b. IV fluids contain 100 g of glucose to prevent ketosis.

c. Adequate nourishment should be delivered to the client within 3 days.

d. Clients progress from clear liquids to full liquids, a soft diet, and then a regular diet as soon as possible.

e. Avoid red liquids after surgery on the mouth or throat so that vomitus is not mistaken for blood.

B. Disorders of the esophagus
   1. Achalasia
      a. Avoid spicy foods and minimize dietary bulk.
      b. Plenty of liquids with small, frequent meals may help.
   2. Gastroesophageal reflux disease (GERD)
      a. Small, frequent meals help.
      b. Protein is associated with tightening of the cardiac sphincter.
      c. Avoid fat, alcohol, caffeine, peppermint, spearmint, and chocolate because they relax the sphincter.
      d. Avoid decaffeinated coffee and pepper because they stimulate gastric secretions.
      e. Acidic juices, such as citrus juices and tomato juice, may be irritating.
   3. Hiatal hernia
      a. Care is same as for GERD
C. Disorders of the stomach
   1. Gastritis
      a. Eat at regular intervals.
      b. Chew food, especially fibrous food, slowly and thoroughly.
      c. Avoid foods that cause pain.
      d. Avoid foods that cause gas, especially vegetables in the cabbage family, including broccoli, cauliflower, and Brussel sprouts.
      e. Avoid gastric irritants such as caffeine, alcohol, NSAIDs, aspirin, strong spices, including nutmeg, pepper, garlic, and chili powder.
      f. Eat in a relaxed manner.
   2. Peptic ulcers
      a. Eat three regular meals with no smoking between because food, including milk, stimulates gastric secretion.
      b. Avoid or limit spices or foods that are not well tolerated.
   3. Dumping syndrome
      a. Limit the intake of simple sugars, consuming frequent meals, and limiting fluids with meals.
      b. Avoid very hot or cold foods.
      c. Lying down for 30–60 minutes after eating retains the meal in the stomach longer.
D. Disorders of the intestine
   1. Irritable bowel syndrome
      a. Most common foods identified are lactose and gluten.
      b. A high-fiber diet provides symptomatic relief.
   2. Diarrhea
      a. Foods perilous for travelers include raw vegetables, raw meat, raw seafood, tap water, ice, and unpasteurized dairy products and are best avoided.

   3. Constipation
      a. Increase fiber in diet with adequate amounts of water.
   4. Crohn's disease
      a. Parenteral and tube feedings may be used separately or together.
      b. High kilocalorie, high-protein, low-fat, and sometimes low-fiber or low-residue intake.
      c. Small frequent feedings are encouraged.
      d. Restrict seasonings and chilled foods.
   5. Ulcerative colitis
      a. A 4- to 6-week course of total parenteral nutrition (TPN) achieves complete bowel rest.
      b. Avoid irritating foods.
      c. Restrict foods that produce gas or loose stools.
      d. Parenteral supplements of iron and vitamin B$_{12}$ may be prescribed.
   6. Dietary guidelines for ostomy clients
      a. Soft or general diet postoperatively
      b. Avoid stringy high-fiber foods initially, such as celery, coconut, corn, cabbage, coleslaw, and popcorn.
      c. Some clients avoid fish, eggs, beer, and carbonated beverages because they produce excessive odor.
E. Diseases and conditions of the liver
   1. Hepatitis
      a. High kilocalorie, high protein, moderate-fat diet is frequently prescribed.
      b. Protein in amounts up to 100 g helps heal the liver.
      c. Client may tolerate emulsified fats as dairy products and eggs better than other fats.
F. Gallbladder disease
   1. A full liquid diet with minimal fat is recommended.
   2. Select skim milk dairy products.
   3. Limit fats or oils to 3 tsp/day.
   4. Consume no more than 6 oz of very lean meat per day.
   5. Gas-forming foods are often poorly tolerated.
   6. Avoid fried foods.
G. Disorders of the pancreas
   1. Avoid alcohol.
   2. Eat six small meals/day.
   3. For cystic fibrosis clients, protein needs are double those of other individuals.
   4. Fat content should be as high as possible for cystic fibrosis.
XII. Diet and cancer
   A. Nutritional guidelines for cancer and terminally ill clients
      1. Cancer clients should be encouraged to eat whether they are hungry or not.
      2. For severely anorexic client, offer 1 oz of a complete nutritional supplement every hour.
      3. Oral hygiene before meals freshens the mouth.
      4. Lemon-flavored beverages improve taste sensations.
      5. Eggs, fish, poultry, and dairy products may be better received than beef or pork.
      6. Serving meat cold or at room temperature lessens the bitter taste.

7. Sweet sauces and marinades added to meat improve its palatability.

B. Mouth ulcerations
1. Foods should be soft and mild.
2. Sauces, gravies, and dressings may make foods easier to eat.
3. Cream soups and milk provide much nutrition.
4. Cold foods may be easier to tolerate.
5. Taking liquids with meals helps wash down the food.
6. Avoid hot items, salty and spicy foods, and acidic juices.
7. Sugarless hard candy, chewing gum, or popsicles may stimulate saliva production.

C. Nausea, vomiting, and diarrhea
1. Eating dry crackers before arising may alleviate nausea.
2. Liquids taken between meals, rather than with them, reduce the volume in the stomach.
3. A low-fat diet is digested faster.
4. Adding nutmeg to food decreases gastric motility.
5. Low-residue diet helps reduce intestinal stimulation.

XIII. Diet in HIV and AIDS
A. Malabsorption is primary problem
B. Nutritional guidelines
1. Clients with a from of carbohydrate intolerance may benefit from either a lactose-restricted or a disaccharide-free diet.
2. A lactose-free diet may be sufficient for clients who are deficient only in lactase.
3. A low-fat diet may be necessary to control steatorrhea.
4. Fluids should be encouraged to maintain hydration when large fluid volume is lost in stools.
5. Yogurt and other foods that contain the *Lactobacillus acidophilus* culture may be helpful if bacteria overgrowth is a problem secondary to long-term anti-infective use.
6. Small, frequent meals make the best use of a limited absorptive capacity of the gut.
7. A multivitamin supplement is indicated to increase the amount of vitamin available for absorption.
8. Avoidance of sorbitol, which is used as a sweetening agent in both sugar-free candies and some medications, has been shown to cause diarrhea.

QUESTIONS

Patricia Gauntlett Beare, RN, PhD, Demetrius J. Porche, RN, CCRN, DNS, and Golden M. Tradewell, RN, PhD

1. After a myocardial infarction, a 52-year-old man has been placed on a 1-g sodium diet. Which of the following choices is considered low sodium?

   1. Canned and dry soups
   2. Ketchup, Worcestershire sauce
   3. Bologna and hot dogs
   4. Fresh or frozen meat, whole-grain bread

2. A 52-year-old male client is 3 weeks' post–myocardial infarction. His physician has ordered a diet to lower his blood cholesterol. Which of the following statements indicates a need for further teaching?

   1. "I ate a grilled cheese sandwich and an avocado salad for lunch yesterday."
   2. "I enjoyed broiled chicken, baked potato, and canned peaches for dinner."
   3. "I fixed a loin lamb chop, macaroni, and an apple-raisin salad for dinner."
   4. "I ate red beans and rice with bread sticks yesterday."

3. A client with a history of strokes has been admitted for evaluation of her dysphagia. Which of the following should the nurse encourage?

   1. Thin, clear liquid foods
   2. Eating in an upright position
   3. Using liquids to clear the mouth of food
   4. Talking to the client while eating to facilitate the social aspect of eating

4. A client is being evaluated for chronic "heartburn." When teaching the client to avoid gastroesophageal reflux, which of the following client statements indicates a need for further teaching?

   1. "I will limit my lifting of heavy objects."
   2. "I will try to lose some of my extra weight."
   3. "I will lie down for a half hour after meals."
   4. "I will elevate the head of my bed at night."

5. A 42-year-old male client was admitted with peptic ulcer disease. Which of the following decreases gastric acid secretion or increases gastric healing?

   1. Eating at bedtime so that acid can work on food at night
   2. Eating a bland diet
   3. Eliminating only foods that cause discomfort
   4. Drinking caffeinated beverages instead of milk

6. A 19-year-old woman is being treated for ulcerative colitis. After her symptoms are under control, she has been ordered to follow a low-fiber diet. Which of the following statements indicates a need for further teaching?

   1. "I can drink coffee, tea, or clear fruit juices."
   2. "I can eat pancakes, waffles, Special K, and puffed wheat."
   3. "I can eat chicken, eggs, and potatoes."

   4. "I can eat peanut butter pie, coconut meringue pie, or cherry pie for dessert."

7. A 76-year-old woman is seen at the clinic with chronic constipation. She has been placed on a high-fiber diet. Which of the following presents good food choices for her?

   1. Popcorn, oat bran muffins, brown rice
   2. Grits, Cheerios, corn flakes
   3. Ripe banana, applesauce, fruit cocktail
   4. Well-cooked meat, potatoes, canned vegetables

8. A client with chronic cholecystitis is treated with a fat- and calorie-controlled diet. Which meal is an example for the nurse to help the client choose?

   1. English muffin, fresh fruit, Canadian bacon
   2. Buttermilk, fried potatoes, pork sausage
   3. French toast, chocolate milk, smoked salmon
   4. Croissant, corned beef, skim milk

9. A 42-year-old female client underwent a gastrectomy 4 months ago. She has developed pernicious anemia. The nurse anticipates that the physician will order:

   1. Vitamin B_{12} in a multivitamin
   2. A dietary consultation
   3. Parenteral vitamin B_{12}
   4. A diet high in vitamin B_{12}

10. The nurse is discussing "old wives' tales" with a group of new mothers. Which of the following statements is actually true about breast-feeding?

    1. Limiting nursing time will prevent sore nipples.
    2. Limiting breast-feeding will build up a supply of milk.
    3. Sore nipples are caused by a tight seal from the baby's lips.
    4. A fussy baby should be nursed frequently.

11. A 35-year-old woman is admitted to your unit with nausea and vomiting, cramps, diarrhea, and chills. These symptoms occurred about 30 hours after she ate supper. Which of the following foods is most likely to be the cause?

    1. Salad
    2. Chicken
    3. Gravy
    4. Raw seafood or fish

12. The nurse is helping a client with a new diagnosis of diabetes to select his meals. Which of the following statements indicates a need for further teaching?

    1. "I will weigh my meat before cooking."
    2. "I will trim off visible fat before or after cooking."
    3. "I know that meat does not contain fiber."
    4. "Many processed meats contain large amounts of carbohydrates."

13. The nurse is helping a client with a new diagnosis of diabetes to select his meals. Which of the following indicates a need for further teaching when selected as a vegetable?

1. Corn
2. Beans
3. Carrots
4. Tomatoes

14. The nurse is helping a client with a new diagnosis of diabetes to select his meals. Which of the following indicates a need for further teaching when selected from the cereal and grain list?

1. Grits
2. Pasta
3. Rice
4. Popcorn

15. A 22-year-old primigravida is 5 ft 5 in tall and weighs 128 lb at the beginning of pregnancy. Her expected weight at term gestation would be:

1. 145 lb
2. 148 lb
3. 155 lb
4. 167 lb

16. A client who is a native of the Middle East normally wears a long robe that covers her arms and body, along with a shawl that covers her head and neck. She is pregnant and the nurse is aware that she will need a supplement of:

1. Vitamin D
2. Calcium
3. Vitamin C
4. Zinc

17. A client experiences morning nausea early in her pregnancy. The nurse advises her to:

1. Eat a small amount of dry, carbohydrate-containing food on awakening
2. Increase her intake of fluids in the early morning
3. Increase her intake of fat to provide enough calories
4. Restrict her intake of fluids throughout the day for a few weeks

18. If an iron supplement is prescribed for a pregnant woman, which point should the nurse emphasize in her teaching?

1. She should take the supplement with food to avoid stomach upsets.
2. She should take the supplement with milk to improve absorption.
3. As long as she takes the supplement, she does not have to worry about including iron sources in her diet.
4. She should include food such as citrus fruits, melons, broccoli, or strawberries in her diet each day.

19. In a teaching plan for a pregnant woman, the nurse would advise her on the need to avoid:

1. Cholesterol
2. Sodium
3. Alcohol
4. Saturated fat

20. A 55-year-old man has liver failure caused by cirrhosis and is in impending hepatic coma. The nurse is assisting him with his diet selection. Which of the following choices indicates a need for further teaching?

1. Fruit salad
2. Cooked buttered carrots
3. Boiled potato
4. Cream of chicken soup

21. In evaluating a 10-year-old boy's understanding of his diet for celiac disease, the nurse would expect him to order which of these foods for breakfast?

1. Corn flakes
2. Buckwheat pancakes
3. Oat bran muffins
4. Cereal with wheat germ

22. An 18-year-old female client is admitted to the hospital with acute renal failure. She is oliguric, hypertensive, and hyperkalemic. The nurse would not expect to see which of the following on her meal tray?

1. Canned, drained pears
2. Whole-wheat bread
3. Fresh orange
4. Unsalted butter

23. A 12-year-old girl has a new diagnosis of insulin-dependent diabetes mellitus. The nurse advises the client that some carbohydrates need to be included in her diet because they:

1. Insulate the body to prevent heat loss
2. Furnish the body with energy
3. Build and repair new tissue
4. Provide a source of dietary fiber

24. In evaluating a client's understanding of the exchange diet, the nurse would expect the client to state that part-skim-milk mozzarella cheese is:

1. A milk exchange
2. A meat exchange
3. A fat exchange
4. Either a milk or a meat exchange

25. In teaching the exchange diet to a client with a new diagnosis of diabetes, the nurse would explain that potatoes are:

1. A vegetable exchange
2. A starch-bread exchange
3. A fruit exchange
4. Either a vegetable or a starch-bread exchange

26. A 57-year-old client has undergone resection of the ileum and much of the jejunum. Postoperatively, the client has experienced diarrhea and steatorrhea. The nurse would expect the diet to be restricted in:

1. Protein
2. Fluid
3. Sodium
4. Fat

27. A client complains of constipation. The nurse teaches the client to add fiber to the diet. The teaching was effective if the client has:
    1. Carrot-raisin salad
    2. Hamburger on a sesame seed bun
    3. Mashed potatoes with gravy
    4. Canned fruit cocktail

28. A 68-year-old woman is receiving a nasogastric tube feeding. Tube placement is known to be correct if:
    1. A loud "whoosh" can be heard over the left upper quadrant of the abdomen when air is injected through the tube
    2. No air bubbles appear when the free end of the tube is held under water during exhalation
    3. The client experiences no gagging or respiratory distress
    4. An abdominal radiograph shows the tube to be in the body of the stomach

29. A client who undergoes a gastric resection is most likely to require supplementation with:
    1. Magnesium
    2. Folic acid
    3. Chloride
    4. Vitamin B$_{12}$

30. A 14-year-old boy has third-degree burns over 50% of his body. He is in stable condition. The best snack for him would be:
    1. Peanut butter sandwich and milkshake
    2. Buttered popcorn and soft drink
    3. Orange juice and fresh vegetables with dip
    4. Milk and crackers

31. To promote wound healing in a burn client, the nurse would expect which vitamin or mineral to be supplemented?
    1. Folic acid
    2. Zinc
    3. Iron
    4. Vitamin K

32. The nurse would offer which food to a client on a clear-liquid diet?
    1. Tea
    2. Orange juice
    3. Sherbet
    4. Vegetable soup

33. A client on a full-liquid diet received the following foods on his tray. Which food should be removed?
    1. Chicken noodle soup
    2. Ice cream
    3. Cream of tomato soup
    4. Custard

34. In teaching a client about a low-fat diet, the nurse explains that a food without any limits is:
    1. Avocado
    2. Blueberry muffin
    3. Chocolate bar
    4. Angel food cake

35. A neonate has a diagnosis of phenylketonuria (PKU). Which of the following statements by her mother informs the nurse that more education is needed?
    1. "I must read the ingredient listing on foods before I give them to the baby."
    2. "As the baby grows, her diet will change."
    3. "The baby will need a special infant formula."
    4. "When she becomes a teenager, she won't need a special diet any longer."

36. Which food would the nurse select for a toddler on a low-phenylalanine diet?
    1. Boiled potato
    2. Macaroni
    3. Corn
    4. Applesauce

37. Which food would the nurse select for a child on a galactose-free diet?
    1. Sherbet
    2. Buttered popcorn
    3. Egg noodles
    4. Pancakes

38. A 4-month-old infant is to begin on solid foods. The following are good reasons for starting with infant rice cereal except:
    1. Rice cereal is the most economical infant food.
    2. An infant of this age has developed the ability to digest the carbohydrate provided by the cereal.
    3. Infant cereals are fortified with iron.
    4. Rice cereal is not often associated with allergic reactions.

39. A mother of a 9-month-old infant gave a diet history of feeding the baby the foods listed below. Which food choice indicates that the mother needs further teaching?
    1. Infant formula
    2. Scrambled egg
    3. Toast strips
    4. Cottage cheese

40. A client who has essential hypertension is following a 2-g sodium diet restriction. The nurse would expect the client to avoid:
    1. Fresh flounder
    2. Hard rolls
    3. Peanut butter
    4. Milk

41. When evaluating a client's understanding of a low-sodium diet, the nurse would expect her to state she uses which seasoning?
    1. Worcestershire sauce
    2. Garlic salt
    3. Ketchup
    4. Lemon juice

42. A client has very high blood cholesterol levels. In regard to diet, the nurse implements a teaching plan and encourages the client to reduce intake of:

1. All types of fats
2. Saturated fats
3. Polyunsaturated fats
4. Monounsaturated fats

43. The nurse would encourage a client on a low-cholesterol diet to drink:
   1. Whole milk
   2. 2% low-fat milk
   3. Skim milk
   4. Acidophilus milk

44. A client states that she is a strict vegetarian (consuming no animal products). What food could the nurse recommend as a source of calcium?
   1. Strawberries
   2. Raisins
   3. Mustard greens
   4. Corn

45. In teaching a weight-loss class, the nurse emphasizes that the most effective way for people to achieve and maintain weight loss is:
   1. Low-calorie liquid-formula diet
   2. Increased exercise combined with low-calorie diet
   3. Increased exercise
   4. Low-calorie diet selected from common foods

46. The mother of a 7-lb 6-oz newborn is trying to decide whether to breast-feed or bottle-feed. In discussing the decision with her, the nurse can say that:
   1. Growth is better in formula-fed infants.
   2. Formula feeding is less expensive than breast feeding.
   3. Breast-fed infants are more likely to have colic than formula-fed ones.
   4. Breast-fed infants are less likely to develop allergies.

47. A client would like to breast-feed her newborn son. The nurse knows that he will need a supplement to provide:
   1. Zinc
   2. Vitamin E
   3. Fluoride
   4. Thiamine

48. At a baby's 2-week checkup in the clinic, his mother asks whether it is time to start him on solid foods. The nurse can tell her that:
   1. It is best to start solid foods soon because the baby will be more likely to accept them now than when he is older.
   2. Solid foods should not be started until the infant is at least 4 months old, when it will be less likely to cause allergies.
   3. It is a good idea to start solid foods now because doing so will help the baby to sleep through the night at an earlier age.
   4. Solid foods should be started before 2 months of age because doing so will help to prevent the baby from becoming obese.

49. A mother intends to wean her child from breast feeding at 8 months of age. She asks what he should receive in place of the breast milk. The nurse explains that:

1. Whole cow's milk is an economical and nutritious substitute for breast milk for an infant of this age.
2. An infant of this age can be weaned to skim milk because this helps to reduce the risk of his developing heart disease later in life.
3. Formula without iron is the best choice for a child of this age because it is less likely to cause constipation than a formula with iron.
4. Iron-fortified formula should be used until the infant is 12 months old.

50. A 3-year-old client comes to the clinic. His mother reports that he drinks several cups of milk daily but dislikes most other foods except peanut butter and french fries. The nurse suspects that the child is most likely to have a deficiency of which nutrient?
   1. Calcium
   2. Phosphorus
   3. Protein
   4. Iron

51. A client with acute pancreatitis is receiving a low-fat diet. The best breakfast for her would be:
   1. Orange juice, corn flakes with skim milk, biscuits with jam, coffee
   2. Grape juice, bran flakes with skim milk, toast with honey, tea
   3. Tomato juice, poached eggs on toast, coffee
   4. Grapefruit sections, blueberry muffins, and tea

52. During a health-care visit, the client states that "sometimes my gums bleed." The nurse in diet teaching explains that bleeding gums are usually a sign of inadequate intake of:
   1. Vitamin C
   2. Vitamin D
   3. Vitamin E
   4. Vitamin A

53. When presenting a class on nutrition, the nurse should emphasize that in the United States, the most likely cause of anemia is deficiency of:
   1. Iron
   2. Folic acid
   3. Vitamin B_{12}
   4. Intrinsic factor

54. A client has an esophageal tumor obstruction. The client has a gastrostomy. Which type of diet would be best for this client?
   1. Full liquid
   2. Soft
   3. Low residue
   4. Tube feeding via gastrostomy

55. A client develops pneumonia. The nurse encourages his wife to select which nutrient to assist in producing adequate antibodies to resist the infection?
   1. Protein
   2. Fat
   3. Thiamine
   4. Riboflavin

56. The nurse might expect the physician to write orders for a low-residue diet for a client 2–3 days before he undergoes:
    1. Oral surgery
    2. GI surgery
    3. Head and neck surgery
    4. Any surgery

57. A client undergoes gastric surgery and experiences postoperative difficulty with symptoms of dumping syndrome. The food that would be most likely to worsen her symptoms is:
    1. Fried fish
    2. Hard-cooked egg
    3. Plain bagel
    4. Fruit gelatin

58. A client is experiencing symptoms of dumping syndrome. The nurse advises the client to drink fluids:
    1. Just before meals
    2. Only with meals
    3. Before and during meals
    4. After meals

59. A client notes that he experiences cramping, bloating, and watery stools when drinking milk. A plan of care for the client would be to encourage a reduction in intake of:
    1. Milk protein
    2. Lactose
    3. Sucrose
    4. Galactose

60. A client reports that the following is typical of his usual daily eating habits: 1 cup oatmeal, 2 slices whole-grain toast, 1 cup orange juice, 1 cup 2% fat milk, 5 oz lasagna, 1 cup orange juice, 1 cup 2% fat milk, 1 cup steamed broccoli, 2 bean tacos, 1 cup tossed salad with olive oil and vinegar, and 30 oz of beer. According to the food pyramid and the Dietary Guidelines for Americans, it would be most important for the client to:
    1. Decrease his intake of cholesterol
    2. Decrease his alcohol intake
    3. Increase his fiber intake
    4. Increase his vegetable intake

61. In developing a teaching plan for weight control, the nurse is aware that obesity is usually defined as having a body weight that is at least _____% greater than the desirable body weight.

62. A client is found to be obese. The nurse includes diet teaching and makes the client aware of risk factor(s) for other diseases such as:
    1. Peptic ulcer
    2. Periodontal disease
    3. Scleroderma
    4. Hypertension

63. A 6-ft-tall football player who weighs 300 lb has a diagnosis of hiatal hernia and complains of burning chest pain after eating. Which of the following statements by the client indicates a need for further dietary teaching?

1. "I should lie down and rest after eating."
2. "I should not snack before I go to bed."
3. "I should reduce my weight."
4. "I can use an antacid to relieve the burning."

64. A client is placed on a high-fiber diet. Which of the following does the nurse identify as the best source of dietary fiber?
    1. Pineapple juice
    2. Potatoes au gratin
    3. Popcorn
    4. Roast beef

65. A 6-month-old formula-fed infant has an acute case of diarrhea. In instructing the mother regarding the infant's care, the nurse needs to know and teach that *lactose* refers to:
    1. Fruit sugar
    2. Table sugar
    3. Milk sugar
    4. Corn syrup

66. It is important to observe a 6-month-old child admitted with diarrhea for:
    1. Dry, sticky mucous membranes
    2. Edema
    3. Acute weight gain
    4. Skin rash

67. When teaching a pregnant client, the nurse knows that iron supplements are recommended:
    1. Only during the first trimester of pregnancy
    2. Only during the last trimester of pregnancy
    3. Throughout pregnancy and lactation
    4. Only during lactation

68. If a client's weight before pregnancy was 122 lb, she should aim for a weight of approximately _____ lb at the end of pregnancy.

69. When the nurse is teaching a client with insulin-dependent diabetes, a good rule is:
    1. All foods in the meal plan should be consumed at the planned time each day.
    2. It is safe to omit meat or fat exchanges but not to omit fruits, milk, or breads.
    3. Exchanges may be moved from one meal or snack to the next within the same day.
    4. Extra exchanges from the diabetic diet may be consumed as long as the client takes extra insulin with the food.

70. If a client develops a complete intestinal obstruction postoperatively, which type of feeding is he or she most likely to receive?
    1. Nasogastric tube feeding
    2. Full-liquid diet
    3. Total parenteral nutrition
    4. Low-residue diet

71. A client has been found to have very high blood cholesterol levels. The nurse teaches that, in regard to his diet, he should know that blood cholesterol increases with excessive intake of:

1. All types of fats
2. Saturated fats
3. Polyunsaturated fats
4. Monounsaturated fats

72. A client on a low-cholesterol diet should know that cholesterol is found in:

    1. Lean ground beef
    2. Avocado
    3. Peanuts
    4. Palm oil

73. A 60-year-old man with renal failure is not receiving dialysis. If he is hungry between meals, the nurse can offer him:

    1. Hard candy
    2. Soft drinks
    3. Cheddar cheese
    4. Fresh fruit

74. The best breakfast food for a person following a low-fat, low-cholesterol diet would be:

    1. Biscuits with corn oil margarine
    2. Oatmeal with brown sugar
    3. Eggs Benedict
    4. Bagel with cream cheese

75. The best lunch for someone following a low-sodium diet would be:

    1. Cheeseburger, fries, ketchup, soft drink
    2. Bologna sandwich, carrot and celery sticks, brownies, iced tea
    3. Chicken noodle soup, bran muffins, apple turnover, milk
    4. Tossed salad with turkey and hard-cooked egg, vinegar and oil dressing, bread sticks, pineapple rings, iced tea

76. When the nurse is planning the diet for a child with celiac disease, which could be consumed?

    1. White sauce made with bleached flour
    2. Fried rice
    3. Vegetable-barley soup
    4. Oatmeal muffins

77. The nurse would be most concerned when finding that a pregnant client took excessive amounts of an over-the-counter vitamin supplement containing which of the following?

    1. Vitamin E
    2. Biotin
    3. Folic acid
    4. Vitamin A

78. A 78-year-old client complains of constipation. Which of the following would be most likely to benefit this client?

    1. Increasing the number of rest periods
    2. Increasing protein intake
    3. Decreasing intake of fluids at mealtime
    4. Increasing intake of complex carbohydrates

79. In the mid afternoon, a client with diabetes starts experiencing symptoms of dizziness, weakness, sweating, rapid pulse, and delayed thinking. Which would be the least desirable snack?

    1. Orange juice
    2. Honey
    3. Hard candy
    4. Cheese

80. Which of the following would be the best snack for a client with insulin-dependent diabetes before participating in a 2-hour football game?

    1. Fresh fruit
    2. Orange juice
    3. Cheese and crackers
    4. Soda

81. A nurse is teaching a client about fat-soluble vitamins. Which statement by the client indicates that further teaching is necessary?

    1. "Vitamin A is fat soluble."
    2. "Vitamin D is fat soluble."
    3. "Vitamin K is fat soluble."
    4. "Vitamin B_{12} is fat soluble."

82. In lactose intolerance, which of the following can be substituted for milk products?

    1. Cheese
    2. Ice cream
    3. Soy milk
    4. Goat milk

83. Lactose intolerance is a deficiency of which enzyme?

    1. Lactase
    2. Maltase
    3. Peptase
    4. Amylase

84. A 22-year-old client verbalizes an understanding of a gluten-free diet. Which statement by the client indicates that further teaching is needed to help the client fully understand the features of a gluten-free diet?

    1. "High protein is a feature of a gluten-free diet."
    2. "Low protein is a feature of a gluten-free diet."
    3. "High calories are a feature of a gluten-free diet."
    4. "High vitamins and minerals are features of a gluten-free diet."

85. Which of the following statements by a client indicates that further teaching is necessary related to a clear-liquid diet?

    1. "Milk is a clear liquid."
    2. "Tea is a clear liquid."
    3. "Broth is a clear liquid."
    4. "Apple juice is a clear liquid."

86. A client has experienced third-degree burns on 60%–70% of the body. The client is now in stable condition in a private room. The client's diet should consist of:

    1. High protein
    2. Low protein

3. High carbohydrates
4. Low carbohydrates

87. Which of the following would be consistent with a burn client's dietary needs?

1. Hamburger and coleslaw
2. Peanut butter and milkshake
3. Orange juice and vegetables
4. Milk and crackers

88. Celiac disease requires a gluten-free diet. Which of the following should be eliminated from a gluten-free diet?

1. Milk
2. Beef
3. Green vegetables
4. Wheat bread

89. Which of the following would be a necessary supplemental vitamin for someone with cirrhosis of the liver?

1. Vitamin B_6
2. Vitamin B_{12}
3. Folic acid
4. Vitamin K

90. What is the best instruction a nurse can give for constipation?

1. "Decrease fluid intake."
2. "Get bed rest."
3. "Increase dietary fiber."
4. "Take Kaopectate."

91. What is the best instruction a nurse can give for diarrhea?

1. "Decrease fluid intake."
2. "Increase activity."
3. "Increase fluid intake with essential electrolytes."
4. "Encourage extra intake of milk or milk products."

92. Which of the following is considered a full liquid?

1. Cranberry sauce
2. Oatmeal
3. Gelatin
4. Vegetable soup

93. A client is receiving furosemide therapy. Which of the following foods is a rich source of supplemental potassium?

1. Squash
2. Apricots
3. Oatmeal
4. Cream of wheat

94. A client is discharged home on a 2-g sodium diet. Which statement made by the client indicates poor understanding of the specified diet?

1. "Fresh fruit is part of a 2-g sodium diet."
2. "Potatoes are part of a 2-g sodium diet."
3. "Eggs are part of a 2-g sodium diet."
4. "Ice cream is part of a 2-g sodium diet."

95. A client with CHF has a 1000-mL/day fluid restriction with a 2-g sodium diet. Before serving meals to this client, the nurse should:

1. Check the client's admitting diagnosis
2. Notify the dietitian about the fluid restriction
3. Call the physician to clarify the order
4. Assess the client's total fluid intake up to this meal; then collaboratively decide on the amount of fluid to be consumed with the meal

96. The nurse would expect a 45-year-old male client with renal disease to be placed on a _____ diet.

1. High-potassium
2. Potassium-restricted
3. High-sodium
4. High-protein

97. In a protein-restricted diet, which of the following should be altered to maintain appropriate caloric intake?

1. Increase amount of vitamins and minerals.
2. Increase simple carbohydrates and fats.
3. Increase protein and decrease carbohydrates.
4. Decrease amount of vitamins but increase minerals.

98. A client has a diagnosis of cholelithiasis and cholecystitis. A fat-restricted diet was ordered. Which food would be allowed?

1. Chicken
2. Avocado
3. Pecan pie
4. Liver

99. A client's condition has improved with a fat-restricted diet. The diet has been advanced to a controlled-fat–low-fat diet. What food should the nurse remove from the dinner tray?

1. Liver
2. Baked potato
3. Green beans
4. Chicken

100. Which of the following statements informs the nurse that more education is needed for the mother of a child with PKU?

1. "As my child grows his diet will change."
2. "My child has had phenylketonuria and received a special diet since birth."
3. "I must read the ingredients and nutritional information on foods before I give it to my child."
4. "My child will be on a special diet only until puberty."

101. A client is receiving a fluid-restricted diet of 1000 mL because of CHF. The client's daily intake consists of 3 oz of orange juice, 8 oz of milk, two 8-oz glasses of water, and 6 oz of tea. The client wants to have 8 oz of skim milk for an evening snack. The nurse should:

1. Ask for a physician's order to increase the fluid restriction to 1500 mL.
2. Permit the client to drink the skim milk.
3. Explain to the client that 8 oz of skim milk would exceed the daily fluid restrictions.
4. Substitute the skim milk with a clear liquid.

102. A 53-year-old client with a history of coronary artery disease is admitted to the hospital for angina. The physician orders a low-cholesterol diet. The client should decrease the intake of:

1. Veal
2. Chicken
3. Fish
4. Eggs

103. An 80-year-old man was diagnosed with intermittent claudication. He told the nurse that he was using dietary supplements to help with his condition. The nurse instructed the client to:

1. Increase saturated fat content in the diet.
2. Reduce sodium content.
3. Check with physician before taking dietary supplements.
4. Increase calcium intake.

104. A 50-year-old woman requested information on alternative treatments, such as dietary supplements, for osteoarthritis. The nurse instructed the client to:

1. Drink three glasses of milk each day to increase calcium intake.
2. Take acetaminophen every 6 hours.
3. Decrease calcium intake.
4. Check with physician about taking additional calcium in the form of a dietary supplement.

105. Which of the following statements describing cultural factors which have an effect on health is correct?

1. Hispanic and African American women have lower mortality rates secondary to breast and lung cancers than whites.
2. Some cultures expect the client to provide self-care as soon as possible in the hospital, whereas Western culture supports family members providing the care in the hospital.
3. There are cultural differences regarding nutritional effect on health.
4. Many cultures encourage direct eye contact.

106. A frail older adult lives alone. Which of the following intervention is important to meet the older adult's nutritional needs?

1. Fast foods
2. Home-delivered meals
3. Frozen dinners
4. Restaurant food

107. In caring for a frail older adult living alone, which of the following statements indicates a need for further teaching?

1. "I take a multivitamin daily."
2. "My dentures are too loose."
3. "Certain foods smell so good."
4. "I eat three meals a day."

108. One of the most common herbs used in the United States is:

1. NSAIDs
2. Heparin
3. Vitamin E
4. Garlic

109. A Middle Eastern woman requested herbal treatment for menopausal cramps. The nurse understands that many cultures may use which of the following herbs to treat menopausal cramps?

1. Echinacea
2. St. John's wort
3. Black cohosh
4. Aloe

110. Which of the following dietary supplements is contraindicted when taking Coumadin?

1. Dehydroepiandrosterone (DHEA)
2. Echinacea
3. Hawthorn
4. Ginger

111. Which of the following herbal treatments is used by many cultures to reduce benign prostatic hyperplasia?

1. Zinc
2. St. John's wort
3. Melatonin
4. Saw palmetto

112. A 34-year-old woman was undergoing a hysterectomy. What instructions need to be given if she is taking dietary supplements?

1. Advise client that all dietary supplements are safe.
2. Discontinue dietary supplements 2–3 weeks before surgery.
3. Advise client to discuss health-care needs with employees of health food stores.
4. Keep all dietary supplements in the refrigerator.

113. A hospice client who was taking a large amount of oxycodone for pain was complaining about constipation. The hospice nurse suggested:

1. Decrease water.
2. Eat more fiber.
3. Decrease activity.
4. Take extra laxatives.

114. A frail older adult was observed as not eating a complete meal and not taking a multivitamin. Based on this nutritional assessment, the nurse suspects the client is at risk for:

1. Fever
2. Pressure sores
3. Third-degree burns
4. Obesity

115. What nutritional instructions would the nurse give to a client with a stage II pressure sore?

1. Drink plenty of water.
2. Eat extra fiber.
3. Eat more protein.
4. Eat more vegetables.

ANSWERS

1. **(4)** Integrated processes: nursing process — evaluation; client need: physiological integrity; basic care and comfort; content area: nutrition

   RATIONALE

   (1) Canned and dry soups contain salt. **(2)** Ketchup, sauces, and Worcestershire sauce contain salt. **(3)** Any processed food, such as smoked ham or processed luncheon meat, is high in salt. **(4)** Buttermilk, fresh or frozen meats, whole-grain breads, and fresh, frozen, or canned vegetables without salt are allowed.

2. **(1)** Integrated processes: nursing process — evaluation; teaching/learning; client need: physiological integrity; basic care and comfort; content area: nutrition.

   RATIONALE

   (1) Cheese (American, mozzarella, cheddar) is high in fat. Avocados are also high in fat. **(2)** Lean meats with fat trimmed, potatoes, rice, and canned fruits are low in fat. **(3)** Lean meats, macaroni, and fresh fruits are low in fat. **(4)** Beans, rice, and bread sticks are low in fat.

3. **(2)** Integrated processes: nursing process — implementation; teaching/learning; client need: physiological integrity; basic care and comfort; content area: nutrition.

   RATIONALE

   (1) Thin liquids are more difficult to swallow. **(2)** Eating in an upright position allows gravity to assist the passage of food along the esophagus and helps to prevent choking and aspiration. **(3)** Liquids should be used only after the client has cleared the food from her mouth to prevent choking and aspiration. **(4)** The client should be supervised, but distractions should be avoided so that the client can focus attention on eating the meal.

4. **(3)** Integrated processes: nursing process — evaluation; teaching/learning; client need: physiological integrity; basic care and comfort; content area: nutrition.

   RATIONALE

   (1) Limiting bending over at the waist and wearing constrictive clothing increase intra-abdominal reflux. **(2)** Obesity increases intra-abdominal pressure. **(3)** The goal of medical treatment is to reduce intra-abdominal pressure and reflux and gastric acid production. The client should not lie down for 2 to 3 hours after meals. **(4)** Elevating the head of the bed at night decreases reflux.

5. **(3)** Integrated processes: nursing process — evaluation; client need: physiological integrity; basic care and comfort; content area: nutrition.

   RATIONALE

   (1) Eating at bedtime stimulates acid during sleep. **(2)** A bland diet may have adverse effects from ingesting excessive amounts of milk with antacids, causing milk-alkali syndrome and an increase in gastric acid secretion. **(3)** There is little rationale for completely eliminating particular foods unless they cause repeated discomfort. **(4)** Caffeinated and decaffeinated beverages stimulate gastric acid secretions.

6. **(4)** Integrated processes: nursing process — evaluation; teaching/learning; client need: physiological integrity; basic care and comfort; content area: nutrition.

   RATIONALE

   (1) Coffee, tea, carbonated beverages, strained and clear fruits, juices, and milk are allowed. **(2)** Refined breads, rolls, crackers, waffles, and refined dry and cooked cereals are allowed. **(3)** Chicken, well-cooked meats, fish, eggs, and white and sweet potatoes are allowed. **(4)** Any dessert made with seeds, nuts, coconuts, or fruit or vegetable pulp is not recommended.

7. **(1)** Integrated processes: nursing process — evaluation; client need: physiological integrity; basic care and comfort; content area: nutrition.

   RATIONALE

   (1) Foods high in fiber include whole-grain breads, oat bran muffins, brown rice, popcorn, wheat germ, whole-grain cereals, and beans. **(2)** Refined cooked cereals and dry cereals are low in fiber. **(3)** Canned or cooked fruits and vegetables are low in fiber. **(4)** Most well-cooked meats, canned vegetables, and white and sweet potatoes are low in fiber.

8. **(1)** Integrated processes: nursing process — evaluation; client need: physiological integrity; basic care and comfort; content area: nutrition.

   RATIONALE

   (1) English muffins; any whole-grain bread or bagels; fresh, frozen, or dried fruit; and lean pork such as Canadian bacon are low in fat. **(2)** Buttermilk, pork sausage, and fried potatoes are high in fat. **(3)** French toast and chocolate milk are high in fat. Smoked salmon, if canned in water, is acceptable. **(4)** Croissants are very high in fat, as is corned beef. Skim milk is a good choice.

9. **(3)** Integrated processes: nursing process — evaluation; client need: physiological integrity; basic care and comfort; content area: nutrition.

   RATIONALE

   (1) Pernicious anemia occurs from a deficit in vitamin B_{12}, which cannot be absorbed because of a lack of the intrinsic factor, produced by specialized cells in the stomach. It must be given IM. **(2)** Malabsorption occurs despite adequate dietary intake. **(3)** Because there is no source of intrinsic factor as a result of the gastrectomy, vitamin B_{12} must be given parentally. **(4)** The vitamin cannot be absorbed from food because of the lack of intrinsic factor.

10. **(4)** Integrated processes: nursing process — planning; teaching/learning; client need: physiological integrity; basic care and comfort; content area: nutrition.

    RATIONALE

    (1) Limiting nursing time in the first several days will not prevent sore nipples and may hinder milk production. **(2)** The more a baby nurses, the more milk is produced. **(3)** Sore nipples are usually caused by incorrect nursing position. A tummy-to-tummy position or a football hold is correct. The baby's lips should make a tight seal around the breast. **(4)** A baby undergoes growth spurts at 10 days, 2 weeks, 6 weeks, and 3 months. The baby should nurse frequently. A fussy newborn is probably ready to feed.

11. **(2)** Integrated processes: nursing process — evaluation; client need: physiological integrity; basic care and comfort; content area: nutrition.

RATIONALE

(1) *Staphylococcus aureus* found on skin is transmitted to foods requiring handling in preparation, such as salads. Symptoms occur 2–3 hours after eating the food. (2) Eggs, poultry, and other foods containing the *S. aureus* can cause symptoms 12–24 hours after eating the contaminated food. (3) Meats, gravies, and casseroles can contain *Clostridium perfringens*, which causes cramps or diarrhea from a toxin released by the organism growing in the intestine. (4) Raw seafood or fish can cause vibriosis 2–48 hours after eating the contaminated food. Flu-like symptoms are exhibited.

12. (1) Integrated processes: nursing process — evaluation; teaching/learning; client need: physiological integrity; basic care and comfort; content area: nutrition.

    RATIONALE

    (1) Meat should be weighed after cooking. (2) Visible fat should be trimmed off before or after cooking. (3) Meat does not contain fiber, but dried beans, peas, and lentils are good sources of fiber. (4) Some processed meats, seafood, and soy products contain large amounts of carbohydrates.

13. (1) Integrated processes: nursing process — evaluation; teaching/learning; client need: physiological integrity; basic care and comfort; content area: nutrition.

    RATIONALE

    (1) Corn and peas are considered starches. (2) One-half cup cooked beans is a vegetable. (3) One-half cup carrots is considered a vegetable. (4) One-half cup tomatoes is considered a vegetable.

14. (4) Integrated processes: nursing process — evaluation; teaching/learning; client need: physiological integrity; basic care and comfort; content area: nutrition.

    RATIONALE

    (1) One-half cup grits counts as a cereal and grain. (2) One-half cup pasta counts as a cereal and grain. (3) One-third cup rice counts as a cereal and grain. (4) Three cups of popcorn counts as one starch and one fat.

15. (3) Integrated processes: nursing process — planning; client need: physiological integrity; basic care and comfort; content area: nutrition.

    RATIONALE

    (1) Her weight before pregnancy was appropriate for her height, and a gain of 15–20 lb would be inadequate; inadequate gains increase the risk of delivering a low-birth-weight infant. (2) Her weight before pregnancy was appropriate for her height, and a gain of 15–20 lb would be inadequate; inadequate gains increase the risk of delivering a low-birth-weight infant. (3) A gain of 25–30 lb would be associated with the best pregnancy outcome. (4) A gain of 39 lb would provide no additional advantage to the infant, and excessive weight gained during pregnancy might be hard for the mother to lose afterward.

16. (1) Integrated processes: nursing process — evaluation; client need: physiological integrity; basic care and comfort; content area: nutrition.

    RATIONALE

    (1) The client receives little sun exposure. Unless her diet history indicates that she consumes a quart of milk or other good sources of vitamin D daily, a supplement is indicated. (2) There are no data to indicate the need for a calcium supplement. (3) There are no data to indicate the need for a vitamin C supplement. (4) There are no data to indicate the need for a zinc supplement.

17. (1) Integrated processes; nursing process — implementation; teaching/learning; client need: physiological integrity; basic care and comfort; content area: nutrition.

    RATIONALE

    (1) Plain, dry, carbohydrate-containing foods (e.g., dry toast, crackers) on awakening help to alleviate the nausea experienced by some women. (2) Increased intake of fluids during the morning, when nausea is most common, may worsen the symptoms. (3) Fatty foods may worsen nausea, and carbohydrates can supply most of her caloric needs. (4) Reducing intake of fluids in the early morning may help to reduce nausea, but restricting fluids altogether is inadvisable because the pregnant woman needs increased fluids for expansion of plasma volume, synthesis of amniotic fluid, excretion of wastes, and other vital bodily processes.

18. (4) Integrated processes: nursing process — implementation; teaching/learning; client need: physiological integrity; basic care and comfort; content area: nutrition.

    RATIONALE

    (1) The presence of food in the stomach is likely to inhibit absorption of iron. (2) Milk is an inhibitor of iron absorption. (3) "Heme" iron from meats is better absorbed than iron from most supplements, and thus enhances iron nutrition. Moreover, during pregnancy, the woman is highly interested in nutrition and motivated to eat well, and this is a good time to emphasize the principles of a sound diet. (4) Vitamin C sources such as these enhance the absorption of iron from the supplement.

19. (3) Integrated processes: nursing process — implementation; teaching/learning; client need: physiological integrity; basic care and comfort; content area: nutrition.

    RATIONALE

    (1) Cholesterol intake has no known deleterious effect on the fetus. (2) Pregnant women without hypertension have no need to restrict sodium unduly. (3) Alcohol consumption during pregnancy may result in congenital malformations and learning disabilities. (4) Saturated fat has no deleterious effect on the fetus.

20. (4) Integrated processes: nursing process — implementation; teaching/learning; client need: physiological integrity; basic care and comfort; content area: nutrition.

    RATIONALE

    (1) Fruit is low in protein and sodium and thus would not exacerbate liver failure and fluid retention. (2) Carrots are low in protein, and butter would help to provide needed calories. (3) Boiled potato is low in sodium and protein. (4) Unless low-sodium products are used, soup is high in sodium. In addition, the soup could be included in the diet only if the milk products and poultry contained in the soup were included within the daily protein allowance.

21. (1) Integrated processes: nursing process — evaluation; client need: physiological integrity; basic care and comfort; content area: nutrition.

    RATIONALE

    (1) Corn contains no gluten. (2) Buckwheat is believed by many authorities to contain gluten. In any event, buckwheat pancakes are normally made with added wheat flour, which would be a gluten source. (3) Oats contain gluten. (4) Wheat germ contains gluten.

22. (3) Integrated processes: nursing process — implementation; client need: physiological integrity; basic care and comfort; content area: nutrition.

RATIONALE

(1) Canned pears, drained of their juice, are almost free of sodium and are low in fluid and potassium. **(2)** Bread is low in water content and potassium. **(3)** Oranges are rich in potassium. **(4)** Unsalted butter is almost free of sodium and provides needed calories.

23. **(2)** Integrated processes: nursing process — implementation; teaching/learning; client need: physiological integrity; basic care and comfort; content area: nutrition.

RATIONALE

(1) Fat deposits insulate the body to prevent heat loss. **(2)** The primary role of carbohydrates is to provide energy. Some cells, particularly red blood cells (RBCs) and the central nervous system (CNS) cells, rely primarily on carbohydrates to meet their energy needs. **(3)** Proteins (amino acids) are the primary building blocks for new tissue. **(4)** Some complex carbohydrates do provide fiber, but fiber is not the major reason for consuming dietary carbohydrate.

24. **(3)** Integrated processes: nursing process — evaluation; client need: physiological integrity; basic care and comfort; content area: nutrition.

RATIONALE

(1) Cheese is made from milk, but its protein and fat contents are more similar to those of meat than to the items on the milk exchange list. **(2)** The protein and fat contents of cheese are similar to those of meat. **(3)** Items in the fat exchange list are primarily composed of fat, and cheese is a good source of protein. **(4)** The protein and fat contents of cheese are more similar to those of meat than to the items on the milk exchange list.

25. **(2)** Integrated processes: nursing process — implementation; teaching/learning; client need: physiological integrity; basic care and comfort; content area: nutrition.

RATIONALE

(1) Starchy vegetables such as potatoes are more similar in carbohydrate and protein contents to most foods on the starch-bread exchange list than to other vegetables. **(2)** Potatoes are similar in carbohydrate and protein contents to foods on the starch-bread exchange list. **(3)** Potatoes contain more protein than most foods on the fruit exchange list. **(4)** Starchy vegetables such as potatoes are more similar in their carbohydrate and protein contents to most foods on the starch-bread exchange list than to other vegetables.

26. **(4)** Integrated processes: nursing process — planning; client need: physiological integrity; basic care and comfort; content area: nutrition.

RATIONALE

(1) Protein can be absorbed in the upper portion of the small intestine. Adequate protein is needed to promote healing and hypertrophy (enlargement) of the remaining bowel. **(2)** Fluid is largely absorbed in the colon. Adequate fluid is needed to replace diarrheal losses. **(3)** Sodium is lost in diarrhea and needs to be replaced by dietary intake. **(4)** The ileum is the primary site for fat absorption. After resection of the ileum, fat restriction often reduces the volume of stools and improves client comfort.

27. **(1)** Integrated processes: nursing process — evaluation; teaching/learning; client need: physiological integrity; basic care and comfort; content area: nutrition.

RATIONALE

(1) Fresh and dried vegetables and fruits are among the best dietary sources of fiber, which adds bulk to the stools and helps to prevent constipation. **(2)** Sesame seeds provide some fiber, but the number included on the bun would be inadequate to add bulk to stools. **(3)** Mashed potatoes contain starch but little fiber. **(4)** The heating required in the canning process reduces the fiber content of canned fruits and vegetables.

28. **(4)** Integrated processes: nursing process phase: implementation; client need: physiological integrity; basic care and comfort; content area: nutrition.

RATIONALE

(1) An inrush of air can sometimes be heard over the upper left abdominal quadrant even when the tube is positioned in the bronchus or pleural space. **(2)** If the tube is in the pleural space or lodged against the wall of the bronchus, air bubbles may not be emitted during exhalation. **(3)** New "nonreactive" (polyurethane, silicone rubber, and similar substances) tubes are less irritating than the harder tubes previously used and may not cause gagging or respiratory distress even when located in the pulmonary system. In any event, an obtunded client would be unlikely to display these signs. **(4)** Radiographic evidence is the most certain method of confirming appropriate tube placement.

29. **(4)** Integrated processes: nursing process — planning; client need: physiological integrity; basic care and comfort; content area: nutrition.

RATIONALE

(1) Magnesium absorption is not affected by a gastrectomy. **(2)** Folic acid absorption can be affected, but vitamin B_{12} is a greater concern because of its neurological and RBC formation effects. **(3)** Chloride is a principal body anion in the extracellular fluid whose absorption is not affected by a gastrectomy. **(4)** Hydrochloric acid, produced in the stomach, is required to split vitamin B_{12} away from the proteins to which it is bound in food. Intrinsic factor, produced by the gastric mucosa, must be bound to vitamin B_{12} for the vitamin to be absorbed in the ileum. Adults generally have vitamin B_{12} stores sufficient to last approximately 3 years, but after that time, parenteral vitamin B_{12} will be required.

30. **(1)** Integrated processes: nursing process — implementation; client need: physiological integrity; basic care and comfort; content area: nutrition.

RATIONALE

(1) The client needs a high-protein, high-calorie diet for tissue healing and replacement of blood and tissue proteins lost as a result of the burn. These choices provide the most protein and are also rich in calories. **(2)** These choices are good sources of calories, which the client needs to meet his energy needs, but they provide little protein. **(3)** Orange juice and vegetables are low in calories and protein. **(4)** These choices are lower in protein and calories than a peanut butter sandwich and a milkshake.

31. **(2)** Integrated processes: nursing process — planning; client need: physiological integrity; basic care and comfort; content area: nutrition.

RATIONALE

(1) Folic acid is necessary for forming RBCs, which are lost in burns, but zinc is especially important for increasing the strength of healing wounds. **(2)** Zinc increases the tensile strength (the force needed to separate the edges) of healing wounds. **(3)** Iron is needed to replace blood losses, but zinc is especially important for wound healing. **(4)** Vitamin K is required for formation of clotting factors.

32. **(1)** Integrated processes: nursing process — implementation; client need: physiological integrity; basic care and comfort; content area: nutrition.

RATIONALE
(1) Tea is the only choice that is a clear liquid. (2) This food is not a clear liquid. (3) This food is not a clear liquid. (4) This food is not a clear liquid.

33. (1) Integrated processes: nursing process — implementation; client need: physiological integrity; basic care and comfort; content area: nutrition.

RATIONALE
(1) Neither noodles nor chicken chunks would be liquid at room temperature, which is the criterion for including a food in a full-liquid diet. (2) Ice cream is liquid at room temperature. (3) Cream of tomato soup is liquid at room temperature. (4) Custard is liquid at room temperature.

34. (4) Integrated processes: nursing process — implementation; teaching/learning; client need: physiological integrity; basic care and comfort; content area: nutrition.

RATIONALE
(1) Eighty-eight percent of the kilocalories in avocados are derived from fat. (2) Muffins and other "quick breads" (unless specially prepared) contain oil, butter, or margarine, as well as fat from egg yolk. (3) Chocolate candies contain cocoa butter or other fats. (4) Angel food cake contains no egg yolk or other sources of fat.

35. (4) Integrated processes: nursing process — implementation; teaching/learning; client need: physiological integrity; basic care and comfort; content area: nutrition.

RATIONALE
(1) It is essential to read labels to determine whether foods contain proteins (because proteins provide phenylalanine) or are sweetened with aspartame. (2) Infants are initially fed a low-phenylalanine formula or breast milk. As children mature, they eat a wider variety of foods, which requires more vigilance by the family. (3) With careful supervision, it is possible for infants with PKU to be breast-fed. If the mother chooses not to breast-feed, the baby will require a special low-phenylalanine formula. (4) Individuals with PKU display improved mental function if they continue the phenylalanine-restricted diet indefinitely. It is especially important that women who wish to have children ensure that their phenylalanine levels are controlled before they conceive and during pregnancy.

36. (4) Integrated processes: nursing process — implementation; client need: physiological integrity; basic care and comfort; content area: nutrition.

RATIONALE
(1) Starchy vegetables such as potatoes contain some protein and thus supply phenylalanine. (2) Pasta and other grain products are sources of protein. (3) Corn contains some protein and thus supplies phenylalanine. (4) Fruits, which are generally low in protein, provide little phenylalanine.

37. (3) Integrated processes: nursing process — implementation; client need: physiological integrity; basic care and comfort; content area: nutrition.

RATIONALE
(1) Sherbet generally contains milk and therefore contains galactose. (2) Butter contains traces of lactose. (3) Noodles are made without milk or lactose and therefore are galactose free. Food labels or the product manufacturer should be consulted if there is any question about a product's lactose content. (4) Unless they are specially prepared, pancakes are made with milk.

38. (1) Integrated processes: nursing process — implementation; client need: physiological integrity; basic care and comfort; content area: nutrition.

RATIONALE
(1) Infant cereals from all types of grains are usually equivalent in price. (2) Pancreatic amylase activity increases from low levels at birth to relatively normal levels at 4 months, and this prepares the infant to digest the starch in cereal grains. (3) Infant cereals are a good choice for a first food because they are fortified with iron. Iron stores deposited in utero and in the postnatal period begin to be depleted between 3 and 6 months of age. (4) Rice is considered the least allergenic cereal grain for infants; wheat is among the foods that are most likely to cause allergies in infants.

39. (2) Integrated processes: nursing process — evaluation; teaching/learning; client need: physiological integrity; basic care and comfort; content area: nutrition.

RATIONALE
(1) Iron-fortified infant formula, rather than cow's milk, is recommended until 12 months of age because the infant needs good sources of iron and because cow's milk is likely to cause gastrointestinal (GI) blood loss. (2) Egg white is not recommended for infants younger than 12 months because it is commonly associated with allergy when started earlier. (3) The 9-month-old infant enjoys finger foods such as toast strips. (4) Cottage cheese provides high protein.

40. (3) Integrated processes: nursing process — implementation; self-care; client need: physiological integrity; basic care and comfort; content area: nutrition.

RATIONALE
(1) Fish contains some sodium, but unless it is prepared with added salt, there is no need to avoid it on a 2-g sodium diet. (2) Hard rolls and most other yeast breads are relatively low in sodium and can be included in a 2-g sodium diet. (3) Peanut butter is prepared with salt unless a special salt-free product is used. (4) Milk contains sodium, but at this level of sodium restriction, there is no need to limit its intake unduly.

41. (4) Integrated processes: nursing process — implementation; self-care; client need: physiological integrity; basic care and comfort; content area: nutrition.

RATIONALE
(1) Worcestershire sauce, as well as many other seasonings and condiments, is prepared with salt. (2) Garlic salt, as well as many other seasonings and condiments, is prepared with salt. (3) Ketchup, as well as many other seasonings and condiments, is prepared with salt. (4) Lemon juice is virtually sodium free.

42. (2) Integrated processes: nursing process — evaluation; teaching/learning; client need: physiological integrity; basic care and comfort; content area: nutrition.

RATIONALE
(1) Polyunsaturated and monounsaturated fats do not elevate serum cholesterol. (2) Excessive intake of saturated fats is associated with elevations of serum cholesterol. (3) Polyunsaturated fats tend to reduce cholesterol levels. (4) Monounsaturated fats in the diet tend to reduce serum cholesterol or have a neutral effect on it.

43. (3) Integrated processes: nursing process — evaluation; teaching/learning; client need: physiological integrity; basic care and comfort; content area: nutrition.

RATIONALE
(1) Whole milk is rich in milk fat, which is saturated, and contains cholesterol. (2) Two percent milk contains saturated fat and cholesterol. (3) Skim milk is virtually devoid of saturated fat. (4) Sweet acidophilus milk is usually whole or 2% milk. It contains bacterial cultures, but they do not change the fat content.

44. **(3)** Integrated processes: nursing process — evaluation; teaching/learning; client need: physiological integrity; basic care and comfort; content area: nutrition.

RATIONALE

(1) Strawberries (and most other fruits) are low in calcium. **(2)** Raisins are low in calcium. **(3)** Deep-green leafy vegetables, with the exceptions of spinach and Swiss chard, are fair sources of calcium. Spinach and chard contain calcium, but also contain so much oxalic acid that absorption of their calcium is prevented. **(4)** Corn is a poor calcium source.

45. **(2)** Integrated processes: nursing process — planning; teaching/learning; client need: physiological integrity; basic care and comfort; content area: nutrition.

RATIONALE

(1) Rapid weight loss often occurs with use of liquid-formula diets, but the weight is usually regained. **(2)** A low-calorie diet, in addition to an increase in activity, is the most effective way to promote lasting weight loss. **(3)** Exercise alone tones the body and increases the muscle mass but rarely results in substantial weight loss. **(4)** A low-calorie diet alone will result in gradual weight loss, but the addition of exercise to the regimen often helps to curb the appetite and to take the dieter's mind off food.

46. **(4)** Integrated processes: nursing process — caring; implementation; client need: physiological integrity; basic care and comfort; content area: nutrition.

RATIONALE

(1) Growth in infants receiving breast milk is comparable to growth in those receiving commercial formulas. **(2)** Breast feeding is often less expensive than formula feeding. The only real cost of breast feeding (other than a one-time expense for nursing bras) is that resulting from the mother's need for a modest increase in her caloric and protein intake. If she chooses foods wisely, she can meet these increased needs very inexpensively. **(3)** There is no increase in colic in breast-fed infants. **(4)** Young infants are especially prone to development of allergies. Breast milk is much less likely to cause an allergic reaction than cow's milk or soy, the protein sources used in most infant formulas.

47. **(3)** Integrated processes: nursing process — planning; client need: physiological integrity; basic care and comfort; content area: nutrition.

RATIONALE

(1) Human milk is adequate in zinc to meet the needs of full-term infants. **(2)** Human milk is adequate in vitamin E to meet the needs of full-term infants. **(3)** Human milk provides little fluoride, so the breast-fed infant usually needs a supplement at an early age to ensure proper tooth formation. **(4)** Human milk has adequate thiamine to meet the infant's needs.

48. **(2)** Integrated processes: nursing process — implementation; teaching/learning; client need: physiological integrity; basic care and comfort; content area: nutrition.

RATIONALE

(1) Early initiation of solid foods does not improve later acceptance of foods. **(2)** The young infant is prone to development of allergies, and exposure to a wide variety of antigens from foods is apt to result in allergy. **(3)** Research has shown that infants begin to sleep through the night when they reach approximately 11 lb, and introducing solid foods early does not accelerate the process. **(4)** Early introduction of solid foods does not reduce the risk of obesity. Very young infants are less able to communicate their satiety and may be overfed by zealous caregivers. Older infants communicate by turning their heads away, withdrawing eye contact, drooling out food, or refusing to open their lips.

49. **(4)** Integrated processes: nursing process — planning; teaching/learning; client need: physiological integrity; basic care and comfort; content area: nutrition.

RATIONALE

(1) Cow's milk is not recommended for infants younger than 12 months because it is a poor source of iron and often causes GI blood loss. **(2)** Infants are rapidly growing and need the kilocalories provided by fat; use of skim milk may impair growth. There is no evidence that use of skim milk in infancy has any beneficial effects on later heart disease. **(3)** A reliable source of iron, such as iron-fortified formula, is needed by rapidly growing infants. Use of formula without iron is likely to result is iron-deficiency anemia. **(4)** Iron-fortified formula is recommended until 12 months of age because it provides a reliable source of iron and helps to prevent iron-deficiency anemia.

50. **(4)** Integrated processes: nursing process — evaluation; client need: physiological integrity; basic care and comfort; content area: nutrition.

RATIONALE

(1) Milk is a good source of calcium, phosphorus, and protein. **(2)** Milk is a good source of calcium, phosphorus, and protein. **(3)** Milk is a good source of calcium, phosphorus, and protein. **(4)** Milk is an extremely poor source of iron. Excessive milk consumption by toddlers results in "milk anemia."

51. **(2)** Integrated processes: nursing process — implementation; client need: physiological integrity; basic care and comfort; content area: nutrition.

RATIONALE

(1) Biscuits are prepared with shortening. **(2)** This meal is almost fat free. **(3)** Poached eggs contain 5 g of fat each. **(4)** Muffins are prepared with oil or margarine and eggs.

52. **(1)** Integrated processes; nursing process — evaluation; teaching/learning; client need: physiological integrity; basic care and comfort; content area: nutrition.

RATIONALE

(1) Vitamin C is necessary for maintaining capillary walls; thus deficiency often results in bleeding. **(2)** Vitamin D is involved primarily in regulation of calcium and phosphorus metabolism. **(3)** Vitamin E is an antioxidant and is important in maintaining red cell membranes and in preventing anemia. **(4)** Vitamin A deficiency is commonly associated with deterioration of vision, roughening of the skin, and atrophy of the mucous membranes.

53. **(1)** Integrated processes; nursing process — evaluation; teaching/learning; client need: physiological integrity; basic care and comfort; content area: nutrition.

RATIONALE

(1) Iron-deficiency anemia is the most common nutritional anemia in the United States in virtually all age groups. **(2)** Deficiency of folic acid may occur in malnourished individuals; pregnant women and infants are also at risk, but it is not as widespread as iron deficiency. **(3)** The only individuals at serious risk of dietary deficiency of vitamin B_{12} are strict vegetarians. Also, impaired absorption is likely in individuals with gastric or ileal resection, but this problem affects only a limited number of people. **(4)** Impaired production of intrinsic factor occurs spontaneously in some individuals and also after gastric resection, but this problem affects only a limited number of people.

54. **(4)** Integrated processes: nursing process — evaluation; client need: physiological integrity; basic care and comfort; content area: nutrition.

RATIONALE

(1) If the esophagus is obstructed, no oral feedings would be able to bypass the obstruction. (2) If the esophagus is obstructed, no oral feedings would be able to bypass the obstruction. (3) If the esophagus is obstructed, no oral feedings would be able to bypass the obstruction. (4) Gastrostomy feedings would bypass the obstruction.

55. (1) Integrated processes: nursing process — planning; teaching/learning; client need: physiological integrity; basic care and comfort; content area: nutrition.

RATIONALE

(1) Amino acids derived from proteins are components of antibodies. (2) Fat is not a component of antibodies. (3) Thiamine is not a component of antibodies. (4) Riboflavin is not a component of antibodies.

56. (2) Integrated processes: nursing process — planning; client need: physiological integrity; basic care and comfort; content area: nutrition.

RATIONALE

(1) There is no need to prepare the client for oral surgery with a low-residue diet. (2) Some physicians use a low-residue diet before GI surgery to decrease the fecal content of the GI tract during surgery. (3) There is no need for a low-residue diet before head and neck surgery. (4) A low-residue diet is not indicated for any surgery except surgery of the GI tract.

57. (4) Integrated processes: nursing process — evaluation; client need: physiological integrity; basic care and comfort; content area: nutrition.

RATIONALE

(1) The fat and protein provided by the fish would be slowly digested and might reduce symptoms of dumping syndrome. (2) The fat and protein provided by the egg would be slowly digested and might reduce symptoms of dumping syndrome. (3) The starch provided by the bagel would be less likely than simple carbohydrates to cause dumping because it would be gradually hydrolyzed and would not increase the osmolality of the small bowel as rapidly as simple carbohydrates. (4) Simple carbohydrates such as the sucrose in fruit gelatins enter the small bowel quickly after ingestion and rapidly increase the osmolality of the bowel content. Thus, they are the nutrients most likely to cause symptoms in the person with dumping syndrome.

58. (4) Integrated processes: nursing process — planning; teaching/learning; client need: physiological integrity; basic care and comfort; content area: nutrition.

RATIONALE

(1) Fluids present in the stomach at the same time as food increase the speed of gastric emptying and thus increase the likelihood of dumping syndrome. (2) Fluids present in the stomach at the same time as food increase the speed of gastric emptying and thus increase the likelihood of dumping syndrome. (3) Fluids present in the stomach at the same time as food increase the speed of gastric emptying and thus increase the likelihood of dumping syndrome. (4) Avoiding fluids until at least 0.5–1.0 hour after meals reduces the speed with which foods are emptied from the stomach.

59. (2) Integrated processes: nursing process — teaching/learning; evaluation; client need: physiological integrity; basic care and comfort; content area: nutrition.

RATIONALE

(1) It is unusual to experience maldigestion of milk protein. (2) Many adults lack lactase, the enzyme required to digest lactose (milk sugar). The undigested carbohydrate passes into the

colon, where it draws fluid into the feces and often causes cramping and diarrhea. (3) Select another answer. (4) Select another answer.

60. (2) Integrated processes: nursing process — planning; teaching/learning; client need: physiological integrity; basic care and comfort; content area: nutrition.

RATIONALE

(1) The client's intake of animal products (which are the only sources of cholesterol) is limited to one serving of milk and the meat and cheese contained in the lasagna, so his cholesterol intake should not be excessive. (2) The Dietary Guidelines for Americans recommends only a moderate alcohol intake; defined as no more than two drinks per day. A 12-oz glass of beer is equivalent to one drink, so the client's intake is excessive. (3) Whole-grain breads, oatmeal, legumes (beans), and vegetables provide good sources of fiber in the diet. (4) The broccoli and salad are equivalent to three vegetable servings; three to five are recommended.

61. (2) Integrated processes: nursing process — evaluation; client need: physiological integrity; basic care and comfort; content area: nutrition.

RATIONALE

(1) Individuals at 5% of desirable weight are usually described as "normal weight." (2) Although there are exceptions, individuals whose weight is ≥20% of the ideal or desirable weight for their height are usually considered obese. (3) Individuals whose weights are at least 20% more than the ideal or desirable weight are usually considered obese. (4) Individuals whose weights are at least 20% more than the ideal or desirable weight are usually considered obese.

62. (4) Integrated processes: nursing process —teaching/learning; evaluation; client need: physiological integrity; basic care and comfort; content area: nutrition.

RATIONALE

(1) Obesity does not increase the risk of peptic ulcers. (2) Obesity does not increase the risk of periodontal disease. (3) Obesity does not increase the risk of scleroderma. (4) Obesity is a risk factor for development of hypertension.

63. (1) Integrated processes: nursing process — evaluation; teaching/learning; client need: physiological integrity; basic care and comfort; content area: nutrition.

RATIONALE

(1) Although rest can be important, lying down immediately after eating increases the reflux of acid gastric contents. (2) Snacking at bedtime may cause reflux if the client lies down to sleep shortly afterwards. (3) Obesity is often a precipitating cause of reflux and subsequent pain. (4) Use of antacids may help to control the symptoms.

64. (3) Integrated processes: nursing process — evaluation; client need: physiological integrity; basic care and comfort; content area: nutrition.

RATIONALE

(1) One-half cup pineapple has about 2 g of fiber. (2) Potatoes have about 3.8 g of fiber. (3) Popcorn has about 10 g of fiber. (4) Roast beef has about 5 g of fiber.

65. (3) Integrated processes: nursing process — implementation; teaching/learning; client need: physiological integrity; basic care and comfort; content area: nutrition.

RATIONALE

(1) Fruit sugar is fructose. (2) Table sugar is sucrose. (3) Lactose, or milk sugar, is hydrolyzed or digested by enzymes in the mucosal lining of the GI tract. The concentrations of these

enzymes is very low after acute gastroenteritis, and a formula providing carbohydrates other than lactose may be better tolerated than milk-based formulas. **(4)** Corn syrup is glucose or dextrose.

66. **(1)** Integrated processes: nursing process — data collection; client need: physiological integrity; basic care and comfort; content area: nutrition.
RATIONALE
(1) Dehydration, which can occur relatively rapidly in an infant of this age, is manifested by dry, sticky mucous membranes, poor skin turgor, and an acute weight loss. **(2)** A fluid does not cause edema or weight gain. The infant may get a "diaper" skin rash if not cleaned properly, but observing for a fluid volume deficit is most critical. **(3)** The infant has a fluid loss. **(4)** A fluid does not cause edema or weight gain. The infant may get a diaper skin rash if not cleaned properly, but observing for a fluid volume deficit is most critical.

67. **(3)** Integrated processes: nursing process — planning; teaching/learning; client need: physiological integrity; basic care and comfort; content area: nutrition.
RATIONALE
(1) Iron is recommended throughout pregnancy and lactation. **(2)** Iron is recommended throughout pregnancy and lactation. **(3)** Iron supplements are recommended throughout pregnancy to allow the marked expansion in RBC production. Although lactation does not require large amounts of iron, because little iron is secreted in milk, an iron supplement is recommended during lactation to replenish stores that may have been depleted during pregnancy. **(4)** Iron is recommended throughout pregnancy and lactation.

68. **(2)** Integrated processes: nursing process — planning; self-care; client need: physiological integrity; basic care and comfort; content area: nutrition.
RATIONALE
(1) A weight of 135 lb is less than the optimal weight gain. **(2)** Optimal fetal outcome is achieved with a maternal weight gain of approximately 25–30 lb during pregnancy. **(3)** A weight of 159 lb is over the 25–30 lb weight recommended. **(4)** A weight of 165 lb is over the 25–30 lb weight recommended.

69. **(1)** Integrated processes; nursing process — implementation; teaching/learning; client need: physiological integrity; basic care and comfort; content area: nutrition.
RATIONALE
(1) The diet for the insulin-dependent client is designed to provide carbohydrates at times when insulin is at its peak activity. **(2)** Exchanges should neither be omitted nor shifted from one time of the day to another. **(3)** Exchanges should neither be omitted nor shifted from one time of the day to another. **(4)** Insulin regimens can be adjusted for departures from usual eating and exercise habits, but meal plans are based on an individual's usual food intakes.

70. **(3)** Integrated processes: nursing process — implementation; client need: physiological integrity; basic care and comfort; content area: nutrition.
RATIONALE
(1) When a complete intestinal obstruction develops, particularly one low in the GI tract, enteral feedings are not tolerated. **(2)** When a complete intestinal obstruction develops, particularly one low in the GI tract, enteral feedings are not tolerated. **(3)** Only total parenteral nutrition provides nutrients while bypassing the GI obstruction. **(4)** When a complete intestinal obstruction develops, particularly one low in the GI tract, enteral feedings are not tolerated.

71. **(2)** Integrated processes: nursing process — evaluation; teaching/learning; client need: physiological integrity; basic care and comfort; content area: nutrition.
RATIONALE
(1) Different fats have different effects on blood cholesterol levels. **(2)** Saturated fats tend to increase blood cholesterol. **(3)** Polyunsaturated fats have a neutral effect on, or lower, blood cholesterol. **(4)** Monounsaturated fats have a neutral effect on, or lower, blood cholesterol.

72. **(1)** Integrated processes: nursing process — evaluation; teaching/learning; client need: physiological integrity; basic care and comfort; content area: nutrition.
RATIONALE
(1) Only animal products contain cholesterol. Even if the visible fat in meats is trimmed away, the tissues contain cholesterol. **(2)** Avocado is a nonanimal product. **(3)** Peanuts are a nonanimal product. **(4)** Palm oil is a nonanimal product.

73. **(1)** Integrated processes: nursing process — implementation; client need: physiological integrity; basic care and comfort; content area: nutrition.
RATIONALE
(1) He is probably receiving a low-protein, low-potassium, low-sodium diet. If the nurse wants to provide him with a snack that has not been figured into his diet plan, then hard candy, a simple carbohydrate, is the safest. **(2)** Soft drinks provide fluid, and he probably has a fluid restriction; in addition, they provide phosphorus, which may further reduce kidney function. **(3)** Cheese is rich in sodium and high in protein. **(4)** Most fresh fruits are good or excellent sources of potassium.

74. **(2)** Integrated processes: nursing process — evaluation; client need: physiological integrity; basic care and comfort; content area: nutrition.
RATIONALE
(1) Biscuits and other quick breads are high in fat, as is margarine. **(2)** This choice is the lowest in fat and cholesterol. **(3)** Eggs are rich in cholesterol. **(4)** Cream cheese is high in cholesterol.

75. **(4)** Integrated processes: nursing process — evaluation; client need: physiological integrity; basic care and comfort; content area: nutrition.
RATIONALE
(1) Ketchup is high in sodium. **(2)** Processed meats such as bologna are high in sodium. **(3)** Soups are high in sodium. **(4)** All are low-sodium foods.

76. **(2)** Integrated processes: nursing process — evaluation; client need: physiological integrity; basic care and comfort; content area: nutrition.
RATIONALE
(1) Flour contains wheat, which contains gluten. **(2)** Rice is the only grain listed that does not contain gluten. **(3)** Barley contains gluten. **(4)** Oatmeal contains gluten.

77. **(4)** Integrated processes: nursing process — data collection; client need: physiological integrity; basic care and comfort; content area: nutrition.
RATIONALE
(1) Excessive vitamin E may endanger the cardiovascular system but is less harmful than vitamin A. Vitamin A is more dangerous to the liver in both the mother and neonate. **(2)** Biotin is water soluble and unlikely to be toxic. **(3)** Folic acid is water soluble. **(4)** Vitamin A is toxic when taken in excessive amounts.

78. **(4)** Integrated processes: nursing process — planning; self-care; client need: physiological integrity; basic care and comfort; content area: nutrition.
    RATIONALE
    (1) Increasing the number of rest periods decreases GI motility and aggravates constipation. **(2)** Protein does not affect constipation. **(3)** Decreasing fluids increases the risk of constipation. **(4)** The fiber provided by complex carbohydrates increases fecal bulk and reduces constipation.

79. **(4)** Integrated processes: nursing process — implementation; client need: physiological integrity; basic care and comfort; content area: nutrition.
    RATIONALE
    (1) Orange juice is a simple carbohydrate that makes absorption occur rapidly. **(2)** Honey is a simple carbohydrate that makes absorption occur rapidly. **(3)** Hard candy is a simple carbohydrate that makes absorption occur rapidly. **(4)** A simple carbohydrate is needed for fast digestion and absorption; cheese is the most complex carbohydrate listed.

80. **(3)** Integrated processes: nursing process — planning; client need: physiological integrity; basic care and comfort; content area: nutrition.
    RATIONALE
    (1) Fresh fruit is rapidly absorbed and provides quick energy. This would not help with endurance. **(2)** Orange juice is rapidly absorbed and provides quick energy. This would not help with endurance. **(3)** Cheese and crackers are complex carbohydrates that will be digested and absorbed slowly. This will assist in maintaining the blood glucose level at a stable level during the exercise. **(4)** Soda is rapidly absorbed and provides quick energy. This would not help with endurance.

81. **(4)** Integrated processes: nursing process — planning; teaching/learning; client need: physiological integrity; basic care and comfort; content area: nutrition.
    RATIONALE
    (1) Vitamin A is fat soluble. **(2)** Vitamin D is fat soluble. **(3)** Vitamin K is fat soluble. **(4)** Vitamin B_{12} is not fat soluble.

82. **(3)** Integrated processes: nursing process — planning; client need: physiological integrity; basic care and comfort; content area: nutrition.
    RATIONALE
    (1) Cheese contains lactose. **(2)** Ice cream contains lactose. **(3)** Soybean milk is used as a substitute for milk because it does not contain lactose. **(4)** Goat milk contains lactose.

83. **(1)** Integrated processes: nursing process — planning; client need: physiological integrity; basic care and comfort; content area: nutrition.
    RATIONALE
    (1) Lactase is the enzyme that digests milk products. Lactase is the deficient enzyme in lactose intolerance. **(2)** Maltase is starch sugar. **(3)** Peptase is not a word. **(4)** Amylase is a pancreatic enzyme.

84. **(2)** Integrated processes: nursing process — planning; teaching/learning; client need: physiological integrity; basic care and comfort; content area: nutrition.
    RATIONALE
    (1) A gluten-free diet should be high in protein, calories, vitamins, and minerals to maintain a balanced nutritional state. **(2)** A low-protein diet does not meet the requirement of a gluten-free diet: high protein, high calories, and high vitamins and minerals. **(3)** A gluten-free diet should be high in protein, calo-

ries, vitamins, and minerals to maintain a balanced nutritional state. **(4)** A gluten-free diet should be high in protein, calories, vitamins, and minerals to maintain a balanced nutritional state.

85. **(1)** Integrated processes: nursing process — implementation; teaching/learning; client need: physiological integrity; basic care and comfort; content area: nutrition.
    RATIONALE
    (1) A clear-liquid diet contains foods that are clear and liquid at room temperature. Milk is not clear at room temperature. **(2)** Tea is a clear liquid at room temperature. **(3)** Broth is a clear liquid at room temperature. **(4)** Apple juice is a clear liquid at room temperature.

86. **(1)** Integrated processes: nursing process — implementation; client need: physiological integrity; basic care and comfort; content area: nutrition.
    RATIONALE
    (1) A burn client should be placed on a high-protein diet to assist with tissue repair and restoring a positive nitrogen balance unless otherwise contraindicated. **(2)** This choice does not meet high-protein requirements. **(3)** This choice does not meet high-protein requirements. **(4)** This choice does not meet high-protein requirements.

87. **(2)** Integrated processes: nursing process — implementation; client need: physiological integrity; basic care and comfort; content area: nutrition.
    RATIONALE
    (1) Coleslaw is low in protein content. **(2)** Of the foods listed, peanut butter and milkshake have the highest protein and caloric content. **(3)** Vegetables are low in protein content. **(4)** Crackers are low in protein content.

88. **(4)** Integrated processes: nursing process — implementation; client need: physiological integrity; basic care and comfort; content area: nutrition.
    RATIONALE
    (1) Milk does not contain gluten. **(2)** Beef does not contain gluten. **(3)** Green vegetables do not contain gluten. **(4)** Wheat bread contains glutens, a group of proteins found in grain foods.

89. **(4)** Integrated processes: nursing process — planning; client need: physiological integrity; basic care and comfort; content area: nutrition.
    RATIONALE
    (1) Vitamin B_6 is not dependent on bile. **(2)** Vitamin B_{12} is not dependent on bile. **(3)** Folic acid is not dependent on bile. **(4)** Vitamin K is dependent on the presence of bile for absorption.

90. **(3)** Integrated processes: nursing process — implementation; teaching/learning; client need: physiological integrity; basic care and comfort; content area: nutrition.
    RATIONALE
    (1) Decreasing fluid intake would increase the chance of constipation. **(2)** Bed rest would not stimulate the bowel to empty and would increase the chance of constipation. **(3)** Vegetable fiber provides dietary residue. Increased dietary residue increases the volume of fecal material. The increase in fecal material stimulates the bowel to empty. **(4)** Kaopectate is given for diarrhea.

91. **(3)** Integrated processes: nursing process — implementation; teaching/learning; client need: physiological integrity; basic care and comfort; content area: nutrition.
    RATIONALE
    (1) Decreasing fluid intake could lead to dehydration. **(2)** Increased activity would not decrease the fluidity of the stools

or decrease the rapid bowel emptying. **(3)** Diarrhea causes an increase in the fluidity of stool, with a loss of potassium and sodium. Encourage liquids high in potassium and sodium such as Gatorade, soup, broth, water, and apple, orange, and grapefruit juices. **(4)** Milk and milk products have a laxative effect.

92. **(3)** Integrated processes: nursing process — implementation; client need: physiological integrity; basic care and comfort; content area: nutrition.

    RATIONALE

    (1) Cranberry sauce does not liquefy at room temperature. **(2)** Oatmeal does not liquefy at room temperature. **(3)** Gelatin liquefies at room temperature. **(4)** Vegetable soups do not liquefy at room temperature.

93. **(2)** Integrated processes: nursing process — implementation; client need: physiological integrity; basic care and comfort; content area: nutrition.

    RATIONALE

    (1) Squash is not high in potassium content. **(2)** Apricots are high in potassium. **(3)** Oatmeal is a rich source of iron but not of potassium. **(4)** Cream of wheat is a refined cereal. Refined foods have very little potassium

94. **(4)** Integrated processes: nursing process — implementation; teaching/learning; client need: physiological integrity; basic care and comfort; content area: nutrition.

    RATIONALE

    (1) This choice is low in sodium unless sodium is added during cooking. **(2)** This choice is low in sodium unless sodium is added during cooking. **(3)** This choice is low in sodium unless sodium is added during cooking. **(4)** Of the foods listed, ice cream would have the highest sodium content. Ice cream is a processed food.

95. **(4)** Integrated processes: nursing process — implementation; client need: physiological integrity; basic care and comfort; content area: nutrition.

    RATIONALE

    (1) Checking the admitting diagnosis will not denote fluid restrictions. **(2)** The nurse would notify dietary personnel about the fluid restriction before serving the tray. **(3)** Calling the physician is not necessary for this meal situation. **(4)** The fluid intake should be evaluated before serving all meals. The client should be allowed to participate in the decision-making process.

96. **(2)** Integrated processes: nursing process — implementation; client need: physiological integrity; basic care and comfort; content area: nutrition.

    RATIONALE

    (1) A high-potassium diet is contraindicated in treating renal disease. **(2)** Clients with renal disease are unable to excrete potassium adequately, which causes elevated serum potassium. Therefore, the amount of potassium in the diet must be restricted to prevent complication of hyperkalemia. **(3)** Sodium is restricted in treating renal disease. **(4)** Protein is restricted in treating renal disease.

97. **(2)** Integrated processes: nursing process — implementation; client need: physiological integrity; basic care and comfort; content area: nutrition.

    RATIONALE

    (1) Vitamins and minerals do not increase calories. **(2)** Adequate caloric intake must be maintained to prevent catabolism. This is done by increasing the amount of simple carbohydrates and fats in the diet. **(3)** Decreasing carbohydrates is not recommended. **(4)** Neither vitamins nor minerals increase calories.

98. **(1)** Integrated processes: nursing process — implementation; client need: physiological integrity; basic care and comfort; content area: nutrition.

    RATIONALE

    (1) Lean meat is low in fat. **(2)** Hidden sources of fat, such as nuts, avocado, olives, organ meats, chocolate, and coconut, are eliminated from the diet. **(3)** Hidden sources of fat, such as nuts, avocado, olives, organ meats, chocolate, and coconut, are eliminated from the diet. **(4)** Hidden sources of fat, such as nuts, avocado, olives, organ meats, chocolate, and coconut, are eliminated from the diet.

99. **(1)** Integrated processes: nursing process — implementation; client need: physiological integrity; basic care and comfort; content area: nutrition.

    RATIONALE

    (1) Organ meats are high in fat and cholesterol content. **(2)** Baked potatoes have no fat. **(3)** Green beans have no fat. **(4)** Chicken is low in fat, especially if the skin is removed.

100. **(4)** Integrated processes: nursing process — implementation; teaching/learning; client need: physiological integrity; basic care and comfort; content area: nutrition.

    RATIONALE

    (1) Incorrect options are explained in the rationale for the correct answer. **(2)** Incorrect options are explained in the rationale for the correct answer. **(3)** Incorrect options are explained in the rationale for the correct answer. **(4)** PKU is a genetic defect affecting the metabolism of phenylalanine. The phenylalanine-restricted diet will change with growth needs but will be necessary throughout the life span.

101. **(3)** Integrated processes: nursing process — implementation; client need: physiological integrity; basic care and comfort; content area: nutrition.

    RATIONALE

    (1, 2, 4) Incorrect options are explained in the rationale for the correct answer. **(3)** The client has consumed a total of 990 mL of fluids. If the client had the evening snack of skim milk, the total intake would be 1230 mL. It should be explained to the client that the skim milk would exceed the fluid restriction.

102. **(4)** Integrated processes: nursing process — implementation; client need: physiological integrity; basic care and comfort; content area: nutrition.

    RATIONALE

    (1) Veal is low in cholesterol. **(2)** Chicken is low in cholesterol. **(3)** Fish is low in cholesterol. **(4)** On a low-cholesterol diet, the intake of eggs should be decreased to three egg yolks per week.

103. **(3)** Integrated processes; nursing process — implementation; teaching/learning; client need: physiological integrity; pharmacological therapies; content area: nutrition.

    RATIONALE

    (1) A client with intermittent claudication needs to decrease saturated fat content in the diet. **(2)** It is important for the client to check with his physician before taking dietary supplements to prevent adverse effects with prescribed medications. **(3)** It is important for the client to check with his physician before taking dietary supplements to prevent adverse effects with prescribed medications. **(4)** Taking calcium as a dietary supplement is not used to treat intermittent claudication.

104. **(4)** Integrated processes: nursing process — implementation; teaching/learning; client need: physiological integrity; basic care and comfort; content area: nutrition.

RATIONALE
(1) Drinking three glasses of milk per day does not provide an adequate amount of calcium for a 50 year old. (2) Acetaminophen is not a dietary supplement. (3) Many times calcium supplements needed to be added to an older person's diet to provide the necessary calcium. (4) An older person needs to check with his or her physician about the amount of calcium that is to be provided by dietary supplements.

105. **(3)** Integrated processes; nursing process — data collection; client need: physiological integrity; reduction of risk potential; content area: nutrition.

RATIONALE
(1) Hispanic and African American women have higher mortality rates secondary to breast and lung cancers than whites. (2) Some cultures expect family members to provide care in the hospital, whereas Western culture supports self-care as soon as possible. (3) There are cultural differences regarding nutritional effect on health. (4) Many cultures discourage direct eye contact.

106. **(2)** Integrated processes: nursing process — implementation; client need: physiological integrity; basic care and comfort; content area: nutrition.

RATIONALE
(1) Fast foods are usually higher in fat and sodium content; therefore, they are not the best choice in meeting an older adult's nutritional needs. (2) Home-delivered meals, such as with the Meals-on-Wheels sponsored by the Council on Aging, provides nutritional food as recommended by a dietitian. (3) Frozen dinners are usually higher in sodium and fat content and are not the best choice in meeting an older adult's nutritional needs. (4) Restaurant food is usually expensive and is not the best source of meeting an older adult's nutritional needs.

107. **(2)** Integrated processes: nursing process — implementation; teaching/learning; client need: physiological integrity; basic care and comfort; content area: nutrition.

RATIONALE
(1) Taking a multivitamin daily is recommended by health care professionals, especially for a frail, older adult living alone. (2) Dentures that are too loose places the frail older adult living alone at high risk for malnutrition. (3) Foods that smell good to the frail older adult will help stimulate appetite. (4) Eating three meals a day will help keep a nutritional balance in frail older adults who live alone.

108. **(4)** Integrated processes: nursing process — data collection; client need: physiological integrity; basic care and comfort; content area: nutrition.

RATIONALE
(1) NSAIDS are not herbs. (2) Heparin is a drug, not an herb. (3) Vitamin E is a vitamin, not an herb. (4) Garlic is considered one of the most common herbs in the United States.

109. **(3)** Integrated processes: nursing process — data collection; client need: physiological integrity; pharmacological therapies; content area: nutrition.

RATIONALE
(1) The nurse must understand that echinacea is used to prevent colds during the winter seasons. (2) The nurse must understand that St. John's wort is used to treat depression. (3) Black cohosh is used by many cultures to treat menopausal cramps. (4) The nurse must understand that aloe as a dietary supplement is used to treat stomach problems.

110. **(4)** Integrated processes: nursing process — evaluation; client need: physiological integrity; reduction of risk potential; content area: nutrition.

RATIONALE
(1) Ginger is the dietary supplement that is contraindicated when taking Coumadin. (2) Echinacea has no effect on Coumadin. (3) Hawthorn has not effect on Coumadin. (4) Ginger is the dietary supplement that is contraindicated when taking Coumadin.

111. **(4)** Integrated processes: nursing process — data collection; client need: physiological integrity; reduction of risk potential; content area: nutrition.

RATIONALE
(1) Many cultures use saw palmetto to reduce benign prostatic hyperplasia. (2) Many cultures use St. John's wort to reduce depression. (3) Many cultures use melatonin as a sleep aid. (4) Many cultures use saw palmetto to reduce benign prostatic hyperplasia.

112. **(2)** Integrated processes: nursing process — implementation; teaching/learning; client need: physiological integrity; reduction of risk potential; content area: nutrition.

RATIONALE
(1) Not all dietary supplements are safe. (2) It is important to instruct clients to discontinue dietary supplements 2–3 weeks before surgery. (3) Employees from health food stores are not experts nor licensed to discuss health-care needs with individuals. (4) Dietary supplements need to be maintained in a constant environment—not too hot nor too cold.

113. **(4)** Integrated processes: nursing process — implementation; teaching/learning; client need: physiological integrity; basic care and comfort; content area: nutrition.

RATIONALE
(1) Increasing water will help to reduce constipation. (2) Eating more fiber will help to reduce constipation; however, if the constipation is due to narcotics, laxatives taken morning and evening would be more beneficial. (3) A hospice client may not be able to increase activity. (4) Taking laxatives morning and evening would be more beneficial to reduce the effects of narcotic induced constipation.

114. **(2)** Integrated processes: nursing process — data collection; client need: physiological integrity; reduction of risk potential; content area: nutrition.

RATIONALE
(1, 2, 3, 4) When a frail older adult does not eat a complete meal and does not take a multivitamin, the client is at risk for developing pressure sores.

115. **(3)** Integrated processes: nursing process — implementation; teaching/learning; client need: physiological integrity; reduction of risk potential; content area: nutrition.
(1, 2, 3, 4) A client with a stage II pressure sore needs to be instructed to increase protein intake.

Comprehensive Integrated Practice Tests

TEST 1

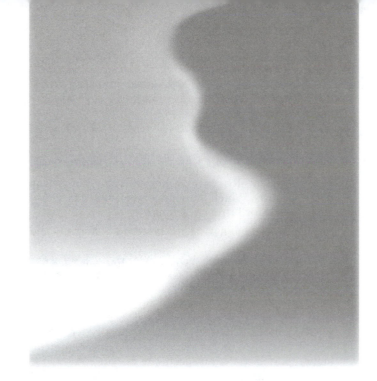

Patricia Gauntlett Beare, RN, PhD
Golden M. Tradewell, RN, PhD

QUESTIONS

1. The nurse is assessing a 70-year-old man. Normal changes that may increase with age include:
   1. Decrease in blood pressure (BP), decrease in cardiac reserve, increase in coronary artery disease
   2. Prostatic hypertrophy, reduced creatinine clearance, increase in renal blood flow
   3. Diminished peristalsis, constipation, reduced gastric acid secretion
   4. Decrease in bone mineral content, loss of height, decrease in number of taste buds

2. An 80-year-old client is being assessed by the nurse. Which of the following occurs as a result of normal aging?
   1. High-frequency hearing loss
   2. Increased susceptibility to postural hypertension
   3. Increased cardiac reserve
   4. Increased adaptation to dark

3. When assessing clients over 65 years old, the nurse would correctly identify which of the following as the most common chronic condition in older Americans?
   1. Arthritis
   2. Hearing impairment
   3. Cataracts
   4. Diabetes

4. The nurse is teaching a group of older people about early signs of aging. Which of the following occur(s) in the early stages of aging? (**Select all that apply.**)
   1. Being able to read fine print without glasses
   2. Osteoarthritic changes of the cervical spine
   3. Osteoarthritic changes in hands
   4. Difficulty staying up at night and working the next day
   5. Difficulty reading fine print without glasses
   6. Being able to stay up at night and work the next day without fatigue

5. A 65-year-old client complains of having trouble sleeping at night. The best response by the nurse is:
   1. "Try to drink some warm milk before you go to bed."
   2. "Try staying up and watching television until you fall asleep."
   3. "I will refer you to Dr. Jones for some sleeping pills."
   4. "Most cases of insomnia are normal as you get older."

6. The nurse is assessing a 70-year-old client. Which of the following symptoms is commonly reported by older persons?
   1. Vaginal bleeding
   2. Reduced urinary frequency
   3. Incontinence
   4. Increased weight gain

7. A 65-year-old client has been taking several aspirins daily for her arthritis. It would be most important for the nurse to observe for (**select all that apply**):
   1. Weight gain
   2. Gastrointestinal (GI) hemorrhage
   3. Oral mucous membrane hypertrophy
   4. Confusion
   5. Decreased neural function
   6. Decreased platelets

8. A 68-year-old client is receiving dietary counseling from the nurse. Which of the following statements indicates a need for further teaching?

1. "I must eat two to four servings of fruit per day."
2. "I must avoid all meats and animal products."
3. "I should use moderation in my sugar and salt consumption."
4. "I must eat 6–11 servings of bread, cereal, and pasta per day."

9. The nurse is doing preoperative teaching with a 26-year-old client for a total hysterectomy for severe endometriosis. Which of the following statements indicates a need for further teaching?

   1. "I'm so glad I'm having this surgery. My husband and I want a large family."
   2. "I should lift no more than 10 lb for the next 4 weeks."
   3. "I can resume normal sexual relations in about 6 weeks."
   4. "I can take Tylenol for pain control."

10. A 50-year-old client is 15 days posthysterectomy. Which of the following symptoms should be immediately reported to the physician?

    1. Serosanguinous vaginal drainage
    2. A temperature of 99.48°F (37.48°C)
    3. Bright-red bleeding from the incisional site or other site
    4. Laboratory findings of 12 g/dL hemoglobin (Hgb) and 36 hematocrit (Hct)

11. A 48-year-old client has a diagnosis of dumping syndrome after gastric surgery. It would be most important for the client to:

    1. Drink concentrated carbohydrates such as milkshakes between meals
    2. Lie down after meals
    3. Eat large well-balanced meals
    4. Drink fluids with meals

12. A 30-year-old woman has just delivered premature twin babies. It is most important for the nurse to inform the parents:

    1. That it is in the twins' best interest to stay in the hospital
    2. How they (the parents) will be incorporated into the twins' care
    3. That they should obtain as much rest as possible in preparation for the twins coming home
    4. Not to call the nursery unless it is an emergency

13. The parents of twin baby girls bring them to the pediatrician's office for their first checkup. The parents have numerous questions. The nurse's response should reflect the fact that:

    1. Twins are very special and need additional attention.
    2. Even though they are twins, each baby needs to be viewed as an individual.
    3. Twins should be treated exactly the same.
    4. Twins should never be separated during this very early period.

14. The nurse is preparing to discharge newborn twins with their parents. It would be most important for the nurse to:

1. Observe the parents feeding, bathing, and dressing the babies
2. Teach the parents what it means when the baby cries
3. Inform the parents when the first immunizations will be given
4. Advise the parents to get help for the first 2 weeks when the twins are at home

15. An 8-year-old child has been hospitalized with a diagnosis of nephrotic syndrome. He has severe edema and proteinuria, and is lethargic. Which of the following nursing measures would be appropriate?

    1. Daily measurement of weight and abdominal girth
    2. A high-carbohydrate diet
    3. Daily exercise and play therapy
    4. Promoting adequate fluid intake

16. A 6-month-old child is admitted to the hospital for evaluation of vomiting. Which of the following would the nurse provide as a toy?

    1. A large puzzle
    2. Push-pull toy
    3. Soft, colorful blocks
    4. A rocking horse

17. A 20-year-old gravida 2, para 2 vaginally delivered a 7-lb 2-oz girl on April 3 at 10:35 PM. She is rubella immune, has a small right sublabial nick, refused ice application to the perineum, is voiding, and has a firm uterus at the level of the umbilicus. She is bottle-feeding her baby. Her blood type is A-negative and her daughter's is A-positive. On the morning of April 4, her lochia is dark red and contains small shreds of tissue. The nurse should describe this discharge as lochia:

    1. Alba
    2. Leuka
    3. Rubra
    4. Serosa

18. At 8 AM on the first postpartum day, a client's fundus is 2 cm above the umbilicus and located on the right side of her abdomen. There is a moderate amount of vaginal blood. The nurse should:

    1. Ask the client if she had any infections during the last 2 weeks of pregnancy.
    2. Notify the registered nurse (RN) or midwife immediately.
    3. Proceed with the data collection and chart the information as noted.
    4. Provide a way for the client to empty her bladder before proceeding with the data collection.

19. A postpartum client asks the nurse how long her vaginal discharge will last. The nurse's best response would be to explain that it will last:

    1. About 3 days
    2. Longer than if she were breast-feeding
    3. Until her checkup in 6 weeks
    4. Until the placental site has healed

20. At 10 AM on the first postpartum day, the nurse notes that a client's fundus is firm and that there is a continuous flow of vaginal blood with no clots. As she gets

out of bed, the client notices a "gushing" from her vagina and passes a small clot. She becomes frightened. The nurse should explain to her that:

1. She probably got up too soon after delivery and needs to take it a little slower.
2. The amount of discharge is increased because she is not breast-feeding.
3. The lochia that pools in the vagina while she is lying in bed drains when she stands.
4. The vaginal opening is edematous and bruised right after delivery.

21. A new mother states that she is afraid to have a bowel movement because she remembers the discomfort she experienced after delivering her other child. The nurse should encourage her to:

1. Eat a low-roughage diet, drink 8 glasses of water per day, and keep physical activity to a minimum.
2. Eat fresh fruits and vegetables, drink six to eight glasses of water per day, and ambulate frequently.
3. Eat small amounts of food for several days so she will be less likely to have a bowel movement until the soreness in her perineum is decreased.
4. Eat whatever she wishes, take a mild laxative for several days, and keep up her Kegel exercises.

22. A client's Rh antibody titer indicates that she has not been sensitized to the Rh factor. The nurse should anticipate that which of the following will be given after delivery?

1. Bromocriptine mesylate (Parlodel)
2. Oxytocin
3. Rho(D) immune globulin (e.g., RhoGAM)
4. Rubella virus vaccine

23. A 22-year-old gravida 1, para 1 delivered a 7-lb 8-oz boy by cesarean birth. She has decided to breast-feed her son. Her abdominal incision is midline and vertical and has a dressing on it. To assess her uterus for position and tone, the nurse should:

1. Ask her how it feels instead of palpating for it.
2. Gently palpate above or below the incision.
3. Gently palpate on each side of the incision.
4. Palpate directly over the incision.

24. When a client breast-feeds her baby after a cesarean birth, the nurse can help by suggesting that she:

1. Bottle-feed the baby after each feeding until she is producing milk in sufficient amount.
2. Lie on her side with the baby lying beside her and turned toward her.
3. Raise the head of her bed and rest the baby high on her abdomen.
4. Wash her nipples with soap and water before and after feeding the baby.

25. As a client's baby starts to breast-feed, the client begins to experience severe abdominal cramps. The nurse should:

1. Assist her to move the baby off her abdominal incision.
2. Explain that breast-feeding does cause discomfort and she should consider bottle-feeding instead.

3. Explain that when the baby sucks, oxytocin, the hormone that causes the uterus to contract, is released.
4. Medicate her for pain and give the baby a bottle for this feeding.

26. A new mother complains that her incision hurts when she has to cough, turn, and breathe deeply. The nurse should teach her to:

1. Breath less deeply, cough gently, and splint her incision to decrease her discomfort.
2. Continue with the exercise because she needs to wear off the anesthetic she received during surgery.
3. Continue with the exercise while splinting her incision because she needs to inflate her lungs fully to prevent pooling of secretions.
4. Discontinue the exercise and inform her physician the next time he or she visits.

27. Students were tested on normal fetal circulation and given the following scenario. A baby was born at term by vaginal birth. She was assessed and placed in her mother's arms. Rapid and radical physiological changes occurred at birth as the baby's body established pulmonary ventilation and her circulatory pattern markedly changed. In the neonate, three structures that were necessary for fetal circulation must close as blood supply is increased to the lungs and liver. Which of the following did the students identify incorrectly?

1. Ductus arteriosus
2. Ductus neonatorum
3. Ductus venosus
4. Foramen ovale

28. Data collection of a newborn at 1 minute after birth reveals a heart rate of 98 bpm, good respiratory effort with crying, active motion, vigorous cry, and pink body with blue extremities. Her Apgar score is _____.

29. When the father of a newborn asks why the baby's hands and feet look blue, the nurse should explain that this condition is common and temporary, and is called:

1. Acrocyanosis
2. Acrodermatosis
3. Cyanoacrylate
4. Vernix caseosa

30. By law, a newborn is given eye drops of a 1% silver nitrate solution or an erythromycin ophthalmic preparation in both eyes. This is done as a prophylactic treatment for:

1. Gonorrheal conjunctivitis
2. Hemorrhagic tendencies
3. Nosocomial infection
4. Staphylococcal infection

31. In the birthing room after the initial data collections are complete, a mother asks to breast-feed her baby. The most appropriate nursing intervention would be to:

1. Ask her to wait until the baby has been thoroughly evaluated in the newborn nursery.
2. Ask her to wait until you give the baby glucose water as the initial feeding.

3. Assist her to breast-feed the baby.
4. Refuse her request.

32. A 2-day-old, full-term newborn infant is of normal weight and length and to this point has had an uncomplicated newborn course. His mother is breast-feeding him. He will be in the neonatal period from the time of his birth through his:

1. Fourteenth day of life
2. Twenty-eighth day of life
3. First year of life
4. Time of discharge from the hospital

33. The intraoperative nurse monitoring a client receiving local anesthesia notices an increase in the heart rate. The change may be caused by the release of:

1. Norepinephrine
2. Glucocorticoids
3. Aldosterone
4. Antidiuretic hormone

34. When assessing a newborn's heart rate (preferably when he is asleep), the nurse should:

1. Auscultate the apical pulse for a full minute.
2. Auscultate the apical pulse for 30 seconds and double it.
3. Auscultate the apical pulse for 15 seconds and multiply by 4.
4. Palpate the brachial pulse for 30 seconds and double it.

35. While he is awake and quiet, a newborn's pulse, in beats per minute, should average _____

36. Of the following findings on data collection, which is most likely to be normal for a newborn infant? (Select all that apply.)

1. Passing meconium during the first 24 hours of life.
2. Failure to void during the first 24 hours of life.
3. Inability to pass a rectal thermometer 1/8 inch into the rectum.
4. Rust-colored or pink stains on a diaper with voiding.
5. Failure to pass meconium during the first 24 hours of life.
6. Voiding immediately after birth.

37. A nurse is preparing to obtain the consent for a client preoperatively. Which of the following is correct?

1. The client's decision to have surgery can be revoked at any time.
2. The consent form may be signed by the client if premedication has been given.
3. A spouse, child, or friend may sign the consent form if the client asks him or her to do so.
4. The perioperative nurse is required to inform the client of all the surgical and anesthetic risks related to the procedure.

38. On the day of birth, a newborn was given an intramuscular (IM) injection of a substance because of a transient blood coagulation deficiency. The substance injected was probably:

1. Aquaphor
2. Cyanocobalamin (vitamin B_{12})
3. Erythromycin
4. Phytonadione (vitamin K)

39. A 68-year-old client had bilateral total knee replacements under general anesthesia. The surgical procedure lasted 4 hours. Preoperatively, the client received instructions on deep-breathing exercises to increase lung ventilation and gas exchange postoperatively. The postsurgical nurse observes correct technique when the client is able to:

1. Take quick, shallow breaths through the mouth, hold them, then cough deeply from the chest.
2. Take a slow, deep breath through the mouth, hold it, exhale, and cough deeply from the throat.
3. Take a slow, deep breath through the nose, hold it, exhale, and cough deeply from the chest.
4. Take a quick, deep breath through the nose, hold it, exhale, and cough deeply from the throat.

40. While teaching a newborn's mother who is breast-feeding about baby care, the nurse informs her that normal stools for her baby are most likely to be:

1. Brown, well-formed, and up to two per day.
2. Dark green, loose, and five to eight per day.
3. Pale yellow, formed, pasty, and every other day.
4. Yellow, loose, and up to 6–10 per day.

41. A newborn's mother asks whether she should feed him foods other than the breast milk. The nurse knows that, according to the American Academy of Pediatrics, breast milk or formula meets all the requirements of growth for the normal infant until the age of:

1. 2 months
2. 6 months
3. 9 months
4. 12 months

42. A 38-year-old woman was hospitalized with a medical diagnosis of cholecystitis. The nurse would expect the history of her present illness to include intolerance to which of the following nutrients?

1. Carbohydrates
2. Fat
3. Protein
4. Vitamin C

43. The preoperative teaching for prevention of postoperative complications includes leg exercises. The nurse teaches leg exercises preoperative to gallbladder surgery to help prevent:

1. Muscle spasms
2. Paralytic ileus
3. Stasis and clot formation
4. Vasogenic shock

44. Before surgery an intravenous (IV) catheter is inserted in a client's forearm. An isotonic solution is administered at a rate sufficient to keep the vein open. The nurse knows that the isotonic solution may be _____.

45. One hour before the scheduled surgery, the nurse gives a client her preanesthetic (preoperative) medication. Which of the following statements by the nurse is most appropriate after the medication is administered?

1. "Please remain in bed and use this call signal if you need anything. I am leaving the side rails up while no one is in the room with you."
2. "Please remember to empty your bladder before you are taken to the operating room."
3. "You may move about in your room as much as you like, but lie down when you begin to feel sleepy."
4. "While you wait to go to the operating room, I will give you a clear explanation of the surgical procedure so you will know what to expect."

46. Rank each of the following postoperative nursing interventions in order of importance:

1. Deep-breathing and coughing exercises
2. Early ambulation
3. Leg exercises (calf, quadriceps, and gluteal)
4. Medication for pain

47. On the morning of the second day after surgery, data collection reveals pain, tenderness, and swelling in a client's left calf. She has not taken the as-needed pain medication ordered for her since the previous day. The nurse's next action should be to:

1. Administer the medication ordered every 4 hours as needed for pain, and include the site of the pain as the intervention is recorded.
2. Allow the client to be up in her room only and elevate her left leg.
3. Immobilize her leg and have her maintain bed rest until the physician examines her leg.
4. Massage her leg to relieve pain and swelling, and ask if she would like her pain medication.

48. A 78-year-old man has been admitted for total joint replacement of his fractured right hip. In conjunction with the hip surgery, the physician orders aspirin 325 mg every day. The nurse is aware that this medication is probably ordered for which of the following effects?

1. Analgesic
2. Antibiotic
3. Anticoagulant
4. Antipyretic

49. To prevent prosthesis dislocation after a total hip replacement, the nurse teaches a client to maintain which of the following leg positions?

1. Abduction
2. Adduction
3. Flexion
4. Internal rotation

50. While evaluating follow-up teaching, the nurse concludes that a client post–hip replacement surgery is beginning to understand after stating that he will have to learn not to cross his legs and not to flex his hip more than 90 degrees. He says, "but I will gradually get back to doing most of my routine daily activities after _____ ":

1. 1 week
2. 3 months
3. 9 months
4. 12 months

51. A 73-year-old man is admitted to the cardiac step-down unit with a diagnosis of congestive heart failure. He has +2 pitting edema bilaterally up to his calves. The physician has ordered bed rest and the following medications: furosemide (Lasix) 80 mg IV bid, digoxin 0.25 mg orally (PO) every morning, theophylline (Slo-bid) 10 mEq (2 tablets) PO tid, aspirin 325 mg PO every day, and nifedipine (Procardia XL) 10 mg PO bid. During data collection, the nurse notes urine output of 10 mL during the last 4 hours, fatigue, slight lethargy, and complaints of visual disturbances. The next action the nurse should take is to:

1. Administer the next dose of furosemide early to increase urine output.
2. Call the physician.
3. Chart data collection data and recheck the client in 30 minutes.
4. Check laboratory values.

52. A client has been placed on furosemide 80 mg IV bid. He has a diagnosis of congestive heart failure. The nurse should be aware that the client's medical diagnosis and treatment put him at risk for potential depletion of which of the following electrolytes?

1. Calcium
2. Chloride
3. Potassium
4. Sodium

53. A 63-year-old woman is admitted to the medical-surgical unit with an exacerbation of symptoms related to ovarian carcinoma. On admission, her BP is 122/82 mm Hg, pulse (P) 88 bpm, respirations (R) 20/min, and temperature 98.2°F (36.7°C). She is expected to return home when the symptoms subside. While she is in the hospital, the physician has ordered morphine sulfate 4 mg IV q3-4 h prn for pain. Her condition worsens. During the nurse's data collection, vital signs include BP 108/64 mm Hg, pulse 63 bpm, and respirations 10/min. Before the nurse leaves the room, tears roll down the client's face as she requests her pain medication. The nurse should:

1. Administer the morphine as ordered.
2. Administer the morphine and offer to sit with her for a few minutes.
3. Report the vital signs to the charge nurse so that a different narcotic analgesic can be ordered.
4. Leave the room to allow her to be alone.

54. A 9-month-old child weighs 20 lb and has sustained a fracture of the right femur. The client is admitted and placed in Bryant's traction. The nurse knows that this type of traction is:

1. Continuous, skeletal
2. Continuous, skin
3. Intermittent, skeletal
4. Intermittent, skin

55. For effective traction, a 9-year-old boy must be maintained in an appropriate position. The nurse is aware that his buttocks must be:

1. Elevated and clear of the bed.
2. Flat on the bed.
3. Supported by a well-padded sling.
4. Supported by a pillow.

56. A 9-month-old infant is hospitalized for a fractured right femur. At this stage, in the infant's development, the nurse should:

1. Apply a Band-Aid after injections to give him the security of wholeness.
2. Have his mother stay and care for her child, if possible.
3. Provide for frequent eye-to-eye contact between parents and child.
4. Set limits and allow him to make choices when possible.

57. A 10-year-old child has a high fever, headache, vomiting, and a scarlatina rash. His throat is sore and dry. Throat culture reveals the presence of group A β-hemolytic streptococcal infection ("strep throat"). When penicillin is prescribed, the nurse should teach the boy or his mother to:

1. Monitor the scarlatina rash to determine when the medication has been effective.
2. Take all the medication even if the symptoms subside several days before it is gone.
3. Take the medication until his temperature is normal.
4. Take the medication until his throat is no longer sore.

58. When a 10-year-old child returns for a follow-up examination after a streptococcal infection, his mother asks why a urinalysis is being done. The nurse explains that:

1. Group A β-hemolytic streptococcal infections can be followed by the complication of glomerulonephritis.
2. Penicillin has the potential side effect of pyelonephritis.
3. The urinalysis will indicate whether a human immunodeficiency virus (HIV) infection is also present.
4. Urinary tract infections are common with streptococcal infections and need to receive prompt treatment.

59. An 8-year-old boy will miss 4 days of school because of illness. He tells his mother that he does not want to go back after he is well. His mother asks the nurse how to handle this situation. The most helpful intervention would probably be to:

1. Allow him to miss a full week of school to provide for continuity when he returns to school.
2. Contact the school counselor for advice.
3. Have the boy's teacher send his school work home and see that he completes the assignments before he returns to school.
4. Obtain special permission for him to return to school earlier than planned and miss only 2 days.

60. A 77-year-old woman has been admitted with occasional urinary incontinence of unknown origin (may be described as functional incontinence). The nurse instructs her on obtaining a clean-catch urine specimen.

Which of the following statements related to collection of a clean-catch urine sample from a female client indicates the need for further teaching?

1. "Separate labia to expose urethral opening."
2. "Cleanse from front to back with antiseptic solution."
3. "Collect entire specimen as I void."
4. "Deliver specimen to the nurse immediately."

61. The nurse caring for a client knows that the average quantity of urine produced by "normal" adult kidney function per 24-hour period is approximately

_____

62. A client's orders include keeping a record of her I & O. During lunch she drank 5 oz of iced tea and ate 4 oz of Jell-O and 2 oz of creamed soup. The nurse would record what number of milliliters as intake?

_____

63. Goals of nursing interventions for clients experiencing temporary incontinence (caused by illness, confusion, or decreased level of consciousness) include (a) prevention of bladder distention and (b) keeping the client dry. Which of the following measures is least likely to help the client to regain voluntary control?

1. Inserting a Foley catheter to keep the client dry.
2. Offering the bedpan or commode on arising and at bedtime.
3. Scheduling toileting every 2 hours.
4. Assisting the client to use the bedpan or toilet about an hour after drinking liquids containing caffeine.

64. A 76-year-old client's urinary incontinence causes her to be subject to alterations in skin integrity. Of the following measures, which would be of fundamental importance in prevention of skin breakdown?

1. Wash with soap and water and dry the perineal area after periods of incontinence.
2. Pad the client's clothing or bed with absorbent material.
3. Apply barrier creams to protect skin from contact with urine.
4. Change wet "diaper" frequently on a regular schedule.

65. Inadequate attention to care of a 76-year-old client who is incontinent and immobile can result in a complication known as a:

1. Flexion contracture
2. Pressure ulcer
3. Dermatologic crisis
4. Pressure point

66. Conservative measures have failed to help a 76-year-old client gain voluntary control of voiding. An order has been given for insertion of a Foley catheter. Which of the following positions would not be used to catheterize a female client? **(Select all that apply.)**

1. Left Sims'
2. Supine (dorsal)
3. Dorsal recumbent
4. Prone
5. Trendelenburg
6. Semi-Fowler's

67. A 76-year-old client's Foley catheter is draining well via a closed system to the drainage bag hanging from the side of the bed. The physician has ordered a urinalysis. While maintaining sterile technique, the nurse will:

    1. Allow the urine to flow into the specimen container from the tube at the lower edge of the drainage bag.
    2. Separate the catheter from the drainage tubing and allow the urine to flow from the catheter into the specimen container.
    3. Withdraw a quantity of urine from the catheter with a sterile needle and syringe inserted into the catheter above the bifurcation.
    4. Using a sterile needle, withdraw a specimen from the port located on the urinary drainage tubing.

68. The nurse recognizes that the single most effective intervention to limit the spread of nosocomial (hospital-acquired) infections is:

    1. Prophylactic anti-infective therapy for susceptible clients.
    2. Correct hand washing technique faithfully observed.
    3. Proper disposal of blood and other body fluids.
    4. Frequent in-service education programs on isolation technique.

69. To implement procedures correctly, the nurse must understand the differences among various invasive procedures, that is, which procedures require sterile technique for performance and which can be carried out using clean technique. Which of the following procedures does not require sterility of equipment and solutions used?

    1. Urinary catheterization
    2. Hyperalimentation
    3. Nasogastric feeding
    4. Tracheostomy suctioning

70. A 48-year-old client is admitted with fever (temperature 102.8°F [38.88°C]) and acute severe pain in several joints of the extremities, especially the large toe. Data collection reveals a family history of gout. The nurse anticipates that the physician may initially order which of the following drugs?

    1. Allopurinol
    2. Colchicine
    3. Probenecid
    4. Sulfinpyrazone

71. Assessment of a client's large toe with gangrene might reveal which of the following characteristics?

    1. Pain
    2. Swelling
    3. Increased heat
    4. Cyanosis

72. Gout results from impaired uric acid production or excretion. The physician has ordered a 24-hour urine collection to begin at 8 AM. The nurse initiating the collection will:

    1. Collect and include the urine specimen voided at 8 AM the day the collection is begun.
    2. Collect all urine voidings after the 8 AM voiding, in-cluding the 8-AM specimen 24 hours after the beginning of the collection.
    3. Maintain the collection in the client's room at room temperature during the 24-hour period.
    4. Collect as many of the client's voidings as possible during the collection period, using clean-catch technique.

73. A client with gout is discharged from the hospital. Which of the following might best describe the dietary regimen on discharge from the hospital?

    1. Decreased fluid intake and high-purine diet
    2. Fasting, crash diets, or both
    3. Shellfish, organ meats, alcohol
    4. Potatoes, milk, increased fluids

74. A nursing diagnosis for a client with gout is alteration in comfort as a result of pain, related to the disease process. When talking about what the client can do to provide comfort and relieve pain, the client gives the following measures. Which one indicates a need for further teaching?

    1. "Apply pressure to the affected joint as ordered."
    2. "Apply cold or heat packs."
    3. "Administer analgesics and anti-inflammatory agents."
    4. "Provide immobilization for the affected joint."

75. When planning care for a client with gout, the nurse identifies the major goal of drug therapy in arthritis and related conditions as:

    1. Providing emotional support.
    2. Curing the underlying cause.
    3. Reducing inflammation of joints.
    4. Preparing the client for surgery.

76. A client has an order for a total of 3000 mL of 5% dextrose in water to be infused over 24 hours. What is the approximate infusion rate in drops per minute? Standard drop factor is 10.

    _____

77. After a client's IV fluids have been infusing for some period, the flow is interrupted. Which of the following measures done by a nurse indicates a need to review the IV procedure for further teaching?

    1. Check for swelling at the needle site.
    2. Move the client's arm to a new position.
    3. Lower the receptacle below the level of the needle.
    4. Flush cannula or needle with sterile saline.

78. A 75-year-old client is receiving IV therapy. Later that night the client begins experiencing headache, flushed skin, rapid pulse, increased BP, increased respirations, coughing, and shortness of breath. These symptoms may indicate possible:

    1. Circulatory overload
    2. Drug overload
    3. Superficial thrombophlebitis
    4. Air embolism

79. A client has a diagnosis of bronchial asthma. Any of the following drugs may be used in the treatment of asthma. Which of the medications is effective in inhibiting the allergic reaction?

1. Epinephrine
2. Terbutaline sulfate
3. Cromolyn sodium
4. Theophylline

80. A 57-year-old client has been experiencing anorexia, weight loss, and diarrhea and is admitted for diagnostic purposes. He has an order for enemas in preparation for a barium enema the next day. Which of the following nursing actions represents the best response appropriate to administration of enemas?

1. Lubricate tip of tubing and insert tubing 2 inches with client lying in the left lateral position with right leg flexed.
2. Expel air from tubing; lubricate and insert tip of tubing 4 inches with client lying in right lateral position with left leg flexed.
3. Open clamp and allow solution to flow moderately fast with container at level of 15 inches above anus.
4. Allow solution to flow slowly until container is empty or until client is unable to take any more; clamp tubing and remove from anus.

81. A 62-year-old client is admitted to the eye unit with a past history of foggy vision, diminished accommodation, nondescript ocular discomfort, and complaint of mild aching in both eyes. Initial data collection is conducted and tonometry (measurement of intraocular pressure) is ordered. Intraocular pressure is 28 mm Hg. The nurse knows that the range for normal intraocular pressure is:

1. 11–22 mm Hg
2. 24–32 mm Hg
3. 34–44 mm Hg
4. 50–75 mm Hg

82. A client is diagnosed as having chronic (open-angle) glaucoma, the most common form of glaucoma. Medical treatment is used initially, and surgery may be required if medical treatment is not successful. Drugs that either increase the outflow of aqueous humor or decrease the production of aqueous humor may be prescribed. The principal objective of drug treatment of glaucoma is:

1. Evaluation for diagnostic purposes
2. Preparation of the client for surgery
3. Education of the client
4. Reduction of intraocular pressure

83. The nurse caring for a client with glaucoma knows that a miotic drug:

1. Dilates the pupil
2. Constricts the pupil
3. Cures glaucoma
4. Anesthetizes the eye

84. Miotic drugs are frequently prescribed for various types of glaucoma. The nurse may administer which of the following drugs to facilitate miosis?

1. Acetazolamide (Diamox)
2. Pilocarpine
3. Mannitol
4. Rimexolone

85. A client's physician has ordered pilocarpine 2%, gtt ii OS qid. To implement the order correctly, the nurse would administer:

1. 2 drops in left eye four times a day
2. 11 drops in left eye four times a day
3. 2 drops in right eye every day
4. 2 drops in both eyes four times a day

86. Regarding instillation of a client's eye drops, the nurse should:

1. Instruct the client to focus gaze straight ahead.
2. Drop the solution gently onto the cornea.
3. Drop medication into the center of the lower lid.
4. Touch the eyedropper gently to the client's lower eyelid.

87. While constructing discharge planning with a client with glaucoma and the family, the nurse teaches the client to occlude the nasolacrimal (tear) duct by applying digital pressure at the inner canthus during administration of eye drops and for 2 minutes afterward. The primary reason for such action is:

1. To prevent excessive systemic absorption of drugs
2. To prevent the client from tearing during administration
3. To prevent blinking of the eyelids during administration
4. To prevent possible loss of medication

88. The nurse caring for the client should teach the client who has glaucoma not to take:

1. Beta blockers
2. Antiemetics
3. Mydriatics
4. Analgesics

89. A 73-year-old client has been admitted to undergo an intraocular lens implant because of a cataract (clouding or opacity of lens) in the right eye. Surgery will be performed under local anesthesia. Plans include the client being discharged home the evening of the day of surgery. Preoperative medication is diazepam (Valium) 10 mg PO. The diazepam supplied consists of scored tablets of 5 mg each. The nurse should administer by mouth _____.

90. The nurse is checking a care plan for a client with cataract surgery. Which of the following is an error in nursing care planning for postoperative measures and discharge teaching?

1. Position the client on the operative side with pillows.
2. Patch operative (right) eye and employ protective shield as ordered.
3. Administer prescribed medications for prevention of nausea and constipation.
4. Instruct client not to lift, pull, or push heavy objects.

91. A neighbor asks you, as a nurse, to recommend eye drops for his mother, who has recently developed an eye irritation. You should recommend:

1. Visine; it is the most commonly prescribed eye medication.
2. Atropine, as it is inexpensive and very effective.

3. Aspirin to decrease inflammation and provide comfort.
4. Professional assessment to help determine the cause of the problem.

92. A 2-year-old child presents holding her ear and rolling her head from side to side. Postauricular and cervical lymph glands are enlarged. Her temperature is 104°F (40°C). Her appetite has been poor, and chewing seems to be painful for her. She has had a cold, and irritability has been characteristic of her temperament for several days. The nurse knows that the client's signs and symptoms may be indicative of which of the following common early childhood health problems?

1. Conjunctivitis
2. Tonsillitis
3. Otitis media
4. Cystitis

93. The nurse knows that several factors predispose infants and young children to otitis media. Which of the following statements related to susceptibility to otitis media is least accurate?

1. Eustachian tubes are short, narrow, and lie in a somewhat vertical plane.
2. Cartilage lining is underdeveloped and may allow eustachian tubes to open inappropriately.
3. Humoral defense mechanisms are still immature.
4. Usual lying-down positions favor pharyngeal pooling, which may hinder eustachian tube drainage.

94. To administer a 2-year-old child's ear medication, the nurse must know that there is one fundamental variation in the method employed for adults and the method for infants and children. Which of the following steps for admininistration of otic medications will be altered for the client?

1. Position the client on the unaffected side.
2. Pull the pinna (auricle) up and back before administration.
3. Direct the drops toward the ear canal.
4. Allow the client to remain positioned for 5–10 minutes (after administration).

95. The nurse is responsible for discharge teaching regarding care of a 2-year-old child with otitis media after the child goes home. To ensure that that the proper technique for administrating otic medication has been learned, the best action the nurse can take is to have the mother or person responsible for administering the eardrops:

1. Repeat the instructions to the nurse verbally.
2. Write down the procedure as given by the nurse.
3. Take a written test to demonstrate mastery of the technique.
4. Perform the procedure in the presence of the nurse.

96. A 68-year-old client has experienced a gradual decline in motor function; after a thorough diagnostic workup, a diagnosis of Parkinson's disease has been made. Parkinson's disease is accompanied by brain cell degeneration and dopamine deficiency. Which of the following statements about the disorder is accurate?

1. Parkinson's disease can be treated with levodopa, which eventually halts the degenerative process.
2. Parkinson's disease can result in a "parkinsonian crisis," caused by extended use of the drugs used to treat the disorder.
3. Parkinson's disease is a familial disease.
4. Parkinson's disease does not usually affect the individual's intellectual faculties.

97. Which of the following drugs used to treat a client's Parkinson's disease may also be used for prevention of lactation and for female infertility?

1. Levodopa
2. Bromocriptine mesylate (Parlodel)
3. Diphenhydramine (Benadryl)
4. Benztropine mesylate (Cogentin)

98. A client with Parkinson's disease may experience constipation resulting from lack of exercise, medication side effects, or loss of saliva in the GI tract. Which of the following client statements regarding promotion of normal elimination would indicate a need for further teaching?

1. "I should increase intake of fluid and dietary fiber."
2. "I should use mild laxatives or stool softeners."
3. "I should establish a regular time for bowel movements."
4. "I should take a 2-hour nap each afternoon."

99. Several medications are prescribed for controlling constipation symptoms in a client with Parkinson's disease. Which of the following statements best describes the appropriate nursing action?

1. When the client needs information about drug therapy, he should be referred to the physician.
2. When medication information is required, the nurse knows that the pharmacist should provide such information.
3. When the client requires drug information, the nurse should contact the physician for an order to give the information.
4. When a drug regimen is begun, the nurse should instruct the client regarding administration, adverse effects, and other fundamental knowledge.

100. A 20-year-old client has a history of epilepsy controlled by medication. Recently, the client ceased taking prescribed drugs and subsequently experienced status epilepticus. The condition can best be described as:

1. A period of remission when the client experiences no seizures.
2. A time of continuous seizures or seizures in rapid succession.
3. A rare degenerative disorder related to epilepsy.
4. A term that is synonymous with petit mal seizures.

101. An ampule of diazepam contains 5 mg/mL. How many minims are required to administer 2 mg? _____

102. Which of the following actions is least likely to occur within the realm of a practical (vocational) nursing responsibility?

1. Administering medications
2. Prescribing drug therapy
3. Gathering data for research
4. Evaluating effectiveness of medications

103. Assessment of the gums of a client with epilepsy reveals gingival hyperplasia (hypertrophy). The condition may result from a long-standing use of which of the following drugs?

    1. Phenytoin (Dilantin)
    2. Primidone (Mysoline)
    3. Clonazepam (Klonopin)
    4. Diazepam

104. A client is given the usual medication of choice for status epilepticus. The drug is administered IV, very slowly, until the seizures stop. The drug described is:

    1. Docusate sodium
    2. Digoxin
    3. Diazepam
    4. Dexamethasone

105. A client is seen in the emergency room with an open sucking chest wound. The first action the nurse would take is to:

    1. Administer oxygen.
    2. Perform chest physiotherapy and coughing.
    3. Administer pain medication.
    4. Seal the wound with sterile petroleum gauze.

106. A client is being treated with chest tubes because of a pneumothorax. The nurse recognizes that chest tubes may be used to:

    1. Regain positive intrapleural pressure.
    2. Prevent pleural irritation.
    3. Remove air and fluid from the intrapleural space.
    4. Establish negative intra-alveolar pressure.

107. Nursing care of the client with closed chest drainage should include:

    1. Clamping chest tube every 2 hours.
    2. Elevating chest tube higher than client's chest.
    3. Milking chest tube only if obstructed by clots.
    4. Clamping chest tube when moving the client.

108. While bathing a client with chest tubes, the nurse notices that there is bubbling in the water-seal chamber. This probably means that:

    1. There is a leak in the system.
    2. The system is functioning properly.
    3. The client is exhaling.
    4. The client needs to be turned to the left side.

109. A 46-year-old oil company manager is admitted via the emergency room to your unit for observation because of epigastric pain and hematemesis. He has a long history of alcohol use. A tentative diagnosis of gastritis secondary to alcoholism is made. To prevent Wernicke's encephalopathy, a neurological disease manifested by confusion and ataxia, the nurse expects the client to be treated with:

    1. Antabuse
    2. Vitamin C

3. Chlordiazepoxide (Librium)
4. Thiamine

110. While assessing a client with alcoholism and related gastritis, it is extremely important for the nurse to try to determine:

    1. How long has the client been sick?
    2. With whom does the client live?
    3. Does the client always have gastric-type pain after he drinks?
    4. When did the client take the last drink?

111. On the second hospital day, the nurse recognizes which signs as impending delirium tremens (DTs) in an alcoholic client?

    1. Elevated BP, visual hallucinations, restlessness
    2. Elevated BP, lowered temperature, seizures
    3. Lowered BP, elevated temperature, restlessness
    4. Lowered BP, elevated temperature, seizures

112. An alcoholic client in DTs becomes belligerent, so the nurse applies four-point leather restraints. It is important to recognize that the nurse needs to do which of the following activities?

    1. Get order for restraints as needed; document every hour; tell him that the restraints are "to put him in his place."
    2. Get as-needed order for restraints; document every half hour; tell him that the restraints are for "disciplinary measures."
    3. Get specific order for restraints; check circulation every 15 minutes and document; tell him that the restraints will be taken off in 1 hour.
    4. Get specific order for restraints; check circulation every 15 minutes and document; tell him that the restraints are to prevent him from hurting himself or others.

113. A 55-year-old plumber suffered a cerebrovascular accident (CVA), or stroke, resulting in right hemiplegia and speech problems. He was admitted to the medical floor of a community hospital, where his wife visits daily. She is very supportive and assists with his care. Progress is slow for the client, and he had difficulty expressing frustration because of his aphasia. His wife tends to overcompensate for this by pampering him and taking over tasks that he does slowly or clumsily. Physical therapy personnel work daily with him on ambulation; after being fitted with a leg brace, he is able to ambulate with a quadripod cane. The rehabilitation process begins with this client when:

    1. He is about to be discharged or transferred to a rehabilitation facility.
    2. The critical period of illness is passed.
    3. He is admitted to the hospital.
    4. He expresses an interest in walking.

114. The nurse is using principles of rehabilitation when he or she:

    1. Encourages a client to dress in street clothes.
    2. Bathes a client and combs hair.

3. Brushes a client's teeth when the client has trouble or forgets.
4. Asks the physician to order a Foley catheter for occasional urinary incontinence.

115. The physician orders active and passive range-of-motion (ROM) exercises to all extremities. For the client, passive ROM exercises are:

1. Done by the nurse or therapist without assistance from the client.
2. Done by the therapist, who instructs the client which way to move and exercise.
3. More effective than active ROM exercises in preventing contractures.
4. Done by the client three times a day.

116. A nurse is administering the Denver Developmental Screening Test (DDST) and recognizes that the test:

1. Assesses the child from birth to 2 years
2. Cannot be adjusted for prematurity
3. Can be administered to all minority ethnic groups
4. Is not an IQ test

117. The nurse is assessing a 2-year-old child. Which of the following toys is suitable for this child?

1. Squeak toy
2. Pull toy
3. Tricycle, Big Wheel
4. Jungle gym

118. The nurse is assessing a 12-month-old infant. Which of the following is appropriate gross motor development seen for the first time?

1. Sits with support, head steady
2. Crawls, creeps, or walks holding on to furniture
3. Walks well, stoops, and recovers
4. Kicks ball forward, walks up steps, walks backward

119. A 24-year-old pregnant client comes into the prenatal clinic. She is complaining of severe headaches, vertigo, and blurred vision. The priority nursing action is to:

1. Encourage her to rest more frequently during the day.
2. Tell her to take Tylenol or aspirin for the headache pain.
3. Immediately notify the physician.
4. Refer her for allergy testing.

120. The nurse teaches an older client who is undergoing an amniocentesis. Which of the following statements by the client indicates a need for further teaching?

1. "This test will determine if my baby's lungs are mature."
2. "This test will tell me if my baby has Down's syndrome."
3. "This test will tell me if there is a problem with my blood reacting to the baby's blood."
4. "This test will determine the fetal age and position."

121. When preparing a pregnant client for an amniocentesis, the client verbalizes understanding of the procedure to the nurse. Which of the following indicates a need for further teaching?

1. "I will drink lots of water and try not to go to the bathroom."
2. "I will sign a consent form."
3. "I must report any vaginal bleeding or fever afterwards."
4. "I will have my BP, pulse, and respirations taken very frequently before and after the procedure."

122. A 22-year-old client is admitted to the emergency room with vaginal bleeding, low abdominal cramping, and a BP of 80/40 mm Hg, P 130 bpm, R 20/min. The nurse correctly suspects these to be symptoms of:

1. Overdose of aspirin
2. Toxic shock syndrome
3. Endometriosis
4. Spontaneous abortion

123. A 26-year-old woman on a psychiatric unit refuses to sleep in her room because she says that it is "bugged." The most appropriate way in which the nurse might initially handle this situation is to:

1. Simply state that the room is not bugged.
2. Change the room.
3. Ask her why she believes the room is bugged.
4. Ignore her delusion.

124. A 31-year-old client is admitted to a psychiatric unit. She thinks that her coworkers are accusing her of indiscretions and spying on her. The initial nursing goal is directed at:

1. Joining in group activities
2. Establishing trust with staff
3. Limiting contacts with other clients
4. Allowing coworkers to visit

125. In teaching a client about the care of a leg brace, the nurse should emphasize:

1. The need to inspect skin daily and to expect some minor irritations.
2. The cleaning and maintenance of the brace, which should be done by a professional therapist.
3. The importance of keeping brace joints free of lint and oiling them once a week.
4. That weight fluctuations have little effect on the fit of the brace.

126. A 28-year-old client was injured in a motorcycle accident. The right leg was amputated above the knee. The nurse explains that a temporary prosthesis will be fitted to the leg. The most important use for a temporary prosthesis immediately after surgery is that it:

1. Allows the client to stand with aid within a few days.
2. Substitutes for a dressing over the stump.
3. Enhances body image.
4. Prevents complications of bed rest.

127. A client is learning to use crutches for the first time. When planning care for this client, which of the following is most important?

1. Heavy padding of the axillary bar so that it can help support body weight

2. Looking down frequently to see the position of the crutches and feet.
3. Having two assistants aid the client
4. Carefully assessing the client's activity level

128. To prepare a client for crutch walking, it would be most important for the nurse to:
1. Refer the client to physical therapy.
2. Initiate muscle-strengthening exercises for arms and shoulders.
3. Urge the client to conserve strength in other activities to avoid tiring.
4. Demonstrate crutch walking: how to sit, stand, and get up from the floor in case of falling.

129. When a client receives a permanent prosthesis, the nurse should teach the client to:
1. Wash the prosthesis daily with soap and water.
2. Wear it only when going out or having company.
3. Inspect the prosthesis daily for loose or worn parts.
4. Oil all joints daily.

130. In the data collection phase of the nursing process, nurses:
1. Make plans to help the client meet treatment goals.
2. Gather, verify, and communicate data about a client's health needs.
3. Identify problems and act to eliminate them.
4. Communicate with the client and formulate realistic goals to meet his or her health needs.

131. An 8-year-old child is admitted to the pediatric unit with a diagnosis of chronic nephrosis. In discussing the plan of care with the client's mother, you share that the purpose of weighing the child is:
1. To measure adequacy of nutritional management.
2. To check the accuracy of the fluid intake record.
3. To impress on the child the importance of eating well.
4. To determine changes in the amount of edema.

132. Causing mental distress by name calling, isolating, ignoring, or ridiculing is an example of:
1. Psychological abuse
2. Physical abuse
3. Active neglect
4. Passive neglect

133. A 90-year-old client is kept locked in a room of a house. The client is diabetic and is fed once a day by relatives. They do not give the client insulin because it is too expensive. The nurse identifies deliberately abandoning an older person or denying health care as an example of:
1. Psychological abuse
2. Physical abuse
3. Passive neglect
4. Active neglect

134. The nurse is observing a physician do a complete examination to rule out appendicitis. Which area of

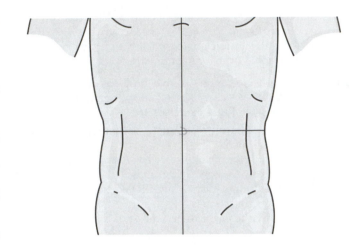

the abdomen would the physician palpate? (Place an X on the correct area in the figure.)

135. The nurse identifies the best way to facilitate growth and development in the acutely ill toddler as:
1. Direct efforts at preparing and teaching parents to ensure nonanxious parenting of the child.
2. Telling the toddler well in advance of a procedure that is to take place.
3. Separating the toddler from parent, especially if there are temper tantrums.
4. Encouraging the child to regress to a previous developmental level for familiarity and comfort.

136. A 7-year-old child has been hospitalized for dehydration and vomiting. It would be most important for the nurse to remember which of the following?
1. Fear is related to body injury, loss of control, and death, and mutilation fantasies are common.
2. A child may view hospitalization as a punishment for thoughts.
3. Fears are related to body image.
4. A child may exhibit regressive behavior such as whining, tantrums, and thumb sucking.

137. According to Maslow's hierarchy, the first priority in nursing actions must be aimed at:
1. Moving toward satisfaction of creative and emotional needs as early as possible.
2. Helping the client gain respect from others to prevent loneliness.
3. Doing first things first: meeting the client's physiological needs before moving on to other needs.
4. Helping the client to establish close relationships with as many persons as possible.

138. The nurse is evaluating a mother's knowledge of steroid therapy because her child is being discharged. It is most important to know whether the mother knows that steroid therapy:
1. Commonly causes hirsutism
2. Aggravates acne
3. Causes cushingoid features to disappear
4. "Masks" infections

139. The first priority of nursing care of the client with a head injury is to:
    1. Check level of consciousness
    2. Evaluate pupils
    3. Protect airway
    4. Evaluate motor function

140. An 80-year-old woman is admitted for cataract surgery. When you are first assessing her, she tells you that she used to be several inches taller than she is now. The best response would be to:
    1. Tell her she can regain her height by practicing better posture.
    2. Disregard her statement because she is probably confused owing to her advanced age.
    3. Acknowledge her statement as being inaccurate because older people do not tend to become shorter with age.
    4. Ask her how tall she used to be, measure her current height, and include both in your data collection.

141. A 64-year-old client frequently complains that the room is too cold. The nurse realizes that the reason for this may be that:
    1. A normal decrease in subcutaneous fat predisposes older people to feeling cold.
    2. Older people often complain because they are lonely.
    3. Sweat glands diminish in size, number, and activity as they become sclerosed.
    4. Older persons are more susceptible to heatstroke.

142. A nursing home resident has a pressure sore exposing the trochanter of the hip. The nurse identifies this as:
    1. Stage I
    2. Stage II
    3. Stage III
    4. Stage IV

143. A chronically debilitated 82-year-old client is admitted to the hospital from a nursing home. The nurse identifies which of the following as risk factors for development of pressure ulcers?
    1. Incontinence, immobility, impaired nutrition
    2. Immobility, incontinence, agitation
    3. Incontinence, impaired nutrition, agitation
    4. Agitation, hyperactivity, thin skin

144. An 80-year-old client is hospitalized for cataract surgery. She tells you she sometimes has "palpitations" when she climbs stairs but that she has never had chest pain on exertion. The nurse should know that:
    1. The heart of the aging person may respond by temporarily beating faster.
    2. She is a candidate for myocardial infarction.
    3. Rapid heartbeat on exertion is a cardinal sign of heart failure.
    4. She probably has mitral stenosis.

145. An 80-year-old client should be encouraged to be up and about during hospitalization for cataract surgery, within prudent limitations imposed by the surgery. This is primarily because:
    1. The older person is at high risk for pneumonia.
    2. The immune system is more efficient in aging persons.
    3. The intercostal muscles become flabby and dilated.
    4. Alveolar atrophy is reversed by early ambulation.

146. A client has had gallbladder "attacks" in the past and is considered at risk for gallstone formation. The nurse should check that the client's diet is:
    1. High in antacids and calcium
    2. Low in cholesterol
    3. High in protein and carbohydrate
    4. Free of electrolytes

147. Antabuse has been ordered for a client to bolster sobriety. In planning discharge teaching sessions, the nurse should include which of the following topics?
    1. Importance of reduced smoking
    2. Limiting exposure to the sun
    3. Medication scheduling and side effects
    4. Restricted sexual and physical activity

148. For communicating with the older hearing-impaired person, the nurse issues the following guidelines:
    1. "Stand at the person's side, and talk loudly in his or her ear."
    2. "Speak at a normal rate."
    3. "Speak in short sentences and allow time for a response."
    4. "Repeat the message using different words, and raise your voice."

149. When planning the dietary needs of a 68-year-old client, the nurse considers that the older person needs:
    1. 800 mg of calcium in the daily diet
    2. 1000–2500 mg of calcium in the daily diet
    3. 1000–1500 g of calcium in the daily diet
    4. 1.0–1.5 g of calcium in the daily diet

150. The nurse is planning fluid intake for a 68-year-old client. The older person should take in the following amount of water daily:
    1. 1000 mL
    2. 2000 mL
    3. 3000 mL
    4. 3000 L

151. A 45-year-old client has recently been placed on a low-sodium diet. The nurse is teaching her how to read food labels on food products.
    1. "List ingredients contained by amounts, in descending order."
    2. "List major ingredients only."
    3. "Always give helpful information about sodium content and fiber."
    4. "Always list the daily requirements."

152. The nurse recognizes that to communicate with the older person:

1. It should be recognized that silence will create tension.
2. Restraints may be necessary to get the older person to listen.
3. Ample time must be allowed for questions to be answered and information given.
4. Eye contact should be avoided because it may make the older person feel self-conscious.

153. When caring for a 68-year-old client, the nurse recognizes that which of the following may contribute to failure to identify the presence of an infection?

   1. The cough reflex is less active.
   2. The skin is thinner with diminished blood supply.
   3. Prostatic hypertrophy reduces the natural ability to flush the bladder.
   4. Absence of fever is not unusual.

154. When assessing the home of a 75-year-old home-health client for safety, the nurse identifies that fatal accidents occur most often in the:

   1. Bathroom
   2. Living room
   3. Bedroom
   4. Kitchen

155. After assessing the environment of a 70-year-old client, the nurse recognizes the need for further teaching when the client says "I will:

   1. Eliminate clutter; ensure a wide pathway."
   2. Carpet all stairways, using throw rugs over slippery areas."
   3. Keep handles of pans on the stove turned in and away from the pathway."
   4. Install and regularly check smoke detectors."

156. A client has a diagnosis of venous thrombosis. The nurse correctly identifies which of the following as a risk factor?

   1. Surgical procedures
   2. Excessive exercises
   3. Decubitus ulcers and a diet low in iron
   4. Immobility

157. A 24-year-old woman is in active labor with contractions coming every 2 minutes and lasting 60 seconds. Fetal heart rate is 150 bpm. Her BP is 70/50 mm Hg and the woman's pulse rate is 120 bpm. The first nursing action is to:

   1. Place the client in lithotomy position.
   2. Elevate the head of the bed.
   3. Ask someone else to check the client's pulse.
   4. Place the client on her left side.

158. A 15-year-old girl believes that she is pregnant. Which of the following symptoms does the nurse recognize as one of the earliest indications of pregnancy?

   1. Amenorrhea
   2. Dysmenorrhea
   3. Pica
   4. Nausea

159. A 15-year-old girl is 4 months pregnant when she comes to the clinic for her routine checkup. Which of the following symptoms would be abnormal?

   1. Urinary frequency
   2. Polyphagia
   3. Nausea
   4. Dysuria

160. A 9-month-old infant is prone to croup. His mother asks what she can do at home to help relieve his symptoms. The nurse suggests:

   1. "Give him cough medicine every 4 hours while he is awake."
   2. "Give him a warm bath."
   3. "Keep the house temperature 80.8°F (26.68°C)."
   4. "Keep the humidity in the house low."

161. A 16-year-old adolescent is 6 hours post-tonsillectomy. Which of the following should the nurse include in the care?

   1. Position client on her back to promote drainage.
   2. Encourage client to cough, clear the throat, or blow the nose frequently.
   3. Have the client use a straw to drink cool fluids.
   4. Offer a liquid diet and cool fluids first 12–24 hours.

162. A 2-year-old child comes with his mother to the clinic. The child is fussy and irritable, and keeps tugging on his right ear. When assessing the child, the nurse suspects:

   1. Ménière's disease
   2. Otitis media
   3. Otosclerosis
   4. Meningitis

163. A 42-year-old client is 5 weeks postileostomy and is beginning to use a permanent appliance. The client is complaining of an odor from the appliance bag. The nurse explains that the best way to prevent odor is to:

   1. Use a commercial deodorizer that is sprayed inside the bag.
   2. Avoid excessive amounts of gas-forming foods.
   3. Thoroughly clean the bag at regular intervals.
   4. Refit the bag because of odor leakage.

164. The nurse has given the Mantoux tuberculin tests to a family in the clinic. To interpret the results correctly, the nurse would need to know which of the following is a positive reaction at 48 hours?

   1. The area of induration
   2. The amount of erythema
   3. The size of the raised wheal
   4. The absence of erythema or induration

165. A 38-year-old client had a cesarean section and delivered premature twins 14 hours ago. She is hungry and wants to start her liquid diet. Before giving a tray to her, the nurse's most important action is to:

   1. Check her dressing
   2. Check bowel sounds

3. Encourage ambulation
4. Give pain medication

166. A client is unconscious with a head injury from a motor vehicle accident. The nurse is observing him for increased intracranial pressure. Which set of vital signs would indicate this? His normal vital signs are BP 140/80 mm Hg, P 80 bpm, and R 18/min.

1. R 18, P 100, BP 170/90
2. R 16, P 80, BP 120/76
3. R 12, P 60, BP 180/120
4. R 24, P 120, BP 60/40

167. When giving an enema to a client, the nurse knows that the correct temperature for an enema is:

1. 70–80°F (21.1–26.6°C)
2. 80–90°F (26.6–32.2°C)
3. 102–105°F (38.8–40.5°C)
4. 110–120°F (43.3–48.8°C)

168. A physician asks you to gather equipment so that he can start an (IV) infusion on a client who is to receive blood. The nurse would set up with which IV needle?

1. No. 16 Angiocath
2. No. 22 Angiocath
3. No. 25 butterfly
4. No. 27 butterfly

169. The correct technique for a nurse to use when suctioning is:

1. To occlude the catheter suction port when withdrawing
2. To occlude the catheter suction port when entering
3. To instill 20 mL of normal saline
4. To open the catheter suction port when withdrawing

170. A client is 5 ft 2 in. tall and weighs 100 lb. The nurse is to administer 4.4 mL of gamma globulin IM. The nurse should:

1. Give one injection into the vastus lateralis.
2. Give one injection into the gluteus maximus.
3. Divide the dosage and give an injection into each deltoid.
4. Divide the dosage and give an injection into each buttock in the gluteal muscle.

171. The nurse is to administer heparin 5000 units into the abdomen, and should be sure to:

1. Massage the site after the injection.
2. Firmly pinch the skin and administer the injection at a 90-degree angle.
3. Aspirate before injecting the medicine.
4. Give subcutaneously (SC).

172. A 12-year-old boy is in a leg cast for a fractured femur. The most important nursing intervention is to:

1. Palpate for a pedal pulse
2. Palpate for a popliteal pulse
3. Report any drainage on the cast
4. Keep traction on the cast at all times

173. A mother calls the clinic and tells the nurse that her 12-year-old daughter has spilled hot grease on her foot and it has two blisters the size of quarters. The nurse initially advises her to:

1. Break the blisters and cover with a clean dressing.
2. Leave the blisters intact and open to air.
3. Break the blisters and place ice on the area.
4. Leave the blisters intact and apply petrolatum.

174. A 3-day-old infant was a healthy newborn. He now has a diagnosis of phenylketonuria (PKU). His mother asks the nurse how the diagnosis was made. Your response is that it was made from which type of specimen?

1. Gastric secretions
2. Arterial blood gases
3. Capillary blood
4. Urine

175. A 14-year-old adolescent is admitted to a behavioral management unit. When planning care, the nurse recognizes that the central task of early adolescence is:

1. Industry versus inferiority
2. Identity versus role confusion
3. Intimacy versus isolation
4. Integrity versus despair

176. While working on a psychiatric unit, the nurse is especially careful to observe depressed clients:

1. In the early morning
2. In the afternoon
3. In the evening
4. At visiting time

177. A 25-year-old client with a diagnosis of schizophrenia is sitting in a corner rocking to and fro, twisting her hands. One of the best initial approaches by the nurse is to:

1. Bring the client some warm milk
2. Hug the client
3. Bring the client a deck of cards
4. Sit quietly by the client

178. Although it is the physician's responsibility to prescribe medication, the nurse should understand the basis for the drug therapy. One of the drugs prescribed is isoniazid for tuberculosis therapy. It would be important for the nurse to know that isoniazid is given with pyridoxine 50–100 mg daily to prevent:

1. Labyrinth damage
2. Peripheral neuritis
3. Renal toxicity
4. GI irritation

179. A client with a diagnosis of tuberculosis has been discharged from the hospital on drug therapy. The most important outcome of the nurse's teaching is for the client to:

1. Take the medications regularly and without interruption.

2. Carry extra medication when traveling.
3. Learn how to discontinue drugs when symptoms of intolerance occur.
4. Wear a Medic Alert bracelet.

180. A 40-year-old client is hospitalized with an extensive myocardial infarction. The client is very frustrated with the limitations imposed, such as bed rest. In addition, the client is always complaining about the food. This is an example of:

1. Compensation
2. Denial
3. Displacement
4. Projection

181. The highest-priority nursing intervention for a 39-year-old client with a prolapsed umbilical cord is to:

1. Leave the room to obtain assistance.
2. Monitor fetal heartbeats.
3. Cover the exposed cord with a sterile dressing.
4. Place in knee-chest or exaggerated Trendelenburg position.

182. A 26-year-old client was admitted to the hospital with a diagnosis of appendicitis. Which of the following signs and symptoms are indicative of appendicitis?

1. Anorexia and high fever
2. Nausea and vomiting after eating
3. Tenderness located in the lower right quadrant
4. Tenderness over McBurney's point

183. Which of the following interventions would be appropriate for a client with suspected appendicitis?

1. Place a heating pad on the tender area to decrease pain.
2. Administer an enema preoperatively.
3. Give the client sips of cool water.
4. Maintain a semi-Fowler's position.

184. The nurse is sitting with a woman who is in active labor in her home. Because of a hurricane, she cannot be taken to the hospital. What is the most important action for the nurse?

1. Time contractions for frequency and duration.
2. Remain calm and support the mother.
3. Boil water and all the equipment.
4. Provide the client with a light meal so that she can maintain her strength.

185. A nurse is on a boat where people are eating and drinking. Someone yells "Help! My wife's choking!" The nurse would initially:

1. Ask the husband, "Can she talk?"
2. Give a back blow.
3. Give an abdominal thrust.
4. Hit her in the chest.

186. The nurse is applying a tourniquet to the upper arm of a client who has sustained a gunshot wound. This is a last resort because:

1. Tourniquets are difficult to apply.
2. Tourniquets must be released every 20 minutes.

3. Tourniquets may be used below the elbow or knee.
4. Tourniquets cause considerable nerve and tissue damage.

187. The nurse is helping to orient a 72-year-old client with organic brain syndrome (OBS) to his room in a nursing home. Which of the following is appropriate?

1. Give him a complete orientation to the unit and its rules.
2. Limit the orientation to small, specific amounts of essential information.
3. Show him only his room to avoid further confusion.
4. Ask him questions to determine what he understands.

188. When planning for a 79-year-old client's activities of daily living (ADLs), it is essential that the nurse:

1. Make the client responsible for own care.
2. Encourage the client to do as much of his or her own care as possible.
3. Assign another resident to show the client the routine.
4. Do as much care as possible for the client.

189. The physician orders a sputum specimen to be collected on a client suspected of having TB. The specimen is best collected:

1. At bedtime.
2. In early morning.
3. Before lunch.
4. Time does not matter.

190. A client starts having a seizure. It would be most important to:

1. Protect the head from injury and turn the head to the side.
2. Place a tongue blade or other object between the teeth.
3. Restrain the client to prevent injury.
4. Move the client to the floor and hold her down.

191. A 24-year-old client has been admitted to the emergency room. The physician suspects a head injury and a skull fracture. Cerebrospinal fluid (CSF) leakage may occur. The nurse assesses for:

1. Watering of the eyes and drainage of mucus from the nose
2. Clear fluid from the nose or ears
3. Purulent, thick yellow drainage from the nose or ears
4. Bleeding from the nose or ears

192. What type of strategy would the nurse teach a 77-year-old client about successful aging?

1. Eat red meat to keep your protein level up.
2. Refrain from sexual activity.
3. Do what makes you happy.
4. Do not keep any pets.

193. What type of basic nursing intervention is useful in assisting an older person with feelings of self-worth and self-esteem?

1. Letting the older person decide on his or her food plan
2. Assisting with hygiene and grooming
3. Not allowing the older person to take a bath or shower
4. Refraining from putting cosmetics on the older woman

194. What nursing intervention is appropriate to help maintain mental-health wellness in older adults?

1. Calling them "honey"
2. Encouraging dependence
3. Referring to their diapers used for incontinence
4. Allowing as much control over care as possible

195. What is the most appropriate response to an older person in teaching about medications?

1. "Take plenty of vitamins."
2. "Use sedatives to help you sleep."
3. "Take daily laxatives."
4. "Take as few medications as possible."

196. What is the responsibility of the hospital nurse in maintaining an older person's mental health?

1. Assess for signs of abuse.
2. Teach instructions for home care to both older person and family.
3. Assess for signs of social isolation.
4. Teach ways to cope with aging.

197. The nurse working in a nursing home identifies which kind of activity that a nursing home resident can have some control over?

1. Administration of routine medications
2. Requesting that certain staff members be assigned to him or her
3. Complete control of the food plan
4. Type and time of bath

198. Which nursing intervention can be used to prevent loneliness in a nursing home resident?

1. Allow clients to wander in other residents' rooms.
2. Provide group learning.
3. Provide individual one-to-one contact.
4. Limit communication for the residents with dementia.

199. What interpersonal impact does humor have on an older person?

1. Humor serves as an outlet for inner tensions and anxieties.
2. Older persons are more likely to be offended when jokes about aging are told by people of their own age group.
3. Humor helps to establish relationships.
4. Humor stimulates alertness.

200. What type of humor intervention can a nurse use in any setting with an older person?

1. Tease the older person even if it is against his or her wishes.
2. Wear scary costumes for effect.
3. Tell grim stories.
4. Use cartoons in teaching materials.

201. A 38-year-old client was diagnosed with endometriosis. The physician ordered danazol 400 mg bid. In stock were 200-mg tablets. How many tablets will the client receive?

1. 1 tablet
2. 1.5 tablets
3. 2 tablets
4. 2.5 tablets

202. A 45-year-old client was seen by her gynecologist with complaints of abnormal uterine bleeding. The physician ordered conjugated estrogens (Premarin) for this breakthrough bleeding. He ordered the nurse to give the client 10 mg IM. On hand was a 25 mg/mL vial. How many milliliters did the nurse draw up?

1. 0.1 mL
2. 0.2 mL
3. 0.3 mL
4. 0.4 mL

203. A 30-year-old was being treated with norethindrone (Micronor) 20 mg for endometriosis. The pharmacist dispensed 5-mg tablets. The nurse instructed the client to take how many tablets?

1. 2 tablets
2. 4 tablets
3. 6 tablets
4. 8 tablets

204. A 17-year-old client was diagnosed with herpes genitalis. The physician ordered acycolovir (Zovirax) 200 mg every 4 hours while awake times 5 days (8 AM, noon, 4 PM, and 8 PM). The nurse instructed the client to have on hand how many 200 mg tablets?

1. 10 tablets
2. 15 tablets
3. 20 tablets
4. 25 tablets

205. A young woman was complaining of burning on urination. The physician diagnoses cystitis and ordered ampicillin 250 mg IM every 6 hours. After reconstitution, the vial contained 500 mg/5 mL. How many milliliters will the nurse administer?

1. 1 mL
2. 1.5 mL
3. 2.0 mL
4. 2.5 mL

ANSWERS

1. **(4)** Integrated processes: nursing process — data collection; client need: health promotion and maintenance; content area: medical-surgical.

   RATIONALE

   (1) BP increases with age. **(2)** Renal blood flow is nearly halved, renal tubules are less able to concentrate urine, and prostatic hypertrophy is almost universal. Creatinine clearance also steadily decreases with age. **(3)** Peristalsis is decreased, gastric acid is reduced, but constipation rarely arises unless there is poor diet, drug effects, decreased mobility, or disease. **(4)** Average loss in height is 2 inches, the number of taste buds decreases by 70%, and bone mineral content is decreased by 10%–15% in men.

2. **(1)** Integrated processes: nursing process — data collection; client need: health promotion and maintenance; content area: medical-surgical.

   RATIONALE

   (1) High-frequency hearing loss, or presbycusis, occurs with particular problems with high-pitched sounds such as *s, z, sh,* and *ch.* **(2)** Increased susceptibility to postural hypotension occurs because of reduced baroceptor responsiveness. **(3)** Decreased cardiac reserve occurs, making the older person more susceptible to fluid overload. **(4)** Decreased adaptation to dark occurs, making night driving more hazardous.

3. **(1)** Integrated processes: nursing process — data collection; client need: health promotion and maintenance; content area: medical-surgical.

   RATIONALE

   (1) Arthritis is the most common chronic condition, occurring in 48 of 100 persons over 65 years old. **(2)** Hearing impairment occurs in 32 of 100 persons over 65 years old. **(3)** Cataracts occur in 17 of 100 persons over 65 years old. **(4)** Diabetes occurs in 16 of 100 persons over 65 years old.

4. **(2, 4, 5)** Integrated processes: nursing process — data collection; teaching/learning; client need: health promotion and maintenance; content area: medical-surgical.

   RATIONALE

   (1) The gradual loss of lens elasticity, or presbyopia, occurs in the early 40s. **(2)** By age 40 years, all adults have osteoarthritic changes in the cervical spine. **(3)** By age 40 years, all adults have osteoarthritic changes in the cervical spine. **(4)** Difficulty staying up at night and working the next day is the most common early sign of aging. **(5)** The gradual loss of lens elasticity, or presbyopia, occurs in the early 40s. **(6)** Difficulty staying up at night and working the next day is the most common early sign of aging.

5. **(4)** Integrated processes: nursing process — data collection; teaching/learning; client need: health promotion and maintenance; content area: medical-surgical.

   RATIONALE

   (1) Although this is a good response because milk helps release hormones and calm the client, it is not the best answer. **(2)** Most older people will not be helped by this. **(3)** Sleep disturbances may occur from nocturia, arthritis, or diabetes. These may require a referral to the doctor; otherwise, sleep disturbance is normal. **(4)** Most older people complain of problems sleeping. A combination of wakefulness, resting, dozing, and sleep is the usual pattern.

6. **(3)** Integrated processes: nursing process — data collection; client need: health promotion and maintenance; content area: medical-surgical.

   RATIONALE

   (1) Vaginal bleeding is never a normal sign in postmenopausal women. **(2)** Urinary frequency occurs because of decreased bladder capacity and decreased ability of the renal tubules. **(3)** Incontinence may occur because of benign prostatic hypertrophy in men, decreased estrogen in women, and loss of sphincter tone. **(4)** Weight increases until the mid 50s, then declines.

7. **(2, 6)** Integrated processes: nursing process — data collection; client need: physiological integrity; pharmacological therapies; content area: pharmacology.

   RATIONALE

   (1) Weight gain from edema is a common side effect of steroids and nonsteroidal anti-inflammatory drugs (NSAIDs). **(2)** GI hemorrhage occurs when aspirin destroys the lining of the stomach. It can also interfere with platelet functioning. **(3)** Anticonvulsants may cause gingival hypertrophy, but aspirin does not. **(4)** Many drugs, especially histamine H2 receptor agents, may cause confusion. **(5)** Many drugs, especially histamine H2 receptor agents, may cause confusion. **(6)** Aspirin interferes with platelet functioning.

8. **(2)** Integrated processes: nursing process — data collection; teaching/learning; client need: physiological integrity; basic care and comfort; content area: medical-surgical.

   RATIONALE

   (1) Fruit and vegetable groups should be increased to two to four servings and three to five servings per day, respectively. **(2)** Meat, animal products, and dried beans and nuts should be eaten in two to three servings per day. **(3)** Sugar and salt intake should be moderate. **(4)** Bread, cereal, and pasta group servings should be 6–11 servings per day.

9. **(1)** Integrated processes: nursing process — evaluation; teaching/learning; client need: psychosocial integrity; content area: medical-surgical.

   RATIONALE

   (1) A total hysterectomy involves removal of the uterus. She will no longer be able to have children. **(2)** Lifting of heavy objects and heavy housework should be avoided for 4 weeks. **(3)** Sexual relations can be resumed in 4–6 weeks with physician's approval. **(4)** Mild analgesics can be taken for pain control.

10. **(3)** Integrated processes: nursing process — implementation, communication and documentation; client need: physiological integrity; reduction of risk potential; content area: medical-surgical.

    RATIONALE

    (1) Serosanguinous vaginal drainage is normal for about 2–4 weeks after an abdominal hysterectomy. **(2)** A temperature of 101.8°F (38.38°C) or more should be immediately reported to the physician. **(3)** Internal hemorrhage from the incision or vagina is a major complication that causes circulating blood volume loss and fluid volume depletion. **(4)** Laboratory findings of 12 g/dL Hgb and 36 Hct are normal values.

11. **(2)** Integrated processes: nursing process — implementation; client need: physiological integrity; reduction of risk potential; content area: medical-surgical.

RATIONALE

(1) The client should avoid concentrated carbohydrates because they increase dumping. **(2)** The client should lie down after meals to decrease the effect of gravity. **(3)** The client should eat small, frequent well-balanced meals. **(4)** The client should avoid drinking fluids during and for about 2 hours after eating.

12. **(2)** Integrated processes: nursing process — implementation; teaching/learning; client need: health promotion and maintenance; content area: maternity nursing.

RATIONALE

(1) It is important to explain to the parents the necessity of keeping the twins in the hospital, but not of most importance. **(2)** Instructing the parents in how they will be incorporated into the twins' care is most important because it facilitates bonding and identifies expectations. **(3)** Rest is important, but not of most importance. **(4)** Parents may call the nursery whenever they need to be reassured or have the need for health teaching.

13. **(2)** Integrated processes: nursing process — implementation; teaching/learning; client need: health promotion and maintenance; content area: pediatrics.

RATIONALE

(1) Twins are two individual babies and each needs attention, but not more than usual. **(2)** Treating the twins as individuals facilitates the future self-identity of each as separate from the other twin. **(3)** Twins should be treated as individuals, each with his or her own unique personality. **(4)** New research shows that newborn twins should be kept together to decrease crying, but they may be separated.

14. **(1)** Integrated processes: nursing process — implementation; client need: health promotion and maintenance; content area: pediatrics.

RATIONALE

(1) A return demonstration of parenting skills validates learning. **(2)** Teaching the parent what to check for when the baby cries is important (i.e., Is the baby wet? Is the baby hungry?). However, safe caregiving is essential. **(3)** The parents will be taking the babies to the physician's office for follow-up visits. The immunization schedule can be reinforced at that time. **(4)** Help is not essential for the first few weeks when the babies are brought home.

15. **(1)** Integrated processes: nursing process — implementation; client need: physiological integrity; physiological adaptation; content area: pediatrics.

RATIONALE

(1) Careful monitoring of fluid intake and output (I&O), along with daily measurement of weight and abdominal girth, is essential. **(2)** A diet high in protein may help to restore the body's normal plasma oncotic pressure. **(3)** The child with severe edema may be placed on bed rest to promote diuresis. **(4)** Fluids are restricted based on client's symptoms. Controlling edema is critical.

16. **(3)** Integrated processes: nursing process — implementation; client need: health promotion and maintenance; content area: pediatrics.

RATIONALE

(1) The child does not have the motor skills or intellectual skills to solve a puzzle. **(2)** The child does not have the motor skills to walk with a push-pull toy. **(3)** Soft, colorful toys are appropriate for the 6-month-old child. **(4)** The child does not have the motor skills to ride a rocking horse.

17. **(3)** Integrated processes: nursing process — data collection; communicaition and documentation; client need: health promotion and maintenance; content area: maternity nursing.

RATIONALE

(1) Lochia alba (10 days, 6 weeks) is yellowish white. **(2)** Leuka is not a valid word. **(3)** Lochia rubra persists from delivery until about the third day. It is dark red and contains blood, debris from the placenta, and decidua and clots. **(4)** Lochia serosa is serous, watery pink to brown, occurring from 3 days to 6–10 days.

18. **(4)** Integrated processes: nursing process — implementation; client need: physiological integrity; physiological adaptation; content area: maternity nursing.

RATIONALE

(1) Infections would cause a rise in temperature and are not related to this situation. **(2)** If it is not an emergency, the midwife or RN does not need to be called. **(3)** This is a good option, but not the best. **(4)** A distended bladder can cause uterine relaxation and displace the uterus from its midline position. Emptying the bladder allows the uterus to resume its contracted position.

19. **(4)** Integrated processes: nursing process — implementation; teaching/learning; client need: physiological integrity; basic care and comfort; content area: maternity nursing.

RATIONALE

(1) Three days is usually too short. **(2)** The response that refers to breast-feeding does not address her question appropriately. **(3)** Although lochia alba may continue normally to the sixth week, it does not always do so. **(4)** The vaginal discharge will continue until the placental site has healed.

20. **(3)** Integrated processes: nursing process — implementation; teaching/learning; client need: physiological integrity; basic care and comfort; content area: maternity nursing.

RATIONALE

(1) Early ambulation is recommended and enhances involution of the uterus. **(2)** Breast-feeding also enhances involution of the uterus but does not prevent pooling of blood in the vagina. **(3)** A gush of blood sometimes occurs when the postpartal mother first arises and is caused by pooling of blood in the vagina, which flows out because of gravity when she stands. **(4)** The vagina does appear edematous and bruised after delivery, but that does not cause the pooling of blood.

21. **(2)** Integrated processes: nursing process — implementation; teaching/learning; client need: physiological integrity; basic care and comfort; content area: maternity nursing.

RATIONALE

(1) Limited physical activity, low-roughage diet, and inadequate fluids may postpone the bowel movement and allow it to harden in the rectum, resulting in greater pain at the time of bowel movement. **(2)** Early ambulation, fluids, and foods with roughage will promote normal evacuation of the bowel, resulting in minimal discomfort as bowel elimination pattern is restored. **(3)** Encourage foods with roughage to promote normal bowel evacuation. **(4)** Laxatives may be necessary but should be used as prescribed by the physician. Kegel exercises are important but for reasons other than promoting peristalsis.

22. **(3)** Integrated processes: nursing process — planning; client need: physiological integrity; reduction of risk potential; content area: maternity nursing.

RATIONALE

(1) Bromocriptine mesylate (Parlodel) may be administered after delivery to suppress lactation by preventing the secretion of prolactin. (2) Oxytocin is used to stimulate labor artificially. (3) The mother's blood is Rh negative, whereas her daughter's is Rh positive. Injection of Rho(D) immune globulin within 72 hours of delivery will prevent her from producing antibodies against the Rh factor, which could harm future pregnancies. (4) Rubella virus vaccine is not related to the Rh factor; it is administered to women who do not already demonstrate immunity.

23. **(3)** Integrated processes: nursing process — data collection; client need: health promotion and maintenance; content area: maternity nursing.

    RATIONALE
    (1) The client should not be asked to provide this information; this could cause the nurse to miss essential data. (2) Above or below the incision is too high or too low. (3) Gentle palpation on the sides of the midline vertical incision should reveal each side of the uterus because the uterus is usually found below the umbilicus and at the midline. (4) To palpate directly over the incision would produce unnecessary pain and trauma to the tissues, and palpation would be hampered by the presence of the dressing material.

24. **(2)** Integrated processes: nursing process — implementation, teaching/learning; client need: health promotion and maintenance; content area: maternity nursing.

    RATIONALE
    (1) The baby will receive sufficient nutrition from the breast, and giving a bottle after each feeding would prevent successful breast-feeding. (2) A side-lying position, with pillows supporting the mother's head and with baby turned toward mother, provides adequate support for both mother and baby and does not increase incisional pain. (3) Holding the baby high on her abdomen would increase the mother's incisional pain and might not permit the baby adequate access to the nipple. (4) Nipples should be cleansed with water before each feeding; soap may be drying to them.

25. **(3)** Integrated processes: nursing process — implementation, teaching/learning; client need: health promotion and maintenance; content area: maternity nursing.

    RATIONALE
    (1) Pain is usually not coming from the abdominal incision. (2) The abdominal discomfort is transitory and will usually be gone in a few days as she continues to breast-feed. (3) The explanation that oxytocin is released and causes the uterus to contract is the response that will promote the mother's understanding, self-care, and breast-feeding success. (4) A mild analgesic may be given 40–60 minutes before the nursing period. Bottle-feeding will interfere with the establishment of successful breast-feeding.

26. **(3)** Integrated processes: nursing process — implementation, teaching/learning; client need: physiological integrity; reduction of risk potential; content area: maternity nursing.

    RATIONALE
    (1) She needs to breathe deeply to prevent atelectasis and pneumonia. (2) She is not wearing off the anesthetic, and there is no need to contact the physician at this time. (3) She must continue with these measures, which prevent pooling of secretions (hypostatic pneumonia) and collapse of alveoli (atelectasis) during the postanesthesia period. Teach her to splint her incision because the support reduces discomfort. (4) There is no need to call the physician.

27. **(1)** Integrated processes: nursing process — evaluation; client need: health promotion and maintenance; content area: maternity nursing

RATIONALE
(1) The ductus arteriosus connects with the main pulmonary artery and the aorta. These two structures allow most of the fetal blood to bypass the lungs. (2) There is no ductus neonatorum. (3) The ductus venosus is a major blood channel that develops through the embryonic liver from the umbilical vein to the inferior vena cava. (4) The foramen ovale is an opening between the two atria of the heart.

28. **(8)** Integrated processes: nursing process — data collection; client need: health promotion and maintenance; content area: maternity nursing.

    RATIONALE
    (1) Guess again! (2) Recalculate! (3) Apgar scoring allows only one point for a heart rate of a 100 and one point for pink body with blue extremities. (For each of these to be given two points, the neonate must have a heart rate of 100 and a pink body including the extremities.) The other three observations are given two points each, for a total score of eight. (4) Guess again!

29. **(1)** Integrated processes: nursing process — implementation, teaching/learning; client need: health promotion and maintenance; content area: maternity nursing.

    RATIONALE
    (1) *Acro* means extremity and *cyanosis* means dark blue. Acrocyanosis of the hands and feet may be normal in an infant within the first few hours after birth. (2) Acrodermatosis is not correct, and refers to a skin disease that affects the hands and feet. (3) Cyanoacrylate adhesives and toxic glues such as Superglue are not related to a description of the infant. (4) Vernix caseosa is a protective sebaceous deposit covering the fetus.

30. **(1)** Integrated processes: nursing process — implementation; client need: physiological integrity; reduction of risk potential; content area: maternity nursing.

    RATIONALE
    (1) Law requires prevention of ophthalmia neonatorum, which is caused by gonococcal organisms, potentially acquired from the mother's birth canal. An erythromycin preparation is preferred over silver nitrate in some institutions. (2) The treatment has no effect on hemorrhagic tendencies. (3) The treatment does not apply to nosocomial infections. (4) The treatment does not apply to staphylococcal infections.

31. **(3)** Integrated processes: nursing process — implementation; client need: health promotion and maintenance; content area: maternity nursing.

    RATIONALE
    (1) There is no reason to wait until the neonatal nursery evaluation is complete or to refuse the request. (2) Even in facilities where sterile water is given as a newborn infant's first feeding, glucose water is not used because, if aspirated, it is dangerous to lung tissue. (3) Putting a baby to the breast after delivery provides both physiological and psychosocial benefits. For example, it stimulates the production of oxytocin, which causes the uterus to contract, assisting with delivery of the placenta and control of bleeding. (4) There is no reason to refuse her request.

32. **(2)** Integrated processes: nursing process — data collection; client need: health promotion and maintenance; content area: maternity nursing.

    RATIONALE
    (1) Select another answer. (2) A neonate is an infant from birth through the first 28 days of life. An infant is a child <1 year of age. (3) Guess again! (4) Guess again!

33. **(1)** Integrated processes: nursing process — implementation; client need: health promotion and maintenance; content area: medical-surgical.

RATIONALE

(1) Norepinephrine is a stimulant that causes peripheral vasocontriction and increased blood pressure and heart rate. **(2)** This hormone causes gluconeogenesis, a negative nitrogen balance, decrease in the immune response, and increased platelet activity resulting in an increase in the amount of available energy fuel, slowing of the tissue repair process, increased risk of infection, and increased clot formation. **(3)** Release of this hormone causes sodium and water reabsorption, leading to decreased urination and an increased circulatory volume. **(4)** The release of antidiuretic hormone causes the physiological changes listed in rationale 3.

34. **(1)** Integrated processes: nursing process — data collection; client need: health promotion and maintenance; content area: maternity nursing.

RATIONALE

(1) The apical pulse rate is most accurate. **(2)** Auscultating for a full minute provides greater opportunity for noting variations and abnormalities. **(3)** Auscultating for a full minute provides greater opportunity for noting variations and abnormalities. **(4)** Peripheral pulses should also be evaluated to detect any lags or unusual characteristics.

35. **(120–150 beats per minute)** Integrated processes: nursing process — data collection; client need: health promotion and maintenance; content area: maternity nursing.

RATIONALE

(1) Rates as low as 70–90 during sleep have been reported as normal. **(2)** Rates of 100–120 are below normal if the baby is awake. **(3)** Rates of 120–150 while the baby is awake are normal. **(4)** Rates may be as high as 180 when the newborn infant is crying.

36. **(1, 4, 6)** Integrated processes: nursing process — data collection; client need: health promotion and maintenance; content area: maternity nursing.

RATIONALE

(1) Normal full-term neonates pass meconium within 24 hours of life, or at least by 48 hours. **(2)** Many newborn infants void immediately after birth, 92% void by 24 hours, and 99% by 48 hours. **(3)** A perforate anus allows passage of a rectal thermometer, so option 3 is never normal. **(4)** Rust-colored or pink stains on a diaper with voiding are most likely to be normal. Large amounts of uric acid are excreted during the newborn period, and these urates appear as pink stains ("brick dust spots" or "brick dust") on a diaper. **(5)** Normal full-term neonates pass meconium within 24 hours of life, or at least by 48 hours. **(6)** Many newborn infants void immediately after birth.

37. **(1)** Integrated processes: nursing process — implementation; communication and documentation; client need: safe, effective care environment; coordinated care; content area: medical-surgical.

RATIONALE

(1) This statement is true. If a client should express a lack of understanding of the procedure or an unwillingness to continue with the surgery, this should be reported to the nursing supervisor and to the client's physician immediately. **(2)** No client should receive preoperative medication until the consent form has been signed. Mind-altering medication renders the client mentally incompetent. When the medication has been given, the drug effects should be allowed to wear off before the consent can be obtained. **(3)** Competent adults should sign their own consent forms. Spouses, children, and friends cannot do so legally. **(4)** The surgeon and the anesthesia care provider, not the perioperative nurse, are required to inform the client of the risks of procedures.

38. **(4)** Integrated processes: nursing process — implementation; client need: physiological integrity; pharmacological therapies; content area: maternity nursing.

RATIONALE

(1) Aquaphor is a trade name for petrolatum. **(2)** Cyanocobalamin does not help produce clotting factors. **(3)** Erythromycin is an antibiotic used for prophylaxis of gonorrheal conjunctivitis. **(4)** The absence of normal flora needed to synthesize vitamin K in the newborn infant's gut creates a transiente blood coagulation deficiency. There are usually no clinical consequences, but an injection of this substance is given prophylactically on the day of birth to combat the deficiency. Aqua-Mephyton is a trade name for phytonadione (vitamin K).

39. **(3)** Integrated processes: nursing process — implementation; client need: physiological integrity; reduction of risk potential; content area: medical-surgical.

RATIONALE

(1) A deep breath through the nose is most effective. **(2)** Breathing in through the nose is recommended. **(3)** After surgery there is a decline in lung ventilation and gas exchange that varies with the individual client, length of anesthesia, and surgical site. The client is taught this technique of sustained maximal inspiration to prevent collapse of alveoli and to mobilize secretions after surgery. **(4)** A slow breath through the nose and coughing from the chest is most effective.

40. **(4)** Integrated processes: nursing process — data collection, teaching/learning; client need: physiological integrity; basic care and comfort; content area: maternity nursing.

RATIONALE

(1) Well-formed brown stools are unusual for newborn infants. **(2)** The stools of a breast-fed newborn infant may be pasty green, but dark green is normal only for meconium. **(3)** Normal newborn stools vary in frequency from up to 10 daily to 1 every 2–3 days. **(4)** Breast-fed infants usually produce stools that are yellow-gold, soft, or mushy. They are more liquid, more frequent, and less pale yellow than those of formula-fed infants.

41. **(2)** Integrated processes: nursing process — implementation, teaching/learning; client need: physiological integrity; basic care and comfort; content area: maternity nursing.

RATIONALE

(1) The American Academy of Pediatrics (2005) recommends breast milk as the optimal food for the first 4–6 months of life. **(2)** The American Academy of Pediatrics (2005) recommends breast milk as the optimal food for the first 4–6 months of life. **(3)** The American Academy of Pediatrics (2005) recommends breast milk as the optimal food for the first 4–6 months of life. **(4)** The American Academy of Pediatrics (2005) recommends breast milk as the optimal food for the first 4–6 months of life.

42. **(2)** Integrated processes: nursing process — data collection; client need: physiological integrity; basic care and comfort; content area: medical-surgical.

RATIONALE

(1) She should have no difficulty with carbohydrates. Select another option. **(2)** Inflammation of the gallbladder (cholecystitis), presence of gallstones (cholelithiasis), or both interfere with movement of bile from the liver or gallbladder into the small intestine, where it promotes the digestion of fats. **(3)** She should have no difficulty with protein. Select another option. **(4)** She should have no difficulty with vitamin C. Select another option.

43. **(3)** Integrated processes: nursing process — implementation, teaching/learning; client need: physiological integrity; reduction of risk potential; content area: medical-surgical.

    RATIONALE

    (1) Leg exercises will not help to prevent muscle spasms. **(2)** Paralytic ileus is paralysis of intestines, which may occur after any abdominal surgery but is not prevented by leg exercises. **(3)** Muscle contractions involved in the leg exercise increase venous return and therefore help prevent stasis of blood and clot formation. If a clot forms and becomes dislodged, the resulting embolus can be life threatening. **(4)** Vasogenic shock results from inadequate vascular tone caused by nerve injury, chemicals, or sepsis and is not affected by leg exercises.

44. **(0.9% sodium chloride)** Integrated processes: nursing process — implementation; client need: physiological integrity; pharmacological therapies; content area: medical-surgical.

    RATIONALE

    (1) Isotonic solutions of the two agents in the question would be 0.9% sodium chloride or 5% dextrose. **(2)** The 0.45% sodium chloride is hypotonic. **(3)** The 10% dextrose is hypertonic. **(4)** The 50% dextrose is hypertonic.

45. **(1)** Integrated processes: nursing process — implementation; client need: physiological integrity; pharmacological therapies; content area: medical-surgical.

    RATIONALE

    (1) Preoperative medications often cause drowsiness or dizziness. After administration, the bed side rails should be up and the room light dim. The calm, drowsy state should be interrupted only when necessary and then briefly and quietly. **(2)** Her bladder should have been emptied before the medication was administered. **(3)** It is not safe to allow the client to move around in the room. **(4)** The nurse should explain the procedure or answer any questions before the client is premedicated.

46. **(2, 1, 4, 3)** Integrated processes: nursing process — implementation; client need: physiological integrity; reduction of risk potential; content area: medical-surgical.

    RATIONALE

    (1) Deep-breathing and coughing mainly affect respiratory function. **(2)** The benefits of early ambulation include improved respiratory, circulatory, and GI function; improved wound healing because of improved circulation; increased comfort and morale; reduced pain; and reduced recovery time, hospital stay, and expenses. **(3)** Leg exercises mainly affect circulatory function. **(4)** Medication for pain increases comfort and rest.

47. **(3)** Integrated processes: nursing process — implementation; client need: physiological integrity; reduction of risk potential; content area: medical-surgical.

    RATIONALE

    (1) The pain medication may reduce the sensation of pain but would not prevent emboli. **(2)** Pain, tenderness, and swelling in the lower extremity may signal the presence of a clot. She must be placed on bed rest. The physician will decide whether to continue the bed rest. The desired outcome is prevention of an embolism. **(3)** Pain, tenderness, and swelling in the lower extremity after surgery signal the potential presence of phlebothrombosis. Immobilization helps to prevent embolus formation by reducing the chances for thrombi to break loose. **(4)** Massage may cause release of a clot into the bloodstream (i.e., formation of an embolism).

48. **(3)** Integrated processes: nursing process — implementation; client need: physiological integrity; pharmacological therapies; content area: medical-surgical.

RATIONALE

(1) Aspirin also reduces pain and fever, but for those effects a higher dosage is usually required. **(2)** Aspirin is not an antibiotic. **(3)** Given in small doses in conjunction with a surgical procedure, aspirin may be used for its prophylactic anticoagulation effect. **(4)** Aspirin also reduces pain and fever, but for those effects a higher dosage is usually required.

49. **(1)** Integrated processes: nursing process — implementation, teaching/learning; client need: physiological integrity; reduction of risk potential; content area: medical-surgical.

    RATIONALE

    (1) Postoperative positioning after total hip replacement varies with the type of prosthesis and its method of insertion. However, positioning is usually directed at maintaining abduction and limiting flexion of the hip. **(2)** Leg adduction can cause dislocation. **(3)** Hip flexion 90 degrees can cause dislocation. **(4)** This cannot be done. Select another option.

50. **(3 months)** Integrated processes: nursing process — implementation, teaching/learning; client need: physiological integrity; reduction of risk potential; content area: medical-surgical.

    RATIONALE

    (1) After total hip replacement, it is important not to flex the hip 90 degrees and to avoid extremes of internal rotation, adduction, and flexion of the hip to prevent dislocation. Routine activities of daily living (ADLs) are not possible in 1 week. **(2)** After total hip replacement, it is important not to flex the hip 90 degrees and to avoid extremes of internal rotation, adduction, and flexion of the hip to prevent dislocation. Other ADLs are usually possible by 3 months after surgery. **(3)** After total hip replacement, it is important not to flex the hip 90 degrees and to avoid extremes of internal rotation, adduction, and flexion of the hip to prevent dislocation. Routine ADLs are possible after 3 months. **(4)** After total hip replacement, it is important not to flex the hip 90 degrees and to avoid extremes of internal rotation, adduction, and flexion of the hip to prevent dislocation. Routine ADLs are possible after 3 months.

51. **(4)** Integrated processes: nursing process — data collection; client need: physiological integrity; pharmacological therapies; content area: medical-surgical.

    RATIONALE

    (1) It is inappropriate to simply administer furosemide (Lasix) when urinary output is insufficient. **(2)** Calling the physician is an inappropriate response. The physician will be unable to diagnose the problem completely if he or she is not presented with all of the facts of the situation. **(3)** The client's symptoms imply a problem requiring immediate attention, not one that may be postponed for 30 minutes. **(4)** Collected data indicate digitalis toxicity; however, additional data regarding blood levels of digoxin are required to determine appropriate action. In this case, the physician would be most likely to withhold the digoxin until blood levels return to the therapeutic range.

52. **(3)** Integrated processes: nursing process — data collection; client need: physiological integrity; pharmacological therapies; content area: medical-surgical.

    RATIONALE

    (1) Calcium should not be significantly affected. Select another option. **(2)** Chloride should not be significantly affected. Select another option. **(3)** Furosemide is a potassium-depleting diuretic. **(4)** Sodium should not be significantly affected. Select another option.

53. **(3)** Integrated processes: nursing process — implementation; client need: physiological integrity; pharmacological therapies; content area: medical-surgical

    RATIONALE

    (1) Administration of additional morphine may result in respiratory arrest. **(2)** Administration of additional morphine may result in respiratory arrest. **(2)** Decreased respiratory rate is an early sign of morphine toxicity. If the client's respiratory rate is 8–10 or less, withhold a repeated dose and consult the physician. Another narcotic may relieve the pain without depression of respiration. **(4)** Leaving the room to allow the client to be alone does not address her current need.

54. **(2)** Integrated processes: nursing process — implementation; client need: physiological integrity; reduction of risk potential; content area: medical-surgical.

    RATIONALE

    (1) Bryant's traction is continuous skin traction. **(2)** Bryant's traction is skin traction applied to both legs to minimize potential trauma to the affected leg while maintaining appropriate position of the bone fragments. It involves bilateral vertical extension of the legs and is continuously applied. **(3)** Bryant's traction is continuous skin traction. **(4)** Bryant's traction is continuous skin traction.

55. **(1)** Integrated processes: nursing process — implementation; client need: physiological integrity; reduction of risk potential; content area: medical-surgical.

    RATIONALE

    (1) With Bryant's traction, the child's weight serves as countertraction to the vertical pull of the weights. It is necessary, then, for his buttocks to be elevated and clear of the bed to allow his weight to pull against the force of the weights. An abdominal restraint is usually necessary to keep him from turning from side to side. **(2)** The buttocks must be elevated to allow countertraction to the vertical pull of the weights. An abdominal restraint is usually necessary to keep him from turning side to side. **(3)** A sling is not appropriate. **(4)** A pillow is not appropriate.

56. **(2)** Integrated processes: nursing process — implementation, caring; client need: health promotion and maintenance; content area: medical-surgical.

    RATIONALE

    (1) The Band-Aid applies to toddlers, not infants. **(2)** Having the mother stay and care for her child helps prevent separation anxiety. **(3)** Eye contact and touch are especially important during the first month of life when bonding between mother and child is beginning. **(4)** The limits and choices apply to toddlers, not infants.

57. **(2)** Integrated processes: nursing process — implementation, teaching/learning; client need: physiological integrity; pharmacological therapies; content area: pediatrics.

    RATIONALE

    (1) The medication is ordered for a set number of days and is given whether or not a rash is present. **(2)** Penicillin G is given for 7–10 days to eradicate the streptococcal infection completely and prevent its complications, although symptoms will usually subside within the first couple of days. **(3)** The medication is ordered for a set number of days whether or not the temperature is normal. **(4)** The medication is ordered for a set number of days whether or not the throat is sore.

58. **(1)** Integrated processes: nursing process — implementation, teaching/learning; client need: physiological integrity; reduction of risk potential; content area: pediatrics.

RATIONALE

(1) Urinalysis allows early diagnosis and treatment of acute glomerulonephritis. Some of the serious complications that can follow infections with group A β-hemolytic streptococci include acute glomerulonephritis, rheumatic fever, peritonsillar abscess, pneumonia, and meningitis. **(2)** Urinalysis is not usually associated directly with pyelonephritis. Select another option. **(3)** Urinalysis is not usually associated with HIV (AIDS). Select another option. **(4)** Urinalysis is not usually associated with urinary tract infections. Select another option.

59. **(3)** Integrated processes: nursing process — implementation, teaching/learning; client need: psychosocial adaptation; content area: pediatrics.

    RATIONALE

    (1) Missing a full week would only add to this problem. **(2)** The school counselor is not needed. **(3)** Because he is an 8-year-old school-age child, the boy's problem is probably concern about falling behind in school, resulting in the loss of his role or position at school. He may fear loss of recently mastered skills, and keeping up with his work could prevent this fear. **(4)** Returning to school early may interfere with his physical recovery.

60. **(3)** Integrated processes: nursing process — implementation, teaching/learning; client need: physiological integrity; reduction of risk potential; content area: medical-surgical.

    RATIONALE

    (1) Labia must remain separated during collection. **(2)** Cleansing is from least contaminated area to most contaminated area, or front to back. **(3)** The initial stream of urine is allowed to flow into the bedpan or toilet, the midstream portion is collected, and the sterile specimen container is removed from the stream while the client is still voiding. **(4)** Examination of urine is most reliable if examined within the hour after voiding.

61. **(1200–1500 mL)** Integrated processes: nursing process — data collection; client need: physiological integrity; physiological adaptation; content area: medical-surgical.

    RATIONALE

    (1) Select another option. **(2)** Urine volume varies depending on fluid intake, cardiac and renal condition of the client, hormonal influences, and loss of fluid in perspiration or exhaled air. **(3)** Select another option. **(4)** Select another option.

62. **(330 mL)** Integrated processes: nursing process — data collection, communication and documentation; client need: physiological integrity; physiological adaptation; content area: medical-surgical.

    RATIONALE

    (1) Select another option. **(2)** Select another option. **(3)** Select another option. **(4)** Jell-O and creamed soup are considered liquids along with the tea. Eleven ounces multiplied by 30 mL/oz yields a total of 330 mL.

63. **(1)** Integrated processes: nursing process — planning; client need: physiological integrity; basic care and comfort; content area: medical-surgical.

    RATIONALE

    (1) Inserting a Foley catheter will not help the client to regain voluntary control of bladder function. **(2)** Nursing interventions are appropriate to goals sought. **(3)** Nursing interventions are appropriate to goals sought. **(4)** Nursing interventions are appropriate to goals sought.

64. **(1)** Integrated processes: nursing process — implementation; client need: physiological integrity; basic care and comfort; content area: medical-surgical.

RATIONALE

(**1**) Proper cleansing and drying are basic to maintenance of skin integrity. (**2**) Padding clothing or bed linen and applying barrier creams may be important but secondary to providing a clean, dry skin surface. (**3**) Padding clothing or bed linen and applying barrier creams may be important but are secondary to providing a clean, dry skin surface. (**4**) Use of diapers should be discouraged because they are demeaning and may convey the impression that incontinence is permissible.

65. (**2**) Integrated processes: nursing process — planning; client need: physiological integrity; physiological adaptation; content area: medical-surgical.

RATIONALE

(**1**) A flexion contracture is a permanent contraction of a muscle resulting from spasm or paralysis. (**2**) A pressure ulcer results from continued pressure, usually over a bony prominence. Skin breakdown can be hastened by improper cleansing or infrequent alteration of position. Massage can promote circulation in the areas of concern, helping to decrease the possibility of skin breakdown. (**3**) A pressure ulcer may be considered a "dermatologic crisis," but this is not the appropriate answer to the question. (**4**) Any pressure point is not itself a "complication."

66. (**1, 4, 5, 6**) Integrated processes: nursing process — planning; client need: physiological integrity; reduction of risk potential; content area: medical-surgical.

RATIONALE

(**1**) The left Sims' position is between a lateral and a prone position and is suitable for vaginal and rectal access. (**2**) In the supine or dorsal position, the client is in a back-lying position with legs extended. This position may be used to catheterize a client if the client is unable to be placed in a dorsal recumbent position. (**3**) In the dorsal recumbent position, the client lies on her back with knees flexed and hips rotated externally, a position that allows access to the urinary meatus in the female client. (**4**) In the prone position, the client is lying flat on her abdomen. (**5**) Trendelenburg position is not used to catheterize a client. (**6**) Semi-Fowler's position obstructs the view of the perineal area and would not be used to catheterize a client.

67. (**4**) Integrated processes: nursing process — implementation; client need: physiological integrity; reduction of risk potential; content area: medical-surgical.

RATIONALE

(**1**) Option 1 is incorrect because a specimen of urine that has been standing in the bag should never be used for examination. Standing urine changes and sterility cannot be ensured at the drainage port. (**2**) Option 2 also is incorrect: a system designed to remain closed should never be opened; again, sterility cannot be ensured. (**3**) As suggested in option 3, puncture above the bifurcation may damage the channel used to inflate the balloon and may lead to deflation; also, some materials used in the manufacture of catheters do not close completely after puncture. (**4**) The port is designed to allow penetration with a sterile system and closure on withdrawal of a needle.

68. (**2**) Integrated processes: nursing process — implementation; client need: physiological integrity; reduction of risk potential; content area: medical-surgical.

RATIONALE

(**1**) Prophylactic therapy is used in some instances. (**2**) Proper hand washing by all personnel and clients is fundamental to the control of all infections. No other measures surpass hand washing in importance for controlling the spread of infection. (**3**) Proper disposal of potentially infective materials is essential. No other measures surpass hand washing in importance for controlling the spread of infection. (**4**) Educational programs may be helpful, but such knowledge is most valuable when applied in practice.

69. (**3**) Integrated processes: nursing process — implementation; client need: safe, effective care environment; safety and infection control; content area: medical-surgical.

RATIONALE

(**1**) To minimize the possibility for infection, no unsterile solutions or equipment should be introduced into the urethra, urinary bladder, or trachea. (**2**) Hyperalimentation is a means of providing nutrients IV. Clients receiving total parenteral nutrition (TPN) are particularly susceptible to catheter-related infections. Strict aseptic technique must be maintained during the TPN procedure and in regard to the dressings at the site. (**3**) The alimentary canal is not sterile; therefore, unsterile (but clean) equipment and solutions can be introduced to that body system. Other procedures carried out using clean technique include gastrostomy feedings, colostomy care, and enemas. (**4**) To minimize the possibility for infection, no unsterile solutions or equipment should be introduced into the urethra, urinary bladder, or trachea.

70. (**2**) Integrated processes: nursing process — data collection; client need: physiological integrity; pharmacological therapies; content area: medical-surgical.

RATIONALE

(**1**) Allopurinol, probenecid, and sulfinpyrazone are maintenance drugs used for chronic gout. The choice among these drugs depends on the physiological mechanism underlying the disorder. (**2**) Decrease in client symptoms on administration of colchicine is useful in establishing a diagnosis of gout or gouty arthritis. (**3**) Allopurinol, probenecid, and sulfinpyrazone are maintenance drugs used for chronic gout. The choice among these drugs depends on the physiological mechanism underlying the disorder. (**4**) Allopurinol, probenecid, and sulfinpyrazone are maintenance drugs used for chronic gout. The choice among these drugs depends on the physiological mechanism underlying the disorder.

71. (**4**) Integrated processes: nursing process — data collection; client need: health promotion and maintenance; content area: medical-surgical.

RATIONALE

(**1**) Pain, swelling, increased heat, and redness are classic manifestations of inflammation such as gout. (**2**) Pain, swelling, increased heat, and redness are classic manifestations of inflammation such as gout. (**3**) Pain, swelling, increased heat, and redness are classic manifestations of inflammation such as gout. (**4**) The toe would exhibit cyanosis.

72. (**2**) Integrated processes: nursing process — implementation; client need: physiological integrity; reduction of risk potential; content area: medical-surgical.

RATIONALE

(**1**) The first voided specimen at 8 AM on the day of collection is discarded. (**2**) Other voided specimens after the 8 AM voiding, including the final voiding at 8 AM on the day the collection ends, must be included in the sample. (**3**) The sample must be kept refrigerated or cooled in the room during collection. (**4**) All urine is saved for 24-hour collections.

73. (**4**) Integrated processes: nursing process — planning; client need: physiological integrity; basic care and comfort; content area: medical-surgical.

RATIONALE

(**1**) Clients with gout should increase fluids to 3000 mL/day unless contraindicated. (**2**) Fasting and crash diets increase the serum uric acid level and should be avoided. (3) High-purine diet (shellfish, liver, organ meats, sardines, anchovies) and excessive alcohol intake should be avoided to avoid precipitation of an acute attack of gout. (4) Increased fluids and alkaline foods such as potatoes or milk increase the urine pH and decrease formation of uric acid crystals, which may lead to formation of kidney stones.

74. **(1)** Integrated processes: nursing process — implementation, teaching/learning; client need: physiological integrity; basic care and comfort; content area: medical-surgical.

RATIONALE

(1) Gout is one of the most excruciatingly painful conditions that the nurse may see. Often a cradle is required to keep the pressure of a sheet from the affected joint. Any or all of the additional measures may be appropriate nursing interventions. Pressure will not relieve pain in the affected joint. **(2)** Cold or heat may relieve pain. **(3)** Analgesics or anti-inflammatory agents may relieve pain. **(4)** Immobilization may decrease pain.

75. **(3)** Integrated processes: nursing process — planning; client need: physiological integrity; pharmacological therapies; content area: medical-surgical.

RATIONALE

(1) Administration of drugs for emotional support is not viable. **(2)** There is no known cure for arthritis. **(3)** Reduction of pain and inflammation is the major purpose of drug therapy. **(4)** Drugs may be given in preparation for surgery, but option 4 is inappropriate for the question asked.

76. **(21 gtt/min)** Integrated processes: nursing process — planning; client need: physiological integrity; pharmacological therapies; content area: medical-surgical.

RATIONALE

The standard drop factor indicates the number of drops per milliliter that the tubing will deliver. Multiplying the drop factor of 10 by the total milliliters gives 30,000, the number of drops to be given in 24 hours. Multiplying 60 minutes by 24 hours calculates the total number of minutes in 24 hours (1440). Dividing 30,000 drops by 1440 minutes comes to 21.5 drops/min. The nurse should set the infusion to administer approximately 21 drops/min to administer 3000 mL in 24 hours.

77. **(4)** Integrated processes: nursing process — data collection, teaching/learning; client need: physiological integrity; pharmacological therapies; content area: medical-surgical.

RATIONALE

(1) Option 1 is appropriate because swelling may demonstrate the presence of edema, suggesting infiltration. **(2)** Option 2 is appropriate because the client may have moved an arm, which may have caused the bevel of the needle to lie against the side of the vein, thereby obstructing the flow of solution. **(3)** Option 3 may be appropriate because patency of the tubing may be assessed by observing return of blood from the client into the IV tubing when the receptacle is lowered. **(4)** Never flush the needle or cannula by injecting saline with a syringe and needle directly into the tubing because such action may force a blood clot into circulation.

78. **(1)** Integrated processes: nursing process — data collection; client need: physiological integrity; pharmacological therapies; content area: medical-surgical.

RATIONALE

(1) In addition to the aforementioned symptoms, a client experiencing circulatory overload may exhibit venous distention, syncope, shock, dyspnea, and cyanosis resulting from pulmonary edema. **(2)** Drug overload may occur from receiving an excessive amount of fluid containing drugs; and symptoms may include dizziness, fainting leading to shock, and symptoms specific to the offending drug. **(3)** Superficial thrombophlebitis may produce tenderness at first with subsequent pain along the course of the vein, edema and redness at injection site, and excessive warmth in the affected arm as compared with the other arm. These signs are characteristic of inflammation. **(4)** An air embolism results when air gets into the circulatory system. Symptoms may include hypotension, cyanosis, tachycardia, increased venous pressure, and loss of consciousness.

79. **(3)** Integrated processes: nursing process — planning; client need: physiological integrity; pharmacological therapies; content area: medical-surgical.

RATIONALE

(1) Epinephrine, terbutaline sulfate, and theophylline each act to relieve bronchospasm. **(2)** Epinephrine, terbutaline sulfate, and theophylline each act to relieve bronchospasm. **(3)** Cromolyn sodium has no bronchodilator, anti-inflammatory, or antihistamine action. Cromolyn is not effective for acute bronchial asthmatic attacks. Cromolyn inhibits the allergic reaction if inhaled before the challenge by the antigen. **(4)** Epinephrine, terbutaline sulfate, and theophylline each act to relieve bronchospasm.

80. **(4)** Integrated processes: nursing process — implementation; client need: physiological integrity; reduction of risk potential; content area: medical-surgical.

RATIONALE

(1) Tubing should be inserted 3–4 inches for an adult (1–2 inches for a child). **(2)** For some radiological procedures (relating to the transverse colon), the client may need to receive the enema while lying on the right side, but unless specified, the left side is the position of choice. **(3)** Solution should not flow moderately fast. **(4)** Fluid should flow slowly, the client should take as much as possible of amount ordered, and tubing should be clamped before removing from anus to prevent leakage. Tip is lubricated and left lateral position is the preferred position for administration of an enema because it facilitates flow of solution by gravity into the sigmoid and descending colon, which are on the left side.

81. **(1)** Integrated processes: nursing process — data collection; client need: health promotion and maintenance; content area: medical-surgical.

RATIONALE

(1) The tonometer is placed directly on the anesthetized cornea. A reading of 11–22 mm Hg indicates intraocular pressure that is within normal limits. **(2)** A reading of 24–32 mm Hg suggests glaucoma. **(3)** A reading of 35–44 mm Hg suggests glaucoma. **(4)** Readings of 50–75 mm Hg can occur with acute attacks in clients with acute (angle-closure) glaucoma.

82. **(4)** Integrated processes: nursing process — planning; client need: physiological integrity; pharmacological therapies; content area: medical-surgical.

RATIONALE

(1) Diagnosis has already been made if treatment has begun. **(2)** Control of intraocular pressure may be desired before surgery, but the primary objective of treatment for glaucoma is reduction of intraocular pressure, which may damage the optic nerve and result in blindness. **(3)** Option 3 has no relationship to the question. **(4)** Reduction of intraocular pressure is the ultimate goal in drug treatment of glaucoma.

83. **(2)** Integrated processes: nursing process — planning; client need: physiological integrity; pharmacological therapies; content area: medical-surgical.

RATIONALE

(1) Dilation of the pupil could obstruct the flow of aqueous humor and thereby increase intraocular pressure. (2) A miotic drug causes the pupil to contract, allowing the iris to draw away from the cornea, thus facilitating the drainage of aqueous humor through lymph spaces in the canal of Schlemm. (3) Glaucoma is a disorder that can be controlled rather than cured. (4) Anesthetic action is needed during tonometry but not for treatment of glaucoma.

84. **(2)** Integrated processes: nursing process — implementation; client need: physiological integrity; pharmacological therapies; content area: medical-surgical.

RATIONALE

(1) Acetazolamide is a carbonic anhydrase inhibitor that decreases production of aqueous humor. (2) Pilocarpine constricts the pupil (miosis) and contracts ciliary musculature, facilitating aqueous outflow. (3) Mannitol reduces intraocular pressure by increasing blood osmolality. (4) Rimexolone is used for postoperative ocular inflammation.

85. **(1)** Integrated processes: nursing process — implementation; client need: physiological integrity; pharmacological therapies; content area: medical-surgical.

RATIONALE

(1) The symbol for the number 2 in the apothecary system of measurement is two lowercase "i's." The abbreviation for left eye is OS. The abbreviation for four times a day is qid. (2) Eleven drops is incorrect. (3) The right eye would be designated OD, and every day is qd. (4) Both eyes would be designated OU.

86. **(3)** Integrated processes: nursing process — implementation; client need: physiological integrity; pharmacological therapies; content area: medical-surgical.

RATIONALE

(1) The client should focus gaze upward toward the forehead. (2) The medication should not hit the sensitive cornea. (3) The nurse pulls the lower lid down gently and drops medication into the center of the lower lid as the client focuses gaze upward toward the forehead. (4) The eyedropper should remain sterile. An eyedropper that touches the lower lid will be contaminated. Bacterial contamination of the solution may result.

87. **(1)** Integrated processes: nursing process — planning; client need: physiological integrity; pharmacological therapies; content area: medical-surgical.

RATIONALE

(1) Excessive absorption of strong drugs (e.g., epinephrine) may occur through the nasolacrimal duct, leading to undesirable effects. (2) This option is not a priority reason. (3) This option does not prevent blinking. (4) Option 4 is also a correct reason for occlusion of the nasolacrimal duct but may be secondary in importance to prevention of systemic absorption of the drug.

88. **(3)** Integrated processes: nursing process — planning, teaching/learning; client need: physiological integrity; pharmacological therapies; content area: medical-surgical.

RATIONALE

(1) Beta blockers may be used to achieve miosis. (2) Antiemetics may be employed to help prevent vomiting in a client with acute glaucoma (which could increase intraocular pressure). (3) Mydriatics (e.g., atropine) in a glaucomatous eye may precipitate an acute glaucoma attack that may result in blindness. (Mydriatics cause pupillary dilation.) It is important also that the client be cautioned against using over-the-counter drugs such as antihistamines, as these may contain mydriatics. (4) Analgesics may be prescribed to alleviate pain of acute glaucoma.

89. **(Two tablets)** Integrated processes: nursing process — implementation; client need: physiological integrity; pharmacological therapies; content area: medical-surgical.

RATIONALE

The ratio and proportion method helps ensure accurate calculation of drug dosages. In this problem, 5 mg is to 1 tablet as 10 mg is to x tablets. Cross-multiplying gives $5x = 10$ mg. Then $x = 10$ mg $\div$ 5 mg. Finally, $x = 2$ tablets.

90. **(1)** Integrated processes: nursing process — implementation, teaching/learning; client need: physiological integrity; reduction of risk potential; content area: medical-surgical.

RATIONALE

(1) The client is positioned on the unoperative side to eliminate pressure on the suture line. (2) The patch and shield protect the eye from accidental injury. (3) Antiemetics and laxatives should be administered as ordered. (4) The client should not lift, pull, or push heavy objects.

91. **(4)** Integrated processes: nursing process — planning, teaching/learning; client need: safe, effective care environment; safety and infection control; content area: medical-surgical.

RATIONALE

(1) The cause of a problem should be determined before treatment is instituted. (2) The cause of a problem should be determined before treatment is instituted. (3) The cause of a problem should be determined before treatment is instituted. (4) Vocational nurses are not licensed to prescribe medications.

92. **(3)** Integrated processes: nursing process — data collection; client need: health promotion and maintenance; content area: pediatrics.

RATIONALE

(1) Conjunctivitis is inflammation of the conjunctiva (lines the eyelids and is reflected onto the eyeball). (2) Otitis media may result from tonsillitis, but the listed characteristics better described otitis media than tonsillitis. (3) The presenting signs and symptoms are characteristic of otitis media. The client may also exhibit signs of vomiting and diarrhea. (4) Cystitis is inflammation of the urinary bladder.

93. **(1)** Integrated processes: nursing process — evaluation; client need: health promotion and maintenance; content area: pediatrics.

RATIONALE

(1) In infants and young children, the eustachian tubes are short, wide, and straight and lie in a somewhat horizontal plane. (2) This statement is accurate. (3) This statement is accurate. (4) This statement is accurate.

94. **(2)** Integrated processes: nursing process — implementation; client need: physiological integrity; pharmacological therapies; content area: pediatrics.

RATIONALE

(1) This intervention is part of the correct procedure. (2) For infants and children, 3 years of age, the nurse pulls the pinna down and back to administer eardrops. Because the external auditory canal is cartilaginous and straight, downward action separates the walls of the canal for instillation. The adult ear canal has more ossification and angles slightly, so a gentle pull upward straightens the canal. Positioning the client on the unaffected side allows medication to flow inward by gravity. Allowing the client to remain in the same position keeps the medication from running out of the canal. The drops are directed toward the ear canal because drops that hit the tympanic membrane directly may cause pain. Two additional measures associated with instillation of eardrops are (a) warm the medication by rolling the bottle in the hands for a few minutes

(cold medication may induce nausea or vertigo), and (b) the nurse's hand should rest on the client's head for stabilization to help prevent injury if the client moves. **(3)** This intervention is part of the correct procedure. **(4)** This intervention is part of the correct procedure.

95. **(4)** Integrated processes: nursing process — evaluation, teaching/learning; client need: physiological integrity; pharmacological therapies; content area: pediatrics.

RATIONALE

(1) Theoretical knowledge of a procedure or memorization of factual information concerning the process may not ensure ability to apply the knowledge in practice. **(2)** Theoretical knowledge of a procedure or memorization of factual information concerning the process may not ensure ability to apply the knowledge in practice. **(3)** Theoretical knowledge of a procedure or memorization of factual information concerning the process may not ensure ability to apply the knowledge in practice. **(4)** Demonstration of the procedure in the presence of the nurse allows the nurse to evaluate the person's ability to apply as well as to comprehend the information. Successful performance of the procedure may also enhance the person's self-confidence to perform the task properly.

96. **(4)** Integrated processes: nursing process — data collection; client need: physiological integrity; physiological adaptation; content area: medical-surgical.

RATIONALE

(1) Currently, no treatment stops the degenerative process of Parkinson's disease. **(2)** Parkinsonian crisis occurs on abrupt withdrawal of prescribed medications or with emotional trauma — this is a medical emergency. **(3)** Parkinson's disease is not familial. **(4)** Intellectual capacity is not lost, although mood disturbances often occur.

97. **(2)** Integrated processes: nursing process — planning; client need: physiological integrity; pharmacological therapies; content area: medical-surgical.

RATIONALE

(1) Select another option. **(2)** All the aforementioned drugs are antiparkinsonian agents. Bromocriptine mesylate is used also for amenorrhea, galactorrhea, prevention of lactation, and female infertility. **(3)** Select another option. **(4)** Select another option.

98. **(4)** Integrated processes: nursing process — planning, teaching/learning; client need: physiological integrity; basic care and comfort; content area: medical-surgical.

RATIONALE

(1) This response is correct. **(2)** This response is correct. **(3)** This response is correct. **(4)** An afternoon nap will not help to facilitate bowel function. Any of the other three choices may help to prevent constipation.

99. **(4)** Integrated processes: nursing process — implementation, communication and documentation; client need: physiological integrity; pharmacological therapies; content area: medical-surgical.

RATIONALE

(1) The nurse may be instructed by the physician on specific knowledge required by the client. **(2)** The pharmacist is not usually contacted to give drug information to the client (although he or she may provide information when the client purchases the drugs). **(3)** The nurse does not need a physician's order to provide information related to the drug regimen. **(4)** The nurse is the person closest to the client. The nurse has knowledge (or can find out) about the medications, and he or she has the responsibility for independent nursing action in discharge teaching.

100. **(2)** Integrated processes: nursing process — data collection; client need: physiological integrity; pharmacological therapies; content area: medical-surgical.

RATIONALE

(1) This answer is not true; select another option. **(2)** Status epilepticus is a medical emergency in which the client has continuous seizures or seizures in rapid succession lasting at least 30 minutes. There are many kinds of status epilepticus. **(3)** This answer is not true; select another option. **(4)** This is not true; select another option.

101. **(6)** Integrated processes: nursing process — planning; client need: physiological integrity; pharmacological therapies; content area: medical-surgical.

RATIONALE

This problem requires conversion of milliliters to minims first. The nurse must know that 1 mL is equivalent to 15–16 minims. The correct dosage can be ascertained by ratio and proportion calculation as follows: 2 mg is to x minims as 5 mg is to 15 minims. Cross-multiplying gives $5x = 30$; then $x = 30 \div 5$. Finally, $x = 6$ minims.

102. **(2)** Integrated processes: nursing process — evaluation; client need: safe, effective care environment; coordinated care; content area: medical-surgical.

RATIONALE

(1) This action is within the standard practice of nursing. **(2)** Only physicians are licensed to prescribe medications. **(3)** This action is within the standard practice of nursing. **(4)** This action is within the standard practice of nursing.

103. **(1)** Integrated processes: nursing process — data collection; client need: physiological integrity; pharmacological therapies; content area: medical-surgical.

RATIONALE

(1) All of the drugs listed are anticonvulsant medications with various side effects. Long-term use of phenytoin has been known to result in hypertrophy of gingival tissue. Special attention to meticulous oral care is important for clients receiving this drug. **(2)** Primidone does not cause gingival hypertrophy. **(3)** Clonazepam does not cause gingival hypertrophy. **(4)** Diazepam does not cause gingival hypertrophy.

104. **(3)** Integrated processes: nursing process — implementation; client need: physiological integrity; pharmacological therapies; content area: medical-surgical.

RATIONALE

(1) Docusate sodium is a stool softener. **(2)** Digoxin is a cardiac glycoside. **(3)** Diazepam is the usual medication of choice. **(4)** Dexamethasone is a synthetic adrenocorticosteroid.

105. **(4)** Integrated processes: nursing process — implementation; client need: physiological integrity; reduction of risk potential; content area: medical-surgical.

RATIONALE

(1) Although oxygen therapy is given to maintain adequate ventilation and oxygenation, it is not the priority action. **(2)** Chest physiotherapy and coughing with support to the chest wall are used primarily for pulmonary contusions to maintain airway clearance, but are not the priority action. **(3)** Pain medication may be administered, but it is not the priority. **(4)** The wound must be sealed immediately to prevent the development of a tension pneumothorax.

106. **(3)** Integrated processes: nursing process — evaluation; client need: physiological integrity; reduction of risk potential; content area: medical-surgical.

RATIONALE

(1) The purpose is to regain normally negative intrapleural pressure. (2) Chest tubes have no effect on plural irritation. (3) Chest tubes are used because the normally negative pressure that causes inspiration has been interrupted. To regain negative intrapleural pressure, a tube is inserted and negative pressure applied with the aid of a water seal and/or negative-pressure pump to remove both air and fluid. (4) The purpose is to establish normal negative intrapleural pressure.

107. (3) Integrated processes: nursing process — planning; client need: physiological integrity; reduction of risk potential; content area: medical-surgical.

RATIONALE

(1) The chest tube may be clamped temporarily to determine whether there is an air leak (bubbling in the water-seal chamber). (2) The chest drainage devices should always be kept lower than the client to prevent reflux into the chest. (3) Gentle milking should be instituted only if a flow becomes obstructed because of clot formation. (4) The chest tube should not be clamped for client transport. When transporting a client, the suction may be disconnected, but the water seal must be maintained.

108. (1) Integrated processes: nursing process — evaluation; client need: physiological integrity; reduction of risk potential; content area: medical-surgical.

RATIONALE

(1) Bubbling means that there is a leak from the pleural cavity or drainage system. (2) Bubbling indicates a leak in the system and that the system is not functioning properly. (3) The water level in the water-seal chamber will rise and fall with inspiration and expiration. (4) Turning on the side does not cause bubbling; a leak in the system does.

109. (4) Integrated processes: nursing process — planning; client need: physiological integrity; basic care and comfort; content area: medical-surgical.

RATIONALE

(1) Antabuse is a drug used to treat alcohol abuse. (2) Vitamin C is not used to prevent encephalopathy. (3) Chlordiazepoxide may be used to treat delirium tremens. (4) Thiamine deficiency may occur with alcoholism because of damaged GI tract and lack of absorption or malnutrition. Wernicke's encephalopathy is caused by thiamine deficiency.

110. (4) Integrated processes: nursing process — planning; client need: health promotion and maintenance; content area: medical-surgical.

RATIONALE

(1) Asking this question is not the most important priority. (2) Asking this question is not the most important priority but will become more important at discharge. (3) Asking this question is not the most important priority. (4) Alcoholics may have seizures or delirium tremens related to withdrawal. Usually, the seizures occur from 12 to 48 hours after the last drink. Some seizures have been reported up to 2 weeks after the last drink.

111. (1) Integrated processes: nursing process — planning; client need: health promotion and maintenance; content area: medical-surgical.

RATIONALE

(1) Alcoholic withdrawal may include visual and tactile hallucinations; auditory hallucinations are more likely to occur in psychosis. The BP is elevated because of an outpouring of norepinephrine-epinephrine. (2) Temperature is usually not affected. (3) BP is elevated because of an outpouring of nor-epinephrine-epinephrine; temperature is not affected. (4) Temperature is usually not affected.

112. (4) Integrated processes: nursing process — implementation, communication and documentation; client need: safe, effective care environment; safety and infection control; content area: medical-surgical.

RATIONALE

(1) Restraints are applied to prevent the client from hurting himself or others, not for punitive measures. (2) Physicians should write a specific order for restraints, not an as-needed order. (3) The restraints may not necessarily be taken off in 1 hour. (4) Because the client is severely immobilized, his circulation should be checked frequently, and documentation should occur every 15 minutes. (A flow sheet is appropriate for this.)

113. (3) Integrated processes: nursing process — implementation; client need: health promotion and maintenance; content area: medical-surgical.

RATIONALE

(1) At discharge, it is too late to encourage the client to become as independent as possible. (2) His needs should be assessed on admission and reevaluated as he progresses. (3) Rehabilitation is best when started at the time of admission. (4) He must be encouraged to exercise and walk as soon as possible.

114. (1) Integrated processes: nursing process — implementation; client need: physiological integrity; basic care and comfort; content area: medical-surgical.

RATIONALE

(1) The nurse should promote activity that allows a client to function and look as normal as possible. (2) Bathing the client and combing hair does not promote independence. (3) The nurse may remind client to brush teeth, but not do it. (4) Foley catheter can introduce bacteria into the urinary tract system. Instituting Kegel's exercises would be more appropriate.

115. (1) Integrated processes: nursing process — implementation; client need: physiological integrity; reduction of risk potential; content area: medical-surgical.

RATIONALE

(1) Passive ROM is the range of movement at a particular joint that is accomplished by the use of a machine or an assistant. (2) Active ROM is the range of movement at a particular joint that a client is able to accomplish without assistance. (3) Active ROM exercises are more effective than passive ROM. (4) With passive ROM, there is no assistance from the client.

116. (4) Integrated processes: nursing process — data collection; client need: health promotion and maintenance; content area: pediatrics.

RATIONALE

(1) The DDST assesses the child from birth to 6 years. (2) The DDST adjusts for premature birth by subtracting the number of weeks of prematurity from the chronological age. (3) The value of the DDST is questionable in minority ethnic groups. (4) The DDST is not an intelligence test but measures four skill areas: gross motor, fine motor, language, and personal-social skills.

117. (3) Integrated processes: nursing process — evaluation; client need: health promotion and maintenance; content area: pediatrics.

RATIONALE

(1) Squeak toys are appropriate for the 6- to 12-month-old child. (2) Pull toys are appropriate for the 12- to 18-month-old child who walks well. (3) By 2–4 years, the child can pedal a

tricycle. (4) A 4- to 6-year-old child has the dexterity and motor skills to play on a jungle gym.

118. **(2)** Integrated processes: nursing process — data collection; client need: health promotion and maintenance; content area: pediatrics.

RATIONALE

(1) By 0–6 months, the infant can sit with support and roll over from side to back. **(2)** At 6–12 months, the infant can crawl, creep, or walk holding on to furniture. **(3)** At 12–18 months, the child can walk well, stoop, and recover. **(4)** At 18–24 months, the child can kick a ball forward, walk up steps, walk backwards, and throw a ball overhand.

119. **(3)** Integrated processes: nursing process — evaluation, communication and documentation; client need: health promotion and maintenance; content area: maternity nursing.

RATIONALE

(1) Although this may be true, these symptoms need to be evaluated by a physician. **(2)** Tylenol or aspirin may relieve the pain, but these symptoms may indicate serious complications and must be evaluated by the physician. **(3)** These signs require immediate notification of the physician, because the pregnancy may be in jeopardy. **(4)** The nurse cannot make a judgment as to whether or not these symptoms are a result of the allergy.

120. **(4)** Integrated processes: nursing process — evaluation, teaching/learning; client need: health promotion and maintenance; content area: maternity nursing.

RATIONALE

(1) The amniocentesis determines the fetal lung maturity with lecithin:sphingomyelin ratio. **(2)** The amniocentesis ascertains the presence of chromosomal aberrations. **(3)** The extent of ABO, Rh can be determined by amniocentesis. **(4)** A sonogram, not an amniocentesis, allows visualization of the fetus, uterus, and placenta.

121. **(1)** Integrated processes: nursing process — evaluation, teaching/learning; client need: physiological integrity; reduction of risk potential; content area: maternity nursing.

RATIONALE

(1) Encouraging bladder fullness is appropriate for a sonogram. Bladder fullness could result in puncture of the bladder in an amniocentesis. **(2)** The client will sign an informal consent. **(3)** Vaginal bleeding and elevated temperature should be observed for and reported. **(4)** Vital signs are taken every 5 minutes during the procedure and every 15 minutes after the procedure.

122. **(4)** Integrated processes: nursing process — evaluation; client need: health promotion and maintenance; content area: maternity nursing.

RATIONALE

(1) Aspirin may cause decreased platelet aggregation, GI bleeding, and abdominal pain. It is not likely to cause vaginal bleeding. **(2)** Toxic shock syndrome is caused by certain strains of *Staphylococcus aureus*. The fever is 102.8°F (38.98°C) or greater; hypotension, GI vomiting, severe myalgia, and alterations in consciousness are some of the symptoms. **(3)** Endometriosis may cause abdominal cramping but not shock symptoms. **(4)** A spontaneous abortion occurs naturally during the second or third month. Symptoms include vaginal bleeding, spotting or hemorrhaging, low abdominal cramping, passing of tissue through the vagina, or shock.

123. **(1)** Integrated processes: nursing process — implementation, caring; client need: psychosocial integrity; content area: psychiatric nursing.

RATIONALE

(1) Psychiatric clients cannot be reasoned with or argued with because they believe a delusion to be true. The best approach is a simple statement of reality. **(2)** Changing her room would feed her delusion. **(3)** Psychiatric clients cannot identify why, but they accept a delusion as being true. **(4)** This option does not point out the reality.

124. **(2)** Integrated processes: nursing process — planning, caring; client need: psychosocial integrity; content area: psychiatric nursing.

RATIONALE

(1) Joining in group activities initially is inappropriate until she is less delusional. **(2)** Establishing trust is of primary importance because she is so paranoid and lacks trust in others. **(3)** Limiting contacts with other clients is important, but developing a sense of trust with staff is the priority. **(4)** Coworkers should not visit until she becomes less delusional.

125. **(1)** Integrated processes: nursing process — implementation, teaching/learning; client need: physiological integrity; basic care and comfort; content area: medical-surgical.

RATIONALE

(1) Inspect skin to monitor for irritation and breakdown. **(2)** This is not a relevant option for care of a brace. **(3)** This is not a relevant option for care of a brace. **(4)** Weight fluctuations may cause the brace to become loose or tight.

126. **(1)** Integrated processes: nursing process — implementation; client need: physiological integrity; basic care and comfort; content area: medical-surgical.

RATIONALE

(1) Allowing the client to stand with aid helps to prevent complications resulting from immobility. **(2)** A prosthesis does not substitute for a dressing. **(3)** A prosthesis does not enhance body image. **(4)** A prosthesis does prevent complications of immobility, but does so because it allows the client to stand.

127. **(4)** Integrated processes: nursing process — data collection; client need: physiological integrity; basic care and comfort; content area: medical-surgical.

RATIONALE

(1) Leaning on an axillary bar may cause nerve damage. **(2)** The client should be taught to walk upright, looking straight ahead. **(3)** Although making sure that adequate help is available to support the client initially, option 3 is not as important as option 4. **(4)** If the client cannot tolerate the physical activity, he or she will not adjust to crutch walking.

128. **(2)** Integrated processes: nursing process — implementation; client need: physiological integrity; basic care and comfort; content area: medical-surgical.

RATIONALE

(1) The nurse cannot order physical therapy. **(2)** The client will need strength before using crutches. **(3)** It is most important for the client to do muscle-strengthening exercises. **(4)** Although option 4 is also correct, it is a physical priority for the client to have the necessary strength to perform crutch walking.

129. **(3)** Integrated processes: nursing process — evaluation, teaching/learning; client need: physiological integrity; basic care and comfort; content area: medical-surgical

RATIONALE

(1) The prosthesis must be kept in working order, and water can cause rusting. **(2)** The client needs to wear the prosthesis all the time. **(3)** The prosthesis should be maintained in good working order. **(4)** The joints should not be oiled.

130. **(2)** Integrated processes: nursing process — data collection, communication and documentation; client need: health promotion and maintenance; content area: medical-surgical.
RATIONALE
(**1**) This action occurs during the planning phase. (**2**) Data collection is the first phase of the nursing process in which nurses establish a database about the client's problems and needs, level of wellness, health practices, and past illnesses. (**3**) This action occurs during the problem identification stage. (**4**) This action occurs during the planning stage.

131. **(4)** Integrated processes: nursing process — planning, teaching/learning; client need: physiological integrity; basic care and comfort; content area: pediatrics.
RATIONALE
(**1**) Although weighing a client is a factor in determining nutritional management, it is not the primary reason for daily weights. (**2**) Weight does not accurately reflect fluid intake, but rather fluid balances. (**3**) This response is not a viable option. (**4**) Measurement of daily weight is the primary way of evaluating edema and fluid shifts.

132. **(1)** Integrated processes: nursing process — evaluation; client need: psychosocial integrity; content area: psychiatric nursing.
RATIONALE
(**1**) Psychological abuse is causing mental distress by name calling, isolating, ignoring, or ridiculing an individual. (**2**) Excessive or improper use of physical force on an individual is physical abuse. (**3**) Active neglect is deliberately denying ordered health care to an individual. (**4**) Passive neglect is the unintentional abuse in which the caregiver does not do something that is required because of a lack of skills, knowledge, or ability.

133. **(4)** Integrated processes: nursing process — evaluation; client need: psychosocial integrity; content area: medical-surgical.
RATIONALE
(**1**) Psychological abuse is causing mental distress by name calling, isolating, ignoring, or ridiculing an individual. (**2**) Physical abuse is the excessive or improper use of physical force on an individual. (**3**) Unintentional abuse in which the caregiver does not do that which is required because of a lack of skills, knowledge, or ability is called passive neglect. (**4**) Active neglect is deliberately denying ordered health care to an individual.

134. **(See figure below)** integrated processes: nursing process — data collection; client need: health promotion and maintenance; content area: medical-surgical.

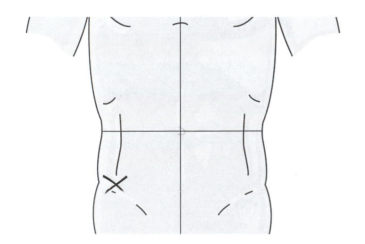

RATIONALE
Palpation is the process of examining by application of the hands or fingers to the external surface of the body to detect evidence of disease or abnormalities in the various organs. Right lower quadrant is the area of the abdomen to be palpated in order to rule out appendicitis.

135. **(1)** Integrated processes: nursing process — planning, teaching/learning; client need: health promotion and maintenance; content area: pediatrics
RATIONALE
(**1**) Toddlers benefit most from having parents who are not overtly anxious and trust the hospital personnel. (**2**) The toddler will not remember well in advance of the procedure. (**3**) Separation anxiety is strongest during the toddler years. Promote care by parents. (**4**) Providing objects such as a blanket or toys from home for familiarity and comfort encourages regression.

136. **(1)** Integrated processes: nursing process — evaluation, caring; client need: health promotion and maintenance; content area: psychiatric nursing.
RATIONALE
(**1**) In the 7-year-old child, fears are related to body injury; allow the child to participate in procedures and prepare the child in advance. (**2**) For the 4- to 6-year-old child, the child's magical thoughts and fantasies may distort the hospital experience. The nurse should explain simply the relationship between cause, illness, and treatment. (**3**) For the 12- to 18-year-old adolescent, fears are related to body image. The nurse should promote privacy, provide detailed information, and promote self-care. (**4**) The 16-month-old to 4-year-old toddler is resistive and exhibits regressive behaviors such as tantrums. Provide for routines and promote care by parents.

137. **(3)** Integrated processes: nursing process — planning; client need: physiological integrity; basic care and comfort; content area: psychiatric nursing.
RATIONALE
(**1**) Physiological needs are first priority. (**2**) This action relates to love and belonging, which come after physiological needs. (**3**) If physiological needs are not met, psychological needs cannot be met. Maslow's hierarchy goes from physical needs to safety and security, to love and belonging, and to self-esteem and self-actualization. (**4**) This action relates to love and belonging and is a lower priority than physiological and safety and security needs.

138. **(4)** Integrated processes: nursing process — evaluation, teaching/learning; client need: physiological integrity; pharmacological therapies; content area: pediatrics.
RATIONALE
(**1**) All options are true, but infections are life threatening and therefore are most important to recognize. (**2**) All options are true, but infections are life threatening and therefore are most important to recognize. (**3**) All options are true, but infections are life threatening and therefore are most important to recognize. (**4**) All options are true, but infections are life threatening and therefore are most important to recognize.

139. **(3)** Integrated processes: nursing process — evaluation; client need: physiological integrity; physiological adaptation; content area: medical-surgical.
RATIONALE
(**1**) The nurse should assess the level of consciousness after the airway is established. (**2**) Pupils are evaluated after an open airway is established. (**3**) The first priority of nursing care is to ensure protection of the airway and to stabilize cervical

injuries. (**4**) Motor function is evaluated after the airway is evaluated.

140. (**4**) Integrated processes: nursing process — data collection; client need: health promotion and maintenance; content area: medical-surgical.

RATIONALE

(**1**) Option 2 is not a true statement. (**2**) Option 2 makes the client seem foolish. (**3**) Option 3 is not true because vertebral column spacing decreases with aging. (**4**) Option 4 is correct and is necessary for a baseline data collection.

141. (**1**) Integrated processes: nursing process — evaluation; client need: health promotion and maintenance; content area: medical-surgical.

RATIONALE

(**1**) Subcutaneous fat works as an insulator against cold. (**2**) This statement may be true, but there is a physical reason. (**3**) There is no change in sweat glands. (**4**) This option does not respond to the question.

142. (**4**) Integrated processes: nursing process — evaluation; client need: physiological integrity; physiological adaptation; content area: medical-surgical.

RATIONALE

(**1**) A stage I pressure sore consists of an area of redness that does not blanch or fade. (**2**) A stage II pressure sore consists of partial-thickness skin loss involving the epidermis or dermis. (**3**) A stage III pressure sore consists of full-thickness loss involving necrosis of subcutaneous tissue. (**4**) A stage IV pressure sore consists of full-thickness loss involving damage to bone, muscle, or supporting structures.

143. (**1**) Integrated processes: nursing process — evaluation; client need: health promotion and maintenance; content area: medical-surgical.

RATIONALE

(**1**) The primary risk factors for pressure ulcers are immobility and limited activity. Other risk factors include altered level of consciousness, incontinence, and impaired nutritional status. (**2**) Immobility and incontinence are risk factors for pressure ulcers; agitation is not. (**3**) Incontinence and impaired nutrition are risk factors; agitation is not. (**4**) Loss of subcutaneous fat support in the skin is a normal process of aging; agitation and hyperactivity are not risk factors.

144. (**1**) Integrated processes: nursing process — data collection; client need: health promotion and maintenance; content area: medical-surgical.

RATIONALE

(**1**) Increased exercise causes BP to increase and the person can feel his or her own heartbeat. (**2**) There is no indication that she is a candidate for myocardial infarction. (**3**) This is not a cardinal sign of heart failure. Dyspnea and edema of the extremities are more likely symptoms. (**4**) There is no indication of mitral stenosis.

145. (**1**) Integrated processes: nursing process — evaluation; client need: physiological integrity; reduction of risk potential; content area: medical-surgical.

RATIONALE

(**1**) Older persons have decreased lung expansion because of rib cage inelasticity, and a decreased immune response, which predisposes older persons to pneumonia. (**2**) There is a decrease in the immune response with aging. (**3**) Aging has little effect on the pulmonary system; respiratory muscle strength remains unchanged. (**4**) Immobile clients are at increased risk for pneumonia postoperatively because of decreased functional reserve and a decreased cough reflex.

146. (**2**) Integrated processes: nursing process — planning; client need: physiological integrity; basic care and comfort; content area: medical-surgical.

RATIONALE

(**1**) A diet high in antacids and calcium has no effect on formation of biliary calculi. (**2**) Biliary calculi are high in cholesterol; therefore, the cholesterol intake of this client needs to be limited. (**3**) A diet high in protein and carbohydrate has no effect on formation of biliary calculi. (**4**) An electrolyte-free diet has no effect on formation of biliary calculi.

147. (**3**) Integrated processes: nursing process — implementation, teaching/learning; client need: physiological integrity; pharmacological therapies; content area: medical-surgical.

RATIONALE

(**1**) Reduced smoking may be healthy, but Antabuse has no effect. (**2**) Antabuse has no effects connected to the sun. (**3**) In a person taking Antabuse, the general physical symptoms experienced after ingesting even a small amount of alcohol may be severe. The drug remains in the body for several days after being discontinued. (**4**) There would be no restricted sexual or physical activity.

148. (**3**) Integrated processes: nursing process — implementation, communication and documentation; client need: health promotion and maintenance; content area: medical-surgical.

RATIONALE

(**1**) Talking loudly distorts sounds. High-frequency-hearing sound loss causes older people to have problems discriminating certain high-pitched sounds. Speak in front of the person so that he or she can see your lip movement. (**2**) Speaking more slowly and distinctly will help the older person to process the information. (**3**) The best communication is face-to-face, using short sentences and talking in a normal voice tone. (**4**) Repeating the message may confuse the client, and raising your voice distorts the sound.

149. (**4**) Integrated processes: nursing process — evaluation; client need: physiological integrity; basic care and comfort; content area: medical-surgical.

RATIONALE

(**1**) The Food and Drug Administration (FDA) recommendation to delay bone degeneration is to include 1.0–1.5 g of calcium in the daily diet. (**2**) The FDA recommendation to delay bone degeneration is to include 1.5–1.5 g of calcium in the daily diet. (**3**) The FDA recommendation to delay bone degeneration is to include 1.0–1.5 g of calcium in the daily diet. (**4**) The FDA recommendation to delay bone degeneration is to include 1.0–1.5 g of calcium in the daily diet.

150. (**3**) Integrated processes: nursing process — planning; client need: physiological integrity; basic care and comfort; content area: medical-surgical.

RATIONALE

(**1**) A 1000-mL intake is inadequate for daily fluid needs. (**2**) A 2000-mL intake is inadequate for daily fluid needs. (**3**) The need for fluid intake does not decrease with age. Three thousand milliliters is approximately 3 quarts of fluid. (**4**) Three thousand liters is approximately 3000 quarts of fluid.

151. (**1**) Integrated processes: nursing process — evaluation, teaching/learning; client need: physiological integrity; basic care and comfort; content area: medical-surgical.

RATIONALE

(**1**) The FDA requirement is to list ingredients by amounts in descending order. (**2**) This statement is not true; select another option. (**3**) This statement is not true; select another option. (**4**) This statement is not true; select another option.

152. **(3)** Integrated processes: nursing process — planning, communication and documentation; client need: psychosocial integrity; content area: medical-surgical.
RATIONALE
(1) Silence allows the person to think and add information. **(2)** Neither chemical nor physical restraints should be used as a punitive measure. **(3)** This is a tenet for good communication with all persons, but it is especially true for the older person, who may take more time to process material. **(4)** Eye contact may aid in the communication process.

153. **(4)** Integrated processes: nursing process — evaluation; client need: health promotion and maintenance; content area: medical-surgical.
RATIONALE
(1) The cough reflex is less active and may contribute to development of an infection, but this is not the question. **(2)** The skin is the body's primary barrier against infection, but this is not the question. **(3)** Prostatic hypertrophy, with increased residual urine, reduces the natural process of flushing the bladder, but this is not the question. **(4)** Absence of fever in the face of bacterial infection is not unusual in older persons.

154. **(1)** Integrated processes: nursing process — evaluation; client need: safe, effective care environment; safety and infection control; content area: medical-surgical.
RATIONALE
(1) Although falls can occur anywhere, most occur in the bathroom because of slippery floors and bath fixtures, as well as inadequate support fixtures such as rails. **(2)** In the living room, many falls occur from throw rugs or from unstable chairs or furniture. **(3)** Many falls occur in the bedroom when the older person gets up during the night to go to the bathroom. **(4)** Burns occur in the kitchen from stoves or hot pots or pans left on the stove.

155. **(2)** Integrated processes: nursing process — evaluation, teaching/learning; client need: safe, effective care environment; safety and infection control; content area: medical-surgical.
RATIONALE
(1) Elimination of clutter promotes safety by decreasing the chances of falling or tripping. **(2)** Carpets, especially throw rugs, increase the chance for tripping or sliding. **(3)** Handles of pans should be turned inward so the client does not accidentally reach for them or knock them off the stove. **(4)** Smoke detector batteries need to be changed regularly. A good method is to change them twice a year when standard time and daylight saving time change.

156. **(4)** Integrated processes: nursing process — evaluation; client need: physiological integrity; reduction of risk potential; content area: medical-surgical.
RATIONALE
(1) Some surgical procedures may cause immobility, but not all. **(2)** Immobility, rather than excessive exercise, is more likely to cause venous thrombosis. **(3)** A low-iron diet or decubitus ulcer will not affect the formation of venous thrombosis. **(4)** Prolonged immobility promotes stasis of blood and subsequent venous thrombosis.

157. **(4)** Integrated processes: nursing process — evaluation; client need: health promotion and prevention; content area: maternity nursing.
RATIONALE
(1) This action will not help; select another option. **(2)** Elevating the head of the bed may actually decrease her BP;

select another option. **(3)** The pulse will not change if another person takes it; reassess the situation. **(4)** Placing the client on her left side relieves pressure on the vena cava to increase venous return and thereby increase BP.

158. **(1)** Integrated processes: nursing process — evaluation; client need: health promotion and maintenance; content area: maternity nursing.
RATIONALE
(1) Amenorrhea is an early sign of pregnancy. **(2)** Dysmenorrhea, or painful menses, is not a sign of pregnancy and may occur at any time during a menstrual period. **(3)** Pica occurs when a pregnant woman has a desire for clay-like substances. **(4)** Nausea is a later sign that can occur.

159. **(4)** Integrated processes: nursing process — evaluation; client need: health promotion and maintenance; content area: maternity nursing.
RATIONALE
(1) Urinary frequency is normal and occurs because of pressure on the bladder. **(2)** Polyphagia, or increased appetite, is common. **(3)** Nausea is common until after the 16th week of pregnancy. **(4)** Dysuria, or painful urination, could indicate a bladder infection.

160. **(2)** Integrated processes: nursing process — data collection, teaching/learning; client need: physiological integrity; basic care and comfort; content area: pediatrics.
RATIONALE
(1) Croup is an inflammation of the larynx, trachea, and bronchi causing narrowing of the air passages from edema. Cough medicine is inappropriate. **(2)** Warm, moist air is required to decrease epiglottal edema. **(3)** Warm, dry heat will make the symptoms worse. **(4)** Warm, dry heat will make the symptoms worse.

161. **(4)** Integrated processes: nursing process — implementation; client need: physiological integrity; basic care and comfort; content area: pediatrics.
RATIONALE
(1) The client should be positioned on her side or stomach to promote drainage. **(2)** Coughing, clearing the throat, or blowing his nose will increase bleeding. **(3)** Using a straw will increase the chance of bleeding. **(4)** Cool fluid and a liquid diet promote fluid intake and healing.

162. **(2)** Integrated processes: nursing process — data collection; client need: health promotion and maintenance; content area: pediatrics.
RATIONALE
(1) Ménière's disease is a chronic disease of adulthood characterized by sudden attacks of vertigo, tinnitus, and hearing loss. **(2)** Otitis media is an infection of the middle ear, primarily the result of a blocked eustachian tube. In infants, there is a tendency to rub, hold, or pull the affected ear. **(3)** Otosclerosis is a disorder of the middle ear characterized by slow formation of spongy bone around the stapes, which causes progressive hearing loss. **(4)** Meningitis is an inflammation of the lining of the brain. Irritability is a symptom, but usually it is accompanied by nuchal pain, fever, vomiting, or headache.

163. **(3)** Integrated processes: nursing process — implementation, teaching/learning; client need: physiological integrity; basic care and comfort; content area: medical-surgical.
RATIONALE
(1) A commercial deodorizer can be used, but there is a better option. **(2)** Gas-forming foods can cause odor, but there is a

better option. (3) Cleaning the bag frequently gets rid of the basis of the odor problem — fecal residue. (4) The bag may need to be refitted, but there is a better option.

164. (1) Integrated processes: nursing process — evaluation; client need: health promotion and maintenance; content area: medical-surgical.

RATIONALE

(1) The area of induration is 10 mm but may vary with HIV infection and close contact with active tuberculosis (TB) cases or persons with a chest radiograph consistent with healed TB. Tuberculin reactions should be measured and recorded in millimeters after 48 hours at the largest diameter of the induration. (2) A normal response to the purified protein derivative (PPD) is erythema; select another option. (3) An intradermal injection of PPD causes a wheal to form; select another option. (4) Absence of erythema or induration is a negative response to the test.

165. (2) Integrated processes: nursing process — data collection; client need: physiological integrity; basic care and comfort; content area: maternity nursing.

RATIONALE

(1) It is important to check her dressing, but this question is related to feeding. (2) You might do all the listed interventions, but the correct answer to the question is option (2). Make sure bowel sounds have returned before providing nourishment after surgery. (3) It is important to encourage ambulation, but the question is related to feeding. (4) It is important to give pain medication, but this question is related to feeding.

166. (3) Integrated processes: nursing process — data collection; client need: physiological integrity; physiological adaptation; content area: medical-surgical.

RATIONALE

(1) Increased BP may not necessarily be a sign of increased intracranial pressure. (2) The vital signs are all normal. (3) Classic signs of increased intracranial pressure are a decrease in respirations, a decrease in pulse rate, and an increase in BP. (4) This information indicates impending shock.

167. (3) Integrated processes: nursing process — evaluation; client need: physiological integrity; basic care and comfort; content area: medical-surgical.

RATIONALE

(1) A temperature range of 70–90°F (21.1–32.2°C) can cause spasm because it is too cold. (2) A temperature range of 80–90°F (26.6–32.2°C) can cause spasm because it is too cold. (3) The temperature should be just greater than body temperature. (4) A temperature of 110°F (43.3°C) will burn.

168. (1) Integrated processes: nursing process — evaluation; client need: physiological integrity; pharmacological therapies; content area: medical-surgical.

RATIONALE

(1) To administer blood, you need a large-bore needle. The only needle listed that can deliver blood is the No. 16 Angiocath. (2) This Angiocath is too small; select another size. (3) This butterfly is too small; select another size. (4) This butterfly is too small; select another size.

169. (1) Integrated processes: nursing process — implementation; client need: physiological integrity; reduction of risk potential; content area: medical-surgical.

RATIONALE

(1) When suctioning, the nurse should occlude the suction port on withdrawal. Other options would either deprive the

client of oxygen or provide an inadequate vacuum. (2) This technique will deprive the client of oxygen. (3) Instilling 20 mL of normal saline may cause a fluid overload if this is instilled each time. (4) Opening the catheter suction port when withdrawing will cause an inadequate vacuum.

170. (4) Integrated processes: nursing process — implementation; client need: physiological integrity; pharmacological therapies; content area: medical-surgical.

RATIONALE

(1) A volume of 4.4 mL is too great for one injection. (2) A volume of 4.4 mL is too great for one injection. (3) A volume of 2.2 mL is too great for administration in the deltoid muscle. (4). Because a volume of 4.4 mL is too great for one injection; the dosage must be divided.

171. (4) Integrated processes: nursing process — implementation; client need: physiological integrity; pharmacological therapies; content area: medical-surgical.

RATIONALE

(1) The skin should not be massaged after the injection. (2) Heparin should be given as an SC injection, not IM. (3) Heparin should not be aspirated because of the possibility of causing bruising or bleeding. (4) Heparin should be given SC.

172. (1) Integrated processes: nursing process — data collection; client need: physiological integrity; reduction of risk potential; content area: pediatrics.

RATIONALE

(1) Absence of a pedal pulse is of the utmost importance because it indicates circulatory compromise. (2) You cannot palpate for a popliteal pulse through a cast. (3) Some drainage is expected. (4) There is no mention that the client is in traction.

173. (2) Integrated processes: nursing process — evaluation, teaching/learning; client need: physiological integrity; basic care and comfort; content area: pediatrics.

RATIONALE

(1) The blisters should be kept intact to prevent infection. (2) Skin should be kept intact to prevent infection. (3) Ice or cool water helps to disperse heat and prevent further damage, but skin should be kept intact. (4) Petrolatum only makes the blister worse by containing the heat and limiting air exposure.

174. (3) Integrated processes: nursing process — evaluation, teaching/learning; client need: health promotion and maintenance; content area: pediatrics.

RATIONALE

(1) Analysis of gastric secretions does not detect PKU. (2) PKU is not detected in arterial blood gases. (3) This test is performed on capillary blood, although the phenylpyruvic acid is excreted in the urine. Phenylketonuria is a hereditary disease caused by the body's failure to oxidize an amino acid because of a defective enzyme. This is called the Guthrie test. (4) Serum phenylalanine levels of 12–15 mg per 100 mL will begin to appear in the urine. By this time, some degree of irreversible mental damage may have occurred.

175. (2) Integrated processes: nursing process — planning; client need: health promotion and maintenance; content area: psychiatric nursing.

RATIONALE

(1) Industry versus inferiority is characteristic of the school-age child. (2) Erikson's stages of development indicate that the early adolescent is achieving role identity. (3) Intimacy versus

isolation is characteristic of the young adult. (4) Integrity versus despair is characteristic of the older adult.

176. (1) Integrated processes: nursing process — evaluation; client need: psychosocial integrity; content area: psychiatric nursing.
    RATIONALE
    (1) Morning-evening variation in symptoms occurs with psychotic depression. The client is most depressed in the morning and experiences a slight elevation of mood as the day progresses. (2) Mood is usually better in the afternoon; select another option. (3) Mood is usually elevated toward evening; select another answer. (4) Visiting time may either increase or decrease mood, depending on the client's relationship with the visitors.

177. (1) Integrated processes: nursing process — implementation, caring; client need: psychosocial integrity; content area: psychiatric nursing.
    RATIONALE
    (1) Because the basic trauma in schizophrenia is a disturbed parent-infant relationship, giving the client some milk will promote trust. (2) Hugging is very intrusive; select another option. (3) Bringing the client a deck of cards is an option, but there are better ones. (4) This is an excellent option; sitting quietly with the client may help to decrease agitation and promotes sharing of feelings. However, there is a better option.

178. (2) Integrated processes: nursing process — evaluation; client need: physiological integrity; pharmacological therapies; content area: medical-surgical.
    RATIONALE
    (1) Streptomycin (not isoniazid) can cause eighth cranial nerve damage, is nephrotoxic, and causes labyrinth damage and hepatitis. (2) Isoniazid can cause peripheral neuritis; pyridoxine is given prophylactically. (3) Streptomycin and ethambutol (not isoniazid) are rarely used with people with renal disease. (4) Para-aminosalicylic acid (PAS) and ethionamide (not isoniazid) can cause gastric disturbance.

179. (1) Integrated processes: nursing process — evaluation, teaching/learning; client need: physiological integrity; pharmacological therapies; content area: medical-surgical.
    RATIONALE
    (1) Discontinuance of even one drug may cause organisms to become drug resistant. (2) This outcome is important, but not the most important. (3) Drugs should never be discontinued by the client, only by the physician. (4) It is important to wear a Medic Alert bracelet, but not of highest importance.

180. (3) Integrated processes: nursing process — evaluation; client need: psychosocial integrity; content area: medical-surgical.
    RATIONALE
    (1) Compensation is covering up a weakness by emphasizing a desirable trait. An example is a physically handicapped individual who is an outstanding scholar. (2) Denial is the refusal to accept reality. (3) Displacement is the discharging of pent-up feelings to a less dangerous object or area. He is displacing his anger about his medical restrictions to a less dangerous one such as diet. (4) Projection is the attribution of one's own undesirable traits to someone else.

181. (4) Integrated processes: nursing process — evaluation; client need: health promotion and maintenance; content area: maternity nursing.

RATIONALE
(1) The nurse should not leave the room. Relieving the pressure is the highest priority. Use the call light to obtain help. (2) Fetal heart rate should be monitored, but this is not the highest priority. (3) This is not an appropriate answer. (4) Cord prolapse is an extremely serious complication that calls for immediate action because pressure on the cord deprives the baby of oxygen. The highest priority is to relieve the pressure of the fetal body or head from the cord.

182. (3) Integrated processes: nursing process — data collection; client need: health promotion and maintenance; content area: medical-surgical.
    RATIONALE
    (1) Clients usually present with a low-grade fever. (2) Nausea and vomiting may occur, but they are not related to eating. (3) Tenderness in the lower right quadrant is a classic sign. It is usually located over McBurney's point. (4) The area of tenderness is McBurney's point.

183. (4) Integrated processes: nursing process — implementation; client need: physiological integrity; basic care and comfort; content area: medical-surgical.
    RATIONALE
    (1) A heating pad may cause the appendix to rupture. (2) An enema is never given preoperatively in appendicitis because it could cause the appendix to rupture, and peritonitis could result. (3) Keep client NPO to decrease peristalsis. (4) A semi-Fowler's position relieves abdominal pain and tension.

184. (2) Integrated processes: nursing process — implementation, caring; client need: health promotion and maintenance; content area: maternity nursing.
    RATIONALE
    (1) Timing contractions is only important to determine when the baby will be delivered. (2) Remaining calm will let nature take its course. (3) Boiling water works in the movies and gives nervous people something to do. (4) She should be NPO because digestion stops when labor begins.

185. (1) Integrated processes: nursing process — implementation; client need: health promotion and maintenance; content area: medical-surgical.
    RATIONALE
    (1) Asking the man if his wife can talk establishes whether she has something in her airway. A victim is unable to talk if she is choking. (2) Giving a blow to the back if the person is choking will cause the food to move further down in the airway. (3) An abdominal thrust is done after the rescuer knows the airway is blocked. (4) Hitting the person on the chest is done after establishing an airway, if cardiopulmonary resuscitation (CPR) is being done. This is not appropriate for this situation.

186. (4) Integrated processes: nursing process — evaluation; client need: physiological integrity; physiological adaptation; content area: medical-surgical.
    RATIONALE
    (1) Tourniquets are not difficult to apply. (2) If a tourniquet is applied, it should be released only by the physician. (3) Direct pressure and elevation usually control bleeding in these areas. (4) Tourniquets can cause a considerable amount of damage, which may be permanent.

187. (2) Integrated processes: nursing process — evaluation, teaching/learning; client need: health promotion and maintenance; content area: medical-surgical.

RATIONALE

(1) Give only essential information because he will not be able to remember a lot of information. (2) The orientation should be limited to small, specific amounts of essential information. He will not be able to remember a lot of facts or details. (3) This is too specific, and will not provide visual clues for him. (4) Questions will further confuse him and add to his anxiety.

188. **(2)** Integrated processes: nursing process — planning; client need: physiological integrity; basic care and comfort; content area: medical-surgical.

RATIONALE

(1) Making the client responsible for his or her own care may not be appropriate based on the client's physiological and psychological functioning. (2) The plan needs to be based on the client's level of functioning with self-care and independence; reinforced as much as possible. (3) Assigning another resident is not appropriate. (4) The client should be encouraged to be independent and care for himself or herself as much as possible.

189. **(2)** Integrated processes: nursing process — implementation; client need: health promotion and maintenance; content area: medical-surgical.

RATIONALE

(1) An early morning specimen contains the most cells and bacteria. (2) The best time to collect a sputum specimen is the first thing in the morning. These specimens are more likely to contain cells and bacteria. (3) Before or after lunch is not conducive to the appetite or digestion and, most important, does not contain the cells or bacteria that an early morning specimen would. (4) Time does matter; select another option.

190. **(1)** Integrated processes: nursing process — implementation; client need: health promotion and maintenance; content area: medical-surgical.

RATIONALE

(1) Protecting the client from injury and decreasing the risk of aspiration are the priorities for client safety. (2) A tongue blade or other object might cause injury to the client's teeth or jaw, but aspiration is the major danger. (3) Restraints during a seizure might cause injury to the client. (4) Trying to move the client to the floor and holding the client down might cause injury.

191. **(2)** Integrated processes: nursing process — data collection; client need: health promotion and maintenance; content area: medical-surgical.

RATIONALE

(1) Clear fluid from the nose or ears is the correct answer. (2) CSF is clear fluid from the nose or ears. The nurse should test the drainage for the presence of glucose. (3) CSF is clear, thin fluid from the nose or ears. (4) Bleeding would indicate intracranial bleeding or skull fracture.

192. **(3)** Integrated processes: nursing process — implementation, teaching/learning; client need: health promotion and maintenance; content area: medical-surgical.

RATIONALE

(1) People who live a long time generally have a modest caloric intake, do not eat a lot of meat or processed foods, and eat fresh vegetables, fruits, and grains. (2) Sexual activity does not have to decline with age, and continued activity may extend life. (3) A little "enlightened selfishness" will make the older person and his or her friends feel better and live longer. (4) Having friends, relatives, or pets increases survival.

193. **(2)** Integrated processes: nursing process — implementation, caring; client need: health promotion and maintenance; content area: medical-surgical.

RATIONALE

(1) Letting the person decide on a food plan may be contrary to physician's orders. (2) Appearance often affects the way people feel. Basic nursing interventions related to cleanliness, hygiene, and grooming are important in helping older people maintain feelings of self-worth and self-esteem. (3) Providing hygiene maintains an older person's feelings of self-worth and self-esteem. (4) Older women often like cosmetics but prefer those that are appropriate for older skin.

194. **(4)** Integrated processes: nursing process — implementation, caring; client need: psychosocial integrity; content area: medical-surgical.

RATIONALE

(1) Call the client by his or her last name preceded by "Mr.," "Mrs.," "Ms.," or "Miss," not by an endearing term such as "honey." (2) Encourage independence. (3) Avoid comments or actions that reflect ageism, such as reference to diapers. (4) Allowing as much control of care and environment as possible is a general nursing intervention that can be used to help maintain mental-health wellness in older adults.

195. **(4)** Integrated processes: nursing process — implementation, teaching/learning; client need: physiological integrity; pharmacological therapies; content area: medical-surgical

RATIONALE

(1) Encourage nutritional diet instead of vitamin pills. (2) Encourage exercise and activities with others instead of sedatives, hypnotics, antianxiety agents, and alcohol. (3) Advise exercise and high-bulk foods instead of laxatives. (4) Discourage misuse of medications by teaching the client to administer as few medications as possible to prevent possible delirium and other complications such as falls.

196. **(2)** Integrated processes: nursing process — implementation, teaching/learning; client need: psychosocial integrity; content area: psychiatric nursing.

RATIONALE

(1) Hospital nurses are not able to view the family dynamics that may indicate abuse during the short stay in the hospital. (2) Hospital nurses have the responsibility in the discharge planning and teaching of older clients and their families to reduce anxiety and promote mental health. (3) Hospital nurses may not be able to assess social isolation during the short stay in the hospital. (4) Because of the short stay in the hospital, the nurse will not be able to teach effective ways to cope with aging.

197. **(4)** Integrated processes: nursing process — implementation, caring; client need: physiological integrity; basic care and comfort; content area: psychiatric nursing.

RATIONALE

(1) Whether to take medications ordered "as needed" is not an example of the kind of activity that a nursing home resident can have some control over. (2) Assignment of staff members is not the responsibility of a nursing home resident. (3) Participating in a partial choice of food plan is an example of the kind of activity that a nursing home resident can have some control over, but the control is not complete. (4) Type and time of bath is an example of the kind of activity that a nursing home resident can have some control over.

198. **(3)** Integrated processes: nursing process — implementation, caring; client need: psychosocial integrity; content area: psychiatric nursing.

RATIONALE

(1) Allowing a resident to wander into another resident's room is inappropriate and does not prevent loneliness. (2) Group activities may be helpful, but one-to-one contact is most beneficial. (3) Group activities may be helpful, but people can feel lonely even in a group without some one-to-one contact and communication. (4) Effective communication, even with patients with dementia, should be a primary goal of all nursing home staff members.

199. **(3)** Integrated processes: nursing process — evaluation, caring; client need: psychosocial integrity; content area: psychiatric nursing.

RATIONALE

(1) Humor serving as an outlet for inner tensions and anxieties is a psychological effect. (2) Older persons are less offended when people of their own age group joke about aging than when younger persons joke about aging. (3) Interpersonally, humor has been referred to as a "social lubricant" because it helps to establish relationships and promote group cohesion. (4) Stimulating awareness is a physiological effect of humor.

200. **(4)** Integrated processes: nursing process — implementation; client need: psychosocial integrity; content area: psychiatric nursing.

RATIONALE

(1) Teasing an older person without his or her consent is a violation of the person's boundaries. (2) Funny costumes, false noses, and hats, not scary costumes, can be worn for visual impact. (3) Funny stories or jokes should be told rather than grim or frightening stories. (4) Post or otherwise share cartoons with clients and their families. Use cartoons as teaching materials.

201. **(3)** Integrated processes: nursing process — implementation; client need: physiological integrity; pharmacological therapies; content area: maternity nursing.

RATIONALE

400 mg divided by 200 mg $\times$ 1 tablet $=$ 2 tablets

202. **(4)** Integrated processes: nursing process — implementation; client need: physiological integrity; pharmacological therapies; content area: maternity nursing.

RATIONALE

25 mg : 1 mL $=$ 10 mg : x $=$ 0.4 mL

203. **(2)** Integrated processes: nursing process — implementation, teaching/learning; client need: physiological integrity; pharmacological therapies; content area: maternity nursing.

RATIONALE

5 mg : 1 tablet $=$ 20 mg : x $=$ 4 tablets

204. **(3)** Integrated processes: nursing process — implementation, teaching/learning; client need: physiological integrity; pharmacological therapies; content area: maternity nursing.

RATIONALE

200 mg : 1 tablet $\times$ 4 tablets/day $\times$ 5 days $=$ 20 tablets

205. **(4)** Integrated processes: nursing process — implementation; client need: physiological integrity; pharmacological therapies; content area: maternity nursing.

RATIONALE

500 mg : 5 mL $=$ 250 mg : x $=$ 2.5 mL

T E S T 2

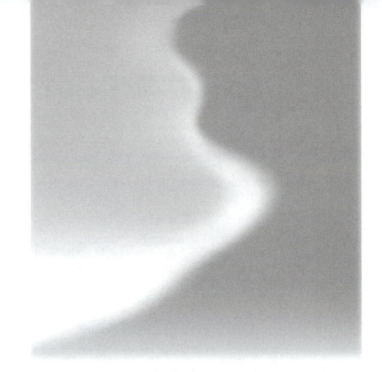

Patricia Gauntlett Beare, RN, PhD
Larry D. Purnell, RN, PhD
Golden M. Tradewell, RN, PhD

QUESTIONS

1. The focus and purpose of health teaching are to:
   1. Resolve the problem
   2. Facilitate teaching methods
   3. Facilitate client's mastery
   4. Facilitate teacher's control

2. When should the nurse begin teaching an older client?
   1. At the time of admission
   2. At the time of discharge
   3. At home
   4. When the older client is physically capable

3. In teaching an older person administration of medications, the nurse's best response would be:
   1. "Take your medications tid."
   2. "The doctor wants you to take your medicine every 6 hours."
   3. "Take your medicine when you go to bed at night."
   4. "Take your medicine ac and hs."

4. The presenting signs and symptoms of disease in the older person are frequently atypical and nonspecific, such as:
   1. An elevated white blood cell (WBC) count and fever in sepsis
   2. Chest pain in myocardial infarction
   3. Apathy in thyrotoxicosis.
   4. Polyuria and polydipsia in diabetic emergencies

5. Which of the following does the nurse need to consider first before setting goals with an older adult?
   1. What does the nurse expect the older person to accomplish?

2. What kind of relaxation time does the older person have?
3. What kind of social support does the older person have?
4. Does the older person enjoy being alone?

6. A 72-year-old client leaving rehabilitation still requires assistance with walking. The physician orders her to relocate to a center that will permit daily assistance in walking. Concerned about leaving her husband, who is in poor health, she tells the nurse that she would rather give up walking than leave her husband. The nurse's response is:
   1. "Your needs come first."
   2. "Your husband would want what is best for you."
   3. "I understand that staying with your husband is more important than walking."
   4. "Are you sure you want to throw all of your success away?"

7. The nurse is orienting a 78-year-old client to her new room in the long-term care facility. The nurse instructs the client to:
   1. Stay away from the men's hall.
   2. Refrain from socializing in the lounge.
   3. Personalize her living space with personal possessions.
   4. Be aware that she will be treated as if she were "sick."

8. How can the nurse intervene to make the dining area and mealtime pleasant in a long-term care facility?
   1. Serve the food quickly and remove the trays on time.
   2. Seat residents alphabetically.
   3. Seat residents according to social preferences.
   4. Have residents eat alone in their rooms.

9. A client is to receive 30 units of neutral prota-mine Hagedorn (NPH) insulin and 4 units of regular insulin at 8 AM. The nurse would: (**Select all that apply.**)

   1. Inject air into the NPH insulin first.
   2. Draw up the insulins in separate syringes.
   3. Draw up the regular insulin first.
   4. Ask the pharmacy for the desired mixture.
   5. Notify physician to change the order to a combined dose.
   6. Inject air into both vials..

10. The physician orders norethindrone (Norlutin) 7.5 mg PO for a young woman experiencing breakthrough bleeding. The pharmacist dispenses 5-mg tablets and instructs the client to take _____ tablet(s).

11. The nurse is doing a physical data collection on a 6-month-old infant. The baby is sitting quietly on the mother's lap. Which of the following parts of the data collection should the nurse do first?

    1. Auscultate heart and lungs.
    2. Examine eyes, ears, and mouth.
    3. Examine head and move toward the feet.
    4. Palpate peripheral pulses.

12. A client who is in mechanical restraints asks the nurse when they can be removed. Which one of the following is the best response by the nurse?

    1. "Please tell me why you were physically violent."
    2. "When apologies are made for creating such a disturbance."
    3. "When your behavior is under control and you are no longer a danger to yourself or others."
    4. "When the medication has calmed your violent behavior."

13. The nurse caring for a 4-year-old child after a tonsillectomy and adenoidectomy monitors for signs and symptoms of hemorrhage. Which of the following would be an early indication of hemorrhage?

    1. Swallowing infrequently
    2. Dark-brown emesis of approximately 25 mL
    3. Pulse rate of 95 bpm
    4. Drooling of bright-red secretions

14. A pregnant client is started on an iron supplement. What information can the nurse give the client to aid in absorption of the supplement?

    1. "Take your iron with milk."
    2. "Take your supplement with your prenatal vitamins."
    3. "Take your iron with orange juice."
    4. "Take your iron in the morning with breakfast."

15. During an otoscopic examination on a 9-year-old child, the nurse pulls the pinna in which direction? (Place an X on the pinna in the figure and then indicate with an arrow the direction in which it is pulled to position for an otoscopic examination.)

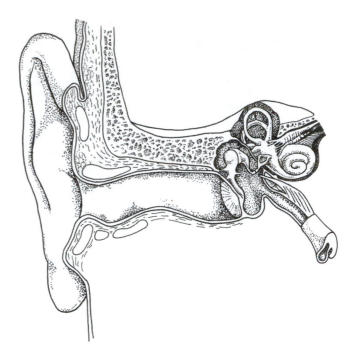

16. After reviewing danger signs during pregnancy that should be reported immediately to the health-care provider, which of the following responses would indicate to the nurse that the client understands?

    1. "Intermittent vomiting."
    2. "Vaginal bleeding."
    3. "Leukorrhea."
    4. "Urinary frequency."

17. A nurse is teaching a 27-year-old, first-time mother of a healthy full-term girl. Which of the following statements by the newborn's mother indicates a need for further teaching?

    1. "I need to place my daughter on her side to sleep."
    2. "I need to place my daughter on her back to sleep."
    3. "I need to place my daughter on her abdomen to sleep."
    4. "I need to place my daughter upright to burp her before I put her to sleep after her bottle."

18. The nurse, in planning program activities for clients in a day treatment setting, should:

    1. Facilitate diversional activities for the lower-functioning clients.
    2. Focus on pathology.
    3. Provide for meaningful social interaction.
    4. Provide for multifaceted needs.

19. A client arrives in the clinic for her first prenatal visit. She states that her last menstrual period was May 12–16. Using Naegele's rule, determine her expected date of confinement.

   _____

20. Which of the following statements indicates to the nurse the best understanding of placental functioning?

1. "The placenta filters out harmful substances."
2. "The placenta is where my blood circulates through my baby."
3. "The umbilical cord has one vein and one artery."
4. "The placenta gives my baby oxygen and nutrients."

21. A 58-year-old client is 4 days postoperative status for a coronary bypass graft surgery. The nurse encourages him to cough and deep breathe to clear the thick secretions from his lungs. The client states that it hurts too much to breathe. Which of the following nursing actions would be appropriate to help this client restore pulmonary function after surgery? (**Select all that apply.**)

    1. Administer morphine sulfate as ordered.
    2. Use incentive spirometer every hour.
    3. Use a pillow to splint the chest.
    4. Teach diaphragmatic breathing to the client.
    5. Provide narcotic-based cough medication.
    6. Log roll the client to the left side.

22. A 33-year-old client is experiencing severe irritability secondary to acute alcohol withdrawal. The physician orders lorazepam (Ativan) 1 mg IV tid. Using a 4-mg/mL vial, how many milliliters does the nurse administer?

23. A 38-year-old client is admitted with fever and dyspnea and is intubated and placed on a ventilator for respiratory distress. After the endotracheal tube has been placed in the client, the nurse would immediately do which of the following?

    1. Check for bilateral breath sounds.
    2. Call for a chest radiograph.
    3. Obtain stat arterial blood gases.
    4. Check the client's vital signs.

24. A 49-year-old client is admitted with signs and symptoms of pulmonary embolism. The nurse is aware that which of the following is a risk factor associated with pulmonary embolism?

    1. Hypervolemia
    2. Arthritis
    3. Long-bone fracture
    4. Osteoporosis

25. A child with neutropenia has just been admitted to the pediatric unit. Which of the following actions by the nurse would take highest priority?

    1. Encourage eating raw vegetables and fruits for their vitamin C content.
    2. Prohibit any activity and maintain strict bedrest.
    3. Report immediately any temperature elevation.
    4. Screen visitors.

26. A 46-year-old client is 3 days postoperative status from a craniotomy. The client develops diabetes insipidus. The nurse realizes that which of the following causes diabetes insipidus?

    1. Increased antidiuretic hormone (ADH) production
    2. Decreased ADH production
    3. Hypovolemia
    4. Renal failure

27. A 78-year-old male client is admitted for shortness for breath on exertion and extreme fatigue. Some time after lunch, he asks the nurse if there are any large-print magazines or books in the hospital to read. He tells the nurse that it is the only type of print he can read. The nurse would identify which of the following conditions as the reason for the client's visual problem?

    1. Cataracts
    2. Presbyopia
    3. Xerostomia
    4. Arcus senilis

28. Which of the following statements by a 23-weeks-pregnant client indicates to the nurse the need for further instruction on improving circulation?

    1. "I should avoid crossing my legs while sitting."
    2. "I should put on my support pantyhose after I have walked to the bathroom."
    3. "I should elevate my legs whenever I sit at work."
    4. "I should dorsiflex my feet if I have been standing for a long period of time."

29. What are effective mechanisms to prevent and control the spread of hepatitis A in any setting? (**Select all that apply.**)

    1. Education
    2. Hand washing.
    3. Avoidance of illicit drug use.
    4. Immunization to prevent hepatitis B virus infection.
    5. Drink the water while visiting other countries.
    6. Do not drink water while visiting other countries.

30. The second stage of labor is complete when:

    1. The cervix is completely dilated.
    2. The client begins the pushing process.
    3. The infant is delivered.
    4. The placenta has been delivered.

31. A 28-year-old client is admitted with Cushing's syndrome. Which of the following physical changes would the nurse expect to observe in a client with this disorder?

    1. Bronzing of the skin, weight loss, and alopecia
    2. Hyperactivity, acne, and ecchymosis
    3. Moon face, hirsutism, and thin extremities
    4. Buffalo hump, thin extremities, and girdle obesity

32. Which of the following information is most important in teaching parents about the hygiene of a preschooler?

    1. The parent should assist with or supervise all of his or her hygienic needs, especially bathing, until age 5 years.
    2. The preschooler is fearful of being pulled down the drain because of the inability to judge size.
    3. The child cannot dress himself or herself completely until age 4 years.
    4. Specific instructions and directions with no options are best to ensure proper bathing and dressing.

33. A client is 4 days after delivery by cesarean section. Which of the following is true regarding uterine involution after a cesarean section?

    1. The uterus involutes 1 cm/day.
    2. Lochia increases about day 5.
    3. Lochia decreases about day 5.
    4. There is less risk for endometritis.

34. A 6-year-old boy has asthma. His mother asks the nurse if he can participate in any sports. The nurse would recommend which of the following sports?

    1. Basketball
    2. Long-distance running
    3. Swimming
    4. Soccer
    5. Baseball
    6. Field hockey

35. A mother has her 12-year-old daughter in the arthritis clinic. The physician prescribes naproxen (Naprosyn)—first dose 500 mg, then 250 mg every 8 hours—for signs and complaints of inflamed joints and pain. The mother asks how long it will take for the naproxen to be effective. Which of the following is the most accurate response by the nurse?

    1. "It is a long-acting drug and will take several months for therapeutic effect."
    2. "Therapeutic effects may not be noticed for 3–4 weeks."
    3. "The medicine works rapidly, so she will be moving her joints better in 24 hours."
    4. "She will have relief of pain after the first dose, but the inflammation will not decrease for several days."

36. A client gave birth 10 minutes ago. The placenta has still not delivered. The nurse should:

    1. Inform the primary health-care provider.
    2. Apply traction to the umbilical cord.
    3. Prepare the client for surgery.
    4. Reassure the client that this is normal.

37. The nurse is caring for a 4-year-old child admitted with a history of spontaneous pneumothorax. The child has a closed-chest drainage system. The purpose of the water in the closed-chest drainage chamber is to:

    1. Decrease the danger of sudden change in pressure in the tube.
    2. Prevent entrance of air into the pleural cavity.
    3. Provide faster removal of chest secretions by capillary action.
    4. Facilitate emptying bloody drainage from the chest.

38. Discharge instructions for a client recovering from severe iron-deficiency anemia should emphasize the need for:

    1. Planned rest periods.
    2. Fluid intake of 3000 mL daily.
    3. A diet high in vitamin B_{12}.
    4. A diet high in folic acid.

39. A 2-year-old girl has a diagnosis of urinary tract infection (UTI). While teaching the mother, the nurse identifies the following factor as having predisposed her daughter to a UTI:

    1. Increased fluid intake
    2. Frequent emptying of the bladder
    3. Ingestion of highly acidic juices
    4. Short urethra in young girls

40. For many women, one of the first signs of pregnancy is fullness or tingling of the breasts. These changes are a result of:

    1. The presence of breast milk
    2. An enhanced sexual drive
    3. A decreased blood supply
    4. Hormonal changes

41. An 8-year-old child was admitted to the hospital with an acute illness. During the admission assessment, the nurse notes the child's religious affiliation as being Mormon. What beliefs about diet and food practices are common to this religion?

    1. Members may not have blood transfusions.
    2. Members may eat meat from animals that are vegetable eaters, have cloven hooves, and chew their cud.
    3. Members should avoid tea, coffee, chocolate, and other products containing caffeine.
    4. Members must fast for 6 hours before receiving Holy Communion.

42. A 15-year-old female client is seen at the clinic and is given a diagnosis of a UTI infection. In preparing to teach her, the nurse would include which of the following in the plan of care?

    1. Inform her that the cause of such infection in adolescents is usually sexual activity.
    2. Tell her that drinking large amounts of carbonated beverages can help to dilute the urine.
    3. Tell her that douching will help to rid the vagina of bacteria.
    4. Tell her that it is best to take showers because baths may contribute to bacterial growth that may predispose a female to a UTI.

43. A 4-year-old boy is admitted to the children's surgical unit for first-stage repair of hypospadias. In considering the level of development of the preschool-age child, which of the following statements accurately describes this stage of development?

    1. He is experiencing the Electra complex.
    2. He is beginning to question his sexuality.
    3. He is anxious about penile size.
    4. He is afraid of mutilation.

44. An alcoholic client is discharged from the inpatient treatment setting on disulfiram (Antabuse). The nurse should instruct the client to avoid the use of:

    1. Vinegar-based dressings, cough elixirs, and cologne.
    2. Cough elixirs, cologne, and acetaminophen.
    3. Cologne, acetaminophen, and penicillin.
    4. Acetaminophen, penicillin, and vinegar-based dressings.

45. A nurse is teaching a 65-year-old client about closed-angle glaucoma. Which of the following statements indicates a clear understanding of closed-angle glaucoma?

1. "I should never take over-the-counter medications without consulting my doctor."
2. "If I forget to take my eye drops, I just wait for the next dose."
3. "I can stop taking my eye drops when my vision improves."
4. "I will return to my eye doctor for a checkup every 2 years."

46. A 17-year-old female client suspects that she is 10 days pregnant. Because she cannot come to the clinic this week, the client tells the nurse that she will use a home pregnancy test. The nurse should emphasize the fact that:

1. Consumer tests have a high rate of false-positive results.
2. Consumer tests are easy to use.
3. A test with a negative result should be repeated in a week if amenorrhea continues.
4. The results of clinic tests are kept private.

47. Which of the following is expected behavior in a 4-year-old child?

1. The child may tell "tall tales" and have imaginary playmates.
2. The child may make extra demands for attention because fear of loss of love is common.
3. The child still clings to the security blanket.
4. The child will be more tranquil than at 3 years old.

48. An 8-year-old child is admitted to the pediatric unit with a diagnosis of acute glomerulonephritis (AGN). A nursing care plan would include which of the following?

1. Forcing fluids
2. Increasing sodium in the diet
3. Weighing daily
4. Taking vital signs once per shift

49. When the client's membranes spontaneously rupture, the nurse's first action is to:

1. Change the client's linen.
2. Notify the primary health-care provider.
3. Assess fetal heart tones.
4. Document the client's response to the event.

50. On the second-day postpartum cesarean section, the nurse notes that a breast-feeding client's uterus is 3 cm below her umbilicus. The nurse would expect this finding to be:

1. Abnormal because her baby weighed 7 lb.
2. Abnormal because this is her first baby.
3. Normal because she has had a cesarean birth.
4. Normal because she is breast-feeding.

51. A 45-year-old client performs the repetitive act of checking the front door of her house to make certain that it is locked. The client feels out of control and requests admission to the hospital. During the initial interview, the nurse observes that the client is restless and has difficulty focusing on a topic. The nurse is aware that the client's behavior represents an effort to:

1. Relieve tension
2. Control her thoughts

3. Seek attention
4. Control a phobia

52. A 20-year-old client has third-degree burns on 9% of the body. The nurse explains to the family that one leg has been burned and that third degree means that:

1. Subcutaneous (SC) tissues and possibly underlying tissues are involved.
2. Destruction of epidermis and dermis has occurred.
3. Only the epidermis has been lost.
4. The leg is covered by erythema and blisters.

53. A 16-year-old girl developed macrocytic anemia secondary to pregnancy. The physician orders 1 mg of folic acid intramuscularly (IM) for 4–5 days. Using a 5-mg/mL vial, the nurse administers how many milliliters?

_____

54. Which finding indicates that a client who takes nitroglycerin (NTG) needs further teaching to prevent complications?

1. Client took six NTGs tablets before notifying the physician.
2. Client places the tablet under the tongue until dissolved.
3. Client stores the medication in an airtight, dark bottle.
4. Client reports that he premedicates before sexual intercourse.

55. A client with diabetes had 30 units of NPH insulin SC at 8 AM. The nurse might plan for this client to have a snack between:

1. 10 AM and 2 PM
2. 12 noon and 4 PM
3. 2 PM and 8 PM
4. 4 PM and 7 PM

56. The descent of the fetal head into the pelvis before delivery is called:

1. Quickening
2. Effacement
3. Lightening
4. Station

57. Which of the following approaches by the nurse is best when administering an IM injection of an antibiotic to a 2-year-old child?

1. Tell the child it will not hurt, secure the child, and administer the antibiotic IM.
2. Tell the child there will be a little stick in the arm and explain that it will hurt a little.
3. Allow the child to assist in drawing up the medication beforehand.
4. Enter the room with medication prepared, briefly state that he or she is giving the child a shot, administer it, and comfort the child.

58. When planning nursing care for a 5-year-old child, which nursing action is most appropriate for the child placed under an oxygen mist tent?

1. Encourage the child to keep stuffed animals in bed with him or her.
2. Encourage the use of a battery-operated tape player for music.
3. Use only synthetic-material blankets under the tent.
4. Use a plastic or vinyl doll for play.

59. A client with newly diagnosed diabetes is being discharged; the client is to give himself insulin when he goes home. Before discharging the client, the nurse ensures that he:

1. Explains all of the details about how to give the insulin.
2. Administers the injection into an orange.
3. Administers the injection to a significant other.
4. Administers the insulin to himself.

60. On afternoon rounds, the nurse sees the mother of a terminal cancer client weeping silently. What would be the most appropriate nursing intervention?

1. Tell her that you (the nurse) know how she feels.
2. Tell her she must not cry and that everything is going to be all right.
3. Go immediately to her and ask her what she is crying about.
4. Sit in the chair beside her, put your hand on her hand, and wait for her to speak.

61. The nursing process is a systematic, rational method of planning and providing nursing care based on a client's actual or potential health-care needs. The step in which the nurse carries out planned nursing interventions is called:

1. Planning
2. Evaluation
3. Implementation
4. Data collection

62. A 4-year-old child is seen in the clinic. She is pulling on her ear and says, "My ear hurts." This statement is an example of:

1. Secondary data
2. Constant data
3. Objective data
4. Subjective data

63. According to Maslow's hierarchy of needs, a client having respiratory distress would fit under the category with the highest priority, called:

1. Safety and security needs
2. Physiological needs
3. Self-actualization
4. Psychosocial needs

64. An 85-year-old client in a skilled nursing care facility is complaining of chest pain. Essential nursing data collection includes:

1. The location, intensity, and duration of the pain
2. How well the client slept last night
3. Whether the pain increases on movement
4. The client's body temperature

65. A 67-year-old client is admitted with pulmonary emphysema. Signs and symptoms that the nurse might expect to note in data collection may include:

1. Severe chest pain, hot dry skin, minimal breath sounds, inspiratory wheezing
2. Exertional dyspnea, cough with copious amounts of mucopurulent sputum, barrel-shaped chest
3. Anxiety, cyanosis, hypotension, dysphagia, chronic respiratory alkalosis
4. Orthopnea, inspiratory wheezing, lack of chest movement on the left side, severe knife-like chest pain

66. Medications often used in the treatment of chronic obstructive pulmonary disease (COPD) include bronchodilators to relax smooth muscle and to increase vital capacity. An example of a bronchodilator is:

1. Spironolactone (Aldactone)
2. Nifedipine (Procardia)
3. Aminophylline
4. Digoxin

67. The nurse needs to monitor clients receiving bronchodilators for side effects or toxic effects of these drugs, which include:

1. Seeing halos around lights and having blurred vision, tachycardia, hypotension, anorexia
2. Dehydration, hypokalemia, urticaria, abdominal or epigastric pain
3. Tachycardia, cardiac arrhythmias, photosensitivity, headache, confusion
4. Restlessness, tachycardia, insomnia, nausea, vomiting, palpitations, seizures

68. A client with pulmonary emphysema has severe difficulty breathing and orthopnea. Orthopnea means that the client:

1. Has respiratory distress
2. Has blood gases that show respiratory acidosis
3. Has periods of apnea
4. Can breathe more easily when sitting upright

69. The flow rate for O_2 administration to a client with severe emphysema (i.e., COPD) will be in low concentrations, 1–2 L/min because:

1. High levels of O_2 will cause tachypnea and hypoxemia.
2. The respiratory center in the brain has adapted to low levels of O_2 as the main stimulus for respiration, and administration of high concentrations of O_2 will depress respirations.
3. COPD clients often need to receive long-term oxygen therapy, and high levels of O_2 could create a dependency.
4. Higher levels of O_2 should be administered only as a last resort to prevent carbon dioxide retention and respiratory alkalosis

70. Safety precautions in the use of oxygen therapy include:

1. Posting "No smoking" signs on the door of the room.
2. Not using any electrical equipment near the oxygen flow meter.

3. Instructing the client that smoking is permitted only when the oxygen is not on.
4. Avoiding use of medications that might interact with oxygen.

71. A client's oral temperature is 102°F (38.8°C). This is:
   1. Within the normal range for an oral temperature
   2. Afebrile
   3. Febrile and higher than normal
   4. An indication that the electronic thermometer needs to be recharged

72. Factors that can affect normal body temperature include:
   1. Diet, blood pressure, time of day.
   2. Medications taken, mood, health status, exercise.
   3. Smoking, environment, weight, medications.
   4. Age, diurnal variations, environment, exercise.

73. A 44-year-old client has type I, or insulin-dependent, diabetes mellitus and is receiving 30 units of Humulin neutral protamine Hagedorn (NPH) insulin every morning. The nurse will observe him for signs and symptoms of hypoglycemia:
   1. 30–60 minutes after administration.
   2. 8–12 hours after administration.
   3. 18 hours after administration.
   4. 2–4 hours after administration.

74. Symptoms of hypoglycemia include:
   1. Hunger, inability to concentrate, tremors, tachycardia, diaphoresis, diplopia, blurred vision
   2. Hypothermia, anorexia, lethargy, increased thirst, nausea, vomiting
   3. Irritability, loss of appetite, dry, hot flushed skin, diplopia
   4. Inability to concentrate, air hunger, headaches, blood glucose level of 140

75. A client is to receive regular and NPH insulin. The nurse will:
   1. Draw up the amount of regular insulin into the syringe first.
   2. Draw up the NPH insulin first because this will enhance mixing of the two insulins.
   3. Inject a volume of air equal to that of medication into the NPH insulin vial first and withdraw the NPH insulin before withdrawing the amount of regular insulin.
   4. Draw up the regular insulin into the syringe first.

76. The normal route of administration of insulin is:
   1. IM
   2. Intradermal
   3. SC
   4. Oral

77. The nurse is assigned to care for a 47-year-old female client who is first-day postoperative cholecystectomy. She will be kept on nothing by mouth (NPO) postoperatively until:

1. She no longer has nausea and her appetite returns.
2. She is fully awake and the effects of the anesthesia have worn off.
3. Her physician writes an order for clear liquids as tolerated.
4. Peristalsis has returned as evidenced by auscultation of bowel sounds and the ability to pass flatus.

78. A postoperative cholecystectomy client is receiving a clear liquid diet. Which of the following foods is allowed?
   1. Jell-O, cream of chicken soup, milk
   2. Oatmeal, orange juice, vanilla pudding
   3. Water, coffee or tea, sherbet, pureed bananas
   4. A grape popsicle, plain gelatin, apple juice, water

79. Medications that may be given to a postoperative client experiencing nausea and vomiting include:
   1. Trimethobenzamide (Tigan) or promethazine (Phenergan)
   2. Glycopyrrolate (Robinul) or diphenhydramine (Benadryl)
   3. Merperidine (Demerol) or pentazocine (Talwin)
   4. Atropine or morphine

80. A most important nursing intervention in which the nurse instructs the client to prevent postoperative respiratory complications is:
   1. To perform range-of-motion and leg exercises as soon as the anesthetic has worn off
   2. To stop smoking and to cough and deep breathe at least every 2 hours
   3. To elevate the feet when sitting up and to wear anti-embolic stockings during postoperative ambulation
   4. To provide low-flow oxygen and to increase vitamin C intake

81. The nursing intervention that will quickly alert the nurse to any changes in a postoperative client's condition is:
   1. Measuring and recording intake and output (I&O)
   2. Assessing pain quality and intensity
   3. Monitoring vital signs
   4. Inspecting the dressing or drainage tubes, or both, for bleeding

82. The nurse has just administered digoxin (Lanoxin) 0.25 mg to a client, and the client asks, "How does this medicine help my heart beat?" The nurse's best response is:
   1. "It helps to dilate the blood vessels, which increases your heart rate."
   2. "It increases the force of the contraction of the heart muscle and also strengthens the heartbeat."
   3. "It constricts the coronary arteries, which helps to supply more blood to your heart."
   4. "It lengthens the number of impulses generated, which in turn slows down your heart rate."

83. The nurse instructs a client in the cardiac unit to take his radial and apical heart rates, and the client asks, "Why is this important?" The nurse's best response is:

1. "It is important for you to know how to take your own pulse."
2. "You will know what your normal pulse rate is."
3. "The physician will want you to call him or her and perhaps omit your digoxin if your pulse rate falls below a certain level."
4. "Knowing your normal pulse rate will alert you to changes, which may require omitting or even increasing the amount of your medication."

84. A 67-year-old executive is hospitalized with a cerebrovascular accident (CVA), or stroke. Blood pressure on admission is 170/110 mm Hg. The executive has some weakness in the left arm and leg. The cause of this left-sided weakness is:

    1. A hemorrhage or clot on the left side of the brain, which has cut off the blood supply to the spinal cord
    2. Hypertension, and it is a temporary condition
    3. A hemorrhage or clot on the right side of the brain
    4. A thrombosis of the spinal cord, which has decreased the blood supply to the extremities

85. A 66-year-old male client's blood pressure of 170/110 mm Hg is:

    1. Within the normal range for a man of his age
    2. Serious hypertension
    3. Slightly higher than normal
    4. Slightly high but probably a result of his hospitalization and diagnosis

86. Some clients with CVAs experience expressive aphasia, which is:

    1. Inability to speak because of intellectual impairment related to brain damage
    2. Inability to read and understand
    3. Difficulty in speaking and swallowing related to neuromuscular impairment and brain damage
    4. Inability to speak, understand, or write because of impairment of the blood supply to the speech center

87. Maintenance of body function and prevention of complications is crucial in the nursing management of a client who has suffered a CVA. Nursing interventions that will aid in recovery and prevent contractures include:

    1. Turning and repositioning client every 2 hours, using a footboard and pillows, and encouraging range-of-motion exercises to all extremities
    2. Elevating the head of the bed 40 degrees; instructing client to turn, cough, and deep breathe every 2–4 hours.
    3. Performing neurological assessment every 2 hours, turning and repositioning client, using flotation mattress, and auscultating lung sounds.
    4. Changing client's position from side-to-side every 2 hours, monitoring vital signs, and observing for signs of dehydration and electrolyte imbalance.

88. Discharge instructions to give a client with a CVA to aid in preventing a recurrence include:

    1. "Use community resources, keep appointments for speech and physical therapy, take medication as ordered, and maintain a diet high in protein and vitamin E."
    2. "Lose weight and stop smoking (if applicable), follow dietary instructions (low salt, low cholesterol, and low fat), keep blood pressure under control, and report any changes in your condition to your physician."
    3. "Keep blood pressure under control, perform aerobic exercises three times a week, and maintain 1500-Kcal American Diabetes Association (ADA) diet."
    4. "Stop smoking (if applicable), avoid overexposure to very cold weather, continue speech and physical rehabilitation, and monitor daily I&O."

89. A 34-year-old woman is first day postappendectomy. The nurse assists her in coughing and deep breathing every 2 hours to:

    1. Prevent pulmonary complications.
    2. Help to remove secretions from the lungs and bronchi.
    3. Prevent postoperative thrombophlebitis.
    4. Mobilize secretions and prevent paralytic ileus.

90. Nursing interventions that help to prevent circulatory problems in postoperative clients include:

    1. Performing leg exercises and early ambulation.
    2. Checking vital signs every 4 hours.
    3. Decreasing fluid intake and assessing for edema.
    4. Administering oxygen via nasal cannula.

91. The appearance of a second postoperative day surgical wound should have:

    1. A slight erythema at the distal portion and slight sanguineous drainage.
    2. Absence of redness or swelling and edges well approximated.
    3. Minimal to moderate swelling and slight purulent discharge.
    4. Slight scar tissue and minimal serous drainage.

92. A 36-year-old male client is experiencing dyspnea and chest pain. This assessment is an alteration in which of his basic needs?

    1. The need for love and belonging
    2. Physiological needs (i.e., oxygen)
    3. Self-esteem
    4. Safety and security (i.e., comfort)

93. Surgical wound infections are the second most frequent type of nosocomial infection found in hospitals. Health personnel could best reduce these infections by:

    1. Leaving incisions open to air to promote healing
    2. Using strict surgical asepsis when changing all dressings
    3. Strictly adhering to the principles of effective hand washing
    4. Always cleansing incisions from bottom to top—from the least contaminated to the most contaminated area

94. An 85-year-old client in a skilled care facility has an infected leg ulcer. Hot moist packs are ordered. The nurse will use extreme caution in applying these packs because many older clients have:

1. Reduced sensitivity to pain
2. Reduced sensation to temperature stimuli
3. Thickened integumentary areas
4. Increased sensation of nerve pathways

95. The nurse is applying an elastic bandage to the sprained ankle of a client in an outpatient clinic. The nurse leaves the toes exposed to:

1. Allow range-of-motion exercises and prevent potential complications
2. Decrease discomfort and potential edema
3. Allow the skin to breathe
4. Check for circulation and sensation of the extremity

96. A 72-year-old client has nausea and vomiting, arrhythmias, diarrhea, and changes in color vision. The client has been taking digoxin 0.25 mg daily for the last 6 months. These symptoms are:

1. Probably a result of something that the client ate
2. A toxic effect of digoxin
3. A side effect of digoxin
4. A result of a dose of digoxin too high for client's age

97. Nursing interventions for a client receiving SC heparin include:

1. Monitoring apical pulse and blood pressure before each administration.
2. Strictly monitoring the client's I&O.
3. Assessing skin, mucous membranes, urine, and other body secretions for possible bleeding.
4. Assessing the client for an electrolyte imbalance.

98. A teenage girl is very angry about a test she failed in school today and accuses the teacher of wanting to make her feel "stupid." This is an example of:

1. Anger
2. Repression
3. Projection
4. Denial

99. A client with pancreatitis has a history of alcohol abuse. The nurse will observe the client for agitation, nausea and vomiting, delirium tremens, and visual, auditory, and tactile hallucinations. These are indications of:

1. Possible cirrhosis of the liver
2. Alcohol withdrawal
3. Depression
4. Suicidal thoughts

100. The nurse is assisting a third-day postoperative client in selecting a dinner menu. Vitamin C is essential in tissue healing. Which of the following menus will best aid in providing vitamin C?

1. Roast chicken, corn on the cob, mashed potatoes, butterscotch pudding
2. Fish fillet, brown rice, green beans, tomato juice, Jell-O with sliced fruit
3. Chicken breast fillet in tomato sauce, potatoes, broccoli, cantaloupe with sliced strawberries
4. Veal parmesan, white rice, carrots, tossed salad, custard pudding

101. The nurse is to administer iron dextran IM to a client with iron-deficiency anemia. Because this drug is irritating to tissues, the nurse will:

1. Carefully inject it into the ventrogluteal site, which has a large muscle mass.
2. Administer it into the ventrogluteal site using the Z-track technique and a 2- to 3-inch long needle.
3. Administer it into a large muscle and massage the area thoroughly for absorption into the muscle.
4. Administer it IV because the nurse knows that it will cause less irritation by this route.

102. The nurse is to administer 500 mg of amoxicillin PO to a client with pneumonia. The medication on hand is labeled in grams. The nurse will give:

_____

103. A 4-year-old child has varicella (chickenpox). In the future, the child should have what type of immunity?

1. Artificially acquired immunity
2. Natural passive immunity
3. Actively acquired immunity
4. Naturally acquired active immunity

104. Hand washing is crucial in preventing the spread of infection. This practice breaks the chain of infection during which phase of the cycle?

1. Portal of entry to host
2. Reservoir
3. Method of transmission
4. Portal of exit from source

105. The data collection phase of the nursing process is best described as:

1. Evaluating whether the problem has been resolved.
2. Putting planned nursing strategies into action.
3. Setting priorities with the client that will resolve the identified problem.
4. Gathering, communicating, and verifying data about health needs of the client .

106. An 86-year-old client is admitted with a diagnosis of hypernatremia. The nurse should expect the blood plasma level to be:

1. High in sodium ions
2. High in calcium levels
3. Low in sodium ions
4. Low in chlorides

107. A 16-year-old adolescent admitted with sickle cell crisis has complaints of dyspnea and leg pain. The pain of sickle cell anemia is caused by:

1. The disturbance in cellular metabolism.
2. Enlargement of the bone marrow and a decrease in the number of circulating RBCs.
3. The sickling (clumping) of the cells, which obstructs the capillary blood flow and causes occlusion and thrombosis.
4. Bleeding into the joints because of the rapid destruction of RBCs by the bone marrow.

108. Genetic counseling is very important in sickle cell anemia because it is:

1. A nonserious condition with a very poor prognosis.
2. A hereditary chronic form of anemia that results in a shortened life span.
3. An acquired immunosuppressive condition resulting in little resistance to infection.
4. A sex-linked inherited coagulation disorder causing spontaneous bleeding.

109. A 20-month-old baby is admitted to the pediatric unit with injuries that could possibly have resulted from child abuse. The mother states that the child "fell down the stairs." Which of the following will provide the nurse with additional information when assessing the baby?

1. Ask the mother why such a young child was left unattended.
2. Talk to the child and ask what happened.
3. Observe the interaction between mother and child.
4. Pick up and examine the child more carefully.

110. A nurse comes upon the scene of an automobile accident. On further investigation, the driver does not appear to be conscious. What is the nurse's first priority?

1. Establish a patent airway.
2. Assess for pulselessness.
3. Assess for unresponsiveness.
4. Call for help.

111. A 52-year-old male client is admitted with a possible myocardial infarction. His wife is very frightened and asks the nurse, "Is he going to die?" Which would be the most appropriate response by the nurse?

1. "I really can't tell you that; you'll have to talk to his doctor."
2. "You have to be brave for your husband now; let's not talk like that."
3. "I know you're scared; would you like to sit and talk for a while?"
4. "Perhaps your husband is not really as sick as he appears. Most people don't die from a heart attack."

112. An adult client's pulse is rapid and irregular; this would be referred to as:

1. Weak and thready
2. Tachycardia and arrhythmia
3. Tachycardia and bounding
4. Tachycardia and hypotension

113. A 4-year-old child is admitted with acute lymphocytic leukemia. Which of the following symptoms are typical of this type of leukemia?

1. Pallor, weakness, fatigue, lymphadenopathy
2. Hypotension, anorexia, thrombosis, alopecia
3. Thrombocytopenia, enlarged cervical lymph nodes, chest pain
4. Anemia, spontaneous bleeding, decreased urinary output

114. The nurse must be extremely careful in protecting a client with leukemia from any source of infection primarily because:

1. If these clients acquire an infection and antibiotics are ordered, they would suffer very serious side effects from such drugs.
2. They might contact pneumonia and become even more ill.
3. Leukemia seriously affects the blood-forming system (WBCs) and its ability to ward off infection.
4. An infection could precipitate spontaneous bleeding and hemorrhage.

115. A 47-year-old client is having surgery to remove gallstones. This surgery is called:

1. Cholelithotomy
2. Cholelithiasis
3. Lithotripsy
4. Cholecystostomy

116. Nurses are responsible for assessing urinary function in their clients. A urinometer is:

1. An instrument used to measure a client's output accurately.
2. A device used to obtain a urine specimen from a client.
3. An instrument used to measure the specific gravity of urine.
4. A device used to test the urine for sugar and acetone.

117. When measuring the specific gravity of the urine of a client who is dehydrated, the nurse would expect:

1. A specific gravity below the norm because of decreased urinary output.
2. An increase in specific gravity because of the concentration of the urine and excess sodium.
3. An increased specific gravity because of increased urinary output.
4. A specific gravity within the normal range, unless the client's output is higher than usual.

118. When doing preoperative and postoperative teaching with a client who is very anxious, the nurse must remember that:

1. The client's stress level is only temporary.
2. The client may not be able to follow directions or explanations given at this time.
3. The client may have a lot of misplaced hostility and may be noncompliant.
4. The client's anxiety is probably not related to fear of the unknown.

119. Nurses can experience anxiety, especially in a new or an unknown situation, such as performing a procedure for the first time. Which of the following will help to decrease the nurse's anxiety in such a situation?

1. Ask another team member to do the procedure.
2. Relax and remain confident, and performance will be effective.
3. Ask questions and review the procedure, because knowledge and competence help to allay anxiety.
4. Assume that anxiety often releases hormones that improve effectiveness and performance.

120. A client has just been told by the physician that his condition is extremely grave and the prognosis very poor. When the nurse enters his room, he says, "The doctor said I am just fine and can go home today." What is the probable rationale for his statement?

    1. He refuses to believe what the doctor has said and is using denial as a means of coping.
    2. He probably misunderstood the doctor's explanation.
    3. He is bargaining in an attempt to be discharged and postpone facing his prognosis.
    4. He is depressed and just wants to go home and pretend he didn't hear what the doctor said.

121. Which of the following is the nurse's first intervention in the treatment of an adult client in respiratory arrest?

    1. Pinch the victim's nose and administer two quick breaths into the mouth.
    2. Administer 100% O_2 with an Ambu bag.
    3. Open the victim's airway using the head-tilt-chin-lift maneuver.
    4. Begin chest compressions at a ratio of 15 compressions:2 ventilations.

122. When a nurse is performing cardiopulmonary resuscitation (CPR) on an adult and is the only rescuer, the compression:ventilation ratio is:

    1. 5 compressions:2 ventilations
    2. 15 compressions:2 ventilations
    3. 5 compressions:1 ventilation
    4. 15 compressions:1 ventilation

123. A client with cancer of the lung is receiving chemotherapy. The nurse will monitor blood values, specifically the WBC count, because:

    1. These drugs cause proliferation of red blood cells (RBCs) and the nurse needs to be aware of any pertinent changes.
    2. These drugs cause polycythemia and could precipitate thrombosis.
    3. These drugs depress the bone marrow, inhibiting the production of blood cells, and a serious decrease in WBCs increases susceptibility to infection.
    4. A serious decrease in WBCs could alter the effects of the drug and even cause bleeding tendencies.

124. Nurses encounter many ethical dilemmas in their practice. Which of the following could be considered an ethical dilemma?

    1. A client refuses to take digoxin as ordered.
    2. A terminally ill client's pain is not being properly managed.
    3. A child is admitted with signs and symptoms of physical abuse.
    4. The nurse observes another nurse on the unit taking a controlled substance that was meant for a client.

125. A licensed practical nurse (LPN) working in a health-care agency is expected to practice:

    1. Within the same standards as other LPNs in a similar setting.
    2. According to the guidelines of the nurse or physician under whose supervision the LPN is practicing.
    3. Within the scope of his or her knowledge and experience.
    4. To the best of his or her ability and experience.

126. Which lunch menu should the nurse recommend for a child with celiac disease?

    1. Hot dog, french fries, milk, and cake
    2. Spaghetti, garlic bread, salad, and pudding
    3. Pizza, cookies, and malt
    4. Baked fish, corn on the cob, and apple

127. A client complains of nausea and headache. This is an example of:

    1. Objective data
    2. Variable data
    3. Constant data
    4. Subjective data

128. When taking an oral temperature with a glass thermometer, to obtain an accurate reading the nurse must leave it in place for:

    1. 5–10 minutes
    2. Approximately 2–4 minutes
    3. 30–60 seconds
    4. Approximately 1.0–1.5 minutes

129. Before administering digoxin, the nurse checks:

    1. The client's blood pressure.
    2. The apical pulse for 60 seconds.
    3. The radial pulse.
    4. The client for pitting edema.

130. When discharging a client with a prescription for warfarin (Coumadin), the nurse instructs the client not to take aspirin because aspirin:

    1. Can cause irritation to the lining of the stomach.
    2. Frequently has delayed effects and is not readily absorbed in the body.
    3. Interferes with clot formation and could precipitate bleeding.
    4. Is not very effective and causes more side effects than most medications.

131. In giving dietary discharge instruction to a client with a recent myocardial infarction, the nurse instructs him to avoid foods that:

    1. Are high in potassium, because this could seriously alter his serum electrolytes.
    2. Contain caffeine, such as chocolate and tomato juice.
    3. Are high in saturated fats.
    4. Are high in sugar and vitamin B.

132. A 53-year-old client with a recent stroke is very frustrated because he will not be able to return to his occupation as an airline pilot. He is very angry today and refuses his medication. What should the nurse understand?

1. Clients who can no longer be as independent as in the past experience a great deal of frustration.
2. His feelings are temporary, and he will soon learn to adapt.
3. He is using his anger and noncompliance to get attention.
4. He is denying his illness and displaying immature behavior.

133. A 24-year-old woman is pregnant for the first time. The term for a first pregnancy is:

1. Primipara
2. Multigravida
3. Primigravida
4. Para

134. A 19-year-old primigravida is admitted with pre-eclampsia. The nurse will monitor her very closely for:

1. Hypotension
2. Nausea
3. Bleeding
4. Evidence of seizure activity

135. A 4-year-old child is admitted with a fever of 105.8°F (40.58°C) and a potential diagnosis of infectious meningitis. The physician has ordered a lumbar puncture. The purpose of this test is:

1. To decrease the pressure on the brain.
2. To bring down fever.
3. To examine the cerebrospinal fluid (CSF) for evidence of bacteria indicative of meningitis.
4. To examine the spinal column for evidence of bleeding.

136. After a lumbar puncture, the nurse will position the client:

1. In semi-Fowler's position to allow for drainage of CSF.
2. Flat for about 6 hours to prevent a possible spinal headache.
3. In a prone position to prevent post-test meningeal irritation.
4. On the side with the head of the bed slightly elevated to prevent aspiration.

137. A neighbor, who is working in the yard burning leaves, suddenly begins screaming for help. His clothing is on fire and he is screaming uncontrollably. The nurse's first action is to:

1. Grab a garden hose and try to put out the fire.
2. Throw dirt on the victim to smother the flames.
3. Place him in a horizontal position and roll him in a blanket or coat to smother the flames.
4. Call the fire department for assistance.

138. On arrival at the hospital, the primary focus for a client with a thermal injury is:

1. Attention to respiratory and emotional problems
2. Maintaining a patent airway, determining respiratory status, assessing the extent of the injury, and meeting fluid needs
3. Determining the cause of the accident

4. Inserting an endotracheal tube and determining potential need for skin grafting

139. The nurse is to make an entry on a client's chart at 4 PM using military time. The time the nurse enters is:

_____

140. Which of the following most accurately exemplifies documentation of objective data?

1. Respirations appear shallow and noisy.
2. The client seems to be depressed today.
3. Dressing was changed, and incision is clean and healing, with 2 cm of serosanguineous drainage.
4. The client has complaints of pain in her left lower quadrant (LLQ), not relieved by medication.

141. Erik Erikson defines the developmental stage of late adulthood (age 60 years or older) as:

1. Generativity versus stagnation
2. Ego integrity versus despair
3. Intimacy versus isolation
4. Retirement versus depression

142. An 18-year-old client sustained a compound fracture of the left tibia while skiing and is admitted to the emergency room (ER). The rationale for cleaning the wound from the area of least contamination to the area of greatest contamination is to:

1. Help to promote wound healing by removing any drainage.
2. Remove any moisture that harbors organisms that may have collected.
3. Prevent introduction of organisms into the wound.
4. Prevent contaminating areas previously cleaned.

143. The Apgar scale is an assessment tool that rates the physiological characteristics of the newborn infant. The maximum total score is:

_____

144. An infant whose respirations are slow and irregular at 1 and 5 minutes after birth will receive an Apgar respiratory score of:

1. 3
2. 10
3. 1
4. 2

145. The most appropriate position for giving a client a back rub at the hour of sleep is:

1. Supine
2. Prone
3. Lateral
4. Semi-Fowler's

146. A frequent site and cause of nosocomial infection is the:

1. Urinary tract, related to placing the drainage bag above the bladder.
2. Incision, related to use of aseptic technique when changing the dressing.

3. Bloodstream, related to self-administration of insulin.
4. Respiratory system, related to clients coughing without covering their mouths.

147. A second-day postoperative client is having incisional pain. The client was medicated an hour ago. Which of the following noninvasive nursing interventions will best aid in decreasing pain at this time?

1. Change position and give a back rub.
2. Assist in range-of-motion exercises.
3. Give an injection of meperidine (Demerol) as ordered.
4. Explain to the client that medication has just been given and to try to relax.

148. A nurse is working in the ER and receives a frantic phone call from a mother whose 2-year-old child has swallowed a bottle of aspirin (about 20 tablets). The nurse instructs her to:

1. Call the poison control center.
2. Induce vomiting if the child is conscious and bring her to the ER.
3. Give the child an antiemetic and observe closely for the next 24 hours.
4. Dilute the aspirin by having the child drink a glass of milk.

149. When positioning a postoperative client who has had a total hip replacement, the nurse is careful to keep the operative leg:

1. Flexed
2. Abducted
3. Adducted
4. Supported by pillows under the knee and foot

150. An adult client with angina has a radial pulse of 58 bpm. This slow rate is considered below normal and is called:

1. Tachycardia
2. Arrhythmia
3. Sinus rhythm
4. Bradycardia

151. A 23-year-old client is 3 months pregnant and has hypertension as a complication of pregnancy. Which food would the nurse encourage her to avoid?

1. Peanut butter
2. Smoked ham
3. Broccoli
4. Chicken

152. A pregnant client who has hypertension is given a prescription for furosemide (Lasix), a potassium-wasting diuretic. The nurse would encourage her to eat:

1. Bananas
2. Apples
3. Rice
4. Grapefruit

153. A client has delivered a healthy 6-lb 2-oz baby. She does not want to breast-feed. The nurse explains to her that she should:

1. Restrict fluids to 1000 mL daily.
2. Increase fluids to 3500 mL daily.
3. Wear a tight bra or binder on her breasts.
4. Apply warm compresses to her breasts.

154. The nursing assistant on a nurse's unit is 8 months pregnant. While in the cafeteria at lunch time, she begins choking on roast turkey. The nurse's first intervention is to:

1. Ask, "Can you talk?"
2. Give her three back blows.
3. Give her three chest thrusts.
4. Perform the Heimlich maneuver.

155. A 22-year-old client prematurely delivered a 5-lb 1-oz baby. She has Rh-negative blood and is to receive Rho(D) immune globulin (RhoGAM). She asks the nurse why. The nurse explains to her that:

1. Rho(D) immune globulin is given to all mothers.
2. Rho(D) immune globulin is given to Rh-negative mothers with Rh-positive babies.
3. Rho(D) immune globulin is given to Rh-negative mothers with Rh-negative babies.
4. Rho(D) immune globulin is given to all Rh-negative mothers.

156. A client does not want to breast-feed her baby. To suppress milk production, the nurse administers:

1. Acetazolamide (Diamox)
2. Hydromorphone (Dilaudid)
3. Dexamethasone (Decadron)
4. Estradiol valerate (Deladumone)

157. A 42-year-old client has had a full-term pregnancy. Her labor is not progressing, and oxytocin (Pitocin) is started. During induction, the nurse observes her to make sure her resting phase is adequate. Her resting phase should be at least:

1. 15 seconds
2. 20 seconds
3. 30 seconds
4. 60 seconds

158. A primigravida who is 3 months pregnant is experiencing nausea. She asks the nurse why she has nausea. The nurse explains that:

1. It is caused by her anxiety over having her first child.
2. It is caused by a change in hormonal levels.
3. A change in diet will relieve the nausea.
4. Adequate rest will relieve the nausea.

159. A 15-year-old client thinks that she is pregnant and wants an abortion. She does not want her parents to know. The nurse's best advice is to:

1. Tell her parents anyway.
2. Encourage her to talk with the father of her child.
3. Encourage her not to have an abortion.
4. Help her to make an appointment with the local clinic.

160. A 30-year-old pregnant client has insulin-dependent diabetes. Her insulin requirements will:

1. Decrease during her pregnancy.
2. Not change during her pregnancy.
3. Vary during her pregnancy.
4. Change the requirement for the type of insulin needed during her pregnancy.

161. Which of the following drains is considered an open drain?

1. Penrose
2. Jackson-Pratt
3. Hemovac
4. Surgivac

162. The nurse is to apply an Ace bandage to a sprained ankle. The nurse would wrap it beginning at the _____ aspect.

1. Medial
2. Distal
3. Lateral
4. Proximal

163. A nurse is going to remove an indwelling catheter from an 80-year-old client. The nurse's first action is to:

1. Deflate the balloon
2. Disconnect the bag and tubing
3. Clamp off the tubing
4. Explain the procedure to the client

164. One method of determining the IM injection site in the gluteal muscle is to imagine that it is divided into four equal quadrants. The injection site is in which quadrant?

1. Inner upper quadrant
2. Upper outer quadrant
3. Lower outer quadrant
4. Lower inner quadrant

165. The angle of the needle for an intradermal injection is:

1. 10 degrees
2. 30 degrees
3. 45 degrees
4. 90 degrees

166. A nurse is going to give an SC injection. An appropriate needle length and size is:

1. 1 inch, 25 gauge
2. 1 inch, 20 gauge
3. 11/2 inches, 18 gauge
4. 5/8 inch, 26 gauge

167. Which of the following is not a purpose of a nasogastric tube?

1. For gastric decompression
2. For gastric feeding
3. To remove flatus from the colon
4. To administer medications

168. Which of the following is not an acceptable position for a client when receiving a tube feeding?

1. Semi-Fowler's on the back
2. Flat or supine
3. Semi-Fowler's on the right side
4. Semi-Fowler's on the left side

169. A client is receiving an IV infusion using a volume-controlled pump. To check to see if it is infusing at the proper rate, the nurse's first step is to:

1. Check the rate on the pump.
2. Count the drops with the door open.
3. Count the drops with the door closed.
4. Position the pump at least 18 inches above the bed.

170. Which of the following is used for urinary diversion?

1. Colostomy
2. Ileostomy
3. Ureterostomy
4. Gastrostomy

171. The preferred IM injection site for a 1-year-old infant is the:

1. Deltoid
2. Gluteus
3. Rectus femoris
4. Triceps

172. A 9-year-old child has a short-leg cast for a fractured ankle. Instruction to the child and mother on discharge from the ER includes:

1. Dry the cast thoroughly with a hair dryer.
2. Use a coat hanger to scratch under the cast.
3. Keep the leg flat for 24 hours.
4. Avoid lifting the cast with the fingertips.

173. Toys to be avoided by a 5-year-old child who has hemophilia include:

1. Tricycle
2. Swings
3. Plastic toys with sharp edges
4. Large Lincoln logs

174. A 7-year-old child has a diagnosis of hypothyroidism. The nurse would suggest that the mother keep the room temperature at:

1. 60°F (15.5°C)
2. 70°F (21.1°C)
3. 75°F (23.8°C)
4. 85°F (29.4°C)

175. An infant client was born with a cleft lip and palate. What method would the nurse use to feed the client?

1. Medicine dropper
2. Metal spoon
3. Soft long nipple
4. Gastrostomy tube

176. A 3-year-old client has just been given a diagnosis of a volvulus. The child's father asks the nurse what it is. The nurse explains that it is:

1. A twisted bowel.
2. The bowel telescoping into itself.

3. The presence of adhesions.

4. A very short large intestine.

177. A 12-year-old client has had surgical correction of a ruptured appendix. Postoperatively the client should be positioned:

1. Flat and side-lying
2. Supine
3. Prone
4. In semi-Fowler's position

178. A 2-year-old child fell from a bicycle and hit her head. On her discharge from the ER, the nurse explains to her parents that they should immediately return her to the ER if she:

1. Has a headache
2. Changes her level of consciousness
3. Does not eat
4. Begins crying

179. A neighbor rushes to a nurse's house because her 6-month-old baby has stopped breathing. The nurse's first response is to establish an airway. Next the nurse tries breathing for the baby. How many breaths does the nurse give initially?

1. One
2. Two
3. Three
4. Four

180. Which of the following congenital disorders is a genetic defect?

1. Congenital hip dysplasia
2. Sickle cell anemia
3. Fetal alcohol syndrome
4. Cerebral palsy

181. The physician has ordered Tylenol 650 mg PO. The nurse has available Tylenol 5 grains. How many tablets would the nurse give?

_____

182. The physician has ordered 1000 mL D$_5$W (5% dextrose in water) plus 80 mEq potassium chloride to run over 12 hours via IV volume-controlled pump. At what hourly rate would the nurse set the pump?

_____

183. The physician has ordered neutral protamine Hagedorn (NPH) insulin 35 units plus regular insulin 10 units. The nurse's first step in drawing up these two insulins into the same syringe is:

1. Injecting air into the regular insulin
2. Injecting air into the NPH insulin
3. Drawing up the regular insulin
4. Drawing up the NPH insulin

184. The physician has ordered gentamicin 1 mg/kg body weight IM. The client weighs 176 lb. How much would the nurse administer?

_____

185. The physician has ordered cephalexin (Keflex) 1 g PO. Cephalexin 250-mg capsules are available. How many capsules would the nurse give?

_____

186. The physician has ordered renal dopamine 1 g/kg body weight. In evaluating the response to dopamine, the nurse would expect the following:

1. Increase in blood pressure
2. Decrease in blood pressure
3. Increase in urine output
4. Decrease in urine output

187. A 38-year-old client received her 20 units of regular insulin at 7:30 AM. She refuses to eat breakfast. The nurse would be sure to observe her for:

1. Diaphoresis
2. Polyuria
3. Polydipsia
4. Polyphagia

188. A 7-year-old child is receiving insulin. He is going to camp tomorrow. He asks the nurse if he should take his insulin before he goes. The nurse suggests that:

1. He increase his daily dose by 5 units
2. He increase his daily dose by 10 units
3. He take the same dose as usual
4. He not take any insulin until after he arrives at camp

189. Which of the following statements reflects a value conflict that may influence interpersonal relationships?

1. The client says, "My pain is worse today."
2. The nurse says, "All alcoholics are manipulative."
3. The nurse's aide says, "Not all drug users are worthless."
4. The client says, "Not all nurses are unfeeling."

190. Unacceptable manipulative behavior is best controlled by:

1. Prevention
2. Controlling
3. Limit setting
4. Firmness

191. A 22-year-old client is admitted to the psychiatric unit with a diagnosis of schizophrenia, which was first diagnosed 2 years ago. The client is disheveled and has not bathed recently. The parents inform you that the client has not left her room for 10 days. On admission, the client tells the nurse, "They lied, I didn't kill my mother. You're the killers." This response is an example of:

1. Grandiose delusions
2. Auditory hallucinations
3. Persecutory hallucinations
4. Paranoid delusions

192. A schizophrenic client tells the nurse, "They lied; I did not kill my mother." The nurse's best response to the client about the mother is:

1. "I just saw your mother; she's fine."
2. "Tell me more about your mother."
3. "I'll put you in an isolation room."
4. "I'll have your mother come to see you now."

193. A client is actively hallucinating and withdrawn. The nurse wants to engage the client in a reality-oriented activity. The best approach is:

1. To state, "I'd like you to be my partner in this game."
2. To insist that the client join a group activity.
3. To explain the benefits of a group activity.
4. To ask, "Would you like to play checkers?"

194. An 80-year-old client had an ileostomy 3 days ago. He is asking the nurse about his ileostomy and wants to know whether he will have to irrigate it as his brother, who has a colostomy, has to. Based on knowledge of the GI tract, the nurse can tell him that:

1. He will need to irrigate it daily.
2. He should ask his physician.
3. Ileostomies do not need irrigating.
4. He could have his brother demonstrate the irrigation.

195. A 57-year-old client is recovering from a peptic ulcer and asks about foods. The nurse's directions include:

1. "Drink lots of milk."
2. "Eat anything that does not seem to bother you."
3. "Drink orange juice for breakfast."
4. "Limit calories to 1500 Kcal daily."

196. A 77-year-old client seeks the nurse's advice on constipation. Which of the following is not good advice?

1. "Take a mild laxative daily at bedtime."
2. "Increase fluids."
3. "Eat bran on a daily basis."
4. "Eat more fruits and vegetables."

197. A female client has an indwelling urinary catheter. The nurse notices that the urine has a strong odor and is cloudy. The nurse's next action is to:

1. Send a urine specimen to the laboratory for routine urinalysis.
2. Send a urine specimen to the laboratory for cultures.
3. Irrigate the catheter.
4. Measure the specific gravity.

198. Classic subjective complaints of a UTI are:

1. Polyuria and frequency
2. Oliguria and pressure
3. Discharge and pressure
4. Frequency and dysuria

199. A 32-year-old client had a cholecystectomy 2 hours ago. The client weighs 250 lb and had general anesthesia. The client is complaining of pain. Priority nursing diagnosis at this time is:

1. Alteration in comfort
2. High risk for airway impairment
3. Alteration in fluid volume
4. Knowledge deficit

200. A 66-year-old client is seen at the clinic. She has had nausea and vomiting for 2 days and is complaining of dizziness. She thinks she has food poisoning. Evaluating her vital signs, the nurse would also include:

1. Taking blood pressure in both arms and legs.
2. Simultaneously taking apical and radial pulses.
3. Assessing orthostatic vital signs.
4. Palpating the bladder.

201. A 3-year-old was admitted with aseptic meningitis. The physician ordered 40 mg of chewable tablets of acetaminophen. On hand were 80 mg tablets. How many tablets will the nurse administer?

1. $^1/_2$ tablet
2. 1 tablet
3. $1^1/_2$ tablet
4. 2 tablets

202. The physician ordered amikacin (Amikin) 40 mg every 8 hours for a 2-year-old child. On hand is a 100-mg/2-mL vial. How many milliliters will the nurse administer?

1. 0.4 mL
2. 0.6 mL
3. 0.8 mL
4. 1.0 mL

203. During an emergency situation, the nurse used a tuberculin syringe to draw up 30 units of Humulin R regular U-100 insulin. How much did the nurse draw up?

1. 0.10 mL
2. 0.20 mL
3. 0.30 mL
4. 0.40 mL

204. The client was diagnosed with strep throat. The physician ordered benzathine penicillin G (Bicillin) 2,400,000 units implementation stat. The pharmacy sent a 10-mL vial of Bicillin containing 600,000 units/mL. How many milliliters will the nurse give?

1. 1 mL
2. 2 mL
3. 3 mL
4. 4 mL

205. The client was experiencing severe pain secondary to a migraine headache. The physician's orders read: "Give morphine sulfate 12 mg IM stat for pain." On hand was morphine 15 mg/mL. How many milliliters did the nurse draw up?

1. 0.2 mL
2. 0.4 mL
3. 0.6 mL
4. 0.8 mL

ANSWERS

1. **(3)** Integrated processes: nursing process — implementation, teaching/learning; client need: health promotion and maintenance; content area: medical-surgical.
   RATIONALE
   (1) The purpose of health teaching is to define the problem. **(2)** The purpose of health teaching is to facilitate client's mastery. **(3)** The focus and purpose of health teaching are to define the problem, suggest coping behaviors, and facilitate client's mastery and control. **(4)** The purpose of health teaching is to facilitate client's control.

2. **(4)** Integrated processes: nursing process — implementation, teaching/learning; client need: health promotion and maintenance; content area: medical-surgical.
   RATIONALE
   (1) Teaching should begin when the older client is physically capable. **(2)** Teaching should begin when the older client is physically capable. **(3)** Teaching should begin when the older client is physically capable. **(4)** Client teaching should not be done at the time of discharge, but as soon as the older person is physically capable, has the energy and stamina, and has minimal anxiety over the illness or control over the anxiety.

3. **(3)** Integrated processes: nursing process — implementation, teaching/learning; client need: physiological integrity; pharmacological therapies; content area: medical-surgical.
   RATIONALE
   (1) Clients do not understand medical jargon "tid." **(2)** Clients may not be able to read a clock and know the time. **(3)** Asking when the client goes to bed at night and gets up in the morning and specifically planning medication to be taken around those times has meaning for the client. **(4)** Clients do not understand medical jargon "ac" and "hs."

4. **(3)** Integrated processes: nursing process — data collection; client need: physiological integrity; reduction of risk potential; content area: medical-surgical.
   RATIONALE
   (1) An older person with sepsis does not have a febrile response. **(2)** An older person with myocardial infarction would present with fatigue and shortness of breath, not chest pains. **(3)** An older person with thyrotoxicosis presents with apathy rather than the hypermetabolic picture typically found in young adults. **(4)** An older person with a diabetic emergency presents with a change in level of consciousness.

5. **(1)** Integrated processes: nursing process — planning; client need: safe, effective care environment; coordinated care; content area: medical-surgical.
   RATIONALE
   (1) The nurse needs to consider what the older person desires from the health-care system, both now and in the future. **(2)** The nurse needs to consider the older person's leisure-time activities. **(3)** The nurse needs to consider the nature of the older person's relationships and social support system. **(4)** The nurse needs to consider the nature of the older person's relationships and social support system.

6. **(3)** Integrated processes: nursing process — implementation, caring; client need: psychosocial integrity; content area: medical-surgical.

   RATIONALE
   (1) Validating an older person's concern is important in the rehabilitation process. **(2)** Validating an older person's concern is important in the rehabilitation process. **(3)** Rehabilitation concepts in a geriatric population help individuals to determine what physical activities have inherent meaning and what choices an older person may make to meet his or her own priorities. **(4)** Validating an older person's concern is important in the rehabilitation process.

7. **(3)** Integrated processes: nursing process — implementation, communication and documentation; client need: psychosocial integrity; content area: psychiatric nursing.
   RATIONALE
   (1) This response is not appropriate. **(2)** The lounge is to be used for socializing. **(3)** Residents and their families should be encouraged to personalize the living space by placing personal possessions. **(4)** The resident is less likely to be labeled as "sick" if she personalizes the living space.

8. **(3)** Integrated processes: nursing process — implementation, caring; client need: physiological integrity; basic care and comfort; content area: psychiatric nursing.
   RATIONALE
   (1) Serve the food to give the resident ample time to eat. **(2)** Meal service times for residents with behavioral problems should be staggered. **(3)** Having to eat with others who behave disruptively during meals is a very unpleasant experience; nurses should seat the residents according to social preference. **(4)** Mealtime can be a time for socializing.

9. **(3, 6)** Integrated processes: nursing process — implementation; client need: physiological integrity; pharmacological therapies; content area: medical-surgical.
   RATIONALE
   (1) If NPH is drawn up first, this intermediate-acting insulin could be mixed with regular insulin. **(2)** The client would receive two injections, and this is not necessary. **(3)** After air is injected into the NPH, the regular insulin is drawn into the syringe first. If some regular insulin should get into the vial of NPH, the action of the NPH would not be greatly affected. **(4)** The nurse can mix the two insulins without the assistance of the pharmacy. **(5)** It is not necessary for the physician to order a combined dose. **(6)** Inject air into both vials; then draw up the regular insulin first.

10. **(1.5 tablets)** Integrated processes: nursing process — implementation, communication and documentation; client need: physiological integrity; pharmacological therapies; content area: maternity nursing.
    RATIONALE
    5 mg : 1 tablet : 7.5 : x = 1.5 tablets

11. **(1)** Integrated processes: nursing process — implementation; client need: physiological integrity; basic care and comfort; content area: maternity nursing.
    RATIONALE
    (1) If an infant is quiet, begin with auscultating the heart, lungs, and abdomen. This is difficult to do if the child is fussing. **(2)** Traumatic data collections, such as from eyes, ears, and mouth, should be completed last or while the infant is crying. **(3)** The

head-to-toe data collection should be altered to meet the developmental needs of the infant. **(4)** Percussion and palpation of areas should follow auscultation.

12. **(3)** Integrated processes: nursing process — planning; client need: safe, effective care environment; safety and infection control; content area: psychiatric nursing.

    RATIONALE

    (1) "Why" questions may put the client on the defensive and increase the agitated state. **(2)** Apologies are no assurance that the client has the ability to control behavior. **(3)** The decision to release the client from mechanical restraints is based on assessment data that indicate the client's ability to control his violent behavior. **(4)** Current medication practice involves a combination of neuroleptics and antianxiety medications. However, there is no assurance that the medication will calm violent behavior.

13. **(4)** Integrated processes: nursing process — assessment; client need: physiological integrity; reduction of risk potential; content area: pediatrics.

    RATIONALE

    (1) Swallowing frequently, not infrequently, would be a sign or symptom of hemorrhage. **(2)** Dark-brown emesis is old blood and is usually present in the emesis after tonsillectomy and adenoidectomy. **(3)** A pulse rate of 95 bpm is normal for a 4-year-old child. **(4)** Drooling of bright-red secretions may be an early indication of hemorrhage after tonsillectomy and adenoidectomy.

14. **(3)** Integrated processes: nursing process — implementation, teaching/learning; client need: physiological integrity; pharmacological therapies; content area: maternity nursing.

    RATIONALE

    (1) Milk and calcium supplements decrease absorption of iron. **(2)** Milk and calcium supplements decrease absorption of iron. **(3)** Research has shown that iron is absorbed best if taken at bedtime with citrus juice. **(4)** Iron is absorbed best at bedtime and on an essentially empty stomach.

15. **(Down and back; see figure below)** Integrated processes: nursing process — data collection; client need: health promotion and maintenance; content area: pediatrics.

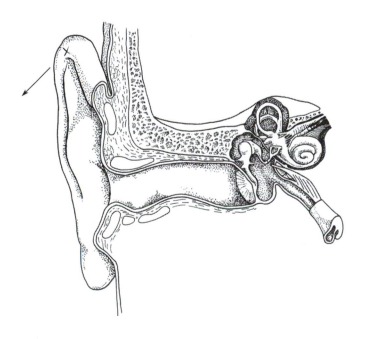

16. **(2)** Integrated processes: nursing process — evaluation, teaching/learning; client need: health promotion and maintenance; content area: maternity nursing.

    RATIONALE

    (1) Intermittent vomiting is not a danger sign; continuous vomiting is. **(2)** Vaginal bleeding is the number one danger sign to be reported because of the high risk of injury to the mother and the fetus. The client should seek health care immediately. **(3)** Leukorrhea, or vaginal discharge, is not a threat to the mother's life or that of her fetus. Vaginal discharge is a common occurrence during pregnancy. **(4)** Urinary frequency is a common discomfort of pregnancy because of the increased pressure on the maternal bladder.

17. **(3)** Integrated processes: nursing process — evaluation, teaching/learning; client need: health promotion and maintenance; content area: pediatrics.

    RATIONALE

    (1) The mother is correct to place the infant on the side as recommended by the American Academy of Pediatrics (AAP). **(2)** The mother is correct to place the infant in a supine position to sleep as recommended by the AAP. **(3)** The mother needs further teaching because the abdomen is no longer recommended as a sleeping position for healthy newborns. Only infants with breathing problems or excessive vomiting should sleep prone. **(4)** The upright position is appropriate for burping, which is indicated after feedings.

18. **(3)** Integrated processes: nursing process — planning; client need: psychosocial integrity; content area: psychiatric nursing.

    RATIONALE

    (1) Diversional activities for lower-functioning clients may precipitate anxiety and regression. **(2)** Program activities should focus on strengths rather than on pathology. This approach may help the client to relinquish the sick role and to demonstrate more adaptive behavior. **(3)** Day treatment centers provide social interaction and recreational and learning activities for persons who might otherwise be isolated. **(4)** Day treatment centers provide social skills training, opportunities for socialization, structure, and support for the client. The remaining needs are provided by significant others.

19. **(February 19)** Integrated processes: nursing process — data collection; client need: health promotion and maintenance; content area: maternity nursing.

    RATIONALE

    Naegele's rule, the most common method of determining a delivery date, is obtained by subtracting 3 months from the first day of the last menstrual period and then adding 1 year and seven days to that date. The correct answer is determined by: May minus 3 months is February. Adding 1 year and 7 days to the 12th results in an EDC of February 19.

20. **(4)** Integrated processes: nursing process — evaluation, teaching/learning; client need: health promotion and maintenance; content area: maternity nursing.

    RATIONALE

    (1) The placenta does not filter out harmful substances. Whatever the mother takes in, the fetus eventually gets. **(2)** The maternal blood and fetal blood do not directly mix. Maternal

RATIONALE

With older children, usually over the age of 3 years, the auricle or pinna is pulled up and back to allow visualization of the tympanic membrane, but in infants the correct direction to straighten the ear canal is down and back.

nutrients and fetal wastes permeate the capillary walls of the placental villi. (3) The umbilical cord has two arteries and one vein. (4) The placenta is the connection between maternal nutrition and fetal waste.

21. **(2, 3, 4)** Integrated processes: nursing process — implementation, teaching/learning; client need: physiological integrity; reduction of risk potential; content area: medical-surgical.

RATIONALE

(1) Morphine sulfate can decrease deep breathing and increase the client's chance of developing pneumonia. (2) An incentive spirometer is used to help the client improve tidal volume and deep breathing. It is used to restore pulmonary function. (3) Using a pillow as a splint helps the client to cough after abdominal or thoracic surgery. This helps to restore pulmonary function. (4) The client can benefit from diaphragmatic breathing by using accessory muscles. The client can deep breathe without placing pressure on the incision. (5) Narcotic-based cough medication can decrease deep breathing and increase the client's chance of developing pneumonia. (6) The client should be turned every 2 hours, alternating both sides.

22. **(0.25 mL)** Integrated processes: nursing process — implementation; client need: physiological integrity; pharmacological therapies; content area: psychiatric nursing.

RATIONALE

Set up the problem using ratio:proportion. 4 mg = 1 mL; 1 mg = x; solve for x = 0.25 mL.

23. **(1)** Integrated processes: nursing process — implementation; client need: physiological integrity; reduction of risk potential; content area: medical-surgical.

RATIONALE

(1) The first action a nurse should take after the placement of an endotracheal tube is check the breath sounds of the client to ensure correct tube placement and bilateral expansion of the lungs. (2) A chest radiograph would be done after the nurse has assessed the client and after the physician has written the order. (3) Obtaining arterial blood gases is a respiratory therapist's function and also needs a physician's orders. However, the nurse is responsible for making sure the physician's orders have been carried out. (4) The nurse would check the client's vital signs only after having assessed the breath sounds and tube placement.

24. **(3)** Integrated processes: nursing process — planning; client need: physiological integrity; reduction of risk potential; content area: medical-surgical.

RATIONALE

(1) Hypovolemia, not hypervolemia, can predispose an individual to pulmonary embolus and can produce hypercoagulability of the blood. (2) Arthritis is an inflammation of the joints and would not predispose a client to pulmonary embolus. (3) A long-bone fracture can predispose a client to pulmonary embolus by causing trauma and a change in the peripheral blood flow. (4) Osteoporosis is the thinning of the density of the bone and does not predispose a client to pulmonary embolus.

25. **(3)** Integrated processes: nursing process — implementation, communication and documentation; client need: physiological integrity; reduction of risk potential; content area: pediatrics.

RATIONALE

(1) Raw vegetables, fruit, and fish should be prohibited because they can introduce bacteria. (2) Total restriction of activity is not necessary. Games or toys that can be disinfected and watching

TV are appropriate activities. (3) Any temperature elevation is significant, and temperature elevations of 100.4°F (38.0°C) or greater are reported to the physician. (4) Persons with colds, sore throats, or infections should be prohibited from visiting, but reporting temperature elevation is more important.

26. **(2)** Integrated processes: nursing process — planning; client need: physiological integrity; physiological adaptation; content area: medical-surgical.

RATIONALE

(1) An increase in the production of ADH would cause fluid retention, leading to syndrome of inappropriate antidiuretic hormone (SIADH) and not diabetes insipidus, which is marked by dehydration. (2) This answer is correct. There is a decrease in the amount of ADH produced by the pituitary. The syndrome is marked by excessive urination, dehydration, and fluid and electrolyte imbalances. (3) Hypovolemia would be a result of diabetes insipidus and not a cause for the disorder. (4) Renal failure would not be a cause of diabetes insipidus.

27. **(2)** Integrated processes: nursing process — data collection; client need: health promotion and maintenance; content area: geriatrics.

RATIONALE

(1) Cataracts cause an opacity of the lens and lead to a gradual loss of vision. Images are usually hazy and the client is bothered by glare. (2) This answer is correct. This condition is marked by the inability to read objects up close and is caused by the loss of elasticity of the lens of the eye. This is a common result of the aging of the eye lens. (3) Xerostomia is a condition seen in older persons in which they suffer from frequent dry mouth. (4) Arcus senilis is the deposition of lipids in the iris of the eye. It is usually seen as a slight yellow ring around the iris and is associated with aging.

28. **(2)** Integrated processes: nursing process — implementation, teaching/learning; client need: health promotion and maintenance; content area: maternity nursing.

RATIONALE

(1) Dependent edema of the lower extremities may occur because of poor venous return related to crossing the legs. (2) To prevent dependent edema, support pantyhose should be put on in the morning before putting the lower extremities in a dependent position such as walking. (3) Sitting with feet elevated facilitates venous return. (4) Dorsiflexion improves circulation and prevents venous stasis.

29. **(1, 2)** Integrated processes: nursing process — implementation; client need: safe, effective care environment; safety and infection control; content area: pediatrics.

RATIONALE

(1) Education of children and parents is important. (2) One effective method of prevention is the use of hand washing. (3) Illicit drug use places individuals at risk for the development of hepatitis B. (4) The current vaccine is effective only against the hepatitis B organism. (5) Refrain from drinking water while visiting other countries. (6) Refrain from drinking water while visiting other countries.

30. **(3)** Integrated processes: nursing process — data collection; client need: health promotion and maintenance; content area: maternity nursing.

RATIONALE

(1) Stage 1 is completed when the cervix is completely dilated. (2) Pushing occurs at the end of stage 1 and beginning of stage 2. (3) Stage 2 begins when the client is fully dilated and is complete on delivery of the infant. (4) From the time the infant

delivers until delivery of the placenta is stage (3) The delivery of the placenta is the beginning of the recovery stage, stage 4.

31. (3) Integrated processes: nursing process — data collection; client need: physiological integrity; physiological adaptation; content area: medical-surgical.

    RATIONALE

    (1) These are physical changes associated with Addison's disease, which is caused by a decrease in glucocorticoid production. (2) Acne and ecchymosis are physical changes seen in Cushing's syndrome; however, hyperactivity is not associated with this disorder. (3) This answer is correct. Cushing's syndrome is a disease in which there is an excessive amount of glucocorticoid and hyperplasia of the adrenal cortex. Other physical symptoms associated with this disease include purplish striae, delayed wound healing, and a buffalo hump noted in the upper back. (4) These are normal physical changes associated with aging.

32. (1) Integrated processes: nursing process — data collection, teaching/learning; client need: health promotion and maintenance; content area: pediatrics.

    RATIONALE

    (1) The parent should supervise or assist with hygiene, especially bathing, until the age of 5 years to prevent injury or drowning and to ensure proper technique. (2) The preschooler is fearful about the drain, but physiological safety takes priority over psychological safety. (3) Usually the 3-year-old child can dress himself or herself, except for back buttons, and should be allowed to do so. (4) Options can be allowed if they exist. The option to bathe and dress should not be allowed.

33. (2) Integrated processes: nursing process — data collection; client need: health promotion and maintenance; content area: maternity nursing.

    RATIONALE

    (1) After a cesarean birth, there is about a 5-day delay in involution. (2) Lochia increases when the uterus begins to involute, around day 5. (3) Lochia is scant the first few days. Then, as involution occurs, the lochia increases. (4) Because of delayed involution, there is an increased risk of an infection (endometritis).

34. (3, 5) Integrated processes: nursing process — implementation, communication and documentation; client need: health promotion and maintenance; content area: pediatrics.

    RATIONALE

    (1, 2, 4, 6) Exercise-induced asthma is common to all persons with asthma. This condition is rare in activities that require only short bursts of energy (e.g., baseball, gymnastics, skiing) compared with those that involve endurance exercise (e.g., soccer, basketball, distance running, and field hockey). (3) Swimming, even long-distance swimming, is recommended because the child breathes air saturated with moisture, and exhaling under water prolongs expiration and increases end-expiratory pressure. (5) Exercise-induced asthma is common to all persons with asthma. This condition is rare in activities that require only short bursts of energy (e.g., baseball, gymnastics, skiing) compared with those that involve endurance exercise (e.g., soccer, basketball, distance running, and field hockey).

35. (2) Integrated processes: nursing process — implementation, communication and documentation; client need: physiological integrity; pharmacological therapies; content area: pediatrics.

    RATIONALE

    (1) The therapeutic effects may not be seen immediately but are apparent in 2–4 weeks. (2) The normal time for the effects to be apparent is anywhere from 2–4 weeks. (3) The naproxen does not work that quickly for the inflammatory response from arthritis. (4) Beneficial effects for arthritis take longer than for other conditions, such as menstrual cramps.

36. (4) Integrated processes: nursing process — implementation, communication and documentation; client need: health promotion and maintenance; content area: maternity nursing.

    RATIONALE

    (1) The primary health-care provider should be present until after the delivery of the placenta. If the physician or midwife is not there at this time, this is a normal finding and would not be an indication to call him or her. (2) The primary health-care provider may sometimes apply tension to the cord to facilitate delivery of the placenta. This is not the role of the nurse, and traction on the cord increases the risk of complications such as uterine inversion. (3) Ten minutes is still within the acceptable time frame for the third stage of labor. If the client does not deliver the placenta within 30 minutes, the physician will explore the uterus and may determine that the client has a placenta accreta, which would require surgical intervention. (4) The normal time frame for delivery of the placenta is 5–30 minutes. Most placentas are delivered within 5 minutes, but 10 minutes is certainly within the expected time frame for this stage.

37. (2) Integrated processes: nursing process — planning; client need: physiological integrity; reduction of risk potential; content area: pediatrics.

    RATIONALE

    (1) The purpose of the water in the closed-chest drainage system is to prevent entrance of air into the pleural cavity. It is not to decrease the danger of sudden change in pressure in the tube. (2) The purpose of the water in the closed-chest drainage system is to prevent entrance of air into the pleural cavity. (3) The purpose of the water in the closed-chest drainage system is to prevent entrance of air into the pleural cavity. It is not the faster removal of chest secretion by capillary action. (4) The purpose of the water in the closed-chest drainage system is to prevent entrance of air into the pleural cavity. It is not to facilitate emptying bloody drainage from the chest.

38. (1) Integrated processes: nursing process — implementation, teaching/learning; client need: physiological integrity; basic care and comfort; content area: medical-surgical.

    RATIONALE

    (1) The client may feel weak and fatigue easily because of tissue hypoxia caused by diminished red blood cells (RBCs) with oxygen-carrying capacity. Rest is indicated. (2) A high fluid intake is desirable, but it is not the priority intervention for a client recovering from iron deficiency. (3) A diet rich in vitamin B_{12} will not necessarily prevent iron-deficiency anemia. (4) A diet high in folic acid is indicated for anemia caused by folate deficiency, not iron-deficiency anemia.

39. (4) Integrated processes: nursing process — implementation, teaching/learning; client need: health promotion and maintenance; content area: pediatrics.

    RATIONALE

    (1) Increased fluid intake leads to diuresis. Diuresis enhances the antibacterial properties of the renal medulla. (2) The single most important factor influencing the occurrence of UTI is urinary stasis. The act of frequently emptying the bladder flushes away organisms causing UTI. (3) Concentrated and alkaline urine predisposes a client to UTI. Ingestion of highly acidic juices, such as cranberry juice, acidify the urine. (4) The short urethra, which measures 3/4 inch in young girls, provides a ready pathway for the invasion of organisms.

40. **(4)** Integrated processes: nursing process — planning; client need: health promotion and maintenance; content area: maternity nursing.

RATIONALE

(1) Breast milk does not develop in the breast early in pregnancy. **(2)** Although some women do experience an increase in sexual drive early in pregnancy, the changes in the breast are not a result of this. **(3)** The tender breasts that occur with early pregnancy result from an increased blood supply. **(4)** The hormones of pregnancy, particularly estrogen and progesterone, prepare the body for breast-feeding. Estrogen has an influence on the development of the ducts, and progesterone causes alveolar and lobular development. Blood vessels enlarge and become prominent, and the darkening and enlargement of the tubercles of Montgomery are related to the action of estrogen.

41. **(3)** Integrated processes: nursing process — data collection; client need: psychosocial integrity; content area: pediatrics.

RATIONALE

(1) This is a belief of the Jehovah Witness faith. **(2)** Particular types of meat are not forbidden. **(3)** The Mormon faith encourages the avoidance of such stimulants as tea, coffee, chocolate, and other products containing caffeine. **(4)** Mormons fast for 24 hours on the first Sunday of each month.

42. **(4)** Integrated processes: nursing process — planning, teaching/learning; client need: health promotion and maintenance; content area: pediatrics.

RATIONALE

(1) Sexual intercourse may produce transient bacteriuria in female adolescents and is associated with increased risk of UTI, but it would not be appropriate to teach that it is usually the cause of UTI in adolescents. **(2)** Drinking large amounts of carbonated beverages would be contraindicated with UTI because this may be a contributing factor to UTI. **(3)** Douching may contribute to bacteriuria in females and is not recommended. **(4)** UTIs have been related to the use of hot tubs or whirlpool baths, and thus, if one is predisposed to UTIs, it is best to avoid tub baths.

43. **(4)** Integrated processes: nursing process — planning; client need: health promotion and maintenance; content area: pediatrics.

RATIONALE

(1) The Electra complex is a phenomenon of female psychological development in which the girl has libidinal feelings directed toward her father. **(2)** Adolescence, not the preschool years, is a period during which individuals commonly question their sexual orientation. **(3)** Penile size is not a concern of a 4-year-old boy. **(4)** Mutilation and castration anxiety are normal according to Freud's Oedipal, or phallic, stage for the preschool child.

44. **(1)** Integrated processes: nursing process — implementation, teaching/learning; client need: physiological integrity; pharmacological therapies; content area: psychiatric nursing.

RATIONALE

(1) Vinegar-based salad dressing, cough elixirs, and cologne all contain alcohol and could cause a severe reaction in the presence of disulfirum. **(2)** Cough elixirs and cologne contain alcohol. **(3)** Cologne contains alcohol; acetaminophen and penicillin do not. **(4)** Acetaminophen and penicillin do not contain alcohol; vinegar-based salad dressing does.

45. **(1)** Integrated processes: nursing process — implementation, teaching/learning; client need: physiological integrity; physiological adaptation; content area: medical-surgical.

RATIONALE

(1) Medications that dilate the pupil could further increase intraocular pressure by blocking drainage from the eye through the canal of Schlemm. **(2)** Doses of eye drops should not be missed. **(3)** Eye drops will probably be given over the client's lifetime. **(4)** Clients with glaucoma should see their ophthalmologist at least yearly.

46. **(3)** Integrated processes: nursing process — implementation, communication and documentation; client need: health promotion and maintenance; content area: maternity nursing.

RATIONALE

(1) Consumer tests actually have higher rates of false-negative results. This is related to the test being performed too soon after a missed period. **(2)** There are many variables that must be controlled for, such as specimen contamination, timing, or movement of sample. The ease of testing is relative. **(3)** Because of the increased chance of false-negative results, it is important to determine pregnancy at the earliest time to provide prenatal care and to minimize fetal risk. **(4)** Home testing does ensure privacy, so the client is the only one who will know the result.

47. **(1)** Integrated processes: nursing process — data collection; client need: health promotion and maintenance; content area: pediatrics.

RATIONALE

(1) Tall tales and imaginary playmates are normal for the 4-year-old child. **(2)** The 3-year-old child is more likely to have a security blanket or other object and to fear loss of love. **(3)** The 3-year-old child is more likely to have a security blanket or other object and to fear loss of love. **(4)** The 4-year-old child is typically more aggressive than the 3-year-old child and will become more tranquil at 5 years old.

48. **(3)** Integrated processes: nursing process — planning; client need: physiological integrity; physiological adaptation; content area: pediatrics.

RATIONALE

(1) Fluid restriction is seldom necessary in the treatment of AGN. Forcing fluids would be contraindicated because of the edema associated with AGN. **(2)** Sodium may be restricted during the edematous phase. Increasing sodium in the diet would be contraindicated. **(3)** A record of daily weight is the most useful means to assess fluid balance in a child with AGN. **(4)** Regular measurements of vital signs, not once a shift, are essential to identify the acute hypertension associated with AGN.

49. **(3)** Integrated processes: nursing process — implementation; client need: health promotion and maintenance; content area: maternity nursing.

RATIONALE

(1) Because of the risk of cord prolapse with the rupture of membranes, the nurse must first ensure fetal well-being before performing comfort measures. **(2)** Because of the risk of cord prolapse with the rupture of membranes, the nurse must first ensure fetal well-being before notifying the physician or midwife. **(3)** The nurse should first evaluate fetal well-being by assessing the fetal heart tones. There is a high risk of cord prolapse with the rupture of the amniotic membranes. **(4)** Because of the risk of cord prolapse with the rupture of membranes, the nurse must first ensure fetal well-being before documenting the client's response.

50. **(4)** Integrated processes: nursing process — data collection; client need: health promotion and maintenance; content area: maternity nursing.

RATIONALE
(1) This finding is not abnormal. (2) This finding is not abnormal. (3) Cesarean section does not affect uterine contraction. (4) Stimulation of the nipple with breast-feeding causes the release of oxytocin, the hormone that causes the uterus to contract. This results in greater uterine muscle tone; consequently, smaller uterine size is possible earlier than if the mother were not breast-feeding. It is not abnormal, nor is it the result of cesarean birth.

51. (1) Integrated processes: nursing process — planning; client need: psychosocial integrity; content area: psychiatric nursing.

RATIONALE
(1) Compulsions are attempts to relieve tension. (2) Obsessions are recurring thoughts that cannot be dismissed from the consciousness. (3) Compulsive behavior is a defense against anxiety. It is not an attention-seeking behavior. (4) The client is suffering from a compulsive disorder, not a phobia.

52. (1) Integrated processes: nursing process — planning; client need: physiological integrity; physiological adaptation; content area: medical-surgical.

RATIONALE
(1) Third-degree burns may extend into SC tissue, muscle, and nerves. (2) Loss of the dermis and epidermis are characteristic of second-degree burns. (3) Loss of only the epidermis would mean that the burns were first degree. (4) Blisters and erythema are seen in second-degree burns.

53. (0.2 mL) Integrated processes: nursing process — implementation; client need: physiological integrity; pharmacological therapies; content area: maternity nursing.

RATIONALE
$5 \text{ mg} : 1 \text{ mL} = 1 \text{ mg} : x = 0.2 \text{ mL}$.

54. (1) Integrated processes: nursing process — evaluation, teaching/learning; client need: physiological integrity; pharmacological therapies; content area: medical-surgical.

RATIONALE
(1) This behavior would indicate a need for further teaching. The client should notify the physician if original pain is unrelieved by three doses of NTG. (2) This action should be taken by the client receiving NTG. It does not indicate a need for further teaching. (3) This action should be taken by the client receiving NTG. It does not indicate a need for further teaching. (4) This action should be taken by the client receiving NTG. It does not indicate a need for further teaching.

55. (3) Integrated processes: nursing process — planning; client need: physiological integrity; pharmacological therapies; content area: medical-surgical.

RATIONALE
(1) NPH insulin SC peaks in 6–12 hours; this is too soon. (2) NPH insulin SC peaks in 6–12 hours; this is too soon. (3) NPH insulin SC peaks in 6–12 hours; this is appropriate. (4) NPH insulin SC peaks in 6–12 hours; this is too late.

56. (3) Integrated processes: nursing process — data collection; client need: health promotion and maintenance; content area: maternity nursing.

RATIONALE
(1) Quickening refers to the first movements of the growing fetus that are felt by the mother. (2) Effacement refers to the shortening and thinning of the cervix that occurs before delivery. (3) Lightening refers to the tilting or dropping of the fetal head forward and downward into the true pelvis. This usually occurs 2–3 weeks before labor in the primigravida but frequently does not occur until the beginning of labor in many multigravidas. (4) Station is defined as the location of the presenting part of the fetus in relation to the ischial spines of the birth canal.

57. (4) Integrated processes: nursing process — implementation, caring; client need: physiological integrity; pharmacological therapies; content area: pediatrics.

RATIONALE
(1) Honesty is preferred. An IM antibiotic will probably hurt. (2) Children take things literally and will assume that the nurse is putting a real stick in the arm. (3) Although seeing and holding supplies may be beneficial in some instances, the child is not able to prepare an IM properly. (4) Brief explanations presented positively and immediately before a procedure are best.

58. (4) Integrated processes: nursing process — implementation; client need: physiological integrity; reduction of risk potential; content area: pediatrics.

RATIONALE
(1) Stuffed animals are not suitable toys because moisture will dampen the toys and make it difficult to keep them dry. (2) The toy may be a source of sparks and a potential fire hazard. (3) Synthetic blankets can initiate sparks, which may cause a fire. (4) Vinyl or plastic items do not absorb moisture and can be easily wiped dry.

59. (4) Integrated processes: nursing process — evaluation; client need: physiological integrity; pharmacological therapies; content area: medical-surgical.

RATIONALE
(1) Knowledge of a psychomotor skill is evaluated best by demonstration. (2) The nurse must see a demonstration of the procedure as it will be done in the home. (3) The client needs to show that fear of sticking one's self, not another, with a needle can be overcome. (4) This is the exact procedure that will be carried out at home.

60. (4) Integrated processes: nursing process — implementation, caring; client need: psychosocial integrity; content area: psychiatric nursing.

RATIONALE
(1) Telling her that you understand how she feels is not an appropriate response. It is a closed statement and does not invite a response. (2) Telling her not to cry and that everything is going to be all right is not an appropriate response. It is a nontherapeutic statement. (3) Going immediately to her and asking her what is she crying about does invite a response; however, it is not as therapeutic as being attentive and letting her know you care by your touch and waiting for her to speak. (4) Sitting in the chair beside her and letting her feel your presence and waiting for her to speak is a therapeutic response.

61. (3) Integrated processes: nursing process — implementation; client need: safe, effective care environment; coordinated care; content area: medical-surgical.

RATIONALE
(1) Planning is the phase that comes before implementation. (2) Evaluation is determining whether needs have been met. (3) Implementation is carrying out the goals and plans. (4) Data collection identifies the need for which implementation strategies are planned.

62. (4) Integrated processes: nursing process — data collection; client need: health promotion and maintenance; content area: medical-surgical.

RATIONALE
(1) Secondary data come from someone other than the client. (2) Constant is not a classification for client data. (3) Objective

data are data that are visible or obtained from laboratory or diagnostic tests. (4) Subjective data come from the client.

63. (2) Integrated processes: nursing process — data collection; client need: physiological integrity; physiological adaptation; content area: medical-surgical.
RATIONALE
(1) Safety and security needs come after physiological needs. (2) A client with respiratory distress has a need for adequate oxygen, which is the most essential physiological need. Physiological needs are given the highest priority in Maslow's hierarchy because they are necessary for survival. (3) Self-actualization is a need that is not reached until later in one's life. (4) Psychosocial needs are not higher than physiological needs.

64. (1) Integrated processes: nursing process — data collection; client need: health promotion and maintenance; content area: medical-surgical.
RATIONALE
(1) The location, intensity, and duration of the pain indicate how life-threatening the pain might be. (2) The nurse may collect this information, but it is not as important as the location, intensity, and duration. (3) The nurse may collect this information, but it is not as important as the location, intensity, and duration. (4) The nurse may collect this information, but it is not as important as the location, intensity, and duration.

65. (2) Integrated processes: nursing process — data collection; client need: physiological integrity; physiological adaptation; content area: medical-surgical.
RATIONALE
(1) Severe chest pain and hot dry skin are not signs and symptoms of pulmonary emphysema. (2) Pulmonary emphysema (i.e., chronic obstructive pulmonary disease) has specific symptoms related to permanent lung changes and chronic acidosis. Exertional dyspnea is the predominant one because of air trapping and loss of lung elasticity; the swelling and overdistention of the alveoli sacs results in a cough producing copious amounts of mucopurulent sputum. Chronic hyperinflation and use of accessory muscles in breathing causes an increase in anteroposterior chest diameter, commonly referred to as "barrel chest." (3) Dysphagia and alkalosis are not signs and symptoms of pulmonary emphysema. Acidosis is a characteristic, not alkalosis. (4) Lack of chest movement on one side and knifelike chest pain are not signs and symptoms of pulmonary emphysema.

66. (3) Integrated processes: nursing process — data collection; client need: physiological integrity; pharmacological therapies; content area: medical-surgical.
RATIONALE
(1) Spironolactone is a potassium-sparing diuretic. (2) Nifedipine is an antihypertensive drug. (3) Aminophylline is a theophylline salt, a common bronchodilator to relax the smooth muscle of the respiratory tract and frequently used in the treatment of COPD. (4) Digoxin is a cardiotonic. Clients with COPD who also have cardiovascular complications frequently receive this medication, but it is not specific for treating the COPD.

67. (4) Integrated processes: nursing process — data collection; client need: physiological integrity; pharmacological therapies; content area: medical-surgical.
RATIONALE
(1) These are not typical side effects of bronchodilators. (2) These are not typical side effects of bronchodilators. (3) These are not typical side effects of bronchodilators. (4) The aim of bronchodilator therapy is to keep the client's theophylline level within the normal range (10–20 mcg/mL). Minor side effects usually decrease after a few days of therapy; serious side effects or

toxic effects are generally related to theophylline serum levels 0.20 mcg/mL.

68. (4) Integrated processes: nursing process — planning; client need: physiological integrity; basic care and comfort; content area: medical-surgical.
RATIONALE
(1) This is not a definition of orthopnea. (2) This is not a definition of orthopnea. (3) This is not a definition of orthopnea. (4) Orthopnea is a respiratory condition in which there is discomfort in breathing in any position except sitting or standing. It is seen in heart failure, pulmonary edema, and severe emphysema. The client may be in respiratory distress, be acidotic, and have periods of apnea as well; but the question asks for a definition of orthopnea.

69. (2) Integrated processes: nursing process — evaluation; client need: physiological integrity; physiological adaptation; content area: medical-surgical.
RATIONALE
(1) High levels of O_2 will not cause tachycardia or hypoxemia. (2) Chronic pulmonary emphysema causes permanent lung damage to the alveolar walls and capillaries, resulting in air trapping, loss of elasticity, and chronic respiratory acidosis. The constant high levels of CO_2 in the blood, tissues, and brain (respiratory center) cause the emphysema client to rely on low levels of O_2 as the stimulus for respiration. Administering high levels of O_2 (0.2 L/min) could decrease the hypoxic drive and result in respiratory depression or arrest. (3) Although some clients on long-term oxygen therapy may become psychologically dependent, this does not answer the question. (4) This may be a true statement, but it does not answer the question.

70. (1) Integrated processes: nursing process — implementation, communication and documentation; client need: physiological integrity; physiological adaptation; content area: medical-surgical.
RATIONALE
(1) Oxygen supports combustion, and even the tiniest spark could cause a fire or explosion if it came in contact with the oxygen. "No smoking" signs should be posted, and the clients and visitors must be told that smoking is not permitted in the room where oxygen is present. (2) Well-grounded electrical equipment can be safely used near the flow meter. (3) Turning off the oxygen does not eliminate the possibility of a spark causing a fire to occur. (4) Medications usually do not interact with oxygen.

71. (3) Integrated processes: nursing process — data collection; client need: health promotion and maintenance; content area: medical-surgical.
RATIONALE
(1) This is above the normal range for a temperature. (2) Afebrile means that there is no temperature elevation. This is a temperature elevation. (3) The temperature of the body taken orally in a healthy individual is 98.6°F (37°C). A higher temperature than that is considered fever. (4) If an electronic thermometer needed to be recharged, it would not register a temperature.

72. (4) Integrated processes: nursing process — data collection; client need: health promotion and maintenance; content area: medical-surgical.
RATIONALE
(1) Diet does not affect the body temperature. (2) Medications and mood do not affect the body temperature. (3) Weight and medications do not affect the body temperature. (4) Factors that can affect the client's body temperature include:

Age: The temperature of the very young is labile because of immature physiological control mechanisms; and that of older persons is labile because of deteriorating control mechanisms.

Diurnal variations: Body temperature is lowest at 1–4 AM and peaks at 4–6 PM.

Environment extremes: These can lower or raise body temperature accordingly.

Exercise: This raises the basal metabolic rate and can also increase body temperature

73. **(2)** Integrated processes: nursing process — data collection; client need: physiological integrity; pharmacological therapies; content area: medical-surgical.

RATIONALE

(1) NPH insulin does not start acting this quickly. Regular insulin starts acting within this time. **(2)** Humulin NPH insulin is the intermediate-acting insulin that peaks at 8–12 hours after administration, which would be a potential time for a hypoglycemic reaction to occur. **(3)** This is too long a period for an insulin reaction to occur. **(4)** This is too soon for an insulin action to occur for NPH insulin.

74. **(1)** Integrated processes: nursing process — data collection; client need: health promotion and maintenance; content area: medical-surgical.

RATIONALE

(1) Hypoglycemia occurs when there is too much insulin in the bloodstream in relation to the available glucose; it can occur during peak insulin administration times, causing symptoms such as hunger, inability to concentrate, tremors, increased pulse rate, diaphoresis, and visual disturbances. **(2)** Hot dry skin, nausea, and vomiting are not signs of hypoglycemia. **(3)** These are not signs of hypoglycemia. **(4)** Hypoglycemia does not occur until the blood glucose is < 80 mg/dL.

75. **(1)** Integrated processes: nursing process — implementation; client need: physiological integrity; pharmacological therapies; content area: medical-surgical.

RATIONALE

(1) Regular insulin does not contain a modifying protein to slow absorption and is the only type of insulin that can be given IV. For that reason, the nurse always draws up the regular insulin first when mixing two types, to prevent possible contamination of the regular insulin with the added protein, which could slow absorption. **(2)** This answer is incorrect; see rationale 1. **(3)** This answer is incorrect; see rationale 1. **(4)** This answer is incorrect; see rationale 1.

76. **(3)** Integrated processes: nursing process — implementation; client need: physiological integrity; pharmacological therapies; content area: medical-surgical.

RATIONALE

(1) Insulin is not given IM. **(2)** Insulin is not given intradermally. **(3)** Insulin is normally given SC 15–30 minutes before breakfast to maintain postprandial blood sugar 80–140 mg/dL. Insulin is never given IM because it would be absorbed too rapidly. Regular insulin can be given IV in acute situation. **(4)** Insulin is destroyed by gastric juices if taken orally.

77. **(4)** Integrated processes: nursing process — implementation; client need: physiological integrity; reduction of risk potential; content area: medical-surgical.

RATIONALE

(1) Having an appetite and no nausea does not mean that bowel sounds have returned. **(2)** She may be awake, but this does not mean that bowel sounds have returned. **(3)** Even though the nurse has an order for clear liquids, this does not ensure that bowel sounds have returned. **(4)** Most general anesthetics and preoperative medications decrease gastric motility. Trauma and manipulation of gastric organs also disturb normal digestion and elimination. Food and fluids are withheld in postoperative clients until bowel sounds and the ability to pass flatus have returned and nausea and vomiting have subsided.

78. **(4)** Integrated processes: nursing process — planning; client need: physiological integrity; basic care and comfort; content area: medical-surgical.

RATIONALE

(1) These items are not on a clear liquid diet. **(2)** These items are not on a clear liquid diet. **(3)** Pureed bananas are not on a clear liquid diet. **(4)** A clear liquid diet includes foods that are clear; it is often limited to water, tea, broth, ginger ale, and plain gelatin. The major objective is to relieve thirst and to prevent dehydration.

79. **(1)** Integrated processes: nursing process — implementation; client need: physiological integrity; pharmacological therapies; content area: medical-surgical.

RATIONALE

(1) Trimethobenzamide is an antiemetic that acts by blocking the chemoreceptor trigger zone, which in turn acts on the vomiting center. Promethazine is an antihistamine that acts on the gastrointestinal (GI) system by blocking histamine to provide sedation and decrease nausea. **(2)** Glycopyrrolate is not an antiemetic; diphenhydramine is an antihistamine that does not decrease nausea. **(3)** Merperidine and pentazocine are analgesics and may cause nausea. **(4)** Morphine is an analgesic, and atropine decreases peristalsis, which does not decrease nausea.

80. **(2)** Integrated processes: nursing process — implementation, teaching/learning; client need: physiological integrity; reduction of risk potential; content area: medical-surgical.

RATIONALE

(1) These exercises may increase activity but are not primary interventions for decreasing respiratory complications. **(2)** Prevention of postoperative respiratory complications begins with teaching coughing and deep breathing and encouraging clients to stop smoking, which immobilizes cilia and impairs oxygenation. **(3)** These activities will not prevent respiratory complications. **(4)** These interventions are not specific to preventing respiratory complications.

81. **(3)** Integrated processes: nursing process — implementation; client need: physiological integrity; reduction of risk potential; content area: medical-surgical.

RATIONALE

(1) Although the nurse may perform these activities on a postoperative client, they will not alert the nurse to an acute problem. **(2)** These symptoms are expected after surgery. **(3)** Vital signs (temperature, pulse, respirations, and blood pressure) are indicators of a person's health status. They are a quick and efficient way of monitoring a client's condition or identifying the presence of problems (especially potential bleeding or shock in a postoperative client). **(4)** These options are appropriate interventions but will not provide an overall health status.

82. **(2)** Integrated processes: nursing process — evaluation, communication and documentation; client need: physiological integrity; pharmacological therapies; content area: medical-surgical.

RATIONALE

(1) Except in toxic doses, digoxin decreases the heart rate. **(2)** Digoxin is a cardiotonic drug that increases the force of contraction of the myocardium, thereby increasing cardiac output. Cardiotonics also depress the sinoatrial node and slow conduction of the electrical impulses to the atrioventricular node, decreasing the number of ventricular contractions per minute. **(3)** Digoxin does not constrict the arteries. **(4)** Digoxin does not lengthen the number of impulses generated.

83. **(3)** Integrated processes: nursing process — evaluation, communication and documentation; client need: health promotion and maintenance; content area: medical-surgical.

    RATIONALE

    (1) This statement is true, but it is not the best response. **(2)** This statement is true, but it is not the best response. **(3)** Digoxin can cause serious side effects or toxic effects, and many physicians want the client to monitor the pulse rate and be given instructions to notify the physician if it falls below or exceeds a certain rate. **(4)** This is a true statement, but it is not the best response.

84. **(3)** Integrated processes: nursing process — evaluation; client need: physiological integrity; physiological adaptation; content area: medical-surgical.

    RATIONALE

    (1) A hemorrhage in the brain does not cut off blood supply to the spinal cord. **(2)** Hypertension may have precipitated the stroke but does not cause the symptoms; the symptoms are brought on by the stroke. **(3)** When a client suffers a stroke, the hemorrhage or clot causes weakness or hemiplegia on the opposite side of the brain, because there is a crossover of nerves in the pyramidal tract as they lead from the brain down the spinal column. **(4)** There is no thrombosis of the spinal cord in a stroke.

85. **(2)** Integrated processes: nursing process — data collection; client need: health promotion and maintenance; content area: medical-surgical.

    RATIONALE

    (1) This blood pressure is not in normal range. **(2)** Normal blood pressure for adults ranges from about 100/60–140/90 mm Hg. A sustained systolic pressure of 150 mm Hg or higher and a sustained diastolic blood pressure of 90 mm Hg or higher is usually considered hypertension. Blood pressure of 170/110 mm Hg is considered serious hypertension and may be directly related to a CVA. **(3)** This blood pressure is more than slightly elevated. **(4)** This blood pressure is more than "slightly high."

86. **(4)** Integrated processes: nursing process — data collection; client need: physiological integrity; physiological adaptation; content area: medical-surgical.

    RATIONALE

    (1) This response meets the criteria for aphasia but is not complete. **(2)** This response meets the criteria for aphasia but is not complete. **(3)** This response does not meet the criteria for aphasia. **(4)** A hemorrhage or clot to the brain often affects the blood supply to the speech center located in the brain, causing various types of aphasia.

87. **(1)** Integrated processes: nursing process — implementation; client need: physiological integrity; basic care and comfort; content area: medical-surgical.

    RATIONALE

    (1) A contracture is a permanent tightening or shortening of a muscle because of a paralysis. Range-of-motion exercises increase circulation, strengthen muscles, and prevent contractures. Position changes, as well as use of footboards and pillows, also help to keep the body in good alignment, prevent foot drop, and hasten recovery by preventing other complications (respiratory, circulatory, and skin breakdown). **(2)** These interventions are appropriate but will not prevent contractures. **(3)** These interventions are appropriate but will not prevent contractures. **(4)** These interventions will not prevent contractures.

88. **(2)** Integrated processes: nursing process — planning, teaching/learning; client need: physiological integrity; reduction of risk potential; content area: medical-surgical.

    RATIONALE

    (1) This is good advice but will not prevent recurrence of a stroke. **(2)** Being overweight and smoking cigarettes decrease blood supply to vital organs and contribute to arteriosclerosis and atherosclerosis, which are etiological factors in stroke. A diet that is too high in salt, fat, or cholesterol also can contribute to another stroke, by causing fluid retention and narrowing of arteries. Alerting the doctor to any changes in physical condition will also help to maintain health and to prevent further complications. **(3)** This is good advice but will not prevent recurrence of a stroke. **(4)** This is good advice but will not prevent recurrence of a stroke.

89. **(2)** Integrated processes: nursing process — evaluation; client need: physiological integrity; reduction of risk potential; content area: medical-surgical.

    RATIONALE

    (1) These exercises will not prevent pulmonary complications. **(2)** Anesthetics impair respiratory function. Coughing and deep breathing postoperatively help to remove secretions from the lungs and bronchi and to prevent respiratory complications of pneumonia and atelectasis. **(3)** Coughing and deep breathing will not prevent thrombophlebitis. **(4)** Coughing and deep breathing will not prevent a paralytic ileus.

90. **(1)** Integrated processes: nursing process — implementation; client need: physiological integrity; reduction of risk potential; content area: medical-surgical.

    RATIONALE

    (1) The decreased mobility after surgery, side effects of anesthesia, and possible electrolyte imbalances all increase the risk of circulatory complications such as thrombophlebitis and pulmonary embolus. Leg exercises aid in preventing the formation of a thrombus. Ambulation stimulates circulation in the lower extremities, preventing venous stasis, thrombophlebitis, and possible pulmonary embolus. **(2)** Checking vital signs will not prevent complications. **(3)** Decreasing fluids may increase complications. Assessing for edema will not prevent complications. **(4)** Oxygen is important but will not prevent circulatory problems.

91. **(2)** Integrated processes: nursing process — data collection; client need: health promotion and maintenance; content area: medical-surgical.

    RATIONALE

    (1) There should be no redness or swelling on a second-day postoperative wound. **(2)** A surgical wound heals by primary intention. Wound edges should be well approximated with no evidence of redness or swelling and with a scant to moderate amount of serosanguineous drainage on the second day after surgery. **(3)** There should not be purulent drainage, indicating that an infection has started on the second day postoperatively. **(4)** Scar tissue would not occur until much later after healing has taken place.

92. **(2)** Integrated processes: nursing process — data collection; client need: physiological integrity; physiological adaptation; content area: medical-surgical.

    RATIONALE

    (1) The need for love and belonging involves physical and emotional relationships. **(2)** Abraham Maslow's hierarchy of human needs is a theory nurses use to understand the relationships of basic human needs. Physiological needs (of which oxygen is the most essential) have the highest priority. The client's chest pain and dyspnea are interfering with basic need for oxygen. **(3)** Self-actualization and self- esteem are higher on the hierarchy (i.e., less important) than physiological needs. (4) Safety and security needs include thirst, hunger, sleep, and rest.

93. (3) Integrated processes: nursing process — implementation; client need: safe, effective care environment; safety and infection control; content area: medical-surgical.

RATIONALE

(1) This option is appropriate, but the best response is hand washing. (2) This option is appropriate, but the best response is hand washing. (3) Research shows that 70% of all nosocomial infections occur in postoperative clients. In a hospital study of 541 nosocomial infections over 7 months, 21% were caused by the same species as that found on hands. Hand washing is considered one of the best ways to prevent the spread of infection. (4) This option is appropriate, but the best response is hand washing.

94. (2) Integrated processes: nursing process — evaluation; client need: physiological integrity; reduction of risk potential; content area: medical-surgical.

RATIONALE

(1) Older clients frequently have decreased sensitivity to pain, but the question refers to the application of heat. (2) Older persons often have sensory impairment and are unable to perceive that heat is damaging the tissues; they are therefore at risk for burns. They also have a low heat tolerance, which puts them at risk for burns, as well as impaired circulation, which puts them at risk for tissue damage. (3) Older persons do not have thickened skin. (4) Older persons have decreased sensation of nerve pathways.

95. (4) Integrated processes: nursing process — implementation; client need: physiological integrity; basic care and comfort; content area: medical-surgical.

RATIONALE

(1) This is not the rationale for leaving the toes exposed. (2) Leaving the toes exposed will not decrease discomfort. (3) This is not the rationale for leaving the toes exposed. (4) When bandaging an extremity, the end of the body part should be exposed whenever possible so that the nurse (or the client) will be able to determine the adequacy of blood circulation to the extremity.

96. (2) Integrated processes: nursing process — evaluation; client need: physiological integrity; pharmacological therapies; content area: medical-surgical.

RATIONALE

(1) Change in color vision would not be caused by something the client ate. (2) These are symptoms of digitalis toxicity. There is a narrow margin of safety between the full therapeutic effects and the toxic effects of cardiotonics. Clients taking digitalis preparations must be instructed in these adverse effects and in how to monitor their pulse rate, and keep all appointments for laboratory (serum levels) or diagnostic tests. (3) These symptoms are a result of toxicity, not side effects. (4) These symptoms are caused by a high dose of digoxin, but they have nothing to do with the client's age. This is not the best answer.

97. (3) Integrated processes: nursing process — data collection; client need: physiological integrity; pharmacological therapies; content area: medical-surgical.

RATIONALE

(1) Heparin per se is not an indication to monitor vital signs. (2) Heparin per se is not an indication to monitor I&O. (3) The principal adverse reaction to heparin, an anticoagulant, is bleeding. The nurse will monitor the client for any evidence of bleeding and take precautions to prevent it. (4) Heparin will not cause an electrolyte imbalance.

98. (3) Integrated processes: nursing process — evaluation; client need: psychosocial integrity; content area: psychiatric nursing.

RATIONALE

(1) An expression of anger would be stating feelings about the self without blaming others. (2) Repression is excluding memories from awareness. (3) Projection, an adaptive mechanism for dealing with inner stress, is the attribution of one's own feelings, ideas, or characteristics (usually undesirable ones) to another person. (4) Denial is ignoring or refusing to accept disagreeable realities.

99. (2) Integrated processes: nursing process — data collection; client need: physiological integrity; physiological adaptation; content area: medical-surgical.

RATIONALE

(1) Alcoholics may have cirrhosis of the liver, but the symptoms listed are not those of cirrhosis. (2) Alcohol is a central nervous system depressant; when alcohol is withdrawn abruptly, the alcoholic may develop alcohol withdrawal syndrome. Alcohol withdrawal symptoms (as listed) are considered a hyperexcitable state or a rebound phenomenon and have been called a "sympathetic storm." Recognition of early signs and symptoms is crucial: delirium tremens is fatal in 15% of clients. (3) There is no indication that the client is depressed, nor are these symptoms of that condition. (4) There is no indication that the client is suicidal, nor are these symptoms of that condition.

100. (3) Integrated processes: nursing process — planning; client need: physiological integrity; basic care and comfort; content area: medical-surgical.

RATIONALE

(1) These foods do not contain any significant amounts of vitamin C. (2) These foods do not contain any significant amounts of vitamin C. (3) Vitamin C is essential in tissue healing. Tomato sauce, potatoes, broccoli, cantaloupe, and strawberries are all excellent sources of vitamin C. (4) These foods do not contain any significant amounts of vitamin C.

101. (2) Integrated processes: nursing process — planning; client need: physiological integrity; pharmacological therapies; content area: medical-surgical.

RATIONALE

(1) This site is acceptable but does not indicate that the nurse is using a Z-track technique. (2) Iron dextran, often used in the treatment of iron-deficiency anemia, is very irritating to SC tissue. The nurse should therefore give it deep IM into a large muscle, with a 2- to 3-inch long needle, using the Z-track technique. This prevents oozing of the drug back into subcutaneous tissue. (3) This answer does not include the Z-track technique. (4) Iron dextran cannot be given IV.

102. (0.5 g) Integrated processes: nursing process — planning; client need: physiological integrity; pharmacological therapies; content area: medical-surgical.

RATIONALE

There are 1000 mg in a gram. Therefore, if the nurse is to administer 500 mg, the nurse will give 0.5 g, or 1/2 g.

103. (4) Integrated processes: nursing process — evaluation; client need: health promotion and maintenance; content area: pediatrics.

RATIONALE

(1) Artificially acquired immunity occurs with immunizations. (2) Natural passive immunity occurs with placental transfer. (3) Active acquired immunity occurs with an injection of human or animal serum. (4) When a person contracts

chickenpox, antibodies are formed in the presence of active infection in the body. This is a naturally acquired type of active immunity, which should produce a lifelong immunity to that disease.

104. **(3)** Integrated processes: nursing process — planning; client need: safe, effective care environment; safety and infection control; content area: medical-surgical.

    RATIONALE

    (1) Intact skin is the main mechanism in the portal of entry. **(2)** The reservoir will not prevent the spread of infection. **(3)** The aim of most hospital precautions is breaking the chain during the mode (method) of transmission phase of the cycle. Hand washing (especially between client contacts), which prevents the spread of infection during the mode of transmission, is the most effective means of controlling and preventing the spread of microorganisms. **(4)** Careful isolation and disposal of waste and waste products (portal of exit) will decrease the spread of infection but will not break the chain.

105. **(4)** Integrated processes: nursing process — evaluation; client need: safe, effective care environment; coordinated care; content area: medical-surgical.

    RATIONALE

    (1) This choice describes the evaluation phase. **(2)** This choice describes the implementation phase. **(3)** This choice describes the planning phase. **(4)** Data collection is the first phase of the nursing process. The nurse gathers, verifies, and communicates data about a client to establish a database about the client's level of wellness, health practices, past illnesses, and related experiences and health-care goals.

106. **(1)** Integrated processes: nursing process — data collection; client need: physiological integrity; physiological adaptation; content area: medical-surgical.

    RATIONALE

    (1) Hypernatremia means sodium excess in the blood plasma. The nurse would therefore expect a sodium level higher than the norm of 135–145 mEq/L (plasma). **(2)** Hypercalcemia is a high blood level of calcium. **(3)** Hyponatremia is a low blood level of sodium. **(4)** Hypochloremia is a low blood level of chlorides.

107. **(3)** Integrated processes: nursing process — data collection; client need: physiological integrity; physiological adaptation; content area: medical-surgical.

    RATIONALE

    (1) Cellular metabolism may be affected, but it does not cause the pain. **(2)** The number of circulating RBCs decreases, but this decrease is not the cause of the pain in sickle cell anemia. **(3)** In sickle cell anemia, the RBCs that contain the sickle cell hemoglobin are deoxygenated, causing them to elongate and become crescent shaped. They are then unable to pass through the bloodstream, causing thrombosis, pain, and infarction because of the decreased blood supply. **(4)** There is no bleeding in the joints with sickle cell anemia.

108. **(2)** Integrated processes: nursing process — implementation; client need: health promotion and maintenance; content area: maternity nursing.

    RATIONALE

    (1) Sickle cell anemia is a serious condition. **(2)** Sickle cell anemia is an inherited severe multisystem disease for which there is no known cure. Genetic counseling is important because the disease can be transmitted to offspring. **(3)** Sickle cell anemia is not an acquired immunosuppressive condition. **(4)** Sickle cell anemia is not sex linked.

109. **(3)** Integrated processes: nursing process — implementation; client need: psychosocial integrity; content area: pediatrics.

    RATIONALE

    (1) Asking the mother why the child was left unattended will put her on the defensive. **(2)** A 20-month-old child cannot describe what happened. **(3)** In a suspected case of child abuse, some additional information may be obtained by observing the parent-child interaction. How does the parent talk to the child? Is verbalization negative or positive? How does the parent respond to the child? Does the child seek comfort from the parent? **(4)** Examining the child will give the nurse more assessment data on physical injuries, but it will not help to determine the interaction between mother and child. This is not the best response.

110. **(3)** Integrated processes: nursing process — implementation; client need: physiological integrity; physiological adaptation; content area: medical-surgical.

    RATIONALE

    (1) This is not the first step in CPR. **(2)** This is not the first step in CPR. **(3)** Before beginning CPR, the nurse should first assess for unresponsiveness and should then look, listen, and feel for any signs of spontaneous respirations. These are the standard steps in CPR. **(4)** This is not the first step in CPR.

111. **(3)** Integrated processes: nursing process — implementation; client need: psychosocial integrity; content area: psychiatric nursing.

    RATIONALE

    (1) This response will not decrease her anxiety. **(2)** This response will not decrease her anxiety. **(3)** Therapeutic communication is crucial at this time. Listen to the client's wife and allow her to ventilate her feelings. Provide the opportunity for her to express her feelings and fears; to ask further questions; and to seek comfort, support, and understanding. This is the best response for the circumstances. **(4)** This response will not decrease her anxiety.

112. **(2)** Integrated processes: nursing process — data collection; client need: health promotion and maintenance; content area: medical-surgical.

    RATIONALE

    (1) "Thready" means a very weak pulse. **(2)** By definition, "tachy" is derived from the Greek *tachys*, meaning swift. "Cardia" is from the Greek *kardia*, meaning heart. The Greek word *rhythmos* means rhythm (measured time or movement; regular occurrence of an impulse). *Arhythmos* means without rhythm or lacking rhythm, or not regular. **(3)** There is no indication that the pulse is bounding. **(4)** There is no indication that there is hypotension. It does not fit the definition of rapid and irregular.

113. **(1)** Integrated processes: nursing process — data collection; client need: health promotion and maintenance; content area: pediatrics.

    RATIONALE

    (1) Early signs and symptoms of acute lymphocytic leukemia include pallor, weakness, fatigue, and lymphadenopathy. Leukemia, a malignant disorder of the bone marrow and lymph nodes, leads to an increase in uncontrollable WBCs, which enlarges lymph tissue (lymphadenopathy) and causes a decrease in other blood cells (RBCs and platelets), resulting in pallor, weakness, and fatigue. **(2)** The symptoms listed are not characteristic of acute lymphocytic leukemia. **(3)** The symptoms listed are not characteristic of acute lymphocytic leukemia. **(4)** The symptoms listed are not characteristic of acute lymphocytic leukemia.

114. **(3)** Integrated processes: nursing process — implementation; client need: safe, effective care environment; safety and infection control; content area: medical-surgical.

    RATIONALE

    (1) Side effects of antibiotics are not more serious in these clients than in other clients. This is not the best response. **(2)** Correct, but with the explanation given in option **(3)**. **(3)** Clients with acute leukemia have an increased potential for infection because they have many immature WBCs that are incapable of fighting infection. **(4)** An infection will not precipitate bleeding.

115. **(1)** Integrated processes: nursing process — implementation; client need: physiological integrity; physiological adaptation; content area: medical-surgical.

    RATIONALE

    (1) Cholelithotomy is the removal of gallstones through an incision. **(2)** Cholelithiasis means the formation or presence of calculi or bile stones in the gallbladder. **(3)** Lithotripsy is the process of crushing stones through shock waves. **(4)** Cholecystectomy is removal of the gallbladder.

116. **(3)** Integrated processes: nursing process — planning; client need: physiological integrity; basic care and comfort; content area: medical-surgical.

    RATIONALE

    (1) A urinometer does not measure output. **(2)** A urinometer is not used to take a specimen. **(3)** A urinometer is an instrument that measures specific gravity of urine, comparing its weight with that of water. **(4)** This is not a device for measuring glucose (sugar) and acetone.

117. **(2)** Integrated processes: nursing process — evaluation; client need: health promotion and maintenance; content area: medical-surgical.

    RATIONALE

    (1) A dehydrated client will have an increased specific gravity. **(2)** When a client is dehydrated or hypovolemic, sodium and other electrolytes are lost through excretion along with water, resulting in urine that is more concentrated. The more concentrated the urine, the higher its specific gravity (and weight) will be. A dehydrated client would have decreased urinary output. **(3)** Dehydrated clients have a decreased urine output. **(4)** Dehydrated clients have a decreased urine output.

118. **(2)** Integrated processes: nursing process — planning; client need: psychosocial integrity; content area: psychiatric nursing.

    RATIONALE

    (1) The anxiety may not be temporary. **(2)** Anxiety is an emotional response to a threat to one's self-esteem or well-being. Clients undergoing a surgical procedure are often highly stressed and unable to follow directions or explanations given. The nurse first needs to listen, allow the client to express any fears, and answer questions before giving teaching or explanation. **(3)** This statement may or may not be true, but it does not address anxiety. **(4)** Anxiety may or may not be related to fear of the unknown. This is not the best response.

119. **(3)** Integrated processes: nursing process — planning, communication and documentation; client need: psychsocial integrity; content area: psychiatric nursing.

    RATIONALE

    (1) This strategy might help to reduce the nurse's anxiety, but it is not the best response. **(2)** The nurse may have confidence, but the anxiety will still remain. **(3)** Anxiety often impairs functioning and can also lead to errors in judgment and performance. Nurses unfamiliar with a procedure need to take time to review it, to ask questions, and to remember that knowledge and competence guard against anxiety and that as knowledge and competence increase, anxiety lessens. **(4)** This statement may be true, depending on the level of anxiety. This is not the best response.

120. **(1)** Integrated processes: nursing process — data collection; client need: psychosocial integrity; content area: psychiatric nursing.

    RATIONALE

    (1) Clients often at first deny the seriousness of their illness and go through elaborate mental "gymnastics" (such as denial) to prove to themselves that this is not really happening to them. This mental mechanism is a means of helping them to cope, until they are able to begin to deal with the reality of their illness. **(2)** It is more likely that he is in denial rather than not hearing the physician. **(3)** Bargaining is a later stage of coping with a grave prognosis. **(4)** Depression is a later stage of coping with a grave prognosis.

121. **(3)** Integrated processes: nursing process — implementation; client need: physiological integrity; physiological adaptation; content area: medical-surgical.

    RATIONALE

    (1) This is not the first intervention in CPR. **(2)** This is not the first intervention in CPR. **(3)** Of the foregoing choices, in a client with respiratory arrest the nurse must first open the airway before proceeding with other interventions. Opening the airway often will aid in spontaneous respirations. This is standard protocol for CPR. **(4)** This is not the first intervention in CPR.

122. **(2)** Integrated processes: nursing process — implementation; client need: physiological integrity; physiological adaptation; content area: medical-surgical.

    RATIONALE

    (1) This ratio does not meet the standards of CPR. **(2)** The American Medical Association and American Health Association guidelines for CPR are 15 chest compressions:2 ventilations in a one-person rescue. **(3)** This ratio does not meet the standards of CPR. **(4)** This ratio does not meet the standards of CPR.

123. **(3)** Integrated processes: nursing process — data collection; client need: physiological integrity; pharmacological therapies; content area: medical-surgical.

    RATIONALE

    (1) These drugs do not cause proliferation of RBCs. **(2)** These drugs do not cause polycythemia. **(3)** Chemotherapy is aimed at destroying cancer cells, which are rapidly dividing cells. In the process, chemotherapy also destroys other rapidly dividing cells (e.g., bone marrow), which could cause a profound decrease in WBCs, putting the client at risk for infection, which he or she may not be able to fight off. **(4)** Chemotherapy does not cause bleeding tendencies.

124. **(4)** Integrated processes: nursing process — implementation; client need: safe, effective care environment; coordinated care; content area: psychiatric nursing.

    RATIONALE

    (1) A client's refusal to take medication is not an ethical dilemma. **(2)** This choice does not meet the definition of an ethical dilemma. **(3)** Physical abuse is reportable by law; thus there is no ethical dilemma. **(4)** An ethical dilemma occurs when there is a conflict of values. Ethics concerns what is right or wrong; values influence how one perceives others and how one acts. In option 4, the nurse's values come into conflict, because the nurse does not want to report the colleague but knows that he or she needs help and that the behavior could endanger clients. As a professional, the nurse is accountable to maintain standards of practice and assumes an ethical responsibility to clients.

125. **(1)** Integrated processes: nursing process — implementation; client need: safe, effective care environment; coordinated care; content area: medical-surgical.
RATIONALE
(1) Nurses are responsible for practicing within the standards of care developed by their licensing agencies and profession. These standards are guidelines for determining whether a nurse has acted as any reasonable prudent nurse with the same level of education and experience would have acted. **(2)** The Board of Nursing sets guidelines for LPNs, not individual nurses or physicians. **(3)** This choice does not meet the criteria for the Board of Nursing. **(4)** This choice does not meet the requirements for the Board of Nursing.

126. **(4)** Integrated processes: nursing process — implementation; client need: physiological integrity; basic care and comfort; content area: pediatrics.
RATIONALE
(1) Hot dogs, bread, and cake contain gluten. This child needs a gluten-free diet. **(2)** All these foods (except salad) contain gluten. **(3)** All these foods contain gluten. **(4)** These foods are gluten-free and should be recommended for this child's diet.

127. **(4)** Integrated processes: nursing process — data collection; client need: health promotion and maintenance; content area: medical-surgical.
RATIONALE
(1) Complaints of nausea and headache are not objective data. **(2)** Variable data are used in research. **(3)** Constant data are used in research. **(4)** Complaints of nausea and headache are subjective data information only — the client's perceptions or feelings about a health problem. Objective data are concrete data that can be palpated, observed, or auscultated.

128. **(2)** Integrated processes: nursing process — implementation; client need: health promotion and maintenance; content area: medical-surgical.
RATIONALE
(1) 5 minutes is longer than necessary. **(2)** The nurse must allow sufficient time for the temperature to register. The recommended time is 2–3 minutes for a glass thermometer. **(3)** 30–60 seconds is not long enough to register a temperature on a glass thermometer. **(4)** 1.0–1.5 minutes is not long enough to register a temperature on a glass thermometer.

129. **(2)** Integrated processes: nursing process — evaluation; client need: physiological integrity; pharmacological therapies; content area: medical-surgical.
RATIONALE
(1) It is not necessary to take the blood pressure before giving digoxin. **(2)** It is necessary to take an apical pulse for a full minute before administering digoxin, a cardiotonic. Changes in pulse quality, rate, and rhythm cannot always be easily assessed by a radial pulse. The physician may want the nurse to hold the drug and notify him or her if the apical pulse rate falls below 60 bpm or the client displays any symptoms of digitalis toxicity (arrhythmias or changes in pulse rhythm). **(3)** Before giving digoxin, the apical pulse is taken, not the radial pulse. **(4)** One does not need to check for pitting edema before giving digoxin.

130. **(3)** Integrated processes: nursing process — implementation, teaching/learning; client need: physiological integrity; pharmacological therapies; content area: medical-surgical.
RATIONALE
(1) This statement is true, but it is not the reason for not taking aspirin with warfarin. **(2)** This statement is true, but it is not the reason for not taking aspirin with warfarin. **(3)** Aspirin interferes with clot formation and potentiates the action of anticoagulants (warfarin) and could cause bleeding or hemorrhage. Clients taking warfarin should be instructed to use acetaminophen instead of aspirin. **(4)** This statement is true, but it is not the reason for not taking aspirin with warfarin.

131. **(3)** Integrated processes: nursing process — planning, teaching/learning; client need: health promotion and maintenance; content area: medical-surgical.
RATIONALE
(1) There is no reason to restrict potassium in the diet of a client who has had a myocardial infarction unless he is on a special medication that can causes retention of potassium. **(2)** Tomato juice is not high in caffeine. **(3)** Following a diet that is high in saturated fats constitutes a risk factor for myocardial infarction and the development of coronary artery disease. **(4)** The client with myocardial infarction does not normally need to be concerned about vitamin B in the diet.

132. **(1)** Integrated processes: nursing process — evaluation; client need: psychosocial integrity; content area: medical-surgical.
RATIONALE
(1) This client's frustration is a natural reaction, especially because his illness interferes with his occupation and his means of earning a living. A change in occupation may be more difficult because of his age and condition. **(2)** His behavior may not be temporary. **(3)** His behavior is not related to a desire for attention. **(4)** His behavior is not related to immaturity.

133. **(3)** Integrated processes: nursing process — data collection; client need: health promotion and maintenance; content area: maternity nursing.
RATIONALE
(1) Primipara means having given birth once. **(2)** Multigravida means having had more than one pregnancy. **(3)** Primigravida is the term used for a woman during her first pregnancy: primi meaning first, or one, and gravida meaning pregnant, or heavy with child. **(4)** Para means past pregnancies.

134. **(4)** Integrated processes: nursing process — data collection; client need: health promotion and maintenance; content area: maternity nursing.
RATIONALE
(1) Clients with preeclampsia have hypertension. **(2)** The client may have nausea, but this does not require frequent monitoring. **(3)** Preeclampsia is not associated with bleeding. **(4)** Preeclampsia, or toxemia of pregnancy, if not monitored and treated promptly, can lead to eclampsia. Symptoms of eclampsia include convulsive seizures and coma — a very grave condition of pregnancy. The nurse may monitor this client for the other conditions as well, but they do not characterize preeclampsia, which is what the question is about.

135. **(3)** Integrated processes: nursing process — data collection; client need: physiological integrity; reduction of risk potential; content area: medical-surgical.
RATIONALE
(1) The purpose of a lumbar puncture is diagnostic, not to relieve pressure on the brain. **(2)** Performing a lumbar punc-

ture will not bring down the temperature. (**3**) In meningitis, an inflammation of the meninges of the brain, CSF surrounds the brain and spinal cord. A lumbar puncture is performed in this instance to examine the CSF for evidence of bacteria (which causes meningitis) or increased WBCs resulting from inflammation or infection. (**4**) The spinal fluid can be examined for blood, but the primary reason for a lumbar puncture in this case is diagnostic in nature.

136. (**2**) Integrated processes: nursing process — implementation; client need: physiological integrity; reduction of risk potential; content area: medical-surgical.
RATIONALE
(**1**) Maintaining the client in a semi-Fowler's position would increase the likelihood of headache. (**2**) Keeping the room dark and the bed flat, as well as increasing hydration, will relieve discomfort and help to prevent headache. (**3**) Keeping the client prone would not prevent meningeal irritation. (**4**) Some clients experience a "spinal" headache after the removal of CSF, and lying on the side would not relieve it.

137. (**3**) Integrated processes: nursing process — implementation; client need: physiological integrity; physiological adaptation; content area: medical-surgical.
RATIONALE
(**1**) This may be a later activity, but it is not the first action. (**2**) This may be a later activity, but it is not the first action. (**3**) At the scene of a fire, the first priority is to prevent further injury to the victim. Laying the victim flat prevents the fire, hot air, and smoke from rising toward the head and respiratory passages. Rolling the victim in a blanket or article of clothing will help to smother the fire. (**4**) This may be a later activity, but it is not a first priority.

138. (**2**) Integrated processes: nursing process — planning; client need: physiological integrity; physiological adaptation; content area: medical-surgical.
RATIONALE
(**1**) Paying attention to emotional needs will come later. (**2**) Maintaining a patent airway should always be the nurse's primary focus. Primary areas of assessment and intervention also include determining the extent of the burn and fluid and electrolyte needs. The extent and depth of injury control the physiological response and the type of treatment required. Fluid replacement is the cornerstone to successful treatment and early survival of the burn client because of massive fluid shifts and potential hemodynamic shock. (**3**) Determining the cause of the accident will come later. (**4**) Assessing the need for skin grafting will occur later.

139. (**1600**) Integrated processes: nursing process — implementation, communication and documentation; client need: safe, effective care environment; coordinated care; content area: medical-surgical.
RATIONALE
To provide continuity and less chance of error in documentation of time, many agencies use military time in their documentation. After 12 noon, time is recorded as 1300 for 1 PM; thus, 4 PM would be recorded as 1600.

140. (**3**) Integrated processes: nursing process — data collection; client need: health promotion and maintenance; content area: medical-surgical.
RATIONALE
(**1**) This choice is objective data but not descriptive or measurable ("appear" is a vague description). (**2**) This choice

is subjective data. (**3**) Objective data are the results of direct observation by the nurse. (**4**) This choice is subjective data.

141. (**2**) Integrated processes: nursing process — planning; client need: health promotion and maintenance; content area: medical-surgical.
RATIONALE
(**1**) Generativity versus stagnation occurs in the middle years. (**2**) Erikson views life development as a continuous struggle for emotional and social equilibrium. The conflict of late adulthood (age 65 years or older) is ego integrity versus despair. During this stage, the older adult struggles to feel a sense of worth about life and achievements. (**3**) Intimacy versus isolation occurs in young adulthood. (**4**) Retirement versus depression is not a stage of Erikson.

142. (**3**) Integrated processes: nursing process — implementation; client need: safe, effective care environment; safety and infection control; content area: medical-surgical.
RATIONALE
(**1**) This is not the rationale for cleaning the wound in this fashion. (**2**) This is not the rationale for cleaning the wound in this fashion. (**3**) Wounds are cleaned from the least contaminated to the most contaminated area to prevent introduction of organisms back into the wound. (**4**) This is not the rationale for cleaning the wound in this fashion.

143. (**10**) Integrated processes: nursing process — data collection; client need: health promotion and maintenance; content area: maternity nursing.
RATIONALE
The Apgar score is a system of assessing the newborn infant's physical condition at 1 minute after birth (and again at 1, 2, or 5 minutes after birth). A score of 0, 1, or 2 is given for the heart rate, respiratory effort, muscle tone, response to stimuli, and color, for a maximum score of 10.

144. (**3**) Integrated processes: nursing process — data collection; client need: health promotion and maintenance; content area: maternity nursing.
RATIONALE
(**1**) This score is too high. (**2**) This score is too high. (**3**) In Apgar scoring of the newborn infant, respiratory effort is given a normal score of 2 for good respirations and in an infant who is crying. A score of 1 is given for slow and irregular respirations, and 0 is given for absence of respirations. (**4**) This score is too high.

145. (**2**) Integrated processes: nursing process — planning; client need: physiological integrity; basic care and comfort; content area: medical-surgical.
RATIONALE
(**1**) The nurse cannot give a back rub in this position. (**2**) Having the client in the prone position when giving a back rub makes it easier to apply necessary pressure to back muscles, to promote relaxation and to relieve muscle tension. (**3**) Prone position is better than lateral. (**4**) This is a difficult position to give a back rub.

146. (**1**) Integrated processes: nursing process — evaluation; client need: safe, effective care environment; safety and infection control; content area: medical-surgical.
RATIONALE
(**1**) A nosocomial infection is one that results from the delivery of health services in a health-care facility. The urinary tract is a

prime site; placing the urinary drainage bag above the level of the bladder allows reflux of urine in the catheter or bag (which could be contaminated) to reenter the bladder and become a source of infection. (2) Aseptic technique would help to prevent nosocomial infections. (3) Self-administration of insulin would not cause a nosocomial infection. (4) Spreading germs by not covering the mouth is not an example of a nosocomial infection.

147. **(1)** Integrated processes: nursing process — implementation; client need: physiological integrity; basic care and comfort; content area: medical-surgical.

RATIONALE

(1) Changing position and giving a back rub are simple noninvasive ways to reduce pain perception and to promote relaxation when it is too soon to administer another pain medication. (2) Range-of-motion exercises would increase pain. (3) Giving another injection of meperidine is an invasive action. (4) Explaining to this client that medication has just been given will not decrease pain.

148. **(2)** Integrated processes: nursing process — implementation, communication and documentation; client need: physiological integrity; pharmacological therapies; content area: pediatrics.

RATIONALE

(1) It is not appropriate to have the mother call the poison control center. (2) The procedure for accidental aspirin poisoning in a conscious client is to induce vomiting and to bring the client to the ER for gastric lavage. Inducing vomiting may not ensure complete emptying of stomach contents, and absorption could cause serious complications. Immediate gastric lavage will clear the stomach of the drug and prevent further absorption. (3) The antiemetic should be given in the ER rather than at home. (4) Diluting the medicine will not prevent further absorption.

149. **(2)** Integrated processes: nursing process — implementation; client need: physiological integrity; reduction of risk potential; content area: medical-surgical.

RATIONALE

(1) Flexion is not the correct position for this client. (2) The leg of a client who has had a total hip replacement must be maintained in a position of abduction in the early postoperative period to prevent adduction and flexion and potential dislocation. (3) Adduction is not the correct position for this client. (4) This positioning alone will not prevent adduction.

150. **(4)** Integrated processes: nursing process — data collection; client need: health promotion and maintenance; content area: medical-surgical.

RATIONALE

(1) Tachycardia is a pulse rate above 100. (2) Arrhythmia means an irregular heartbeat. (3) Sinus rhythm means the heartbeat is initiated from the sinoatrial node. The normal adult pulse rate is 60–100. (4) A pulse rate <60 is called bradycardia, derived from the Greek *bradys*, meaning slow, and *kardia*, meaning heart: slow heart rate.

151. **(2)** Integrated processes: nursing process — planning; client need: health promotion and maintenance; content area: maternity nursing.

RATIONALE

(1) There is nothing in peanut butter that would aggravate hypertension. (2) Smoked ham is high in sodium, which increases fluid retention, which in turn increases blood pressure. (3) There is nothing in broccoli that would contraindicate it during pregnancy. (4) Chicken is allowed for a client with hypertension as long as it is not prepared high in salt.

152. **(1)** Integrated processes: nursing process — planning; client need: physiological integrity; pharmacological therapies; content area: maternity nursing.

RATIONALE

(1) Bananas are high in potassium. (2) Apples are healthy but they will not supply the needed potassium. (3) Rice is healthy but it will not supply the needed potassium. (4) Grapefruit is healthy but it will not supply the needed potassium.

153. **(3)** Integrated processes: nursing process — implementation, teaching/learning; client need: health promotion and maintenance; content area: maternity nursing.

RATIONALE

(1) Do not restrict fluids to 1000 mL/day; the client needs more than this. (2) Increasing fluids will increase milk production. (3) A tight bra or binder will decrease milk production. (4) Applying warm compresses will increase milk production.

154. **(1)** Integrated processes: nursing process — implementation; client need: physiological integrity; physiological adaptation; content area: maternity nursing.

RATIONALE

(1) The first step is to determine how serious the situation is. If she can talk, the choking is not serious. (2) Back blows are a later action. (3) In the late stages of pregnancy, chest thrusts should be performed with the victim standing or sitting; however, this is not the first action. (4) The Heimlich maneuver is contraindicated in pregnancy.

155. **(2)** Integrated processes: nursing process — evaluation, teaching/learning; client need: physiological integrity; pharmacological therapies; content area: maternity nursing.

RATIONALE

(1) Rho(D) immune globulin is not given to all mothers. (2) Rho(D) immune globulin is given only to Rh-negative mothers who have Rh-positive babies. (3) Rho(D) immune globulin is not given in this situation. (4) Rho(D) immune globulin is not given in this situation.

156. **(4)** Integrated processes: nursing process — implementation; client need: physiological integrity; pharmacological therapies; content area: maternity nursing.

RATIONALE

(1) Acetazolimide is a diuretic and is not given to suppress milk production. (2) Hydromorphone is an analgesic and is not given to suppress milk production. (3) Dexamethasone is a steroid and is not given to suppress milk production. (4) Estradiol valerate is the only drug listed that suppresses milk production.

157. **(3)** Integrated processes: nursing process — data collection; client need: physiological integrity; pharmacological therapies; content area: maternity nursing.

RATIONALE

(1) To be adequate, a resting phase must be at least 30 seconds long. (2) To be adequate, a resting phase must be at least 30 seconds long. (3) To be adequate, a resting phase must be at least 30 seconds long. This meets the criteria. (4) To be adequate, the resting phase must be at least 30 seconds long. Sixty seconds is more than required.

158. (2) Integrated processes: nursing process — implementation, teaching/learning; client need: health promotion and maintenance; content area: maternity nursing.

RATIONALE

(1) Nausea during pregnancy is not caused by anxiety. (2) Nausea during pregnancy has a physiological basis because of hormone levels and is independent of rest, anxiety, or foods. (3) A change in diet will not stop her nausea. (4) Adequate rest will not relieve her nausea.

159. (4) Integrated processes: nursing process — data collection, communication and documentation; client need: psychosocial integrity; content area: psychiatric nursing.

RATIONALE

(1) Telling her parents would not be respecting her privacy or confidentiality. (2) The nurse might suggest this, but the nurse does not know whether the client knows who the father is or whether she has an ongoing relationship with him. (3) The nurse remains nonjudgmental regarding a client's abortion. (4) The clinic staff will help her with counseling and explore reasons for the abortion. The nurse respects the confidentiality of the client.

160. (3) Integrated processes: nursing process — data collection; client need: physiological integrity; pharmacological therapies; content area: medical-surgical.

RATIONALE

(1) Insulin needs will increase during certain phases of pregnancy. (2) Insulin requirements change during pregnancy. (3) Insulin requirements change during pregnancy during each trimester and with weight gain. (4) Pregnancy does not alter the type of insulin needed.

161. (1) Integrated processes: nursing process — implementation; client need: physiological integrity; reduction of risk potential; content area: medical-surgical.

RATIONALE

(1) A Penrose drain is an open drain. (2) A Jackson-Pratt is a closed drain. (3) A Hemovac is a closed drain. (4) A Surgivac is a closed drain.

162. (2) Integrated processes: nursing process — implementation; client need: physiological integrity; reduction of risk potential; content area: medical-surgical.

RATIONALE

(1) An Ace bandage cannot be wrapped medially. (2) Ace bandages are wrapped from distal to proximal to increase venous return. (3) An Ace bandage cannot be wrapped laterally. (4) Wrapping a bandage beginning at the proximal site decreases venous return.

163. (4) Integrated processes: nursing process — implementation, communication and documentation; client need: physiological integrity; basic care and comfort; content area: medical-surgical.

RATIONALE

(1) The nurse would deflate the balloon, but this is not the first step. (2) The nurse does not have to disconnect the bag and tubing. (3) The nurse might clamp off the tubing, but this is not the first step. (4) The first step of any procedure is to explain it to the client even if he or she is confused.

164. (2) Integrated processes: nursing process — data collection; client need: physiological integrity; pharmacological therapies; content area: medical-surgical.

RATIONALE

(1) In this area the nurse might hit the sciatic nerve. (2) This is the quadrant without major blood vessels or nerves. (3) This quadrant is painful and has many blood vessels. (4) This quadrant has major nerves and blood vessels.

165. (1) Integrated processes: nursing process — implementation; client need: physiological integrity; pharmacological therapies; content area: medical-surgical.

RATIONALE

(1) An intradermal injection is just under the skin. (2) This angle would go too deep. (3) This angle would go too deep. (4) This angle would go too deep.

166. (4) Integrated processes: nursing process — implementation; client need: physiological integrity; pharmacological therapies; content area: medical-surgical.

RATIONALE

(1) This needle is too long for an SC injection. (2) This needle is too long and has too large a gauge for an SC injection. (3) This needle is too long and has too large a gauge for an SC injection. (4) SC needle length is 1/2–5/8 inch. Acceptable gauges are 25, 26, or 27.

167. (3) Integrated processes: nursing process — evaluation; client need: physiological integrity; reduction of risk potential; content area: medical-surgical.

RATIONALE

(1) A nasogastric tube can be used for decompression of the stomach. (2) A nasogastric tube can be used for gastric feeding. (3) A nasogastric tube can remove air from the stomach but not from the colon. (4) A nasogastric tube can be used for administering medications.

168. (2) Integrated processes: nursing process — evaluation; client need: physiological integrity; reduction of risk potential; content area: medical-surgical.

RATIONALE

(1) This is an acceptable position to help prevent regurgitation in most clients. (2) This position increases chances for regurgitation and aspiration. (3) This is an acceptable position to help prevent regurgitation in most clients. (4) This is an acceptable position to help prevent regurgitation in most clients.

169. (1) Integrated processes: nursing process — implementation; client need: physiological integrity; pharmacological therapies; content area: medical-surgical.

RATIONALE

(1) The first step is to look at the pump. (2) Counting drops will not give an accurate rate with a pump. (3) Counting drops will not give an accurate rate with a pump. (4) The height of the pump will not affect volume-controlled pumps.

170. (3) Integrated processes: nursing process — implementation; client need: physiological integrity; reduction of risk potential; content area: medical-surgical.

RATIONALE

(1) A colostomy is a fecal diversion. (2) An ileostomy is a fecal diversion. (3) A utereostomy is used for urinary diversion. (4) A gastrostomy tube is used for gastric feeding.

171. (3) Integrated processes: nursing process — implementation; client need: physiological integrity; pharmacological therapies; content area: medical-surgical.

RATIONALE

(1) Only the leg is used for children this age. (2) Only the leg is used for children this age. (3) Only the leg is used for

IM injections in children 2 years old. Other muscles are not fully developed. (4) Only the leg is used for children this age.

172. (4) Integrated processes: nursing process — implementation, teaching/learning; client need: health promotion and maintenance; content area: medical-surgical.

RATIONALE

(1) It is preferable for casts to air dry. (2) One should not put anything down a cast. (3) The leg should be elevated to prevent edema. (4) To prevent pressure on the underlying tissue, the cast should be lifted with the flat part of the hand.

173. (3) Integrated processes: nursing process — evaluation; client need: health promotion and maintenance; content area: pediatrics.

RATIONALE

(1) Preventing cuts is important because hemophilia is a disorder that leads to easy bleeding. A tricycle is a relatively safe toy. (2) Preventing cuts is important because hemophilia is a disorder that leads to easy bleeding. Swings are relatively safe. (3) Preventing cuts is important because hemophilia is a disorder that leads to easy bleeding. This is an unsafe toy for a child with hemophilia. The sharp edges can cause cuts leading to bleeding. (4) Lincoln logs are a relatively safe toy.

174. (3) Integrated processes: nursing process — implementation, communication and documentation; client need: physiological integrity; basic care and comfort; content area: pediatrics.

RATIONALE

(1) A client with hypothyroidism gets cold easily. This room temperature is too cold. (2) A client with hypothyroidism gets cold easily. This room temperature is too cold. (3) Persons with hypothyroidism have a tendency to be cold. A temperature of 75.0°F (23.8°C) is warmer than usual and is a good temperature for a child with hypothyroidism. (4) A temperature of 85.0°F (29.4°C) is too warm.

175. (3) Integrated processes: nursing process — implementation; client need: physiological integrity; basic care and comfort; content area: pediatrics.

RATIONALE

(1) A medicine dropper is inappropriate; the child needs a nipple to stimulate the sucking reflex. (2) The child with a cleft lip and palate cannot use a metal spoon. (3) This child cannot drink fluids normally. She needs a long soft nipple for best results to prevent injury and to promote oral feeding. (4) A gastrostomy tube is not a good choice if food can be provided orally.

176. (1) Integrated processes: nursing process — implementation, teaching/learning; client need: physiological integrity; physiological adaptation; content area: pediatrics.

RATIONALE

(1) A twisted bowel is the pathology of volvulus. (2) Telescoping is known as intussusception. (3) Adhesions are scar tissue formations. (4) A volvulus does not affect the length of the intestine.

177. (4) Integrated processes: nursing process — implementation; client need: physiological integrity; reduction of risk potential; content area: medical-surgical.

RATIONALE

(1) Lying flat will pull on the incision and increase pain. (2) A supine position would increase the pain. (3) A prone position would increase the pain. (4) A semi-Fowler's position would prevent contaminated abdominal contents from ascending above the diaphragm.

178. (2) Integrated processes: nursing process — evaluation, communication and documentation; client need: health promotion and maintenance; content area: medical-surgical.

RATIONALE

(1) A headache is to be expected. (2) The most significant serious finding in head injury is an alteration in consciousness that would signify increased intracranial pressure. (3) Not eating is not of great concern at this time. (4) It is normal for a 2-year-old child to cry.

179. (4) Integrated processes: nursing process — implementation; client need: physiological integrity; physiological adaptation; content area: maternity nursing.

RATIONALE

(1) The recommendation of the American Heart Association is four initial breaths. (2) The recommendation of the American Heart Association is four initial breaths. (3) The recommendation of the American Heart Association is four initial breaths. (4) This is the American Heart Association guideline.

180. (2) Integrated processes: nursing process — evaluation; client need: physiological integrity; physiological adaptation; content area: maternity nursing.

RATIONALE

(1) This is a nongenetic congenital disorder. It is not passed on genetically. (2) Sickle cell anemia B is an inherited chronic form of anemia in which abnormal sickle or crescent-shaped RBCs are present. (3) Fetal alcohol syndrome is a nongenetic congenital disorder. It is not passed on genetically. (4) Cerebral palsy is a nongenetic congenital disorder. It is not passed on genetically.

181. (2 tablets) Integrated processes: nursing process — implementation; client need: physiological integrity; pharmacological therapies; content area: medical-surgical.

RATIONALE

1 grain = 65 mg. 5 grains = 325 mg, or 1 tablet : 325 mg :: x : 650 mg. x = 650 mg/325 mg, or 2 tablets.

182. (83 mL/hr) Integrated processes: nursing process — implementation; client need: physiological integrity; pharmacological therapies; content area: medical-surgical.

RATIONALE

1000 mL/12 hr = 83.3, or 83 mL/hr.

183. (2) Integrated processes: nursing process — implementation; client need: physiological integrity; pharmacological therapies; content area: medical-surgical.

RATIONALE

(1) Air is drawn into the NPH insulin to prevent contamination of the regular insulin, as it is pure insulin. See correct steps in rationale 2. (2) The correct steps to complete mixing are to (a) draw air into the NPH vial, (b) draw air into the regular insulin vial and draw up the insulin, and (c) reenter NPH vial and draw up required amount. (3) See correct steps in rationale 2. (4) See correct steps in rationale 2.

184. (80 mg) Integrated processes: nursing process — implementation; client need: physiological integrity; pharmacological therapies; content area: medical-surgical.

RATIONALE

1 lb = 2.2 kg. 176 lb/2.2 kg = 80 kg = 1 mg/kg = 80 mg.

185. **(4)** Integrated processes: nursing process — implementation; client need: physiological integrity; pharmacological therapies; content area: medical-surgical.
     RATIONALE
     1 g = 1000 mg. 1000 mg/250 = 4 capsules.

186. **(3)** Integrated processes: nursing process — evaluation; client need: physiological integrity; pharmacological therapies; content area: medical-surgical.
     RATIONALE
     (1) Low-dose renal dopamine does not affect blood pressure. **(2)** Low-dose renal dopamine does not affect blood pressure. **(3)** Vasodilation will increase urine output. **(4)** Low-dose dopamine will increase urine output, not decrease it.

187. **(1)** Integrated processes: nursing process — data collection; client need: physiological integrity; pharmacological therapies; content area: medical-surgical.
     RATIONALE
     (1) Diaphoresis is a symptom of hypoglycemia, which can result from taking insulin without eating. **(2)** Polyuria results from a high blood glucose level. **(3)** Polydipsia results from a high blood glucose level. **(4)** Polyphagia results from a high blood glucose level.

188. **(3)** Integrated processes: nursing process — evaluation, teaching/learning; client need: physiological integrity; pharmacological therapies; content area: pediatrics.
     RATIONALE
     (1) He will not go to camp until tomorrow; therefore, he should take the same dose today. **(2)** He will not go to camp until tomorrow; therefore, he should take the same dose today. **(3)** Because of increased exercise at camp, the need for insulin will be decreased. **(4)** He should take his insulin when he eats breakfast and before leaving for camp.

189. **(2)** Integrated processes: nursing process — implementation, caring; client need: psychosocial integrity; content area: psychiatric nursing.
     RATIONALE
     (1) There is no value statement here. The client is making a subjective comment. **(2)** The nurse is being judgmental when he or she classifies people into groups and assumes that all people are the same. **(3)** There is no value conflict in this statement. The aide is being respectful of people. **(4)** There is not a value conflict in this statement.

190. **(3)** Integrated processes: nursing process — implementation; client need: psychosocial integrity; content area: psychiatric nursing.
     RATIONALE
     (1) The nurse cannot prevent manipulative behavior. **(2)** The nurse cannot control manipulative behavior. **(3)** It is essential that the nurse enforce limit setting to help control manipulative behavior. **(4)** Firmness is not as successful in controlling manipulative behavior as limit setting.

191. **(3)** Integrated processes: nursing process — evaluation; client need: psychosocial integrity; content area: psychiatric nursing.
     RATIONALE
     (1) This is an example of persecutory hallucinations, not grandiose delusions, such as thinking that the person is a superior being. **(2)** This is an example of persecutory hallucinations, not auditory hallucinations, such as hearing voices that do not exist. **(3)** Persecutory hallucinations occur when people think that someone is after them for something they did not do or that is not reality based. **(4)** Paranoid delusions occur when the individual thinks that someone is blaming him or her incorrectly.

192. **(2)** Integrated processes: nursing process — evaluation; client need: psychosocial integrity; content area: psychiatric nursing.
     RATIONALE
     (1) The client may not believe this statement by the nurse. **(2)** The best intervention is to get the client to talk about her mother and her feelings. **(3)** Isolation will not be beneficial in this situation. **(4)** If the client is hallucinating, the presence of the mother may encourage more erratic behavior.

193. **(1)** Integrated processes: nursing process — implementation; client need: psychosocial integrity; content area: psychiatric nursing.
     RATIONALE
     (1) The client needs simple, straightforward directions. **(2)** To insist on the client's joining may aggravate the condition. **(3)** Explaining the benefits will not be successful. The client is too ill at this time. **(4)** The client is not ready to make decisions at this time.

194. **(3)** Integrated processes: nursing process — implementation, teaching/learning; client need: physiological integrity; reduction of risk potential; content area: medical-surgical.
     RATIONALE
     (1) Ileostomies have continuous liquid to semiliquid drainage and normally do not need irrigating. **(2)** The nurse can answer the question; it does not need to be referred to the physician. **(3)** Because ileostomies do not need irrigation, the client does not need anyone to show him the irrigation procedure. **(4)** There is no need for demonstrating the irrigation procedure. Ileostomies do not need irrigating.

195. **(2)** Integrated processes: nursing process — implementation, teaching/learning; client need: health promotion and maintenance; content area: medical-surgical.
     RATIONALE
     (1) Milk may irritate ulcers and may increase acid production. **(2)** Clients with ulcers can eat anything that does not bother them. **(3)** Juice may irritate ulcers. **(4)** There is no need to reduce calories according to this scenario.

196. **(1)** Integrated processes: nursing process — implementation; client need: physiological integrity; basic care and comfort; content area: medical-surgical.
     RATIONALE
     (1) This is not good advice. Diet control should be tried first before depending on laxatives. **(2)** Increasing fluids will help to prevent constipation. **(3)** Including bran (bulk) on a daily basis will help to prevent constipation. **(4)** Eating more fruits and vegetables will help to prevent constipation.

197. **(2)** Integrated processes: nursing process — data collection; client need: physiological integrity; reduction of risk potential; content area: medical-surgical.
     RATIONALE
     (1) The client has symptoms of a bladder infection. Sending a routine urinalysis to the laboratory will not help to diagnose a bladder infection. **(2)** Client has symptoms of a UTI, so the specimen must be cultured. **(3)** Irrigating the catheter will not help a bladder infection. **(4)** Measuring the specific gravity will not help the client's bladder infection.

198. **(4)** Integrated processes: nursing process — data collection; client need: physiological integrity; physiological adaptations; content area: medical-surgical.

RATIONALE
(1) Polyuria and frequency may be caused by increased fluid intake. (2) Oliguria and pressure may be caused by decreased fluid intake. (3) Discharge and pressure are more diagnostic of a vaginal infection. (4) Classic symptoms of a UTI are frequency and dysuria.

199. **(2)** Integrated processes: nursing process — data collection; client need: physiological integrity; reduction of risk potential; content area: medical-surgical.

RATIONALE
(1) Airway problems have priority over comfort. (2) The airway is of highest priority in postoperative clients after general anesthesia. (3) There is a potential for fluid volume alteration, but airway management takes priority. (4) The client may have a knowledge deficit, but airway problems have the highest priority.

200. **(3)** Integrated processes: nursing process phase: data collection; client need: physiological integrity; reduction of risk potential; content area: medical-surgical.

RATIONALE
(1) The nurse may take blood pressure in both arms for comparison, but the essential need here is for orthostatic vital signs. (2) There is no indication that the priority is for taking both the apical and radial pulse simultaneously. (3) Change in orthostatic vital signs (e.g., blood pressure) will indicate severity of dehydration. (4) Palpating the bladder will not help assess for fluid volume deficit.

201. **(1)** Integrated processes: nursing process — implementation; client need: physiological integrity; pharmacological therapies; content area: pediatrics.

RATIONALE
80 mg : 1 tablet = 40 mg : x = 0.5 tablet

202. **(3)** Integrated processes: nursing process — implementation; client need: physiological integrity; pharmacological therapies; content area: pediatrics.

RATIONALE
100 mg : 2 mL = 40 mg : x = 0.8 mL

203. **(3)** Integrated processes: nursing process — implementation; client need: physiological integrity; pharmacological therapies; content area: medical-surgical.

RATIONALE
30 units divided by 100 units $\times$ 1 mL = 0.30 mL

204. **(4)** Integrated processes: nursing process — implementation; client need: physiological integrity; pharmacological therapies; content area: medical-surgical.

RATIONALE
2,400,000 units divided by 600,000 units $\times$ 1 mL = 4 mL

205. **(4)** Integrated processes: nursing process — implementation; client need: physiological integrity; pharmacological therapies; content area: medical-surgical.

RATIONALE
12 mg divided by 15 mg $\times$ 1 mL = 0.8 mL

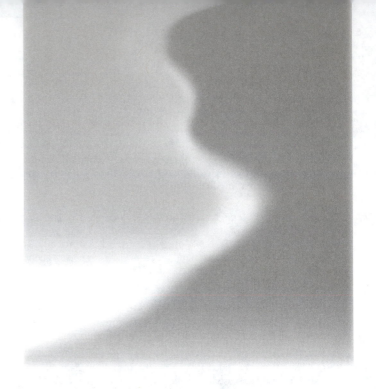

TEST 3

Larry D. Purnell, RN, PhD
Golden M. Tradewell, RN, PhD

QUESTIONS

1. The most common cause of myocardial infarction is:
   1. Atherosclerosis
   2. Synergistic effects
   3. Pulmonary embolism
   4. Blows to the chest

2. An 80-year-old client is recovering from cardiogenic shock. She has a urinary catheter for continuous drainage. Urinary output in this stage should be:
   1. 20 mL/hr
   2. 30 mL/hr
   3. 100 mL/hr
   4. 50 mL/hr

3. The mother of a 5-year-old child calls the emergency room and tells the nurse that her husband is bringing the child in because of a wasp sting, to which the child is allergic. What is the first medicine the nurse would have available?
   1. Diphenhydramine (Benadryl)
   2. Methylprednisolone (Solu-Medrol)
   3. Epinephrine
   4. Sodium bicarbonate

4. Objective signs that a client is in shock are:
   1. An increase in blood pressure and a decrease in pulse.
   2. An increase in blood pressure and an increase in pulse.
   3. A decrease in blood pressure and a decrease in pulse.
   4. A decrease in blood pressure and an increase in pulse.

5. An 80-year-old client has third-degree burns on 25% of the body. The priority nursing diagnosis is:
   1. Alteration in comfort
   2. Fluid volume deficit
   3. Alteration in nutrition
   4. Circulation, altered

6. A 47-year-old client had a supratentorial craniotomy after a motorcycle accident. Positioning after surgery is:
   1. Semi-Fowler's
   2. Flat
   3. Prone
   4. Lateral

7. A client is experiencing an increase in intracranial pressure. The nurse would expect his blood pressure to be:
   1. Systolic up, diastolic down
   2. Systolic down, diastolic down
   3. Systolic up, diastolic up
   4. Systolic down, diastolic up

8. A 77-year-old client who is taking Lanoxin (digoxin) has a low blood potassium level. The nurse would be especially sure to monitor:
   1. Pulse
   2. Blood pressure
   3. Urinary output
   4. Specific gravity

9. A client has acute pancreatitis. To determine its severity, the nurse would look at which laboratory test?
   1. Serum transaminase
   2. Serum amylase
   3. Serum sodium
   4. Serum magnesium

10. A 59-year-old client has a nasogastric tube for suction. Which of the following would be contraindicated for this client? (Select all that apply.)

    1. Ice chips
    2. Glycerine swabs
    3. Hard candies
    4. Peroxide gargles
    5. Soft candies
    6. Cold water

11. An 80-year-old client with unconsciousness of unknown etiology has just been admitted. The priority nursing diagnosis is:

    1. Airway maintenance
    2. Alteration in nutrition
    3. Alteration in consciousness
    4. Alteration in elimination

12. A client with acute renal failure now has an hourly urine output of 150 mL. The client is in what stage of renal failure?

    1. Oliguria phase
    2. Initial phase
    3. Diuretic phase
    4. Recovery phase

13. The most serious electrolyte abnormality for a client in chronic renal failure is: (Select all that apply.)

    1. Hypokalemia
    2. Hyperkalemia
    3. Hyponatremia
    4. Hypernatremia
    5. Hypercalcemia
    6. Hypocalcemia

14. A 38-year-old client has chronic cirrhosis and is jaundiced. To decrease pruritus from the jaundice, the nurse would:

    1. Use wool blankets.
    2. Keep the room temperature above 75.8°F (23.88°C).
    3. Keep the room temperature below 70.8°F (21.18°C).
    4. Use lots of soap in the bath water.

15. The most likely side effect of chemotherapy is:

    1. Fatigue
    2. Nausea
    3. Dehydration
    4. Skin ulceration

16. A 77-year-old client with thrombocytopenia and dementia likes to talk about her younger days and occasionally confabulates. This behavior:

    1. Prevents aggression
    2. Gains attention
    3. Indicates acute psychosis
    4. Maintains self-esteem

17. For which condition must the nurse notify the state health department?

    1. Chlamydial infection
    2. Syphilis
    3. Nonspecific urethritis
    4. Herpes

18. Oxygen is transported in which component of the blood?

    1. Serum
    2. Plasma
    3. Red blood cells (RBCs)
    4. White blood cells (WBCs)

19. The charge nurse asks the nurse to bring a 1000-mL intravenous (IV) bag of 5% dextrose (D_5) and normal saline (NS). The nurse selects:

    1. D5/0.33 NS
    2. D5/0.45 NS
    3. D5/0.9 NS
    4. D5/0.2 NS

20. Which of the following is not a complication of IV therapy?

    1. Extravasation
    2. Phlebitis
    3. Infiltration
    4. Renal shutdown

21. Uses of a tracheostomy tube include:

    1. Promotion of nutrition
    2. Relief of flatus
    3. Achievement of an artificial airway
    4. Increasing dead space

22. A 32-year-old client has a thoracotomy tube in place. To best promote drainage, the nurse should:

    1. Keep the client on the unaffected side.
    2. Keep water seal at chest level.
    3. Reposition the client every 2 hours.
    4. Turn him on his affected side.

23. A complication that can occur during the insertion of a subclavian catheter is:

    1. Arterial spasm
    2. Pulmonary infection
    3. Phlebitis
    4. Air embolism

24. A 22-year-old client just had a leg cast applied. Which symptom would be of most concern to the nurse?

    1. Swelling of the toes
    2. Blood drainage on the cast
    3. Toes cool to the touch
    4. Loss of sensation in the toes

25. Hypertension is called a "silent health problem." Which of the following is not a symptom of hypertension?

    1. Headache
    2. Nausea
    3. Vertigo
    4. Epistaxis

26. Collection of fluid in the pleural cavity is called pleural effusion. Place an X in the area in the figure where this occurs:

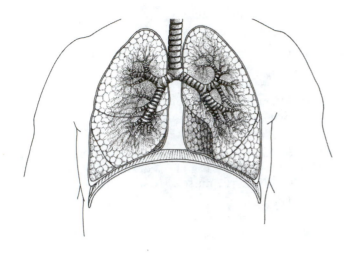

27. Generalized edema is called:
    1. Anasarca
    2. Pitting
    3. Ascites
    4. Lymphedema

28. What is the name of the hormonal dysfunction that causes increased growth in the hands, feet, and facial bones?
    1. Myxedema
    2. Acromegaly
    3. Gigantism
    4. Addison's disease

29. A 43-year-old client has a hormonal disturbance characterized by hirsutism, truncal obesity, and a buffalo hump. These are symptoms of the disease called:
    1. Acromegaly
    2. Myxedema
    3. Cushing's disease
    4. Graves' disease

30. In which of the following situations is reading the temperature orally contraindicated?
    1. A 45-year-old client with a duodenal ulcer
    2. A client who has recently suffered a heart attack
    3. An adult client with an elevated temperature
    4. A confused older client

31. Which of the following groups is most susceptible to extreme changes in environmental temperature?
    1. Toddlers
    2. Newborn infants
    3. Young adults
    4. Adolescents

32. Which of the following pulse sites can be used in measuring blood pressure in adults? Select all that apply.
    1. Brachial
    2. Femoral
    3. Carotid
    4. Radial
    5. Popliteal
    6. Jugular

33. Which of the following terms means an irregular pulse?
    1. Tachycardia
    2. Diastole
    3. Arrhythmia
    4. Bradycardia

34. What is the appropriate site for taking the pulse of an infant?
    1. Apical
    2. Radial
    3. Femoral
    4. Temporal

35. The difference in pressure during relaxation of the left ventricles and that which remains constant is called:
    1. Pulse pressure
    2. Maximal pressure
    3. Systolic pressure
    4. Diastolic pressure

36. A 35-year-old client is hospitalized with a fractured right femur. Which of the following blood pressures would be considered within the normal range for him?
    1. 88/50 mm Hg
    2. 124/80 mm Hg
    3. 180/110 mm Hg
    4. 144/92 mm Hg

37. A 45-year-old auto accident victim has fractures of both arms. The client is in bilateral (both sides) casts from the shoulders to the hands. Appropriate sites to take the client's pulse include:
    1. Temporal or brachial
    2. Brachial or femoral
    3. Radial or carotid
    4. Carotid or femoral

38. A 15-year-old client is admitted with a fever of 103°F (39.4°C). The client is flushed and complains of a headache. The nurse also notes that the skin is warm and dry and the lips and oral membranes are parched. This represents which part of the nursing process?
    1. Planning
    2. Implementation
    3. Data collection
    4. Evaluation

39. A client has a fever that is possibly the result of a throat infection. This would be which part of the nursing diagnosis statement?
    1. P—the problem
    2. E—the etiology or cause
    3. E—the evaluation of the problem
    4. S—the signs and symptoms manifested

40. The nurse administers acetaminophen (Tylenol), 10 grains, for a client's fever, as ordered by the physician. The administration of acetaminophen represents which phase of the nursing process?
    1. Implementation
    2. Evaluation
    3. Planning
    4. Reassessment

41. Twenty minutes after giving acetaminophen to a client with an elevated temperature, the nurse notes her response to the medication (decreased temperature). This represents which phase of the nursing process?
    1. Planning
    2. Data collection
    3. Analysis
    4. Evaluation

42. Assessment of a client's dry skin and parched oral mucous membranes is an example of what type of data?
    1. Constant
    2. Objective
    3. Subjective
    4. Modifiable

43. Which of the following is considered one client strength?
    1. Shallow respirations
    2. Irregular pulse rate
    3. History of bronchial asthma
    4. Weight within normal range

44. Which of the following conditions could cause a decrease in blood pressure? (Select all that apply.)
    1. Fever
    2. Hemorrhage
    3. Stress
    4. Obesity
    5. Anaphylactic shock
    6. Increased intracranial pressure

45. When measuring a client's blood pressure, the first faint clear tapping sounds the nurse hears on release of the hand valve indicate:
    1. Diastolic pressure
    2. Venous pressure
    3. Pulse pressure
    4. Systolic pressure

46. When a nurse makes an error in charting, which of the following nursing actions should be taken?
    1. Draw a line through the error, and begin again.
    2. Use white correction fluid, rewrite the data, and initial the corrections.
    3. Draw a line through the error, initial above it, and write "error."
    4. Draw a line through the error and write the correct data above.

47. Using a "source-oriented" medical record, the nurse will find a client's age, address, and other biographical data on the:
    1. Graphic sheet
    2. Admission sheet
    3. Progress notes
    4. Nurses' notes

48. One of the orders written on a client's chart is abbreviated NPO. This means:
    1. Normal physical observations
    2. Normal preoperative orders
    3. Nothing by mouth
    4. No physician orders written

49. When a new client is admitted to the hospital, which of the following actions should the nurse take first?
    1. Collect a urine specimen.
    2. Assist the client to undress and record items on a clothing list.
    3. Take and record vital signs.
    4. Greet the client, identify himself or herself, explain hospital routine, and identify reason for admission.

50. An 87-year-old client with pneumonia is assigned to a nurse's care. Which of the following assessments takes first priority?
    1. Rapid, irregular respirations of 32/min
    2. Skin warm, flushed, and dry
    3. Temperature of 99.4°F (37.4°C)
    4. Dry unproductive cough

51. The data collection on a client with pneumonia identifies dyspnea. This means:
    1. Respirations are shallow.
    2. The client is breathing very rapidly.
    3. The client cannot breathe in a supine position.
    4. Breathing has become difficult and labored.

52. The optimal position to enhance optimal ventilation for a client with pneumonia is:
    1. In Fowler's position.
    2. Lying on the unaffected side.
    3. In Sims' position.
    4. In the dorsal recumbent position.

53. The physician has ordered O_2 via nasal cannula at 3 L/min. Safety precautions when oxygen is in use include:
    1. Avoiding use of all types of lotions for skin care.
    2. Placing "No smoking" signs in prominent places in the client's room.
    3. Keeping the flow rate 4 L/min to prevent toxicity.
    4. Making sure that the room is well ventilated.

54. When teaching health care to an older client with osteoporosis, the nurse would:
    1. Remind the client to take anti-inflammatory medication to prevent joint stiffness.
    2. Remind the client of the importance of a yearly physical examination.
    3. Instruct the client to eat foods rich in calcium and to increase physical activity.
    4. Encourage the client to avoid long walks and becoming fatigued.

55. Constipation is frequently a problem among older persons. Which of the following is a means of prevention?
    1. Good attention to nutrition and avoidance of enriched foods
    2. Increased exercise; a low-bulk and low-fat diet
    3. A diet high in calcium and carbohydrates
    4. Increased fluid intake, increased exercise, and adequate bulk in the diet

56. The nurse is to administer an injection of vitamin B_{12} to an adult client. Which of the following nursing interventions will decrease irritation to subcutaneous (SC) tissue?
    1. Injecting the medication into the deltoid muscle
    2. Using the Z-track method of intramuscular (IM) injection into the ventrogluteal muscle
    3. Changing the needle before injection into the gluteus maximus
    4. Injecting the medication into the gluteus medius and firmly massaging the area after the injection

57. The nurse enters a client's room to administer her oral medications and the client states that one of the medications is different from what she has taken in the past. Which of the following nursing interventions will prevent a medication error?
    1. Recheck the medication in question against the physician's order before proceeding.
    2. Tell the client that it must be a new medication that her physician has ordered.
    3. Leave her medications at the bedside and tell her that they are what her physician has ordered.
    4. Omit the medication and record the fact that it was refused.

58. Symptoms that the nurse would expect to find in collecting data on a client with pulmonary emphysema include:
    1. Hemoptysis, unproductive cough, cardiac arrhythmias, and pedal edema.
    2. Exertional dyspnea, cough, increased mucous production, and wheezing.
    3. Chronic cough, diminished breath sounds, bradycardia, and epistaxis.
    4. Chest pain, hemoptysis, inspiratory wheezing, and right-sided atelectasis.

59. The nurse would expect the blood gases of a client with emphysema to show:
    1. Hypoxia, respiratory alkalosis, elevated PaO_2
    2. Hypoxemia, hypercapnia, respiratory acidosis
    3. Elevated SaO_2, hypocapnia, respiratory acidosis
    4. Increased SaO_2, hypocapnia, respiratory acidosis

60. A 75-year-old male client is admitted with a diagnosis of left-sided cerebrovascular accident (CVA). A nursing priority in caring for this client is:
    1. Assessing level of consciousness and neurological functioning at frequent intervals
    2. Passive range-of-motion exercises to prevent contractures
    3. Administration of laxatives to prevent constipation
    4. Minimal neurological stimulation to prevent a change in condition

61. When communicating with a post-CVA client with expressive aphasia, the nurse would understand that:
    1. The client may have difficulty in understanding what is being said.
    2. Communication in writing might be necessary.
    3. It might be difficult to understand the client.

4. The client will have difficulty in speaking and in writing.

62. In collecting data on a client with a urinary tract infection, the nurse would expect symptoms to include:
    1. Abdominal pain, nocturia, elevated temperature
    2. Frequency, urgency, dysuria, suprapubic pressure
    3. Flank pain, hematuria, abdominal distention
    4. Urinary retention, elevated pulse rate, crystalluria

63. Nursing interventions and teaching in caring for a client with a urinary tract infection include:
    1. Increasing fluid intake, cleansing the perineal area from front to back after elimination, administering medications ordered to acidify the urine
    2. Administering anti-inflammatory drugs, measuring intake and output (I&O) and specific gravity of urine
    3. Monitoring blood pressure, assessing for fluid retention, measuring I&O
    4. Increasing fluid intake, administering diuretics, monitoring electrolytes

64. A high-risk factor in a potential suicide client is:
    1. Increased physical activity
    2. A recent change in mood
    3. Hypersomnia
    4. Crying; increased verbal activity

65. A gravida 2 obstetrical client is Rh negative. There could be a complication to the fetus if:
    1. The mother received Rho(D) immune globulin (RhoGAM) after her first delivery.
    2. The father is Rh negative.
    3. The father is Rh positive.
    4. The baby is Rh negative.

66. The best source of dietary calcium to recommend to a pregnant client is:
    1. Milk
    2. Bananas
    3. Salad greens
    4. Orange juice

67. In which client care situation on a general care unit should surgical asepsis be used?
    1. Before removing a dressing
    2. When inserting a urinary catheter
    3. When administering a saline enema
    4. When giving perineal care

68. The single most important means of preventing the spread of infection is:
    1. Effective hand washing
    2. Use of clean gloves in performing client care
    3. Isolation precautions
    4. Disinfectants

69. After assessing a client's pulse and finding it to be 124 bpm and rapid, the nurse would chart this as:
    1. Bradycardia
    2. Pulse paradox
    3. Arrhythmia
    4. Tachycardia

70. Nursing interventions for hyperthermia should increase heat loss and decrease heat production, such as:
    1. Increasing fluids and increasing physical activity
    2. Providing extra blankets and offering acetaminophen as ordered
    3. Increasing fluids and administering tepid sponge baths
    4. Offering warm fluids and reducing physical activity

71. In collecting data on a client and documenting subjective data, the nurse charts data that:
    1. The nurse assessed and observed, including interpretations and conclusions drawn.
    2. The client perceives, and the way he or she expresses it.
    3. The nurse observed, including responses to treatment.
    4. The nurse perceived and gathered in the client assessment.

72. The nursing process should be integrated into the documentation because:
    1. It includes observations made and problems identified.
    2. It is the best means of communicating with other members of the health-care team and is the foundation of nursing practice.
    3. It includes the nurse's assessment and information that should be charted.
    4. It is pertinent data and should be charted on the Kardex and kept updated.

73. A client is terminally ill. When the nurse enters the room, it is evident that the client has been crying. A statement to enhance communication would be:
    1. "You seem sad and depressed today; what is the problem?"
    2. "How are you feeling today?"
    3. "Come on, cheer up, I'm sure things will look brighter tomorrow."
    4. "I see that you have been crying. Would you like to talk about it?"

74. To listen attentively to a client, the nurse needs to:
    1. Respond quickly to statements made and questions asked so the client knows that the nurse is interested.
    2. Listen to what the client says and ask why he or she feels that way.
    3. Listen with all of the senses and maintain eye contact with the client.
    4. Sit down, lean back in the chair, and cross the arms.

75. What is the nurse's first action when discovering a hospitalized client who appears to have ceased breathing?
    1. Determine unresponsiveness.
    2. Begin cardiac compression.
    3. Give two quick breaths.
    4. Call for help.

76. Which is the best indicator to use to determine that external cardiac compressions should be started?
    1. Unresponsiveness
    2. Absence of carotid pulse
    3. Cessation of respirations
    4. Fixed and dilated pupils

77. The steps of the nursing process, in the correct order, are:
    1. Data collection, discrimination, planning, evaluation, reevaluation
    2. Data collection, analysis, intervention, planning, diagnosis
    3. Data collection, discovering, evaluation, planning, reassessment
    4. Data collection, planning, implementation, and evaluation

78. The basic four food groups are:
    1. Fruits and vegetables, milk and cheese, breads and cereals, vitamins and minerals
    2. Fruits and vegetables, milk and milk products, breads and cereals, meats and poultry and alternates
    3. Milk and milk products, breads and cereals, carbohydrates and protein, vitamins and minerals
    4. Milk and milk products, fruits, vegetables, cheese and poultry

79. The "five rights" for safe administration of medications are:
    1. Right drug, right dose, right client, right amount, right route.
    2. Right drug, right client, right order, right route, right time.
    3. Right drug, right dose, right time, right route, right client.
    4. Right client, right drug, right strength, right time, right documentation.

80. A 66-year-old client is admitted with dehydration and hypernatremia. Clinical signs and symptoms for which the nurse will observe the client include:
    1. Cool moist skin, hypotension, elevated serum sodium, hypothermia.
    2. Extreme thirst; dry, sticky mucous membranes; flushed skin; elevated temperature; elevated sodium serum.
    3. Agitated behavior, hyperpyrexia, decreased specific gravity of urine, hypotension.
    4. Anorexia, cool moist skin, fatigue, elevated serum sodium, personality changes.

81. Normal serum potassium concentration levels range from:
    1. 3.2–4.5 mEq/L
    2. 2.5–4.5 mEq/L
    3. 3.5–5.5 mEq/L
    4. 3.5–4.0 mEq/L

82. A client with dehydration and hypokalemia is to receive an IV infusion of 1000 mL of D_5/0.33 sodium chloride with 20 mEq of potassium chloride. It is to be administered over an 8-hour period. The administration set has a drop factor of 20 gtt/mL. The nurse will set the flow rate at: _____.

83. A 27-year-old client is scheduled for an appendectomy. The nurse will be certain that the client has emptied the bladder before surgery primarily because:

    1. A full bladder preoperatively could cause postoperative urinary retention.
    2. A full bladder could very easily be injured during the surgical procedure (surgical trauma).
    3. A full bladder could cause urinary stasis and a potential postoperative urinary tract infection.
    4. The nurse will need to obtain a urinalysis before surgery.

84. The nurse will be certain that a surgical client has been given informed consent. Informed consent means that:

    1. The client has given full consent for the surgical procedure.
    2. A properly informed and fully competent client has given full consent to the surgical procedure.
    3. The client has been prepared for surgery and given full consent to the procedure.
    4. The physician has fully explained the surgical procedure to the client.

85. Food and fluids are withheld before a surgical procedure primarily:

    1. Because the client may experience nausea and vomiting because of anxiety.
    2. To reduce postoperative nausea and vomiting.
    3. To reduce preoperative and postoperative discomfort.
    4. Because food or fluids in the stomach increase the possibility of aspiration of stomach contents while the client is anesthetized.

86. In some instances, the surgical area is shaved of hair before surgery. The primary rationale for this is:

    1. To prevent postoperative discomfort.
    2. To destroy microorganisms and to reduce the chance of infection.
    3. To prevent pain and discomfort during postoperative dressing changes.
    4. To provide a better view of the surgical site.

87. The physician orders 5000 units of heparin every 12 hours SC for the first 48 hours postoperatively. The rationale for this medication is:

    1. To decrease the risk of postoperative emboli
    2. To prevent the risk of postoperative hemorrhage
    3. To increase blood coagulation
    4. To prevent possible postoperative paralytic ileus

88. Which of the following signs could indicate a possible wound infection?

    1. Elevated body temperature, erythema, swelling surrounding the suture line, increased abdominal pain
    2. Diaphoresis, anorexia, serosanguineous drainage, diminished bowel sounds
    3. Swelling around the incision, serosanguineous drainage, skin edges well approximated
    4. Elevated body temperature, bright-red drainage, increased urine output

89. A nurse arrives on the scene of an automobile accident and finds the driver unconscious and bleeding from a head laceration. The first action the nurse will take is:

    1. Ensure that the victim has a patent airway.
    2. Try to stop the bleeding by applying pressure to the nearest artery and by elevating the extremity above the heart.
    3. Go to the nearest telephone and activate the emergency medical system.
    4. Elevate the victim's head, and begin cardiopulmonary resuscitation (CPR).

90. A client is to undergo ionizing radiation treatment for breast cancer. To explain this to the client, the nurse understands that radiation attempts to kill cancer cells by:

    1. Dissolving the cell nucleus via heat and destroying cancer cells.
    2. Altering the normal pattern of normal cells which in turn will kill off the cancer cells.
    3. Radiation passing through living tissues and inhibiting cell division protein.
    4. Disrupting cancer cells via magnetic resuscitation.

91. A nurse is caring for a client with a radioactive uterine implant. Nursing interventions will focus on:

    1. Observing the principles of time, distance, and shielding
    2. Keeping at least 12 ft away from the source of radiation
    3. Keeping the client on protective isolation and allowing the client to do as much self-care as possible
    4. Wearing a radiation film badge and spending only 10 minutes at a time at the bedside

92. A nurse and community health educator can teach prevention of chest injuries by:

    1. Teaching clients that both passive and active smoking contribute to chest injuries.
    2. Encouraging the use of passenger seat belts in motor vehicles.
    3. Teaching clients to drive at or below the speed limit to prevent potential automobile accidents and resultant chest injuries.
    4. Teaching that children must be placed in the back seat of moving vehicles to prevent chest injury in the event of an accident.

93. A 68-year-old client is admitted to the hospital with increased breathlessness, a productive cough, and fever and chills. His arterial blood gas values are PaO_2 58 mm Hg, $PaCO_2$ 55 mm Hg, and pH 7.0. These are indicative of:

    1. Hypoventilation and respiratory alkalosis
    2. Metabolic alkalosis resulting from uncompensated respiratory alkalosis
    3. Respiratory acidosis resulting from hypoventilation
    4. Respiratory alkalosis resulting from pulmonary disease

94. With early signs of hypoxia, the nurse would expect to assess a chronic obstructive pulmonary disease client for:

    1. Dyspnea, neurological changes, hypertension, diminished breath sounds
    2. Increased rate and depth of respirations, headache, changes in behavior, decreased judgment, drowsiness

3. Orthopnea, use of accessory muscles to breathe, cyanosis of nail beds
4. Labored breathing, crowing respirations, inspiratory wheezing

95. A 45-year-old client is post-myocardial infarction. The client is placed on a low-salt, low-cholesterol diet. Some foods that the nurse will instruct the client to decrease in amounts include:

1. Green leafy vegetables, citrus fruits
2. Bananas, whole-grain breads, nuts
3. Potatoes, cruciferous vegetables, raisins
4. Organ meats, whole milk, egg yolks, shellfish

96. A 66-year-old client takes a potassium-depleting diuretic. Foods that will help to keep the client's potassium level within normal limits include:

1. Dairy products, whole-grain cereals, starchy vegetables
2. Citrus fruits, liver and organ meats, dark-green vegetables
3. Bananas, oranges, cantaloupe, fish, spinach, whole-grain cereals
4. Nuts, dairy products, citrus fruits, enriched bread

97. Medications usually used in the treatment of rheumatoid arthritis include:

1. Anti-inflammatory agents
2. Antilipemic agents
3. Antibiotics
4. Sympatholytic agents

98. A 24-year-old woman is admitted in labor at 39 weeks' gestation. The nurse will position her in the Sims' position because:

1. It increases fetal activity.
2. It facilitates descent of the presenting part through the birth canal.
3. It enhances maternal and placental circulation and promotes relaxation.
4. It decreases the intensity of the labor pains, especially in back labor.

99. A fetal heart rate of 132 bpm in a client who is in labor should be interpreted as:

1. Abnormal.
2. Fetal distress.
3. Within the normal limits.
4. Slightly above the norm.

100. The nurse times the frequency of a client's labor contractions from the:

1. Beginning of one contraction until relaxation of the uterus
2. Beginning of one contraction until the beginning of the next
3. Peak of one contraction until the beginning of the next
4. Contraction of the uterus until its relaxation

101. The third stage of labor is defined as:

1. The stage when the placenta and membranes are delivered.

2. The beginning of the first contraction, ending with the birth of the baby.
3. The time when the cervix is fully dilated, lasting until the delivery of the baby.
4. The period when the baby is delivered, ending with the delivery of the placenta and membranes.

102. A 3-month-old infant is admitted with possible pyloric stenosis. A classic sign of this condition is:

1. Anemia
2. Projectile vomiting
3. Diarrhea
4. Anorexia

103. While caring for a client with acute glomerulonephritis, an important nursing intervention would be:

1. Monitoring and assessing I&O
2. Monitoring pulse and respirations
3. Forcing fluids
4. Increasing ambulation

104. Which of the following would be the best food choice to select for a post-tonsillectomy 4-year-old child?

1. Ice slush
2. A glass of milk
3. Orange juice
4. Decaffeinated soda pop

105. The primary purposes of changing a postoperative client's dressing are:

1. To inspect the dressing
2. To inspect the incisional area for healing and for evidence of infection
3. To inspect the dressing and to provide comfort for the client
4. To chart the type and amount of drainage

106. A client will be ambulatory on the first day after surgery. The primary benefits of early ambulation are:

1. To improve circulation, stimulate elimination, and prevent dependence
2. To facilitate the normal functioning of all body organs and systems, and reduce the danger of potential postoperative complications
3. To improve appetite, prevent nausea and vomiting, and prevent potential evisceration
4. To prevent formation of emboli, promote ventilation, and stimulate diaphoresis

107. A client, aged 75 years, is admitted to the hospital with a diagnosis of congestive heart failure (CHF). This condition develops as a result of:

1. Increased cardiac output resulting from hypovolemia
2. Increased metabolic needs of the body
3. Accumulation of serous fluid in the pleural space
4. The heart's inability to pump effectively to meet the demands of the body

108. A client is receiving chemotherapy for treatment of breast cancer. She has begun to experience alopecia (loss of hair). It is important to inform her that the alopecia is:

1. Temporary and that hair will grow again soon after chemotherapy is discontinued

2. Permanent but that wearing a wig will help her overall self-concept and cosmetic appearance
3. Not life threatening and the hair may even begin to grow again when she is in remission
4. Never permanent and that it will aid her in finding ways to improve her appearance

109. A client, aged 52 years, has a diagnosis of hypertension. Admission blood pressure is 200/110 mm Hg, and the client is complaining of a severe headache and dizziness. The licensed practical nurse's (LPN's) first priority is to:

1. Document the blood pressure in the admission notes.
2. Report this immediately to the registered nurse (RN).
3. Give the client acetaminophen as prescribed for headache.
4. Ask the client if there is a history of hypertension in the family.

110. A client who is a two-pack/day cigarette smoker changes the topic of conversation whenever her smoking is brought up. This psychological defense mechanism is called:

1. Sublimation
2. Repression
3. Denial
4. Compensation

111. A 22-month-old infant is admitted with gastroenteritis, hyperthermia, and dehydration. Which nursing intervention will most effectively aid in reducing fever?

1. Giving 5 gr of aspirin
2. Sponging the client with alcohol
3. Applying extra blankets
4. Giving the client a tepid sponge bath

112. When instilling eardrops in the left ear of a 3-year-old child, the nurse will:

1. Ask the child to sit in an upright position.
2. Pull the auricle upward and forward during instillation.
3. Pull the pinna upward and backward during instillation.
4. Straighten the ear canal by grasping the pinna and gently pulling it down and backward.

113. Which of the following side effects are commonly seen during initial treatment with nitrates (vasodilators)?

1. Flushing, hypotension, bradycardia
2. Headache, postural hypotension, flushing
3. Drowsiness, anorexia, hypertension
4. Tachycardia, hypertension, hypokalemia

114. Two days after her cholecystectomy, a client has been experiencing nausea and vomiting. The client has a T-tube in place. For what electrolyte imbalance will the nurse monitor?

1. Hypernatremia
2. Hyperkalemia

3. Hypervolemia
4. Hypokalemia

115. Before administering an antihypertensive agent, the nurse will:

1. Check all extremities for any pitting edema.
2. Measure and record the client's blood pressure.
3. Weigh the client.
4. Take an apical pulse reading.

116. A client is receiving regular insulin according to 6-hour fasting blood sugar levels. The nurse will observe her for side effects within:

1. 2–4 hours
2. 30–60 minutes
3. 15–20 minutes
4. 2–3 hours

117. The nurse is caring for a client with thrombophlebitis. A medication that may be administered in the treatment of this condition is:

1. Ampicillin
2. Heparin
3. Propranolol (Inderal)
4. Nitroglycerin

118. A 22-year-old primipara has had a cesarean delivery. The nurse will observe her for possible postpartum hemorrhage by:

1. Monitoring her pulse rate and checking her dressing
2. Monitoring her vital signs and palpating the level of the fundus
3. Checking her blood pressure and the color of her nail beds
4. Monitoring the color and amount of her flow

119. Pulmonary tuberculosis is on the increase. Signs and symptoms of this condition for which the nurse will assess a client include:

1. Elevated WBC count, diaphoresis, hypertension, anorexia
2. Anorexia, fatigue, low-grade afternoon fever, weight loss, cough, possible hemoptysis
3. Chest pain, tachycardia, enlarged cervical lymph nodes, joint pain, fatigue
4. Bradycardia, weight gain, subnormal temperature, general malaise, elevated sedimentation rate

120. A 34-year-old client has been recently admitted to the hospital for the third time this past month with anxiety, nausea and vomiting, and a tentative diagnosis of hypochondriasis. Which of the following statements correctly defines this disorder?

1. The outward manifestation of anger that the client is not able to express directly and that is manifested in physical symptoms.
2. The inability to acknowledge thoughts or feelings in oneself and attributing them to another.
3. A defense used by the ego when it does not wish to remember a painful feeling or emotion
4. A defense by the ego when it feels severely threatened or during periods of internal psychic stress

121. A nurse in a long-term psychiatric unit finds that a client with depression has not showered for a week and is very unkempt in appearance. The nurse would:

1. Do nothing and wait until the client is ready to shower on his or her own.
2. Tell the client to go and shower now.
3. Assist the client in gathering the necessary items to bathe.
4. Obtain physical help and carry the client to the shower.

122. A 22-year-old computer programmer was admitted last night with schizophrenia. He is watching television in the day room. As the nurse approaches him, he says, "Leave me alone, don't bother me." The nurse would:

1. Introduce himself or herself and stay with him for a while.
2. Stay at his side for an hour to let him know that he is not in control.
3. Leave with plans to return in 1 hour.
4. Gently touch his hand and offer help.

123. A 34-year-old client is scheduled for major surgery. Since admission, the client has been very demanding, continuously calling the nurse to straighten a pillow and pour a glass of water. The nurse identifies this as an example of which defense mechanism?

1. Regression
2. Conversion
3. Denial
4. Projection

124. A single father brings his 17-year-old daughter to the clinic because she refuses to leave the house for fear of meeting someone she does not know. He wants to know what this condition is called. The nurse explains that it is called:

1. Acrophobia
2. Xenophobia
3. Claustrophobia
4. Agoraphobia

125. During change of shift report, the nurse reports that a new admission has bulimia. The nurse recognizes that bulimia is:

1. A phobia of obesity.
2. A disorder associated with starvation.
3. A disorder associated with vomiting.
4. A disorder associated with bingeing and vomiting.

126. A 78-year-old client with senile dementia is wandering the halls in a long-term care facility. He is looking for his 5-year-old son. The nurse would:

1. Ask him when he last saw his son.
2. Remind him that his son is now a grown man.
3. Ask him to describe his son.
4. Help him back to his room.

127. A home-health nurse is caring for a client with a colostomy. Her family asks the nurse for advice on coping with their father, who has organic brain syndrome. He is very forgetful and gets angry when the family reminds him that he should remember. The nurse's best advice for the family is that they should:

1. Place him in a long-term care facility because he is potentially dangerous to himself.
2. Give detailed instructions to him when he does something wrong.
3. Reorient him when he loses contact with reality.
4. Provide flexibility in his daily activities.

128. A 22-year-old client with an antisocial personality refuses to participate in group activities and makes fun of other clients, calling them "nut cases." Which of the following nursing plans would be most effective for the staff to follow?

1. Isolate the client from the other clients to avoid disturbing them with the name calling.
2. Set ground rules.
3. Call a team meeting to discuss the treatment plan.
4. Require the client's participation in all group activities.

129. A 44-year-old paranoid client is admitted for corrective orthopedic surgery. He refuses oral medication, saying that the nurse is trying to poison him. The nurse would:

1. Insist that he take the medicine because it is not poison.
2. Skip the medicine and report the behavior to the physician.
3. Give him the choice of taking it orally or IM.
4. Ask him why he thinks it is poison.

130. A 24-year-old female client has refused to get out of bed for 3 days. Her mother brings her to the hospital. The client is given a diagnosis of depression. After 4 days on the unit, she refuses to take her oral medicine because she says it is causing her to have difficulty seeing. The nurse would:

1. Administer the medication IM.
2. Hold the medicine until the client is evaluated further.
3. Insist that she take the medicine orally.
4. Confine her to her room until she is ready to take her medicine.

131. A home-health nurse gives the mother of the 9-month-old child instructions for recurrent attacks of croup. The nurse recommends to the mother that when the child begins to cough, she should:

1. Give an additional dose of the prescribed expectorant.
2. Keep the child warm.
3. Turn the child upside down and give gentle back blows.
4. Turn the shower on and create a warm mist.

132. A 45-year-old client has just had electroconvulsive therapy. The nurse would:

1. Take his vital signs every 5–10 minutes.
2. Observe the client for nausea and vomiting.
3. Reorient the client to time and place.
4. Place the client on bed rest for the next 24 hours.

133. A woman who is 8 months pregnant is at the clinic for her regular appointment. She confides in the nurse that her husband wants her to bottle-feed the baby. He thinks that breast-feeding will distort her breasts. She asks the nurse's opinion. The nurse's response is:

1. "To please your husband, you should bottle-feed."
2. "Have you tried talking with your mother about the problem?"
3. "You should discuss this with your doctor."
4. "What would you like to do?"

134. An 18-year-old mother delivers a healthy full-term baby boy. Three days later, he is given a diagnosis of phenylketonuria (PKU). The mother asks the nurse if this condition will affect the child's eating habits when he gets older. The nurse tells her that the child will have to avoid eating:

1. Foods high in protein
2. Fruit juices
3. Leafy green vegetables
4. Foods with caffeine

135. It is apparent that a 24-year-old client is going to abort. She is very apprehensive. Which of the following statements is best to give the client support?

1. "Just try to stay calm; everything will be all right."
2. "Is this your first spontaneous abortion?"
3. "It is best to abort now rather than later on in your pregnancy."
4. "I will stay with you to help you through this."

136. A 19-year-old female client is admitted to the psychiatric unit because she talks to herself, is suspicious of other people, laughs inappropriately, and hears voices telling her to kill herself. She is sitting in the lounge quietly talking to a card table. The nurse would:

1. Ignore the behavior; she is not bothering anyone.
2. Try to engage her in some physical activity.
3. Tell her to stop talking.
4. Ask her with whom is she talking.

137. A 48-year-old male client is in restraints for severe agitation. The best way to assess whether he is ready to have the restraints removed is:

1. Give him a sedative, wait 30 minutes, and then remove the restraints.
2. Check his pupils for dilation.
3. Observe him for tense muscles.
4. Ask him if he is in control now.

138. A 34-year-old primipara has just had her water break. The nurse's next action is to:

1. Complete a vaginal exam.
2. Ask her husband to leave the room.

3. Take her vital signs.
4. Check the fetal heart rate.

139. A newborn has an elevated bilirubin and phototherapy is ordered. The nurse would:

1. Cover the baby with a blanket to prevent chilling.
2. Keep the baby NPO during the therapy.
3. Cover the baby's eyes to prevent retinal damage.
4. Prepare for an IV infusion.

140. To evaluate the effects of phototherapy for an infant with increased bilirubin, the nurse would expect that the:

1. Infant's appetite will increase.
2. Infant will become less irritable.
3. Skin color will become less jaundiced.
4. Photophobia will decrease.

141. In an automobile manufacturing plant, coworkers bring a woman who is about to deliver a baby to the nurse's office. The nurse has the secretary call for help and assists with the impending delivery. The nurse would:

1. Apply gentle pressure to the delivering head.
2. Have her cross her legs to delay the delivery until help arrives.
3. Discourage the mother from pushing.
4. Encourage the mother to hold her breath.

142. The nurse in the delivery room has just been handed a newborn baby. The nurse's first action is to:

1. Gently slap the baby's bottom to stimulate breathing.
2. Hold the baby's head down to help the mucus drain.
3. Place the baby on the mother's abdomen.
4. Take the baby's vital signs.

143. A 54-year-old client is having delusions. It is important that the nurse:

1. Correct the delusions
2. Not talk about the delusions
3. Tell the client to think about something else
4. Not disagree with the client about the delusions

144. A 62-year-old client with glaucoma is reluctant to have surgery. He asks the nurse what will happen if he does not have the surgery. The nurse explains that he:

1. Could get a detached retina
2. Will become nearsighted
3. Will become farsighted
4. May become blind

145. A 2-year-old is admitted with bacterial meningitis. The priority nursing intervention is to:

1. Complete neurological checks
2. Take vital signs
3. Administer antibiotics
4. Encourage good nutrition

146. A nurse enters the room of a 36-year-old client who is speaking as if someone else is in the room. He wants to introduce the nurse to his friend. The nurse's best response is to:

1. Offer to give him some medication.
2. Tell him that no one is there except the client and nurse.
3. Ask him what the person's name is.
4. Ask him to describe his friend.

147. A delusional client thinks the rest of the clients are "out to take his things." The best nursing response to this behavior is:

1. Ignore it because it is not hurting anyone.
2. Correct the thinking each time the client says it.
3. Involve the client in a physical activity.
4. Ask the client to clarify what he means.

148. A 22-year-old client is admitted for emergency surgery because of an ectopic pregnancy. Priority nursing intervention for this client is:

1. Getting a signed consent for sterilization
2. Obtaining a type and cross-match for blood replacement
3. Giving her postoperative instructions
4. Obtaining a thorough obstetrical history

149. A 42-year-old client has just delivered a stillborn infant. She is rather upset and quietly crying. The nurse's best response to comfort her is:

1. Assure her that everything will be okay.
2. Ask her if she would like to talk about why she is crying.
3. Tell her to not worry; she can have another baby.
4. Tell her that this is best because the baby would have had other problems.

150. A 10-year-old child is admitted to the pediatric unit with glomerulonephritis. The first nursing priority is:

1. Checking blood pressure
2. Checking stool for occult blood
3. Preparing for a urinary catheterization
4. Preparing for insertion of a gastrointestinal (GI) tube

151. A 6-month-old client is brought to the pediatric clinic with diarrhea. The nurse would be sure to check:

1. Blood pressure
2. Skin turgor
3. For decreased respirations
4. For decreased pulse

152. A nurse is visiting the home of a 4-year-old client with hemophilia. A priority area to check for bleeding is the:

1. Thorax
2. Abdomen
3. Skull
4. Joints

153. A 3-month-old client has congenital hip dysplasia. The nurse would teach the parents to:

1. Keep the child's hips wrapped in blankets.
2. Keep the child's hips aligned with the feet.
3. Carry the child straddling the hip.
4. Carry the child in a manner that keeps the legs straight.

154. A 2-year-old has had diarrhea for 2 days. Which of the following would the nurse instruct the parents to avoid?

1. Apple juice
2. Cooked carrots
3. Creamed soup
4. Applesauce

155. The nurse is teaching the parents of a 1-year-old child to administer eardrops for otitis media. The nurse instructs them to:

1. Pull the pinna up and back before giving the drops.
2. Pull the pinna down and back before giving the drops.
3. Pull the pinna forward and down after giving the drops.
4. Pull the pinna straight toward them before giving the drops.

156. The 19-year-old parents of a 3-week-old newborn bring their child to the clinic because he is vomiting every time he eats. The physician determines that this is normal newborn regurgitation. The nurse reassures the parents by explaining that this normal because the:

1. Formula is richer than breast milk
2. Stomach is very small
3. Cardiac sphincter is not fully mature
4. Stomach lining is easily irritated

157. A 2-month-old client has had surgical repair of a cleft lip. The nurse teaches the parents to feed the baby using a:

1. Teaspoon
2. Small plastic cup
3. Bottle with a soft nipple
4. Syringe with a soft catheter

158. A 15-month-old child has tetrology of Fallot and will have surgery in 2 months. What toy does the nurse recommend for the child?

1. Stacking blocks
2. A pull toy
3. A horn
4. Bouncing balls

159. A 7-year-old client has a diagnosis of hypothyroidism and is placed on levothyroxine. The nurse instructs the parents to give the medicine:

1. Until symptoms disappear
2. Daily in the morning
3. Until constipation develops
4. Until weight is stabilized

160. A mother brings her 9-year-old daughter to the clinic because she is overweight. What is the best advice to give the mother to help her child lose weight?

1. As she progresses in school, she will become more active and lose weight naturally.
2. Eliminate all sweets from the diet.
3. Give her large doses of supplemental vitamins to suppress the appetite.
4. Begin a program of activity and exercise.

161. The nurse is monitoring the blood pressure of a 23-year-old client in active labor. The nurse takes her blood pressure:

1. During contractions
2. Between contractions
3. Immediately after contractions
4. At the peak of contractions

162. A newborn with meningomyelocele is delivered to the nursery. In what position would the nurse place the child?

1. Side-lying
2. Prone
3. Dorsal
4. Fowler's

163. A 28-year-old woman who has been raped presents herself in the emergency room. The nurse's first action is to:

1. Report it to the police.
2. Report it to the supervisor.
3. Determine her most immediate needs.
4. Call her family for support.

164. Three hours after delivery, a 22-year-old client complains of severe perineal pain. Which nursing strategy has priority?

1. Give her an ordered pain medicine.
2. Check her fundus.
3. Inspect her perineum.
4. Give a sitz bath.

165. Percussion and postural drainage are ordered for a 6-month-old child with tracheobronchitis When is the best time to schedule this intervention?

1. Immediately after meals
2. Immediately before meals
3. Just before play time
4. Midway between meals

166. A 6-year-old child being seen at the school clinic has a diagnosis of lead poisoning. Lead poisoning can lead to:

1. Increased urination
2. Decreased urination
3. Malnutrition
4. Anemia

167. A nurse's 17-year-old neighbor admits to having sexual activity and is now having a thick white discharge. The nurse tells her to:

1. Drink lots of water and if it does not go away in 2 days, go to the clinic.
2. Not to worry about it just yet; this is a natural occurrence and will go away on its own.

3. Suggest that she be seen as soon as possible in the clinic; she may have a sexually transmitted disease.
4. Tell her mother.

168. As part of the school health clinic staff, a nurse notices that a 12-year-old child has illegible handwriting and continuously transposes figures. The nurse refers him for further testing because she suspects:

1. Aphasia
2. A learning disability
3. Visual problems
4. A neurological disorder

169. An 8-year-old client has a seizure disorder. In preparing the environment to protect the child from injury during a seizure, the nurse would:

1. Place a wooden tongue blade near the bedside.
2. Place a plastic bite block near the bedside.
3. Keep restraints near the bedside to be used in case of a seizure.
4. Keep a syringe of antiseizure medication at the bedside.

170. The nurse is giving medication instructions to a 45-year-old client with minimal English skills. The best way to ensure compliance is to:

1. Speak slowly.
2. Exaggerate the words.
3. Speak loudly.
4. Provide written instructions.

171. A 12-year-old client needs a leg operation. Who should sign the consent form?

1. The mother
2. The father
3. Both the mother and father
4. Let the parents decide

172. A 68-year-old Islamic male client needs to have a urinary catheter inserted. Who is the best person to do the procedure?

1. A female registered nurse
2. A male orderly
3. The client's wife
4. A male LPN

173. An 82-year-old traditional Native American female client does not maintain eye contact with the nurse when the nurse is giving discharge instructions. The nurse should interpret this behavior to mean that:

1. She does not understand the instructions.
2. She is not interested in the instructions.
3. This is probably normal in her culture.
4. She prefers a physician to give the instructions.

174. The father of a Vietnamese child with bronchitis is rubbing the child's back with a coin. The coin leaves red marks. The nurse should:

1. Suspect the possibility of child abuse.
2. Recognize this as a traditional healing method among Vietnamese.
3. Not allow the father to be alone with his child.

4. Forbid this practice while the child is in the hospital.

175. A 45-year-old client is scheduled for knee surgery. Because he does not like the hospital food, his wife brings food from home. He is on a regular diet. The nurse's first response is to:

1. Ask her to not do this. It is against hospital policy.
2. Make a referral to the dietitian.
3. Allow the client to eat the food.
4. Take the food away.

176. A 67-year-old Japanese client has been given a diagnosis of cancer of the liver. The family does not want the client to know. Which of the following is the most appropriate initial action?

1. Tell him anyway; it is his right to know.
2. Respect the family's wishes.
3. Refer the situation to the ethics committee.
4. Insist that the family tell the client.

177. A 57-year-old Mexican client with a myocardial infarction has been transferred to the cardiac step-down unit. The extended family comes to visit. The most appropriate action is to:

1. Restrict visitors to two at a time.
2. Ask for a family member to help control visitors on a rotational basis.
3. Ask the physician to speak with the family.
4. Act as the control person.

178. A 35-year-old client in a long-term care facility has terminal breast cancer. She is taking herbal tea for her indigestion. The nurse's first action is to:

1. Carefully explain that herbal teas are not permitted.
2. Report the situation to her physician.
3. Report the situation to the pharmacist.
4. Allow her to take the herbal teas.

179. A 34-year-old client with a new diagnosis of insulin-dependent diabetes refuses to take insulin when she goes home. She tells the nurse that God will take care of her. The nurse's most appropriate action is to:

1. Ask her physician to prescribe an oral hypoglycemic agent.
2. Have the chaplain talk with her.
3. Ask her physician to talk with her about this "nonsense."
4. Explain to her that God cannot heal diabetes.

180. A 72-year-old Filipino client is in the long-term care facility for cancer of the lung. The client is reluctant to cough and deep breathe, maintains a rigid position in bed, and refuses needed pain medication. The best initial approach is to:

1. Give the pain medication.
2. Ask the physician to order the medicine around the clock instead of on an as-needed basis.
3. Explore the reasons for not taking the pain medication.
4. Report the situation to the nursing supervisor.

181. A 63-year-old client being prepared for surgery becomes visibly upset when the nurse tries to remove a beaded bracelet from the client's wrist. The nurse should:

1. Tape the bracelet in place.
2. Encourage the family to remove the bracelet.
3. Delay the surgery until the bracelet is removed.
4. Enclose the hand and wrist in a mitten.

182. A 42-year-old laminectomy client is discharged home. He tells the nurse that he still has pain and is going to see an acupuncturist when he gets home. What is the nurse's best response?

1. "The acupuncturist may ruin the surgery."
2. "Be sure to tell your physician that you are seeing an acupuncturist, and be sure to tell the acupuncturist that you have had a laminectomy."
3. "The acupuncture cannot do as much good as the surgery."
4. "I do not think that is a good idea."

183. A 45-year-old home-care client on crutches is demonstrating her crutch walking for the nurse. The nurse knows that she is using the crutches correctly if she:

1. Has both feet far apart
2. Places her weight on the axilla
3. Places her weight on the palms of her hands
4. Does not swing her weight through the crutches

184. During a home visit to a client, her husband tells the nurse that he is experiencing urinary frequency, extreme thirst, and blurred vision. What is the nurse's best advice?

1. Encourage him to make an appointment with his physician as soon as possible; he may have diabetes mellitus.
2. Instruct him to go to the emergency room immediately.
3. Tell him it is probably nothing to worry about, but if it continues, he should make an appointment with his physician.
4. Call the supervisor and ask for advice.

185. A 22-year-old client had an allergic reaction to a home permanent. She is being discharged from the emergency room with a prescription for methylprednisolone tablets. The nurse stresses the importance of:

1. Taking the pills as long as her symptoms continue.
2. Completing the medication exactly as instructed or some serious complications can develop.
3. Taking the medicine at bedtime.
4. Taking the medicine before breakfast.

186. A 60-year-old client has a 15-year history of heavy alcohol abuse. The nurse's priority intervention is to:

1. Increase nutritional status
2. Increase fluid intake
3. Monitor neurological status
4. Monitor vital signs

187. The nurse is giving discharge instructions in the emergency room to a client with cholecystitis. What foods are important for the client to avoid?

    1. Meats
    2. Fruits high in sugar
    3. Fatty foods
    4. Vegetables high in fiber

188. As part of a community health fair, a nurse is teaching residents to do breast self-examinations. The best time to conduct the breast self-examination is:

    1. First of the month
    2. End of the month
    3. 3 days before the menses begins
    4. 3 days after the menses begins

189. A 56-year-old client with cirrhosis and renal failure has pruritus. To help decrease the itching, the nurse suggests:

    1. Taking a bath with very warm water
    2. Keeping his bedroom temperature between 80 and 85°F (26.6 and 29.4°C)
    3. Avoiding soap in the bath water as much as possible
    4. Using perfumed lotion after bathing

190. The nurse is evaluating the hemodialysis shunt on a 54-year-old client. A functioning shunt would:

    1. Be cool to touch
    2. Have a visible pulsation
    3. Have a palpable rush of blood
    4. Be outlined with erythematous skin

191. A 42-year-old ambulatory client who has had abdominal surgery just had the wound edges separate. What is the nurse's priority action?

    1. Put the client back to bed.
    2. Place moist saline gauze over the wound.
    3. Call the physician.
    4. Medicate the client for pain.

192. A 76-year-old client with CHF has just expired. Several family members are at the bedside. One of the daughters sits on the floor and begins to wail. The nurse would:

    1. Tell her that everything will be okay.
    2. Help her to sit in a chair.
    3. Call the physician for a tranquilizer.
    4. Stay close to her and ask if she needs anything.

193. An 87-year-old client in the long-term care facility has chronic constipation. The first priority is dietary control. Which of the following foods will help to decrease constipation?

    1. Lean meat and meat by-products
    2. Fruits and vegetables
    3. Poultry and fish
    4. Rice and potatoes

194. A 76-year-old home-care client has angina pectoris. When he has an attack, he should first:

    1. Take a nitroglycerin tablet
    2. Call the rescue squad
    3. Stop all activity
    4. Ignore the pain for at least 3 minutes before taking nitroglycerin

195. A 24-year-old client is in hypovolemic shock secondary to hemorrhage. The most significant change in vital signs that indicates worsening of the condition includes:

    1. A decrease in pulse rate.
    2. An increase in respirations.
    3. A decrease in respirations.
    4. An increase in pulse rate.

196. A 54-year-old client who has had major abdominal surgery has been returned to the nursing unit from the recovery room. The best position for comfort is:

    1. High-Fowler's position
    2. Semi-Fowler's position
    3. Prone
    4. Supine

197. A 52-year-old home-care client is 3 days' postprostatectomy. Priority teaching includes:

    1. Drinking at least 3000 mL of fluid each day
    2. Avoiding citrus drinks
    3. Avoiding milk and milk products
    4. Drinking only cranberry and apple juices

198. A 53-year-old mastectomy client has a Hemo-Vac in place. After emptying the Hemo-Vac, the nurse would:

    1. Place it in a dependent position to improve drainage.
    2. Completely collapse the Hemo-Vac before reinserting the air plug.
    3. Milk the tubing every 2 hours to prevent clotting.
    4. Reattach it to the wall suctioning unit.

199. A 33-year-old client is recovering from an endoscopy. Before giving fluids, the most important assessment is determining:

    1. A gag reflex
    2. Thirst
    3. Bowel sounds
    4. Degree of alertness

200. The nurse in an endocrine referral clinic is reviewing the records for the day's appointments. One of the clients has Cushing's syndrome. The nurse would expect this client to have the following appearance:

    1. Truncal obesity and hirsutism
    2. Enlarged hands and feet
    3. A large jaw and large feet
    4. A buffalo hump and large hands

201. The client was diagnosed as having hypothyroidism. The physician placed her on levothyroxine (Synthroid) 0.3 mg PO every day. The tablets are

labeled 300 μg. How many tablets would the nurse give the client?

1. ¹/₂ tablet
2. 1 tablet
3. 2 tablets
4. 3 tablets

202. The client was having grand mal seizures. The physician ordered phenytoin (Dilantin) suspension 150 mg PO tid to be given via the nasogastric tube. The stock supply was labeled 75 mg/7.5 mL. How many milliliters need to be given to fulfill the order?

1. 7.5 mL
2. 10 mL
3. 15 mL
4. 20 mL

203. A 90-year-old nursing home resident developed a severe cough that was accompanied by pleurisy pain. The physician ordered the cough with hydromorphone (Dilaudid) cough syrup 1 mg prn. Using a 1-mg/5-mL elixir, how many milliliters did the nurse administer?

1. 2 mL
2. 3 mL
3. 4 mL
4. 5 mL

204. Your client, age 68 years, is a newly diagnosed non–insulin-dependent diabetic. The physician ordered chlorpropamide (Diabinese) 150 mg PO bid. The pharmacy sent Diabinese 0.1-g tablets. The nurse will administer how many tablets to the client?

1. 1 tablet
2. 1.5 tablets
3. 2 tablets
4. 2.5 tablets

205. A 76-year-old nursing home resident was complaining about not sleeping at night. The physician ordered chloral hydrate (Noctec) 500 mg 30 minutes before sleep. Using a 250-mg/5-mL elixir, how many milliliters did the nurse administer?

1. 6 mL
2. 8 mL
3. 10 mL
4. 12 mL

1. **(1)** Integrated processes: nursing process — evaluation; client need: physiological integrity; physiological adaptation; content area: medical-surgical.

   RATIONALE
   (1) Although other factors may rarely cause myocardial infarction, the most common cause is atherosclerosis. **(2)** The primary cause of myocardial infarction is atherosclerosis. **(3)** The primary cause of myocardial infarction is atherosclerosis. **(4)** The primary cause of myocardial infarction is atherosclerosis.

2. **(2)** Integrated processes: nursing process — data collection; client need: physiological integrity; physiological adaptation; content area: medical-surgical.

   RATIONALE
   (1) Less than 20 mL/hr is not enough to keep renal perfusion within normal parameters. **(2)** The minimum expected hourly urine output in shock is 30 mL/hr. **(3)** This amount is too great to expect from a client recovering from cardiogenic shock. **(4)** This amount is too great to expect from a client recovering from cardiogenic shock.

3. **(3)** Integrated processes: nursing process — evaluation; client need: physiological integrity; pharmacological therapies; content area: medical-surgical.

   RATIONALE
   (1) Diphenhydramine is the second medicine to have available. **(2)** Methlyprednisolone may or may not be given; determined by the allergic reaction. **(3)** The first emergency drug in an allergic reaction is epinephrine. **(4)** Sodium bicarbonate is not used as a first-line drug in anaphylaxis.

4. **(4)** Integrated processes: nursing process — data collection; client need: physiological integrity; physiological adaptation; content area: medical-surgical.

   RATIONALE
   (1) In shock, the blood pressure drops and the pulse increases to compensate. **(2)** In shock, the blood pressure drops and the pulse increases to compensate. **(3)** In shock, the blood pressure drops and the pulse increases to compensate. **(4)** In shock, the blood pressure drops and the pulse increases to compensate.

5. **(2)** Integrated processes: nursing process — data collection; client need: physiological integrity; physiological adaptation; content area: medical-surgical.

   RATIONALE
   (1) There is no pain in third-degree burns. **(2)** As large areas of skin are burned, large amounts of fluids are lost. **(3)** Nutrition is important but not the highest priority. **(4)** Circulation, altered is not an acceptable nursing diagnosis.

6. **(1)** Integrated processes: nursing process — implementation; client need: physiological integrity; physiological adaptation; content area: medical-surgical.

   RATIONALE
   (1) The physician should order the client's positioning; however, the semi-Fowler's is used to decrease intracranial pressure. **(2)** This position will not decrease intracranial pressure. **(3)** This position will not decrease intracranial pressure. **(4)** This position will not decrease intracranial pressure.

7. **(1)** Integrated processes: nursing process — evaluation; client need: physiological integrity; physiological adaptation; content area: medical-surgical.

   RATIONALE
   (1) Widened pulse pressure is indicative of increased intracranial pressure. **(2)** This pattern is not a widened pulse pressure. **(3)** This pattern is not a widened pulse pressure. **(4)** This pattern is not a widened pulse pressure; it is a narrowed pulse pressure, which occurs in shock.

8. **(1)** Integrated processes: nursing process — implementation; client need: physiological integrity; pharmacological therapies; content area: medical-surgical.

   RATIONALE
   (1) Electrolyte imbalance of potassium affects the conduction system of the heart, causing abnormal rates or rhythm. **(2)** Potassium does not have a direct effect on the blood pressure. **(3)** Potassium does not have an effect on urinary output. **(4)** Potassium does not have a primary effect on the urine specific gravity.

9. **(2)** Integrated processes: nursing process — evaluation; client need: physiological integrity; reduction of risk potential; content area: medical-surgical.

   RATIONALE
   (1) Serum transaminase is not diagnostic of pancreatitis. **(2)** Severity of pancreatitis is directly correlated to level of amylase, a pancreatic enzyme. **(3)** Serum sodium is not diagnostic of pancreatitis. **(4)** Serum magnesium levels are not diagnostic of pancreatitis, although clients with pancreatitis frequently have low magnesium levels.

10. **(1, 5, 6)** Integrated processes: nursing process — evaluation; client need: physiological integrity; reduction of risk potential; content area: medical-surgical.

    RATIONALE
    (1) Ice chips deplete electrolytes by washing out stomach fluid contents. **(2)** Glycerine can be comforting to the client. **(3)** Hard candies can be comforting to the client, although they should be limited in quantity. **(4)** Peroxide gargles can be comforting to the client without depleting electrolytes. **(5)** Hard candies, not soft candies, can be comforting to the client. **(6)** Excessive cold water depletes electrolytes by washing out stomach fluid contents.

11. **(1)** Integrated processes: nursing process — data collection; client need: physiological integrity; reduction of risk potential; content area: medical-surgical.

    RATIONALE
    (1) Establishing an airway always has highest priority. **(2)** This option is appropriate but does not have the highest priority. **(3)** This option is appropriate but does not have the highest priority. **(4)** This option is appropriate but does not have the highest priority.

12. **(3)** Integrated processes: nursing process — evaluation; client need: physiological integrity; physiological adaptation; content area: medical-surgical.

    RATIONALE
    (1) In the oliguric stage, the client does not put out much urine. **(2)** In the initial phase, the client is usually oliguric. **(3)** The

abnormally large amount of urine output indicates the diuretic phase. (4) The recovery phase is not a recognized term for urinary output for clients in renal failure.

13. (2, 6) Integrated processes: nursing process — data collection; client need: physiological integrity; physiological adaptation; content area: medical-surgical.

RATIONALE
(1) Renal failure clients have problems with hyperkalemia, not hypokalemia. Hypokalemia does not occur with renal failure. (2) Hyperkalemia causes cardiac rhythm problems because of retention of potassium. (3) Hyponatremia is not a common problem with renal failure. (4) Hypernatremia is not as serious as hyperkalemia. (5) Bone disease due to renal osteodystrophy from hyperphosphatemia and hypocalcemia occurs in chronic renal failure. (6) Bone disease due to renal osteodystrophy from hyperphosphatemia and hypocalcemia occurs in chronic renal failure.

14. (3) Integrated processes: nursing process — implementation; client need: physiological integrity; basic care and comfort; content area: medical-surgical.

RATIONALE
(1) Wool blankets increase pruritus. (2) Keeping a room at this temperature increases perspiring and increases pruritus. (3) A decrease in sweating decreases pruritus. (4) Soap residue can increase sweating or cause further skin irritation and pruritus.

15. (2) Integrated processes: nursing process — data collection; client need: physiological integrity; pharmacological therapies; content area: medical-surgical.

RATIONALE
(1) Fatigue may be a side effect of chemotherapy, but the most common side effect is nausea. (2) Nausea is the most common side effect of chemotherapy. (3) Dehydration may be a side effect of chemotherapy, but the most common side effect is nausea. (4) Skin ulceration may be a side effect of chemotherapy, but the most common side effect is nausea.

16. (4) Integrated processes: nursing process — evaluation; client need: psychosocial integrity; content area: psychiatric nursing.

RATIONALE
(1) Confabulation does not prevent aggression. (2) The person does not confabulate to get attention but confabulates for self-esteem. (3) Confabulation does not denote acute psychosis. (4) Confabulation increases self-esteem.

17. (2) Integrated processes: nursing process — implementation; client need: safe, effective care environment; coordinated care; content area: medical-surgical.

RATIONALE
(1) Chlamydial infection is not reportable to the health department. (2) Syphilis is federally mandated to be reported in all states. (3) Nonspecific urethritis is not reportable to the health department. (4) Herpes is not reportable to the health department.

18. (3) Integrated processes: nursing process — evaluation; client need: physiological integrity; physiological adaptation; content area: medical-surgical.

RATIONALE
(1) The majority of oxygen is carried in the RBCs, not the serum. (2) The majority of oxygen is carried in the RBCs, not the plasma. (3) RBCs carry oxygen to the tissues in the body and give up carbon dioxide when passing through the lungs. (4) WBCs do not carry oxygen.

19. (3) Integrated processes: nursing process — evaluation; client need: physiological integrity; pharmacological therapies; content area: medical-surgical.

RATIONALE
(1) NS is 0.9. (2) NS is 0.9. (3) NS is 0.9. (4) NS is 0.9.

20. (4) Integrated processes: nursing process — evaluation; client need: physiological integrity; pharmacological therapies; content area: medical-surgical.

RATIONALE
(1) Extravasation is a common complication of IV therapy. (2) Phlebitis is a common complication of IV therapy. (3) Infiltration is a common complication of IV therapy. (4) Renal shutdown is a result of hypovolemic states; it is not a complication of IV therapy.

21. (3) Integrated processes: nursing process — implementation; client need: physiological integrity; reduction of risk potential; content area: medical-surgical.

RATIONALE
(1) A tracheostomy tube cannot be used for nutrition. (2) A tracheostomy tube cannot be used to relieve flatus. (3) A tracheostomy is defined as creation of an artificial airway. (4) Tracheostomy decreases dead space.

22. (4) Integrated processes: nursing process — implementation; client need: physiological integrity; reduction of risk potential; content area: medical-surgical.

RATIONALE
(1) Keeping the client on the unaffected side deters drainage. (2) Keeping a water seal is a function of the drainage system, not the level of the system. (3) Repositioning will help drainage only when the client is on the affected side. This is not the best response. (4) Turning the client on the affected side is the best way to promote drainage.

23. (4) Integrated processes: nursing process — evaluation; client need: physiological integrity; reduction of risk potential; content area: medical-surgical.

RATIONALE
(1) A subclavian catheter goes into a vein; therefore, it cannot cause an arterial spasm. (2) A subclavian catheter cannot cause a pulmonary infection. (3) Phlebitis is a later complication, not one that can occur on insertion. (4) Air embolism can occur on insertion of a subclavian catheter if the entry port is not occluded.

24. (4) Integrated processes: nursing process — evaluation; client need: physiological integrity; reduction of risk potential; content area: medical-surgical.

RATIONALE
(1) Some swelling of the toes is expected. (2) Depending on the reason for the cast, some blood drainage is expected. (3) Toes may be cool (not cold) from inactivity. (4) Loss of sensation in the toes may indicate that the cast is too tight and should be reported to the physician.

25. (2) Integrated processes: nursing process — data collection; client need: health promotion and maintenance; content area: medical-surgical.

RATIONALE
(1) Headache is a common symptom of hypertension. (2) Nausea is not a symptom of hypertension. (3) Vertigo is a common symptom of hypertension. (4) Epistaxis is a common symptom of hypertension.

26. (See figure) Integrated processes: nursing process — data collection; client need: physiological integrity; physiological adaptation; content area: medical-surgical.

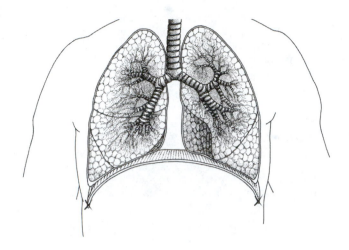

RATIONALE
Pleural effusion is defined as fluid in the pleural cavity between the visceral and parietal pleura.

27. **(1)** Integrated processes: nursing process — data collection; client need: physiological integrity; physiological adaptation; content area: medical-surgical.

RATIONALE
(1) Anasarca is defined as severe, generalized edema. **(2)** Pitting is a term to describe the degree of edema. **(3)** Ascites is fluid in the abdomen. **(4)** Lymphedema describes fluid in the lymphatic drainage system but is not generalized.

28. **(2)** Integrated processes: nursing process — evaluation; client need: physiological integrity; physiological adaptation; content area: medical-surgical.

RATIONALE
(1) Myxedema is a thyroid disorder. **(2)** Acromegaly is the disorder that causes these symptoms in adults. **(3)** Gigantism is a disease of children that causes abnormal long bone growth. **(4)** Addison's disease is a disease of the adrenal glands that causes mineralocorticoid abnormalities.

29. **(3)** Integrated processes: nursing process — evaluation; client need: physiological integrity; physiological adaptation; content area: medical-surgical.

RATIONALE
(1) Acromegaly is a disorder that causes enlargement of the hands, feet, and facial bones. **(2)** Myxedema is a hypothyroid disorder. **(3)** In Cushing's disease, a hypersecretion of the adrenal cortex occurs with an excessive production of glucocorticoids, resulting in these symptoms. **(4)** Graves' disease is a hyperthyroid condition.

30. **(4)** Integrated processes: nursing process — implementation; client need: physiological integrity; reduction of risk potential; content area: medical-surgical.

RATIONALE
(1) There are no contraindications to taking an oral temperature in this client. **(2)** There are no contraindications to taking an oral temperature in this client. **(3)** There are no contraindications to taking an oral temperature in this client. **(4)** Taking an oral temperature reading is contraindicated in older, confused clients because of potential injury.

31. **(2)** Integrated processes: nursing process — implementation; client need: health promotion and maintenance; content area: maternity nursing.

RATIONALE
(1) These clients have well-developed temperature-regulating mechanisms. **(2)** A newborn infant's body temperature-regulating mechanism is immature, and infants are greatly influenced by environmental temperatures and must be protected from extreme changes. **(3)** These clients have well-developed temperature-regulating mechanisms. **(4)** These clients have well-developed temperature-regulating mechanisms.

32. **(1, 4, 5)** Integrated processes: nursing process — implementation; client need: physiological integrity; reduction of risk potential; content area: medical-surgical.

RATIONALE
(1) The upper arm (site of brachial artery) is usually used for measuring blood pressure. **(2)** The femoral artery cannot be used for measuring blood pressure. **(3)** The carotid artery is not usually used for measuring the blood pressure. **(4)** The radial artery is sometimes used to measure the blood pressure, especially in hypotensive clients. **(5)** The popliteal pulse behind the knee can be used to measure the blood pressure, especially in hypotensive clients. **(6)** This is a vein, not an artery.

33. **(3)** Integrated processes: nursing process — implementation; client need: physiological integrity; physiological adaptation; content area: medical-surgical.

RATIONALE
(1) Tachycardia is a term meaning a fast heart rate. **(2)** Diastole is the period of time that the heart is at rest. **(3)** Pulse rhythm is the pattern of the beats and the intervals between beats. An irregular rhythm is called an arrhythmia, taken from the Latin word for "without rhythm." **(4)** Bradycardia is a term meaning a slow heart rate.

34. **(1)** Integrated processes: nursing process — implementation; client need: physiological integrity; reduction of risk potential; content area: medical-surgical.

RATIONALE
(1) The apical site is routinely used to assess the pulse of infants and children up to 3 years of age. The average pulse of an infant is 125 bpm or more, and a rapid rate is more accurately determined when the pulse is taken apically. **(2)** The radial pulse is not the preferred site for taking a pulse in an infant. **(3)** The femoral pulse is not the preferred site for taking a pulse in an infant. **(4)** The temporal pulse is not the preferred site for taking a pulse in an infant.

35. **(4)** Integrated processes: nursing process — implementation; client need: physiological integrity; physiological adaptation; content area: medical-surgical.

RATIONALE
(1) Pulse pressure is the difference between the systolic and diastolic pressures. **(2)** Maximal pressure is not an acceptable term. **(3)** Systolic pressure is the pressure exerted on the vessel wall at the end of ventricular contraction. **(4)** Blood moves in waves, and the *diastolic pressure* is the pressure when the ventricles are at rest—the lower pressure, present at all times within the arteries.

36. **(2)** Integrated processes: nursing process — implementation; client need: physiological integrity; reduction of risk potential; content area: medical-surgical.

RATIONALE
(1) This blood pressure is considered low. **(2)** The average blood pressure of a healthy young adult is 120/80 mm Hg. **(3)**

This blood pressure indicates hypertension. (4) This blood pressure indicates hypertension.

37. (4) Integrated processes: nursing process — implementation; client need: physiological integrity; reduction of risk potential; content area: medical-surgical.
RATIONALE
(1) Both arms are in long casts; the nurse cannot take a brachial pulse. (2) Both arms are in long casts; the nurse cannot take a brachial pulse. (3) Both arms are in long casts; the nurse cannot take a radial pulse. (4) There are nine common peripheral pulse sites. Because of the bilateral casts in this situation, only the carotid or femoral arteries are accessible for palpation.

38. (3) Integrated processes: nursing process — data collection; client need: physiological integrity; physiological adaptation; content area: medical-surgical.
RATIONALE
(1) Planning is the second stage of the nursing process. (2) Implementation is the third stage of the nursing process. (3) Data collection is the first stage of the nursing process; it includes gathering objective and subjective data and verification. (4) Evaluation is the last stage of the nursing process.

39. (2) Integrated processes: nursing process — data collection; client need: physiological integrity; physiological adaptation; content area: medical-surgical.
RATIONALE
(1) The problem is the stem. (2) The etiology of the problem or contributing factors is the second part of a nursing diagnosis statement. (3) Evaluation occurs as the result of nursing interventions. (4) Signs and symptoms are the contributing factors.

40. (1) Integrated processes: nursing process — implementation; client need: physiological integrity; pharmacological therapies; content area: medical-surgical.
RATIONALE
(1) Implementation is putting nursing strategies into action in this situation, a dependent nursing action (physician's order). (2) Evaluation occurs after the acetaminophen has been given and is based on a reassessment of the contributing factors. (3) Planning occurs after a nursing diagnosis is formulated. (4) Reassessment occurs as a result of evaluation findings.

41. (2) Integrated processes: nursing process — data collection; client need: physiological integrity; physiological adaptation; content area: medical-surgical.
RATIONALE
(1) Planning occurs after the nursing diagnosis is formulated. (2) Data collection is collecting objective and subjective data and verification. (3) Analysis occurs to formulate the diagnosis. (4) To evaluate is to judge or appraise; in this case, the client's response to the medication given.

42. (2) Integrated processes: nursing process — data collection; client need: health promotion and maintenance; content area: medical-surgical.
RATIONALE
(1) Constant data do not change. (2) Objective data are data that are detectable by the observer, in this case, dry skin and parched oral mucous membranes. Objective data can be seen, heard, felt, or smelled. (3) Subjective data are data that the client tells the nurse about. (4) Modifiable data are data that can

be changed. This is not a commonly used term in nursing data collection.

43. (4) Integrated processes: nursing process — data collection; client need: health promotion and maintenance; content area: medical-surgical.
RATIONALE
(1) Shallow respirations are a client weakness. (2) Irregular pulse is a client weakness. (3) A history of bronchial asthma is a client weakness. (4) Normal weight is one client strength. Nurses need to assess strengths as well as weaknesses.

44. (2, 5) Integrated processes: nursing process — implementation; client need: physiological integrity; physiological adaptation; content area: medical-surgical.
RATIONALE
(1) Fever is likely to cause an increase in blood pressure. (2) Hypotension may be caused by excessive blood loss (hemorrhage), as a result of the decreased blood volume. When circulating blood volume falls, as in hemorrhage, the blood pressure falls. (3) Stress is likely to increase blood pressure. (4) Obesity is likely to cause an increase in blood pressure. (5) Anaphylactic shock can result in hypotension. (6) Although increased intracranial pressure causes a widening of the pulse pressure, it may not result in hypotension.

45. (4) Integrated processes: nursing process — implementation; client need: physiological integrity; reduction of risk potential; content area: medical-surgical.
RATIONALE
(1) The diastolic pressure is the last sound heard on release of pressure. (2) Venous pressure is not a term used in measuring blood pressure. (3) Pulse pressure is the difference between the systolic and diastolic readings. (4) The point on the manometer when the first clear Korotkoff sound is heard (contraction of the ventricles) indicates systolic blood pressure.

46. (3) Integrated processes: nursing process — implementation; client need: safe, effective care environment; coordinated care; content area: medical-surgical.
RATIONALE
(1) There is no acceptable method of making a correction in a medical record as stated other than option 3. (2) There is no acceptable method of making a correction in a medical record other than option 3. (3) If an error is made in charting, the nurse should not erase it or scratch it out but should draw a line through the error, write the word "error," and sign or initial it above. (4) There is no acceptable method of making a correction in a medical record other than option 3.

47. (2) Integrated processes: nursing process — implementation; client need: safe, effective care environment; coordinated care; content area: medical-surgical.
RATIONALE
(1) The graphic sheet is a record of vital signs. (2) Information is grouped according to the source or the health-care department in this type of record. (3) Progress notes contain the physician's recording. (4) Nurses' notes contain nurses' documentations.

48. (3) Integrated processes: nursing process — implementation; client need: safe, effective care environment; coordinated care; content area: medical-surgical.
RATIONALE
(1) There is no standard abbreviation for this phrase. (2) There is no standard abbreviation for this phrase. (3) WPO is a uni-

versal abbreviation. Many abbreviations are taken from root Latin or Greek words (*per ora*). (**4**) There is no standard abbreviation for this phrase.

49. (**4**) Integrated processes: nursing process — implementation; client need: safe, effective care environment; coordinated care; content area: medical-surgical.
   RATIONALE
   (**1**) Collecting a urine specimen would come later. (**2**) Assisting the client to undress is a later priority. (**3**) Taking and recording vital signs would be a second priority. (**4**) One of the most important steps in the admission procedure is to make the client feel welcome, orient him or her to the new surroundings, and allay any anxieties.

50. (**1**) Integrated processes: nursing process — implementation; client need: physiological integrity; reduction of risk potential; content area: medical-surgical.
   RATIONALE
   (**1**) The ABCs (airway, breathing, circulation) are always the first priority. Rapid, irregular respirations of 32/min needs immediate intervention. (**2**) Skin warm, flushed, and dry does not take as high a priority as increased respirations. (**3**) This slight temperature elevation is not a priority. (**4**) Dry, unproductive cough is not a priority.

51. (**4**) Integrated processes: nursing process — implementation; client need: physiological integrity; physiological adaptation; content area: medical-surgical.
   RATIONALE
   (**1**) Shallow respirations do not necessarily mean that the client is compromised. (**2**) Rapid breathing is called tachypnea and could be a physiological compensatory mechanism. (**3**) Fowler's position enhances breathing by promoting lung expansion. (**4**) Dyspnea means difficult breathing (taken from the Greek *dys* for "difficult" and *pnea* for "breath").

52. (**1**) Integrated processes: nursing process — implementation; client need: physiological integrity; reduction of risk potential; content area: medical-surgical.
   RATIONALE
   (**1**) In Fowler's position the head and knees are elevated, facilitating breathing. (**2**) Lying on the side is not as effective as the semi-Fowler's or Fowler's position and may aggravate the client's dyspnea. (**3**) Sims' position will aggravate the client's dyspnea. (**4**) The dorsal recumbent position will aggravate the client's dyspnea.

53. (**2**) Integrated processes: nursing process — implementation; client need: physiological integrity; reduction of risk potential; content area: medical-surgical.
   RATIONALE
   (**1**) Skin lotions do not interfere with oxygen. (**2**) Oxygen is a highly combustible gas that can easily ignite on contact with a spark. The nurse should promote the client's safety by posting "No smoking" signs and by explaining that smoking is not permitted when oxygen is in use. (**3**) The flow rate is 3 L, not 4 L. (**4**) All rooms should be well ventilated.

54. (**3**) Integrated processes: nursing process — implementation, teaching/learning; client need: health promotion and maintenance; content area: medical-surgical.
   RATIONALE
   (**1**) A client who takes anti-inflammatory medications may be increasing his or her chance of developing osteoporosis.

(**2**) All clients should have a yearly checkup, but this does not answer the question in relation to osteoporosis. (**3**) Adequate calcium intake and exercise have been found to delay some of the bone mineral loss associated with osteoporosis and aging. (**4**) Encouraging walking would help calcium absorption.

55. (**4**) Integrated processes: nursing process — implementation; client need: physiological integrity; basic care and comfort; content area: medical-surgical.
   RATIONALE
   (**1**) Avoidance of enriched foods may not meet the requirements for decreasing constipation. (**2**) A low-bulk diet increases the chances for constipation. (**3**) A diet high in calcium and carbohydrates will increase constipation. (**4**) Increased daily fluid intake, extra bulk in the diet, and regular exercise help to stimulate normal motility of the intestines.

56. (**2**) Integrated processes: nursing process — implementation; client need: physiological integrity; pharmacological therapies; content area: medical-surgical.
   RATIONALE
   (**1**) The deltoid muscle should not be used for administering irritating medications. (**2**) Z-track injection of IM medications is recommended for medications that could be irritating to tissues. Retracting the skin and SC tissue to one side and maintaining that traction for 10 seconds after injection interrupts the needle track, preventing the medication from seeping into the needle track or SC tissue and causing irritation. (**3**) Changing the needle will not help to prevent irritating SC tissue. (**4**) Do not massage the injection site after injecting irritating medications; it increases the irritation.

57. (**1**) Integrated processes: nursing process — implementation; client need: safe, effective care environment; safety and infection control; content area: medical-surgical.
   RATIONALE
   (**1**) Always recheck the medication against the physician's order when the client notes a discrepancy. Most often the client is correct, and this will avoid a medication error. (**2**) It may not be a new medication; check to make sure. (**3**) Never leave the medication at the client's bedside. (**4**) Do not omit the medication; the client did not refuse it but has questioned it.

58. (**2**) Integrated processes: nursing process — data collection; client need: physiological integrity; physiological adaptation; content area: medical-surgical.
   RATIONALE
   (**1**) Hemoptysis occurs in clients with pulmonary edema. (**2**) Exertional dyspnea, chronic cough, wheezing, and increased mucus production are symptoms of pulmonary emphysema as a result of specific morphologic changes in lung tissue: distention of the alveolar sacs, rupture of the alveolar walls, and destruction of the alveolar capillary bed. (**3**) Epistaxis is not a symptom of pulmonary emphysema. (**4**) Not all of these are symptoms of emphysema.

59. (**2**) Integrated processes: nursing process — implementation; client need: physiological integrity; physiological adaptation; content area: medical-surgical.
   RATIONALE
   (**1**) Alkalosis is not consistent with pulmonary emphysema. (**2**) The chronic damage to the alveolar walls and capillaries and their decreased elasticity result in a decrease in the exchange of gases between the bloodstream and the air and a retention of carbon dioxide (hypercapnia). (**3**) Elevated SaO_2

and hypocapnia are not associated with pulmonary emphysema. (4) Hypocapnia is not a symptom of emphysema.

60. (1) Integrated processes: nursing process — data collection; client need: physiological integrity; reduction of risk potential; content area: medical-surgical.
RATIONALE
(1) During the initial stages of a CVA, it is imperative to maintain cerebral circulation. This can best be done by frequent monitoring of neurological functioning and level of cosciousness. (2) Range-of-motion exercise could be done but would not have first priority. (3) Laxatives may be administered if listed therapy did not control constipation, but this is not the priority. (4) Some neurological stimulation is encouraged.

61. (4) Integrated processes: nursing process — implementation; client need: physiological integrity; physiological adaptation; content area: medical-surgical.
RATIONALE
(1) Aphasic clients do not have difficulty in understanding. (2) Writing is not an option with aphasia. (3) The nurse may have difficulty understanding the client but will be able to communicate using alternative methods, depending on the client. (4) When a CVA affects the left hemisphere of the brain, damage to the speech center may occur. In expressive aphasia, the client has difficulty speaking and writing.

62. (2) Integrated processes: nursing process — implementation; client need: physiological integrity; physiological adaptation; content area: medical-surgical.
RATIONALE
(1) There is suprapubic pressure in urinary tract infections, but not abdominal pain. (2) When pathogens invade the urinary tract, the bladder loses its elasticity. Its filling capacity becomes ineffective, and a moderate stretching of the bladder results in symptoms mentioned in option 2. (3) There is not usually distention. (4) Elevated pulse rate is not a symptom of urinary tract infection.

63. (1) Integrated processes: nursing process — implementation, teaching/learning; client need: physiological integrity; physiological adaptation; content area: medical-surgical.
RATIONALE
(1) Practicing good perineal care can prevent contamination from the vagina and rectum. Acidifying the urine via medication or drinking cranberry or prune juice is believed to discourage bacterial multiplication. Increased fluid intake helps to flush out the bacteria present. (2) These would not be taught to a client with a urinary tract infection. (3) These would not be taught to a client with a urinary tract infection. (4) These would not be taught to a client with a urinary tract infection.

64. (2) Integrated processes: nursing process — implementation; client need: psychosocial integrity; content area: psychiatric nursing.
RATIONALE
(1) Increased physical activity is not specific for suicide. (2) Most suicidal persons give verbal or behavioral (mood change) warnings before committing suicide. They feel and act less depressed because they have come to terms with a decision to end their lives. (3) Hypersomnia is not specific for suicide. (4) Increased verbal activity is not specific for suicide.

65. (3) Integrated processes: nursing process — implementation; client need: physiological integrity; reduction of risk potential; content area: maternity nursing.
RATIONALE
(1) If the mother received Rho(D) immune globulin after her first pregnancy, there would be no complication. (2) If the father is Rh negative, there would be no complication. (3) In a second pregnancy, an Rh negative mother may produce antibodies against the Rh factor (Rh-positive baby), which cross the placenta and attack the fetus's RBCs if she has not been given Rho(D) immune globulin within 72 hours after delivery of her first baby. The possibility exists that if the father is Rh positive, the infant may also be Rh positive. (4) The baby being Rh negative is not a complication.

66. (1) Integrated processes: nursing process — implementation; client need: health promotion and maintenance; content area: maternity nursing.
RATIONALE
(1) Pregnancy increases calcium requirements by nearly 50%. Milk is the single most important source of this nutrient. (2) Bananas are high in potassium but not in calcium. (3) Salad greens also contain calcium but not as much as milk contains. (4) Orange juice does not contain any significant amount of calcium.

67. (2) Integrated processes: nursing process — implementation; client need: safe, effective care environment; safety and infection control; content area: medical-surgical.
RATIONALE
(1) Surgical aseptic technique is not required to remove a dressing. (2) Urinary catheterization is an invasive procedure, and surgical asepsis is crucial to prevent introduction of bacteria and a subsequent urinary infection. (3) Administering an enema does not require surgical aseptic technique. (4) Giving perineal care does not require surgical aseptic technique.

68. (1) Integrated processes: nursing process — implementation; client need: safe, effective care environment; safety and infection control; content area: medical-surgical.
RATIONALE
(1) Research has proved that most microorganisms are transferred by direct contact and that effective hand washing is considered one of the most effective infection-control measures. (2) This option will help to reduce the spread of infection, but the single most important measure is hand washing. (3) This option will help to reduce the spread of infection, but the single most important measure is hand washing. (4) This option will help to reduce the spread of infection, but the single most important measure is hand washing.

69. (4) Integrated processes: nursing process — implementation, communication and documentation; client need: safe, effective environment; coordinated care; content area: medical-surgical.
RATIONALE
(1) Bradycardia is a slow pulse rate. (2) Pulse paradox is reduction of amplitude of the pulse during inspiration. (3) Arrhythmia is an irregular pulse. (4) A pulse rate of 100 bpm is called tachycardia (taken from the Greek *tachys*, meaning "swift" or "rapid," and *kardia*, meaning "heart").

70. (3) Integrated processes: nursing process — implementation; client need: physiological integrity; reduction of risk potential; content area: medical-surgical.
RATIONALE
(1) Increasing physical activity will increase heat production. (2) Providing extra blankets will increase heat production. (3) Increasing fluid intake will counteract potential dehydration,

and giving tepid sponge baths will increase heat loss through conduction. **(4)** Offering warm fluids will not increase heat loss.

71. **(2)** Integrated processes: nursing process — data collection, communication and documentation; client need: safe, effective care environment; coordinated care; content area: medical-surgical.
    RATIONALE
    (1) This option is objective data. **(2)** Subjective data are data resulting from the feelings or temperament of the subject (client)—data apparent only to the person affected, which can be described or verified only by that person. **(3)** This option is objective data. **(4)** This option is objective data.

72. **(2)** Integrated processes: nursing process — implementation, communication and documentation; client need: safe, effective care environment; coordinated care; content area: medical-surgical.
    RATIONALE
    (1) This is only part of the reason for using the nursing process. **(2)** The nursing process provides a framework of accountability, and the client's record serves as the vehicle by which different members of the health-care team communicate assessments, interventions, and evaluations. **(3)** This is only part of the reason for using the nursing process. **(4)** This is only part of the reason for using the nursing process.

73. **(4)** Integrated processes: nursing process — implementation, caring; client need: psychosocial integrity; content area: psychiatric nursing.
    RATIONALE
    (1) This option does not display an open communication system. **(2)** This option does not display an open communication system. **(3)** This option does not display an open communication system. **(4)** This is an open-ended statement that shows that the nurse has observed the client's distress and allows verbalization of feelings.

74. **(3)** Integrated processes: nursing process — implementation, caring; client need: psychosocial integrity; content area: medical-surgical.
    RATIONALE
    (1) This behavior does not display open attentive listening. **(2)** This behavior does not display open attentive listening. **(3)** Attentive listening requires all the senses and skills; maintaining eye contact helps the nurse to interpret the nonverbal as well as the verbal message and lets the client know the nurse is listening and involved. **(4)** This behavior does not display open attentive listening.

75. **(1)** Integrated processes: nursing process — implementation; client need: physiological integrity; physiological adaptation; content area: medical-surgical.
    RATIONALE
    (1) The first intervention when the nurse arrives on the scene if the client appears to have "ceased breathing" is to determine whether he or she is responsive. This is the first step of basic CPR. **(2)** This is not the first step of CPR. **(3)** This is not the first step of CPR. **(4)** This is not the first step of CPR.

76. **(1)** Integrated processes: nursing process — data collection; client need: physiological integrity; physiological adaptation; content area: medical-surgical.
    RATIONALE
    (1) The first step of CPR is to establish unresponsiveness. **(2)** Absence of the carotid pulse determines pulselessness and cardiac arrest. It is essential to assess the carotid pulse accurately because performing external chest percussions on a client with a pulse can lead to serious medical complications. **(3)** The second step of CPR is to determine cessation of respirations. **(4)** Fixed and dilated pupils are not an indication to start or stop breathing or compressions.

77. **(4)** Integrated processes: nursing process — implementation; client need: safe, effective care environment; coordinated care; content area: medical-surgical.
    RATIONALE
    (1) This is not the correct order for the nursing process. **(2)** This is not the correct order for the nursing process. **(3)** This is not the correct order for the nursing process. **(4)** The nursing process consists of a four-step process of data collection, analysis or planning, implementation, and evaluation. The nursing process uses a systematic, rational, and logical manner to plan, provide, and evaluate nursing care.

78. **(2)** Integrated processes: nursing process — implementation; client need: physiological integrity; basic care and comfort; content area: medical-surgical.
    RATIONALE
    (1) Vitamins and minerals are essential in the diet, but they are not one of the four basic food groups. **(2)** The "basic four" food guide was introduced by the U.S. Department of Agriculture (USDA) in 1956. This plan is based on four basic groups for sound nutrition: milk and milk products, meats and alternates, breads and cereals, and fruits and vegetables. **(3)** Vitamins and minerals are not one of the four basic food groups. **(4)** Poultry by itself is not one of the four basic food groups.

79. **(3)** Integrated processes: nursing process — implementation; client need: physiological integrity; pharmacological therapies; content area: medical-surgical.
    RATIONALE
    (1) Right amount and right dose are the same thing. **(2)** Right order is not one of the five rights. **(3)** The five rights are the essential guidelines for safe administration of medications. **(4)** Right documentation is important, but it is not one of the five rights.

80. **(2)** Integrated processes: nursing process — data collection; client need: physiological integrity; physiological adaptation; content area: medical-surgical.
    RATIONALE
    (1) Cool moist skin and hypothermia are not indicative of dehydration. **(2)** Sodium excess can occur with dehydration when water loss exceeds sodium loss, manifesting these symptoms because of hyperosmolarity of the extracellular fluid. **(3)** Decreased specific gravity of urine is not a symptom of dehydration. **(4)** Anorexia and cool moist skin are not symptoms of dehydration.

81. **(3)** Integrated processes: nursing process — data collection; client need: physiological integrity; reduction of risk potential; content area: medical-surgical.
    RATIONALE
    (1) A potassium level of 3.2 is too low. **(2)** A potassium level of 2.5 is too low. **(3)** Potassium is a major cation of intracellular fluid, in which 98% of this electrolyte is found. Serum potassium levels, however, are based on the portion of potassium in the extracellular fluid, where the normal range is 3.5–5.5 mEq/L. **(4)** A potassium level of 4 is not the upper range of normal.

82. **(42 gtt/min)** Integrated processes: nursing process — implementation; client need: physiological integrity; pharmacological therapies; content area: medical-surgical.

RATIONALE

The formula for calculating drops per minute of an IV infusion is: Total infusion volume/ Number of hours × drops per minute. 1000 mL/ 8 hr = 125 mL. 125 mL/60min = 2.08 mL/min. 2.08 mL/min × 20gtt/min = 41.6, or 42 gtts/mL/min.

83. **(2)** Integrated processes: nursing process — implementation; client need: physiological integrity; reduction of risk potential; content area: medical-surgical.

RATIONALE

(1) This may be correct, but it is not the primary purpose for emptying the bladder before surgery. **(2)** The primary purpose of emptying the bladder before surgery is to prevent inadvertent injury to the bladder during the surgical procedure. **(3)** This may be correct, but it is not the primary purpose for emptying the bladder before surgery. **(4)** This option may be correct, but it is not the primary reason for emptying the bladder before surgery.

84. **(2)** Integrated processes: nursing process — implementation, communication and documentation; client need: safe, effective care environment; coordinated care; content area: medical-surgical.

RATIONALE

(1) This option does not cover the entire extent of informed consent. **(2)** Informed consent is an agreement by a client to accept a course of treatment or a procedure after complete information, including the risks of treatment and facts relating to it, has been provided by the physician. It is a part of the Patient's Bill of Rights. This protects clients from having any surgical procedure they do not want or do not know about, and it also protects the hospital and health personnel from a claim by a client or family that permission was not granted. **(3)** This option does not cover the entire extent of informed consent. **(4)** This option does not cover the entire extent of informed consent.

85. **(4)** Integrated processes: nursing process — implementation; client need: physiological integrity; reduction of risk potential; content area: medical-surgical.

RATIONALE

(1) This may be a true statement for some clients but is not the reason why food and fluids are withheld before surgery. **(2)** This may be a true statement for some clients but is not the reason why food and fluids are withheld before surgery. **(3)** This may be a true statement for some clients but is not the reason why food and fluids are withheld before surgery. **(4)** Anesthesia depresses GI functioning, and because of the danger that the client may vomit during induction of anesthesia, the client should be NPO for at least 6–8 hours before surgery to prevent possible aspiration of food or fluids.

86. **(2)** Integrated processes: nursing process — implementation; client need: physiological integrity; reduction of risk potential; content area: medical-surgical.

RATIONALE

(1) Shaving before a surgical procedure does not prevent postoperative discomfort. **(2)** The primary purpose of removing hair from the surgical area is to destroy microorganisms and thus to reduce the chance of infection. **(3)** Shaving before a surgical procedure does not prevent pain. **(4)** Shaving before a surgical procedure does not provide a better view of the surgical area.

87. **(1)** Integrated processes: nursing process — implementation, communication and documentation; client need: physiological integrity; pharmacological therapies; content area: medical-surgical.

RATIONALE

(1) Heparin (an anticoagulant) is often used postoperatively to prevent thromboembolic complications arising from surgery. **(2)** Heparin use would increase the risk of postoperative hemorrhage. **(3)** Heparin would decrease blood coagulation. **(4)** Heparin does not prevent postoperative paralytic ileus.

88. **(1)** Integrated processes: nursing process — implementation; client need: physiological integrity; physiological adaptation; content area: medical-surgical.

RATIONALE

(1) The clinical signs of wound infection include redness, swelling, pain, induration, fever, and leukocytosis. **(2)** Anorexia, diminished bowel sounds, and serosanguineous drainage are not symptoms of a wound infection. **(3)** Well-approximated edges and serosanguineous drainage are not signs of a wound infection. **(4)** Bright-red drainage is abnormal but not indicative of wound infection.

89. **(1)** Integrated processes: nursing process — implementation; client need: physiological integrity; physiological adaptation; content area: medical-surgical.

RATIONALE

(1) The ABCs of CPR are airway, breathing, and circulation. **(2)** Airway and circulation need to first be assessed before definitive treatment is implemented. **(3)** This is not the first action in this scenario. **(4)** The nurse would not elevate the client's head to begin CPR.

90. **(3)** Integrated processes: nursing process — implementation; client need: physiological integrity; physiological adaptation; content area: medical-surgical.

RATIONALE

(1) Radiation does not kill by heat. **(2)** This is not how radiation works. See rationale 3. **(3)** Ionizing radiation is energy in the form of waves or particles transmitted to rapidly dividing cancer cells, which are radiosensitive. Radiation chemically alters tissue protein and disrupts the cancer cells by inhibiting their division. **(4)** There is no such thing as magnetic resuscitation.

91. **(1)** Integrated processes: nursing process — implementation; client need: physiological integrity; reduction of risk potential; content area: medical-surgical.

RATIONALE

(1) To prevent overexposure to radiation when caring for clients with radioactive implants, close-contact time should not exceed 15 minutes daily. As the distance from the source of radiation is increased, exposure is decreased. Shielding is necessary for safe protection, especially when the principles of time and distance cannot always be adhered to. **(2)** One does not have to stay 12 ft away. **(3)** The client does not have to be on protective isolation. **(4)** One does not have to wear a film badge, and one can stay in the room for 15 minutes.

92. **(2)** Integrated processes: nursing process — implementation, teaching/learning; client need: health promotion and maintenance; content area: medical-surgical.

RATIONALE

(1) Passive and active smoking do not cause chest injuries. **(2)** A significant number of chest injuries result from passengers being unrestrained (without seat belts) in automobile accidents and are caused by the forces of acceleration and deceleration. **(3)** Driving below the speed limit may increase the opportunity for accidents. **(4)** Placing children in the back seat does not decrease chest injury unless they are also restrained in seat belts.

93. **(3)** Integrated processes: nursing process — data collection; client need: physiological integrity; physiological adaptation; content area: medical-surgical.
RATIONALE
(1) Hypoventilation causes acidosis. **(2)** The client is acidotic, not alkalotic. **(3)** The client's PaO_2 is far less than the norm of 80–95 mm Hg; his $PaCO_2$ is elevated from the norm of 35–45 mm Hg; and his pH is well below the norm of 7.35–7.45. These indicate respiratory acidosis, and hypoventilation is the primary factor. **(4)** This is acidosis, not alkalosis.

94. **(2)** Integrated processes: nursing process — data collection; client need: physiological integrity; physiological adaptation; content area: medical-surgical.
RATIONALE
(1) Hypertension is a late sign of hypoxia. **(2)** Hypoxia is a diminished oxygen supply to the cells of the body, resulting in the symptoms listed. The respiratory control center is located in the brain; therefore, judgment can also be impaired. **(3)** Cyanosis is a late sign of hypoxia. **(4)** Crowing respirations are characteristic of obstruction.

95. **(4)** Integrated processes: nursing process — implementation; client need: health promotion and maintenance; content area: medical-surgical.
RATIONALE
(1) There is no need to decrease these foods in the diet. **(2)** There is no need to decrease these foods in the diet. **(3)** There is no need to decrease these foods in the diet. **(4)** Foods high in cholesterol, especially in low-density lipoproteins such as those mentioned in option 4, are believed to contribute to the occurrence of myocardial infarction and other coronary and vascular disorders. The other foods listed are not high in cholesterol.

96. **(3)** Integrated processes: nursing process — implementation; client need: physiological integrity; basic care and comfort; content area: medical-surgical.
RATIONALE
(1) These foods are not high in potassium. **(2)** These foods are not high in potassium. **(3)** These are potassium-rich foods that will help to keep potassium levels within normal limits when clients are receiving potassium-depleting diuretics. **(4)** These foods and nuts are not high in potassium.

97. **(1)** Integrated processes: nursing process — implementation; client need: physiological integrity; pharmacological therapies; content area: medical-surgical.
RATIONALE
(1) Anti-inflammatory agents are used to treat arthritis because they counteract inflammation. **(2)** Antilipemic drugs are not beneficial in treating arthritis. **(3)** Antibiotics are not useful in treating arthritis, especially on a long-term basis. **(4)** Sympatholytic agents are not beneficial in treating arthritis.

98. **(3)** Integrated processes: nursing process — implementation; client need: health promotion and maintenance; content area: medical-surgical.
RATIONALE
(1) This position does not increase fetal activity. **(2)** This position does not facilitate the descent into the birth canal. **(3)** The Sims' position promotes conscious relaxation, facilitates focusing and breathing techniques, and enhances fetal and maternal circulation, as well as preventing supine hypotension (which can occur in the supine position). **(4)** This position does not decrease the intensity of labor pains.

99. **(3)** Integrated processes: nursing process — data collection; client need: health promotion and maintenance; content area: maternity nursing.
RATIONALE
(1) This is not an abnormal heart rate for an infant. **(2)** This heart rate does not indicate distress. **(3)** A normal fetal heart rate is 120–160 bpm. **(4)** This heart rate is not above the norm.

100. **(2)** Integrated processes: nursing process — implementation; client need: health promotion and maintenance; content area: maternity nursing.
RATIONALE
(1) This response defines duration. **(2)** The frequency of contractions refers to the time interval from the beginning of one contraction to the beginning of the next. **(3)** This is not a method for measuring the frequency of contractions. **(4)** This is not a method for measuring the frequency of contractions.

101. **(4)** Integrated processes: nursing process — data collection; client need: health promotion and maintenance; content area: maternity nursing.
RATIONALE
(1) This is a part of stage 3 but not the entire stage. **(2)** This is part of stage 1. **(3)** This is a part of stage 2. **(4)** The process of labor is traditionally divided into three stages. The third stage begins when the baby is delivered and ends with the delivery of the placenta and membranes. Currently, a fourth stage has been added to allow for full evaluation of the newly delivered mother.

102. **(2)** Integrated processes: nursing process — data collection; client need: physiological integrity; physiological adaptation; content area: pediatrics.
RATIONALE
(1) Anemia may occur as a result of poor nutrition but is not a classic sign. **(2)** Pyloric stenosis (narrowing) is a disorder of the digestive tract caused by an overgrowth of the circular muscles of the pylorus. This narrowing causes partial blockage that prevents food from properly emptying into the duodenum, resulting in forceful (projectile) vomiting. **(3)** Diarrhea is not a classic symptom of pyloric stenosis. **(4)** Anorexia is not a classic symptom of pyloric stenosis.

103. **(1)** Integrated processes: nursing process — implementation; client need: physiological integrity; physiological adaptation; content area: medical-surgical.
RATIONALE
(1) In acute glomerulonephritis, urinary output is decreased, specific gravity is high, and fluid restriction may be necessary (because of possible impaired renal function); therefore, keeping I&O in balance and assessing color and character of the urine is important. **(2)** Monitoring pulse and respirations is important but is not the most important intervention. **(3)** Fluids are to be restricted rather than encouraged. **(4)** Ambulation does not affect glomerulonephritis.

104. **(1)** Integrated processes: nursing process — implementation; client need: physiological integrity; basic care and comfort; content area: medical-surgical.
RATIONALE
(1) Clear liquids are given to a postoperative tonsillectomy client. An ice slush may be more appealing to a 4-year-old child. Many ice slushes contain synthetic fruit juices, which are not as irritating as natural juices. **(2)** Milk is not a clear liquid.

(3) Orange juice is not a clear liquid. (4) Decaffeinated soda pop still has carbonation.

105. **(2)** Integrated processes: nursing process — implementation; client need: safe, effective care environment; safety and infection control; content area: medical-surgical.
RATIONALE
(1) The nurse would perform this intervention, but it is not the primary reason for changing the dressing. (2) Inspection and assessment of the incisional area and prevention of potential problems (infection, dehiscence, bleeding) are the main reasons why a client's dressing is changed. (3) Dressings do not necessarily prevent an infection or provide comfort. (4) Charting is important but is not the reason for changing a dressing.

106. **(2)** Integrated processes: nursing process — implementation; client need: physiological integrity; reduction of risk potential; content area: medical-surgical.
RATIONALE
(1) Early ambulation does not prevent dependence. (2) Research has shown that early postoperative ambulation helps to restore all body systems to normal and prevents potential postoperative complications. (3) Early ambulation does not prevent nausea and vomiting. (4) Diaphoresis is not a desirable outcome.

107. **(4)** Integrated processes: nursing process — data collection; client need: physiological integrity; physiological adaptation; content area: medical-surgical.
RATIONALE
(1) Increased cardiac output does not usually result from hypovolemia. (2) Increased metabolic needs do not cause CHF. (3) Accumulation of serous fluid in the pleural space does not lead to CHF. (4) With CHF the heart fails, becomes filled with fluid, and no longer can adequately pump blood throughout the body.

108. **(1)** Integrated processes: nursing process — implementation, teaching/learning; client need: physiological integrity; pharmacological therapies; content area: medical-surgical.
RATIONALE
(1) Hair cells (like other rapidly dividing cells) are very sensitive to chemotherapeutic drugs. Clients should be assured that hair loss is temporary but that the texture and color of the regrowth may differ from the original. (2) Alopecia from chemotherapy is rarely permanent. (3) This statement about alopecia being "not life threatening" will not help the client's self-esteem. (4) One should not tell the client that alopecia is never permanent; the rest of this statement will not help the client's self-esteem.

109. **(2)** Integrated processes: nursing process — implementation, communication and documentation; client need: safe, effective care environment; coordinated care; content area: medical-surgical.
RATIONALE
(1) The nurse would document the blood pressure in the chart, but this is not the priority action. (2) A LPN always reports to the RN significant changes in vital signs as well as subjective or objective symptoms that indicate a change in the client's condition. A blood pressure reading of 200/110 mm Hg and the accompanying symptoms bear immediate reporting. (3) Giving acetaminophen is the next action after notifying the registered nurse. (4) A LPN would inquire about family history of hypertension, but this is not of the highest priority.

110. **(3)** Integrated processes: nursing process — data collection; client need: psychosocial integrity; content area: psychiatric nursing.
RATIONALE
(1) Sublimation is acceptance of a socially approved substitute. (2) Repression is involuntary exclusion of an undesirable thought from the memory. (3) Denial is a refusal to admit the reality of or to acknowledge the presence of something painful. (4) Compensation is the process by which a person makes up for a deficiency by emphasizing an asset.

111. **(4)** Integrated processes: nursing process — implementation; client need: physiological integrity; basic care and comfort; content area: medical-surgical.
RATIONALE
(1) Giving aspirin is not the first priority. (2) Sponging with alcohol would be done if the tepid bath did not work. (3) Applying blankets would increase the child's temperature. (4) A tepid sponge bath increases heat loss through conduction and is the first measure used to reduce fever in a young child.

112. **(4)** Integrated processes: nursing process — implementation; client need: physiological integrity; pharmacological therapies; content area: pediatrics.
RATIONALE
(1) Having the child sit upright would make it more difficult to instill eardrops. (2) This is not the correct technique for instilling eardrops in a child. (3) This is not the correct technique for instilling eardrops in a child. (4) To straighten the auditory canal of an infant or toddler (which is shorter than that of an adult), gently pull the pinna down and backward.

113. **(2)** Integrated processes: nursing process — data collection; client need: physiological integrity; pharmacological therapies; content area: medical-surgical.
RATIONALE
(1) Bradycardia is not commonly seen in vasodilator therapy. (2) Vasodilators (antihypertensives) lower the blood pressure by dilating arterial blood vessels. These agents stimulate central adrenergic receptors, resulting in the adverse effects listed. (3) Hypertension is not commonly seen in vasodilator therapy. (4) Hypokalemia is not commonly seen in vasodilator therapy.

114. **(4)** Integrated processes: nursing process — data collection; client need: physiological integrity; physiological adaptation; content area: medical-surgical.
RATIONALE
(1) Gastric suction may cause hyponatremia, not hypernatremia. (2) Gastric suction would cause hypokalemia, not hyperkalemia. (3) Gastric suctioning would not cause hypervolemia; fluid is being lost. (4) Gastric secretions are high in potassium.

115. **(2)** Integrated processes: nursing process — implementation; client need: physiological integrity; pharmacological therapies; content area: medical-surgical.
RATIONALE
(1) This option constitutes assessment data collected in patients with cardiac disease but is not of first priority when administering antihypertensive medications. (2) Because the purpose of giving an antihypertensive agent is to lower arterial blood pressure, it is always crucial first to measure the client's blood pressure to establish a baseline and also to be

certain the blood pressure is not too low, in which case the administration of an antihypertensive agent would result in serious adverse effects. **(3)** This option constitutes assessment data collected in patients with cardiac disease but is not of first priority when administering antihypertensive medications. **(4)** This option constitutes assessment data collected in patients with cardiac disease but is not of first priority when administering antihypertensive medications.

116. **(2)** Integrated processes: nursing process — data collection; client need: physiological integrity; pharmacological therapies; content area: medical-surgical.
RATIONALE
(1) This is too late for a regular insulin reaction. **(2)** Regular insulin is a rapid-acting insulin, reaching its onset within 30–60 minutes, which might precipitate adverse effects (hypoglycemia) because of too much insulin in the bloodstream. **(3)** This is too soon for regular insulin to peak. **(4)** This is past the peak of regular insulin.

117. **(2)** Integrated processes: nursing process — implementation; client need: physiological integrity; pharmacological therapies; content area: medical-surgical.
RATIONALE
(1) Ampicillin is an antibiotic. **(2)** Heparin is an anticoagulant and inactivates several of the factors necessary for the clotting of blood. It is often ordered to treat thrombophlebitis (inflammation of a vein with formation of a thrombus) to prevent a potential embolus that could lodge in the lungs, heart, or brain, causing serious complications or death or both. **(3)** Propranolol is used for cardiac conditions, not phlebitis. **(4)** Nitroglycerin is used for cardiac conditions.

118. **(2)** Integrated processes: nursing process — data collection; client need: health promotion and maintenance; content area: medical-surgical.
RATIONALE
(1) This is an activity the nurse would do, but it is not the best answer because the signs may not be detected before significant bleeding occurs. **(2)** Significant changes in vital signs will quickly alert the nurse to potential hemorrhage. Assessment and palpation of the fundus is one way to check for height and tone, presence of clots, and possible uterine atony to prevent a potential hemorrhage. **(3)** Nail bed color change is a late sign of hemorrhage. **(4)** Monitoring color and amount of flow will not necessarily indicate hemorrhage.

119. **(2)** Integrated processes: nursing process — data collection; client need: physiological integrity; physiological adaptation; content area: medical-surgical.
RATIONALE
(1) *Mycobacterium* does not cause hypertension or anorexia. **(2)** Presence of the *Mycobacterium* acid-fast gram-positive bacillus causes symptoms as listed. Initial symptoms are related to the infectious process. Cough and hemoptysis occur if there is pulmonary involvement. **(3)** *Mycobacterium* does not cause enlarged lymph nodes. **(4)** *Mycobacterium* does not cause bradycardia or weight gain.

120. **(1)** Integrated processes: nursing process — data collection; client need: psychosocial integrity; content area: psychiatric nursing.
RATIONALE
(1) Hypochondriasis is a defense used by the ego when it has real or imagined aggressive, critical feelings toward others. The critical feelings are turned back on the ego and are experienced as guilt, often transformed into physical complaints. **(2)** This is projection. **(3)** This is suppression. **(4)** This is repression.

121. **(3)** Integrated processes: nursing process — implementation, caring; client need: psychosocial integrity; content area: psychiatric nursing.
RATIONALE
(1) Doing nothing will not meet the client's basic grooming needs. **(2)** Telling the client to bathe may not accomplish the task. **(3)** Clients with depression frequently do not have the energy to take care of their personal grooming needs. The nurse assists with these needs without fostering dependence. **(4)** This option will not promote independence.

122. **(1)** Integrated processes: nursing process — implementation, caring; client need: psychosocial integrity; content area: psychiatric nursing.
RATIONALE
(1) The nurse will stay with the client initially for a short period to begin developing trust. **(2)** It is not necessary to stay for an hour; besides, this is not a matter of control. **(3)** The best plan is to stay a short while and then return later. **(4)** Therapeutic touch is not appropriate until trust is established.

123. **(1)** Integrated processes: nursing process — planning, caring; client need: psychosocial integrity; content area: psychiatric nursing.
RATIONALE
(1) Regression is adopting behavioral patterns characteristic of an earlier stage to reduce stress. **(2)** Conversion is channeling psychological stress into physical symptoms. **(3)** Denial occurs when the anxiety-producing situations are rejected as they actually are. **(4)** Projection is attributing undesirable symptoms to other people or objects.

124. **(2)** Integrated processes: nursing process — planning, teaching/learning; client need: psychosocial integrity; content area: psychiatric nursing.
RATIONALE
(1) Acrophobia is fear of height. **(2)** Xenophobia is fear of strangers. **(3)** Claustrophobia is fear of enclosed spaces. **(4)** Agoraphobia is fear of open spaces.

125. **(4)** Integrated processes: nursing process — planning; client need: psychosocial integrity; content area: psychiatric nursing.
RATIONALE
(1) Bulimia is not a phobia. **(2)** Anorexia is a disorder involving starving oneself. **(3)** Bulimia is more than just vomiting. **(4)** Bulimia is eating massive amounts of food and then purging by either vomiting or taking laxatives.

126. **(4)** Integrated processes: nursing process — planning, caring; client need: psychosocial integrity; content area: psychiatric nursing.
RATIONALE
(1) This action will only reinforce his confusion. **(2)** This is a short-term solution and may initiate a defense mechanism. **(3)** If he can describe his son, this reinforces his confusion. He does not have a 5-year old son. **(4)** This action will help to orient him to his surroundings.

127. **(3)** Integrated processes: nursing process — implementation, teaching/learning; client need: psychosocial integrity; content area: psychiatric nursing.

RATIONALE

(1) He may be potentially dangerous to himself, but the family is not asking to have him placed in a long-term care facility. (2) Giving detailed instructions to clients with organic brain syndrome will only increase their confusion. (3) Organic brain syndrome clients need frequent reality orientation. (4) This will only increase his anxiety and confusion.

128. **(3)** Integrated processes: nursing process — planning, communication and documentation; client need: psychosocial integrity; content area: psychiatric nursing.

RATIONALE

(1) This approach will reinforce the antisocial behavior. (2) Setting ground rules does not mean the client will follow them. (3) This approach ensures that all team members are engaged in the treatment plan. (4) Requiring participation does not mean that the client will participate.

129. **(3)** Integrated processes: nursing process — implementation; client need: physiological integrity; pharmacological therapies; content area: psychiatric nursing.

RATIONALE

(1) The nurse is pitting himself or herself against the client. (2) This is not an option; he needs his medication or his behavior will get worse. (3) Giving him a choice allows him to have some control. (4) The client is paranoid; he does not know why he thinks this. This approach will only reinforce his paranoid thoughts.

130. **(2)** Integrated processes: nursing process — evaluation; client need: physiological integrity; pharmacological therapies; content area: psychiatric nursing.

RATIONALE

(1) The client needs her symptoms evaluated; giving the medicine IM is inappropriate at this time. (2) Holding the medicine until the client's symptoms can be evaluated is the correct choice. (3) Insisting that she takes her medicine will not control her visual problems. (4) The client needs to be evaluated, not confined to her room.

131. **(4)** Integrated processes: nursing process — implementation, teaching/learning; client need: physiological integrity; physiological adaptation; content area: pediatrics.

RATIONALE

(1) This action could potentially overdose the child. (2) Keeping the child warm would increase the cough. (3) Turning the child upside down might increase epiglottal edema and make the child worse. (4) This is the best choice because a warm mist reduces epiglottal edema and relieves coughing.

132. **(3)** Integrated processes: nursing process — implementation; client need: physiological integrity; reduction of risk potential; content area: psychiatric nursing.

RATIONALE

(1) It is not necessary to take vital signs every 5–10 minutes after electroconvulsive therapy. (2) Nausea and vomiting are not usual side effects of electroconvulsive therapy. (3) Clients undergoing electroconvulsive therapy are usually confused after therapy and need reorientation. (4) Bed rest is not required after electroconvulsive therapy.

133. **(4)** Integrated processes: nursing process — planning; client need: health promotion and maintenance; content area: psychiatric nursing.

RATIONALE

(1) The nurse should be a client advocate. This statement is the nurse's opinion. (2) The problem is between the husband and wife, not the woman's mother. (3) The woman is asking the nurse for help. This is not the best response. (4) This statement will help the client to discuss her feelings before any decision is made.

134. **(1)** Integrated processes: nursing process — planning, teaching/learning; client need: health promotion and maintenance; content area: pediatric nursing.

RATIONALE

(1) Children with PKU must restrict the amount of protein in their diet because accumulation of phenylalanine is toxic to the brain. (2) Juices are not restricted in children with PKU. (3) Leafy green vegetables do not have to be restricted in children with PKU. (4) Caffeine does not have to be restricted in children with PKU.

135. **(4)** Integrated processes: nursing process — implementation, caring; client need: health promotion and maintenance; content area: psychiatric nursing.

RATIONALE

(1) The nurse does not know that everything will be all right. This is false reassurance. (2) This statement will not help to ease the client's apprehension. (3) This statement may increase the client's apprehension. (4) Remaining with the client will help to provide support through the aborting process.

136. **(2)** Integrated processes: nursing process — implementation; client need: psychosocial integrity; content area: psychiatric nursing.

RATIONALE

(1) Ignoring the behavior reinforces the hallucinations. (2) Engaging the client in physical activity helps to decrease hallucinations. (3) Telling her to stop talking may increase her agitation. (4) She probably does not know with whom she is talking, and this response reinforces the hallucinations.

137. **(3)** Integrated processes: nursing process — data collection; client need: safe, effective care environment; safety and infection control; content area: psychiatric nursing.

RATIONALE

(1) Giving a sedative may be an unnecessary intervention. (2) Dilated pupils will not tell the nurse if the client is agitated. (3) A client with relaxed muscles is not agitated. (4) He may say yes, but he is not in control and may then hurt himself or someone else.

138. **(1)** Integrated processes: nursing process — implementation; client need: health promotion and maintenance; content area: maternity nursing.

RATIONALE

(1) Completing a vaginal examination to check for a prolapsed cord is the next action. (2) The husband does not need to leave the room; he is a support. (3) This may be a nursing action, but it is not the first action. (4) This may be a nursing action, but it is not the first action.

139. **(3)** Integrated processes: nursing process — implementation; client need: physiological integrity; reduction of risk potential; content area: maternity nursing.

RATIONALE

(1) The baby should not be covered in order to get maximum exposure to the light. (2) The baby needs fluids to eliminate the bilirubin. (3) The baby's eyes should be covered to prevent retinal damage. (4) An IV infusion is not necessary. The baby can take fluids orally.

140. **(3)** Integrated processes: nursing process — evaluation; client need: physiological integrity; reduction of risk potential; content area: maternity nursing.

     RATIONALE

     (1) Phototherapy does not usually affect the infant's appetite. **(2)** Phototherapy does not increase an infant's irritability. **(3)** The phototherapy light should decrease the jaundice in the infant, thereby allowing the nurse to know that it is effective. **(4)** Phototherapy does not cause photophobia.

141. **(1)** Integrated processes: nursing process — implementation; client need: health promotion and maintenance; content area: maternity nursing.

     RATIONALE

     (1) Applying gentle pressure to the head prevents tearing of the perineum. **(2)** The nurse should not encourage the mother to cross the legs to impede the delivery. **(3)** The nurse should not discourage the delivery. **(4)** The nurse should do nothing that will impede the delivery.

142. **(2)** Integrated processes: nursing process — implementation; client need: health promotion and maintenance; content area: maternity nursing.

     RATIONALE

     (1) The nurse should not slap the baby's bottom; this could cause cardiac problems. **(2)** Holding the head in a dependent position helps the mucus to drain and stimulates breathing. **(3)** The first action is to clear the baby's airway. **(4)** Vital signs will be taken later.

143. **(4)** Integrated processes: nursing process — implementation; client need: psychosocial integrity; content area: psychiatric nursing.

     RATIONALE

     (1) Correcting the delusions will make them more fixed. **(2)** Avoiding talking about the delusions is not therapeutic. **(3)** This response is not therapeutic. **(4)** If the nurse disagrees with the client, the delusions become more fixed.

144. **(4)** Integrated processes: nursing process — implementation, teaching/learning; client need: physiological integrity; reduction of risk potential; content area: medical-surgical.

     RATIONALE

     (1) Glaucoma does not cause a detached retina. **(2)** Glaucoma does not affect nearsightedness. **(3)** Glaucoma does not affect farsightedness. **(4)** If left untreated, glaucoma can lead to blindness.

145. **(3)** Integrated processes: nursing process — implementation; client need: physiological integrity; physiological adaptation; content area: medical-surgical.

     RATIONALE

     (1) This is an appropriate nursing strategy but not the first priority. **(2)** This is an appropriate nursing strategy but not the first priority. **(3)** The first priority is administering antibiotics. **(4)** This is an appropriate nursing strategy but not the first priority.

146. **(2)** Integrated processes: nursing process — implementation; client need: psychosocial integrity; content area: psychiatric nursing.

     RATIONALE

     (1) Giving him medication right now will not stop his delusions. **(2)** This is therapeutic without reinforcing his delusions. **(3)** This response would reinforce his delusions. **(4)** This response would reinforce his delusions.

147. **(3)** Integrated processes: nursing process — implementation; client need: psychosocial integrity; content area: psychiatric nursing.

     RATIONALE

     (1) Ignoring the behavior reinforces the delusions. **(2)** Correcting the behavior may lead to an argument and reinforce the delusions. **(3)** Physical activity may help the delusions to diminish. **(4)** This approach reinforces the delusion.

148. **(2)** Integrated processes: nursing process — implementation, communication and documentation; client need: physiological integrity; physiological adaptation; content area: maternity nursing.

     RATIONALE

     (1) The sterilization consent is not always necessary for an ectopic pregnancy. **(2)** Blood replacement is crucial in case of hemorrhage. **(3)** This is a nursing action but not the priority. **(4)** This is appropriate but not the first priority.

149. **(2)** Integrated processes: nursing process — implementation, caring; client need: psychosocial integrity; content area: psychiatric nursing.

     RATIONALE

     (1) This response is false reassurance. **(2)** Asking the client if she wishes to talk about the event is therapeutic. **(3)** This is not a therapeutic response, and the nurse does not know the client's wishes at this time. **(4)** This is not a therapeutic response.

150. **(1)** Integrated processes: nursing process — data collection; client need: physiological integrity; reduction of risk potential; content area: pediatrics.

     RATIONALE

     (1) Acute hypertension may occur in children with glomerulonephritis. The nurse must check the blood pressure to prevent complications. **(2)** Clients with glomerulonephritis do not usually have occult bleeding. **(3)** A urinary catheterization may be ordered, but this is not the priority nursing action. **(4)** There is no indication for GI intubation.

151. **(2)** Integrated processes: nursing process — data collection; client need: health promotion and maintenance; content area: pediatrics.

     RATIONALE

     (1) Blood pressure is not a reliable measure of dehydration in small children. **(2)** Skin turgor is decreased in clients with dehydration. **(3)** Clients with dehydration have increased respirations. **(4)** Clients with dehydration have an increased pulse rate.

152. **(4)** Integrated processes: nursing process — data collection; client need: health promotion and maintenance; content area: pediatrics.

     RATIONALE

     (1) Although bleeding can occur in the thorax, this is not the most common site for bleeding in children with hemophilia. **(2)** Although bleeding can occur in the abdomen, this is not the most common site for bleeding in children with hemophilia. **(3)** Although bleeding can occur in the skull, this is not the most common site for bleeding in children with hemophilia. **(4)** The most common site of bleeding in children with hemophilia is the joints.

153. **(3)** Integrated processes: nursing process — implementation, teaching/learning; client need: health promotion and maintenance; content area: pediatrics.

RATIONALE
(1) This practice limits hip abduction. (2) This practice limits hip abduction. (3) This position promotes hip abduction. (4) This position limits hip abduction.

154. **(3)** Integrated processes: nursing process — implementation, teaching/learning; client need: physiological integrity; physiological adaptation; content area: pediatrics.
RATIONALE
(1) Apple juice is permitted in children with diarrhea. (2) Cooked carrots are permitted in children with diarrhea. (3) Milk and milk products should be avoided because they aggravate diarrhea. (4) Applesauce is permitted in children with diarrhea.

155. **(1)** Integrated processes: nursing process — implementation, teaching/learning; client need: physiological integrity; pharmacological therapies; content area: pediatrics.
RATIONALE
(1) To straighten the ear canal in a child, the pinna is pulled up and back. (2) This method is used to straighten the ear canal in an adult. (3) This method will not straighten the ear canal. (4) This method will not straighten the ear canal.

156. **(3)** Integrated processes: nursing process — implementation, teaching/learning; client need: health promotion and maintenance; content area: pediatrics.
RATIONALE
(1) This is not the reason for normal regurgitation in the newborn. (2) Although the stomach is small, this is not the reason for normal newborn regurgitation. (3) Because the cardiac sphincter is not fully mature, newborns have frequent regurgitation. (4) There is no scientific evidence to support this statement.

157. **(4)** Integrated processes: nursing process — implementation, teaching/learning; client need: physiological integrity; reduction of risk potential; content area: pediatrics.
RATIONALE
(1) A teaspoon is too hard and may injure the surgical repair. (2) The child is too young to drink from a cup. (3) A soft nipple may stimulate the sucking reflex and injure the surgery. (4) A syringe with a soft catheter allows feedings to be given to the side and back of the mouth without injuring the surgery.

158. **(1)** Integrated processes: nursing process — implementation; client need: health promotion and maintenance; content area: pediatrics.
RATIONALE
(1) Stacking blocks is a quiet activity that does not increase oxygen needs. (2) A pull toy is a physical activity that increases oxygen demands. (3) A horn increases oxygen demands. (4) Bouncing balls increase physical activity and therefore increase oxygen demands.

159. **(2)** Integrated processes: nursing process — implementation; client need: physiological integrity; pharmacological therapies; content area: pediatrics.
RATIONALE
(1) The medicine will need to be continued for the rest of the child's life. (2) This medicine should be given daily in the morning. (3) A symptom of toxicity from this medicine includes diarrhea, not constipation. (4) The child should continue to gain weight; otherwise, toxicity may be present.

160. **(4)** Integrated processes: nursing process — implementation, teaching/learning; client need: health promotion and maintenance; content area: pediatrics.
RATIONALE
(1) Progressing in school does not automatically mean that she will lose weight. (2) Not all sweets have to be eliminated from the diet. (3) Large doses of vitamins are inappropriate and will not suppress her appetite. (4) A planned program of activity and physical exercise will help her to lose weight.

161. **(2)** Integrated processes: nursing process — implementation; client need: health promotion and maintenance; content area: maternity nursing.
RATIONALE
(1) Taking the blood pressure during a contraction will give an inaccurate reading. (2) Taking blood pressure between contractions will give the most accurate blood pressure. (3) Taking the blood pressure immediately after a contraction will give an inaccurate blood pressure. (4) Taking the blood pressure at the peak of a contraction will give an inaccurate blood pressure.

162. **(2)** Integrated processes: nursing process — implementation; client need: physiological integrity; physiological adaptation; content area: pediatrics.
RATIONALE
(1) The side-lying position is a difficult position to maintain in an infant. (2) The prone position will prevent injury to the affected area. (3) The dorsal position will harm the affected area. (4) The Fowler's position will harm the affected area.

163. **(3)** Integrated processes: nursing process — implementation; client need: psychosocial integrity; content area: psychiatric nursing.
RATIONALE
(1) Although the nurse would notify the police, this is not the first priority. (2) Although the nurse may report it to the supervisor, this is not the first priority. (3) The first priority is to determine the client's immediate needs so she can establish a sense of control. (4) The nurse would not call her family until she has agreed to their being called.

164. **(3)** Integrated processes: nursing process — data collection; client need: health promotion and maintenance; content area: maternity nursing.
RATIONALE
(1) Although the nurse may administer a pain medicine, the first priority is assessment. (2) Although the nurse may check her fundus, the first priority is to inspect the perineum. She may have a hematoma. (3) Assessment of the perineum is the first priority. She may have a hematoma. (4) A sitz bath may be given later, but assessment of the perineum has priority.

165. **(2)** Integrated processes: nursing process — planning; client need: physiological integrity; reduction of risk potential; content area: pediatrics.
RATIONALE
(1) Percussion and postural drainage after meals may cause the child to vomit. (2) Percussion and drainage immediately before meals will decrease congestion and improve the appetite. (3) It is too difficult to schedule this activity between unpredictable playtimes. (4) Midway between meals will not improve her appetite.

166. **(4)** Integrated processes: nursing process — planning; client need: physiological integrity; physiological adaptation; content area: pediatrics.
RATIONALE
(1) Lead poisoning does not cause increased urination. **(2)** Lead poisoning does not cause decreased urination. **(3)** Lead poisoning does not usually cause malnutrition. **(4)** One of the initial signs of lead poisoning is anemia.

167. **(3)** Integrated processes: nursing process — implementation, teaching/learning; client need: health promotion and maintenance; content area: medical-surgical.
RATIONALE
(1) Drinking lots of water will not help the discharge. She needs antibiotics. **(2)** Thick white discharge is not a normal occurrence. She needs to see a health provider at the clinic or her private physician. **(3)** She needs treatment as soon as possible to prevent long-range damage to the urinary and reproductive systems. **(4)** Do not tell her mother. She may not want her mother to know.

168. **(2)** Integrated processes: nursing process — implementation; client need: health promotion and maintenance; content area: pediatrics.
RATIONALE
(1) This is not aphasia. Aphasia is having difficulty expressing oneself. **(2)** Transposing figures is one of the symptoms that the child has a learning disability. **(3)** Transposing figures is not consistent with visual problems. **(4)** There are no indications that there is a neurological disorder. Many 12-year-olds have illegible handwriting.

169. **(2)** Integrated processes: nursing process — planning; client need: physiological integrity; physiological adaptation; content area: medical-surgical.
RATIONALE
(1) Do not use wooden tongue blades during a seizure; they can splinter and cause damage. **(2)** Hard plastic bite blocks are preferred to prevent biting the tongue. **(3)** Restraining a person during a seizure can cause more harm. **(4)** It is an unsafe practice to keep a syringe of medicine near the bedside.

170. **(1)** Integrated processes: nursing process — implementation, teaching/learning; client need: health promotion and maintenance; content area: medical-surgical.
RATIONALE
(1) Speak slowly so that the client has a better chance of understanding. **(2)** Exaggerating the words causes increased confusion. **(3)** The client is not hard of hearing; she does not understand the language. **(4)** Written instructions do not ensure understanding. She may not be able to read the language either.

171. **(4)** Integrated processes: nursing process — implementation, communication and documentation; client need: safe, effective care environment; coordinated care; content area: medical-surgical.
RATIONALE
(1) Although the mother may sign, it is best to let both parents decide. **(2)** Although the father may sign, it is best to let both parents decide. **(3)** There is no need for both parents to sign the consent form. **(4)** Letting both parents decide avoids cultural imposition.

172. **(4)** Integrated processes: nursing process — implementation, caring; client need: psychosocial integrity; content area: medical-surgical.

RATIONALE
(1) It is usually unacceptable for a woman to touch a male's body in the Islamic culture. **(2)** Although the orderly is a male, he may not be permitted to insert a catheter. The male nurse is the best person to insert the catheter. **(3)** It is preferable to have a trained person do the procedure. **(4)** The male LPN is the best person to do the procedure.

173. **(3)** Integrated processes: nursing process — implementation; client need: psychosocial integrity; content area: medical-surgical.
RATIONALE
(1) Just because someone does not maintain eye contact does not mean that he or she does not understand. **(2)** Just because someone does not maintain eye contact does not mean that he or she is not interested in the conversation. **(3)** Not maintaining eye contact with superiors (the nurse in this case) is common among some Native Americans. **(4)** Not maintaining eye contact does not mean that the client prefers a physician to give the instructions.

174. **(2)** Integrated processes: nursing process — planning; client need: psychosocial integrity; content area: medical-surgical.
RATIONALE
(1) This is not child abuse; coining is a traditional Vietnamese treatment. **(2)** Coining is a traditional Vietnamese treatment that is used for respiratory conditions. **(3)** The practice is not harmful; the father can stay with his child. **(4)** There is no reason to discontinue this practice while the child is in the hospital; it does not interfere with other therapies.

175. **(3)** Integrated processes: nursing process — implementation; client need: physiological integrity; basic care and comfort; content area: psychiatric nursing.
RATIONALE
(1) Although it may be against hospital policy, it should not be and the client should be allowed to eat the food. **(2)** A dietitian should be consulted at a later time. The immediate priority is to let the client eat the food. **(3)** The client is on a regular diet; he can eat the food. **(4)** Do not take the food away.

176. **(2)** Integrated processes: nursing process — planning; client need: psychosocial integrity; content area: medical-surgical.
RATIONALE
(1) The client may eventually be told, but initially the nurse should respect the family's wishes. **(2)** Respect the family's wishes initially. In the Japanese culture, to give the client a terminal diagnosis means to give up hope. **(3)** This may be a later action. **(4)** Insisting that the family tell the client about the terminal diagnosis is cultural imposition.

177. **(2)** Integrated processes: nursing process — planning; client need: psychosocial integrity; content area: psychiatric nursing.
RATIONALE
(1) Restricting visitors in this cultural group may not help the situation. **(2)** Eliciting the help of family members will give the client and family some autonomy. In the Mexican culture, it is a family obligation for all family members to visit the hospitalized family member. **(3)** Control of visitors is a nursing function, not a physician function. **(4)** Acting as the control person will not give the family autonomy.

178. **(4)** Integrated processes: nursing process — implementation; client need: physiological integrity; basic care and comfort; content area: psychiatric nursing.
RATIONALE
(1) There is no reason why the client cannot take herbal teas. They do not interfere with other treatments. **(2)** The nurse may report the situation to the physician later, but the first action is to let her drink her herbal tea. **(3)** The nurse may report the situation to the pharmacist later so it can be added to her profile, but the initial action is to let the client drink her herbal tea. **(4)** Herbal tea gives the client some relief and autonomy.

179. **(2)** Integrated processes: nursing process — planning, caring; client need: psychosocial integrity; content area: psychiatric nursing.
RATIONALE
(1) Oral hypoglycemic medications do not work for insulin-dependent diabetes mellitus. **(2)** Because this is a spiritual and religious issue, the chaplain may have more influence with the client. **(3)** Clients' beliefs should never be labeled as nonsense. **(4)** This statement is an example of cultural imposition.

180. **(3)** Integrated processes: nursing process — planning, caring; client need: psychosocial integrity; content area: psychiatric nursing.
RATIONALE
(1) This action negates client autonomy and rights. **(2)** The physician may eventually order the medicine around the clock, but this is not the first action. **(3)** Exploring the reason for not taking the medicine is the first action. Many Filipino clients are stoical about pain because "it is God's will." **(4)** Although the nurse may report the situation to the nursing supervisor, the first action is to explore the client's reasons for not taking the pain medication.

181. **(1)** Integrated processes: nursing process — implementation, caring; client need: psychosocial integrity; content area: psychiatric nursing.
RATIONALE
(1) Tape the bracelet in place. The bracelet provides for spiritual needs. **(2)** It is not necessary to have the family remove the bracelet. **(3)** It is not necessary to delay the surgery. **(4)** Do not enclose the hand in a mitten. The nail beds will be used in surgery to help determine oxygenation.

182. **(2)** Integrated processes: nursing process — implementation; client need: physiological integrity; reduction of risk potential; content area: medical-surgical.
RATIONALE
(1) It is unlikely that the acupuncturist will ruin the surgery. **(2)** Both the physician and the acupuncturist should be made aware of each other's involvement. **(3)** In some cases, the acupuncture may be as effective as the surgery. **(4)** This statement is judgmental and does not promote client autonomy.

183. **(3)** Integrated processes: nursing process — evaluation; client need: physiological integrity; reduction of risk potential; content area: medical-surgical.
RATIONALE
(1) The feet should not be far apart; this increases the chances of catching her feet on the crutches. **(2)** Placing weight on the axilla can cause damage to the nerves in the axilla. **(3)** Proper crutch walking is placing the weight on the palms of the hands. **(4)** Proper crutch walking includes a swing-through gait.

184. **(1)** Integrated processes: nursing process — implementation, teaching/learning; client need: health promotion and maintenance; content area: medical-surgical.
RATIONALE
(1) The nurse should recognize these symptoms as being consistent with diabetes. She should encourage him to make an appointment with his physician as soon as possible. **(2)** The nurse would encourage him to go to the emergency room only if he gets significantly worse or is unable to obtain an appointment with his physician. **(3)** These symptoms, consistent with diabetes, should not be taken lightly. **(4)** The nurse does not need to notify the supervisor at this time.

185. **(2)** Integrated processes: nursing process — implementation, teaching/learning; client need: physiological integrity; pharmacological therapies; content area: medical-surgical.
RATIONALE
(1) She will continue the medicine even after the symptoms have disappeared. **(2)** The methylprednisolone prescription will include instructions for taking a different number of tablets each day on a decreasing basis. Serious adrenal complications may occur if she does not take the medication exactly as instructed. **(3)** The client will be taking the medication several times each day in the beginning. **(4)** The client will be taking the medication several times each day in the beginning.

186. **(4)** Integrated processes: nursing process — implementation; client need: health promotion and maintenance; content area: medical-surgical.
RATIONALE
(1) Although increasing nutritional status is important, the first priority is to monitor vital signs. **(2)** Although increasing fluid intake is important, the first priority is to monitor vital signs. **(3)** Although monitoring neurological status is important, the first priority is to monitor vital signs. **(4)** A change in vital signs is the most sensitive indicator of a change in status of the client with alcohol abuse.

187. **(3)** Integrated processes: nursing process — implementation; client need: health promotion and maintenance; content area: medical-surgical.
RATIONALE
(1) Meats are allowed as long as they are not fatty. **(2)** Fruits of all kinds are permitted. **(3)** Fatty foods will increase the pain associated with cholecystitis. **(4)** Vegetables of all kinds are permitted.

188. **(4)** Integrated processes: nursing process — implementation, teaching/learning; client need: health promotion and maintenance; content area: medical-surgical.
RATIONALE
(1) Accurate assessments cannot be made on this schedule. **(2)** Accurate assessments cannot be made on this schedule. **(3)** Three days before the menses begins is not the preferred timing for breast self-examinations. **(4)** The preferred timing for breast self-examinations is 3 days after the menses begin because this is the time with the least amount of breast engorgement.

189. **(3)** Integrated processes: nursing process — implementation, teaching/learning; client need: physiological integrity; basic care and comfort; content area: medical-surgical.

RATIONALE
(1) Taking a bath in very warm water will increase perspiration and increase itching. (2) Keeping the room this warm will increase perspiration and increase itching. (3) Avoiding soap whenever possible will decrease itching. The residue left by soaps will increase itching. (4) Perfumed lotions can irritate the skin and increase itching.

190. **(3)** Integrated processes: nursing process — implementation; client need: health promotion and maintenance; content area: medical-surgical.
RATIONALE
(1) The shunt should be warm to the touch. (2) It is unlikely that a visible pulsation would be seen. (3) A normally functioning shunt has a palpable rush of blood. (4) An outline of erythematous skin would denote a possible infection.

191. **(1)** Integrated processes: nursing process — implementation; client need: physiological integrity; reduction of risk potential; content area: medical-surgical.
RATIONALE
(1) The priority action is to place the client back in bed to prevent evisceration. (2) There is no need for a moist dressing. (3) Calling the physician is the next priority. (4) The client may need pain medication, but the first priority is to put the client back to bed.

192. **(4)** Integrated processes: nursing process — implementation, caring; client need: psychosocial integrity; content area: psychiatric nursing.
RATIONALE
(1) This statement is an attempt to console the client but is inappropriate. (2) She may not want to sit in a chair. (3) Calling the physician is not a first priority. (4) This behavior may be culture bound, and the most appropriate action at this time is to remain close to her and offer support.

193. **(2)** Integrated processes: nursing process — implementation; client need: physiological integrity; basic care and comfort; content area: medical-surgical.
RATIONALE
(1) Lean meats and meat by-products will not help to alleviate constipation. (2) Fruits and vegetables provide fiber and help to alleviate constipation. (3) Poultry and fish will not help to alleviate constipation. (4) Rice and potatoes will make the constipation worse.

194. **(3)** Integrated processes: nursing process — implementation; client need: physiological integrity; physiological adaptation; content area: medical-surgical.
RATIONALE
(1) Taking nitroglycerin is the second priority. (2) He would call the rescue squad only if he does not get relief after repeated doses of nitroglycerin. (3) His first priority is to stop all activity to reduce oxygen needs to the myocardium. (4) He should not ignore the pain; he could be having a myocardial infarction.

195. **(4)** Integrated processes: nursing process — planning; client need: physiological integrity; physiological adaptation; content area: medical-surgical.
RATIONALE
(1) The pulse rate would increase if the condition worsens. (2) Although respirations may increase, the most sensitive indicator that the condition is worsening would be indicated by an increase in pulse rate. (3) Respirations would increase if his condition were worsening. (4) The most sensitive indicator of shock is an increase in pulse rate.

196. **(2)** Integrated processes: nursing process — implementation; client need: physiological integrity; reduction of risk potential; content area: medical-surgical.
RATIONALE
(1) High Fowler's position may impede the airway in clients immediately postoperatively. (2) Semi-Fowler's position will help to decrease pull on the incision and to improve ventilation. (3) This position would increase pain and impede ventilation immediately postoperatively. (4) The supine position would cause pull on the incision.

197. **(1)** Integrated processes: nursing process — implementation, teaching/learning; client need: physiological integrity; reduction of risk potential; content area: medical-surgical.
RATIONALE
(1) The priority is to drink at least 3000 mL of fluid each day to prevent clotting. (2) There is no need to eliminate citrus drinks. (3) There is no need to eliminate milk and milk products from the diet. (4) Although cranberry and apple juices are recommended postoperatively, any liquid is okay to drink.

198. **(2)** Integrated processes: nursing process — implementation; client need: physiological integrity; reduction of risk potential; content area: medical-surgical.
RATIONALE
(1) The position of the Hemo-Vac is not important; drainage is maintained by negative pressure within the unit. (2) Completely collapsing the unit before the air plug is inserted will ensure a proper negative pressure within the unit. (3) There is no need to milk the tubing. (4) Negative pressure in a Hemo-Vac is maintained within the unit; it should not be attached to the wall unit.

199. **(3)** Integrated processes: nursing process — data collection; client need: physiological integrity; reduction of risk potential; content area: medical-surgical.
RATIONALE
(1) The presence of a gag reflex does not ensure that the client can take fluids. (2) The client's thirst is not an indicator of ability to tolerate fluids. (3) The presence of bowel sounds is the most reliable indicator that the client can tolerate fluids without aspirating. (4) Degree of alertness does not ensure the presence of bowel sounds.

200. **(1)** Integrated processes: nursing process — planning; client need: physiological integrity; physiological adaptation; content area: medical-surgical.
RATIONALE
(1) Clients with Cushing's syndrome have truncal obesity and hirsutism. (2) Enlarged hands and feet are consistent with acromegaly. (3) A large jaw and large feet are consistent with acromegaly. (4) Clients with Cushing's syndrome have a buffalo hump, but they do not have large hands.

201. **(2)** Integrated processes: nursing process — implementation; client need: physiological integrity; pharmacological therapies; content area: medical-surgical.
RATIONALE
0.3 mg $= 300$ μg $= 1$ tablet

202. **(3)** Integrated processes: nursing process — implementation; client need: physiological integrity; pharmacological therapies; content area: medical-surgical
RATIONALE
150 mg divided by 75 mg $\times$ 7.5 mL = 15 mL

203. **(4)** Integrated processes: nursing process — implementation; client need: physiological integrity; pharmacological therapies; content area: medical-surgical.

RATIONALE

1 mg : 5 mL = 1 mg : x = 5 mL

204. **(2)** Integrated processes: nursing process — implementation; client need: physiological integrity; pharmacological therapies; content area: medical-surgical.

RATIONALE

150 mg divided by 100 mg × 1 tablet = 1.5 tablets

205. **(3)** Integrated processes: nursing process — implementation; client need: physiological integrity; pharmacological therapies; content area: medical-surgical.

RATIONALE

250 mg : 5 mL = 500 mg : x = 10 mL

TEST 4

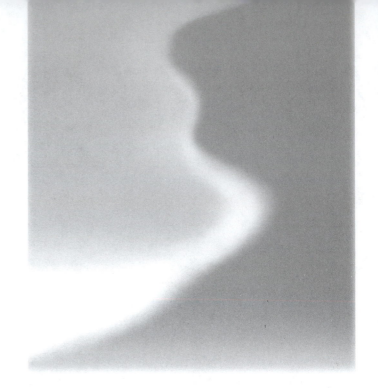

Patricia Gauntlett Beare, RN, PhD
Golden M. Tradewell, RN PhD

QUESTIONS

1. A 45-year-old man returned to his room an hour ago following a gastroscopy. He is requesting some water. The nurse must:

   1. Keep the client nothing by mouth (NPO) until an order is written.
   2. Check the vital signs first.
   3. Check the gag and swallowing reflexes.
   4. Encourage coughing and deep breathing.

2. A client was admitted to the emergency department experiencing grand mal seizures. He was placed on seizure precautions. The nurse knows that an appropriate intervention for a grand mal seizure is:

   1. Insert a tongue blade between the teeth to prevent biting the tongue.
   2. Apply restraints to prevent injury to the self.
   3. Place the client in a supine position.
   4. Place the head in a lateral position.

3. A 30-year-old woman fractured her tibia and several metatarsal bones during a fall while she was jogging. A cast was applied extending from the knee to the toes. The nurse makes frequent observations of which of the following:

   1. Quality of the popliteal and femoral pulses
   2. Color, temperature, and sensation in the toes
   3. Movement of the toes on both feet
   4. The pedal pulses in both lower extremities

4. A client is receiving heparin sodium for a pulmonary embolus. The nurse evaluates which of the following laboratory reports of partial thromboplastin time as indicative of effective heparin therapy?

   1. Within normal range
   2. One to one and one-half times the control (normal) value
   3. Two to two and one-half times the control (normal) value
   4. Three times the control (normal) value

5. A client is on a heparin drip (intravenously). The nurse would keep which of the following drugs available as an antidote?

   1. Vitamin K
   2. Protamine sulfate
   3. Epinephrine
   4. Norepinephrine

6. An 80-year-old client has been taking digoxin (Lanoxin) and furosemide (Lasix) daily for congestive heart failure symptoms. The nurse would want to know the results of the following laboratory test:

   1. Complete blood count
   2. Blood urea nitrogen and creatinine
   3. Coagulation times
   4. Electrolyte panel

7. A nurse assesses an intravenous site of a client and finds it red, swollen, and painful. There is no blood return. The nurse should:

   1. Remove the IV at once.
   2. Watch to see if the swelling gets worse.
   3. Report it to the physician.
   4. Apply an antibiotic ointment to the site.

8. A client diagnosed with insulin-dependent diabetes mellitus (IDDM) becomes irritable and confused; the skin is

cool and clammy, and the pulse rate is 110. The first action of the nurse would be:

1. Give a half-cup of orange juice.
2. Check the serum glucose.
3. Administer regular insulin.
4. Call the physician.

9. A client with IDDM is recovering from diabetic ketoacidosis. The nurse will monitor which of the following serum levels?

1. Sodium
2. Calcium
3. Potassium
4. Magnesium

10. A 29-year-old client has been taking prednisone 60 mg daily for an inflammatory condition for the past 6 months. The physician just wrote an order to discontinue the medication. The nurse should:

1. Stop the medication as ordered.
2. Continue the medication until the physician is available.
3. Call the physician and question the order.
4. Hold the medication until the physician is available.

11. A 26-year-old client is having a chest tube inserted into the left upper chest wall posteriorly. The nurse anticipates that which of the following will be used to cover the incision?

1. Sterile gauze
2. Kerlix
3. A sterile sealant
4. Sterile petrolatum (Vaseline) gauze

12. A client is recovering from a gastrectomy. The nurse will have to administer medication through a nasogastric tube. Prior to giving the medications, the nurse will:

1. Irrigate the tube with saline.
2. Reposition the tube and reapply the tube.
3. Check the tube for placement.
4. Insert the tube 1 inch farther

13. A client is to have a nasogastric tube removed. To prevent aspiration as the tube is pulled past the epiglottis, the nurse teaches the client to:

1. Use a cascade cough
2. Take a deep breath
3. Exhale and hold it
4. Use the Valsalva maneuver

14. A 17-year-old client has nasal congestion, a temperature of 103°F, malaise, and aching muscles. A nurse recommends that the following medication be taken to lower the temperature:

1. Aspirin
2. Enteric-coated aspirin
3. Tylenol
4. Anacin

15. A nurse admits a 23-year-old client to the emergency department in a status epilepticus state. The nurse anticipates that the following drug will be needed:

1. Phenytoin (Dilantin)
2. Phenobarbital
3. Valproic acid
4. Diazepam (Valium)

16. A 44-year-old client has just had a uric acid stone removed from the ureter. The nurse teaches the client that prevention of another stone formation can be aided by forcing fluids and a diet that is:

1. High in vitamin C
2. Low in calcium
3. High in fiber
4. Low in purines

17. An elderly client returns to the nursing unit following a barium enema. The nurse should see that the client:

1. Has an order for a laxative
2. Drinks plenty of fluids
3. Has a dinner high in fiber
4. Takes a sitz bath

18. A client begins having difficulty in breathing and experiences a drop in blood pressure after an injection of penicillin. The nurse's first priority is:

1. Effective heart beat
2. Effective tissue perfusion
3. Normal acid-base balance
4. Open airway

19. A client has narrow-angle glaucoma. The nurse screens the client's medications for the following side-effect:

1. Dilatation of the pupil
2. Constriction of the pupil
3. Constriction of blood vessels
4. Decreased heart rate

20. A nurse assumes the responsibility for the care of an elderly client at 7 AM. The physician had ordered neutral protamine Hagedorn (NPH) insulin to be given at 7:30 AM. Before giving the insulin, the nurse checks to see if the client will eat that day and for the:

1. Signs and symptoms of hypoglycemia
2. Previous sites of injection
3. Serum glucagon level
4. Serum glucose level

21. Diazepam (Valium) is ordered IV for a procedure on an elderly woman. Upon seeing the order, the nurse expresses a concern about:

1. Tolerance
2. Respiratory depression
3. Addiction
4. Anaphylaxis

22. A prescription for diazepam (Valium) is written for a client who is being discharged from the hospital. The nurse teaches the client to:

1. Avoid alcoholic drinks
2. Take the pulse rate frequently
3. Drive only in the daylight
4. Decrease consumption of caffeine

23. A nurse takes an order for a cough medication for her client who has pneumonia. This cough medication should contain a(an):

    1. Mucolytic agent
    2. Depressant for the cough reflex
    3. Expectorant
    4. Bronchiole relaxant

24. The physician has left an order for a laxative prn for a client. The nurse knows that this order should not be carried out for a client who is:

    1. Experiencing abdominal pain of unknown origin
    2. Recovering from an episode of congestive heart failure
    3. Showing signs of hepatic or renal failure
    4. Showing signs of fluid or electrolyte imbalance

25. A client is receiving digoxin (Lanoxin) daily. Prior to giving any preparation of digoxin, the nurse should assess the:

    1. Blood pressure
    2. Respirations
    3. Radial pulse
    4. Apical pulse

26. Which laboratory tests are usually repeated at each prenatal visit?

    1. Hematocrit
    2. Urinalysis for glucose and albumin
    3. Syphilis and gonorrhea screening
    4. Blood typing and antibody titers

27. In most pregnant women, urinary frequency is most problematic:

    1. At 20 weeks' gestation
    2. Following "lightening"
    3. Following "quickening"
    4. During the second trimester

28. The vaginal discharge during pregnancy is characteristically:

    1. Whitish and thick
    2. Yellow and frothy
    3. Thin and blood-tinged
    4. No different than nonpregnant state

29. Your patient is being prepared for an amniocentesis. Before the procedure is performed, it is most important for the nurse to obtain:

    1. The heart rate of the fetus
    2. The mother's body temperature
    3. A urine specimen from the mother
    4. A blood specimen from the mother

30. Of the following assessment findings, which be the most concerning to the nurse during a postpartum examination?

    1. A temperature of 99.8°F
    2. A positive Homan sign
    3. Edema of the perineal area
    4. Uterine contractions during breast-feeding

31. When an epidural is given during the first stage of labor, important nursing interventions in monitoring this client are to: (**Select all that apply.**)

    1. Position the woman flat in bed to avoid a postanesthesia headache.
    2. Monitor the client's blood pressure for hypertension.
    3. Monitor the client's blood pressure for hypotension.
    4. Ensure that the client voids frequently.
    5. Monitor the client's respiratory rate.
    6. Refrain the client from standing.

32. Your client is 25 weeks' pregnant. Her glucose screening test shows a blood sugar level of 180 mg/dL. What follow-up care, if any, would be indicated for this client?

    1. No follow-up is required because the blood sugar is within normal limits.
    2. A glucose tolerance test is indicated.
    3. She should be placed on insulin injections.
    4. She will need weekly nonstress tests to validate fetal well-being.

33. A fetal ultrasound is done prior to an amniocentesis in order to:

    1. Ensure the fetus is mature enough to withstand the amniocentesis.
    2. Evaluate the amount of amniotic fluid.
    3. Locate the fetus and implantation site of the placenta.
    4. Evaluate fetal lung maturity.

34. The client is 10 weeks' pregnant and you are providing her with nutritional education that will be important throughout her pregnancy. She is of average weight for her height. Based on the recommended weight gain during pregnancy, you will advise her that she should gain:

    1. 10–20 lb
    2. 15–22 lb
    3. 25–35 lb
    4. 38–50 lb

35. The client states she is experiencing gastrointestinal discomforts. Your recommended intervention should be:

    1. Lie down for a short time after each meal.
    2. Always include coffee or tea as a beverage with meals.
    3. Eat six or eight small meals per day instead of three large ones.
    4. Take over-the-counter antacids whenever these episodes occur.

36. A laboring client who is pregnant for the second time becomes very anxious as transition progresses. She begins to cry and hyperventilate, which upsets her husband. Your best intervention at this point would be:

    1. Have the client explain what happened in her previous labor and delivery.
    2. Scold her for losing control and assist her in controlling her breathing.
    3. See if she is ready for the epidural.
    4. Explain to both of them that she is making good progress and assure them that you will remain there to assist them both.

37. To ensure a safe outcome for a client who has been placed on oxytocin for induction of labor, the nurse should assess the client for:

1. Nausea, hyperstimulation of the uterus, and poor urine output
2. Hypertension, headache, and arrhythmias
3. Nervousness, diarrhea, and hypertonic contractions
4. Fluid overload, hypertension, and elevated temperature

38. Kegel's exercises are important for mothers following birth because they:

1. Assist in relieving perineal pain
2. Tone the abdominal muscles
3. Assist in preventing postpartal hemorrhage
4. Tone the perineal muscles and promote healing

39. The client explains that her menstrual period is 2 weeks late and she believes she is pregnant. You respond based on your knowledge that the positive signs of pregnancy are:

1. Amenorrhea, nausea, breast changes, and urinary frequency
2. Uterine enlargement and a positive pregnancy test
3. Demonstration of fetal heart tones and verification of fetal movement by someone other than the mother
4. Braxton Hicks contractions, urinary frequency, and a positive pregnancy test

40. Which of the following statements by the client, during a health history, would indicate the need for more information?

1. At 22 weeks' gestation: "My husband and I have enrolled in some parenting education classes."
2. At 16 weeks' gestation: "I know it's about time for me to feel the baby moving and I can hardly wait."
3. At 26 weeks' gestation: "I can still get by with my regular clothes and I don't think I'm going to have to buy any maternity clothes."
4. At 20 weeks' gestation: "My husband came with me for my check-up today. He wants to hear the baby's heartbeat."

41. In assessing a postpartum client, the nurse discovers a boggy uterus with increased lochia flow. Your first nursing intervention should be to:

1. Increase her oxytocin (Pitocin) flow rate.
2. Encourage her to ambulate to the bathroom to empty her bladder.
3. Gently massage the fundus.
4. Examine her cervix for lacerations.

42. The nurse enters the room of a crying client who is 3 days postpartum. She tells the nurse that she doesn't know why she is crying, but she can't seem to stop. Her behavior would indicate:

1. Disappointment in the gender of her new baby
2. Dissatisfaction with the care she is receiving in the hospital
3. Postpartum psychosis
4. Postpartum blues

43. A client with late third trimester bleeding would not receive a digital vaginal examination due to an increased risk of:

1. Initiating undesired labor
2. Separating a low-lying placenta

3. Infection for the mother and fetus
4. Fetal distress prior to labor

44. The client states that she is very disappointed that she cannot breast-feed her baby since her breasts are so small. The nurse's best response would be:

1. "You are probably right. It would be very difficult for you to produce enough milk."
2. "I understand your concern. Perhaps you could provide some breast milk occasionally and provide formula for all the other feedings to ensure that your baby receives enough calories."
3. "The size of the breasts really doesn't have anything to do with it. However, formula is much easier and less stressful for you."
4. "The size and shape of the breast are related to the amount of fatty tissue and are not what influence your milk production. The amount of glandular tissue is what is important. You should be successful with breast-feeding."

45. The client has come to a clinic to have an intrauterine device (IUD) inserted. In explaining this contraceptive method, the nurse tells the client that a common problem is:

1. Painful intercourse
2. Repeated vaginal and uterine infections
3. Spontaneous expulsion of the IUD
4. Cessation of menstrual flow

46. A client was admitted to the emergency department complaining of a sharp lower right abdominal pain. During the nursing history, she reports to the nurse that her last menstrual period was 7 weeks ago. A question the nurse would ask is:

1. "Are you experiencing any shoulder pain?"
2. "Have you ever been pregnant before?"
3. "How many children do you have?"
4. "Can you feel a hard mass on your right side?"

47. The client came for her first prenatal visit. The results of her blood work showed a physiologic anemia. The nurse knows that:

1. Her diet is poor without iron intake.
2. Her liver is not able to keep up with the increased demands of pregnancy.
3. Her blood volume is increased, causing hemodilution.
4. Her blood work needs to be repeated because of a probable laboratory error.

48. The nurse is discussing the labor process with a client who is pregnant for the first time. The nurse explains that the client should come to the hospital when:

1. She loses her mucous plug and has a bloody show.
2. She is having regular contractions that are very uncomfortable.
3. Her membranes rupture or her contractions are regular at 5–7 minutes.
4. Her contractions are 10–15 minutes apart.

49. A client is admitted to the labor and delivery room with contractions that are regular, last 50 seconds, and are 3–5 minutes apart. She reports that she had a bloody show early this morning. Vaginal examination reveals that her cervix is 100% effaced and 8 cm dilated. The nurse knows that this information indicates that the client is in which phase of labor?

1. Active phase
2. Latent phase
3. Retention phase
4. The fourth stage

50. The nurse realizes that the client who is 12 hours postpartum and successfully breast-feeding her new son needs additional instructions when she states:

1. "I must remember to keep lotion handy for my breasts so they won't dry out."
2. "I must remember to wash my hands real good each time before I put the baby to my breast."
3. "I plan to put a large safety pin on my bra after each feeding so that I can remember which breast the baby nursed from at each feeding."
4. "I know how important it is to drink lots of fluid now."

51. The nurse is careful to fold the diaper down to lie below the level of the clamped umbilical cord in a newborn. What is the correct reason for this action?

1. To prevent infection at the cord site
2. To prevent pain at the cord site
3. To facilitate the dry gangrene process to less than 7 days
4. To avoid irritation and prevent wetness on the cord site

52. What is the purpose of covering the genitals of an infant under phototherapy with a bikini diaper made from a face mask?

1. To prevent burning of the genitals
2. To prevent gonadal complications
3. To protect the skin from diarrhea
4. To measure urine output

53. Which of the following statements by the mother of an 8-month-old indicates a need for further teaching?

1. "I should avoid regular, adult canned foods for the baby to prevent possible exposure to lead."
2. " I should use fresh, home-prepared foods for the infant as much as possible."
3. "I can use frozen, home-prepared foods for the infant."
4. "I can add honey or corn syrup to food to increase the infant's acceptance of it."

54. Which of the following statements by the nurse is most accurate when teaching the 6-month-old client's mother about infant nutrition?

1. Introduce combination rice-fruit cereals first along with formula.
2. Begin whole milk with solid foods.
3. Large quantities of fruit juices can be used between feedings.
4. Breast milk and/or formula should continue as the primary source of nutrition.

55. In determining the proper location to initiate chest compressions on an infant, which is the best technique for the nurse to use? (Place an X in the figure on the area of the chest.)

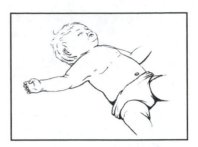

56. Which of the following activities by the mother of an infant would indicate a need for additional teaching?

1. Testing the warmed formula on the inner wrist
2. Testing the warmed formula on her tongue
3. Testing the warmed formula on the top of her hand
4. Providing formula cool to the touch

57. Which of the following statements would indicate that the client had adequate teaching regarding use of baby powder?

1. All forms of baby powder should be avoided in the diaper area.
2. The powder should be placed in the hand and then applied to the diaper area.
3. Talc powder is safer than corn starch products.
4. Powder does not help to keep the skin dry.

58. The physician has ordered topical corticosteroids for a client's atopic dermatitis. The nurse correctly identifies the purpose of applying topical corticosteroids to atopic dermatitis is:

1. To dry the area
2. To moisten the area
3. To decrease inflammation
4. To decrease pruritus

59. The nurse explains to a mother the purpose of waiting until 18–24 months to initiate toilet training for her infant as:

1. The toddler is not psychologically ready until that age.
2. The toddler is not physiologically ready until that age.
3. The toddler is not psychologically or physiologically ready until that age.
4. The toddler is not able to hold urine for a full hour until that time.

60. Which of the following statements by the nurse is most accurate in teaching about the typical play behavior of a toddler?

1. They prefer solitary play.
2. They prefer parallel play.
3. They prefer associative play.
4. They prefer team sports.

61. To promote optimal health for the deciduous teeth, the nurse should instruct the parents in which dental care techniques for their preschoolers? (Select all that apply.)

1. Begin dental care when the first tooth erupts.
2. Take the child for yearly dental examinations once school starts.

3. Supervise brushing and assist with flossing throughout the preschool years.
4. Allow the child to assume self-care for brushing and flossing.
5. Don't worry about the baby teeth, begin brushing the permanent ones.
6. Don't worry about dental examinations until permanent teeth are in.

62. Which approach by the nurse is best in obtaining a health history of a 13-year-old girl?

1. Direct all questions to the mother.
2. Direct all questions to the child.
3. Allow the parent to stay in the room to decrease the child's fear.
4. Question the mother and child together and separately.

63. The nurse correctly identifies that the most common of the opiate-induced side effects in a child is:

1. Constipation
2. Respiratory depression
3. Nausea and vomiting
4. Anaphylaxis

64. The nurse should teach the family and child at risk for hyperlipidemia and hypercholesterolemia that the diet should include which of the following substitutes?

1. Red meat
2. Hot dogs
3. Turkey
4. Regular milk

65. Which of the following statements would indicate that the parent of a child with a newly applied cast needs further instructions?

1. "I should allow the cast to air-dry."
2. "I should use my fingertips to handle the cast."
3. "I should check distal extremities for temperature and color."
4. "I should keep the affected extremity elevated."

66. To prevent sports injuries, the nurse should recommend which one of the following sports as less likely to produce an injury?

1. Football
2. Gymnastics
3. Running
4. Golf

67. Which of the following statements is most important in promoting hydration in a client with a fever and upper respiratory infection?

1. Oral rehydration solutions such as Pedialyte should be considered for infants.
2. Sports drinks such as Gatorade should be considered for children.
3. Parents should be encouraged to measure all intake and output.
4. Liquids should not be forced or the child awakened for fluids.

68. Which of the following statements by the nurse is most accurate when teaching the client about asthma?

1. It is an irreversible airway obstruction.
2. It is a reversible airway obstruction.
3. It is more prevalent in boys than girls.
4. It has usually an onset at 4 to 5 years of age.

69. The nurse correctly identifies the purpose of giving the client with asthma a corticosteroid as:

1. The anti-inflammatory effects
2. To decrease bronchospasms
3. To prevent infection
4. To provide nonsteroidal properties

70. The nurse should teach the client with any type of upper respiratory infection (URI), which of the following?

1. Allergies cause many URLs, and shots are always indicated.
2. Prevention of attacks is not possible.
3. Children will outgrow URIs.
4. Avoid active and passive smoking.

71. The nurse correctly identifies which of the following as usually the earliest detectable sign of dehydration?

1. Tachycardia
2. Dry skin and mucous membranes
3. Sunken fontanelles
4. Delayed capillary refill

72. Which of the following statements by the nurse is most accurate when teaching the parents of a dehydrated child about replacement fluids?

1. Any cola or juice is considered a clear liquid.
2. Diluted formula is considered clear liquid.
3. Water is the only true clear liquid.
4. Clear fluid is one through which newsprint can be read.

73. Which of the following interventions is the first therapeutic management approach in the treatment of mild acute diarrhea in the pediatric client?

1. Parenteral fluids
2. Oral rehydration therapy (ORT)
3. A BRAT diet (bananas, rice, applesauce, toast, and tea)
4. Antidiarrheal agents

74. In preparing to apply a topical preparation over a burn, the nurse would question the application of which agent to a child allergic to sulfa?

1. Silver nitrate
2. Silver sulfadiazine (Silvadene)
3. Povidone-iodine (Betadine)
4. Bacitracin

75. Which of the following statements is most accurate to teach parents in regard to nutrition for toddlers?

1. A rigid schedule of meals and snacks should be provided.
2. The toddler should sit and eat every entire meal with the family.
3. Skim milk or low-fat milk may be used.
4. Serve 1 tablespoon of solid food per year of age per serving.

76. Nursing care for the substance abuse client experiencing alcohol withdrawal delirium includes:

1. Maintaining seizure precautions
2. Restricting fluid intake
3. Increasing sensory stimuli
4. Applying ankle and wrist restraints

77. The nurse is aware that many clients admitted to a psychiatric unit are concerned about:

1. Confidentiality
2. Anonymity
3. Insanity defense
4. Moral distress

78. Many clients have difficulty expressing anger. Which one of the following nursing interventions would assist a client with expressing anger appropriately?

1. Isolate from others
2. Encourage acting out
3. Encourage verbalization
4. Introduce self-care improvement

79. The client reported to the nurse that the therapy session was a failure and a waste of time. The client then remarked, "The next time, I'll just sit there and be a nonparticipant." What defense mechanism is the client demonstrating?

1. Compensation
2. Identification
3. Rationalization
4. Projection

80. During the initial interview, the client tells the nurse that he grew up on the "wrong side of the tracks." He feels rejected by his family, socially unacceptable, and works hard to become the meanest fighter in his block. Which of the following defense mechanisms is the client exhibiting?

1. Projection
2. Compensation
3. Reaction formation
4. Rationalization

81. A 10-year-old girl hit a playmate with a baseball bat. The school nurse intervened in the incident. The girl shouted, "He hit me. He hit me. He hit me." Which of the following defense mechanisms is the girl exhibiting?

1. Displacement
2. Projection
3. Rationalization
4. Sublimation

82. A 3-year-old girl was excited about having a new brother and welcomed him home with a hug and a kiss. After a few days, she started wetting her pants and told her mother that she wanted a diaper. This is most suggestive of:

1. Regression
2. Undoing
3. Repression
4. Reaction formation

83. A psychiatric nurse was instructed by the attending psychiatrist to administer 10 mg of haloperidol (Haldol) to a severely dysfunctional client. The client refused all medications. Which was the best nursing action?

1. Restrain the client and give the medication IM.
2. Accept the client's decision.
3. Plead with the client to reconsider.
4. Obtain a discharge order for noncompliance.

84. On admission to a psychiatric unit, a 22-year-old male client signed a voluntary admission form. After a period of 12 hours, the client informs the nurse of his desire to leave by yelling, "I don't need to be here. Let me out." What is the best response by the nurse?

1. "You can't leave the hospital."
2. "Think about staying for 1 week."
3. "Please sign this legal form indicating your intentions and wait 24 hours."
4. "Ask your doctor about discharge so he can start legal procedures."

85. Disclosure of information, beyond members of the multidisciplinary team, without the consent of the client is a breach of:

1. Anonymity
2. Confidentiality
3. Duty
4. Habeas corpus

86. Psychiatric clients have a right to refuse treatment. When persuasion and manipulation are used to get the client engaged in treatment, the nurse is aware that:

1. The client has no fundamental right to refuse treatment.
2. There is a responsibility to complete treatment once it is started.
3. Paternalism is operating.
4. Constitutional rights are abused.

87. A 29-year-old man client admitted himself for psychiatric treatment. The nurse determines that this admission is:

1. Voluntary
2. Judicial
3. Informal
4. Involuntary

88. The most effective nursing interventions to assist a client who is experiencing moderate anxiety are to:

1. Focus on anxiety reduction.
2. Probe the cause.
3. Investigate decompensation behaviors.
4. Accept the level of anxiety.
5. Support health coping behaviors.
6. Monitor levels of consciousness

89. At the time of admission, a female client suffered from insomnia, shortness of breath, and a rapid pulse. The client was agitated and stated that she was going crazy and losing control. The diagnosis was panic disorder. The nursing plan of care should include:

1. Large doses of antianxiety medications
2. Family education
3. The etiology and management of panic disorders
4. Cognitive restructuring

90. After a complete diagnostic work-up for a client with neurobiological changes, it was determined that the client was experiencing post-traumatic stress disorder (PTSD). In planning care for the client, the nurse should be aware that:

1. The symptoms are a mechanism, which help him cope with an unacceptable situation.
2. The symptoms are a mechanism, which help him cope and support his dependence.
3. The symptoms are a means to manipulate others.
4. The symptoms develop from a nonspecific psychic event.

91. A 25-year-old female client tells the nurse that she has an irrational fear of spiders and goes out of her way to avoid them. In planning care for the client, it is important for the nurse to know that:

1. The client has displaced a conscious conflict to an object symbolically related to the conflict.
2. The anxiety is free-floating.
3. The client accepts the source of distress.
4. The behavioral style of phobic clients is avoidance.

92. During the multidisciplinary team conference, the client explained that she was terrified of rain and practiced avoidance. The team members understand that the client is:

1. Controlling the intensity of the anxiety
2. Fearful of the internal source of distress
3. Aware of the basic source of the anxiety
4. Attempting to undo the source of anxiety

93. A female client continues to exhibit seductive behavior, pressured speech, and psychomotor agitation. Which of the following is the best nursing intervention?

1. Provide a safe environment.
2. Indicate that the behavior is not acceptable.
3. Encourage group activity.
4. Promote highly competitive activities.

94. A scantily dressed client approached the nurse, saying "I am a striptease dancer and I am ready for visitors." Which action by the nurse would be most appropriate?

1. Inform the client that all privileges will be suspended indefinitely.
2. Assure the client that her behavior is appropriate.
3. Redirect the client to her room and assist her with a change of clothes.
4. Allow the client to remain as dressed.

95. The activity therapist is implementing an individualized program for a manic client exhibiting hostility and excessive energy. Which of the following activities would be most appropriate?

1. Writing short stories
2. Team sports

3. Ping-pong
4. Walking

96. A 40-year-old male client discharged from a psychiatric unit 4 days ago presented at the clinic talking loudly, cursing, and crying. Family members stated that they are unable to cope with the behavior and alternative living arrangements must be made. Which living arrangement is most suitable?

1. Long-term psychiatric hospitalization
2. Nursing home placement
3. Group home placement
4. Independent living

97. The physician orders fluoxetine (Prozac) for a depressed client. Which of the following should the nurse remember about fluoxetine?

1. Because fluoxetine is a tricyclic antidepressant, it may precipitate a hypertensive crisis.
2. The therapeutic effect of the drug occurs 2–4 weeks after treatment is begun.
3. Foods such as aged cheese, yogurt, soy sauce, and bananas should not be eaten with this drug.
4. Fluoxetine may be administered safely in combination with monoamine oxidate (MAO) inhibitors.

98. The nurse is caring for a 38-year-old man who was in an automobile accident 3 months ago. He complains of neck pain and brags about the pending insurance settlement. The nurse suspects that the client is:

1. Malingering
2. Suffering from conversion reaction
3. Exhibiting somatization disorder
4. A hypochondriac

99. A 58-year-old client is admitted to the psychiatric unit. During the nursing assessment, the client states, "My mother just walked by the window and I saw her go into the nurse's station." This behavior is an example of:

1. Hallucinations
2. Fantasies
3. Delusions
4. Derealization

100. In caring for a 39-year-old client who acknowledges noncompliance and demonstrates bizarre behaviors, neologism, and thought insertion, the nurse should:

1. Convey acceptance of the client.
2. Spend time focusing on thought insertion.
3. Ignore the behaviors.
4. Assist with identification of target symptoms.

101. How does a nurse develop a culturally appropriate care plan for an older person?

1. By listening to the family's perception of the client's problem.
2. By allowing family members time to discuss their perception of the client's problem.
3. By acknowledging the older person's viewpoint.
4. By recommending a treatment plan based on the physician's recommendation.

102. What term is used to describe professional misconduct, negligent care or treatment, or failure to meet the standards of care, resulting in harm to a person?

1. Civil wrongs
2. Torts
3. Malpractice
4. Informed consent

103. Which of the following is not an element of negligence that must be present to substantiate a malpractice claim?

1. Duty
2. Breach of duty
3. Damages
4. Unrelated causal effect

104. Documentation is the best method of defense in a malpractice suit involving an older person. In addition to the malpractice defense, documentation has what other use?

1. Increases the potential areas of legal exposure
2. Describes client education and discharge instructions
3. Relates conversations of nurses among themselves
4. Refrains from recording untoward events such as falls

105. What aspects of documentation about restraints ensure that the nurse acted competently?

1. Failure to document the need for restraints
2. Failure to monitor client's condition properly
3. Documenting client's response to restraints
4. Failure to try alternatives before using restraints

106. What is the nurse's responsibility in obtaining informed consent before surgery?

1. To obtain the informed consent
2. To witness the signature of the client on the informed consent sheet
3. To read the client his or her rights
4. To sign for the client if he or she is unable to do so

107. Clients can exercise their right to refuse treatment in the form of a "do not resuscitate" (DNR) order. How does the nurse ensure that the client's wishes are carried out?

1. Obtain a telephone order from the physician.
2. Request that the physician write a DNR order on the chart.
3. Resuscitate the client on family members' request.
4. Resuscitate the client regardless of the order.

108. To preserve the older person's wishes and protect the health-care providers, the nurse must see that the following is included in the chart:

1. "Slow code" orders
2. Copies of living will and medical durable power of attorney
3. Telephone order for DNR
4. Physician's request for DNR without family input

109. Which of the following is a common nursing area of legal exposure in caring for older persons?

1. Undermedication
2. Overmedication
3. Reporting complications
4. Assessing the older person's condition every 8 hours

110. While administering medication to a client via a nasogastric tube, the nurse suspects that the tube has become clogged. Which of the following actions are acceptable? (**Select all that apply.**)

1. Aspirate the tube.
2. Remove and replace the tube.
3. Flush with warm water.
4. Flush with a carbonated beverage.
5. Remove nasogastric tube and replace.
6. Flush with normal saline.

111. The nurse is admitting an elderly woman from the local nursing home with severe abdominal pain. Which of the following steps should the nurse implement? (**Select all that apply.**)

1. Ask the client to point to the pain location.
2. Ask the caregiver to point to the location of the pain.
3. Monitor symptoms of pain by taking blood pressure.
4. Ask the client to rate the intensity of the pain by using a pain scale.
5. Observe for indicators of pain, such as restlessness.
6. Observe for indicators of pain, such as cool, dry skin.

112. You are caring for a 40-year-old man with diabetes who has had his right foot amputated for gangrene. He is perspiring, restless, and moaning. Another nurse tells you to give only one-half of the ordered doses of narcotics because of the side effects of respiratory depression and addiction. What would you do? (**Select all that apply.**)

1. Give one-half of the ordered dose and document in the chart.
2. Give the full dose of ordered pain medication.
3. Request the physician to order the dose in oral form instead of intramuscular injection.
4. Refuse to give the pain medication.
5. After pain medication has been given, change the bed linens.
6. Ask the client if he would like to have relaxing music to help distract him from the severe pain.

113. The older adult is at risk for fluid volume deficit from which of the following factors? (**Select all that apply.**)

1. Perception of thirst increases with aging.
2. Muscle tissue declines with age.
3. The amount of total body water increases.
4. Keeping the room environment too cool.
5. Body temperature regulation is less effective with aging.
6. The ability to concentrate urine decreases.

114. A hypertensive client was being seen at the local community clinic. Her blood pressure was 200/140 mm Hg. When asked to give a 24-hour recall of her diet, the client stated that she had had an egg and bacon with a glass of milk for breakfast; bologna sandwich with chips, an orange, and bottled water for lunch; and a tuna fish salad for supper with low-fat yogurt. Which of the following foods have a high sodium content? (**Select all that apply.**)

1. Orange
2. Chips
3. Bologna
4. Bread
5. Tuna fish
6. Milk

115. Because the hypertensive client is taking Lasix, the nurse asked the client if she knew which of the following foods are high in potassium. (**Select all that apply.**)

1. Orange
2. Chips
3. Bologna
4. Bacon
5. Milk
6. Applesauce

116. In teaching the client ways to decrease edema, the nurse suggested which of the following ways? (**Select all that apply.**)

1. Drink at least one soft drink daily.
2. Walk barefoot as often as possible.
3. Change your position in the chair or bed frequently.
4. Wear supportive hose or stockings.
5. Elevate feet and legs when sitting.
6. Wear underwear that helps to hold in abdominal muscles.

117. The nurse plans to administer potassium chloride through the client's enteral feeding tube. What steps should the nurse take to ensure safety? (**Select all that apply.**)

1. Mix the medication with the feeding.
2. Flush the feeding tube before administering the medication.
3. Push air into the feeding tube after administering the medication.
4. Resume the tube feeding as soon as the medication is given.
5. Check for gastric residual before administering the medication.
6. Flush the feeding tube before and after administering the medication.

118. The nurse is completing an intake and output record for a nursing home client who has been hospitalized for pneumonia. The client was NPO. At the beginning of the shift, the nurse hung a 1000-mL bag of D$_5$W (5% dextrose in water) with normal saline. The physician ordered the IV to infuse at 100 mL/hr. How

much fluid was left by the end of the nurse's 8-hour shift?

_____

119. The client who had been hospitalized with pneumonia was receiving enteral feeding at 50 mL/hr. How much formula did the client receive during the nurse's 8-hour shift?

_____

120. The physician ordered a client to receive 250 mL of Glucerna as a bolus feeding. The nurse was checking the gastric residual before administering the noon bolus feeding. After checking the residual, the nurse decided to hold the bolus feeding until 1 PM. How much gastric residual was aspirated out of the stomach when the nurse was checking?

_____

121. The nurse was preparing to administer liquid Tylenol (acetaminophen) to a client who had a percutaneous endoscopic gastrostomy (PEG) tube. What is the minimum amount of water that the nurse should use to dilute the medication?

_____

122. The nurse was establishing a care plan for a client with end-stage renal disease on dialysis. The nurse understands that a combined fluid 24-hour intake for a client with end-stage renal disease on dialysis is:

_____

123. An elderly nursing home client was admitted with a diagnosis of "failure to thrive" syndrome. The client weighed 85 lb upon admission. The physician ordered vitamin B$_{12}$ injections to help stimulate the client's appetite. What type of needle would be appropriate for the client's body size?

_____

124. The nurse preparing to administer an intramuscular injection using the Z-track method knows the correct angle to inject is:

_____

125. The physician ordered 0.25 gr of morphine sulfate to the oncology client. The nurse administering the medication knows that 0.25 gr is equivalent to:

_____

126. Which of the following is not a risk factor for the development of cardiovascular disease?

1. Being underweight
2. Smoking
3. Having hypertension
4. Maintaining a sedentary lifestyle

127. When administering transdermal NTG, it is most important to:

1. Check blood pressure before each dose.
2. Check pulse after administration.

3. Have the client in the sitting position.
4. Check the client's potassium level.

128. A 53-year-old client is following a low-sodium diet. A dinner tray arrives. Which food would the nurse remove?

1. Pears
2. Baked chicken
3. Olives
4. Baked potato

129. A 76-year-old client has left-sided congestive heart failure (CHF). Physical assessment findings to be expected include:

1. Dependent edema
2. Distended neck veins
3. Lower left quadrant (LLQ) pain
4. Dyspnea on exertion

130. A 46-year-old construction worker has arterial insufficiency of the lower extremities. Expected physical findings include:

1. Lymphedema
2. Pedal edema
3. Absence of pedal pulses
4. Bluish cast to extremities

131. The master endocrine gland is controlled by the:

1. Pineal gland
2. Sympathetic nervous system
3. Hypothalamus
4. Pituitary gland

132. A 44-year-old client has had a thyroidectomy. Planning for return from the recovery room, which item would the nurse have ready?

1. Jackson-Pratt drain
2. Tracheostomy tray
3. Salem sump tube
4. IV potassium infusion

133. A term used to describe an infection that develops as a result of a hospital stay is:

1. Pathogenic
2. Synergistic
3. Diagnostic
4. Nosocomial

134. An 80-year-old was being discharged after a below the knee amputation. He told the nurse that his wife had Alzheimer's disease. Which action should the nurse take?

1. Notify hospice coordinator.
2. Notify respiratory therapist.
3. Notify physician to obtain home health consult.
4. Notify elderly protective services.

135. During a home-health visit, the nurse assessed the client's medication. She found that the client had two medications for pain relief. One was an over-the-counter drug, Aleve. The other medication was a prescription, naproxen. Both were 200 mg in strength. What instructions need to be given to the client?

1. Take both medications as ordered.
2. Aleve and naproxen are both the same drug.
3. Use Aleve one day and naproxen the next day.
4. Combine both medications in one bottle.

136. A home-health nurse was assessing an elderly client with osteoporosis. Which of the following would indicate further need for teaching?

1. Properly installed electrical outlets.
2. Bathtub does not have nonslip mats on bottom of tub.
3. Newspapers neatly piled up in a corner.
4. Handrails in place in bathroom.

137. The nurse was assessing a client who had been admitted for diabetes. Which of the following statements indicate that the diabetic client needs more information?

1. "I store my insulin in a warm environment."
2. "I see my physician for follow up exams routinely."
3. "I use my plastic insulin syringes only once."
4. "I check my feet daily for sores."

138. A terminal cancer client, receiving large doses of narcotics for pain control, attempted to get out of bed. In order to reduce the risk of falling, which type of restraint would be most beneficial?

1. Mechanical restraints
2. Leg restraints
3. Using medications to relax the client
4. Using a sheet to tie him to the bed frame

139. A 45-year-old client, receiving a kidney transplant, was in reverse isolation postoperatively. The purpose for this type of isolation is:

1. To protect the client from his own bacteria.
2. To protect the other clients on the nursing unit.
3. To protect the client from outside infections from others on the unit.
4. To protect the hospital staff from the client.

140. A client being discharged to home under the services of home health had an aged deaf parent living with him in the same house. Which of the following programs would help the client with financial assistance?

1. Aid to Families with Dependent Children
2. Meals on Wheels
3. Council on Aging
4. Supplemental Security Income (SSI)

141. The nurse was assisting in a health fair for a group of teenage girls. Preventing pregnancy was a topic of concern for these adolescents. Which of the following statements indicate that the teenage girls need more information on this topic?

1. "I can get pregnant even if my boyfriend withdraws before he comes."
2. "I cannot get pregnant on the first time we have sex."
3. " I can get pregnant anytime I have unprotected sex."

4. "I can get pregnant even though my menstrual cycle is not regular yet."

142. Screening for tuberculosis is done for:
    1. Identification of infected children
    2. HIV-positive clients
    3. Individuals infected with hepatitis B
    4. Individuals who have been compliant with their medication use

143. Tuberculin skin testing is the standard method of identifying persons infected with *Mycobacterium tuberculosis*. This is done by:
    1. Mantoux test by subcutaneous injection
    2. Mantoux test by IM injection
    3. Mantoux test by IV method
    4. Mantoux test by intradermal injection

144. The Centers for Disease Control and Prevention (CDC) recommends preventive therapy for which of the following clients?
    1. Clients with active tuberculosis
    2. Clients with normal chest radiographs
    3. Clients who are HIV positive
    4. Clients with no contact to active tuberculosis

145. A nurse working in home health has both direct and indirect care functions. Which of the following is an example of indirect care functions? (**Select all that apply.**)
    1. Teaching the care provider how to take a blood pressure
    2. Participating in a team conference regarding the client
    3. Teaching the care provider how to read a food label for sodium content
    4. Discussing client needs with the dietitian
    5. Performing wound care as ordered by the physician
    6. Requesting an extension of home health services from the physician

146. The nurse is weighing a pregnant woman at the obstetrics office. The woman was concerned about how much alcohol she could ingest. Which of the following statements indicate that the woman may be at high risk for fetal alcohol syndrome?
    1. "I just snort cocaine once or twice a day."
    2. "I smoke marijuana with my boyfriend and his friends."
    3. "I drink a few beers a day to settle my nerves."
    4. "I don't feel like anyone loves me."

147. The psychosocial climate which the pediatric nurse should try to establish when dealing with suspected family violence is:
    1. Judgmental attitude
    2. Disgust and avoidance
    3. Supportive treatment
    4. Punitive

148. The licensed practical nurse/licensed vocational nurse (LPN/LVN) arrives on the unit with only one registered nurse and one nursing assistant. There are

10 clients to use functional nursing to best care for these 10 clients. Using functional nursing to care for the 10 clients, what is the LPN/LVN's first priority?
    1. Pass out breakfast trays.
    2. Hang four IV medications.
    3. Introduce yourself to patients.
    4. Check medication cards/sheets against the Kardex.

149. The LPN/LVN notices that one of the clients is unable to eat without assistance. Which action is the most appropriate?
    1. Stop and assist the client with his meal.
    2. Ask the team leader to assist the client with his meal.
    3. Ask the nursing assistant to help the client with his meal.
    4. Notify the dietitian that the client cannot eat.

150. A 32-year-old female client is receiving dexamethasone (Decadron). While planning nursing care, the nurse would be sure to include the client's predisposition to:
    1. Renal calculi
    2. Infection
    3. Gallstones
    4. Hypotension

151. A 37-year-old client has been returned to her room after a thyroidectomy. In what position would the nurse place the client?
    1. Right side
    2. Left side
    3. Semi-Fowler's
    4. Low-Fowler's

152. A 57-year-old client with a parathyroidectomy is being returned to the room postoperatively. What tray would the nurse have at the bedside?
    1. Thoracotomy
    2. Tracheostomy
    3. Paracentesis
    4. Pericardiocentesis

153. A 27-year-old client enters the emergency room and has a screwdriver protruding from the right flank. The nurse would:
    1. Remove the screwdriver and apply manual pressure.
    2. Leave it in place and help the client to a stretcher.
    3. Tether the screwdriver in place.
    4. Remove the screwdriver and put on a sterile dressing.

154. A 16-year-old adolescent with a deep, bleeding laceration on the leg enters the clinic. The nurse's first action is to:
    1. Clean the wound of debris.
    2. Apply a tourniquet above the bleeding site.
    3. Apply a tourniquet below the bleeding site.
    4. Apply direct pressure to the wound.

155. An 87-year-old client is scheduled for an above-the-knee amputation (AKA). To best prepare the client for postoperative therapy, the nurse would:

1. Explain phantom limb pain
2. Demonstrate dressing changes
3. Teach crutch walking
4. Teach leg exercises on the unaffected leg

156. A 53-year-old client with arthritis is having difficulty sleeping because of anxiety. The most appropriate activity to promote sleep is:

1. Administer a tranquilizer.
2. Administer a sleeping pill.
3. Help the client to explore feelings.
4. Provide a snack with warm milk.

157. A 36-year-old client with hemorrhoids will be having surgery in 3 days. Before surgery, the nurse would instruct the client to follow what kind of diet?

1. High fiber
2. Low fiber
3. High fat
4. High carbohydrate

158. A client was taking clindamycin (Cleocin) 150 mg every 12 hours for a wound infection. On hand is Cleocin 300 mg/2 mL. How many milliliters are required to deliver each of the two doses?

1. 1
2. 2
3. 3
4. 4

159. The client was diagnosed with Parkinson's disease. The physician ordered levodopa (L-dopa) 750 mg tid. What is the total 24-hour dose for this client?

1. 1500 mg
2. 2000 mg
3. 2200 mg
4. 2250 mg

160. The client was having pruritus secondary to severe anxiety. The physician ordered diphenhydramine (Benadryl) 75 mg. Available is Benadryl injection 25 mg/mL in a 10-mL multiple-dose vial. How many milliliters should be administered to the client?

1. 0.5
2. 1
3. 1.5
4. 3

161. A client was to be given morphine sulfate 3–5 mg IV for pain. The physician ordered the morphine to be titrated. The morphine was supplied in a 10-mg/mL single-dose vial. The nurse needed to titrate the morphine with how much normal saline in order to deliver 1 mg/mL?

1. 1 mL
2. 5 mL
3. 7.5 mL
4. 9 mL

162. A child was to be given an injection of penicillin V (V-Cillin K). The dosage was in a 2-mL syringe. What is the maximum dosage to be administered per intramuscular injection to a child 5 years of age?

1. 1 mL
2. 2 mL
3. 3 mL
4. 4 mL

163. A 79-year-old client with osteoarthritis is scheduled to have an arthroplasty (joint replacement) surgery to the right hip. The client has been active since retirement and is in good health. In the preoperative teaching, the nurse instructs the client that the physician will most likely begin ambulation on the third postoperative day. The rationale for early ambulation following joint replacement is:

1. Prolonged inactivity in an older adult increases the chance of venous thrombosis.
2. Prolonged bed rest increases the chance of developing decubitus ulcers.
3. Late ambulation fosters dependence upon the nursing staff.
4. Early ambulation ensures the client will return to the baseline functional status.

164. Preoperative instructions to arthroplasty clients include hip precaution measures. The nurse correctly instructs the client:

1. Do not sit with your hips at a 90-degree or greater angle.
2. Bend forward using correct body mechanics and use your knees.
3. Do not bend to put on your shoes; use a long shoe horn.
4. Do not keep pillows between legs when lying on your back.

165. The client begins physical therapy for the first time on the third postoperative day. Although she has been resting for 30 minutes after the active physical therapy session, she continues to have elevated vital signs: blood pressure 160/94 mm Hg and pulse rate of 94 bpm. The most appropriate nursing action at this time is to:

1. Do nothing and reevaluate her in an hour.
2. Order a stat electrocardiogram (ECG).
3. Call the physician.
4. Call physical therapy and see if an error was made in therapy.

166. A general rule of thumb for nurses to remember when administering medications to an older adult is:

1. Drugs are given more frequently in the older adult.
2. Drugs are less effective in the older adult.
3. Most medications do more harm than good.
4. Most medications should be given in lower dosages.

167. A 75-year-old client is admitted with gangrene of the right leg. The physician discusses the need for an AKA of the extremity. The initial approach by the nurse following this discussion is:

1. Spend time with the client and allow him to verbalize feelings.
2. Share with the client other persons who have had amputations.

3. Talk with the client's family about how to be supportive after surgery.
4. Explain the procedure for an above-the-knee amputation and answer questions.

168. During a home health visit, the nurse observes that a client's AKA wound was completely healed 1 month postoperative. The most appropriate action by the nurse following this observation is:

1. Discontinue wrapping the stump.
2. Provide a protective cushion to the stump.
3. Discuss the management of phantom pain.
4. Provide strengthening exercises to all limbs.

169. A diabetic client is to receive diabetic diet instructions prior to discharge. When working with the client in meal planning, the nurse allows the client to have occasional "forbidden foods" such as ice cream or other sweets. The rationale for this nursing action is:

1. Knowledge that diabetics rarely follow dietary instructions to the letter.
2. Knowledge that rigid control of diet is less likely to promote compliance.
3. Knowledge that the new insulin therapy more easily maintains blood glucose levels.
4. Knowledge that clinicians occasionally need to assess client's risk for hyperglycemia.

170. A client complains of abdominal cramping shortly before lunch. The nurse questions the client to obtain data related to the abdominal pain and then palpates the abdomen for constipation. The action by the nurse was:

1. Appropriate because constipation is a common problem for older adults.
2. Inappropriate because palpation in the gastrointestinal assessment is performed following percussion.
3. Inappropriate because the client did not complain of constipation.
4. Appropriate because abdominal pain is the first symptom of constipation.

171. The nurse refers the client to his family physician because she fears he has an intestinal obstruction. The nurse bases this decision upon the following assessment data:

1. Abdominal cramps and high-pitched bowel sounds.
2. Diffuse pain with low-grade temperature.
3. Absence of bowel sounds with hyperactivity.
4. Nausea with marked abdominal tenderness.

172. The nursing action most appropriate in assisting an incontinent client to remain dry during the night would be to:

1. Use an absorbent garment such as an adult diaper.
2. Provide a bedside commode and leave the night light on.
3. Talk with the client to determine any life stressors.
4. Insert a Foley catheter and maintain intake and output.

173. In planning nursing care for the client who has experienced a cerebrovascular accident, the nurse must keep in mind that clients with left hemisphere infarctions may have:

1. Dramatic mood swing
2. Impaired judgment
3. Labile affect
4. Aggressive potential

174. The nurse correctly identifies that the most important need for the client with left hemisphere infarction is:

1. Maintenance of nutritional status
2. Diversional activities
3. Prevention of injury
4. Psychological counseling

175. The client is discharged following a CVA, but will continue with physical and speech therapy daily. Which statement by the family best demonstrates a supportive environment?

1. "I just don't know if we can manage mother at home."
2. "We have widened the bathroom door for the wheelchair."
3. "We have a sitter who will be staying with mother at night."
4. "Mother will be back to her old self once we get her home."

176. A client's medications upon discharge are potassium chloride (K-Dur) 20 mEq once daily and bumetanide (Bumex) 1 mg once daily. The nurse prepares to teach the client about his medications and has prepared several handouts that describe the things he will need to know about each drug. Before beginning discharge teaching, the nurse needs to be aware of:

1. The client's attitude toward illness.
2. The client's educational level.
3. The client's past compliance to medications.
4. The client's usual activities of daily living.

177. The nurse recognizes the need to evaluate the client's understanding of his medications. Which response by the client best demonstrates to the nurse that the client has adequate knowledge?

1. "I will take K-Dur with my meals."
2. "I will call the doctor immediately if I get a headache."
3. "I will have my cholesterol level checked every 3 months."
4. "I will take Bumex shortly before bedtime."

178. The client is scheduled for an appointment with the physician for a check-up. Which complaint by the client is most likely to be associated with an adverse reaction to potassium chloride (K-Dur)?

1. "I have had a headache for the past 2 days."
2. "I have trouble remembering things lately."
3. "I noticed my stools were dark and tarry this morning."
4. "I have trouble seeing things up close lately."

179. The nursing assistant asks the nurse how to get the client to assist with her own personal hygiene. The nurse correctly informs the nursing assistant to:

1. Follow the procedure book when bathing.
2. Give her short, specific instructions for what to do next.
3. Provide written, step-by-step directions.
4. Explain ahead of time what you expect her to do.

180. The nursing assistant reports that the client has been incontinent twice during the shift. To assist the client to remain continent the nurse would:

1. Limit fluid intake to within 1000 mL daily.
2. Insert an indwelling catheter.
3. Set up a regular toileting schedule.
4. Label the bathroom door in large letters.

181. The most appropriate nursing action to ensure that a cognitively impaired client receives adequate nutrition is:

1. Weigh the client weekly and maintain a log.
2. Assign a staff member to feed her.
3. Offer high protein liquids between meals.
4. Provide several menus and allow the client to select.

182. The client is confused during the day, but this becomes much worse at night and often she calls "Mama" in a very loud voice. The most appropriate nursing action is:

1. Restrain her at night.
2. Close the door tightly to keep her from awakening the other clients.
3. Have the physician order a stronger sleeping medication.
4. Leave the lights on the in the room.

183. The increasing irritability and anxiety experienced by dementia clients during the early evening hours is referred to as:

1. Agnosia
2. Apraxia
3. Sundowner's syndrome
4. Phase three dementia

184. A physician prescribes estrogen therapy to prevent osteoporosis. The nurse correctly advises the client to:

1. Take the estrogen with meals.
2. Have a yearly mammogram.
3. Have monthly fasting blood glucose.
4. Monitor blood pressure for hypotension.

185. A client with breast cancer completed a round of chemotherapy several days ago. She has been nauseated and vomiting for the past 24 hours. The nurse will include the following intervention in the care of this client:

1. Teach distraction techniques.
2. Teach relaxation exercises.
3. Play music the client enjoys.
4. Minimize sensory stimuli.

186. A client with esophageal varices is brought to the emergency room bleeding profusely from the mouth. Immediately, the nurse will assist the physician with the insertion of a central line and:

1. Hanging packed red blood cells.
2. Insert a Foley catheter.
3. Insert a nasogastric tube through the nose.
4. Draw blood for the hemoglobin and hematocrit.

187. A client with esophageal varices is being treated in the emergency room. The nurse anticipates that the physician will attempt to stop the bleeding by:

1. Insertion of a Sengstaken-Blakemore tube
2. Gastric lavage with iced saline
3. Endoscopic procedure
4. Local application of epinephrine

188. A client with gastrointestinal bleeding is started on oral neomycin. The nurse explains that the purpose of this drug is prevention of:

1. Infection
2. Stress ulcer
3. Constipation
4. Encephalopathy

189. A client has ascites caused by cirrhosis of the liver. Part of the care of this client includes measuring the abdomen daily. The nurse will:

1. Mark the place of measurement.
2. Measure the same time each day.
3. Have the client empty the bladder prior to measuring.
4. Use the same tape measure each time.

190. A client has been admitted to the hospital for treatment of gastric ulcers. The nurse assesses this client for risk factors. One such risk factor is:

1. Highly seasoned food
2. Alcoholic beverages
3. Acid ash diets
4. Nonsteroidal anti-inflammatory drugs

191. A client with peptic ulcers is taking amoxicillin, tamotidine (Pepcid), and Maalox. The nurse teaches the client to take the Maalox:

1. One to 2 hours before meals
2. One-half hour before meals
3. With meals
4. 1 or 2 hours after meals

192. A client is admitted to the hospital with a small-bowel obstruction. When planning the care of this client, the nurse will include observation for signs and symptoms of:

1. Hemorrhage and mesenteric adenitis
2. Perforation and peritonitis
3. Electrolyte imbalance and fluid volume deficit
4. Volvulus and inflammatory bowel disease

193. A client is being discharged from the hospital following an incisional cholecystectomy. A T-tube is in place. The nurse teaches the following preparation for discharge:

1. The T-tube should never be clamped.
2. Keep the bile drainage bag below the insertion site at all times.
3. Clean technique may be used when changing the dressing.
4. There are no restrictions on activity.

194. A client with varicose veins tells the nurse, "I am afraid they will burst while I am walking." Which response by the nurse would be the best?

1. "The only way to prevent rupture is to have surgery."
2. "You must find another job, one that requires less walking."
3. "If that happens, you could bleed to death."
4. "Rupture of varicose veins rarely occurs."

195. A client has a new ileostomy following surgery for ulcerative colitis. The nurse assesses the stoma and reports the following abnormality to the physician:

1. Moderate edema
2. Oozing of blood on touching the stoma
3. Dark red color
4. Pale color

196. A client with an ileostomy is being discharged from the hospital. The nurse would screen the client's medication and request that the physician change the following:

1. Liquid preparations
2. Time-released preparations
3. Oral antibiotics
4. Suppositories

197. A client is taking piperacillin for bacterial pneumonia. Today, the client has diarrhea. The nurse would recommend:

1. Gatorade and a clear liquid diet
2. A low-fiber diet
3. Yogurt, cottage cheese, and buttermilk
4. Omitting milk products

198. A client is diagnosed with hepatitis A. The nurse teaches the client's significant others that they can prevent infection with the virus by:

1. Careful hand washing and good sanitation.
2. Using fluid precautions around the client.
3. Wearing a mask when entering the client's room.
4. Using safe sexual practices.

199. A 22-year-old client is comatose following involvement in a motor vehicle accident. When planning the care of this client, the nurse will include the following outcome:

1. The environment will remain quiet.
2. The cornea will remain intact.
3. Score on the Glasgow Coma Scale will steadily decrease.
4. The head of the bed will remain flat.

200. A client is on seizure precautions. The nurse would see that the client is on bed rest with side rails up. Diazepam (Valium) or lorazepam (Ativan) would be available. An additional precaution would be:

1. Having a sitter at the bedside
2. Having a padded tongue blade available
3. Having an oral airway available
4. Padding the side rails

201. A depressed client was found to have type III hyperlipidemia. The physician ordered gemfibrozil (Lopid) 600 mg bid 30 minutes before meals. On hand were 300 mg capsules. The nurse instructed the client to take how many capsules?

1. 1 capsule
2. 2 capsules
3. 3 capsules
4. 4 capsules

202. Which of the following communication techniques would be most effective for the nurse to use during a nurse-client interaction?

1. Facilitative
2. Nonverbal
3. Public
4. Intrapersonal

203. The nurse enters the room of a 50-year-old client, who is lying in a fetal position with his head covered, and says, "How are you feeling this morning?" The client responds, "I'm feeling fine." The behavior exhibited by the client is:

1. Assertive
2. Aggressive
3. Passive
4. Passive-aggressive

204. Accurate and complete documentation in a client's record in mental health facilities:

1. Should reflect the nursing process.
2. Should be available to all hospital personnel
3. Make it an illegal document
4. Guarantee pertinent and accurate information

205. An 18-year-old newly diagnosed schizophrenic client exhibits withdrawn, regressive, and isolative behaviors. The nurse's initial approach should be to:

1. Speak in realistic, literal terms.
2. Use self-disclosure.
3. Demand information.
4. Explain in depth the rules and regulations.

ANSWERS

1. **(3)** Integrated processes: nursing process — implementation; client need: physiological integrity; physiological adaptation; content area: medical/surgical.
   RATIONALE
   (1) It is not necessary for the client to be NPO if his gag and swallowing reflexes are intact. **(2)** The vital signs should have been checked frequently during the past hour; it is more important to be certain that the client can swallow without aspirating. **(3)** If the gag and swallowing reflexes are not intact, the client is in danger of aspirating. **(4)** Coughing and deep breathing could initiate hemorrhage immediately following a bronchoscopy. There is no effect following a gastroscopy.

2. **(4)** Integrated processes: nursing process — implementation; client need: safe, effective care environment; safety and infection control; content area: medical/surgical.
   RATIONALE
   (1) The client could be injured more by inserting a tongue blade into the mouth. **(2)** A client who is restrained and thrashing about in a grand mal seizure could sustain body injury. **(3)** An unconscious client should not be on his back unless the client is intubated. **(4)** Placing the client in a lateral position helps to maintain an open airway and allows drainage of secretions.

3. **(2)** Integrated processes: nursing process — data collection; client need: physiological integrity; physiological adaptation; content area: medical/surgical.
   RATIONALE
   (1) The femoral and popliteal pulses are between the heart and the cast; therefore, they do not require frequent assessment. **(2)** The cast could interfere with circulation or nerve supply to the toes. **(3)** No data have been provided to indicate that the toes may be removed. A physician must approve any movement in a fractured extremity. **(4)** The pedal pulses are covered by the cast in the affected extremity.

4. **(3)** Integrated processes: nursing process — evaluation; client need: physiological integrity; reduction of risk potential; content area: medical/surgical.
   RATIONALE
   (1) A normal value for the partial thromboplastin time (PTT) does not indicate that the therapy is being effective. **(2)** A PTT only one to one and a half times normal indicates that the therapy is not as effective as it could be. **(3)** The best indicator that heparin therapy is being effective is a PTT of two to two and a half times normal. **(4)** If the PTT is three times the control, the client is in danger of hemorrhaging.

5. **(2)** Integrated processes: nursing process — planning; client need: physiological integrity; pharmacological therapies; content area: medical/surgical.
   RATIONALE
   (1) Vitamin K is an antidote for warfarin but not heparin. **(2)** Protamine sulfate neutralizes heparin. **(3)** Epinephrine is used only to arrest local bleeding. **(4)** Norepinephrine is not used to treat bleeding disorders.

6. **(4)** Integrated processes: nursing process — data collection; client need: physiological integrity; reduction of risk potential; content area: medical/surgical.
   RATIONALE
   (1) The cells of the blood are not usually affected by the drugs being taken. **(2)** The data do not indicate that kidney function is compromised. **(3)** Blood coagulation should not be affected, nor will it affect the medications. **(4)** Electrolyte imbalances may be caused by Lasix; such imbalances can cause digoxin toxicity even when serum levels of digoxin are within normal range.

7. **(1)** Integrated processes: nursing process — implementation; client need: physiological integrity; physiological adaptation; content area: medical/surgical.
   RATIONALE
   (1) The IV is infiltrated and should be removed. **(2)** This would result in injury to the client. **(3)** This action would cause a delay and injury to the client. **(4)** This action would not correct the problem.

8. **(1)** Integrated processes: nursing process — implementation; client need: physiological integrity; physiological adaptation; content area: medical/surgical.
   RATIONALE
   (1) The signs of hypoglycemia are evident and prompt action is needed before the blood glucose level goes lower. **(2)** The serum glucose could continue to drop while the serum glucose is being checked. **(3)** Insulin would lower the blood glucose level even more. **(4)** This action also would cause delay; therefore, it would not be the first action to be taken. If brain cells are deprived of glucose, then brain damage results.

9. **(3)** Integrated processes: nursing process — data collection; client need: physiological integrity; reduction of risk potential; content area: medical/surgical.
   RATIONALE
   (1) The risk of sodium imbalance is not as great as the risk for potassium imbalance. **(2)** Calcium imbalance is not usually associated with diabetic ketoacidosis. **(3)** During the acidotic phase, potassium left the cells in exchange for hydrogen ions and was subsequently lost from the body. **(4)** The risk of a magnesium imbalance is not as great as the risk of a potassium imbalance.

10. **(3)** Integrated processes: nursing process — implementation; client need: physiological integrity; pharmacological therapies; content area: medical/surgical.
    RATIONALE
    (1) Stopping the medication would cause further damage to the endocrine system. **(2)** Continuing the medication would be contradictory to the physician's order. Stopping prednisone too quickly can cause further problems. **(3)** Calling the physician would be the best action. The dosage should be decreased gradually so that the adrenocorticotropic hormone (ACTH) could build up again and stimulate the adrenal gland to function. **(4)** Adrenal insufficiency could develop. The best action would be to call the physician.

11. **(4)** Integrated processes: nursing process — implementation; client need: physiological integrity; reduction of risk potential; content area: medical/surgical.
    RATIONALE
    (1) Sterile gauze would not put a seal around the catheter. **(2)** Kerlix would not provide a seal. **(3)** This would not be neces-

sary. **(4)** This dressing provides sterility and a seal around the catheter.

12. **(3)** Integrated processes: nursing process — implementation; client need: physiological integrity; reduction of risk potential; content area: medical/surgical.

    RATIONALE

    (1) Nasogastric tubes should be checked for placement before anything is put into them. **(2)** Clients with nasogastric tubes following a gastrectomy should not have the tube repositioned. **(3)** Nasogastric tubes should be checked for placement. Most institutions require a radiograph to check for placement. **(4)** These tubes should not be inserted farther after placement has been verified by a radiograph.

13. **(4)** Integrated processes: nursing process — implementation, teaching/learning; client need: physiological integrity; reduction of risk potential; content area: medical/surgical.

    RATIONALE

    (1) This would open the respiratory tract. **(2)** The respiratory tract would be open. **(3)** Aspiration could result. **(4)** The epiglottis would be covering the respiratory tract.

14. **(3)** Integrated processes: nursing process — implementation, teaching/learning; client need: physiological integrity; pharmacological therapies; content area: medical/surgical.

    RATIONALE

    (1) If aspirin is given to anyone who has influenza-like symptoms and who is under the age of 18 years, Reye's syndrome can occur. **(2)** Enteric-coated aspirin would not prevent Reye's syndrome. **(3)** Tylenol can be safely given to lower the temperature. **(4)** All products containing aspirin must also be avoided.

15. **(4)** Integrated processes: nursing process — implementation; client need: physiological integrity; pharmacological therapies; content area: medical/surgical.

    RATIONALE

    (1) Dilantin is used to treat seizure activity on a daily basis. **(2)** Phenobarbital is used to treat seizure activity on a daily basis. **(3)** Valproic acid is used for absence seizures. **(4)** Valium is the drug of choice to terminate seizures of status epilepticus.

16. **(4)** Integrated processes: nursing process — implementation, teaching/learning; client need: physiological integrity; basic care and comfort; content area: medical/surgical.

    RATIONALE

    (1) Vitamin C would help render the urine acid; therefore, it would not help prevent formation of another uric acid stone. **(2)** Low calcium would not help prevent a uric acid stone. **(3)** Fiber is not known to be helpful in preventing stones. **(4)** An end product of purine metabolism is uric acid. A low-purine diet would help prevent formation of another uric acid stone.

17. **(1)** Integrated processes: nursing process — implementation; client need: physiological integrity; basic care and comfort; content area: medical/surgical.

    RATIONALE

    (1) A laxative is needed to clean the barium out of the gastrointestinal system. **(2)** The barium needs to be cleaned out of the body. **(3)** High fiber would not be sufficient to clean out the barium. **(4)** A sitz bath would not remove the barium from the body.

18. **(4)** Integrated processes: nursing process — implementation; client need: physiological integrity; physiological adaptation; content area: medical/surgical.

RATIONALE

(1) An open airway is the highest priority in anaphylactic shock because brain cells will die within 6 minutes of anoxia. **(2)** An open airway is the highest priority in anaphylactic shock because brain cells will die within 6 minutes of anoxia. **(3)** An open airway is the highest priority in anaphylactic shock because brain cells will die within 6 minutes of anoxia. **(4)** An open airway is the highest priority in anaphylactic shock because brain cells will die within 6 minutes of anoxia.

19. **(1)** Integrated processes: nursing process — data collection; client need: physiological integrity; pharmacological therapies; content area: medical/surgical.

    RATIONALE

    (1) Dilatation of the pupil is contraindicated because the canal of Schlemm could be blocked. Blockage of this canal would lead to even greater pressure in the eye. **(2)** Constriction of the pupil would not close the route of drainage from the eye. **(3)** Constriction of blood vessels to the eye would help decrease the pressure in the eye. **(4)** A decreased heart rate could lead to a decreased blood pressure; this might help decrease pressure in the eye.

20. **(4)** Integrated processes: nursing process — implementation; client need: physiological integrity; reduction of risk potential; content area: medical/surgical.

    RATIONALE

    (1) The nurse needs to check the blood glucose level to establish a baseline to reduce the risk of hypoglycemia. **(2)** It is more important to check the serum glucose. If injection sites are not rotated, a local reaction in the tissues is the worst thing that could happen. **(3)** The serum glucose level does not give the information needed. **(4)** If insulin is given when the serum glucose is too low, hypoglycemia can occur.

21. **(2)** Integrated processes: nursing process — implementation, communication and documentation; client need: physiological integrity; pharmacological therapies; content area: medical/surgical.

    RATIONALE

    (1, 2, 3, and 4) An elderly client is at high risk for respiratory depression when given Valium IV.

22. **(1)** Integrated processes: nursing process — implementation, teaching/learning; client need: physiological integrity; pharmacological therapies; content area: medical/surgical.

    RATIONALE

    (1) Alcohol is a central nervous system depressant and can cause death if combined with another central nervous system depressant. **(2)** Taking the pulse rate is not part of the standard procedure for clients on central nervous system depressants. **(3)** Clients should not drive at all while taking central nervous system depressants. **(4)** Tolerance develops to the effects of caffeine; it is not necessary to decrease consumption.

23. **(3)** Integrated processes: nursing process — implementation; client need: physiological integrity; pharmacological therapies; content area: medical/surgical.

    RATIONALE

    (1) Cough medications do not usually contain a mucolytic agent. **(2)** Depressing the cough reflex does not help remove infectious material from the lungs. **(3)** An expectorant is needed to promote removal of secretions from the lungs. **(4)** Relaxing the bronchioles would not promote removal of secretions.

24. **(1)** Integrated processes: nursing process — implementation; client need: physiological integrity; reduction of risk potential; content area: medical/surgical.

RATIONALE
(1) Because the origin of the pain is not known, it is not safe to give a laxative. A complication of the pain, such as a ruptured appendix, could occur. (2) The data do not support a contraindication for a laxative. (3) Laxatives are not contraindicated for either renal or hepatic failure. (4) Fluid and electrolyte balance might be affected by a laxative, but rationale 1 is the best.

25. **(4)** Integrated processes: nursing process — data collection; client need: physiological integrity; reduction of risk potential; content area: medical/surgical.

RATIONALE
(1) A change in blood pressure is not an early sign of digoxin toxicity. (2) A change in respirations is not an early sign of digoxin toxicity. (3) The radial pulse is not the most accurate reflection of cardiac activity. (4) The apical pulse is the best reflection of cardiac activity, especially arrhythmias.

26. **(2)** Integrated processes: nursing process — data collection; client need: health promotion and maintenance; content area: maternity.

RATIONALE
(1) The hematocrit is done at the first prenatal visit and generally not repeated until the 32nd to 36th week. (2) A urine specimen is obtained and a urine dipstick test is done during each prenatal visit. Screening is done for glucose and protein. (3) Sexually transmitted diease (STD) screenings are done at an early prenatal visit but are not routinely repeated throughout the pregnancy unless the client is symptomatic. (4) Blood typing is done early in pregnancy. Coombs' test should be repeated at 28 weeks in Rh-negative women.

27. **(2)** Integrated processes: nursing process — data collection; client need: health promotion and maintenance; content area: maternity.

RATIONALE
(1) During the second trimester, the uterus rises out of the pelvic cavity, reducing the weight on the bladder. (2) During the third trimester, with descent of the presenting part of the enlarged uterus compresses the bladder, causing urinary frequencies. (3) Quickening, the time when the mother may feel fetal movement, will not have any influence on urinary frequency. (4) During the second trimester, when the uterus rises out of the pelvic cavity, the woman's feeling of urinary urgency usually disappears.

28. **(1)** Integrated processes: nursing process — data collection; client need: health promotion and maintenance; content area: maternity.

RATIONALE
(1) Due to hormonal changes that occur during pregnancy, there is an increased sloughing of cells from the cervical and vaginal walls, causing an increase in the amount of vaginal mucus or leukorrhea. The discharge may be thin and milky or thick and sticky but should not cause irritation to tissues. (2) Yellow discharge may indicate the presence of an infection. (3) Blood-tinged mucus would be of concern because this may indicate preterm labor. (4) There is a definite difference in the vaginal discharge during pregnancy. The degree of change varies from woman to woman.

29. **(1)** Integrated processes: nursing process — data collection; client need: health promotion and maintenance; content area: maternity.

RATIONALE
(1) Prior to an amniocentesis, the fetal heart tones are monitored for a baseline. (2) Maternal vital signs are monitored prior to and following this procedure. (3) There is no connection between a urine specimen and an amniocentesis. (4) There is no need for a maternal blood specimen.

30. **(2)** Integrated processes: nursing process — data collection; client need: health promotion and maintenance; content area: maternity.

RATIONALE
(1) A slightly elevated temperature during the first hours after birth is common due to dehydration. A temperature above 100.4°F would be concerning due to the possibility of infection. (2) A positive Homan's sign indicates the possibility of a blood clot. Postpartal clients are predisposed to the formation of phlebitis and thrombo-embolisms due to the decreased venous return, increased viscosity from fluid loss, and the temporary elevation in clotting factors that occur in the time following delivery. (3) Edema of the perineal area is common following a vaginal delivery and would not be of unusual concern. (4) During breastfeeding, uterine contractions are normal as a result of the release of oxytocin.

31. **(3, 5, 6)** Integrated processes: nursing process — implementation; client need: physiological integrity; reduction of risk potential; content area: maternity.

RATIONALE
(1) Headache is not common after epidural administration, though it may occur as a result of poor technique. (2) Elevated blood pressure is not a common side effect of epidural anesthesia. (3) Major complications after an epidural are uncommon; however, because of initial vasodilation following administration, hypotension is always expected due to pooling of blood in the legs. (4) There is no relationship between frequent voiding and epidural anesthesia. (5) Respiratory depression results if the block travels too far upward. (6) As the block wears off, clients feel that their legs are very heavy and numb, resulting in decreased mobility.

32. **(2)** Integrated processes: nursing process — data collection; client need: health promotion and maintenance; content area: maternity.

RATIONALE
(1) A normal blood sugar level would be less than 140 mg/dL. (2) A glucose tolerance test is indicated for any glucose screening result of 140 mg/dL or greater. (3) The need for insulin control cannot be determined based on a glucose screening test. (4) Although nonstress tests may be indicated later in pregnancy to determine the well-being of the fetus, the priority at this gestational age is to achieve euglycemia.

33. **(3)** Integrated processes: nursing process — data collection; client need: health promotion and maintenance; content area: maternity.

RATIONALE
(1) Amniocentesis can be safely performed as early as 15–17 weeks. (2) Ultrasound evaluates amniotic fluid volume, which may be used to determine congenital anomalies. (3) With amniocentesis, a needle inserted through the abdominal wall is guided by ultrasound to evaluate the position of the placenta and the fetus to avoid needle injuries.

34. **(3)** Integrated processes: nursing process — implementation, teaching/learning; client need: health promotion and maintenance; content area: maternity.

RATIONALE
(1) A 10- to 20-lb weight gain would not allow for an adequate growth of the fetus and the maternal organs. (2) A 14- to 22-lb weight gain would not allow for an adequate growth of the fetus

and the maternal organs. (**3**) A 25- to 35-lb weight gain will allow for adequate growth of the fetus and the maternal organs. (**4**) Above a 35-lb weight gain is not the recommended amount.

35. (**3**) Integrated processes: nursing process — implementation, teaching/learning; client need: physiological integrity; basic care and comfort; content area: maternity.
RATIONALE
(**1**) Sitting up for an hour after meals is recommended to assist in decreasing the incidence of heartburn. (**2**) Coffee, tea, alcohol, chocolate, and acidic juices should be avoided because they are gastric irritants that increase GI discomforts. (**3**) Eating several small meals per day, separating solid foods from liquids, not overfilling the stomach, decreasing gastric irritants, and limiting gas-producing foods will assist the client in reducing GI discomforts. (**4**) Antiemetics are not recommended unless prescribed by the physician.

36. (**4**) Integrated processes: nursing process — implementation, caring; client need: pyschosocial integrity; content area: maternity.
RATIONALE
(**1**) Because each labor experience is different, knowing what happened in previous experiences would not be helpful at this time. (**2**) During transition, it is important that the woman receive a great deal of encouragement from her caregivers. Monitoring her breathing will help to decrease the incidence of hyperventilation. (**3**) An epidural is generally administered after the cervix has dilated to at least 4 cm. It is generally not placed this late in the laboring process. (**4**) Transition is a time when the laboring client requires a great deal of support. The nurse should interpret the progress and labor to both members of the couple and affirm their coping abilities.

37. (**1**) Integrated processes: nursing process — data collection; client need: physiological integrity; pharmacological therapies; content area: maternity.
RATIONALE
(**1**) Nausea, hyperstimulation of the uterus, and poor urine output are common side effects of oxytocin. (**2**) Hypotension, headaches, and arrhythmias are common side effects of oxytocin. (**3**) Hypertonic contractions are a common side effect of oxytocin. It does not cause nervousness or diarrhea. (**4**) Because of the antidiuretic effect of oxytocin, it may cause fluid overload. Hypertension and elevated temperature are not side effects.

38. (**4**) Integrated processes: nursing process — data collection; client need: health promotion and maintenance; content area: maternity.
RATIONALE
(**1**) Kegel's exercises themselves do not relieve perineal pain, but because they promote healing they may result in less pain overall. (**2**) Kegel's exercises do not assist in toning the abdominal muscles. (**3**) Postpartal hemorrhage is not prevented by the toning of the pelvic floor muscles. (**4**) Because Kegel's exercises increase the flow of circulation to the episiotomy area, they will assist in the healing process.

39. (**3**) Integrated processes: nursing process — data collection; client need: health promotion and maintenance; content area: maternity.
RATIONALE
(**1**) These signs are considered presumptive signs of pregnancy because they may be caused by conditions other than pregnancy. (**2**) These are considered probable signs of pregnancy. These signs strongly suggest pregnancy, but do not confirm it. (**3**) Fetal heart tones and fetal movement documented by some-one other than the mother as well as visualization of the fetus with ultrasound are considered positive signs of pregnancy. (**4**) Frequency of urination may be caused by an infection and the accuracy of a pregnancy test may vary depending on the time it is done. Other signs of pregnancy such as Braxton Hicks contractions may occur with pseudopregnancy, a condition in which a woman believes very strongly that she is pregnant.

40. (**3**) Integrated processes: nursing process — data collection, teaching/learning; client need: health promotion and maintenance; content area: maternity.
RATIONALE
(**1**) This is good time for couples to begin to evaluate their parenting skills. (**2**) Quickening occurs between the 16th and 18th weeks of pregnancy. (**3**) A woman's uterus should have enlarged enough by 26 weeks' gestation that she should be requiring maternity clothes. If she continues to attempt to wear her pre-pregnancy clothes, it may indicate a denial of the pregnancy or a financial hardship. (**4**) Toward the end of the first trimester, the woman and her family can be offered the opportunity to hear the fetal heart beat.

41. (**3**) Integrated processes: nursing process — implementation; client need: health promotion and maintenance; content area: maternity.
RATIONALE
(**1**) This is not within the scope of practice for a PN. Changes in the flow rate of a medication require a physician's order. (**2**) A full bladder results in the uterus deviated to the side. It does not tone the uterus. (**3**) Gently massaging the fundus will usually increase the uterine tone. (**4**) Cervical tears or lacerations generally present as a firm uterus with persistent, moderate bright red flow.

42. (**4**) Integrated processes: nursing process — implementation; client need: health promotion and maintenance; content area: maternity.
RATIONALE
(**1**) Bonding and attachment begin prior to the infant's birth and, usually, discovering that they have a healthy infant removes any doubts that they may feel about the gender. (**2**) Her expression that she doesn't know why she is crying and is unable to stop does not indicate that she is dissatisfied with the care she is receiving. (**3**) Postpartum psychosis is characterized by acute psychotic behavior generally characteristic of other disorders such as schizophrenic, affective, or organic disorders. (**4**) Postpartum blues, or postpartum depression, is common in the first few days following delivery. This is considered to be a normal mild, transient mood disturbance lasting a few days or more.

43. (**2**) Integrated processes: nursing process — implementation; client need: health promotion and maintenance; content area: maternity.
RATIONALE
(**1**) Labor occurring late in the third trimester is not of great concern because this is close to the term for the pregnancy. (**2**) Painless bleeding late in the third trimester might indicate a placenta previa where the implantation site of the placenta occurs over the cervical os. (**3**) When done correctly, the examination should not result in an infection. (**4**) A vaginal exam could lead to increased fetal distress prior to labor if the exam causes the low-lying placenta to separate further.

44. (**4**) Integrated processes: nursing process — implementation, teaching/learning; client need: health promotion and maintenance; content area: maternity.

RATIONALE

(1) The size of the client's breast does not influence her ability to produce enough milk. (2) The size of the client's breast does not influence her ability to produce enough milk. (3) Although breast size does not influence milk production, this statement infers that formula is a better choice for infants and more convenient for mother. (4) If there are no complications that influence this mother's ability to breast-feed, she should not be unsuccessful based on the size of her breasts.

45. (3) Integrated processes: nursing process — implementation, teaching/learning; client need: health promotion and maintenance; content area: maternity.

RATIONALE

(1) Women with IUDs do not report painful intercourse as a result of the IUD. (2) There is no evidence that IUDs increase the occurrence of these infections. (3) The IUD may cause contraction of the uterus because of an increased irritability. These contractions may cause spontaneous expulsion of the IUD. (4) Following insertion, many women report an excessive menstrual flow for several months.

46. (1) Integrated processes: nursing process — data collection; client need: physiological integrity; physiological adaptation; content area: maternity.

RATIONALE

(1) Because of the rupture of the fallopian tube during an ectopic pregnancy and the subsequent blood loss, pressure on the diaphragm may cause referred shoulder pain. (2) Ectopic pregnancy is not related to the number of times a woman has been pregnant. (3) The number of children is not related to an ectopic pregnancy. (4) Assessing a mass is not the client's responsibility.

47. (3) Integrated processes: nursing process — data collection; client need: physiological integrity; physiological adaptation; content area: maternity.

RATIONALE

(1) Maternal dietary iron intake is not related to physiological anemia. (2) Liver dysfunction does not explain physiological anemia of pregnancy. (3) During the first trimester of pregnancy, maternal blood volume increases approximately 50%, causing a decrease in the concentration of hemoglobin and erythrocytes. This is known as physiological anemia. (4) Physiological anemia is normal, not a laboratory error.

48. (3) Integrated processes: nursing process — implementation, teaching/learning; client need: health promotion and maintenance; content area: maternity.

RATIONALE

(1) Losing her mucus plug and a bloody show usually occurs several hours prior to delivery. (2) The nurse needs to be more specific about the frequency of contractions. (3) Regular contractions that are 5 to 7 minutes apart would indicate a need for the mother to come to the hospital. She is in true labor and cervical changes are probably occurring. (4) With intact membranes, contractions of 10 to 15 minutes' frequency would be too early for a primigravida to come to the hospital.

49. (1) Integrated processes: nursing process — data collection; client need: health promotion and maintenance; content area: maternity.

RATIONALE

(1) The first stage of labor including the active phase is from 3 cm to full cervical dilation. Contractions are strong, closer together and usually last 30 to 60 seconds. (2) The latent phase begins with the onset of true labor and continues to a cervical dilation of 3 cm. Contractions are 15 to 30 minutes in frequency and mild to moderate in intensity. (3) This terminology does not refer to a phase of labor. (4) The fourth stage of labor occurs up to and through 4 hours after the delivery of the fetus and placenta. It is considered a stabilization phase of the mother.

50. (1) Integrated processes: nursing process — data collection, teaching/learning; client need: health promotion and maintenance; content area: maternity.

RATIONALE

(1) Washing the breast prior to each feeding or applying lotions or creams to the breast are not recommended. (2) Good hand washing prior to each feeding is encouraged. There is no need to wash the nipple prior to each feeding, although good hygiene is encouraged. (3) Mothers are encouraged to alternate breasts at each feeding or alternate the breast is used first at each feeding. Placing some type of reminder on the bra, such as a safety pin or ribbon, is a good way for mothers to remember which breast was used first at the previous feeding. (4) Lactating women should have approximately 2500–3000 mL of fluid daily to produce a sufficient amount of breast milk.

51. (4) Integrated processes: nursing process — implementation; client need: physiological integrity; basic care and comfort; content area: pediatrics.

RATIONALE

(1) It is true that infection should be prevented, but many other factors contribute to infection besides diaper placement. (2) There are no nerves in the umbilicus to cause pain. (3) The dry gangrene process takes 7–14 days, depending on the preparations applied to the cord, other perinatal events, and type of delivery. (4) The wetness from diaper soiling and subsequent irritation can be prevented by securing the diaper below the cord.

52. (2) Integrated processes: nursing process — implementation; client need: physiological integrity; reduction of risk potential; content area: pediatrics.

RATIONALE

(1) The Plexiglas shield protects from undesirable ultraviolet rays from the phototherapy lights. (2) Because no long-term research has studied the gonadal function of men treated with phototherapy, many health-care providers seek to protect the gonads. (3) A small diaper is used for absorbency if diarrhea is a real problem. (4) Although hydration status may be monitored by weighing diapers in some clients, the mask would not effectively absorb all of the urine for an accurate measurement.

53. (4) Integrated processes: nursing process — evaluation, teaching/learning; client need: physiological integrity; basic care and comfort; content area: pediatrics.

RATIONALE

(1) Unless the canned food was especially prepared for infants, excessive sodium, salt, and additives may be transferred to the infant. (2) Home-prepared foods, fresh or frozen, are the preferred foods to decrease the risk of unwanted additives. (3) Home-prepared foods, fresh or frozen, are preferred foods to decrease the risk of unwanted additives. (4) Refined sugar may be used, but honey and corn syrup should be avoided because of the risk of botulism.

54. (4) Integrated processes: nursing process — implementation, teaching/learning; client need: physiological integrity; basic care and comfort; content area: pediatrics.

RATIONALE

(1) New foods should be introduced one at a time. Usually, plain rice cereal is the suggested first solid food. (2) Whole milk

should not be introduced within the first year. (3) Large quantities of juice may cause abdominal pain, bloating, or diarrhea. (4) Breast milk and/or formula are primary sources of nutrition for infants up to 12 months.

55. **(See figure)** Integrated processes: nursing process — implementation; client need: physiological integrity; physiological adaptation; content area: pediatrics.

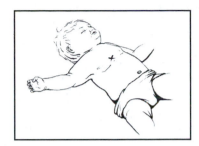

RATIONALE
The drawing of an imaginary line between the nipples and placing two or three fingers below the line is appropriate for infants.

56. **(3)** Integrated processes: nursing process — evaluation, teaching/learning; client need: physiological integrity; basic care and comfort; content area: pediatrics.

RATIONALE
(1) Testing of the formula temperature is always indicated. The inner wrist is not an appropriate site for accurate measurement. (2) The mother's own tongue or back of her hand should be used to test formula temperature. (3) The mother's own tongue or back of her hand should be used to test formula temperature. (4) Formula should be cool to the touch. Warming formula to touch often makes it too hot to be served.

57. **(2)** Integrated processes: nursing process — evaluation, teaching/learning; client need: physiological integrity; basic care and comfort; content area: pediatrics.

RATIONALE
(1) Powder, especially talc, may be dangerous, but corn starch products may be useful in keeping skin dry. (2) Proper technique is to avoid "puffs of powder" in the air, risking aspiration. It is appropriate to put small amounts of powder in the hand first. (3) Talc is very dangerous if inhaled, but corn starch–based products are safer. (4) Powder, especially talc, may be dangerous, but corn starch products, especially, may keep skin dry.

58. **(3)** Integrated processes: nursing process — implementation; client need: physiological integrity; pharmacological therapies; content area: pediatrics.

RATIONALE
(1) Nonlipid hydrophilic agents, such as Cetaphil, and baths may be used in the dry method of treatment. (2) Frequent oil or oil-based oatmeal baths may be used to moisten skin. (3) Corticosteroids decrease inflammation, which may then decrease itching. Cream products may add moisture. (4) Hydroxyzine (Atarax) and diphenhydramine (Benadryl) are often used to decrease pruritus.

59. **(3)** Integrated processes: nursing process — implementation, teaching/learning; client need: physiological integrity; basic care and comfort; content area: pediatrics.

RATIONALE
(1) Both physiological and psychological readiness are needed to determine if toddlers are ready for toilet training. (2) Both physiological and psychological readiness are needed to determine if toddlers are ready for toilet training. (3) Toddlers should be assessed individually for readiness and not hurried. (4) The toddler may be able to hold urine for 2 hours as evidenced by staying dry for that long and/or waking up dry from naps before that age.

60. **(2)** Integrated processes: nursing process — implementation, teaching/learning; client need: health promotion and maintenance; content area: pediatrics.

RATIONALE
(1) Infancy is the period of solitary play. (2) Toddlers prefer parallel play. This is play alongside another child but not with that child. (3) Early childhood is the time for associative play in groups, but limited formal structural rules are needed. (4) Team sports with more rigid rules occur later in childhood.

61. **(1, 3)** Integrated processes: nursing process — implementation, teaching/learning; client need: health promotion and maintenance; content area: pediatrics.

RATIONALE
(1) Cleaning and brushing should begin with the first tooth. (2) Dental examinations are recommended twice per year. (3) Parents should supervise brushing and assist with flossing because fine motor skills are not refined. (4) Parents should supervise brushing and assist with flossing because fine motor skills are not refined. (5) Cleaning and brushing should begin with the first tooth. (6) Cleaning and brushing should begin with the first tooth.

62. **(4)** Integrated processes: nursing process — implementation, caring; client need: psychosocial integrity; content.

RATIONALE
(1) The mother can provide or place most of the information needed, but not all. (2) The child can provide a lot of the needed information, but possibly not all of the historical or other background needed. (3) The parent may remain if the child wants, but should be asked to leave at some point to interview the child further. (4) Do interview the parent and child together and separately to allow each to share any "confidential" information that the other has not heard.

63. **(1)** Integrated processes: nursing process — implementation; client need: physiological integrity; pharmacological therapies; content area: pediatrics.

RATIONALE
(1) Constipation is such a common side effect that ordering prophylactic laxatives for someone in need of long-term therapy is understood. (2) Respirations may decrease but not usually to a state of respiratory depression. (3) Nausea and vomiting are side effects that are less common than constipation. (4) Anaphylaxis is rare.

64. **(3)** Integrated processes: nursing process — implementation, teaching/learning; client need: physiological integrity; basic care and comfort; content area: pediatrics.

RATIONALE
(1) Red meat is high in cholesterol and saturated fats. (2) Low-fat hot dogs are a good substitute, but not regular hot dogs. (3) Turkey, skinless chicken, or tofu is a good substitute for red meat. (4) Skim milk is a better choice than regular milk, which is 4% fat.

65. **(2)** Integrated processes: nursing process — implementation, teaching/learning; client need: physiological integrity; basic care and comfort; content area: pediatrics.

RATIONALE

(1) Heated fans or dryers are not used to dry the cast because then the cast will be dry on the outside and wet underneath, which will cause mold to form. (2) The palms should be used to prevent indentations. (3) Distal area should be checked for signs of impaired blood flow and neurological integrity (4) To prevent swelling, the extremity should not be in a dependent position for greater than 30 minutes at a time.

66. (4) Integrated processes: nursing process — implementation, teaching/learning; client need: health promotion and maintenance; content area: pediatrics.

RATIONALE

(1) According to the AAP, sports have been divided into categories based on how strenuous the sport is and the probability of collision. Collision sports have the greatest risk of injury, followed by contact sports. Football is a collision contact sport. (2) Gymnastics is a limited-contact and collision sport. (3) Running is a strenuous noncontact sport. (4) Golf is a nonstrenuous noncontact sport, and would hence have the least likely chance of causing an injury.

67. (4) Integrated processes: nursing process — implementation; client need: physiological integrity; basic care and comfort; content area: pediatrics.

RATIONALE

(1) Drinks such as Pedialyte or Infantile can be used in infants. (2) Sports drinks such as Gatorade or Exceed can be used for children. (3) Parents should observe the frequency of voiding and notify the practitioner if input appears to be insufficient. (4) It is important to remember that forcing fluids creates the difficulties of trying to force food. Gentle persuasion with preferred or favorite liquids is sufficient. The child should not be awakened for fluids.

68. (2) Integrated processes: nursing process — implementation, teaching/learning; client need: physiological integrity; physiological adaptation; content area: pediatrics.

RATIONALE

(1) Asthma is reversible with treatment or spontaneously. (2) Asthma is reversible with treatment or spontaneously. Chronic obstructive pulmonary disease (COPD) or emphysema is irreversible. (3) Asthma is not influenced by sex. (4) Asthma usually begins before the age of 4 or 5 years.

69. (1) Integrated processes: nursing process — implementation; client need: physiological integrity; pharmacological therapies; content area: pediatrics.

RATIONALE

(1) Corticosteroids have anti-inflammatory properties. (2) B-2 agonists decrease spasms and bronchodilation. (3) Antibiotics prevent and reduce infection. (4) Cromolyn provides non-steroidal anti-inflammatory effects.

70. (4) Integrated processes: nursing process — implementation, teaching/learning; client need: health promotion and maintenance; content area: pediatrics.

RATIONALE

(1) Allergies are a factor in many URIs, but shots are not always indicated. Testing helps determine allergies. (2) Prevention of attacks may be possible if triggers are identified and avoided or prophylactic medications are given. (3) Children do have decreased URIs by age 5 years. Infant infections soar at 3–6 months. But people of all ages may get URIs. (4) Smoking of any type should be avoided because it is not beneficial.

71. (1) Integrated processes: nursing process — implementation, teaching/learning; client need: physiological integrity; physiological adaptation; content area: pediatrics.

RATIONALE

(1) Tachycardia is the earliest sign of dehydration. (2) The order of clinical signs of dehydration is tachycardia, dry skin and mucous membranes, sunken fontanelles, circulatory failure, loss of elasticity, and delayed capillary refill. (3) Tachycardia is the earliest sign of dehydration. (4) Tachycardia is the earliest sign of dehydration.

72. (4) Integrated processes: nursing process — implementation, teaching/learning; client need: physiological integrity; basic care and comfort; content area: pediatrics.

RATIONALE

(1) Many colas are dark, and a newspaper cannot be read through them. (2) Formula and milk products are not considered a liquid because they curd on contact with resin in the stomach. (3) Other fluids such as commercial sport drinks or fluid replacers are considered clear. (4) Any liquid that is clear enough for a newspaper to be read through it is considered to be clear.

73. (2) Integrated processes: nursing process — implementation: client need: physiological integrity; basic care and comfort; content area: pediatrics.

RATIONALE

(1) Parenteral fluids are used for severe dehydration. (2) ORT is first-line treatment as long as the child can take fluids orally. (3) The BRAT diet is low in electrolytes and has little nutritional value since it is low in protein and energy. (4) Antidiarrheal agents are usually not given to infants or toddlers because of the potential adverse effects.

74. (2) Integrated processes: nursing process — implementation; client need: physiological integrity; pharmacological therapies; content area: pediatrics.

RATIONALE

(1) Silvadene contains sulfa and should not be used in those who are allergic to sulfa. Silver nitrate would be used. (2) Silvadene contains sulfa and should not be used in those who are allergic to sulfa. (3) Betadine would be contraindicated in those allergic to iodine. (4) Bacitracin may be used in those allergic to Silvadene.

75. (4) Integrated processes: nursing process — implementation, teaching/learning; client need: physiological integrity; basic care and comfort; content area: pediatrics.

RATIONALE

(1) A rigid schedule should not be enforced. The toddler may eat more or less each day. (2) A toddler is not developmentally ready to sit through long meals. (3) Skim milk and low-fat milk may be used for children more than 2 years old, but the toddler period is 12–36 months. Whole milk is needed at 12–24 months. (4) In general, 1 tablespoon for each year is adequate for a solid food serving. This is in accordance with the number of servings per food group.

76. (1) Integrated processes: nursing process — implementation; client need: physiological integrity; physiological adaptation; content area: psychiatric.

RATIONALE

(1) These clients are at high risk for seizures during the first week after cessation of alcohol intake. (2) Fluid intake should be increased to prevent dehydration. (3) Environmental stimuli should be decreased to prevent precipitation of seizures. (4) Application of restraints may cause the client to increase his or her physical activity and may eventually lead to exhaustion.

77. (1) Integrated processes: nursing process — implementation; client need: safe, effective care environment; coordinated care; content area: psychiatric.

RATIONALE

(1) Because of the stigma associated with a mental illness, many clients are fearful of rejection and reprisal. The nurse protects the psychological space of the client through confidentiality. (2) It is impossible for clients to be anonymous during a hospital stay. (3) Insanity defense is a concern for only those mentally ill hospitalized clients diagnosed as criminally insane. (4) The health-care provider, not the mentally ill client, experiences moral distress during an ethical dilemma.

78. **(3)** Integrated processes: nursing process — implementation; client need: psychosocial integrity; content area: psychiatric.

RATIONALE

(1) Isolation from others may lead to more hostility. (2) Acting out indicates aggressiveness, which is not a healthy behavior. (3) Encourage clients to communicate anger without abridging the rights of others. (4) Improving self-care may increase self-esteem but will not decrease anger.

79. **(3)** Integrated processes: nursing process — data collection; client need: psychosocial integrity; content area: psychiatric.

RATIONALE

(1) Compensation is the process by which a person attempts to make up for real or perceived deficits by strongly emphasizing some other feature that he or she regards as an asset. (2) Identification operates unconsciously and is an attempt to modify behavior and to pattern oneself after another person. (3) Rationalization is used to justify ideas, actions, or feelings with seemingly acceptable reasons or explanations. (4) Projection enables a person to justify his or her own unacceptable feelings and impulses by attributing the behaviors to others.

80. **(2)** Integrated processes: nursing process — data collection; client need: psychosocial integrity; content area: psychiatric.

RATIONALE

(1) Projection enables a person to justify his or her own acceptable feelings and impulses by attributing the behaviors to others. (2) Compensation is the process by which a person attempts to make up for real or perceived deficits by strongly emphasizing some other features that he regards as an asset. (3) Reaction formation is the development of attitudes and behaviors that are opposite to what one really feels or would like to do. (4) Rationalization is used to justify ideas, actions, or feelings with seemingly acceptable reasons or explanations.

81. **(1)** Integrated processes: nursing process — data collection; client need: psychosocial integrity; content area: psychiatric.

RATIONALE

(1) Displacement is a shift of emotions from a person or object to another neutral or less-threatening person or object. (2) Projection enables a person to identify his or her own unacceptable feelings and impulses by attributing the behaviors to others. (3) Rationalization is used to justify ideas, actions, or feelings with seemingly acceptable reasons or explanation. (4) Sublimation allows a person to divert unacceptable impulses and motives into personally and socially acceptable channels.

82. **(1)** Integrated processes: nursing process — data collection; client need: psychosocial integrity; content area: psychiatric.

RATIONALE

(1) Regression is partial or symbolic return to earlier stages of development. (2) Undoing is used to amend or reverse previous thoughts, feelings, or actions. (3) Repression is an involuntary exclusion of unacceptable feelings or thoughts that are automatically pushed into one's unconscious. (4) Reaction formation enables a person to adopt attitudes and behaviors that are opposite to his or her own impulses.

83. **(2)** Integrated processes: nursing process — implementation; client need: psychosocial integrity; content area: psychiatric.

RATIONALE

(1) The client has the right to refuse treatment. Restraining and forcing the medication is against the client's constitutional rights and "The Patient Self-Determination Act." (2) The client has a right to self-determination. Accept the client's decision. (3) Pleading is not a therapeutic nursing intervention. Paternalism is operating and may not be beneficial. (4) This response is not a good choice.

84. **(3)** Integrated processes: nursing process — implementation; client need: psychosocial integrity; content area: psychiatric.

RATIONALE

(1) Psychiatric clients have the right to leave the hospital if they are not a danger to self or others. (2) The nurse may ask the client to remain hospitalized, but this is not the best response. (3) When clients demand discharge from a psychiatric unit, they are asked to put their intentions in writing. They may be detained against their will for a period of time depending on the laws of the state. (4) This is not the best response. However, a client may discuss discharge with the physician.

85. **(2)** Integrated processes: nursing process — implementation; client need: safe, effective care environment; coordinated care; content area: psychiatric.

RATIONALE

(1) Anonymity is a situation in which the name is not disclosed. (2) Disclosure of information by psychiatric professionals is limited to authorized individuals. (3) It is not a duty to provide information to anyone unless the client has provided authorization. (4) Habeas corpus provides for patients held against their will to be discharged immediately, if judged sane.

86. **(3)** Integrated processes: nursing process — implementation; client need: safe, effective care environment; coordinated care; content area: psychiatric.

RATIONALE

(1) Psychiatric clients have the right to refuse treatment under the U.S. Constitution. (2) Clients have the right to refuse treatment once started. (3) Paternalism is operating when the nurse uses persuasion and manipulation to get the client actively engaged in treatment that is believed best for the client. (4) There is no indication that the client's constitutional rights have been abused.

87. **(1)** Integrated processes: nursing process — data collection; client need: safe, effective care environment; coordinated care; content area: psychiatric.

RATIONALE

(1) The client voluntarily admitted himself for psychiatric care. (2) A state determines judicial commitment. (3) Informal admission resembles an admission to a general hospital. (4) Involuntary admission is characterized by an unwilling and forceful admission.

88. **(1, 5)** Integrated processes: nursing process — implementation; client need: psychosocial integrity; content area: psychiatric.

RATIONALE

(1) The first priority is to reduce the anxiety to a tolerable level to prevent pathological behavior. (2) Probing the cause of anxiety is recommended only if the client is experiencing mild or well-controlled anxiety. (3) In moderate anxiety, the perceptual field narrows and the person remains alert. Decompensation is unlikely at this level. (4) Anxiety is on a continuum that becomes problematic if there is no appropriate intervention. (5) Instructing the client on healthy coping behaviors can help

reduce anxiety. **(6)** In moderate anxiety, the perceptual field narrows and the person remains alert.

89. **(3)** Integrated processes: nursing process — planning; client need: psychosocial integrity; content area: psychiatric.

    RATIONALE

    (1) Antianxiety medications should be used cautiously and sparingly because of the addictive properties. The medications may alleviate the symptoms of anxiety but they interfere with understanding the source of the anxiety. **(2)** Anxiety that is communicated interpersonally often affects family members. The immediate focus should be on the client. **(3)** Educating clients is one of the essential nursing responsibilities. **(4)** Cognitive restructuring is associated with community-based therapy.

90. **(1)** Integrated processes: nursing process — planning; client need: psychosocial integrity; content area: psychiatric.

    RATIONALE

    (1) Physical symptoms are a defense mechanism that absorbs and neutralizes the anxiety generated by unacceptable, unconscious impulses. **(2)** The symptoms are not voluntarily controlled. Dependence is not a key issue. **(3)** Symptoms arise from anxiety and are not used to manipulate others. **(4)** The symptoms develop from exposure to a specific traumatic event.

91. **(4)** Integrated processes: nursing process — planning; client need: psychosocial integrity; content area: psychiatric.

    RATIONALE

    (1) The development of phobic behavior is fear that arises through a process of displacing an unconscious conflict to an external object symbolically related to the conflict. **(2)** Free-floating anxiety is not tied to a specific stimulus. **(3)** The client is seeking help for her phobic behavior. **(4)** Persons suffering from phobic behaviors use avoidance.

92. **(1)** Integrated processes: nursing process — planning; client need: psychosocial integrity; content area: psychiatric.

    RATIONALE

    (1) The phobic person controls the intensity of the anxiety by avoiding the object with which the anxiety is associated. **(2)** The phobic person fears a specific external object rather than the internal source of distress. **(3)** Because phobias are displaced fears and at an unconscious level, the basic source is out of awareness. **(4)** This is not a good choice because the source of anxiety is an internal conflict at an unconscious level.

93. **(1)** Integrated processes: nursing process — implementation; client need: psychosocial integrity; content area: psychiatric.

    RATIONALE

    (1) Promoting client safety by providing a quiet environment may calm the hyperactive client. **(2)** This intervention shows little understanding of the disease. **(3)** Because of the psychomotor agitation, the client may have difficulty remaining in a group activity. Constant disruptions create distractions. **(4)** Avoid highly competitive activities because they may bring out hostility and aggressive behaviors.

94. **(3)** Integrated processes: nursing process — implementation; client need: psychosocial integrity; content area: psychiatric.

    RATIONALE

    (1) Matter-of-fact intervention, rather than an angry approach, is more effective. **(2)** Providing false assurances is not an appropriate form of treatment. **(3)** Keep the client's dignity in mind at all times. **(4)** The lack of an appropriate intervention is a form of rejection. Inappropriate behaviors may cause future embarrassment.

95. **(4)** Integrated processes: nursing process — implementation; client need: psychosocial integrity; content area: psychiatric.

    RATIONALE

    (1) A person with excessive energy is unable to sit and concentrate for any length of time. **(2)** Team sports will provide a release of excess energy, but may create unnecessary external stimuli. **(3)** Competition is to be discouraged during the manic phase because it may cause overly aggressive behaviors. **(4)** Walking is the best choice because it is less competitive and provides an opportunity for the release of energy.

96. **(3)** Integrated processes: nursing process — implementation; client need: psychosocial integrity; content area: psychiatric.

    RATIONALE

    (1) Long-term psychiatric care fosters dependence. The goal of therapy is to promote independence. **(2)** A nursing home client becomes dependent on the system. **(3)** A group home will assist the client with structure and help him to develop a level of independence. **(4)** The client requires some form of structure, which is not available with independent living.

97. **(2)** Integrated processes: nursing process — implementation; client need: physiological integrity; pharmacological therapies; content area: psychiatric.

    RATIONALE

    (1) Fluoxetine is not a tricyclic antidepressant. It is an atypical antidepressant. **(2)** This statement is true. **(3)** These foods are high in tyramine and should be avoided when the client is taking MAO inhibitors. Fluoxetine is not an MAO inhibitor. **(4)** Fatal reactions have been reported in clients receiving fluoxetine in combination with MAO inhibitors.

98. **(1)** Integrated processes: nursing process — planning; client need: psychosocial integrity; content area: psychiatric.

    RATIONALE

    (1) Because the client is complaining of neck pain and bragging about an insurance settlement, the nurse suspects he is feigning pain. **(2)** Conversion is a defense mechanism operating unconsciously. The client clearly states his motive. **(3)** Somatization disorder applies to clients who have sought medical attention for recurrent and multiple somatic complaints. **(4)** Hypochondriasis is characterized by constantly worrying about health or fear of having some disease.

99. **(1)** Integrated processes: nursing process — data collection; client need: psychosocial integrity; content area: psychiatric.

    RATIONALE

    (1) A hallucination is a false sensory perception in the absence of an actual external stimulus. **(2)** Fantasies are a defense mechanism used in an attempt to resolve an emotional conflict. **(3)** A delusion is a false belief based on incorrect inference about external reality even with evidence to the contrary. **(4)** Derealization is a perception that the immediate environment is suddenly strange.

100. **(1)** Integrated processes: nursing process — implementation; client need: psychosocial integrity; content area: psychiatric.

    RATIONALE

    (1) Conveying acceptance shows that the nurse is willing to meet the client's needs. **(2)** Thought insertion is only one symptom that contributes to the client's behavior. **(3)** Ignoring the behaviors may create a nontherapeutic relationship because it does not convey acceptance. **(4)** Before attempting to probe for the target symptoms, the client should show improvement in the disease process.

101. **(3)** Integrated processes: nursing process — implementation, communication and documentation; client need: safe, effective care environment; coordinated care; content area: psychiatric nursing.

RATIONALE

(1) The nurse should listen with understanding to the older person's own perception of the problem, not the family's. **(2)** The nurse needs to explain his or her own perception of the problem. **(3)** The nurse should acknowledge and discuss the differences and similarities between the older person's and the nurse's viewpoint. **(4)** The nurse should recommend a treatment plan within the constraints of his or her own ideas and those of the client.

102. **(3)** Integrated processes: nursing process — evaluation; client need: safe, effective care environment; coordinated care; content area: medical-surgical.

RATIONALE

(1) Civil wrongs are the same as torts. **(2)** Torts are civil wrongs that cause harm or damage to a person or party. **(3)** Malpractice is defined as professional misconduct, negligent care or treatment, or failure to meet the standards of care, resulting in harm to a person. **(4)** Informed consent is not an area of legal action of negligence.

103. **(1)** Integrated processes: nursing process — evaluation; client need: safe, effective care environment; coordinated care; content area: medical-surgical.

RATIONALE

(1) Duty is not an element of negligence. **(2)** Breach of duty is an element of negligence. **(3)** Damage is an element of negligence. **(4)** The court must find a causal connection between the breach and the damages, if any, to substantiate the claim.

104. **(2)** Integrated processes: nursing process — evaluation, communication and documentation; client need: safe, effective care environment; coordinated care; content area: medical-surgical.

RATIONALE

(1) Documentation decreases the potential areas of legal exposure. **(2)** Documentation describes client education and discharge instructions. **(3)** Documentation relates physicians' conversations, family comments, and client's concerns and feelings. **(4)** Documentation records untoward events such as falls.

105. **(3)** Integrated processes: nursing process — implementation, communication and documentation; client need: safe, effective care environment; safety and infection control; content area: medical-surgical.

RATIONALE

(1) Document the need for restraints (describe the client's specific behavior and the type of restraints used). **(2)** For a client check, document skin integrity, circulation, respiratory status, client's verbal response, reasons based on client behavior for continued restraints, and physician's orders. **(3)** Documenting client's response to restraints ensures that a nurse is operating from a standard of care. **(4)** Document alternatives used before restraints.

106. **(2)** Integrated processes: nursing process — implementation, communication and documentation; client need: safe, effective care environment; coordinated care; content area: medical-surgical.

RATIONALE

(1) The physician usually has the duty to obtain the informed consent. **(2)** The nurse's responsibility is to witness the signature of the client on the informed consent sheet. **(3)** Clients are read their rights on entering the hospital, not when an informed consent is obtained before surgery. **(4)** If the client is confused, is mentally incompetent, or cannot give informed consent, the next person who is legally permitted to consent must be given the elements of informed consent.

107. **(2)** Integrated processes: nursing process — implementation, communication and documentation; client need: safe, effective care environment; coordinated care; content area: medical-surgical.

RATIONALE

(1) The physician may refuse to sign the telephone order, thus exposing the nurse to liability. **(2)** The attending physician must write a DNR order on the chart to protect the health-care providers legally. **(3)** Competent clients have the right to refuse resuscitation even if family members request it. **(4)** If there is a signed physician's order not to resuscitate, the nurses are covered legally.

108. **(2)** Integrated processes: nursing process — implementation, communication and documentation; client need: safe, effective care environment; coordinated care; content area: medical-surgical.

RATIONALE

(1) "Slow code" orders must not be accepted because they are not legal and have ethical implications. **(2)** Copies of the living will and medical durable power of attorney should be included in the client's chart. **(3)** DNR orders must be written as an order in the client's chart. **(4)** Discussions with the client and family should be documented.

109. **(2)** Integrated processes: nursing process — implementation; client need: safe, effective care environment; coordinated care; content area: medical-surgical.

RATIONALE

(1) Overmedication, not undermedication, is an area of legal exposure. **(2)** Areas of legal exposure include decubitus ulcers, overmedication, falls, and restraints. **(3)** Reporting complications is not an area of legal exposure. **(4)** Assessing an older person's condition every 8 hours is not an area of legal exposure.

110. **(1, 2, 3, 4, 5)** Integrated processes: nursing process — implementation; client need: physiological integrity; reduction of risk potential; content area: medical-surgical.

RATIONALE

(1) If a nasogastric tube becomes clogged, the first action for a nurse to take would be to try to unclog the tube by aspirating it. **(2)** If all methods to unclog the tube fail, the last resort would be to remove and replace the nasogastric tube. **(3)** If aspiration does not work, a small amount of warm water could be used to try to flush the tube. **(4)** If agency policy allows, carbonated beverages can be used to dissolve any clogged medications. **(5)** If all methods to unclog the tube fail, the last resort would be to remove and replace the nasogastric tube. **(6)** If aspiration does not work, a small amount of warm water could be used to try to flush the tube.

111. **(2, 4, 5)** Integrated processes: nursing process — data collection; client need: physiological integrity; physiological adaptation; content area: medical-surgical.

RATIONALE

(1) Ask the caregiver about the client's pain. An older adult may not be able to point to the location. **(2)** Ask the caregiver about the client's pain. An older adult may not be able to point to the location. (**3**) Temperature, pulse, and respiration are indicators of pain. (**4**) If the client is able to communicate, it is best to ask the client to rate the intensity of the pain by using a pain scale. (**5**) Clients usually demonstrate excessive perspiration, clammy skin, and restlessness as indicators of pain. (**6**) Clients usually demonstrate excessive perspiration, clammy skin, and restlessness as indicators of pain.

112. (**2, 5, 6**) Integrated processes: nursing process — implementation; client need: physiological integrity; pharmacological therapies; content area: medical-surgical.

RATIONALE

(**1**) When a client is in pain, administer the full dose of ordered pain medication. (**2**) When a client is in pain, administer the full dose of ordered pain medication. (**3**) Oral pain medication is absorbed slower than intramuscular pain medication. (**4**) It is a breach of duty to refuse to give the medication. (**5**) After the pain has subsided, change the bed linens to aid in comfort. (**6**) Sometimes, relaxing music can be used to help distract from the pain. However, this is should be done in conjunction with giving pain medication.

113. (**2, 5, 6**) Integrated processes: nursing process — data collection; client need: physiological integrity; pharmacological therapies; content area: medical-surgical.

RATIONALE

(**1**) Older adults have a decreased perception of thirst resulting in fluid volume deficit. (**2**) Muscle tissue declines in older adults leaving them at risk for fluid volume deficit. (**3**) The amount of total body water decreases in the older adult. (**4**) Keeping the room environment too hot will increase the risk of fluid volume deficit, especially during hot weather. (**5**) Body temperature is less effective with aging. (**6**) In older adults, the kidney function decreases; the ability to concentrate the urine decreases.

114. (**2, 3**) Integrated processes: nursing process — data collection; client need: physiological integrity; basic care and comfort; content area: medical-surgical.

RATIONALE

(**1**) Oranges do not have high sodium contents. (**2**) Chips are usually high in sodium content. (**3**) Bologna is high in sodium content. (**4**) Bread is not considered a food high in sodium. (**5**) Tuna fish is a good source of protein. This is not the best choice. (**6**) Buttermilk and cheeses have high sodium contents, whereas whole or skim milk does not.

115. (**1, 5**) Integrated processes: nursing process — data collection, teaching/learning; client need: physiological integrity; basic care and comfort; content area: medical-surgical.

RATIONALE

(**1**) Oranges have high potassium contents. (**2**) Chips have high sodium contents, not high potassium contents. (**3**) Bologna, as a processed food, has high sodium contents, not high potassium contents. (**4**) Bacon has high sodium contents, not high potassium contents. (**5**) Milk has potassium content, not a high sodium content. (**6**) Applesauce is a low-potassium food.

116. (**3, 4, 5**) Integrated processes: nursing process — implementation, teaching/learning; client need: physiological integrity; basic care and comfort; content area: medical-surgical.

RATIONALE

(**1**) Soft drinks are high in sodium and will increase edema. (**2**) Walking barefoot increases the risk of injury to feet, especially if feet are swollen. (**3**) Change position if sitting in a chair or bed frequently will help to reduce edema. (**4**) Supportive hose or stockings helps decrease venous stasis, thus reducing swelling. (**5**) Elevate feet and legs when sitting will help reduce edema. (**6**) Avoid restrictive clothing around the abdomen.

117. (**3, 5, 6**) Integrated processes: nursing process — implementation; client need: physiological integrity; basic care and comfort; content area: medical-surgical.

RATIONALE

(**1**) Medications should be diluted with water before administering via feeding tube. (**2**) Flush the tube feeding with water before and after administering medication. (**3**) Push air into the feeding tube after administering medication to ensure that all the medication has been emptied from the tube. (**4**) Keep tube feeding off for 30 minutes after administering medications to ensure absorption. (**5**) Check for gastric residual before administering the medication. (**6**) Flush the feeding tube before and after administering the medication.

118. (**200 cc**) Integrated processes: nursing process — implementation; client need: physiological integrity; pharmacological therapies; content area: medical-surgical.

RATIONALE

If the physician orders the IV to infuse at 100 mL/hr, then 800 mL should have infused in an 8-hour period. Subtract 800 mL from 1000 mL and the remaining total is 200 mL.

119. (**400 mL**) Integrated processes: nursing process — implementation; client need: physiological integrity; pharmacological therapies; content area: medical-surgical.

RATIONALE

If the physician orders the enteral feeding to be administered at 50 mL/hr, then multiply 50 mL × 8 = 400 mL in the 8-hour period.

120. (**100–150 mL**) Integrated processes: nursing process — implementation; client need: physiological integrity; pharmacological therapies; content area: medical-surgical.

RATIONALE

The usual rule is to withhold the feeding and recheck the residual in 1 hour if the residual exceeds 100–150 mL.

121. (**10–30 mL**) Integrated processes: nursing process — implementation; client need: physiological integrity; pharmacological therapies; content area: medical-surgical.

RATIONALE

Diluting drugs with 10–30 mL of tap water and flushing the tube before and after administering each drug can decrease the viscosity of the drug.

122. (**500–1000 mL**) Integrated processes: nursing process — implementation; client need: physiological integrity; basic care and comfort; content area: medical-surgical.

RATIONALE

Five hundred to 1000 mL/day is the recommended 24-hour intake for a client with end-stage renal disease who is undergoing dialysis.

123. (**28-gauge, 1-inch needle**) Integrated processes: nursing process — implementation; client need: physiological integrity; pharmacological therapies; content area: medical-surgical.

RATIONALE

The viscosity of the medication and body size of the client help the nurse determine which gauge and size of needle to use to administer intramuscular injections.

124. (**90 degrees**) Integrated processes: nursing process — implementation; client need: physiological integrity; pharmacological therapies; content area: medical-surgical.

RATIONALE

When administering medication using the Z-track method, the needle should be at a 90-degree angle.

125. **(15 mg)** Integrated processes: nursing process — implementation; client need: physiological integrity; pharmacological therapies; content area: medical-surgical.

RATIONALE

1 gr is equivalent to 60 mg; therefore, if 60 mg = 1 gr, then x mg = 0.25 gr (0.25 mg). Calculate for x = 15 mg.

126. **(1)** Integrated processes: nursing process — data collection; client need: health promotion and maintenance; content area: medical-surgical.

RATIONALE

(1) Being underweight is not a risk factor. **(2)** Smoking is a risk factor for the development of cardiovascular disease. **(3)** Having hypertension is a risk factor for the development of cardiovascular disease. **(4)** Maintaining a sedentary lifestyle is a risk factor for the development of cardiovascular disease.

127. **(1)** Integrated processes: nursing process — implementation; client need: physiological integrity; pharmacological therapies; content area: medical-surgical.

RATIONALE

(1) NTG causes vasodilation, which can cause significant hypotension. **(2)** The nurse may also check the pulse, but it is most important to check the blood pressure. **(3)** The client does not have to be in a sitting position. **(4)** NTG does not directly affect blood potassium level.

128. **(3)** Integrated processes: nursing process — implementation; client need: physiological integrity; basic care and comfort; content area: medical-surgical.

RATIONALE

(1) Pears are not high in sodium. **(2)** Baked chicken is not high in sodium unless specifically prepared with salt. **(3)** Olives are high in sodium. **(4)** Baked potatoes are not high in sodium unless salt is added by the client.

129. **(4)** Integrated processes: nursing process — data collection; client need: physiological integrity; reduction of risk potential; content area: medical-surgical.

RATIONALE

(1) This is an expected finding in right-sided heart failure. **(2)** This is an expected finding in right-sided heart failure. **(3)** LLQ pain is not a sign of CHF. **(4)** Dyspnea is a classic symptom of congestive failure resulting from fluid backup into the lungs.

130. **(3)** Integrated processes: nursing process — data collection; client need: physiological integrity; reduction of risk potential; content area: medical-surgical.

RATIONALE

(1) Lymphedema is a sign of venous insufficiency. **(2)** Pedal edema is a sign of venous insufficiency. **(3)** The absence of pedal pulses indicates arterial insufficiency. **(4)** A bluish cast to the extremities is suggestive of venous insufficiency.

131. **(3)** Integrated processes: nursing process — evaluation; client need: physiological integrity; physiological adaptation; content area: medical-surgical.

RATIONALE

(1) The pineal gland does not control the pituitary gland. **(2)** The sympathetic nervous system does not control the pituitary gland. **(3)** The master endocrine gland is the pituitary gland and is controlled by the hypothalamus. The pituitary gland has sympathetic nervous system innervation but does not control it. **(4)** The master endocrine gland is the pituitary gland.

132. **(2)** Integrated processes: nursing process — implementation; client need: physiological integrity; reduction of risk potential; content area: medical-surgical.

RATIONALE

(1) A Jackson-Pratt drain would be placed in surgery if needed. **(2)** Edema in the neck can lead to respiratory distress. A tracheostomy set should be available for this emergency. **(3)** There is no indication for a Salem sump tube. **(4)** There is no reason to have an IV potassium infusion at the bedside.

133. **(4)** Integrated processes: nursing process — evaluation; client need: safe, effective care environment; safety and infection control; content area: medical-surgical.

RATIONALE

(1) *Pathogenic* means having organisms capable of causing disease. **(2)** *Synergistic* means working together. **(3)** *Diagnostic* means pertaining to a disease. **(4)** *Nosocomial* pertains to a hospital- or infirmary-acquired infection.

134. **(3)** Integrated processes: nursing process — implementation; client need: safe, effective care environment; coordinated care; content area: older adult.

RATIONALE

(1) The elderly client will need home health services, not hospice services. **(2)** The elderly client will need home health services, not respiratory therapist services. **(3)** The elderly client will need home health services. **(4)** The elderly client will need home health services, not elderly protection services.

135. **(2)** Integrated processes: nursing process — implementation, teaching/learning; client need: physiological integrity; pharmacological therapies; content area: older adult.

RATIONALE

(1) Aleve and naproxen are both the same drug. If both are taken together, it could contribute to an overdose. **(2)** Aleve and naproxen are both the same drug. Take only one or the other, but not both drugs. **(3)** This is not the best answer. The client needs to be instructed that the two medications are the same drug. **(4)** This is not the best answer. It is dangerous to have the client combine over-the-counter medications with prescription drugs in the same bottle.

136. **(2)** Integrated processes: nursing process — data collection, teaching/learning; client need: safe, effective care environment; safety and infection control; content area: older adult.

RATIONALE

(1) Properly installed electrical outlets do not pose a safety risk for a home-bound client. **(2)** A home-health nurse would check the bathtub for safety. The client needs to be instructed to have a nonslip mat on the bottom of the tub. **(3)** Newspapers neatly piled in a corner are not a safety issue; however, if the newspapers were scattered throughout the client's room, there is an increased risk of falls. **(4)** Handrails placed in the bathroom prevent the client from falling.

137. **(1)** Integrated processes: nursing process — data collection, teaching/learning; client need: physiological integrity; pharmacological therapies; content area: medical-surgical.

RATIONALE

(1) Insulin needs to be stored in a cool place, preferably a refrigerator, unless otherwise directed. Avoid freezing. **(2)** Diabetic clients need to see the physician for follow-up exams routinely. **(3)** Plastic insulin syringes are to be used only once and discarded. **(4)** Diabetics are prone to sores in the feet and require daily assessment for sores.

138. **(3)** Integrated processes: nursing process — planning; client need: safe, effective care environment; safety and infection control; content area: medical-surgical.
RATIONALE
(1) Mechanical restraints would interfere with a terminal cancer client's comfort. **(2)** Leg restraints would possibly increase the changes of the client falling. **(3)** Using adjunct medications to help the client relax is the safest way to prevent the client from trying to get out of bed. **(4)** Tying the client to the bed with a sheet is dangerous and reduces dignity.

139. **(3)** Integrated processes: nursing process — implementation; client need: safe, effective care environment; safety and infection control; content area: medical-surgical.
RATIONALE
(1) Reverse isolation is used to protect the client from outside infections. **(2)** Isolation is used to protect other clients on the nursing unit from an infectious client. **(3)** Reverse isolation is used to protect the client from outside infections. **(4)** Reverse isolation is used to protect the client from outside infections.

140. **(4)** Integrated processes: nursing process — planning; client need: safe, effective care environment; coordinated care; content area: older adult.
RATIONALE
(1) Aid to Families with Dependent Children provides services for families with children, not the elderly. **(2)** Meals on Wheels provide meals for home-bound individuals, not financial assistance. **(3)** Council on Aging provides a variety of services; one service would be to refer the client to the Social Security Office to submit an application for Supplemental Security Income. **(4)** The Social Security Office helps an elderly client to apply for Supplemental Security Income.

141. **(2)** Integrated processes: nursing process — implementation; client need: health promotion and maintenance; content area: maternity.
RATIONALE
(1) Pregnancy can occur even if the male partner withdraws before ejaculation. **(2)** Unprotected sex can result in pregnancy regardless of whether it is the first time. **(3)** Teens are at high risk for pregnancy with unprotected sex. **(4)** Pregnancy occurs even when the menstrual cycle is not regular.

142. **(2)** Integrated processes: nursing process — data collection; client need: health promotion and maintenance; content area: medical-surgical.
RATIONALE
(1) Screening for tuberculosis is done in groups that experience disease and infection rates higher than normal, such as HIV-positive clients. **(2)** Screening for tuberculosis is done in groups that experience disease and infection rates higher than normal, such as HIV-positive clients. **(3)** Screening for tuberculosis is done in groups that experience disease and infection rates higher than normal, such as HIV-positive clients. **(4)** Screening for tuberculosis is done in groups that experience disease and infection rates higher than normal, such as HIV-positive clients.

143. **(4)** Integrated processes: nursing process — implementation; client need: health promotion and maintenance; content area: medical-surgical.
RATIONALE
(1) Mantoux test is done by intradermal injection, not subcutaneous injection. **(2)** Mantoux test is done by intradermal injection, not by IM injection. **(3)** Manoux test is done by intradermal injection, not by IV method. **(4)** Mantoux test is done by intradermal injection.

144. **(3)** Integrated processes: nursing process — implementation; client need: health promotion and maintenance; content area: medical-surgical.
RATIONALE
(1) CDC recommends preventive therapy for recent tuberculin converters. **(2)** CDC recommends preventive therapy for inadequately treated persons with abnormal chest radiographs. **(3)** CDC recommends preventive therapy for clients who are HIV positive. **(4)** CDC recommends preventive therapy for persons who are HIV positive.

145. **(2, 4, 6)** Integrated processes: nursing process — implementation; client need: safe, effective care environment; coordinated care; content area: older adult.
RATIONALE
(1) Teaching the care provider how to take a blood pressure is an example of direct care. **(2)** Participating in a team conference regarding the client is an example of indirect care. **(3)** Teaching is an example of direct care. **(4)** Discussing the client's needs with a dietitian is an example of indirect care. **(5)** Performing wound care is an example of direct care. **(6)** This is an example of indirect care.

146. **(3)** Integrated processes: nursing process — implementation, teaching/learning; client need: health promotion and maintenance; content area: maternity.
RATIONALE
(1) Ingestion of cocaine places the client at high risk for narcotic abuse. **(2)** Ingestion of marijuana places the client at high risk for narcotic abuse. **(3)** Ingestion of alcoholic beverages during pregnancy places the client at high risk for delivering an infant with fetal alcohol syndrome. **(4)** Low self-esteem places the client at high risk for addictions.

147. **(3)** Integrated processes: nursing process — implementation, caring; client need: psychosocial integrity; content area: psychiatric.
RATIONALE
(1) Being judgmental is nontherapeutic in dealing with suspected family violence. **(2)** Disgust and avoidance is nontherapeutic in dealing with suspected family violence. **(3)** Creating a supportive environment is important in dealing with suspected family violence. **(4)** Punitive treatment is nontherapeutic in dealing with suspected family violence.

148. **(4)** Integrated processes: nursing process — implementation; client need: safe, effective care environment; coordinated care; content area: management of care.
RATIONALE
(1) The nursing assistant can pass out the breakfast trays. **(2)** In functional nursing, the registered nurse will administer IV medications. **(3)** The registered nurse will make brief walking rounds to assess the night shift report and introduce herself to the client. **(4)** In functional nursing, the LPN/LVN will be assigned oral and IM medications. The first priority will be to check the medication cards/sheets against the Kardex.

149. **(3)** Integrated processes: nursing process — implementation; client need: safe, effective care environment; coordinated care; content area: management of care.
RATIONALE
(1) Delegating to the nursing assistant to help the client with his meal is the best way to manage time. **(2)** Delegating to the nursing assistant to help the client with his meal is the best

way to manage time. (3) Delegating to the nursing assistant to help the client with his meal is the best way to manage time. (4) Delegating to the nursing assistant to help the client with his meal is the best way to manage time.

150. (2) Integrated processes: nursing process — planning; client need: physiological integrity; pharmacological therapies; content area: medical-surgical.

RATIONALE

(1) Clients on dexamethasone are not prone to renal calculi. (2) Clients on dexamethasone are prone to infection. (3) Clients on dexamethasone are not prone to gallstones. (4) Clients on dexamethasone are not prone to hypotension.

151. (3) Integrated processes: nursing process — implementation; client need: physiological integrity; reduction of risk potential; content area: medical-surgical.

RATIONALE

(1) This position will not facilitate breathing. (2) This position will not facilitate breathing. (3) This is the best position. (4) Semi-Fowler's is better than low-Fowler's.

152. (2) Integrated processes: nursing process — planning; client need: physiological integrity; reduction of risk potential; content area: medical-surgical.

RATIONALE

(1) A thoracotomy tray is used for the insertion of a chest tube. (2) A tracheostomy tray is needed in case of breathing difficulties. (3) A paracentesis tray is used for an abdominal tap. (4) A pericardiocentesis tray is used for draining fluid from the pericardium.

153. (2) Integrated processes: nursing process — implementation; client need: physiological integrity; physiological adaptation; content area: medical-surgical.

RATIONALE

(1) Do not remove the screwdriver; it may be tamponading a bleeding site. (2) Leave the screwdriver in place until adequate medical help is in place. (3) This is a later action. (4) Do not remove the screwdriver; it may be tamponading a bleeding site.

154. (4) Integrated processes: nursing process — implementation; client need: physiological integrity; physiological adaptation; content area: medical-surgical.

RATIONALE

(1) Cleaning the wound is a second priority. (2) Using a tourniquet is a last resort. (3) If a tourniquet is needed, it would be applied above the laceration. (4) Apply direct pressure first to control the bleeding.

155. (3) Integrated processes: nursing process — implementation, teaching/learning; client need: physiological integrity; reduction of risk potential; content area: medical-surgical.

RATIONALE

(1) Not all clients have phantom limb pain. (2) Demonstrating dressing changes is a later activity. (3) Teaching crutch walking is the best activity to prepare him for postoperative therapy. (4) Teaching leg exercises has a lower priority than teaching crutch walking.

156. (3) Integrated processes: nursing process — implementation; client need: psychosocial integrity; content area: psychiatric nursing.

RATIONALE

(1) This intervention does not help the client to understand the anxiety. (2) This intervention does not help the client to understand the anxiety. (3) The most appropriate initial intervention is to help the client to understand the anxiety. (4) This activity may help the client to sleep, but it does not help the client to understand the anxiety.

157. (1) Integrated processes: nursing process — implementation, teaching/learning; client need: physiological integrity; reduction of risk potential; content area: medical-surgical.

RATIONALE

(1) A high-fiber diet will help to ensure a soft stool and to decrease the chance for bleeding and pain postoperatively. (2) A low-fiber diet will cause bowel irritation. (3) A high-fat diet may cause diarrhea postoperatively. (4) A high-carbohydrate diet may cause constipation postoperatively.

158. (1) Integrated processes: nursing process — implementation, teaching/learning; client need: physiological integrity; pharmacological therapies; content area: medical-surgical.

RATIONALE

Correct calculation: 150 mg divided by 300 mg x 2 mL = 1 mL

159. (4) Integrated processes: nursing process — implementation; client need: physiological integrity; pharmacological therapies; content area: medical-surgical.

RATIONALE

Correct calculation: 750 mg $\times$ 3 doses = 2250 mg

160. (4) Integrated processes: nursing process — implementation; client need: physiological integrity; pharmacological therapies; content area: medical-surgical.

RATIONALE

Correct calculation: 75 mg $\div$ 25 mg $\times$ 1 mL = 3 mL

161. (4) Integrated processes: nursing process — implementation; client need: physiological integrity; pharmacological therapies; content area: medical-surgical.

RATIONALE

Correct calculation: It takes 9 mL of normal saline to be mixed with 1 mL of morphine sulfate (10 mg) to deliver 1 mg/mL.

162. (1) Integrated processes: nursing process — implementation; client need: physiological integrity; pharmacological therapies; content area: pediatric.

RATIONALE

The muscle of a 5-year-old can absorb only 1 mL of medication.

163. (1) Integrated processes: nursing process — implementation, teaching/learning; client need: physiological integrity; reduction of risk potential; content area: medical-surgical.

RATIONALE

(1) Immobilization or even a relatively sedentary existence favors stasis of blood in the veins and predisposes the elderly client to thrombosis. (2) Although prolonged bed rest does increase the chance of developing decubitus ulcers, this is not the rationale for early ambulation following a hip replacement. (3) There is no evidence to support the statement that late ambulation fosters dependence. (4) Although this is a nursing goal, there is no assurance that early ambulation will return the client to baseline functional status.

164. (3) Integrated processes: nursing process — implementation, teaching/learning; client need: physiological integrity; reduction of risk potential; content area: medical-surgical.

RATIONALE

(1) Hip precaution teaching includes instructions to maintain the hip in a position of abduction and neutral rotation. Sitting with the hips at a 90-degree or greater angle is necessary to

maintain the hips in this position. (2) Although use of correct body mechanics is usually a proper instruction to clients, arthroplasty clients should not bend forward more than 90 degrees. (3) Use of a long shoe horn will assist the client to continue to do activities of daily living such as putting on shoes and prevent the necessity of bending forward greater than 90 degrees. (4) Use of pillows between the legs while in bed will assist in maintaining abduction to the hips.

165. **(1)** Integrated processes: nursing process — implementation; client need: physiological integrity; reduction of risk potential; content area: medical-surgical.

RATIONALE

(1) Exercise increases the body's need for oxygen and requires the cardiovascular and respiratory systems to increase the workload to meet this demand. (2) Normal aging changes in the cardiovascular and respiratory systems require a longer period of time to regain homeostasis. (3) Normal aging changes in the cardiovascular and respiratory systems require a longer period of time to regain homeostasis. (4) Normal aging changes in the cardiovascular and respiratory systems require a longer period of time to regain homeostasis.

166. **(3)** Integrated processes: nursing process — implementation; client need: physiological integrity; pharmacological therapies; content area: older adult.

RATIONALE

(1) Drugs given more frequently would result in a greater amount of the medication to the client. Greater amounts of medication place the client at high risk for toxicity because of the decreased renal function that is a normal aging change. (2) Administering medications more frequently places the client at high risk for toxicity because of the decreased renal function that is a normal aging change. (3) Medications, when administered properly and individualized to client needs, are seldom harmful. (4) In clinical practice, the doses of many drugs are excreted primarily by the kidneys are routinely adjusted for older adults to compensate for alteration in renal function.

167. **(1)** Integrated processes: nursing process — implementation, caring; client need: pyschosocial integrity; content area: older adult.

RATIONALE

(1) Knowledge that one is about to lose a limb, no matter what age, is anxiety producing. Spending time with the client and allowing him to verbalize feelings is important to decrease anxiety and to increase coping and acceptance. (2) Allowing the client to interact with persons who have similar conditions may be helpful during rehabilitation; however, it minimizes the feelings of the client and decreases verbalization initially. (3) Although the family should be included in the plan of care for this client, this action by the nurse initially negates nursing responsibility and may potentially decrease successful coping that can be explored. (4) Explanation of the surgical procedure is an important nursing action, but is not the primary concern for the client initially. This action does little to assist the client in resolving emotional issues.

168. **(4)** Integrated processes: nursing process — implementation; client need: physiological integrity; basic care and comfort; content area: older adult.

RATIONALE

(1) Stump wrapping is continued until the client is fitted with the prosthesis. (2) Protective cushioning prevents the stump from becoming hard and firmly shaped and is contraindicated. (3) Phantom pain should be discussed prior to surgery because the sensation usually occurs early on and disappears over a period of weeks or months. (4) Before the prosthesis

is prescribed, the client's general strength must be improved through general conditioning and resistive exercises.

169. **(2)** Integrated processes: nursing process — implementation; client need: physiological integrity; basic care and comfort; content area: medical-surgical.

RATIONALE

(1) This statement is a generalization and is stereotypical. (2) Through careful meal planning, adults who are diabetic may occasionally have sweets or alcoholic beverages. A reasonable, collaborative approach in diabetic teaching is much more likely to result in compliance than rigid control. (3) The goal of insulin therapy is to maintain blood glucose levels within normal parameters, but often a great deal of adjustment is required to achieve a balance. (4) Many clinicians allow more flexibility in blood sugar levels and allow them to rise above normal to determine that the client is not at risk for hypoglycemia, not hyperglycemia.

170. **(2)** Integrated processes: nursing process — data collection; client need: physiological integrity; reduction of risk potential; content area: medical-surgical.

RATIONALE

(1) This question refers to the technique of doing physical examination of the gastrointestinal system. The technique used by the nurse is inappropriate. (2) Because of the bowel activity that can be initiated by the use of palpation, the correct assessment technique sequence in the gastrointestinal examination includes inspection, auscultation, and percussion, followed finally by palpation. (3) The question refers to the technique used by the nurse in performing physical examination of the gastrointestinal system. (4) The question refers to the technique used by the nurse in performing physical examination of the gastrointestinal system.

171. **(1)** Integrated processes: nursing process — data collection, communication and documentation; client need: physiological integrity; reduction of risk potential; content area: medical-surgical.

RATIONALE

(1) Acute intestinal obstruction is characterized by rapid onset of abdominal cramping, vomiting, and distention. Cramps are associated with high-pitched bowel sounds due to peristalsis. (2) Diffuse pain and low-grade temperature are symptoms of appendicitis. (3) Hyperactivity is associated with bowel sounds and is not present in the absence of bowel sounds. (4) Nausea and marked abdominal tenderness are symptoms of cholecystitis.

172. **(2)** Integrated processes: nursing process — implementation; client need: safe, effective care environment; safety and infection control; content area: medical-surgical.

RATIONALE

(1) Absorbent pads do assist in keeping the client dry, but are demoralizing to the client who has cognitive awareness and should not be used unless other approaches prove unsatisfactory. (2) Because the client is only incontinent at night, the use of toilet supplements such as bedside commode, urinal, or bedpan can assist in remaining continent. The use of a night light also assists the client to orient himself to a new environment more quickly and reduce the chance of accidents. (3) Stress is not known to cause incontinence at night. (4) A Foley catheter allows for the introduction of bacteria and predisposes the client to urinary tract infection.

173. **(2)** Integrated processes: nursing process — planning; client need: safe, effective care environment; safety and infection control; content area: medical-surgical.

RATIONALE

(1) Cerebrovascular accident clients do have dramatic mood swings; however, safety is the most important need for the clients at this time. (2) Clients with left hemisphere infarctions tend to have poor judgment and to overestimate physical abilities. In addition, they react quickly and impulsively and are at high risk for injury. Because there is the potential for injury, this is a safety need and thus is a priority plan. (3) Cerebrovascular accident clients do have labile affect; however, safety is the most important need for the client at this time. (4) Aggression would be individualized and is not necessarily a problem with cerebrovascular accident clients.

174. (3) Integrated processes: nursing process — planning; client need: safe, effective care environment; safety and infection control; content area: medical-surgical.

RATIONALE

(1) Although it is important to maintain nutritional status, impaired judgment makes safety the most important need for the client with left hemisphere infarction. (2) Although diversional activity is important, safety is the most important need for the left hemisphere infarction client. (3) Clients with left hemisphere infarctions have poor judgment, overestimate physical abilities, and react quickly and impulsively. These behaviors make them at high risk for injury. (4) Although psychological counseling may be part of the treatment plan for the client, impaired judgment makes safety the most important need.

175. (2) Integrated processes: nursing process — evaluation; client need: psychosocial integrity; content area: medical-surgical.

RATIONALE

(1) This response casts doubt on the ability of the family to function and places feelings of burden on the loved one. (2) This response indicates acceptance of the change in the loved one and changing the environment so that she can function more easily within the home. (3) This response may be supportive but shows no indication of family interaction. (4) This response may indicate unrealistic expectations that may not be reachable.

176. (2) Integrated processes: nursing process — planning, teaching/learning; client need: physiological integrity; reduction of risk potential; content area: medical-surgical.

RATIONALE

(1) Attitude toward illness is important for the nurse to be aware of but is not a key ingredient in the teaching process. (2) Because the nurse has prepared written information regarding his medication, these instructions should be reflective of the client's educational level. (3) Past compliance with medical regimen is important information but may be due to numerous causes. Past compliance is not a key ingredient to the teaching plan, but will require follow-up. (4) The client's usual activities of daily living are not important in looking at medications ordered as a daily dose. Daily dose schedule allows flexibility in administration.

177. (1) Integrated processes: nursing process — evaluation, teaching/learning; client need: health promotion and maintenance; content area: medical-surgical.

RATIONALE

(1) Potassium chloride (K-Dur) should not be taken on an empty stomach because of its potential for gastric irritation. (2) Headache may be important to monitor but is not associated with the discharge medications ordered for the client. (3) Cholesterol may be important to monitor but is not associated with the discharge medications ordered for the client. (4)

Bumetanide (Bumex) is a rapid-acting diuretic and should be taken during awakening hours.

178. (3) Integrated processes: nursing process — data collection; client need: physiological integrity; pharmacological therapies; content area: medical-surgical.

RATIONALE

(1) Headaches are not a normal occurrence but are not indicative of adverse reactions to K-Dur. (2) Impairment in cognition is not a normal occurrence, but is not indicative of adverse reactions to K-Dur. (3) Tarry stools may indicate gastrointestinal bleeding from gastric irritation and an adverse reaction to K-Dur. (4) Difficulty seeing things close up (presbyopia) is a normal aging change.

179. (2) Integrated processes: nursing process — implementation, teaching/learning; client need: safe and effective care environment; coordinated care; content area: management of care.

RATIONALE

(1) Following hospital procedure for bathing is appropriate for nursing staff to remember, but does little to get the client involved in personal hygiene. (2) Giving the client short, specific instructions of what to do allows the client to process the information and aids in following directions. (3) Written, step-by-step instructions may be difficult for the client to comprehend and produce frustration. (4) Explaining what is expected ahead of time requires increased cognitive ability and will not assist to get the client involved in personal hygiene.

180. (3) Integrated processes: nursing process — implementation; client need: physiological integrity; basic care and comfort; content area: medical-surgical.

RATIONALE

(1) Limiting fluids to 1000 mL daily could cause the client to be at risk for electrolyte imbalance, dehydration, and infections. (2) An indwelling catheter provides a medium for urinary tract infections and is not appropriate for incontinence associated with dementia. (3) A regular, consistent schedule of toileting provides an environment that decreases anxiety and frustration. (4) Although labeling the door may help the client to find the bathroom, there is no assurance that this will increase continence.

181. (1) Integrated processes: nursing process — implementation; client need: physiological integrity; basic care and comfort; content area: medical-surgical.

RATIONALE

(1) Weighing the client weekly will provide data that best indicate whether the client is receiving adequate nutrition. (2) Having the staff feed her decreases the ability of the client to perform self-care. While this may be easier than allowing the client to feed herself, it will not provide a measure by which nutritional status can be consistently measured. (3) Selection of a menu requires cognitive ability and may increase the client's frustration. (4) Providing high-protein liquids is an appropriate nursing action, but will not provide a measure by which nutritional status can be consistently measured.

182. (4) Integrated processes: nursing process — implementation; client need: physiological integrity; basic care and comfort; content area: medical-surgical.

RATIONALE

(1) The use of restraints is not recommended for clients with dementia because they are attributed to complications such as increased confusion and injury. (2) Closing the door may help

the other residents to rest but does little to help the client and may increase agitation as she tries to gain orientation in an unfamiliar environment. **(3)** Strong medications for sleep are not recommended for dementia clients because they contribute to complications such as increased confusion and injury. **(4)** Leaving the lights on assists the client to gain orientation to the environment and research suggests that light decreases irritability seen later in the evening hours.

183. **(3)** Integrated processes: nursing process — data collection; client need: physiological integrity; physiological adaptation; content area: medical-surgical.

    RATIONALE

    (1) Agnosia is a disturbance in the recognition of objects. **(2)** Apraxia is the inability to carry out a learned movement voluntarily. **(3)** Sundowner's syndrome is a condition that is seen in dementia clients in the early evening hours and is characterized by insomnia, restlessness, agitation, wandering, and increased confusion. **(4)** Irritability is not seen in stage or phase three dementia. This phase is characterized by emaciation and the client is often bedridden.

184. **(2)** Integrated processes: nursing process — implementation, teaching/learning; client need: health promotion and maintenance; content area: medical-surgical.

    RATIONALE

    (1) There is no evidence of the need to take the drug with meals. **(2)** It is especially important that women receiving estrogen therapy undergo yearly mammography because estrogen increases the risk of breast cancer. **(3)** Estrogen has not been associated with glucose intolerance. **(4)** Estrogen has not been associated with hypotension.

185. **(4)** Integrated processes: nursing process — implementation, caring; client need: physiological integrity; physiological adaptation; content area: medical-surgical.

    RATIONALE

    (1) All sensory stimuli should be minimized as much as possible to avoid stimulation of the vomiting center in the brain stem. **(2)** Relaxation would help, but probably not as much as absence of stimuli. **(3)** Minimizing stimuli reduces the chance of stimulating the vomiting center in the brain stem. **(4)** Minimizing stimuli reduces the chance of stimulating the vomiting center in the brain stem.

186. **(2)** Integrated processes: nursing process — implementation; client need: physiological integrity; basic care and comfort; content area: medical-surgical.

    RATIONALE

    (1) Packed cells would not contain coagulation factors. **(2)** A Foley catheter would be inserted so that the urinary output could be measured every hour to prevent renal failure. **(3)** A large tube would be needed for gastric lavage, and a large tube could more easily be inserted through the mouth. **(4)** It would be more important to insert the Foley catheter; it would take time for the effect of the hemorrhage to show up in the values of the hemoglobin and hematocrit.

187. **(3)** Integrated processes: nursing process — planning; client need: physiological integrity; reduction of risk potential; content area: medical-surgical.

    RATIONALE

    (1) Various procedures administered through an endoscope are the preferred method of treating varices. **(2)** Gastric lavage with saline could be used, but procedures administered through an endoscope are usually more effective. **(3)** Direct visualization of the varices makes it easier for the physicians to arrest the hemorrhage. **(4)** A sclerosing agent would most likely be used.

188. **(4)** Integrated processes: nursing process — implementation, teaching/learning; client need: physiological integrity; pharmacological therapies; content area: medical-surgical.

    RATIONALE

    (1) Neomycin would do little to help prevent infection because it is poorly absorbed from the gastrointestinal tract. **(2)** Stress ulcers would not be prevented. **(3)** Neomycin would not prevent constipation. **(4)** The drug would reduce bacterial flora in the gastrointestinal tract, and thus decrease the production of ammonia. High levels of ammonia produce encephalopathy.

189. **(1)** Integrated processes: nursing process — planning; client need: physiological integrity; reduction of risk potential; content area: medical-surgical.

    RATIONALE

    (1) In order to standardize measurement of an irregularly shaped object such as the abdomen, it would be necessary to measure in the same place each day. Accurate measurement would be important in assessing the status of ascites. **(2)** If the client were eating, the time of day might be important but would not be as important as a standard place for measurement. **(3)** The amount of fluid in the bladder should not affect the measurement of the abdomen unless the measurements were taken directly over the bladder. Measuring over the symphysis pubis would not be a good location for assessing ascites. **(4)** Tape measures are standardized.

190. **(4)** Integrated processes: nursing process — data collection; client need: physiological integrity; reduction of risk potential; content area: medical-surgical.

    RATIONALE

    (1) No evidence exists that highly seasoned foods cause ulcers. **(2)** Alcoholic beverages in moderation probably do not cause ulcers. **(3)** Acid ash diets do not cause ulcers. **(4)** Nonsteroidal anti-inflammatory drugs are an identified risk factor for gastric ulcers. They inhibit prostaglandins, which help to form a protective barrier on the gastric mucosa.

191. **(4)** Integrated processes: nursing process — implementation, teaching/learning; client need: physiological integrity; pharmacological therapies; content area: medical-surgical.

    RATIONALE

    (1) Antacids on an empty stomach are passed through the gastrointestinal tract without coming into contact with much acid. **(2)** Antacids are most effective when given 1–2 hours following a meal. **(3)** Antacids are most effective when given 1–2 hours following a meal. **(4)** Antacids are most effective when given 1–2 hours following a meal.

192. **(3)** Integrated processes: nursing process — data collection; client need: physiological integrity; physiological adaptation; content area: medical-surgical.

    RATIONALE

    (1) Hemorrhage and mesenteric adenitis would not be as likely to occur as hypovolemia and electrolyte imbalance. **(2)** Perforation and peritonitis are not very likely to occur. **(3)** The increased pressure in the lumen of the intestine (proximal to the obstruction) will force fluid and electrolytes from the capillaries in the intestinal wall into the peritoneal cavity. Fluid volume deficit and electrolyte imbalances are likely to occur unless the obstruction is treated. **(4)** Volvulus would be possible but not as likely as hypovolemia and electrolyte imbalances.

193. **(2)** Integrated processes: nursing process — implementation, teaching/learning; client need: physiological integrity; reduction of risk potential; content area: medical-surgical.
RATIONALE
(1) The T-tube can be clamped for meals to allow bile into the duodenum to digest fat. **(2)** The bile drainage bag should be kept below the insertion site at all times to prevent back flow of bile into the common bile duct. **(3)** Sterile technique should be used to dress a cholecystectomy incision. **(4)** The client should not lift anything heavy for 4–6 seeks to prevent wound dehiscence. Sexual activity might also be restricted.

194. **(4)** Integrated processes: nursing process — implementation, teaching/learning; client need: health promotion and maintenance; content area: medical-surgical.
RATIONALE
(1) Varicose veins rarely rupture and this would not be the purpose of surgery. **(2)** Walking is not related to varicose veins. **(3)** If a vein ruptures, it is not a life-threatening emergency because venous pressure is low. **(4)** Varicose veins rarely rupture.

195. **(3)** Integrated processes: nursing process — implementation, communication and documentation; client need: physiological integrity; reduction of risk potential; content area: medical-surgical.
RATIONALE
(1) Moderate edema is normal for the first few days after surgery. **(2)** The stoma is very vascular; oozing of blood on touching it would be normal. **(3)** Dark red color would indicate a problem with blood supply; this should be reported at once. **(4)** Pale color could indicate anemia.

196. **(2)** Integrated processes: nursing process — implementation, communication and documentation; client need: physiological integrity; pharmacological therapies; content area: medical-surgical.
RATIONALE
(1) Research does not indicate a need to change liquid preparations because they would be absorbed in the small intestines. **(2)** Time-released preparations would need to be changed because of possible problems with absorption. **(3)** Research does not indicate a need to change oral antibiotics. **(4)** Suppositories to stimulate bowel elimination would not be used (or ordered), but other medications via the rectum would be possible.

197. **(3)** Integrated processes: nursing process — implementation, teaching/learning; client need: physiological integrity; basic care and comfort; content area medical-surgical.
RATIONALE
(1) The bacterial flora of the intestines needs to be restored. **(2)** A low-residue diet will not restore the bacterial flora in the intestines. **(3)** Yogurt, cottage cheese, and buttermilk contain *Lactobacillus acidophilous*, which helps to restore the normal bacterial flora in the intestines. This restoration will help restore the stool to its normal consistency. **(4)** Research does not indicate that antibiotics cause lactose intolerance; therefore, omitting milk products would not help.

198. **(1)** Integrated processes: nursing process — implementation, teaching/learning; client need: safe, effective care environment; safety and infection control; content area: medical-surgical.
RATIONALE
(1) Hepatitis A is spread through feces, contaminated water, or contaminated food. **(2)** The virus is not spread through body fluids. **(3)** The virus is not spread via the respiratory tract. **(4)** It would be most unusual to spread the virus through sex.

199. **(2)** Integrated processes: nursing process — planning; client need: physiological integrity; reduction of risk potential; content area: medical-surgical.
RATIONALE
(1) The environment should be quiet, but the client also needs sensory stimulation. **(2)** The cornea does need regular care to prevent ulceration; the client does not have a blink reflex. **(3)** Score on the Glasgow Coma Scale should steadily increase. **(4)** If the head of the bed is flat, intracranial pressure could increase.

200. **(4)** Integrated processes: nursing process — planning; client need: physiological integrity; reduction of risk potential; content area: medical-surgical.
RATIONALE
(1) Having a sitter at the bedside would not be necessary. **(2)** A padded tongue blade is no longer recommended because more damage is usually done when inserting it during a seizure. **(3)** An oral airway is not recommended for the same reason the tongue blade is not recommended. **(4)** The side rails should be padded to prevent injury during a seizure.

201. **(2)** Integrated processes: nursing process — implementation, teaching/learning; client need: physiological integrity; pharmacological therapies; content area: medical-surgical.
RATIONALE
300 mg : 1 capsule = 600 mg : x = 2 capsules

202. **(1)** Integrated processes: nursing process — implementation; client need: psychosocial integrity; content area: psychiatric.
RATIONALE
(1) Facilitative communication moves beyond social chitchat and into an interpersonal relationship. Interpersonal communication plays a major role in psychiatric nursing. **(2)** Nonverbal communication does not include the spoken word. However, it may influence the outcome of the interaction. **(3)** Public communication occurs when speaking to a group. **(4)** Intrapersonal communication occurs when persons communicate between themselves.

203. **(3)** Integrated processes: nursing process — implementation; client need: psychosocial integrity; content area: psychiatric.
RATIONALE
(1) Assertive behavior is an accurate statement about feelings, beliefs, and opinions. It is stated in a manner that promotes self-respect and respects others. **(2)** Aggressive behavior is inconsiderate, offensive, and violates the basic rights of others. **(3)** Passive behavior is a response that discounts one's own rights in order to avoid conflict. **(4)** Passive-aggressive behavior is expressed through sarcasm, resistance, manipulation, procrastination, and the use of covert aggression instead of words.

204. **(1)** Integrated processes: nursing process — implementation, communication and documentation; client need: psychosocial integrity; content area: psychiatric.
RATIONALE
(1) Documentation related to delivery of care must reflect the use of the nursing process. **(2)** Information in a client's record is confidential and available to authorized person-

nel only. (3) The client's record is a legal document. (4) There is no guarantee that documentation is pertinent or accurate.

205. **(1)** Integrated processes: nursing process — implementation; client need: psychosocial integrity; content area: psychiatric.

RATIONALE
(1) When addressing a client with schizophrenic disorder, use realistic and concrete terms. (2) The use of self-disclosure is inappropriate if the client cannot benefit from it. (3) Demanding information is a barrier to communication. (4) It is important to keep the conversation simple until the client has a better understanding of his disease process.

APPENDIX

State Boards of Nursing

Alabama Board of Nursing
770 Washington Avenue
RSA Plaza, Suite 250
Montgomery, AL 36130–3900
Phone: (334) 242–4060
FAX: (334) 242–4360
Web site: www.abn.state.al.us

Alaska Board of Nursing
550 W. 7th Avenue, Suite 1500
Anchorage, AK 99501–3567
Phone: (907) 269–8161
FAX: (907) 269–8156
Web site: www.dced.state.ak.us/occ/
    pnur.htm

American Samoa Health Services
    Regulatory Board
LBJ Tropical Medical Center
Pago Pago, AS 96799
Phone: (684) 633–1222
FAX: (684) 633–1869

Arizona State Board of Nursing
1651 E. Morton Avenue, Suite 210
Phoenix, AZ 85020
Phone: (602) 889–5150
FAX: (602) 889–5155
Web site: www.azboardofnursing.org

Arkansas State Board of Nursing
University Tower Building
1123 S. University, Suite 800
Little Rock, AR 72204–1619
Phone: (501) 686–2700
FAX: (501) 686–2714
Web site: www.state.ar.us/nurse

California Board of Vocational Nurse and
    PsychiatricTechnician Examiners
2535 Capitol Oaks Drive, Suite 205
Sacramento, CA 95833
Phone: (916) 263–7800

FAX: (916) 263–7859
Web site: www.bvnpt.ca.gov

Colorado Board of Nursing
1560 Broadway, Suite 880
Denver, CO 80202
Phone: (303) 894–2430
FAX: (303) 894–2821
Web site: www.dora.state.co.us/nursing

Connecticut Board of Examiners for Nursing
Dept. of Public Health
410 Capitol Avenue, MS # 13PHO
P.O. Box 340308
Hartford, CT 06134–0328
Phone: (860) 509–7624
FAX: (860) 509–7553
Web site: www.state.ct.us/dph

Delaware Board of Nursing
861 Silver Lake Boulevard
Cannon Bldg., Suite 203
Dover, DE 19904
Phone: (302) 739–4522
FAX: (302) 739–2711
Web site:www.professionallicensing.
    state.de.us/boards/nursing/index.shtml

District of Columbia Board of Nursing
Dept. of Health
825 N. Capitol Street, NE, 2nd floor
Room 2224
Washington, DC 20002
Phone: (202) 442–4778
FAX: (202) 442–9431
Web site: www.dchealth.dc.gov

Florida Board of Nursing
4042 Bald Cypress Way
Room 120
Tallahassee, FL 32399
Phone: (850) 245–4125
FAX: (850) 245–4172
Web site: www.doh.state.fl.us/mqa

Georgia State Board of Licensed Practical
    Nurses
237 Coliseum Drive
Macon, GA 31217–3858
Phone: (478) 207–1620
FAX: (478) 207–1363
Web site: www.sos.state.ga.us/plb/lpn

Guam Board of Nurse Examiners
P.O. Box 2816
Hagatna, Guam 96932
Phone: (671) 735–7406 or (671) 725–7411
FAX: (671) 735–7413

Hawaii Board of Nursing
King Kalakaua Bldg.
335 Merchant, 3rd Floor
Honolulu, HI 96813
Phone: (808) 586–3000
FAX: (808) 586–2689
Web site: www.state.hi.us/dcca/pvl/areas_
    nurse.html

Idaho Board of Nursing
280 N. 8th Street, Suite 210
P.O. Box 83720
Boise, ID 83720
Phone: (208) 334–3110
FAX: (208) 334–3262
Web site: www.state.id.us/ibn/ibnhome.htm

Illinois Department of Professional
    Regulation
James R. Thompson Center
100 W. Randolph, Suite 9–300
Chicago, Il 60601
Phone: (312) 814–2715
FAX: (312) 814–3145
Web site: www.dpr.state.il.us

Indiana State Board of Nursing
Health Professions Bureau
402 W Washington Street, Room W066

Indianapolis, IN 46204
Phone: (317) 234–2043
FAX: (317) 233–4236
Web site: www.state.in.us/hpb/boards/isbn

Iowa Board of Nursing
Riverpoint Business Park
400 SW 8th Street
Suite B
Des Moines, IA 50309–4685
Phone: (515) 281–3255
FAX: (515) 281–4825
Web site: www.state.ia.us/government/
nursing

Kansas State Board of Nursing
Landon State Office Bldg.
900 SW Jackson, Suite 1051
Topeka, KS 66612
Phone: (785) 296–4929
FAX: (785) 296–3929
Web site: www.ksbn.org

Kentucky Board of Nursing
312 Whittington Parkway, Suite 300
Louisville, KY 40222
Phone: (502) 329–7000
FAX: (502) 329–7011
Web site: www.kbn.ky.gov

Louisiana State Board of Practical Nurse
Examiners
3421 N Causeway Boulevard, Suite 505
Metairie, LA 70002
Phone: (504) 838–5791
FAX: (504) 838–5279
Web site: www.lsbn.state.la.us

Maine State Board of Nursing
158 State House Station
Augusta, ME 04333
Phone: (207) 287–1133
FAX: (207) 287–1149
Web site: www.maine.gov/boardofnursing

Maryland State Board of Nursing
4140 Patterson Avenue
Baltimore, MD 21215
Phone: (410) 585–1900
FAX: (410) 358–3530
Web site: www.mbon.org

Massachusetts Board of Registration in
Nursing
Commonwealth of Massachusetts
239 Causeway Street, Suite 500
Boston, MA 02114
Phone: (617) 727–9961
FAX: (617) 727–1630
Web site: www.mass.gov/dpl/boards/rn/
index.htm

Michigan/DCH/Bureau of Health
Professionals
Ottawa Towers North
611 W. Ottawa, 1st Floor
Lansing, MI 48933
Phone: (517) 335–0918

FAX: (517) 373–2179
Web site: www.michigan.gov/healthlicense

Minnesota Board of Nursing
2829 University Avenue SE
Minneapolis, MN 55414
Phone: (612) 617–2270
FAX: (612) 617–2190
Web site: www.nursingboard.state.mn.us

Mississippi Board of Nursing
1935 Lakeland Drive, Suite B
Jackson, MS 39216–5014
Phone: (601) 987–4188
FAX: (601) 364–2352
Web site: www.msbn.state.ms.us

Missouri State Board of Nursing
3605 Missouri Boulevard
P.O. Box 656
Jefferson City, MO 65102–0656
Phone: (573) 751–0681
FAX: (573) 751–0075
Web site: www.ecodev.state.mo.us/pr/
nursing

Montana State Board of Nursing
301 S Park
P.O. Box 200513
Helena, MT 59620–0513
Phone: (406) 841–2340
FAX: (406) 841–2343
Web site: www.discoveringmontant.com/dli/
bsd/license/bsd_boards/nur_board/board_
page.htm

Nebraska Department of Health and Human
Services Regulation and Licensure
Nursing and Nursing Support
301 Centennial Mall South
Lincoln, NE 68509–4986
Phone: (402) 471–4376
FAX: (402) 471–1066
Web site: www.hhs.state.ne.us/crl/nursing/
nursingindex.htm

Nevada State Board of Nursing
2500 W. Sahara Avenue, Suite 207
Las Vegas, NV 89102–4392
Phone: (702) 486–5800
FAX: (702) 486–5803
Web site: www.nursingboard.state.nv.us

New Hampshire Board of Nursing
21 South Fruit Street, Suite 16
Concord, NH 03301–2341
Phone: (603) 271–2323
FAX: (603) 271–6605
Web site: www.state.nh.us/nursing

New Jersey Board of Nursing
P.O. Box 45010
124 Halsey Street, 6th Floor
Newark, NJ 07101
Phone: (973) 504–6586
FAX: (973) 648–3481
Web site: www. state.nj.us/lps/ca/medical/
nursing.htm

New Mexico Board of Nursing
6301 Indian School Road, NE
Suite 710
Albuquerque, NM 87110
Phone: (505) 841–8340
FAX: (505) 841–8347
Web site: www.state.nm.us/clients/nursing

New York State Board of Nursing
Education Bldg.
89 Washington Avenue
2nd Floor West Wing
Albany, NY 12234
Phone: (518) 474–3817 Ext. 280
FAX: (518) 474–3706
Web site: www.nysed.gov/prof/nurse.htm

North Carolina Board of Nursing
3724 National Drive, Suite 201
Raleigh, NC 27612
Phone: (919) 782–3211
FAX: (919) 781–9461
Web site: www.ncbon.com

North Dakota Board of Nursing
919 S. 7th Street, Suite 504
Bismarck, ND 58504
Phone: (701) 328–9777
FAX: (701) 328–9785
Web site: www.ndbon.org

Northern Mariana Islands
Commonwealth Board of Nurse Examiners
P.O. Box 501458
Saipan, MP 96950
Phone: (670) 664–4812
FAX: (670) 664–4813

Ohio Board of Nursing
17 S High Street, Suite 400
Columbus, OH 43215–3413
Phone: (614) 466–3947
FAX: (614) 466–0388
Web site: www.nursing.ohio.gov

Oklahoma Board of Nursing
2915 N. Classen Boulevard, Suite 524
Oklahoma City, OK 73106
Phone: (405) 962–1800
FAX: (405) 962–1821
Web site: www.youroklahoma.com/
nursing

Oregon State Board of Nursing
800 NE Oregon Street, Box 25
Suite 465
Portland, OR 97232
Phone: (503) 731–4745
FAX: (503) 731–4755
Web site: www.osbn.sate.or.us

Pennsylvania State Board of Nursing
P.O. Box 2649
Harrisburg, PA 17105–2649
Phone: (717) 783–7142
FAX: (717) 783–0822
Web site: www. dos.state.pa.us/bpoa/cwp/
view.asp?a=1104&q=432883

Commonwealth of Puerto Rico
Board of Nurse Examiners
800 Roberto H. Todd Avenue
Room 202, Stop 18
Santurce, PR 00908
Phone: (787) 725–7506
FAX: (787) 725–7903

Rhode Island Board of Nurse Registration
and Nursing Education
105 Cannon Boulevard
Three Capitol Hill
Providence, RI 02908
Phone: (401) 222–5700
FAX: (401) 222–3352
Web site: www.healthri.org/hsr/professions/
nurses.htm

South Carolina State Board of Nursing
110 Centerview Drive, Suite 202
Columbia, SC 29210
Phone: (803) 896–4550
FAX: (803) 896–4525
Web site: www.llr.state.sc.us/pol/nursing

South Dakota Board of Nursing
4305 South Louise Avenue, Suite 201
Sioux Falls, SD 57106–3115
Phone: (605) 362–2760
FAX: (605) 362–2768
Web site: www.state.sd.us/dcr/nursing

Tennessee State Board of Nursing
425 Fifth Avenue North
1st Floor, Cordell Hull Building
Nashville, TN 37247
Phone: (615) 532–5166

FAX: (615) 741–7899
Web site: www.tennessee.gov/health

Texas Board of Nurse Examiners
333 Guadalupe Street, Suite 3–460
Austin, TX 78701
Phone: (512) 305–7400
FAX: (512) 305–7401
Web site: www.bne.state.tx.us

Utah State Board of Nursing
Heber M. Wells Bldg., 4th floor
160 E. 300 S.
Salt Lake City, UT 84111
Phone: (801) 530–6628
FAX: (801) 530–6511
Web site: www.commerce.state.ut.us

Vermont State Board of Nursing
81 River Street
Heritage Bldg.
Montpelier, VT 05609
Phone: (802) 828–2396
FAX: (802) 828–2484
Web site: www.vtprofessionals.org/opr1/
nurses

Virgin Islands Board of Nurse Licensure
Veterans Drive Station
St. Thomas, VI 00803
Phone: (340) 776–7397
FAX: (340) 777–4003

Virginia Board of Nursing
6603 W. Broad Street
5th Floor
Richmond, VA 23230–1712

Phone: (804) 662–9909
FAX: (804) 662–9512
Web site: www.dhp.state.va.us

Washington State Nursing Care Quality
Assurance Commission
Department of Health
HPQA # 6
310 Israel Road SE
Tumwater, WA 98501–7864
Phone: (360) 236–4700
FAX: (360) 236–4738
Web site: https://wws2.wa.gov/doh/
hpqa-licensing/HPS6/Nursing/default.htm

West Virginia State Board of Examiners for
Licensed Practical Nurses
101 Dee Drive
Charleston, WV 25311
Phone: (304) 558–3572
FAX: (304) 558–4367
Web site: www. pnboard.state.wv.us

Wisconsin Department of Regulation and
Licensing
1400 E Washington Avenue, Room 173
Madison, WI 53708
Phone: (608) 266–0145
FAX: (608) 261–7083
Web site: www.drl.state.wi.us

Wyoming State Board of Nursing
2020 Carey Avenue, Suite 110
Cheyenne, WY 82002
Phone: (307) 777–7601
FAX: (307) 777–3519
Web site: www.nursing.state.wy.us

INDEX

Numbers followed by a "t" indicate tabular material.

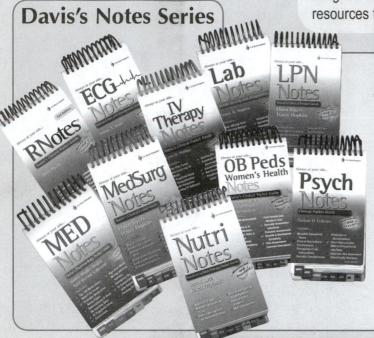
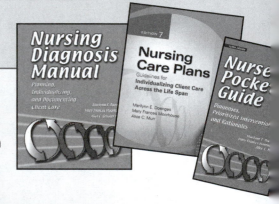
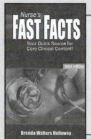
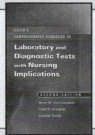
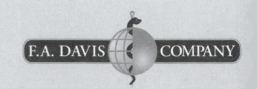